The Circulatory System

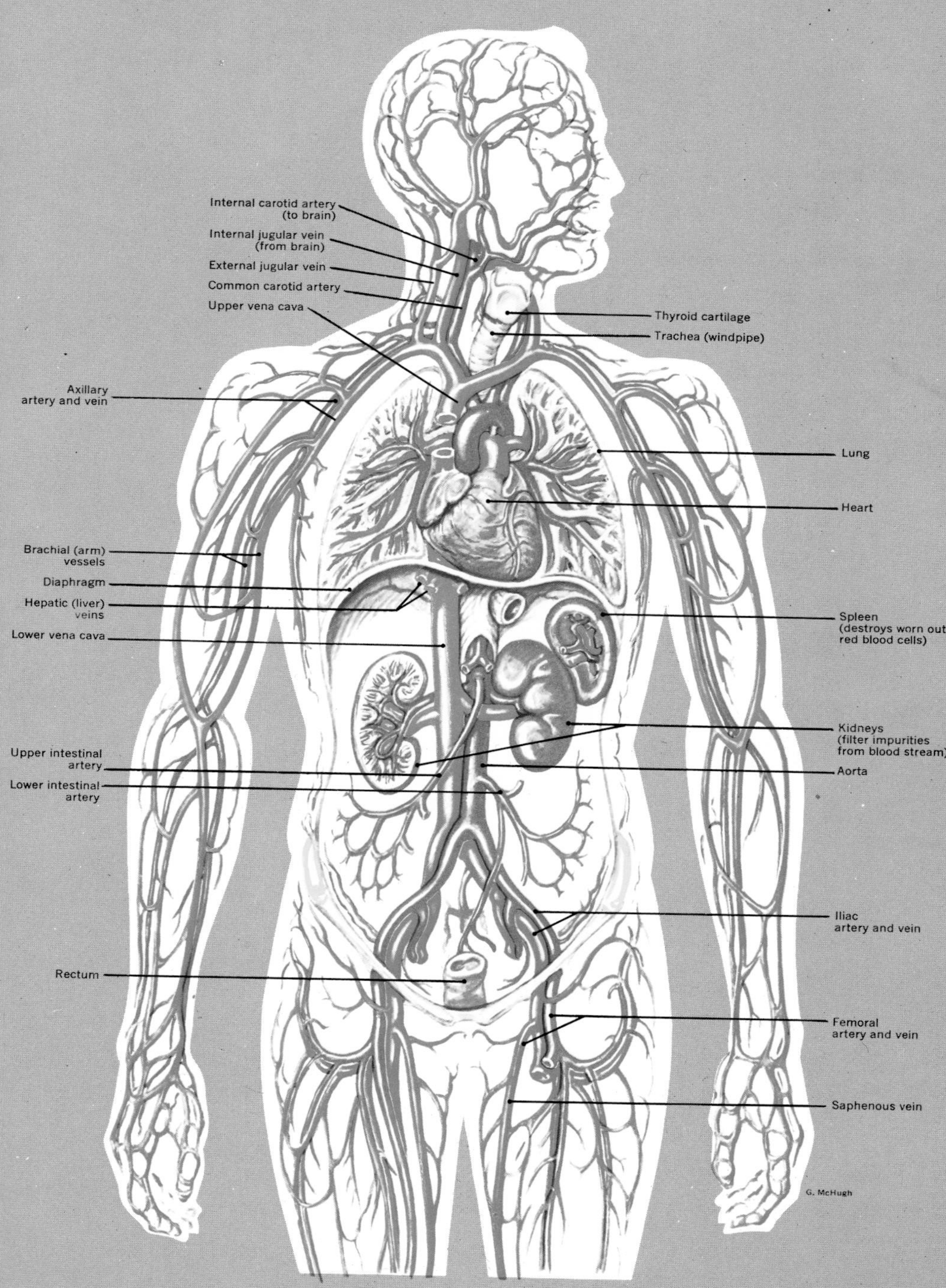

From The New Illustrated Medical and Health Encyclopedia.

PLATE 1

Muscles of Front of Body in Relation to Skeleton

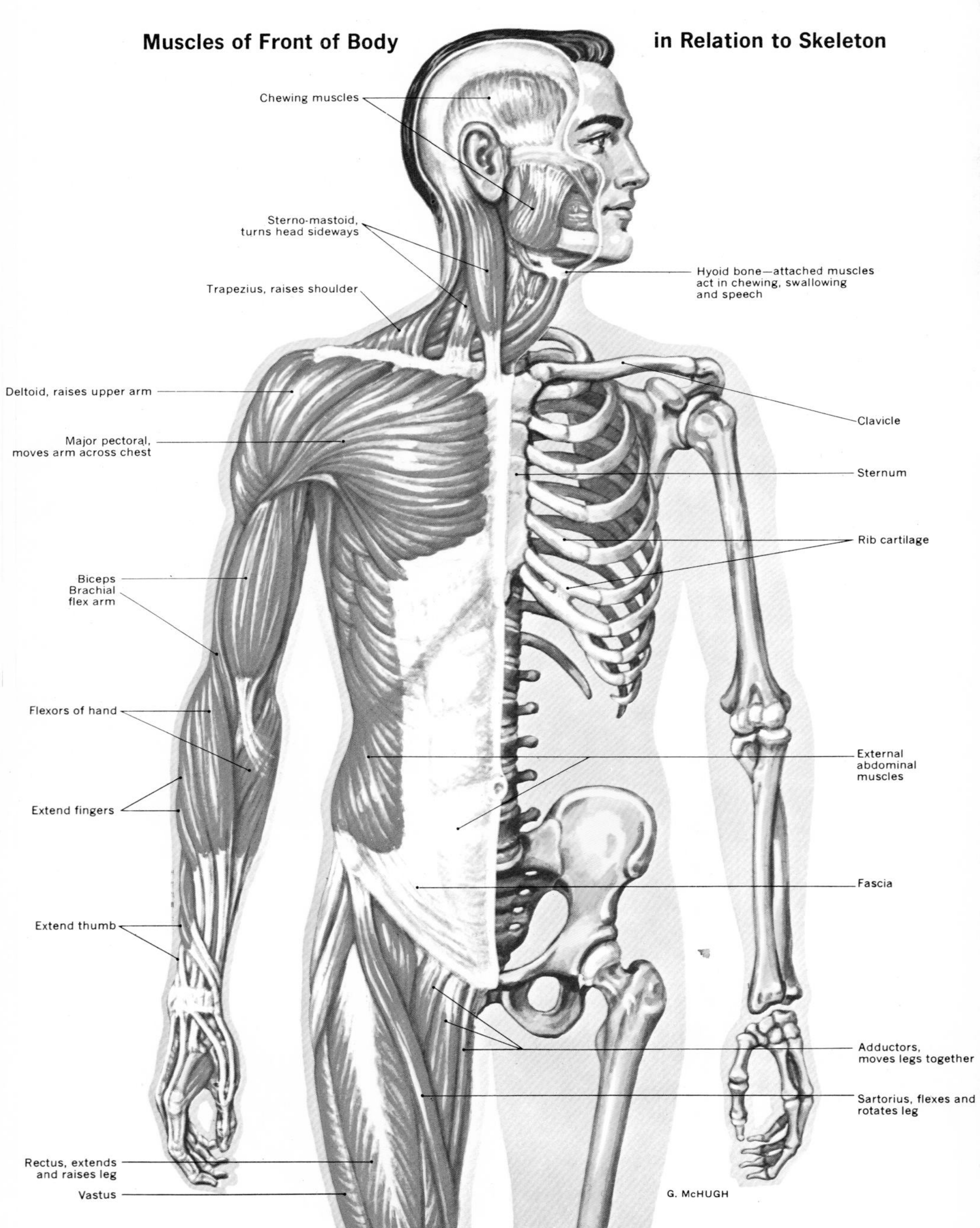

From The New Illustrated Medical and Health Encyclopedia.

The Voluntary Nervous System

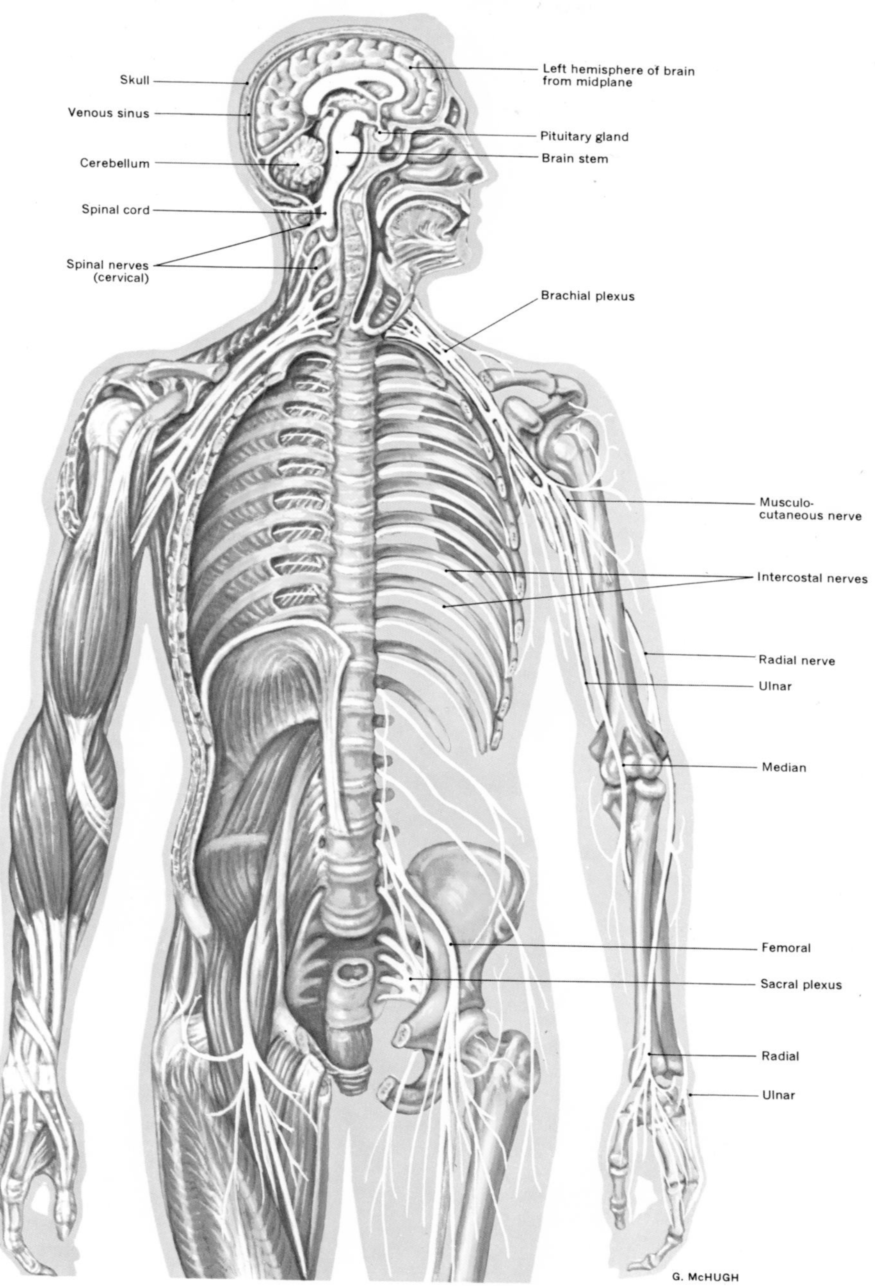

From The New Illustrated Medical and Health Encyclopedia.

Front View of Skeleton

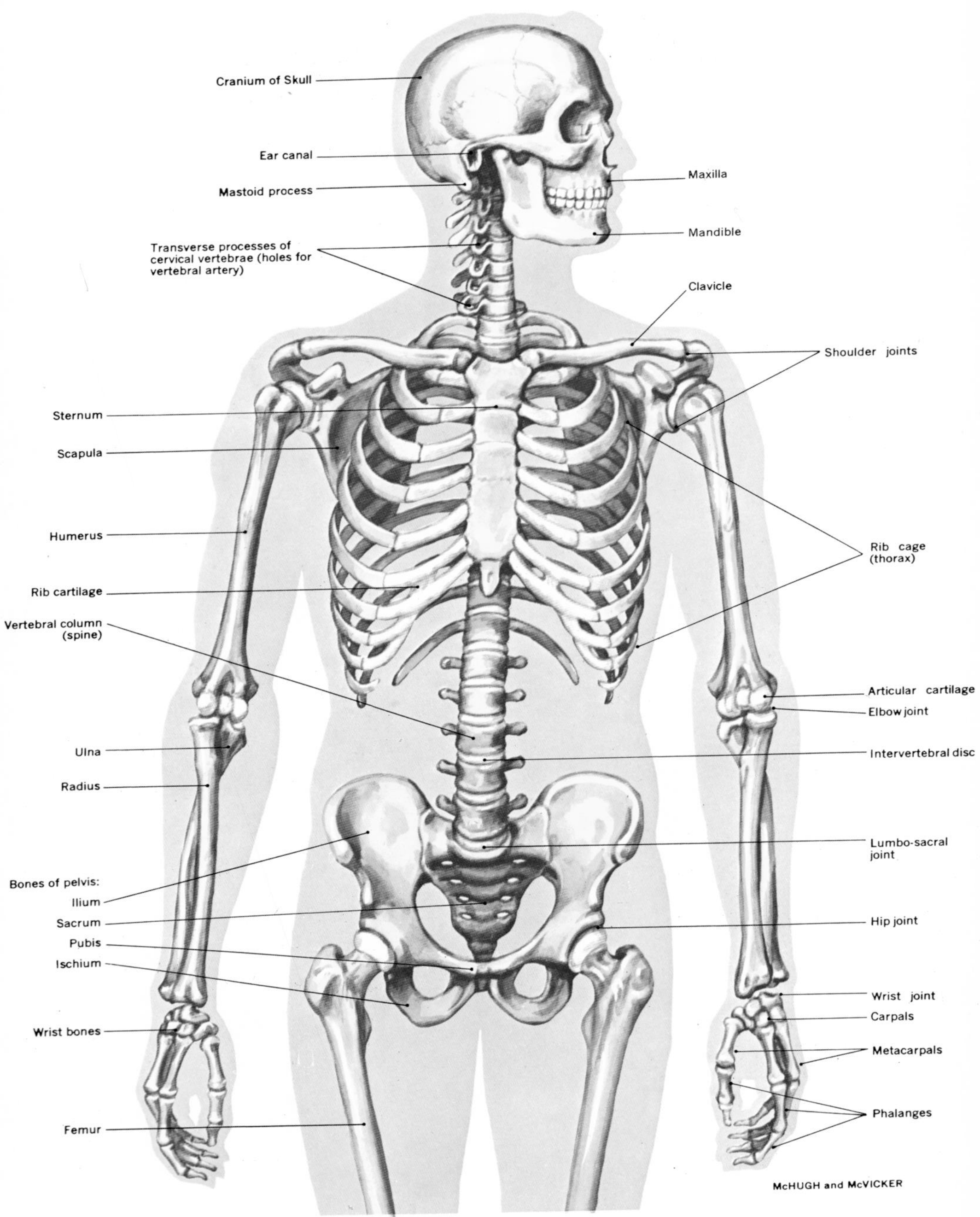

PLATE 4

From The New Illustrated Medical and Health Encyclopedia.

MODERN HOME MEDICAL ADVISER

BOOKS BY MORRIS FISHBEIN, M.D.

AUTHOR:

Handbook of Therapy (1925) with Dr. Oliver T. Osborne
The Medical Follies (1925) Mirrors of Medicine (1925)
The New Medical Follies (1927) The Human Body and Its Care (1929)
An Hour of Health (1929) Doctors and Specialists (1930)
Shattering Health Superstitions (1930)
Fads and Quackery in Healing (1932)
Frontiers of Medicine (1933) Syphilis (1937)
Your Diet and Your Health (1937)
Do You Want to Become a Doctor? (1939) The National Nutrition (1942)
First Aid Training (1943), with Leslie W. Irwin
Health and First Aid (1944), with Leslie W. Irwin
Popular Medical Encyclopedia (1961)
History of the American Medical Association (1947)
Medical Writing: The Technic and the Art (1957)
The Handy Home Medical Adviser (1952)
New Advances in Medicine (1956)
Handy Home Medical Adviser and Concise Medical Encyclopedia (1957)
in Dutch and Portuguese also
Modern Home Remedies and How to Use Them (1966)

EDITOR:

Your Weight and How to Control It (1927; 1962)
Why Men Fail (1928) with William A. White
Common Ailments of Man (1945) Doctors at War (1945)
Medical Uses of Soap (1946) Successful Marriage (1955)
Reducing: Your Weight and How to Control It (1951)
Tonics and Sedatives (1949)
Medical Progress (1953, 1954, 1955, 1956, 1957) Editions in
England and Holland
Children for the Childless (1954) Modern Marriage and Family Living (1957)
Modern Family Health Guide (1959; 1968) Heart Care (1961)
Proceedings of the International Congresses on Poliomyelitis and
on Congenital Malformations, National Foundation
Illustrated Medical and Health Encyclopedia, 14 vols. (1964)
Modern Home Medical Adviser (new, revised edition 1969),
editions in Spanish, Icelandic, and Afrikaans

RECORDS AND MANUALS:

Dr. Fishbein Talks to a Growing Boy Dr. Fishbein Talks to a Growing Girl
Dr. Fishbein's Growing-Up Manual:
A Frank Discussion for Children and Their Parents

NEW, REVISED EDITION

MODERN HOME MEDICAL ADVISER

Your Health and How to Preserve It

EDITED BY Morris Fishbein, M.D.

GARDEN CITY, NEW YORK

Doubleday & Company, Inc.

Library of Congress Catalog Card Number: 69–10978

Printed in the United States of America

Preface

The speed of medical progress continues to be one of the marvels of our scientific century. A comparison of what was known five or ten years ago with the knowledge of today indicates ten or more great discoveries each year.

This book is offered to answer significant questions concerning the common and even some of the extraordinary illnesses that may develop in any family. Included are the infectious diseases caused by viruses and bacteria and parasites, deficiency diseases, diseases of metabolism and digestion, disorders of the glands, allergy, industrial diseases and conditions affecting the skin, eyes, ears, nose and throat.

Prevention is better than cure! Here also are adequate considerations of first aid, prenatal care, care and feeding of the child, sex hygiene, suitable diet, care of the feet, posture, mental hygiene and old age.

The book provides the considerations in choosing a family doctor and the materials that ought to be regularly available in the family medicine chest.

A knowledge of the structure of the body and the way it works–anatomy and physiology–is necessary for understanding. This is provided through charts, diagrams and descriptions.

The years of use of the MODERN HOME MEDICAL ADVISER have indicated possibilities for improving it as a tool for teaching and furnishing information. Many of the articles and most of the pictures are entirely new; all of them are thoroughly revised.

Many new and brilliant young authors have kindly associated themselves with me in this work. I express appreciation to them.

MORRIS FISHBEIN, M.D.

COLLABORATORS

VICTOR ABRAMSON, M.D.
Attending Ophthalmologist, Michael Reese Hospital, Chicago.

RAYMOND D. ADAMS, M.D.
Chief Neurological Service and Neuropathologist, Massachusetts General Hospital, Bullard Professor of Neuropathology, Harvard Medical School, Boston.

HOWARD T. BEHRMAN, M.D.
Professor of Clinical Dermatology and Director of Dermatologic Research, New York Medical College.

ERNEST BEUTLER, M.D.
Chairman, Department of Medicine, City of Hope Medical Center, Duarte, California; Clinical Professor of Medicine, U.S.C.

LOUIS D. BOSHES, M.D.
Clinical Associate Professor of Neurology and Director Consultation Clinic for Epilepsy, Neuropsychiatric Institute, University of Illinois at the Medical Center, Chicago.

LEO H. CRIEP, M.D.
Associate Professor in Medicine and Chief of the Allergy Clinic, University of Pittsburgh School of Medicine; Director of Allergy Laboratory, Veterans Administration, Pittsburgh.

HAROLD S. DIEHL, M.D.
Senior Vice President for Research and Medical Affairs, American Cancer Society, Inc., New York City.

MORRIS FISHBEIN, M.D.
Former Editor, Journal American Medical Association; Contributing Editor, Postgraduate Medicine; Medical Editor, Britannica Book of the Year; Member Chief Editors, Excerpta Medica; and Editor, Medical World News.

CLIFFORD F. GASTINEAU, M.D.
Section of Medicine, Mayo Clinic and Assoc. Prof. Mayo Graduate School of Medicine, Rochester, Minnesota.

J. P. GREENHILL, M.D.
Senior Attending Obstetrician and Gynecologist, Michael Reese Hospital; Professor of Gynecology, Cook County Graduate

School of Medicine; Editor, Yearbook of Obstetrics and Gynecology. Chicago.

HENRY F. HOWE, M.D.
Director, Department of Occupational Health, American Medical Association, Chicago.

ROBERT M. KARK, M.D.
Professor of Medicine, University of Illinois; Physician, Presbyterian-St. Luke's Hospital, Chicago.

JOSEPH B. KIRSNER, M.D.
Professor, Department of Medicine, University of Chicago.

RICHARD P. LASSER, M.D.
Assistant Attending Cardiologist, Mount Sinai Hospital, New York City.

ARTHUR M. MASTER, M.D.
Consultant in Cardiology, U. S. Navy Hospital; Cardiologist, Mount Sinai Hospital, New York City.

ROBERT D. MOORE, M.D.
Former Professor, Department of Surgery, Section of Orthopedics, University of Chicago; Attending Orthopedic Surgeon at Christ Community Hospital, Oaklawn, Ill. and Evangelical Hospital, Chicago, Ill. Consulting Orthopedic Surgeon at Illinois Central Hospital, Chicago, Ill.

JOEL F. PANISH, M.D.
Adjunct in Medicine, Cedars-Sinai Medical Center; Instructor in Medicine, University of Southern California School of Medicine; Attending Physician (Gastroenterology), Veterans Administration Wadsworth Hospital, Los Angeles.

OGLESBY PAUL, M.D.
Chief, Division of Medicine, Passavant Memorial Hospital; Professor of Medicine, Northwestern Univ., Chicago.

HOWARD F. POLLEY, M.D.
Professor of Medicine, Mayo Graduate School of Medicine, University of Minnesota; Chairman of Rheumatology, Mayo Clinic, Rochester, Minnesota.

ALWIN C. RAMBAR, M.D.
Senior Attending Physician, Sarah Morris Hospital for Children, Michael Reese Hospital, Chicago; Chief of Pediatrics, Highland Park Hospital, Highland Park, Illinois.

HOWARD F. ROOT, M.D. (Deceased)
President, Joslin Clinic, Diabetes Foundation, Inc., and International Diabetes Federation, Boston.

MANUEL L. STILLERMAN, M.D.
Clinical Assistant Professor of Ophthalmology, University of Illinois College of Medicine; Chairman Department of Ophthalmology, Michael Reese Hospital, Chicago.

SHELDON S. WALDSTEIN, M.D.
Director, Division of Medicine, and Chairman, Department of Endocrinology, Cook County Hospital; Director of Endocrinology, Hektoen Institute for Medical Research; Professor of Medicine, Northwestern University, Chicago.

Contents

Illustrations

PLATES

MODERN HOME MEDICAL ADVISER

CHAPTER 1

The Choice of a Physician

MORRIS FISHBEIN, M.D.

THE FAMILY DOCTOR

Of all the problems that concern the average family, probably no other is more important for health and happiness than the choice of the family physician. The family doctor before 1900 was mostly learned in the school of experience. In many instances he had studied with a preceptor and perhaps had a course of lectures in some medical school lasting six months and devoted but slightly to the practical side of medicine. Such knowledge he obtained by studying cases with his preceptor. He did develop an intimate personal relationship with those whom he served, which is recognized today as the basic feature of the best type of medical practice.

The family loved, indeed almost worshiped, the family doctor. He was their guide in health as well as in sickness. He alone, of all the community, knew the family secrets, and he could be depended on to keep the faith. True, his remedies were occasionally harsh and his diagnosis largely guesswork, but his record of cures is surprising. He was especially known for his ability to practice the art of scientific observation, using to the utmost his five senses. The physician of today has available innumerable scientific devices for aiding, prolonging, and extending these senses, but unless brains are carefully mixed with the application of the devices the end result may be confusion rather than scientific diagnosis, and the cost far beyond the necessary cost for first-class medical practice. The general practitioners of modern times still serve as family doctors. Often, however, families come to rely on internists and pediatricians to fulfill this function. The center of medical practice has moved from home and the doctor's office to the hospital.

GRADUATION FROM A MEDICAL COLLEGE

In choosing a physician be sure you know the answers to the following questions: First, is he a graduate of a recognized medical school that requires at least four years of thorough training? There was a time when there were more medical schools in the United States than in all the rest of the world. We had almost 200 medical schools in this country around 1900. In September 1968 there were 97 medical colleges that had graduated medical students; 88 of these have been accredited by the Joint Commission on Hospital Accreditation of the Council on Medical Education and Hospitals of the American Medical Association. The remaining 9 are not eligible for consideration for accreditation until after they graduate more medical students. An accredited college is one with a minimum number of full-time teachers and with a well-established graded curriculum. At least two years of college education are required previous to studying medicine, four years of medical education of approximately nine months each, and around one year or two years of internship after graduation.

LICENSE BY THE STATE

Is the doctor licensed to practice medicine in the state in which he has his office? The majority of the states conduct regular examinations for a license to practice, these examinations being given by a group of physicians known as the State Medical Board of Registration and Licensure. In some states the doctor is required to renew his license every year. Before he can get a license he must usually show evidence of his graduation and also undergo a written and practical examination in the basic medical subjects. He must also present certificates of good moral character from at least two physicians who know him.

THE DOCTOR'S INTERNSHIP

Has the doctor had actual training as an intern in a hospital? Or has he been associated with a practicing physician long enough to obtain practical education in medicine? Has he at the time of consultation a direct connection with a good hospital? According to the National Center for Health Statistics in Washington, D.C., there are in the United States 8894 hospitals listed with the center. In September 1967, 7172 of these were registered with the American Hospital Association, and 4763 were accredited by the Joint Commission on Accreditation of Hospitals of the American Hospital Association, the American Medical Association, the American College of Physicians and the American College of Surgeons. Of the 308,630 physicians in the United States at the end of 1967 more than 200,000 are directly affiliated with these hospitals as members of the staff. The appointment of a physician to the staff of a good hospital indicates that he has been passed upon according to his qualifications by the medical staff of the hospital and frequently also by the board of directors of the institution.

MEMBERSHIP IN THE COUNTY MEDICAL SOCIETY

Is the doctor a member of his county medical society, of his state medical society, of the American Medical Association, or of any other recognized, organized body of physicians? The American Medical Association is organized like the United States government. It has county societies which pass carefully on physicians who wish to join. Before a man can belong to his state medical society he must belong to his county medical society. Before he can belong to the American Medical Association he must belong to both county and state medical societies. Before he can belong to any of the recognized special societies, such as those in surgery, diseases of the eye, ear, nose and throat, skin, and other specialties, he must belong to the American Medical Association or to his state and county medical societies.

While membership in a medical society is not an absolute guarantee of honesty or of good faith, the physician who belongs to such a society is subject to the criticism of his colleagues and subject also to being called before special committees to explain actions that are not considered ethical or satisfactory. A patient is much better off with a doctor who belongs to a recognized medical society than in the hands of one who is utterly independent of such organizational control. There are, of course, numerous medical organizations which are not recognized or established or scientific. There is even an organization composed of innumerable quacks who practice all sorts of strange medical cults and promote many unestablished notions.

CHARACTERISTICS OF AN ETHICAL DOCTOR

An ethical physician may be differentiated from a quack by certain well-established characteristics. An ethical physician does not advertise his methods or cures in a newspaper. He does not give out circulars concerning his work or his fees. He does not indiscriminately distribute his picture. He does not put large signboards on his windows or outside his office, advertising his extraordinary merits, or otherwise promoting his wares. A competent ethical physician seldom finds it necessary to travel from town to town to secure patients. He usually has an established place of residence and of work to which patients come when they require his services or to which they send, requesting his attendance when they themselves are unable to travel. The traveling doctor who moves from town to town is not to be consulted or to be considered a safe family physician.

There has been for years a tradition in medicine that new discoveries are freely published to the profession in the various medical periodicals and are not held as secrets by certain men which only they can apply. The public may therefore well beware of any doctor or group of doctors who advertise or publish broadcast the fact that they have discovered a new cure or method of treatment that other doctors do not know about, or who claim they can cure such serious conditions as cancer, tuberculosis, the venereal diseases, or rheumatic disease in a short time by some secret manipulation or by some unestablished method.

THE SCIENTIFIC ADVANCEMENT OF MEDICINE

The advancement of medicine has been associated with the introduction of innumerable complicated devices used not only in the diagnosis of disease but also in treatment. The sense of vision is aided by the microscope which enlarges invisible objects so that they may be seen. There are other instruments such as the cystoscope, the otoscope, the laryngoscope, and the ophthalmoscope which enable the physician competent in their use to look directly into various body cavities. By means of the X ray, opaque tissues are brought into the field of vision, and by the use of various dye substances combined with the X ray most of the organs and tissues of the body can now be seen during life.

The development of physics, of chemistry, of bacteriology, and of many sciences on which medicine rests has made it possible for physicians to determine to the thousandth of a gram the content of the blood and of various secretions and excretions of the body, determining thus the presence of sugar, of protein, of various salts, and of other substances related to the functions of the body in health and in disease. In surgery new devices have been developed for cutting tissues without hemorrhage, for keeping the patient quiet or anesthetized during operation, and for keeping conditions so clean that there is no danger of infection.

New methods have been discovered which aid the specialist in diseases of the nose and throat in looking into the sinuses, in determining their contours, in examining the ear externally and internally, and in peering into the very depths not only of the larynx but even of the lungs.

DEVELOPMENT OF SPECIALISTS

The employment of the special devices used in medical practice requires hours of study and practice for the development of proper technic. As a result of the tremendous expansion of medical knowledge specialization entered the field. Not only is medicine practiced by general practitioners who, it has been determined, can easily take care of eighty-five per cent of the conditions for which patients consult physicians, but also in some thirty or more specialties of various types, such as those which concern themselves wholly with internal medicine and diagnosis; surgery, which is divided into orthopedic surgery, genito-urinary surgery, brain surgery, abdominal surgery, and similar branches. There are also specialists in diseases of the skin, in diseases of women, in diseases of children, in obstetrics, in nervous and mental diseases, in diseases of the stomach and intestines, in industrial medicine, in preventive medicine, in anesthesia, and in several other more confined branches.

There is not as yet any method established by law for determining who shall be considered competent to practice a specialty in medicine and who shall not. Any physician who wishes to do so may set himself up as a specialist in any medical field. The rewards of specialization are usually beyond those of general practice in the form of shorter hours of work, more time for research, higher pay for work accomplished and, no doubt, much more interest in the work. Various means have been developed by the medical profession itself for limiting, if possible, entrance of unworthy men into various specialties. Some of the specialistic societies will not admit any man until he has had at least five years of experience in a specialty and until he has done sufficient research work and published enough scientific papers to prove his competence.

Moreover, the medical profession has itself established examining and certifying boards which now undertake, after a young man has been at least five years in practice, to give him both a written and a practical examination and, provided he is qualified, to issue to him a certificate of competence.

CONSULT THE FAMILY DOCTOR FIRST

In the vast majority of cases people who wish to consult a specialist will do well to go first to their family doctor or general practitioner so that he may, after a study of the case, select for the patient such specialists as may be necessary for consultation as to diagnosis or for specialistic treatment. In this way the patient may save himself a great deal of time and money. Numerous instances are recorded in which a patient with a pain in some portion of the body went directly to a specialist, only to find out that the pain which concerned him was not due to an organ within the field of that specialist but perhaps to some entirely different cause.

For instance, such a condition as ordinary dizziness may be due to causes arising in the digestive tract, in the heart and circulation, in the internal ear, or in the brain. Only a careful study of the history of the case, the nature of the symptoms, and similar factors, will enable a physician to see which one of these organs or systems may be concerned. Similarly, bleeding from the throat may be due to conditions in the throat, in which case a general practitioner or a specialist in diseases of the throat might be consulted. On the other hand, it might be due to tuberculosis of the lungs, to a tumor of the esophagus or to hemorrhage taking place in the stomach, in which case a specialist concerned with those organs might be needed. Hence, for the vast majority of complaints the patient should first of all consult a family physician, preferably one to whom he has gone for some time. He may confidently be guided by his advice.

PICKING A FAMILY DOCTOR

When coming into a community you may select your physician in various ways. If you will call the secretary of the county medical society, the secretary will probably be willing to give you a list of general practitioners in your vicinity. You may then determine by meeting these men and by inquiry into their qualifications whether or not you care to commit the illnesses of yourself and of your family to their care. If you are a member of any well-established fraternal organization or church, association of commerce, business organization, or similar group, you may on inquiry among your associates in these groups find out who are the competent physicians in the community, and then, by making your own inquiries as to competence along the lines of the questions that have been suggested earlier in this chapter, determine which of those that have been recommended is suitable to your needs.

Once a physician has been selected and has been found competent to give not only the type of scientific advice needed for ordinary cases, but also to give the personal intimate attention that is the distinguishing characteristic of the best type of family doctor, you will do well to cling to that family physician and to recognize in him a friend and a counselor. Remember also that the servant is worthy of his hire. Far too often physicians' bills are the last to be paid because the very nature of the profession has in the past made the physician willing to wait until the bills for food, for clothing, for shelter, for fuel, and the other necessities of life have been taken care of. The physician must himself provide these things for his family. A physician who receives from his patient conscientious and responsible treatment is likely to return to that patient even more conscientious and responsible attention than he himself has received.

PERIODIC HEALTH EXAMINATIONS

The modern infant is frequently brought to the office of the pediatrician or family doctor for a periodic examination which surveys his growth and development and provides preventive medicine. The adolescent receives periodic studies in schools and particularly when engaged in sports and

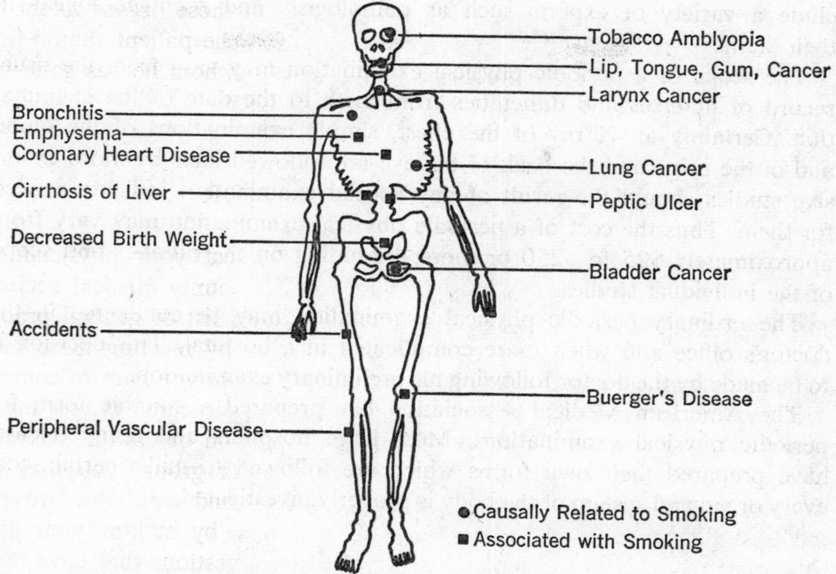

Fig. 1. Distribution of Diseases Associated with Smoking. The National Clearing House for Smoking and Health (a subdivision of the National Center for Chronic Disease Control) is a "prevention measure program." Since cigarette smoking is associated with approximately 300,000 premature deaths and millions of cases of chronic disease annually, they conduct a research and educational program aimed at reducing death and disability associated with smoking. The clearinghouse also works with the communications media as well as school, health, civic, and youth groups to inform the public of the hazards of smoking. In addition, it both conducts and supports social and psychological research into smoking behavior, and distributes scientific information on smoking and smoking-related disease to physicians and research scientists. U. S. Department of Health, Education and Welfare, Public Health Service.

athletics. Most colleges and universities have school physicians and health departments where studies can be made. Some universities examine every student at the time of admission and then conduct periodic studies. When, however, the man or woman goes into industry, or into the household, and grows older the tendency is to abandon this important measure for the prolongation of life.

Many illnesses begin insidiously; the person may not even be aware of them until they have already progressed so far as to make treatment and cure difficult. Such conditions as rheumatoid arthritis, cancer, anemia, and diabetes, which are conspicuous examples, may begin to develop and become worse for months before their presence is detected. The medical profession has cooperated for more than fifty years with the people in the

United States to develop and to urge periodic physical examinations. Some organizations have been developed particularly for this purpose and include a variety of experts such as pathologists and roentgenologists in their staffs.

The scope of a periodic physical examination may vary from the usual record of illnesses and difficulties from birth to the date of the examination. Certainly an X ray of the chest, simple examinations of the blood and of the urine and the back of the eye are followed later by more extensive studies should the result of any special examination indicate a need for them. Thus the cost of a periodic physical examination may vary from approximately $25 to $250 or more depending on the number and scope of the individual studies.

The ordinary periodic physical examination may be conducted in the doctor's office and when more complicated in a hospital. This decision is to be made by the doctor following his preliminary examination.

The American Medical Association has prepared a suitable form for periodic physical examinations. Most large hospitals and many doctors have prepared their own forms which are followed to make certain that every organ and system of the body is properly investigated.

IN AN EMERGENCY

Practically every county in the United States has a medical society. There are now about 100 medical colleges in the United States. Approximately 9000 hospitals of considerable size are available in addition to many smaller institutions including the dispensaries of many industries. Everyone ought to be aware of the medical facilities in the community in which he lives and the best way to contact such facilities when they are needed.

One may determine from any medical school, hospital, or dispensary the names of physicians who are available. In the larger cities, the telephone companies keep available lists of physicians who may be reached in an emergency.

Often the secretary, telephone operator, or receptionist may wish to know something of the nature of the condition for which the call is being made. The person who calls should be prepared to describe briefly what happened. Did the person collapse? Did the person faint and regain consciousness? Was there a blow or a wound? Is there difficulty in breathing? In other chapters in this book, the symptoms of most common diseases are fully described. The questions that will be asked of the person who calls will probably require minimum information as to whether the temperature has been recorded, is the throat sore, is there difficulty in swallowing. A few simple statements relative to such conditions will be most helpful.

COMMUNITY HEALTH AND MEDICAL SERVICES

In the United States the growth of voluntary health agencies has been one of the conspicuous marvels of the present century. Not only are there large organizations concerned with the major disease problems but innumerable institutions for the care of a wide variety of health problems and diseases. The largest telephone directories list such agencies under health and welfare organizations, social services and welfare organizations, and under similar headings. The classified directories list hospitals and homes and the providers of many varieties of nursing services. Similarly, physicians are listed as well as other types of medical practitioners. The associations concerned with heart, cancer, mental health, tuberculosis, and the Red Cross also provide advice and referral to suitable agencies. Both mother and father in any household should look into the availability of this information; best is to keep closely adjacent to the telephone a list of the important agencies with their telephone numbers to be used when needed.

GOING TO THE HOSPITAL

The hospital was once used primarily for poor people in times of emergency or acute sickness. In modern times, the hospital is indispensable from birth to death and even before. Of nearly 200 million people in the United States, more than three-fourths are protected against the cost of hospitalization by membership in Blue Cross or some other form of hospital insurance. When the doctor sends the patient to the hospital, the admitting office will wish to see evidence of such insurance and to make inquiry for information necessary to admission. Practically every hospital has an admittance form which will require answers as to full name, place of residence, name of nearest relative or other person to be notified when necessary, and often even financial information. Furthermore, the Social Security number will be needed and perhaps even records of membership in various social service or similar organizations. Every adult should be aware of this necessity and make certain the necessary information is easily available.

CHAPTER 2

The Family Medicine Chest

MORRIS FISHBEIN, M.D.

Most Americans, being independent and individualistic, feel themselves competent to fix defects in the plumbing and almost equally competent to take care of their own disturbances of health, as well as to prescribe for more complicated disturbances which really ought to have prompt medical attention.

A household remedy should be one with a certain definite action; usually it should contain but one active ingredient. A drug worth keeping in the medicine chest should be something which is used fairly frequently. Dangerous poisons have no place in the family medicine chest. A dangerous poison is one which is likely to produce serious symptoms or death if taken in even moderate amounts. Prescriptions ordered by the family doctor for a certain illness should never be kept for the future. If any of the material remains in the bottle it should be poured promptly into a safe place of disposal. Since useful bottles are rare around most homes, the bottle may be thoroughly washed with hot water, dried, and stored away. Few people realize that most drugs deteriorate with age and that a prescription for a certain illness is not likely to be useful for the future.

The wise person will go over the family medicine chest at least once every three months and at that time discard all materials not constantly in use. The family doctor can be asked to look at the materials once in a while to offer his advice as to those worth keeping.

TAKING MEDICINE

Medicines rightly used can be of immense aid and comfort to the afflicted; wrongly used, they may cause serious damage to the human body. When a doctor prescribes medicines for a patient, they are for that particular patient and not for anybody else in the family. Hence, old prescriptions should not be saved but should be disposed of as soon as possible after they are no longer necessary for the patient for whom they were prescribed.

The doctor usually writes on his prescription, and the druggist recopies on the label, the directions for taking the medicine. When giving medicine to a sick person be sure you know exactly what is on the label of the bottle. If necessary, take the bottle into another room to read the label so as not to be disturbed by conversation with the patient or with anyone else.

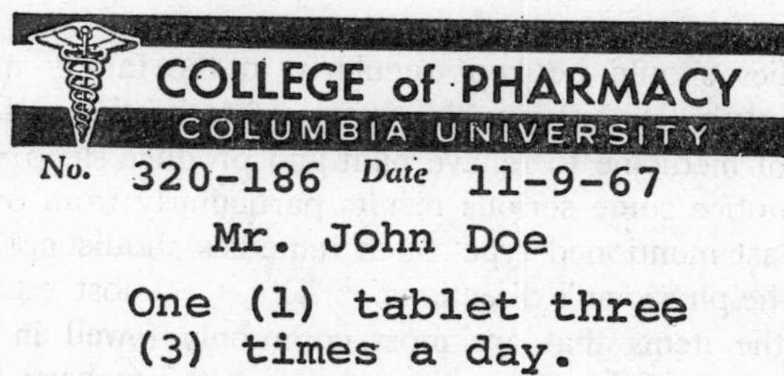

Fig. 2. This prescription was ordered by Dr. Smith for Mr. John Doe for a very definite purpose. It could save John Doe's life. On the other hand, Mr. Doe's life might be jeopardized if he decided to take this potent medication six months later for a *seemingly* similar ailment. The prescription number and date identify this drug in the pharmacist's file. He can advise Mr. Doe as to the stability and potency of the medication if Dr. Smith recommends that it be taken again or renewed. College of Pharmaceutical Sciences, Columbia University.

Then, when you measure out the medicine, think of what you are doing and pay no attention to anything else. Medicines are usually prescribed in dosages of drops, teaspoons, fractions of teaspoons, and spoons of larger sizes. Because spoons are nowadays in many fanciful shapes and sizes, each family should have a medicine glass with measures of various spoons recorded. When a doctor says any number of drops, the drops should be measured with a medicine dropper and not by guesswork.

If liquid medicine is being prescribed, the bottle should be thoroughly shaken each time before the medicine is measured. When medicine is poured out of the bottle, the cork should be deposited with its top down on the table and immediately put back in the bottle after the medicine has been poured.

Most liquid medicine should be mixed with a little water when taken, but sometimes the medicine may be put in the mouth and washed down with a swallow of water. Pills and capsules should either be handed to the patient from the original package so that he may help himself, putting the pill or capsule on the back of the tongue and washing it down with a drink of water, or else brought to the patient on a spoon so that he may take the pill or capsule from the spoon. In other words, the person who is waiting on the patient should not carry the capsules or pills in the palm of the hand, where they may be softened or disintegrated by moisture or contaminated from the hands.

Several ways are recommended in which medicines of unpleasant taste may be made more palatable. If cold water is taken, it will serve to cover the taste. Do not give medicine to children in foods, particularly in milk, as this may create a distaste for the food or milk which may last for a long time thereafter.

Few remedies should be kept regularly in the family medicine chest. American people suffer today with overuse of cathartics and laxatives, and with overuse of medicine to relieve pain and produce sleep. Physicians are beginning to notice some serious results particularly from overdosing with drugs of the last mentioned type. Such remedies should not be used regularly without the physician's directions.

What are the items that are most commonly found in any first-class family medicine chest? Most families want something to use for moving the bowels in the occasional case of temporary obstruction or slowness of action. Under certain circumstances any laxative or cathartic may be exceedingly dangerous. The most conspicuous example is appendicitis. This is at first just an infected spot on a little organ which comes off the large bowel and which apparently has no serious function in the human body. If this infection develops the way a boil develops from a pimple, it may burst and spread throughout the body. When infection is spread in the abdomen the result is peritonitis. Therefore, a laxative or cathartic should never be taken when the abdomen is exceedingly painful.

The most common laxatives found in family medicine chests include liquid petrolatum, or mineral oil, a mechanical lubricant that may interfere with absorption of vitamin A; castor oil, seidlitz powders, milk of magnesia, Epsom salts, sodium phosphate, phenolphthalein, aromatic cascara, and bulk formers like cellulose and psyllium seed preparations. For the people who use the medicine chest a large sign should be placed indicating that none of these preparations is ever to be used for abdominal pain of unknown cause.

The next most commonly found preparations in a family medicine chest, aside from the cosmetics, are pain relievers. Most of these are used for headaches, although sometimes they are used for what are called neuritis, neuralgia, toothache, and other pains of unknown origin, as well as to produce sleep. Most headache powders bought under patent trade marks contain phenacetin or aspirin. Moreover, people tend to form the habit of taking such preparations, and such habits are dangerous, since they temporize with what may eventually become a serious condition. Least harmful of the pain relievers is aspirin.

Other drugs much used to produce sleep nowadays are derivatives of barbituric acid of which some of the best examples are phenobarbital, seconal, nembutal, and ipral. In most states druggists are not permitted to sell such preparations to anyone without a physician's prescription. This should be sufficient indication of their danger as used by many people without medical knowledge. The family medicine chest should not include preparations of this character. The possibilities for harm are sufficiently great to suggest that these preparations be not used except on medical advice. Thousands of deaths have resulted from accidental overdosage.

The most commonly used general pain reliever throughout the country today is acetylsalicylic acid, commonly called aspirin. It is relatively harmless except for a few people who are especially sensitive to it. Such people cannot take even small doses. One aspirin is as good as another, provided it is up to the standard of the United States Pharmacopeia. Special claims are made for aspirins that dissolve more quickly in the stomach. Old tablets become dry and harden and may not be absorbed. Some mixtures of aspirin with other drugs may be more palatable or easier to take.

Among the strongest of medicinal preparations are the narcotics and anesthetics. Narcotics should never be used by anyone without a physician's prescription and, indeed, no drug that has to be administered with a hypodermic syringe should find a place in the average family medicine chest. Some people with diabetes have been taught by their doctors to inject themselves with insulin. Even these people should keep their syringe outfit separate from the materials in the family medicine chest.

All sorts of antiseptics are available for use on the skin, in first aid and also for gargling and for washing various portions of the body. The Council on Drugs of the American Medical Association is not opposed to advertising recognized antiseptics for first aid to the public, and tincture of iodine and mercurochrome are included among the preparations that may be so advertised. Others commonly used are merthiolates, metaphen, and zephiran.

Scientific evidence has not been available to prove that any of the widely advertised antiseptic solutions used as gargles, sprays, or in any other manner will prevent the onset of a common cold. Some mouth washes and gargles do kill germs with which they are sufficiently long in contact. Some make the throat feel better.

The family medicine chest may also contain aromatic spirits of ammonia which is sometimes given when a prompt stimulant is needed following fainting. Half a teaspoonful in water, in a sudden fainting spell, is a fairly safe thing to give in most cases of emergency. The widely publicized milk of magnesia and sodium bicarbonate, or baking soda, are two preparations which can safely be kept in the family medicine chest and which are frequently advised by physicians for alkaline purposes. Some families keep paregoric as a useful preparation in case of cramps that disturb women at periodic intervals.

SURGICAL SUPPLIES

In these days when everybody takes the chance of needing emergency first-aid treatment because of the common use of the automobile and wide indulgence in sports and gardening, some useful supplies should be available in the home.

Among the materials needed for first aid are packages of adhesive tape of various widths, sterile cotton, sterile gauze bandages, sterile gauze pads, scissors which should be kept in the medicine chest and not used for the family sewing or for other purposes around the home, and the ready-made combinations of a piece of adhesive tape with a tiny piece of sterilized bandage that can be used to cover small wounds or wounds after they have been treated with iodine or mercurochrome.

Most people should know that the proper way to stop bleeding of small wounds on the surface of the body is simply to press upon them with a sterile piece of gauze. In case of very serious wounds affecting arteries, and thereby difficult to control, it may be necessary to put a tourniquet around the limb. The tourniquet should be fastened just tight enough to stop the bleeding. An ordinary piece of rubber tubing or a narrow towel tied and twisted with a stick will serve most purposes satisfactorily. It should be temporarily released every ten or fifteen minutes.

In addition to the materials used for first aid, most families will have bed pans for use in cases of illness, glass drinking tubes, syringes for giving enemas, atomizers, and sometimes special devices for creating steam to be medicated with small amounts of tincture of benzoin for relief in various forms of hoarseness or other conditions affecting the larynx and the lungs.

The final materials to be included are the cosmetics. Most modern women prefer to keep their cosmetics in their own boudoirs or sleeping apartments. The man of the house is likely to put his into the family medicine chest. They should include, in most instances, a razor which should be kept in its box and not permitted to lie around loose; also some shaving soap or cream, some face lotion, which may be either witch hazel or any special lotion that he prefers.

Do not use a styptic in the form of a stick of alum to stop slight bleeding points after shaving. Much better are any of the stringent surgical powders, of which a small amount may be taken from the box at each occasion and applied directly to the bleeding point.

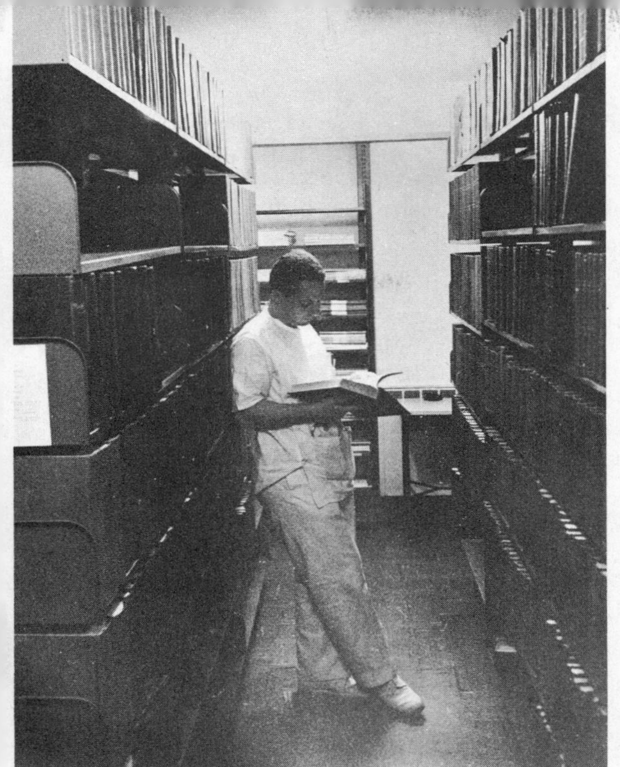

PLATE **1.** Medical student doing research in the medical library. *(Courtesy of Montefiore Hospital and Medical Center, New York/United Hospital Fund of New York.)*

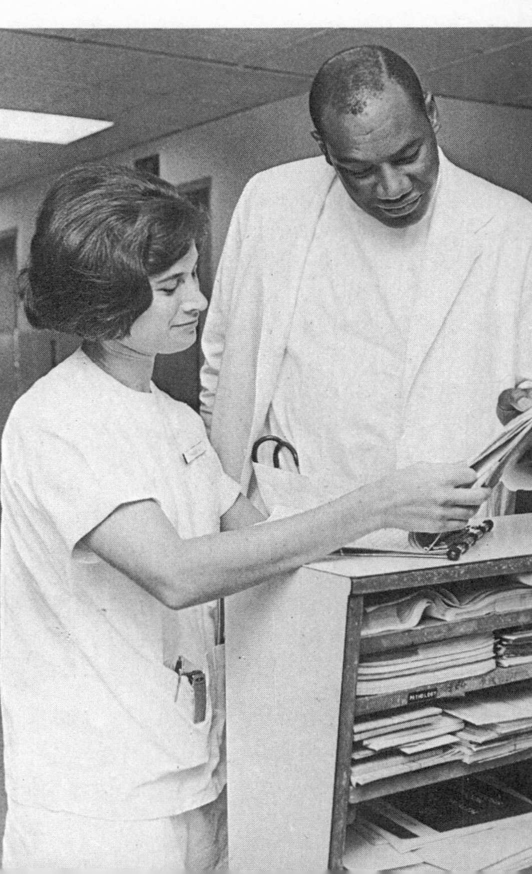

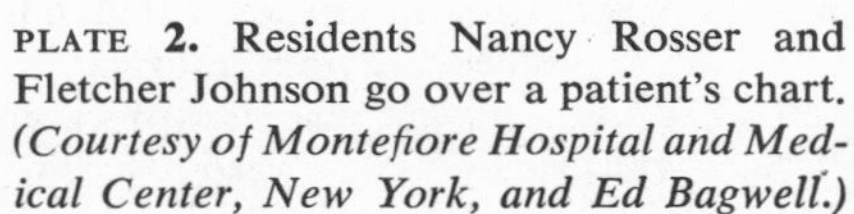

PLATE **2.** Residents Nancy Rosser and Fletcher Johnson go over a patient's chart. *(Courtesy of Montefiore Hospital and Medical Center, New York, and Ed Bagwell.)*

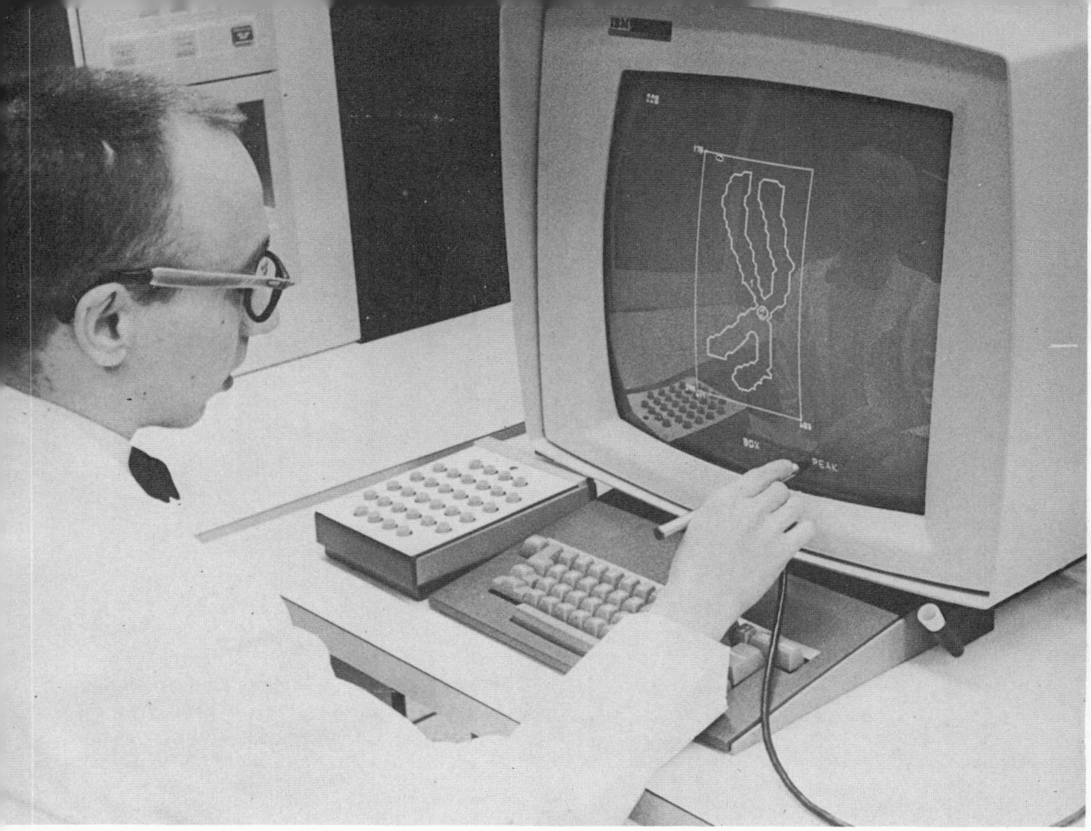

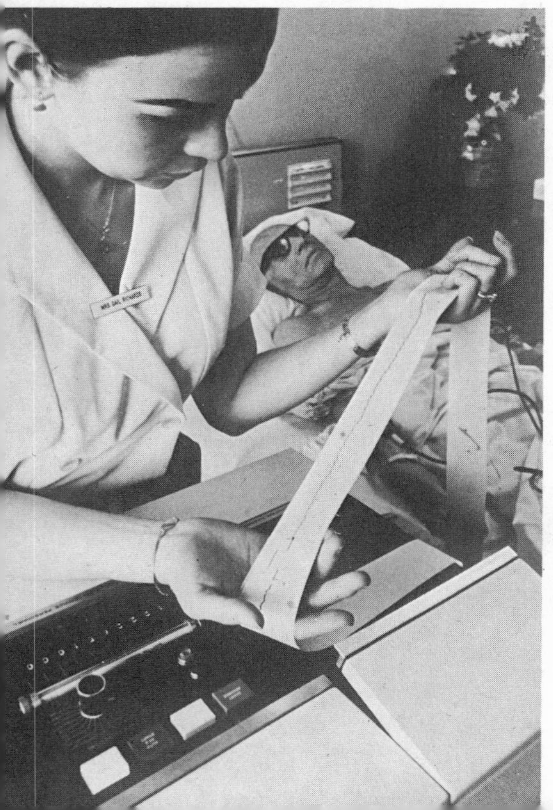

PLATE **3.** Computer helps physician interpret X rays. Dr. Harvey Frey, of UCLA's Radiology Department, studies a microscopic X ray of a chromosome. The computer classifies the chromosomes in various groups so that they may be correlated to various diseases and genetic disorders. *(International Business Machines Corporation.)*

PLATE **4.** In New York City's Mount Sinai Hospital, laboratory technician, Mrs. Gail Richards, views heart rhythm information recorded from patient via experimental bedside electronic system. Electrocardiogram (EKG) signals are captured on a standard strip chart recorded for visual interpretation by a physician. *(International Business Machines Corporation.)*

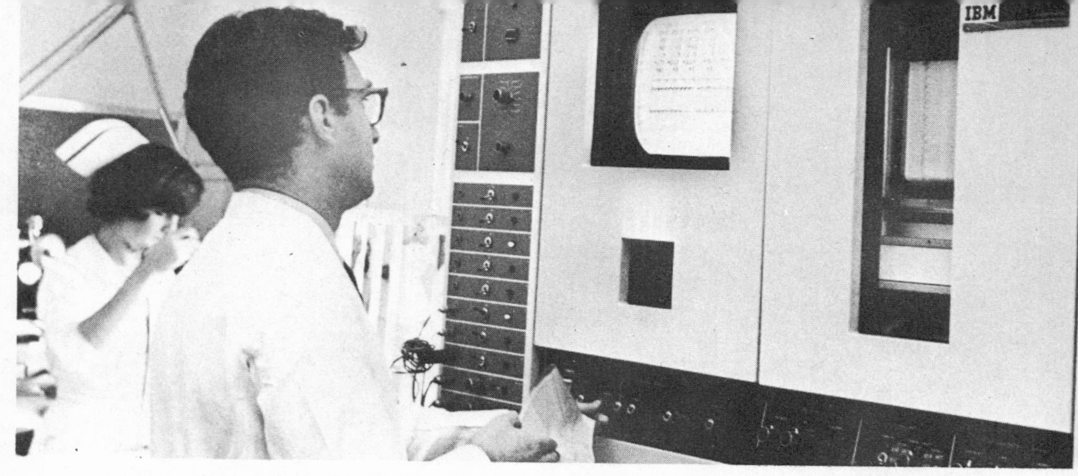

PLATE **5.** Television screen gives Dr. Robert W. Popper a window into new "early warning system" that is helping physicians and nurses at Presbyterian Medical Center (San Francisco) watch over people recovering from open heart-surgery as well as other critically ill patients. This computer accepts basic data from physiological sensors and calculates up to twenty-five factors relating to a patient's condition. The computer automatically interrupts routine summary displays with an alert message to help physicians predict complications. *(International Business Machines Corporation.)*

PLATE **6.** A televisionlike terminal linked to this system displays medical data for IBM systems engineer Jane McBride and Dr. Allan H. Levy, Director of Computer Operations at Baylor University College of Medicine. Terminals like this will enable doctors, nurses, and technicians to process vital medical information immediately. *(International Business Machines Corporation.)*

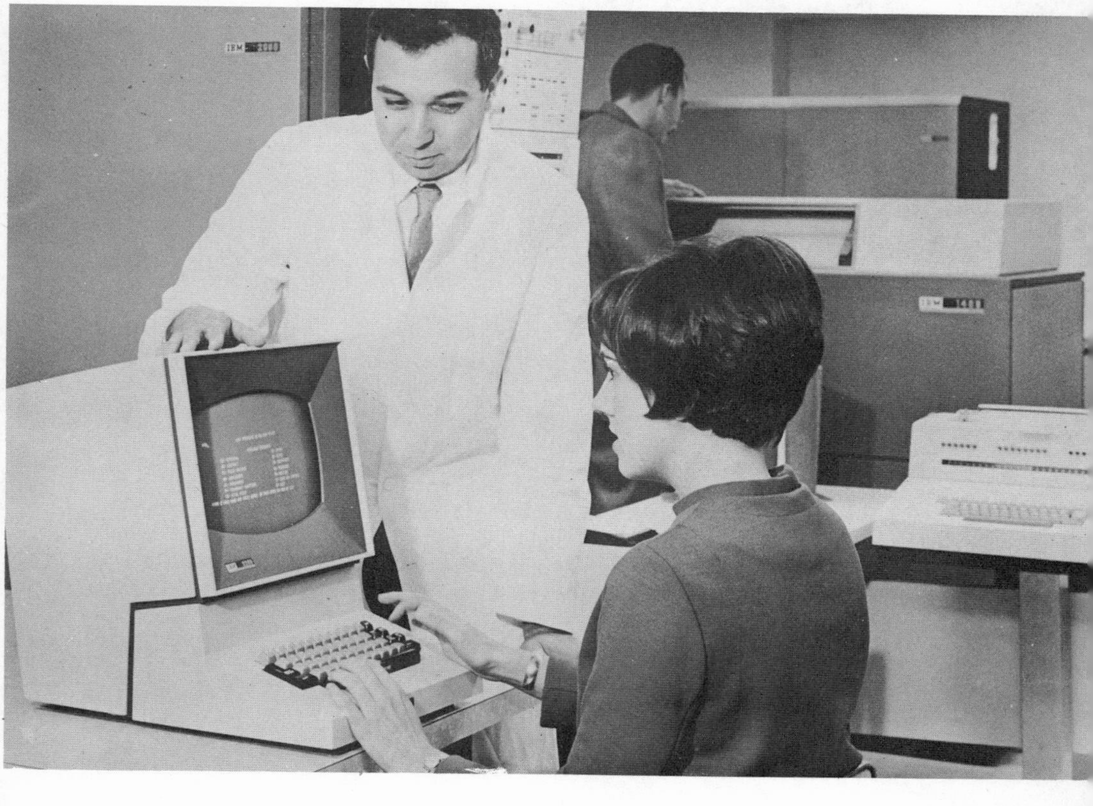

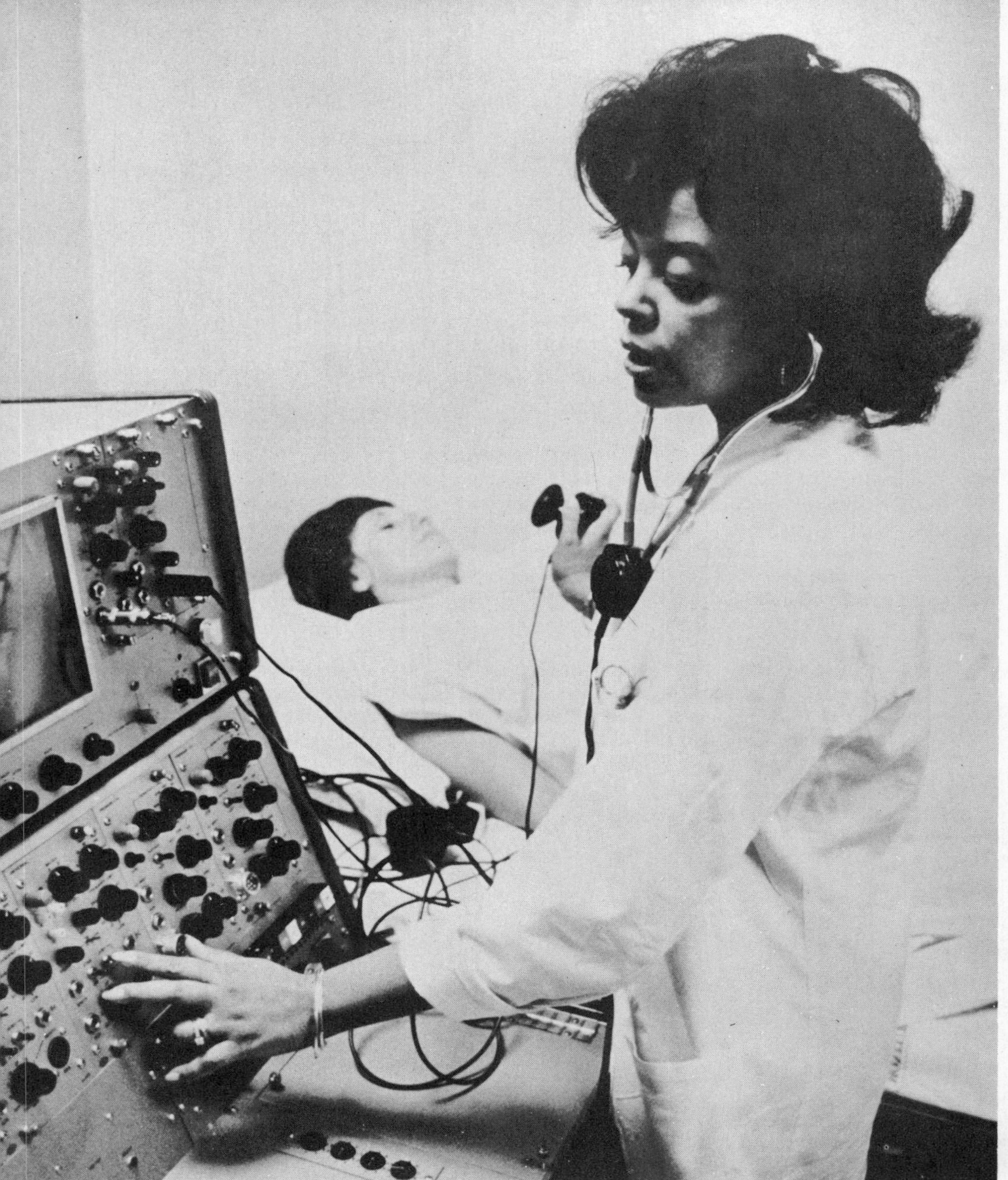

PLATE 7. Patient is being given a phonocardiogram—a diagnostic procedure in which a machine takes pictures of the sounds of the heart and registers them on a graph so that the physicians can pinpoint the source of any unusual sounds or murmurs. Operating the machine is Mrs. Carmen Oxendine, a highly specialized technician who has been trained to do this procedure which, in most hospitals, is performed by a doctor. *(Courtesy of Montefiore Hospital and Medical Center, New York, and Vernon Smith.)*

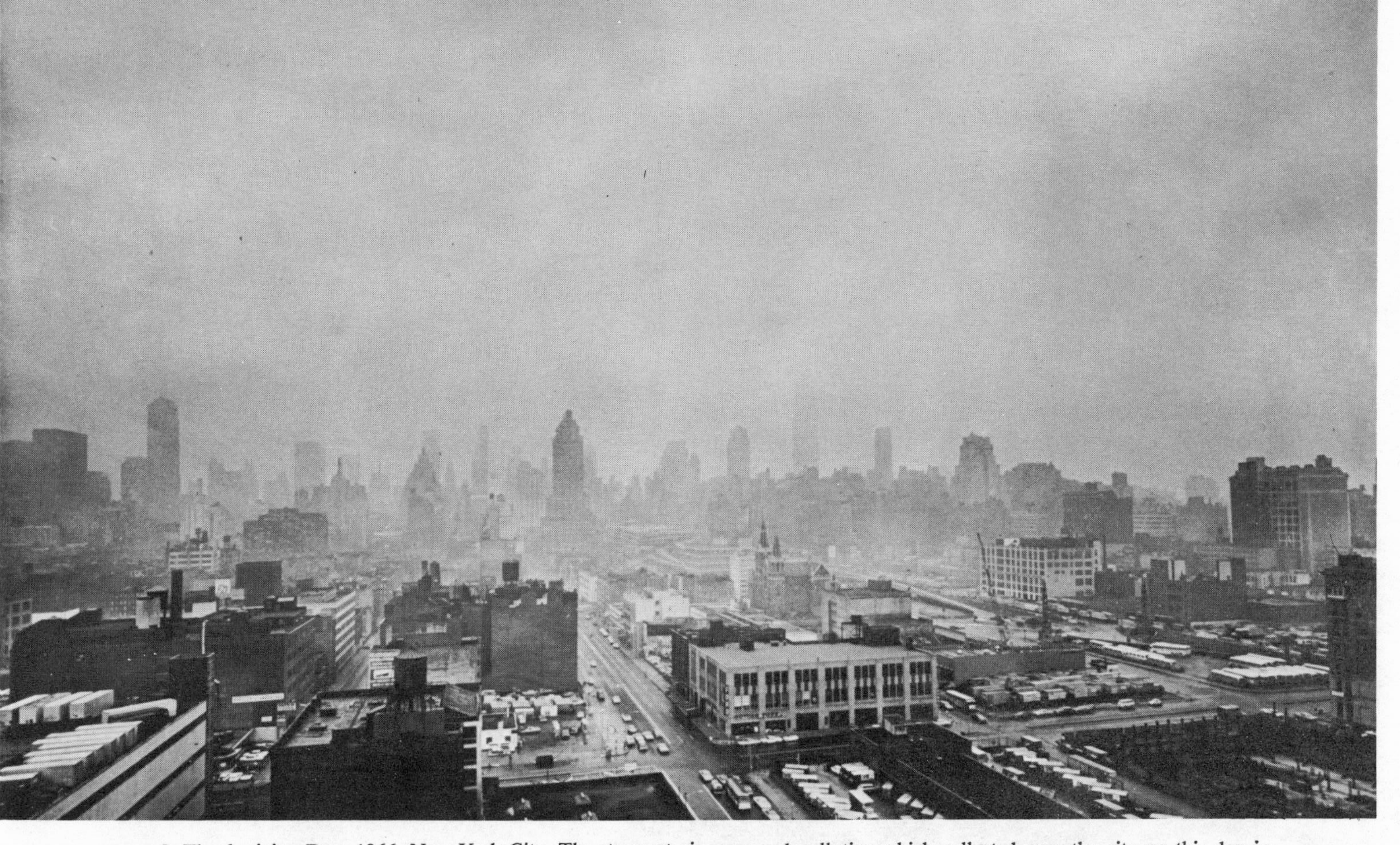

PLATE **8.** Thanksgiving Day, 1966, New York City. The stagnant air mass and pollution which collected over the city on this day in particular threatened human health. Air pollution contributes to the increase of emphysema; aggravates bronchial asthma; does untold damage to plants and animals; and accelerates the deterioration of materials, structures, and machines of all kinds. *(National Center for Air Pollution Control, Bureau of Disease Prevention and Environmental Control.)*

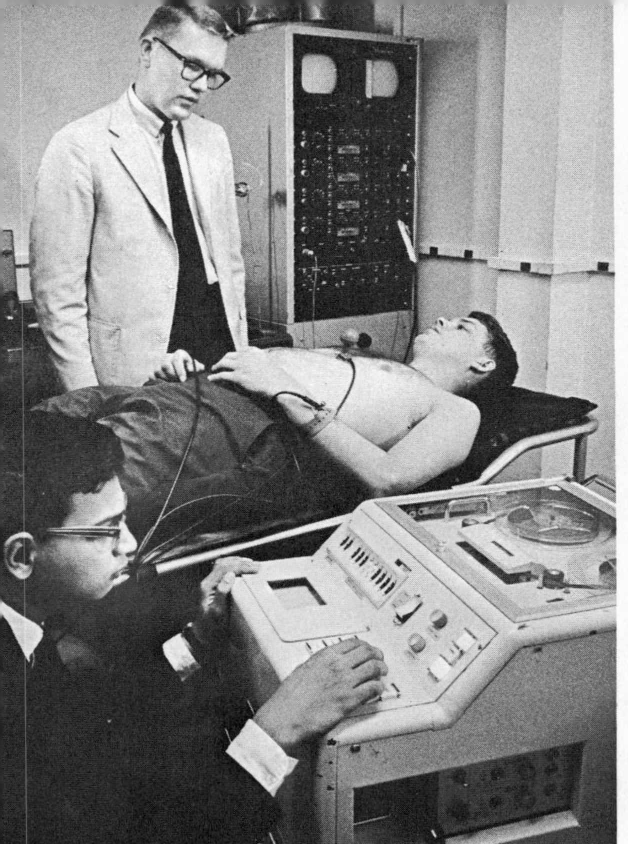

PLATE **9.** Recording electrocardiograms for processing by computer. This is one part of the research program conducted for preventing and controlling cancer, heart disease, kidney disease, chronic respiratory disease, diabetes, arthritis, and neurological and sensory diseases. Programs are also conducted on nutrition, health protection systems development, and the National Clearinghouse for Smoking and Health. *(National Center for Chronic Disease Control, Bureau of Disease Prevention and Environmental Control.)*

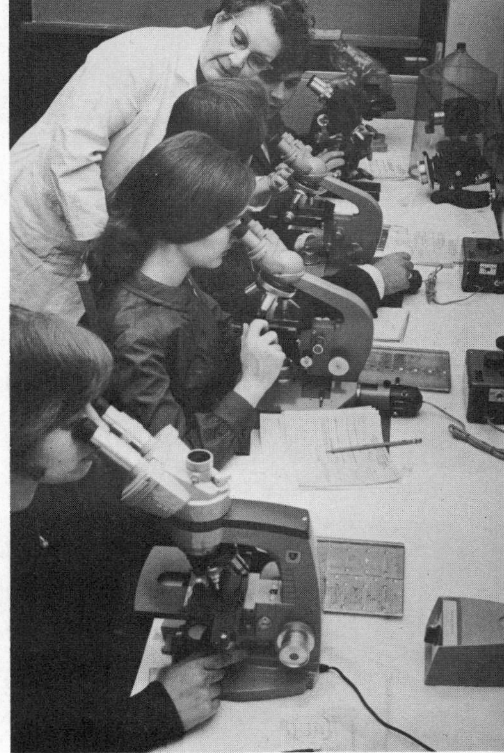

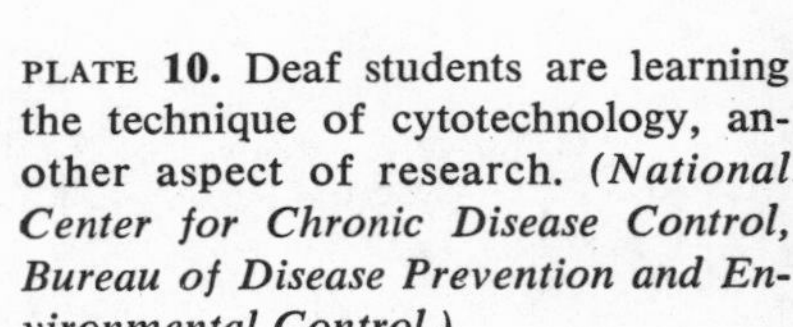

PLATE **10.** Deaf students are learning the technique of cytotechnology, another aspect of research. *(National Center for Chronic Disease Control, Bureau of Disease Prevention and Environmental Control.)*

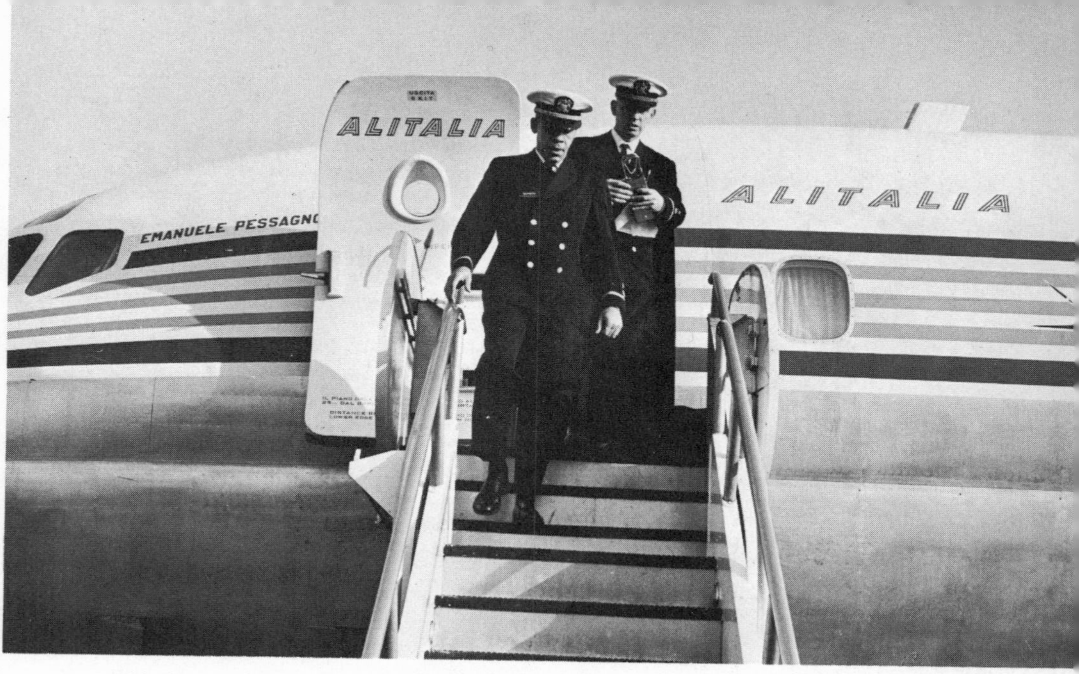

PLATE **11.** Quarantine officers at Kennedy Airport. This is only one part of the work of the Public Health Service's agency for control of infections and certain other preventable diseases. *(National Communicable Disease Center, Bureau of Disease Prevention and Environmental Control.)*

PLATE **12.** Doctors study tissue sections of dead miner. The work of this Public Health Service's agency is concerned with urban sanitation, food and water supplies, injury and occupational health hazards, and other problems affecting the health of people in an urban industrial environment. *(National Center for Urban and Industrial Health, Bureau of Disease Prevention and Environmental Control.)*

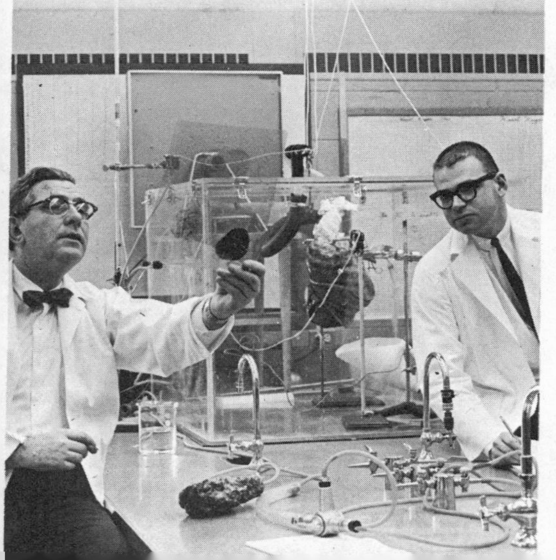

PLATE **13.** Surveying environmental radiation levels. This Public Health Service agency measures radiation in the environment, estimates human exposure, conducts research on the effects of such exposure and leads a nationwide program to protect the public from radiation hazards. *(National Center for Radiological Health, Bureau of Disease Prevention and Environmental Control.)*

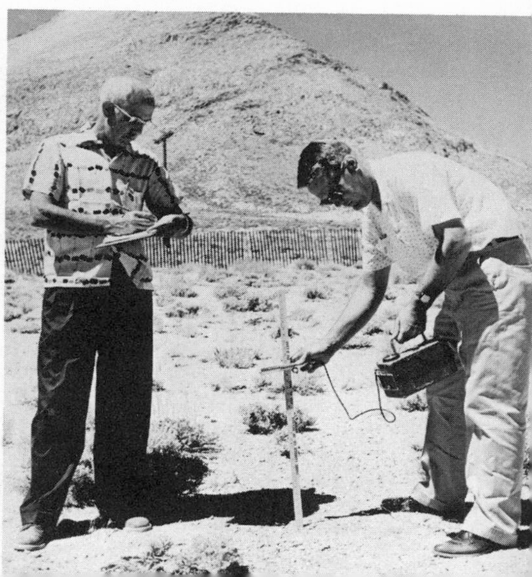

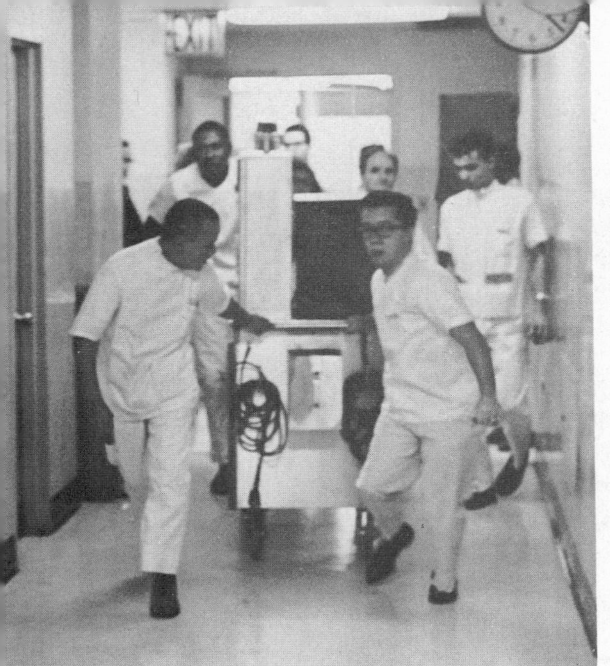

PLATE **14.** Cardiac Arrest Cart, containing every piece of equipment and medication needed to restore a patient's heart and respiration to normal, is sped to the scene of the emergency. *(Courtesy of Montefiore Hospital and Medical Center, New York, and Richard Saunders.)*

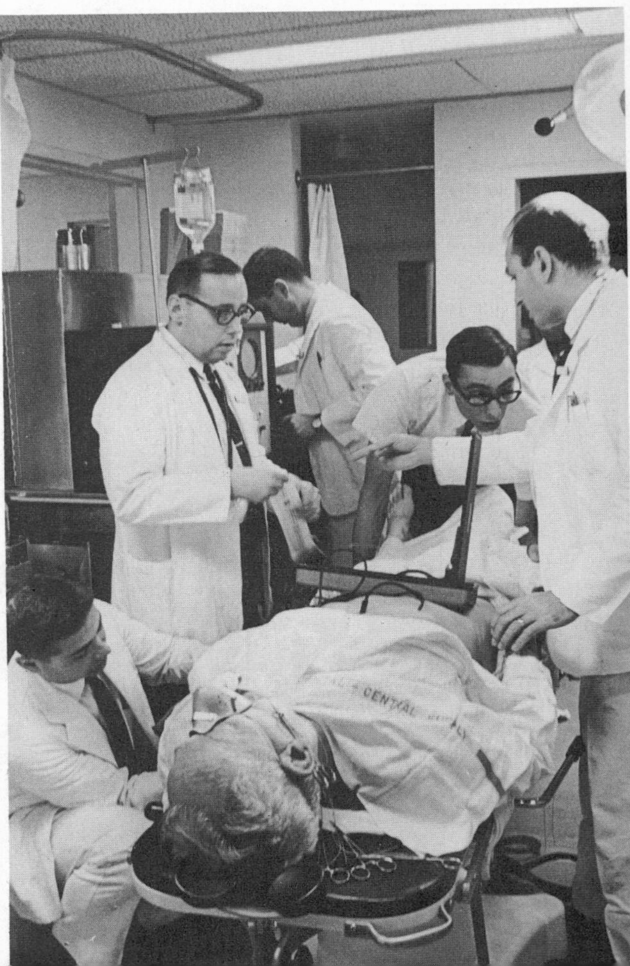

PLATE **15.** Patient has suffered cardiac arrest (sudden and complete cessation of the body's vital functions) and Montefiore's Cardiac Arrest Team, responding to a special emergency signal, has arrived at the scene and is beginning resuscitation. Hospital procedure for handling cardiac arrests is so precisely timed that the team, composed of doctors, nurses, and technicians, arrive at any point in the hospital within 120 seconds (average time is 57 seconds) after the emergency signal is given. *(Courtesy of Montefiore Hospital and Medical Center, New York, and Richard Saunders.)*

Finally, any good talcum powder may be used with satisfaction after shaving and after bathing, according to the individual preferences of the users.

Every modern household should have a good clinical thermometer, a hot-water bottle, and an ice bag. When these are available in an emergency the comfort they give is tremendous.

WARNINGS

Do not save poisonous preparations of any kind, including particularly bichloride of mercury, pills containing strychnine, or solutions containing wood alcohol. Do not keep samples of patent medicines of unknown composition recommended beyond their actual virtues. Never permit any preparation of opium or morphine to be loose in the family medicine chest. Never save any prepared prescription after the specific use for which it was ordered by the physician has disappeared.

EQUIPMENT OF THE FAMILY MEDICINE CHEST

A fountain syringe: This should be of rubber or of metal with a capacity of about two quarts, a long rubber tube and several nozzles of assorted sizes.

A bed pan: In many illnesses it is not safe for the patient to get up even to attend to the usual body needs.

A rubber sheet: This is to be placed under the sheet to prevent soiling of the mattress. A piece of oilcloth will serve the purpose satisfactorily for a short time.

Bandages: These are cheaply purchased. They should be in various sizes from one-inch width to three-inch width.

Adhesive tape: This can also be purchased in spools of various widths and lengths.

Scissors: These should always be kept available in the medicine chest.

Thermometer: A good clinical thermometer should be available, and preferably two, one for taking temperature by mouth and another for temperature by rectum.

Ice bag: The ice bag applied to the sore throat is frequently recommended by doctors.

Atomizer: For spraying nose and throat.

GRADUATED MEDICINE GLASS for measuring dosages.

THE DRUGS AND MEDICAL SUPPLIES

CATHARTICS AND LAXATIVES:

Epsom salts: An old-fashioned remedy with lots of power. Best taken in the morning on arising. About a tablespoonful in a half-glass of warm water.

Citrate of magnesia: A milder saline laxative. Order a bottle from the druggist

Take a half bottle on arising and the rest later if needed. Anywhere from six to twelve ounces of the solution of magnesium citrate is a dose.

Castor oil: An effective and prompt cathartic but likely to be followed by constipation and therefore not indicated in chronic constipation. A dose is four teaspoonfuls. This can now be had in tasteless and flavored forms.

Mineral oil: A lubricant much used in chronic cases of constipation. Dose: One or two tablespoonfuls. Mineral oil should not be used habitually since it absorbs vitamin A.

Other cathartics: Other cathartics and laxatives much used include sodium acid phosphate, phenolphthalein, which is the active substance of such advertised laxatives as Feenamint, Ex-lax, and similar products, also the Hinkle pill, the compound cathartic pill, and other mixtures. Bulk laxatives are psyllium seed, agar, cellothyl. It is not well to develop a cathartic habit. It is not safe to take cathartics in the presence of undiagnosed pains in the abdomen.

GENERAL DRUGS AND SUPPLIES:

Glycerine: Useful for many purposes. A few drops warmed and dropped into the ear are frequently advised for earache.

Vaseline petroleum jelly, cold cream, zinc oxide ointment: These are useful for abrasions of the skin, chafing, sunburn, etc.

Tincture of iodine: An ideal antiseptic for application to cuts or small wounds of the skin. It is usually painted on, using a toothpick wrapped with cotton.

Boric acid: A concentrated solution is a good home antiseptic solution.

Hydrogen peroxide solution: Diluted about one half with water makes a good cleansing wash for wounds. Diluted one to three with water, can be used as a gargle.

Sodium bicarbonate: Baking soda. Useful as a gargle. Much used for so-called "sour stomach." Good in the bath for itching of the skin.

Aspirin: The great American pain reliever. Much used for headaches. Much safer than pyramidon, barbituric acid derivatives, acetanilid, phenacetin, and all the other coal-tar derivatives. Dosage: one or two five-grain tablets, repeated in about three hours.

Aromatic spirits of ammonia: Used to bring about recovery after fainting spells.

Surgical powder: A styptic powder, best used on small cuts after shaving.

Petrolatum eucalyptus menthol compound: A nice mixture for use in the nose as a spray.

Paper towels, paper handkerchiefs: Most useful in sickness. Can be destroyed after use.

The medicine chest should always be kept out of reach of the children. Prescriptions in current use may be kept in the chest, but should be destroyed after the patient is well. Every bottle and package should be clearly labeled. Do not stock up with a lot of cathartics and laxatives, cough and cold remedies. Keep only those regularly used and called for by members of the family.

CHAPTER 3

First Aid

MORRIS FISHBEIN, M.D.

When illness or accidents occur in any home someone should know what can be done immediately. The certainty of knowledge will avoid the confusion, alarm, and distress that inevitably occur when no one knows just what to do in an emergency.

The emergencies that may occur range alphabetically from accidents to zebra-kick. No one can be fully prepared for all of these any more than any family is fully prepared for twins or triplets. Certain supplies may be kept in every home pending the occurrence of various accidents. The knowledge of the availability of these supplies and what to do with them by the mother, father, or the nurse will be found exceedingly helpful when the emergency arises.

ACCIDENTS

In the United States almost one hundred thousand people lose their lives in accidents each year, and some fifteen million people every year have accidents sufficiently severe to take them from their work. Of the accidents which occur in the home, falls constitute 40 per cent of the total; after falls come accidents from burns, scalds, and explosions; then asphyxiation or strangulation and, finally, cuts and scratches. Most of these accidents are preventable with care.

FALLS

When a person is injured in a fall the first step should be a consideration of the extent of the injury. It is necessary to determine whether or not bones have been broken, if there is bruising or hemorrhage and, finally, the extent to which the skin has been damaged. A broken bone usually reveals itself by inability to function. However, the only safe procedure is to call a physician who will take an X-ray picture and ascertain the actual extent of the damage.

Pending the arrival of a doctor it is well to place the injured part completely at rest and, if necessary, to hold it quiet with some suitable splint. A good splint is frequently made by wrapping a large-size magazine, or a newspaper folded many times, with handkerchiefs around the arm or leg to hold the tissues in place. However, unless the person who is applying

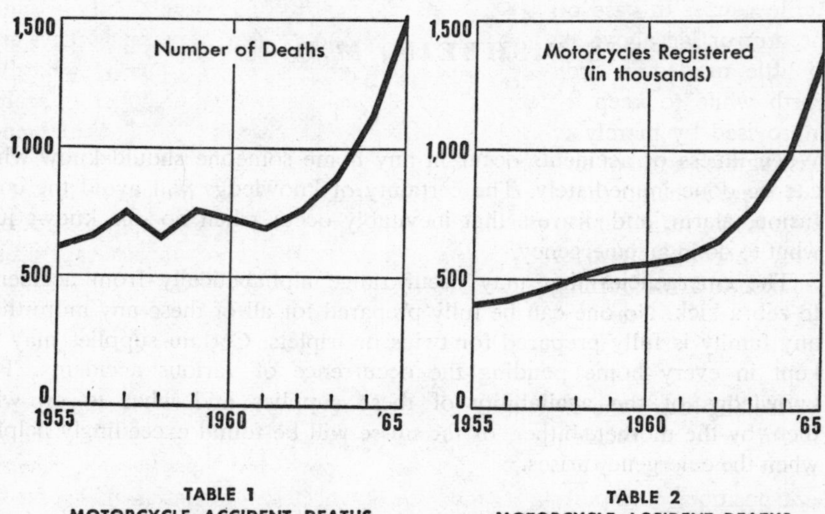

TABLE 1
MOTORCYCLE ACCIDENT DEATHS
UNITED STATES, 1955-1965

Year	Number of Deaths	Deaths per 100,000 Vehicles Registered
1965	1,534	111.1
1964	1,132	114.9
1963	891	113.3
1962	769	116.4
1961	702	117.8
1960	737	128.4
1959	770	136.2
1958	665	127.6
1957	759	161.9
1956	666	154.3
1955	625	151.6

Data include motorscooters and motorized bicycles. Table 2 does not include 19 deaths in motorcycle collisions with railroad trains.

Source of basic data: Reports of Division of Vital Statistics, National Center for Health Statistics; Interstate Commerce Commission; and U.S. Bureau of Public Roads.

TABLE 2
MOTORCYCLE ACCIDENT DEATHS
BY AGE, UNITED STATES, 1965

Age	Number of Deaths	Deaths per 100,000 Population
All Ages	1,515	0.8
Under 1	—	—
1-4	3	0.0
5-9	7	0.0
10-14	82	0.4
15-19	513	3.0
20-24	387	2.9
25-29	203	1.8
30-34	111	1.0
35-39	60	0.5
40-44	40	0.3
45-49	42	0.4
50-54	27	0.3
55-59	11	0.1
60-64	12	0.2
65-69	11	0.2
70-74	5	0.1
75+	1	0.0

Fig. 3. Motorcycle Accident Deaths and Motorcycle Registrations in the United States, 1955–65. *Statistical Bulletin*, Metropolitan Life Insurance Company.

the first-aid measure knows exactly what he or she is doing, it is better merely to put the injured person at rest and to keep him quiet.

BLEEDING OR HEMORRHAGE

In the case of bleeding certain measures may be undertaken at once. Ordinary wounds can be controlled by pressure with a clean piece of sterile gauze. In case of severe hemorrhages, wrap a cloth tightly around the arm or leg above the place of the bleeding. However, tourniquets are so little needed in ordinary accidents about the home that it is hardly worth while to keep a constant supply on hand. A tourniquet is easily improvised by merely tying a loop in a small towel or handkerchief and twisting with a rod of any kind.

If there is hemorrhage from a tooth socket following the extraction of a tooth it can usually be controlled by plugging the socket with sterile cotton or by the application of hot water. Under such circumstances care must be taken to avoid burning or scalding.

NOSEBLEED

Bleeding from the nose is fairly frequent, due either to a purposeful "sock" or to an accident such as running into a door. The simplest measure to stop bleeding from the nose is to place the bleeder in a recumbent position, preferably with the face down. The application of ice water or of hot water to the nose or temporarily packing with sterile clean gauze will help. It will not help particularly, except to distract attention, to pass a key down the back, to inhale smoke, to apply ice to the back of the neck, or to collect cobwebs and stuff them into the nose. If bleeding from the nose is frequent or continuous, a physician should make a careful examination of the blood to determine whether or not clotting, or coagulation, of the blood is delayed because of some deficiency. There is no way to strengthen blood vessels to prevent hemorrhage. If there is frequent hemorrhage from the nose a competent specialist in diseases of the nose will be able to look directly into it and to find out whether a dilated blood vessel or an ulcer of any kind is responsible. He can control such a condition by cauterizing the bleeding point or otherwise modifying the conditions responsible.

CONTROL OF BLEEDING

In addition to bleeding from the nose, there may be oozing from wounds elsewhere in the body. If this is continuous it can usually be controlled by pressure with a pad of sterile gauze. Sometimes the application of hydrogen peroxide will stop such oozing. Water as hot as can be borne may be tried, but merely washing with lukewarm water will frequently increase the bleeding.

Sometimes there is bleeding from a varicose vein of the leg. Under such circumstances the person should lie down, the foot be well elevated, a clean pad of gauze applied and compressed lightly with a bandage. Such a condition, however, is one which demands good medical attention, and a physician should be obtained for handling the condition as soon as possible.

In severe wounds of any kind packing may be attempted, a sufficient amount of sterile gauze being put into the wound and held in place, but obviously medical attention is demanded immediately when available.

Loss of blood is weakening. People who have lost large amounts of blood should be kept in bed and all possible movements avoided. They should be given plenty of nutritious food and plenty of fluids. A physician will prescribe suitable drugs and medicinal preparations for building up the blood after a hemorrhage.

One of the most serious accidents that may occur is sudden hemorrhage from the lungs which occurs occasionally in tuberculosis. Under such circumstances the person affected should be put immediately to bed, kept absolutely quiet, and an ice bag applied to the chest. Obviously, such hemorrhages demand most careful study as to the presence of tuberculosis at the earliest available time.

Whenever there is bleeding from the scalp, which is severe, because the scalp is richly supplied with blood vessels, an attempt should be made to stop the blood by applying a pad of gauze. If this does not work satisfactorily a tight band may be applied around the forehead to compress the blood vessels. Tourniquets applied or kept on too long may do much more harm than good.

Almost anyone can wrap a piece of gauze from a roller bandage around an arm or a leg or the forehead. To put on a bandage that will stay in place, that will be sterile during the process of application and after it is on, and that will serve the purpose satisfactorily is really a job for an expert. The average person should not attempt to learn bandaging, which is as much an artistic performance as playing the piano and probably more artistic than playing the saxophone.

BRUISES

Whenever the tissues of the body are struck with sufficient force there is likely to be bruising. This may come from a blow applied directly or from a fall in which the body moves and strikes against a fixed surface. The first symptom of a bruise is pain; usually this is followed by redness and swelling. Later, due to the blood that has poured out from the blood vessels into the skin, the tissues become black and blue. As the blood is gradually absorbed this changes from brown to yellow and gradually disappears. For most bruises little immediate treatment is necessary. The application of pads wrung out of ice water will lessen pain. Some enzyme preparations can now be prescribed which aid dissolving of blood clots.

A black eye is a form of bruise especially unsightly and likely to arouse ridicule. The application of iced compresses to the eye will stop the pain and perhaps, to some extent, prevent discoloration. After the blackness appears, the application of heat in the form of hot compresses kept on for half an hour three times a day will hasten the disappearance of the swelling and discoloration. Among things that are not to be done to a black eye are the application of a slice of raw beefsteak, pressure with the handle of a knife, and the application of any kind of strong medicinal lotion or solution.

The danger of injury to the eyeball is far more serious than either the mental or physical pain associated with the ordinary black eye. It is well to have the eye looked at promptly to make certain that the eyeball has not been injured in any way.

FOREIGN BODIES

Among the emergencies demanding first aid is the presence of foreign bodies in the eye, ear, nose, throat, or esophagus. Regardless of how careful mothers may be, children occasionally push foreign substances into various body cavities. When a child chokes there is no time to call a doctor. The mother must act promptly. The mother should remember that the attempt to remove any object in the throat by rough methods may do more harm than good. If the baby is small it should be put face downward, or head downward, and given an opportunity to cough the object out. A very large object can, of course, be pulled out with the finger. A physician removes objects from the throat by the use of special devices developed for this purpose. He has "scopes" of every type with which he may look into the various cavities. He has also special lighted tubes with forceps and hooks for the withdrawal of foreign substances.

When foreign substances get into the nose, more harm is usually done by attempts to dislodge them with improper instruments than by letting them alone until competent advice can be had. If blowing the nose will not remove a foreign substance, sneezing may accomplish it. The physician may wash out foreign substances or by the use of proper forceps seize and remove them.

Another type of emergency is the foreign substance in the ear, particularly an insect. An insect in the ear may be removed by turning the head to one side and filling the ear with warm sweet oil poured into it by means of a spoon. The insect is unable to live in the oil, and it promptly dies, and then can be floated out with warm water. In syringing the ear with warm water it is best to spray the water against the side at the entrance of the ear rather than directly against the eardrum.

If a child swallows any sharp-pointed object, such as a piece of glass, a bone, or a pin, relief is sometimes had by eating mashed potatoes and bread thoroughly chewed, which aid the passage of the substance down the gullet into the stomach. It is well then to obtain medical advice immediately. By the use of the X ray the substance may be located and a decision made as to the best method for its removal. Experience shows that in many instances foreign substances that are swallowed will pass from the body by way of the bowel without undue harm.

Foreign substances in the eyes are particularly annoying. With experience, it is possible to locate such foreign substances on the lower or upper lid and to remove cinders or tiny specks with the point of a clean pocket handkerchief. With a little experience it becomes possible for anyone to turn back the upper lid. The simplest method is, first to wash the hands thoroughly; then, with a small matchstick or some similar rod laid across the lid, the patient looks down, the attendant grasps the eyelashes, and turns the lid upside down by pulling the eyelashes over the matchstick or rod.

Do not attempt to remove a foreign substance from the surface of the eyeball without special training in such first aid measures. It is safer, pending the arrival of expert attention, to merely place a small pad of wet gauze over the eye and to restrain the motion of the eye until attention is available. If any foreign substance has been removed from the eye it may be washed out with a saturated solution of boric acid, made by adding a flat teaspoonful of boric acid powder to a glassful of warm water and stirring until dissolved.

The simplest way to put drops in the eye is with the use of an eye dropper. A small quantity of the drops is drawn into the dropper, the patient sits on a chair facing a good light, the person who is putting the drops in stands in front, pulls down the lower lid, and, while the patient looks away, places one or two drops of the fluid on the outer edge of the lower lid. This will run across the eye and wash the surface. The patient looks away in order to avoid seeing the dropper and jumping when it approaches the eye.

All sorts of suggestions are made for the removal of cinders or other specks from the eye, including rubbing the other eye, blowing the nose, and indulging in similar manipulations. The chief advantage of these manipulations is to avoid harm to the eye from too much inexpert attention.

FIREWORKS AND TOY FIREARMS

Among frequent emergencies demanding prompt attention are explosions of fireworks. Hundreds of people used to be killed or injured in celebrating the independence of the United States. Following great campaigns of education this type of celebration has been largely displaced by pageants, plays, and exhibits of fireworks under the control of expert showmen.

Air rifles, BB guns, shotguns, and other small-caliber rifles, blank cartridges and cap pistols, sling shots and rubber band flippers, arrows and stones, are responsible for one third of the accidents resulting in loss of eyesight to children. Firecrackers, torpedoes, bombs, and various types of fireworks are responsible for one fourth of the cases of blindness.

Lockjaw or tetanus is discussed elsewhere in this book. The germs of lockjaw develop in soil and in manure and on dirty clothing. Any time an injury occurs in which dirt is forced into a wound and sealed in there is danger of lockjaw. There is the kind of accident that occurs in explosions of cannon crackers, blank cartridges, and toy cannon. The size of the wound is not significant. The tiniest puncture may admit germs into the body.

Whenever an injury from fireworks occurs, get a doctor as soon as possible. He will open the wound, clean it, and treat it with suitable antiseptics, and in questionable cases inject the antitoxin against lockjaw to prevent that disease. Never wait until lockjaw develops. After the disease has developed it is one of the most serious affecting a human being. So serious is the possibility of lockjaw that in many cases health departments provide antitoxin without charge to make certain that cases of lockjaw do not develop.

WOUNDS

Whenever the skin is opened, torn, or punctured the injury is called a wound. Wounds may thus vary from the tiniest puncture, such as that of a needle, to severe injuries tearing open several inches of skin and penetrating into body cavities. The greatest danger from wounds, after the immediate danger of hemorrhage, lies in infection. Therefore, the first step of importance in first aid is to prevent infection. Infection may be prevented by disinfection.

In taking care of a wound be certain that your own hands are as clean as possible. Surgeons wash the hands thoroughly with soap and water and then wash them in antiseptics, and thereafter wear rubber gloves which have been sterilized by steam under pressure. In taking care of any small wound at home, be certain that the hands of the person who is taking care of the wound are as clean as possible. Hence they should be washed thoroughly with soap and water and perhaps also in alcohol. All materials applied to the wound should be sterilized. Such materials are now available in any drugstore in packages. If a sterile package of material is not available, it may be made by boiling thoroughly materials available in the home. A freshly laundered handkerchief or towel is likely to be relatively free from germs because laundering, heating, and ironing kill organisms on the surface.

Hundreds of antiseptic substances are now available and are widely advertised. Among the best of the antiseptics is alcohol. Tincture of iodine is widely used as a first-aid dressing, as are also mercurochrome, saturated solution of boric acid, hexachlorophene, metaphen, merthiolates, zephiran, and hexylresorcinol solution. When a wound has been contaminated with dirt this should be washed out with a suitable solution. Do not apply hydrogen peroxide to a fresh wound because it may cause pain and unnecessary crusting with destruction of tissue.

After the wound has been disinfected by the application of a suitable antiseptic it should be covered with clean sterile gauze and suitably bound. No one should attempt to sew a wound unless he has had medical training. Whenever pus or infection occurs in a wound it should have prompt medical attention. If a person is far removed from medical attention he should realize that it is of the greatest importance to release the pus by opening the wound and then to apply the antiseptic. Wet dressings of concentrated boric acid solution applied for several days are helpful.

Certain types of wounds represent unusual emergencies, among them splinters entering the skin. Small splinters are best removed by using a needle which has been passed through a flame in order to sterilize it; large splinters by the use of a knife blade sterilized in a similar manner, and perhaps also with the aid of a tweezers.

When a fishhook gets into the skin don't try to pull it out. In order to avoid tearing the tissues push the point onward and forward and let the end of the fishhook follow the point. The barbed end may then be cut off with a wire cutter, and when this is removed the fishhook may be removed by reversing the process.

BURNS

Burns of the skin may be produced by many different methods including the heat from a flame or hot iron, the heat from scalding water or steam, and the heat from electricity. Burns which involve more than one half of the surface of the body are usually fatal. When a person has been suddenly or severely burned he may suffer from shock. This demands immediate attention in order to stimulate him and to save life. He should, of course, be put at rest and the burn suitably covered to prevent continued irritation. Almost everyone now knows that when a person's clothing is actually burning it is well to smother the flames by the use of a blanket, a rug, or any other heavy material that is handy. A tub may be filled with lukewarm water and the burned person put in the tub. The skin under water will suffer less pain from the burn.

In the presence of slight burns or scalds it is preferable to cover the burned portion immediately with cold water, which will check the effect of the heat and stop the pain. Some recommend application of ordinary vinegar. If the foot or hand has been burned by spilling hot water, soup, or coffee over it, put the part burned immediately under water and keep it submerged until the first effects of the injury have passed. Thereafter it may be covered with Vaseline petroleum jelly. Loose cotton should not be put on a burn, nor should wide pieces of gauze be applied. It is practically impossible to remove such materials without great injury to the tissues. The gauze may be applied in narrow strips.

Modern methods of treating burns include application of liquid petrolatum, or the application of melted petrolatum, which hardens and covers the burn.

Burns from acids are among the most serious, particularly nitric and sulfuric acids. The first treatment following a burn by acid is to wash off the acid as quickly as possible with a solution of bicarbonate of soda and to leave the wound in the soda solution for some time. People who work in acids regularly should wear gloves whenever possible. Electric burns are usually deep and severe. They should be treated as are other burns.

RESUSCITATION

Among the most serious of emergencies which may occur, demanding first aid, is resuscitation after asphyxiation, which may result from drowning, from electric shock, and from exhaust-gas poison. Occasionally also there may be asphyxiation from other sources, such as gas escaping from electric refrigerators.

It has been estimated that 25 per cent of men and boys past twelve years of age do not know how to swim, and there are few women who would be capable of swimming long enough or far enough to save themselves in an emergency. When a person has been under water long enough to become unconscious—about four or five minutes—first-aid measures are of greatest importance to save life. There are numerous devices for artificial resuscitation, but it is usually not well to wait until these come. Until 1952 the most commonly practiced method was the Schaefer technique. Then the American Red Cross, the American Medical Association and other agencies after extended research adapted a method called the Holger. Now recommended is mouth-to-mouth resuscitation. This new technique has the distinct advantage of allowing the rescuer to provide enough pressure immediately to inflate the lungs of the victim. Here are the steps recommended by Dr. Peter Safar and his associates at the Department of Anesthesiology, Baltimore City Hospitals.

Method 1 is recommended for adults and large children.

1. When the victim is found, place him on his back and kneel close to his left ear. If foreign material is visible at the mouth, turn the victim's head to the side and quickly clean the mouth and throat with your fingers or a piece of cloth. This should take only a few seconds. If the mouth appears clean, tilt the head back so that the chin is pointing upward. Repeat cleaning procedure during mouth-to-mouth breathing whenever necessary.

2. Extend victim's head, insert your left thumb (which may be wrapped for protection) between his teeth, grasp the lower jaw at midline, and hold it forcefully forward (upward), so that the lower teeth are leading.

3. Close the victim's nose with your right hand. Take a deep breath, place your mouth firmly over his mouth, and blow forcefully. Watch the victim's chest, and when it rises, take your mouth off his mouth and let him exhale passively. Repeat the blowing effort at the rate of about 12 to 20 breaths per minute.

Method 2 is recommended for adults whose mouths cannot be opened and for small children.

1. Extend the victim's head and grasp the lower jaw with both hands, just beneath the ear lobes and hold the jaw forcefully forward (upward), so that the lower teeth are leading. Prevent lip obstruction by retracting the victim's lower lip with your thumbs, but never flex the victim's head.

2. Maintain your support of the jaw. Take a deep breath, place your mouth firmly over the victim's mouth and blow. Cover the nose with your right cheek to prevent air leakage. Blow forcefully. When you see his chest rise, take your mouth off the victim's mouth and let him exhale passively. Repeat the blowing about 12 to 20 times per minute. Blow forcefully in adults, gently in children. Use only puffs from the cheeks in newborn

babies. When you see the victim's chest rise, take your mouth off his mouth and let him exhale passively.

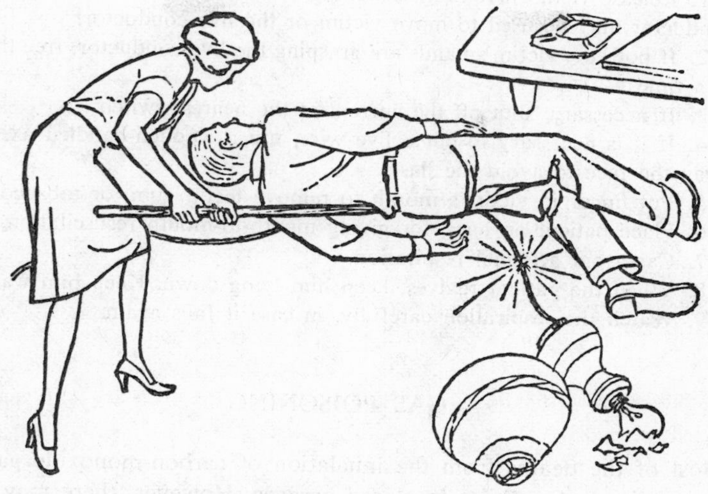

Fig. 4. Electric shock. Remove victim from wire or shut off current. American Red Cross illustration from *First Aid Textbook.*

ELECTRIC SHOCK

Following electric shock it is first necessary to remove the electrocuted man from the electric conductor. Employees of electrical corporations do not stop to shut off the current. They take off a coat or wrap and throw it around the patient's body so as to pull him away from the contact. They are told never to put their hands near the pockets of an electrified man nor near his shoes, because the presence of metal materials or nails in the shoes will cause severe shock to the rescuer.

When a person has been shocked by electricity, death may occur instantaneously from paralysis of the centers of circulation of the heart because of overexcitation of the heart muscle, perhaps due to suffocation from the forcible contraction of the muscles of breathing. Sometimes death occurs from burning, and sometimes the person who has been shocked by electricity falls and dies from the fall.

The person is first removed from contact with the electrical current. Artificial respiration is started at once by the method similar to that described for drowning. A physician should be called immediately who may stimulate the heart by the injection of suitable drugs or by the use of methods of massage applied to the heart. The director of one of the largest first-aid services for electrical corporations makes the following suggestions:

1. Release victim, avoiding sustaining a shock to one's self. Any dry nonconductor may be used to move victim or the live conductor.
2. If both the victim's hands are grasping the live conductor, free them one at a time.
3. If necessary, shut off the current at the nearest switch.
4. If it is necessary to cut a live wire, use a wooden-handled ax, turning away the face to avoid the flash.
5. Put finger in victim's mouth to remove teeth, gum, or tobacco.
6. Place patient on back for giving mouth-to-mouth resuscitation.
7. Carry out artificial respiration.
8. When the patient revives, keep him lying down. Keep him warm.
9. Watch the respiration carefully, in case it fails again.

GAS POISONING

Most of the deaths from the inhalation of carbon-monoxide gas occur from running automobiles in closed garages. However, there may be suffocation from illuminating gas in the home or from working with various types of machines in which carbon monoxide develops. In order to prevent poisoning by automobile-exhaust gas, the following instructions are important.

1. Keep windows open as much as possible.
2. Do not permit the engine to run and discharge exhaust gas directly into the air of the workroom. Every workroom should have a flexible tube which can be attached to the exhaust pipe and through which the exhaust gas may then be carried out of doors.
3. Remember that carbon-monoxide gas has no smell. You cannot, therefore, know if carbon-monoxide gas is in the air by the smell of the room or by the cloudiness of the air. These are produced by burning oil and gasoline.
4. If you suffer with headaches report this fact at once so that the condition of the air may be investigated and proper ventilation established.
5. If you do not feel well, see a doctor at once. You may be particularly sensitive to carbon-monoxide gas, more so than the others. In that case you had better change your occupation. It is not safe for you to be exposed to even very small amounts of the gas.

The Bulletin of the New York State Department of Labor recommends these first-aid measures:

If you get a headache, or feel faint, nervous, or irritable, go out into the fresh air at once and stay there until you feel better. When you go out go out slowly and when you get out sit down quietly. Do not go for a walk. You may not have enough oxygen in your blood to permit you to take any additional exercise or exert yourself in any way. Any added exertion at such a time is dangerous and may be sufficient to cause you to become unconscious. Wrap up warmly, therefore, and sit down out of doors until you feel better.

Do not hurry around unnecessarily at your work. The more exercise you take, the more carbon monoxide will get into your blood.

If one of your comrades faints, get him out into the fresh air at once. Put blankets under and over him and surround him with hot-water bottles or hot bricks. Keep him warm at all costs, or he may develop pneumonia. Persons who become asphyxiated with carbon-monoxide gas are peculiarly susceptible to pneumonia. Call up the gas company and the fire department inhalator squad at once. You must always call both of these, because ambulances are not equipped with resuscitation apparatus. In the meantime the patient should be given artificial respiration. Everyone working in industries where there is a possibility of exposure to carbon-monoxide gas should be familiar with this method of resuscitation. It is very easily carried out. Anyone can learn how to do it. He may thus by his knowledge be able to save someone's life.

Injections of methylene blue has been offered as a scientific means for treating patients with carbon-monoxide poisoning. In the presence of such poisoning a physician should be called immediately. He will then determine whether or not any remedies are to be injected. Of the greatest importance is the immediate application of the methods of artificial respiration already described.

FAINTING AND UNCONSCIOUSNESS

Few persons have the slightest idea of what is to be done when another person suddenly becomes unconscious. There are numerous causes for this condition: a blow on the head; pressure on the brain from a large blood clot; a lack of blood supply to the brain; the effects of such drugs as opium, ether, chloroform, or alcohol; or carbon-monoxide gas; but practically all of these are related in some manner to the brain, since the brain is the seat of consciousness.

A physician who is called to see a person who has suddenly become unconscious makes his decision as to the cause of unconsciousness from a number of factors. He feels the pulse to determine whether, by its rate and strength, the difficulty is affecting the circulation of the blood. If the pulse rate is between 76 and 90 and strong, he realizes that there is no immediate danger of death from failure of respiration. He studies the color of the face. If there is great pallor or blueness or a purple color he realizes that there are difficulties with the blood. He observes also if the skin is hot or cold and determines the presence or absence of perspiration. The eyes are noted to observe if the pupils are equal or unequal, if they are dilated or contracted. Unequal size of the pupils is a common symptom of injury to the brain, such as a brain hemorrhage. It may also be desirable to feel the skull to determine whether or not there is a fracture or crushing injury beneath the surface of the scalp.

In the presence of excessive heat, sunstroke may be the cause of unconsciousness. The odor of the breath may indicate the presence of acidosis or the fact that the person has taken a large dose of alcohol or of ether.

Associated with the onset of fainting there may be dizziness or lightheadedness. The average human being walks erect and pays no attention to his sense of balance because that is controlled by a number of reflex sensations coming to the brain from various places. The semicircular canals of the internal ear give the human being a sense of his position in space. There is also a feeling associated with the muscles which aids the determination of presence in space. If the body tends to accumulate acid, dizziness is a prominent symptom. Anything that interferes with the coördination between the sense of vision, the muscle sense, and the sensations coming from the semicircular canals will produce dizziness.

If the sense of dizziness merely comes and goes and yields quickly to proper hygiene such as suitable attention to the diet, the digestion, the action of the kidneys, and correction of disorders of vision, one need not be disturbed. However, if dizziness is repeated again and again it may be due to insufficient blood supply to the brain, insufficient action of the heart, a tumor growing in connection with the semicircular canals, or some hidden disturbance elsewhere. A feeling of dizziness and fainting, if repeated, demands careful scientific study. Of course, some people faint more easily than do others. Some faint from the slightest emotional shock. Some people faint at the sight of blood, others faint quickly from exhaustion, weakness, lack of air, or similar conditions.

A person who is about to faint realizes it from a feeling of weakness, a blurring of vision, a failure of circulation so that the face becomes pale, and the presence of cold perspiration. The moment a person faints he should be placed flat on the back and his head lowered. The color of the face is an indicator to some extent of the blood supply to the brain. If the face is pale the head should be lowered until the color of the face improves. If, on the other hand, the face is extremely red, it may be desirable to keep the head raised.

A person who has fainted should have plenty of fresh, cool air, cold water applied to the face or chest as a stimulant to recuperative action. Sometimes the inhalation of smelling salts serves to stimulate the breathing of the patient and in that way to aid his recovery. The usual first-aid remedy, found in most family medicine chests, for attacks of fainting is half a teaspoonful of aromatic spirits of ammonia given in water. A person who has fainted should be kept quiet and recumbent until fully recovered. If permitted to get up and walk too soon, serious results may follow.

HEAT STROKE

Heat stroke occurs not only in tropical countries and in extremely hot weather in the temperate zone, but also at any time in factories, engine rooms, laundries, and kitchens, where people work in extreme heat associated with considerable moisture. For prevention, tablets of common salt may be taken every few hours in extremely hot weather.

The symptoms of heat stroke may come on suddenly but most frequently come on gradually. The person who is about to become affected feels weak and tired, gets dizzy and drowsy. The digestion may be disturbed, and there may even be pain in the abdomen. The temperature rises, the fever increases, the pulse becomes rapid, the skin dry, burning, and flushed; the pupils of the eyes are usually contracted, and the breathing fast and noisy. Just before death the pupils may dilate. It is important to be certain of a diagnosis of heat stroke and to make positive that the unconsciousness is not due to drugs, hemorrhage, epilepsy, or diabetes.

The ability to keep cool depends on common sense. One should wear light clothing, loose and porous. Cool baths at frequent intervals aid in making one feel much better. Adequate amounts of sleep keep the body prepared for unusual stress and strain. One should take plenty of water, because evaporation of water from the surface of the body aids the control of temperature. Traveling in hot weather is extremely difficult. It is better, under conditions of extreme heat, to sit in an open coach with a free circulation of air than in the smaller compartments and drawing rooms without air conditioning.

In case of heat exhaustion, the first thing to do is to get the person into a cool place and absolutely at rest, flat on the back. Sponging with cool water helps to control the temperature. It may be necessary to stimulate the circulation with stimulating drugs or coffee to help the patient over the acute condition. Tropical authorities recommend that the person be placed as soon as possible on a bed covered with a large rubber sheet, and then that ice and cold water be rubbed over the body. At the same time that the ice is rubbed, the friction or massage encourages the circulation.

The temperature should be taken regularly and when it falls to 101 degrees, as taken by the rectum instead of by the mouth, one stops the application of cold, covers the patient with blankets, and makes certain that collapse does not follow. If breathing stops it may be necessary to apply artificial respiration. After recovery from heat stroke, small quantities of nutritious food may be given repeatedly in order to aid recovery.

BITE WOUNDS

The bites of insects, snakes, cats, dogs, and other small animals frequently demand some attention in first aid. The stinger of a bee, yellow jacket, or other wasp, should be pulled out, if still in the flesh, and a drop or two of diluted ammonia water applied to the wound. The application of cold compresses will help to stop pain. The sting of a centipede, spider, or scorpion may be more severe than that of a wasp or bee. Bleeding should be encouraged to wash out any material deposited by the bite; then tincture of iodine may be applied and a cold compress used to stop pain. Antihistaminic ointments have a slightly antiseptic effect, relieve itching and act against the sensitization to insect poisons.

Most spider bites in the United States are due to the shoe-button spider or the black widow. It is called shoe button because it looks like a black button; and black widow because the female frequently eats the male. The sting of a scorpion is not frequent. A physician usually treats such stings by injecting some anesthetic solution around the bite, including some adrenalin solution to constrict the blood vessels and prevent absorption of the poison.

Flea bites, if painful, may be treated with weak solutions of menthol or camphor.

Dog bites, or the bites of any small animal, must always be investigated to determine the possibility of hydrophobia in the animal that bites. The treatment of the bite itself is ordinarily the same as that for any infected wound. If it seems certain, however, that the animal has rabies, or hydrophobia, the wound should be thoroughly cauterized by a physician.

The scabies, or itch mite, travels rapidly from one person to another. The handling of infestation with the itch mite is really a problem for a physician. It demands thorough cleansing, the application of suitable drugs, and care of the clothing as well.

The bite of the bedbug seldom becomes infected but is an annoyance. The itching is, of course, easily treated by solutions of weak ammonia or very weak menthol.

In the case of every type of insect, prevention is far better than cure. It is necessary to know, first of all, the presence of the insects; second, their breeding habits; and third, special methods for destroying them. If they are once completely destroyed by fumigation or disinfestation methods they are not likely to return soon again, particularly if sufficient watchfulness is exercised to attack them while they are few in number.

HICCUPS

Hiccups to most people is just a temporary disagreeable symptom, but to the scientist who knows of all of the possible relationships of the hiccup as a symptom of various diseases, it constitutes a phenomenon of considerable significance. Between the chest and the abdomen lies a great muscular structure called the diaphragm. Above the diaphragm are the heart and lungs; below it, the stomach, intestines, liver, pancreas, spleen and other organs.

When one breathes, the diaphragm contracts, enlarging the chest cavity and helping the lungs to expand. In order for any muscle tissue to contract, a stimulus comes to it through a nerve. The nerve that controls the contractions of the diaphragm passes from the upper part of the spinal cord in the region of the neck. If this nerve is irritated at any spot it becomes stimulated, and the stimulation causes a sudden spasmodic contraction of the diaphragm that is called a hiccup.

In many cases hiccup is due to some infection involving the portion of the brain associated with the stimulation of contraction of the diaphragm. In such cases, the condition affects chiefly men more than forty-five years of age and it tends to follow operation on the colon, the prostate gland, the gall bladder, or the stomach. If there is an infection of the brain at the basis of an attack of hiccups, early diagnosis may mean the saving of life. Such diagnosis demands the services of a specialist in neurology.

Then there are cases which can be classed as chemical hiccup. In these cases hiccup occurs following the eating of highly irritating foods or liquids. Generally such hiccups last only a short time. It is also recognized that tumors of the brain, pressing on the areas associated with stimulation of the diaphragm, may produce hiccup. It is also possible by a sudden dilatation of the stomach to produce an irritation which will result in this symptom. Finally, there are cases of hiccup that have a nervous basis, exactly as hysteria may duplicate almost any disease known to medical science. Then there are cases of hiccup in which the origin cannot be easily determined even with the most careful study.

Everybody has his own cure for ordinary hiccups. In most instances it involves something that will fix the attention on anything except the hiccup. The physician who treats such cases may carry out certain procedures in persistent hiccups which frequently bring relief. One of these is to wash out the stomach; another to prescribe certain narcotics and sedatives that will give temporary relief; a third is to treat the specific infection from which the patient seems to be suffering. Another method involves the giving of enemas and doses of oil to clean out the entire intestinal tract. Breathing into a paper bag is also a helpful method.

In the case of a baby, it may be held on the shoulder and patted on the back, which will cause it to expel the air which may be distending its stomach or esophagus and thus leading to hiccups. In some cases the stimulation of the nerve results from poisons associated with infections such as infantile paralysis or epidemic encephalitis. The latter condition has been called American sleeping sickness. In these cases the hiccups may be severe and go on for long periods of time; indeed, actually to the point of exhaustion. The treatment of such conditions is a long and serious matter and it is only by the treatment of the fundamental condition that the hiccups are to be controlled.

When every method of treating hiccups has failed and the symptom persists there may, of course, be danger to life. In such cases the surgeon may expose the phrenic nerve and either cut it or place pressure upon it. This will invariably cause the hiccup to stop by interfering with the passing of the stimulus from the irritated center along the nerve to the diaphragm.

MIGRAINE OR SICK HEADACHE

Migraine or sick headache is often called recurrent headache. It is called sick headache because it is sometimes accompanied with nausea or vomiting. Sometimes it is found to be dependent on uncorrected errors of vision or sinus disease or on various poisonings of the body. In other words, it seems to be associated with sensitivity to food of one kind or another, or even to serious diseases of the stomach and other organs of the body. On occasion, severe headache is associated with disturbance of the brain, such as tumor or hardening of the arteries. In some instances, the headaches may be wholly on a mental basis.

Every case of persistent headache should be carefully studied so that the physician may evaluate all of the different factors that may be concerned. The headache or the pain is the symptom of a disorder of the human body rather than a disease in itself.

Sometimes the headache is associated with the type of nausea that has been mentioned; sometimes with disturbances of vision in the form of blindness, dullness of vision, blinding flashes of light, or dizziness. In certain cases there are, associated with the pains in the head, emotional disturbances such as a feeling of depression or melancholia. In other cases the headaches are associated with restlessness and irritability, and in still another group with confusion, absent-mindedness, or a sense of unreality. In some cases there are pains in the abdomen which are of the same type as the pain in the head.

Women have their symptoms chiefly at the time of menstruation. In many cases the headaches occur frequently, but in the majority about once in two weeks. The type of headache called migraine occurs most often between the ages of eighteen and thirty-five, but may appear at any age. There was a time when it was thought primarily to be a disease affecting women, and some writers have said that it occurs four times as often in women as in men. More recently careful studies seem to show that headaches of this type occur just about as often in men as in women. The reason why it has seemed to be more frequent in women is that they are more likely to consult a physician about the condition than are men, and that the attacks in them may seem to be more severe.

Sometimes the headaches come on without any warning, but in most cases they are preceded by a feeling of depression, by an unwillingness to work or to go about the daily affairs of life. Since there seem to be many possible causes for headaches of this type, the attack on them must be made from various points of view. It is believed that they may on occasion be associated, as has been said, with eye strain or disease of the sinuses. Obviously in such cases careful examination must be made by a competent specialist in diseases of the eye to make certain that the vision is properly corrected with suitable glasses. It should be made certain that the eyes are not abused by working under conditions of improper illumination. The nose must be examined most carefully and, if necessary, X-ray pictures made of the sinuses to make certain that they do not contain polyps or infection.

The physician will use the ophthalmoscope to look in the back of the eye in order to make certain that there is no pressure within the skull due to any disorder. Sometimes it is necessary to X ray the skull for possible observation of an abnormality in the brain.

It is believed that migraine is associated with such disorders of hypersensitivity as hay fever, eczema, asthma, and similar conditions. It is possible in such cases to test the reaction of the patient to various foods and proteins by skin sensitivity tests or perhaps to try elimination diets, in which food substances are eliminated from the diet when their consumption seems to be followed by an attack. Apparently not all cases are due to such sensitivity, but a considerable number may be.

In some instances the attacks seem to come on when the digestion of the person concerned is not working properly. In these instances, it is well to have a thorough study of the gastrointestinal tract to make certain that there is neither constipation nor a residue of putrefactive matter in the bowel.

In other cases the glands of internal secretion may be involved, and it is necessary to make a thorough study of the body with a view to determining that all of the glands are neither overfunctioning nor underfunctioning. This is merely an indication of the necessity for studying every case of recurrent sick headache with all of the means known to modern medical science.

Almost every method of treatment known to medical science has been applied at one time or another in the treatment of recurrent headaches. In many instances some definite change should be made in the life habits of such a patient based on a complete survey of his work, his play, his food, his mental attitude, and his philosophy of life. An inequality of emphasis in the patient's interests and activities should be corrected. He should live a moderate existence, and all excesses should be prevented. This applies particularly to excess in work involving the eyes and to overeating.

A patient who is constantly indoors and gets insufficient exercise should change his habits in the right direction. Rest and change are particularly valuable for people who are constantly under physical, mental, or emotional pressure. Persons who suffer from recurrent sick headaches should not try to work all the time. They will do well to take at least one afternoon and one day a week for rest or recreation, and perhaps both winter and summer vacations.

In controlling the immediate attack, the room in which the patient rests should be darkened and everything be kept quiet. Most such patients are so intensely uncomfortable that they do not want to be touched or interfered with. In some instances, an ice bag to the head or a hot-water bottle to the feet may give relief.

The physician who is actively in charge of the treatment of such a patient can do much by controlling the diet, eliminating the substances to which the patient seems to respond with headache. The use of various glandular preparations to overcome deficiencies in glands or, in some instances, to oppose overactivity of certain glands is again experimental but is worthy of trial.

When drugs are given to control the pain, the constant attention of a physician who is thoroughly familiar with the patient, his habits, his emotional reactions, and particularly his headaches is desirable. It is easy to fall into the habit of taking strong drugs constantly, and the physician who understands the patient and his reactions will know how to avoid the danger of such habits. The drug called ergotamine in various forms, for instance, combined with caffeine as in "cafergone" has been found helpful. The drug is powerful and should be used only when prescribed and in the manner prescribed by the doctor.

METALLIC AND FOOD POISONING

The human being is subject to various kinds of possible poisoning from foods and drugs, from mushrooms, and all sorts of similar toxic substances. There are poisons constantly used in industry which may get into the body and thereby produce severe illness.

In any case of poisoning certain procedures are immediately desirable. First, try to ascertain the nature of the poison taken. An empty bottle in the vicinity, the presence of some of the substance in a cup or utensil, or the presence of the poison on the tablecloth or floor or clothing may be a valuable sign. By smelling the breath and examining the mouth of the patient, the physician may determine the presence of stains or burns characteristic of the action of certain poisons. If the patient has taken the poison accidentally and is conscious, he will probably be willing to tell the physician what he has taken.

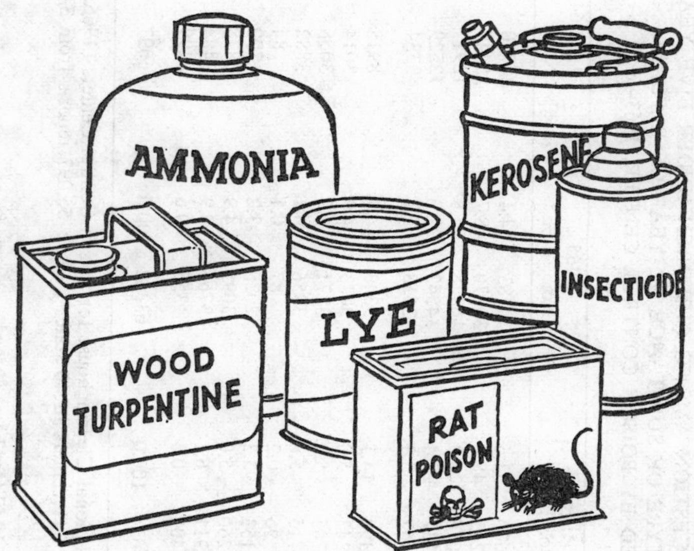

Fig. 5. Commonly used household products which are poisonous. American Red Cross illustration from *First Aid Textbook.*

If poisoning is suspected, a physician should be called immediately. Before the doctor comes, it is well to give white of eggs, milk, or strong tea, which are antagonistic to many poisons. In order to get the poison out of the system as rapidly as possible one should provoke vomiting, either by tickling the back of the throat, by giving a cup of warm water mixed with salt, or by washing out the stomach with a stomach tube, if one understands how this is done. If one puts a heaping teaspoonful of salt in a cupful of lukewarm water, stirs until dissolved, and has the patient drink the mixture, repeating the dose every ten minutes until three or four cupfuls have been taken, vomiting takes place promptly, serving to wash out the stomach.

Thereafter the person must be treated as in any case of fainting, dizziness, or shock, the symptoms being treated according to the nature of the

ACCIDENTAL INGESTION AMONG CHILDREN UNDER FIVE YEARS OF AGE. TYPE OF SUBSTANCE BY YEAR OF REPORT. REPORTED BY POISON CONTROL CENTER, 1963–66.

Type of Substance	1966		1965		1964		1963	
	No.	%	No.	%	No.	%	No.	%
Medicines	34670	53.6	34483	54.4	28780	51.3	24335	51.8
Internal	31213	48.3	30870	48.7	25446	45.4	21588	46.0
Aspirin	16076	24.9	16328	25.8	12917	23.0	10808	23.0
Other	15137	23.4	14542	22.9	12529	22.3	10780	23.0
External	3457	5.3	3613	5.7	3334	5.9	2747	5.9
Cleaning and Polishing Agents	9398	14.5	9343	14.7	8918	15.9	7520	16.0
Petroleum Products	3243	5.0	3073	4.9	3014	5.4	2601	5.5
Cosmetics	3785	5.9	3271	5.2	3058	5.5	2459	5.2
Pesticides	3715	5.8	3856	6.1	3882	6.9	3370	7.2
Gases and Vapors	96	0.2	87	0.1	84	0.1	64	0.1
Plants	2153	3.3	2028	3.2	1700	3.0	1350	2.9
Turpentine, Paints, etc.	3260	5.0	3095	4.9	2878	5.1	2373	5.1
Miscellaneous	3911	6.1	3766	5.9	3484	6.2	2541	5.4
Not Specified	403	0.6	350	0.6	299	0.5	341	0.7
Total	64634	100.0	63352	100.0	56097	100.0	46954	100.0

Source: Individual reports submitted to the National Clearinghouse for Poison Control Centers (1966: 64,634 reports from 356 centers in 41 states[1]; 1965: 63,352 reports from 341 centers in 40 states[1]; 1964: 56,097 reports from 341 centers in 40 states[1]; 1963: 46,954 reports from 335 centers in 40 states[1]).

[1] Includes District of Columbia, Canal Zone, and Military bases abroad.

National Clearing House for Poison Control Centers, United States Department of Health, Education and Welfare, Public Health Service.

case. If the patient is greatly weakened or prostrated he must be kept warm, recumbent, and his general strength sustained.

For many of the common poisons there are special antidotes. However, these are seldom present in the average home, and even when present, few people have time to consult tables of antidotes or know where the antidote is to be found. For poisoning with carbolic acid it is customary to wash out the mouth with whisky or alcohol diluted with water, to have the patient swallow three or four tablespoonfuls of diluted whisky or alcohol diluted with water, and to give a heaping tablespoonful of Epsom salts dissolved in water.

Bichloride of mercury is one of the most dangerous of poisons. The physician should be called at the earliest possible moment in order that he may supply antidotes and do everything possible to sustain the patient's circulation and elimination.

In case of poisoning by various narcotic drugs it is customary to provoke vomiting and then to give strong black coffee, at the same time doing everything possible to keep the patient awake. Sometimes it is necessary to walk him about forcefully. As long as he is awake he will continue to breathe, but if he is permitted to sleep, breathing may stop.

There follows a table of poisonings and methods of treatment summarized by the health department of San Francisco:

SYMPTOMS AND TREATMENT OF ACUTE POISONING

SYMPTOMS	ANTIDOTES AND TREATMENT
Acetanilid, Antipyrin, Acetophenetidin (Phenacetin)	
Vomiting (sometimes). Face cyanosed. Skin: cold; profuse sweat; sometimes rash simulating measles, scarlatina, or pemphigus. Collapse; feeble and irregular pulse; slow respiration.	Lavage or emetic. External heat; recumbent position. Caffeine, digitalis. Carbon dioxide-oxygen inhalation, if needed.
Aconite	
Tingling and numbness of tongue and mouth and sense of formication of the body. Nausea and vomiting; diarrhea with epigastric pain. Dyspnea. Pulse irregular and weak. Skin cold and clammy; features bloodless. Giddiness, staggering walk; feeling of heaviness. The mind remains clear.	Avoid emetics. Gastric lavage–stomach to be washed with 0.1 per cent (1:1000) potassium permanganate, 250 cc. Reflex stimulants: ether, alcohol (whisky), aromatic spirits of ammonia. Caffeine or atropine. Carbon dioxide-oxygen inhalation, if necessary. External heat; recumbent position with head lower than feet.

Symptoms	Antidotes and Treatment
	Alcohol (Ethyl Alcohol)
Ataxia, cramps, coma, decreased respiration. Abolition of the superficial and deep reflexes.	Gastric lavage. Coffee enema. Carbon dioxide-oxygen inhalation. External heat. Aromatic spirits of ammonia, caffeine or atropine.
	Alkalies, Fixed and Caustic (Sodium and Potassium Hydroxide—Lye), Sodium Carbonate (Washing Soda)
Burning pain from mouth to stomach; difficulty in swallowing; sloughed tissues in mouth; vomiting and purging of mucus and blood. Collapse; skin cold and clammy; pulse feeble; anxious countenance; rapid exhaustion; dyspnea. Convulsions. Unconsciousness or coma.	Do not use stomach tube! Give from 100 to 500 cc. of 0.5 per cent hydrochloric acid. Eight ounces of olive oil by mouth. Demulcents such as gelatin, acacia, or flour in water. Caffeine or digitan hypodermically, if necessary. External heat.
	Ammonia
Gastrointestinal symptoms, as in corrosive poisoning. Purging usual, with pain and straining. Body cold, with cold sweat. Countenance anxious. Pulse rapid and weak.	Eight ounces of olive oil by mouth. Large quantities of water. Neutralization with from 100 to 500 cc. of 0.5 per cent hydrochloric acid. *Do not use stomach tube.*
	Anesthetics, Volatile (Chloroform, Ether, Nitrous Oxide)
Rapid heart rate, abolition of reflexes, stoppage of heart or respiration.	Withdrawal of anesthetic. If circulatory collapse persists, ouabain intravenously; epinephrine intravenously or intracardially. If respiration stops, artificial respiration; carbon dioxide-oxygen inhalation; caffeine given intravenously or intramuscularly; atropine hypodermically.
	Arsenic
Symptoms usually appear in from a quarter of an hour to one hour. Vomiting profuse, painful diarrhea; thirst; sense of constriction in throat, rendering swallowing difficult; cyanosis; coma.	Abundant gastric lavage with warm water. External heat. Opiate for diarrhea and colic. Infusion of solution of sodium chloride containing sodium bicarbonate (5 per cent), if necessary. Milk diet. Treat patient as potential nephritic patient.

Symptoms	Antidotes and Treatment
Atropine, Belladonna	
Dryness of mouth. Difficulty in swallowing and articulation; thirst. Skin flushed. Temperature raised. Pulse quick. Pupils widely dilated. Purging. Delirium.	Purified animal charcoal as antidote (2 tablespoonfuls in 250 cc. of water). Evacuation of stomach. Caffeine. Potassium permanganate in 1:1,000 solution, 250 cc.; lavage with the same preparation. Catheterization if necessary. If excitation persists, barbital or paraldehyde. Physostigmine.
Barbituric Acid Derivatives (Phenobarbital, Barbital, etc.)	
Coma, circulatory collapse, pulmonary edema, cold skin, cyanosis. Sometimes delirium, twitching and increased reflexes.	Cover patient warmly; apply hot-water bottles. Gastric lavage. Caffeine. Ephedrine. Carbon dioxide-oxygen inhalation.
Bichloride of Mercury	
Metallic taste, choking sensation. Pain in stomach, vomiting and purging of stringy mucus and blood. Tongue may be white and shriveled. Skin cold and clammy. Pulse feeble and rapid.	*Treatment in Emergency Room:* Antidote (by mouth): 10 cc. of 10 per cent sodium hypophosphite in water and then add 5 cc. hydrogen peroxide for each gram (15 grains) of bichloride of mercury. One glass of water. Lavage with antidote (one dose per hundred cubic centimeters of water). Two egg whites, or liberal dry egg albumin in water, and one glass of milk, followed by lavage with water. *Treatment in the Ward:* Gastric lavage twice a day with 6 quarts of sodium bicarbonate solution. Sodium acetate by mouth (amount to keep urine alkaline). Use low pressure colonic irrigation twice a day with 6 quarts of solution. (2 drams sodium acetate to 1 pint of water.) Send urine, vomitus and colonic washings to the laboratory daily for examination for mercury (500 cc. of each). Daily specimens of urine to interns' laboratory. Daily chemical examination of the blood. Administration of stimulants and sedatives as indicated. Treatment continued until

Symptoms	Antidotes and Treatment
Bichloride of Mercury (continued)	
	symptoms have abated and mercury has disappeared from urine and colonic and gastric washings.
Boron (Boric Acid, Borax Solutions)	
Epigastric pain, abdominal cramps, vomiting, diarrhea, weak pulse, cold clammy skin, sometimes cyanosis and collapse. (Boric acid, 3 to 6 gm., has been fatal to infants, and 15 grams has been fatal to adults. Thirty gm. of borax, likewise, has been fatal to adults.)	Keep patient warm, in recumbent position. If taken by mouth, gastric lavage; or, if given by rectum in enema, rectal lavage, warm water. Caffeine may be given, and the kidneys should be protected by the administration of alkali (1.0 to 5.0 gm. sodium bicarbonate and alkaline drinks or fruit juices) and by the administration of sodium thiosulphate.
Camphor (Camphor Oil; Spirit of Camphor)	
Characteristic odor of breath; burning pain in stomach; colic; giddiness; pulse rapid and weak. Impulsive movements; delirium. Face flushed. Sometimes convulsions. Collapse. Coma.	Apomorphine, hypodermically. Gastric lavage repeatedly with warm water. Inhalation anesthesia to check convulsions; then barbital by mouth or intramuscularly to check excitation. Caffeine or digitan hypodermically, if necessary. External heat. Artificial respiration, if required. Convalescence may be prolonged.
Cantharides	
Burning pain in throat and stomach; difficulty in swallowing. Vomiting and diarrhea; mucus and blood may contain shining particles of the powder. Salivation and swelling of the salivary glands. Burning in urethra; frequent micturition. Urine contains albumin, casts, and blood. Pulse weak and slow; collapse.	Gastric lavage; mucilaginous drinks; opiate for pain. No oil by mouth. Treat as for potential nephritis (alkalies and milk diet).
Chloral Hydrate	
Vomiting, collapse, delirium, fall of temperature, cyanosis, dyspnea or slow respirations. Coma.	Gastric lavage with potassium permanganate 1:1,000, 250 cc. External heat. Caffeine, then digitalis. Carbon dioxide-oxygen inhalation, or artificial respiration, as needed.

SYMPTOMS	ANTIDOTES AND TREATMENT
Cinchophen (Atophan)	
Poisoning generally subacute or chronic, but toxic symptoms may become rapidly severe during or in absence of administration of drug. Symptoms of cinchonism; nausea and vomiting; persistent abdominal pain; diarrhea. Jaundice; liver pain or tenderness; stupor. Urine colored red to brown. Collapse. Coma.	Gastric lavage. Magnesium sulphate. Withdrawal of administration of drug. Camphor oil, caffeine or digitan, if necessary. Continue with treatment for hepatitis; injections of dextrose and insulin; carbohydrate diet; bicarbonate by mouth for acidosis.
Cocaine and Procaine Hydrochloride	
Anxiety, fainting, pallor, dyspnea, brief convulsions and apnea. With smaller doses, confusion, laughter, vertigo, motor excitement, tachycardia, irregular respiration, pallor, dilated pupils and exophthalmos, paresthesia, delirium and dyspnea. If death does not occur in a few minutes, recovery always follows.	Gastric lavage with 1 liter of 0.1 per cent (1:1,000) potassium permanganate (if taken by mouth). One-half per cent potassium permanganate solution if stomach is empty; otherwise, tannic acid (5 gm.). Soluble barbital intravenously.
Cyanides (Sodium or Potassium; Hydrocyanic Acid)	
Characteristic odor of poison. Dyspnea; rapid pulse; unconsciousness; tremors; violent convulsions; dilated pupils; absence of cyanosis. If patient survives an hour, recovery may occur.	If poison has been swallowed, give sodium thiosulphate, 10 per cent in water, 500 cc., using stomach tube if necessary. Inject intravenously 50 cc. methylene blue (1 per cent in 1.8 per cent sodium sulphate solution), repeat in 15 minutes, if necessary. Or, try sodium nitrite, 10 to 20 mgm. per kg. body weight (12 to 24 cc. 5 per cent sodium nitrite solution) intravenously. Epinephrine into heart.
Digitalis	
Vomiting; diarrhea. Slow pulse; cardiac irregularity. Lassitude; muscular and sensory derangements.	Gastric lavage with potassium permanganate 0.1 per cent (1:1,000) or tannic acid, 1 per cent. Horizontal position. External heat. Atropine hypodermically. Quinidine for cardiac irregularity.

Symptoms	Antidotes and Treatment
Ergot	
Pale skin, small and rapid pulse, constricted arteries. Hallucinations. Cyanosis of the finger tips and toes. Sensory disturbances. Ascending gangrene of the extremities.	Gastric lavage in acute poisoning; withdrawal of administration of ergot. Nitrites. Warm room. Periodic inhalation of carbon dioxide and oxygen.
Fluoride (Roach and Insect Powders)	
Nausea and vomiting; burning, cramplike abdominal pains; diarrhea. Sometimes tremors or convulsions. Grayish blue cyanosis. Urine and blood show presence of fluoride.	Copious gastric lavage with limewater or weak calcium chloride solution. Calcium gluconate intramuscularly, or calcium chloride, 10 cc. of 10 per cent in water, intravenously. Digitan hypodermically; artificial respiration, if necessary. External heat.
Formaldehyde	
Odor. Sore mouth. Dysphagia. Severe abdominal pain. Unconsciousness and collapse. Later diarrhea and tenesmus.	Swallow a tumblerful of 0.2 per cent ammonia. Lavage with dilute ammonia followed by raw egg, or egg albumin in water.
Gas (Garage Gas, or from Defective Flue Fumes, Carbon Monoxide)	
Giddiness and singing in the ears. Lividity of face and body. Loss of muscular power. Unconsciousness and collapse.	Carbon dioxide-oxygen inhalation, or artificial respiration, if needed. Bleeding followed by transfusion if indicated. External heat. Oxygen tent if available. Digitalis.
Hydrochloric Acid	
Gastrointestinal symptoms, coffee-ground vomitus. Purging usual, with pain and straining. Body cold, with cold sweat. Countenance anxious. Pulse rapid and weak.	Magnesia magma 100 to 400 cc. White of egg or olive oil as a demulcent; external heat; camphor oil, caffeine or digitan hypodermically, if necessary.
Iodine	
Pain and heat in throat and stomach. Vomiting and purging, vomitus being yellow or blue if starchy matter is present in the stomach. Stools may contain blood. Intense thirst. Giddiness, faintness and convulsions.	Sodium thiosulphate by mouth (1 to 10 gm. in water) as an antidote. Then lavage with 1 per cent sodium thiosulphate. Later, thin starch paste or flour soup. External heat; camphor oil, caffeine or digitan hypodermically, if necessary.

SYMPTOMS	ANTIDOTES AND TREATMENT
Lead	
Metallic taste, dry throat, intense thirst. Abdominal colic. Constipation, dark feces. Vomiting may occur. Giddiness, stupor, convulsions, coma.	Magnesium sulphate in solution as antidote. Lavage with 1 per cent sodium sulphate, mucilaginous (acacia) or egg albumin drinks. External heat. Cathartic after lavage. Calcium gluconate intramuscularly. Opiate for colic.
Morphine, Opium	
Coma, gradual in onset. Symmetrical pinpoint pupils that dilate terminally. Respiration slow and shallow. Body cold. Cyanosis; convulsions.	Potassium permanganate 0.1 per cent (1:1,000), 250 cc. by mouth. Gastric lavage with some solution of potassium permanganate. Black coffee. Try to keep the patient awake by suggestion. Carbon dioxide-oxygen inhalation. Artificial respiration, if necessary. External heat. Caffeine or atropine hypodermically, if respiration fails to improve.
Mushrooms	
Colic, vomiting, purging. Mental excitement followed by coma. Extremities cold. Pulse slow. Respiration stertorous. Pulmonary edema. Pupils dilated.	Gastric lavage. External heat. Atropine.
Nicotine and Tobacco	
Severe depression, prostration and muscular weakness; severe nausea and vomiting. Marked dyspnea. Weak rapid pulse. Pupils first contracted then dilated. Muscular tremors, followed rapidly by convulsions. Coma.	If free vomiting has not occurred, wash out stomach repeatedly with potassium permanganate, 0.1 per cent (1:1,000), and warm water. Strong coffee. Caffeine or digitan hypodermically, if necessary. External heat. Artificial respiration, if necessary.
Nitric Acid	
Pain in throat and stomach. Vomiting of whitish, flaky matter that blackens on exposure to light.	Magnesia magma, from 100 to 400 cc. White of egg, or egg albumin in water, or olive oil (250 cc.) as a demulcent. External heat. Camphor oil, caffeine or digitan hypodermically, if necessary.

SYMPTOMS	ANTIDOTES AND TREATMENT
Nitrites and Nitroglycerine	
Collapse, unconsciousness, cyanosis or pallor, low blood pressure, slow pulse, irregular respiration. Sometimes vomiting and convulsions. Persistent cyanosis. Methemoglobinuria.	Recumbent position. Gastric lavage if poison has been swallowed. Guaiacol 0.5 gm. and Berlin blue 0.5 gm. together, gastrically or orally, 3 to 6 times daily. If necessary, epinephrine intravenously; digitan hypodermically; oxygen inhalation. External heat.
Oils, Volatile and Ecbolic (Tansy, Pennyroyal, Santal, Absinthe, Turpentine)	
Characteristic odor of breath; burning, nausea, vomiting; eructations; colic; diarrhea. Skin rash; jaundice. Convulsions; dilated pupils; rapid stertorous respiration; pulse slow and feeble. Unconsciousness. Coma. Sometimes, uterine hemorrhage, abortion, hematuria.	If vomiting has not occurred, repeatedly wash out stomach with warm water. Demulcents: acacia, starch, or flour in water. Magnesium sulphate unless diarrhea is present. Opiate for colic. Camphor oil, caffeine or digitan, if necessary. External heat. Barbital for excitation. Later, treatments for nephritis and hepatitis; abortion.
Oxalic Acid	
Gastrointestinal symptoms as in corrosive poisoning. Purging, in most cases, with pain and straining. Body cold, with cold sweat. Countenance anxious. Pulse rapid and weak.	Calcium lactate (10 to 20 gm. in 250 cc. of water). Potassium permanganate, 0.1 per cent (1:1,000), 250 cc. by mouth. Gastric lavage with same permanganate solution. Demulcents. Heat applied to abdomen. Camphor oil, caffeine or digitan hypodermically, if necessary.
Paris Green	
Symptoms usually appear in from a quarter of an hour to one hour. Burning heat and constriction or choking in throat, rendering swallowing difficult. Nausea and incessant vomiting and purging. The vomiting matter may be green from bile, or, in the case of arsenic, black from the admixture of soda, or blue from indigo. Pain in the stomach and abdomen. Cramps in the calves of the legs. Urine may be suppressed. There may be delirium or	Abundant gastric lavage with warm water. Infusion of solution of sodium chloride if necessary. Tincture of opium for diarrhea and colic. Caffeine, strychnine or atropine, as needed, for circulatory and respiratory stimulation. Milk diet. Treat as for potential nephritis.

SYMPTOMS — ANTIDOTES AND TREATMENT

paralysis. Collapse; skin cold and clammy, sometimes showing eczematous rash. Pulse small, quick and irregular, or imperceptible.

Phenols (Carbolic Acid, Lysol, Cresols, "Sheep-Dip")

Symptoms	Antidotes and Treatment
Characteristic odor present. Burning sensation in mouth and throat; burns on lips and in mouth; nausea and vomiting. Abdominal pain. Faintness; collapse; pulse slow and weak; face livid; cold sweat; respiration depressed; unconsciousness. Coma. Urine scanty with smoky color.	Gastric lavage with 10 per cent ethyl alcohol in water, 1 quart; continuous lavage with warm water. Infusion of physiological salt solution; epinephrine intravenously or intracardially. Caffeine or digitan hypodermically. External heat. Artificial respiration if necessary. Later treatment same as for aftereffects of corrosives.

Phosphorus

Symptoms	Antidotes and Treatment
Symptoms usually appear in three stages: (1) A few hours after administration, there develops a garlic taste, gastrointestinal irritation, burning pain, thirst, swelling of the abdomen and vomiting of blood (green or black). The vomit has a garlic odor and in the dark may be phosphorescent. The patient may die, or there may be: (2) An intermission of symptoms for three days or more, with a feeling of malaise followed by: (3) The final stage, characterized by intense jaundice, enlarged liver and distended abdomen; great prostration, cold sweat, an anxious look, feeble pulse, muscular twitching, coma.	Two hundred cubic centimeters of 0.2 per cent solution of copper sulphate by mouth. Lavage with from 5 to 10 liters of the same solution followed by lavage with 1 liter of 0.1 per cent potassium permanganate; followed by the administration of 100 cc. of liquid petrolatum. No fats or oils should be given, as they aid absorption. External heat. Treatment continued for liver injury—high carbohydrate diet; dextrose and insulin.

Quinine and Quinidine

Symptoms	Antidotes and Treatment
Ringing in ears, disturbed vision, photophobia. (Later deafness and blindness.) Nausea; vomiting. Faintness. Difficulty of speech, somnolence; unconsciousness, alternating with delirium and coma. Pulse slow and feeble. Sometimes convulsions.	Tannic acid by mouth. Gastric lavage with potassium permanganate 0.1 per cent (1:1,000). Epinephrine intravenously or intracardially, if necessary. Caffeine or digitan hypodermically. If excitation persists, barbital by mouth.

SYMPTOMS	ANTIDOTES AND TREATMENT
	Strychnine, Nux Vomica
Feeling of suffocation and lividity of the face. Tetanic convulsions, with short intermission, causing sweating and exhaustion, opisthotonus, risus sardonicus, staring eyes, fixed chest, and hard abdominal muscles. Hearing and sight are acute, and consciousness is retained. The muscles of the jaw are not affected until late.	*Early:* Give by mouth or with stomach tube purified animal charcoal, from 1 to 2 tablespoonfuls in a glass of water. Gastric lavage with potassium permanganate, 0.1 per cent solution (1:1,000). *Later (with muscular hypertonicity):* Arrest hyperexcitability or convulsions with inhalation anesthesia (ether or chloroform) and then inject intramuscularly soluble barbital, 1 gm. (20 cc. of 5 per cent), later by mouth; or pentobarbital, 1/10 gr. (6 mgms.) per pound body weight as the first dose and one half this amount for succeeding doses. Do not use any methods that excite spasm, such as attempting intravenous injection. The patient should be isolated and kept absolutely quiet. Ether inhalation should be given if convulsions continue. Artificial respiration, if respiration fails.
	Thallium (Depilatories; Rodent Poisons—"Thalgrain")
Abdominal colic, nausea, vomiting, and diarrhea; constipation; stomatitis; alopecia; peripheral neuritis; central nervous involvement (ptosis, strabismus, convulsions, choreiform movements, optic atrophy). Evidences of liver damage, nephritis; sometimes pulmonary edema. Thallium in urine.	*Early:* If emesis has not occurred, copious gastric lavage with 1 per cent sodium or potassium iodide (in water); catharsis (avoid sulphates). If shock is present, 25 gm. (50 cc. of 50 per cent) dextrose intravenously; external heat; reflex stimulants, epinephrine, caffeine, or digitan hypodermically; artificial respiration if necessary. *Later:* Rest in bed; control mobilization of thallium in body by daily intravenous injections of sodium iodide, about 15 to 40 cc. of 2.3 per cent, in water (freshly prepared) (about 0.3 to 1 gm. NaI) until urine test shows absence of thallium; dose of iodide may gradually be doubled. Daily chemical examination of urine: collect and evaporate to dryness 24-hour urines for thallium test—ab-

sence of, or only slight, green color on flaming residue. When symptoms of thallitoxicosis subside, proceed cautiously to increase elimination of thallium by intravenous injection of sodium thiosulphate, 0.3 to 1 gm. (6 to 20 cc. of 5 per cent in water; freshly prepared) for adult, alternating with sodium iodide solution intravenously, if necessary. Pilocarpine (promotes secretion), calcium lactate, if necessary; dilute with hydrochloric acid for achlorhydria; bland ointments for dermatitis; barbital or codeine for restlessness and pain; treatments for liver injury and nephritis, if necessary.

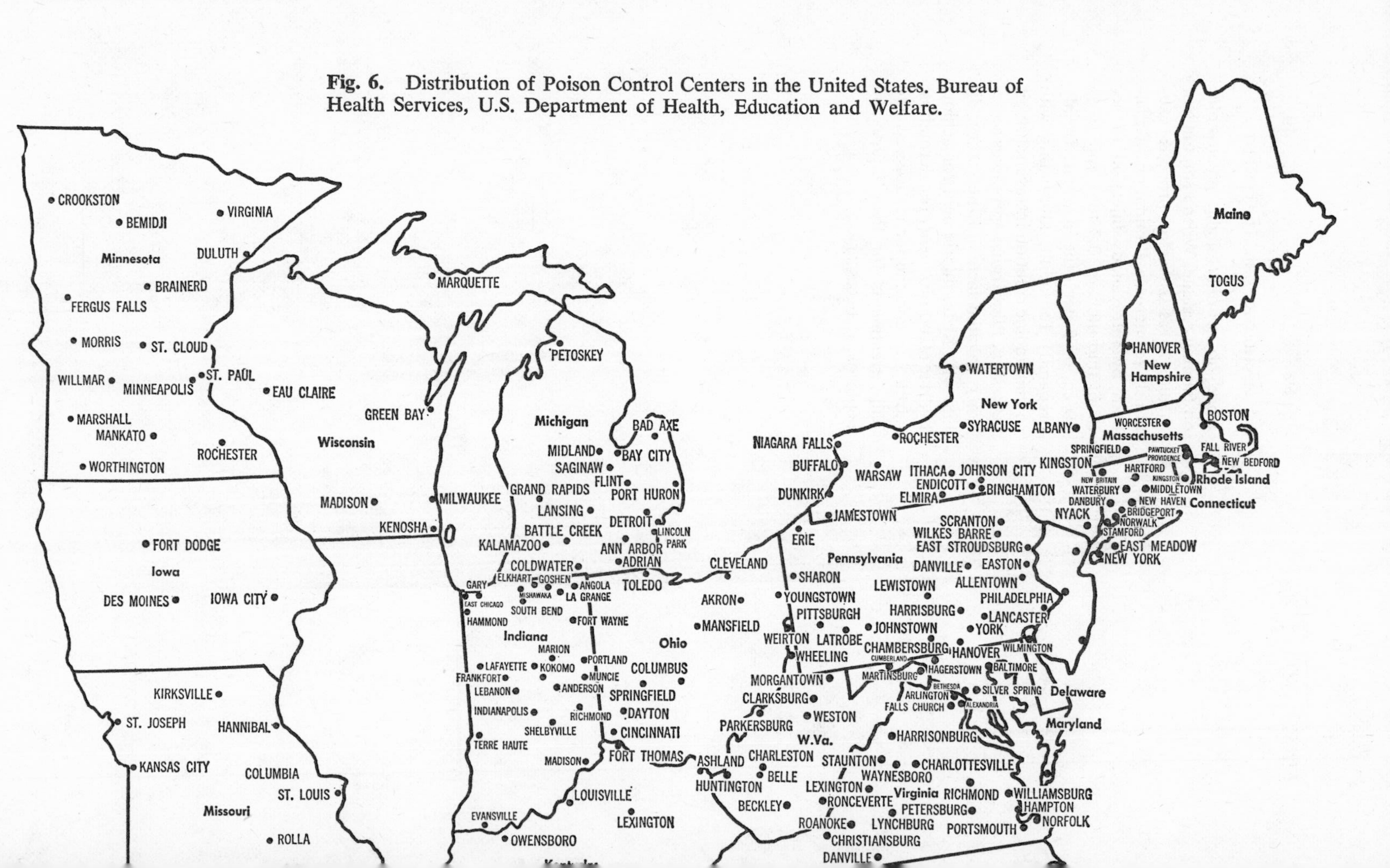

Fig. 6. Distribution of Poison Control Centers in the United States. Bureau of Health Services, U.S. Department of Health, Education and Welfare.

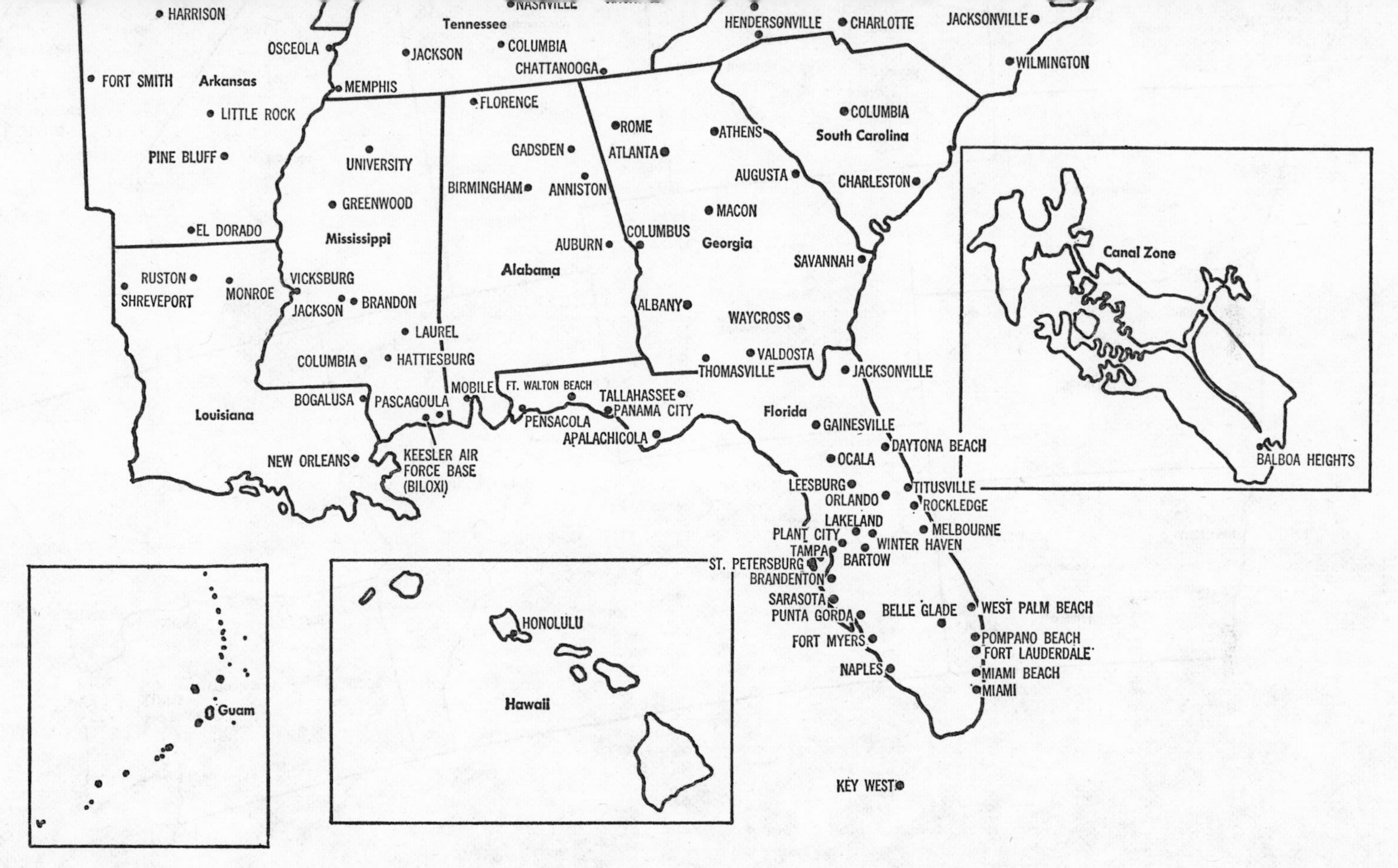
HARRISON
NASHVILLE
Tennessee
HENDERSONVILLE
CHARLOTTE
JACKSONVILLE
OSCEOLA
JACKSON
COLUMBIA
CHATTANOOGA
WILMINGTON
FORT SMITH
Arkansas
MEMPHIS
LITTLE ROCK
FLORENCE
COLUMBIA
South Carolina
ROME
ATHENS
PINE BLUFF
UNIVERSITY
GADSDEN
ATLANTA
AUGUSTA
CHARLESTON
BIRMINGHAM
ANNISTON
GREENWOOD
MACON
EL DORADO
Mississippi
COLUMBUS
Georgia
AUBURN
Alabama
SAVANNAH
Canal Zone
RUSTON
SHREVEPORT
MONROE
VICKSBURG
JACKSON
BRANDON
ALBANY
WAYCROSS
LAUREL
VALDOSTA
COLUMBIA
HATTIESBURG
THOMASVILLE
JACKSONVILLE
MOBILE
FT. WALTON BEACH
BOGALUSA
PASCAGOULA
TALLAHASSEE
PANAMA CITY
Florida
Louisiana
PENSACOLA
GAINESVILLE
APALACHICOLA
DAYTONA BEACH
NEW ORLEANS
KEESLER AIR
FORCE BASE
(BILOXI)
OCALA
BALBOA HEIGHTS
LEESBURG
TITUSVILLE
ORLANDO
ROCKLEDGE
LAKELAND
MELBOURNE
PLANT CITY
WINTER HAVEN
TAMPA
ST. PETERSBURG
BARTOW
BRANDENTON
SARASOTA
WEST PALM BEACH
BELLE GLADE
PUNTA GORDA
HONOLULU
POMPANO BEACH
FORT MYERS
FORT LAUDERDALE
NAPLES
MIAMI BEACH
MIAMI
Hawaii
Guam
KEY WEST

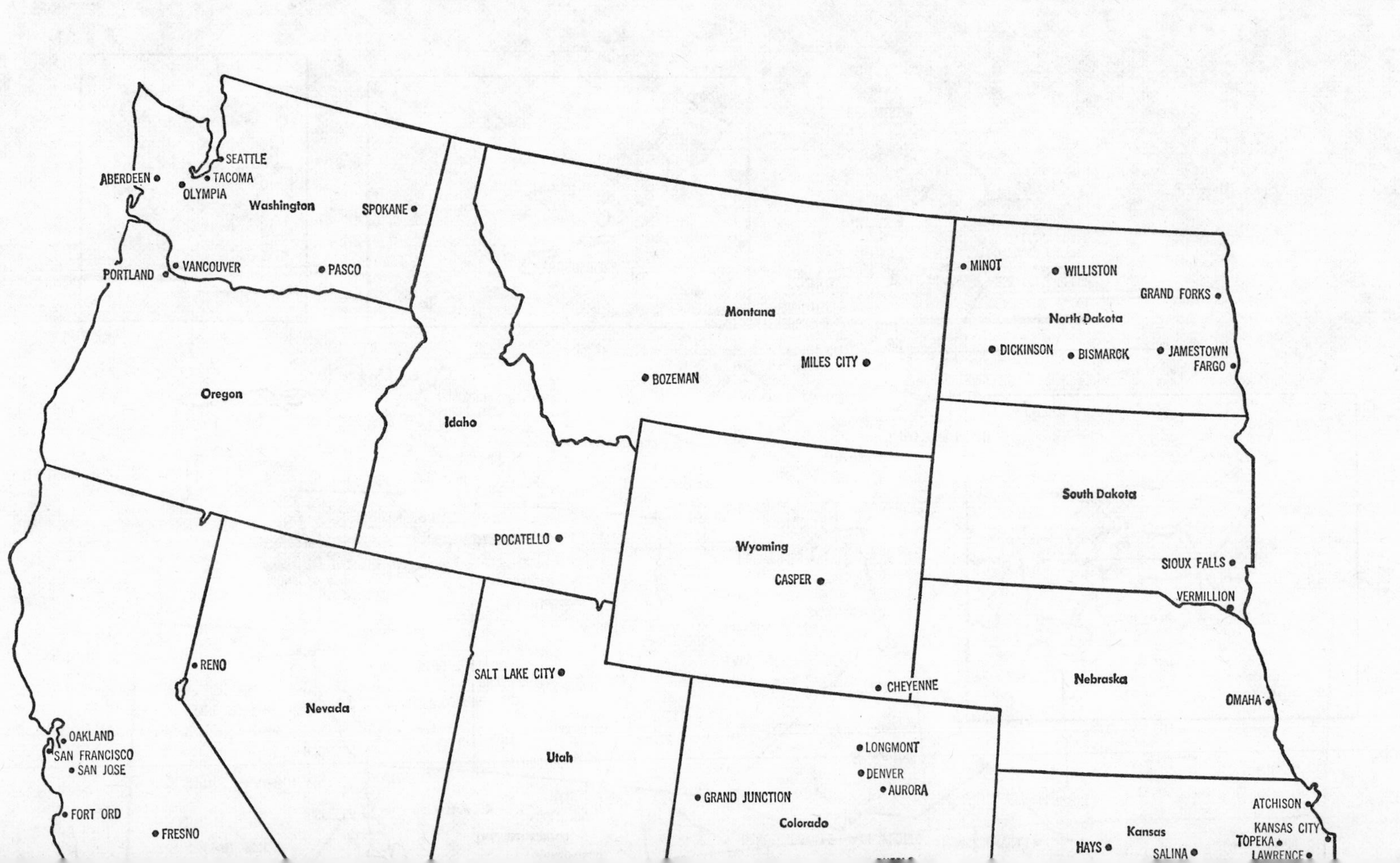
SEATTLE
ABERDEEN
TACOMA
OLYMPIA
Washington
SPOKANE
PORTLAND
VANCOUVER
PASCO
Oregon
Idaho
Montana
BOZEMAN
MILES CITY
MINOT
WILLISTON
GRAND FORKS
North Dakota
DICKINSON
BISMARCK
JAMESTOWN
FARGO
South Dakota
SIOUX FALLS
VERMILLION
POCATELLO
Wyoming
CASPER
RENO
SALT LAKE CITY
CHEYENNE
Nebraska
OMAHA
Nevada
OAKLAND
SAN FRANCISCO
SAN JOSE
Utah
LONGMONT
DENVER
AURORA
GRAND JUNCTION
Colorado
FORT ORD
FRESNO
ATCHISON
KANSAS CITY
TOPEKA
LAWRENCE
Kansas
HAYS
SALINA

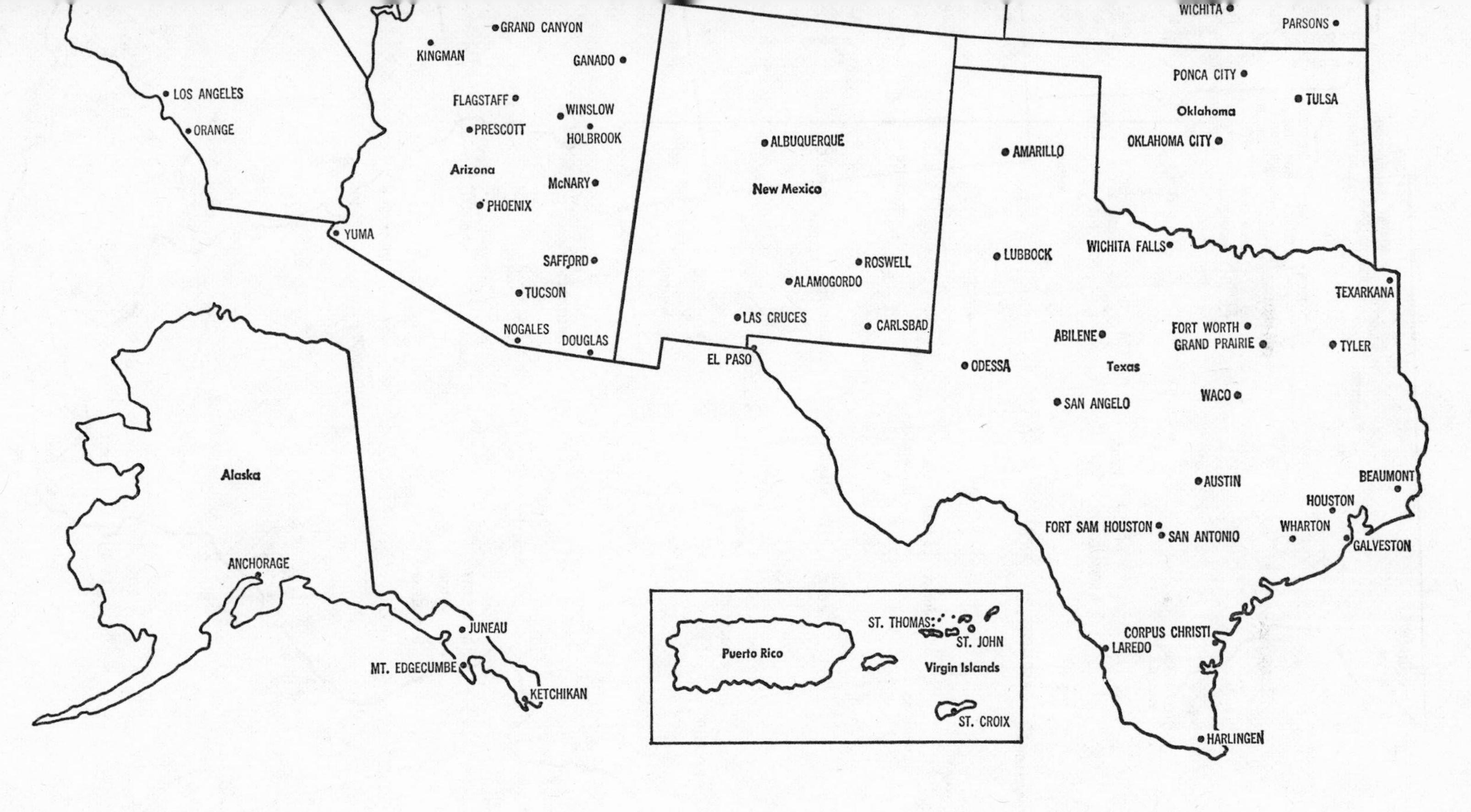
LOS ANGELES
ORANGE
KINGMAN
GRAND CANYON
GANADO
FLAGSTAFF
WINSLOW
PRESCOTT
HOLBROOK
Arizona
McNARY
PHOENIX
YUMA
SAFFORD
TUCSON
NOGALES
DOUGLAS
ALBUQUERQUE
New Mexico
ROSWELL
ALAMOGORDO
LAS CRUCES
CARLSBAD
EL PASO
WICHITA
PARSONS
PONCA CITY
TULSA
Oklahoma
OKLAHOMA CITY
AMARILLO
LUBBOCK
WICHITA FALLS
TEXARKANA
FORT WORTH
GRAND PRAIRIE
TYLER
ABILENE
ODESSA
Texas
WACO
SAN ANGELO
AUSTIN
BEAUMONT
HOUSTON
WHARTON
GALVESTON
FORT SAM HOUSTON
SAN ANTONIO
CORPUS CHRISTI
LAREDO
HARLINGEN
Alaska
ANCHORAGE
JUNEAU
MT. EDGECUMBE
KETCHIKAN
Puerto Rico
ST. THOMAS
ST. JOHN
Virgin Islands
ST. CROIX

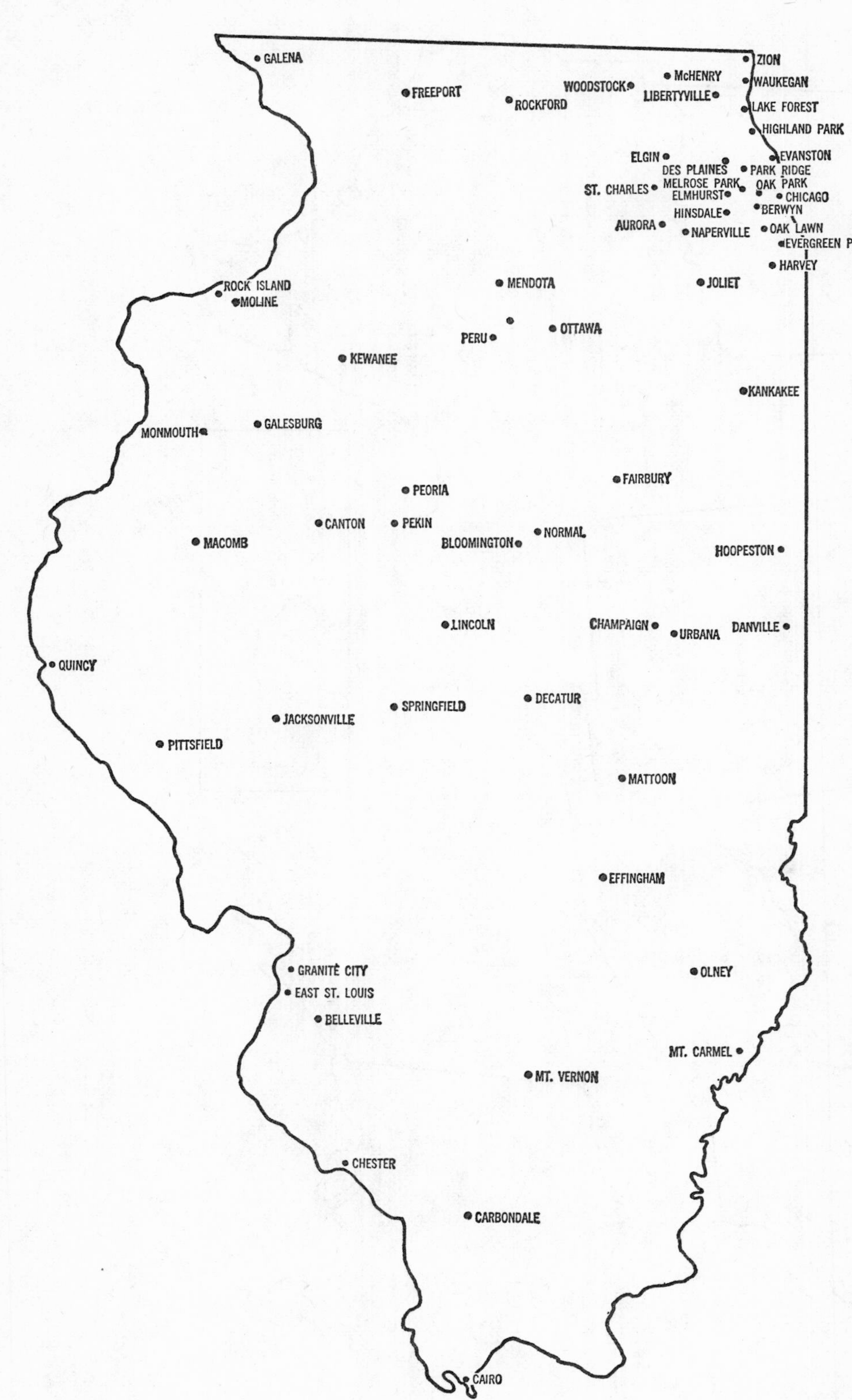

GALENA
FREEPORT
ROCKFORD
WOODSTOCK
McHENRY
LIBERTYVILLE
ZION
WAUKEGAN
LAKE FOREST
HIGHLAND PARK
ELGIN
EVANSTON
DES PLAINES
PARK RIDGE
MELROSE PARK
OAK PARK
ST. CHARLES
ELMHURST
CHICAGO
BERWYN
HINSDALE
AURORA
NAPERVILLE
OAK LAWN
EVERGREEN PARK
HARVEY
ROCK ISLAND
MOLINE
MENDOTA
JOLIET
PERU
OTTAWA
KEWANEE
KANKAKEE
MONMOUTH
GALESBURG
FAIRBURY
PEORIA
CANTON
PEKIN
NORMAL
MACOMB
BLOOMINGTON
HOOPESTON
LINCOLN
CHAMPAIGN
URBANA
DANVILLE
QUINCY
SPRINGFIELD
DECATUR
JACKSONVILLE
PITTSFIELD
MATTOON
EFFINGHAM
GRANITE CITY
EAST ST. LOUIS
OLNEY
BELLEVILLE
MT. CARMEL
MT. VERNON
CHESTER
CARBONDALE
CAIRO

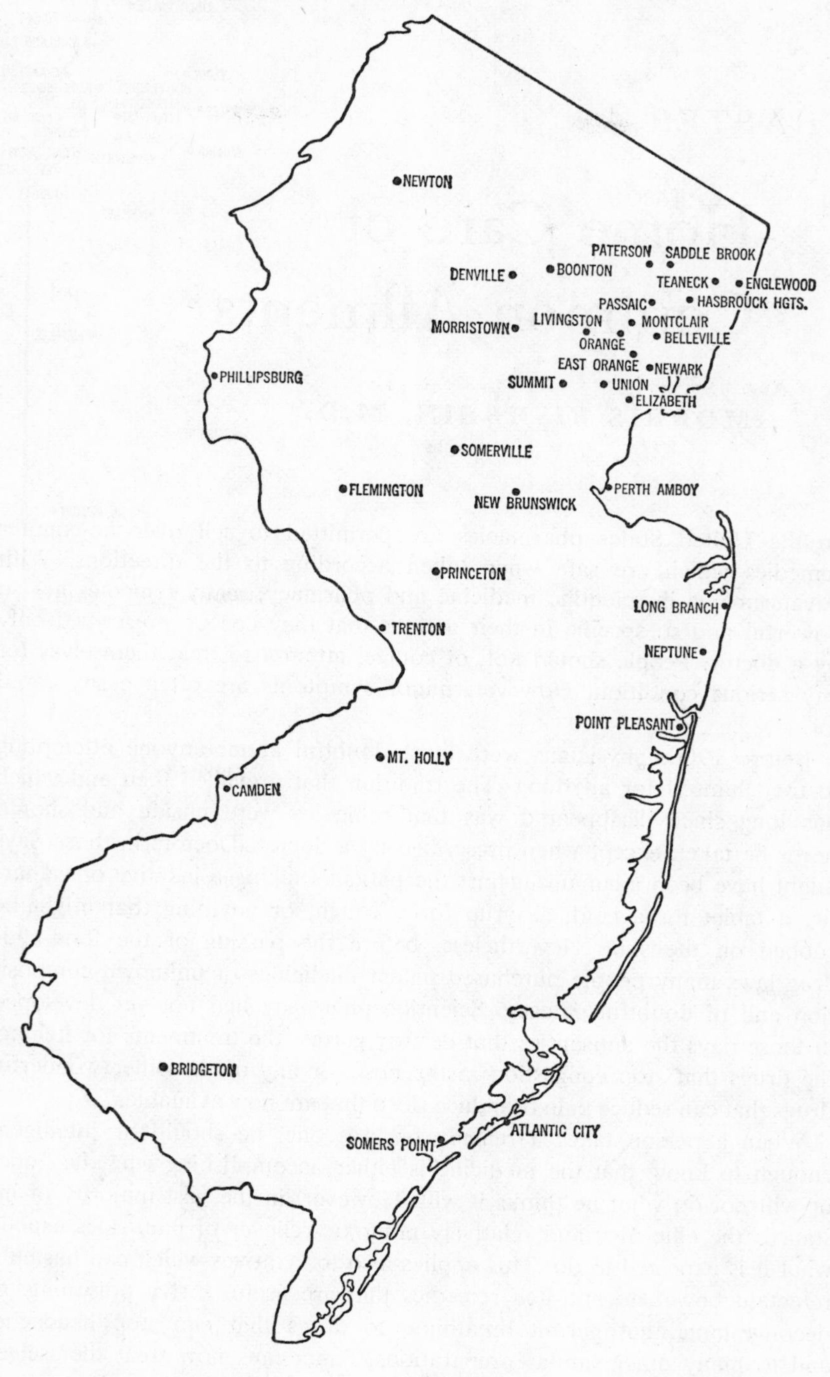
NEWTON
PATERSON
SADDLE BROOK
DENVILLE
BOONTON
TEANECK
ENGLEWOOD
PASSAIC
HASBROUCK HGTS.
LIVINGSTON
MONTCLAIR
MORRISTOWN
ORANGE
BELLEVILLE
EAST ORANGE
NEWARK
PHILLIPSBURG
SUMMIT
UNION
ELIZABETH
SOMERVILLE
FLEMINGTON
PERTH AMBOY
NEW BRUNSWICK
PRINCETON
LONG BRANCH
TRENTON
NEPTUNE
POINT PLEASANT
MT. HOLLY
CAMDEN
BRIDGETON
ATLANTIC CITY
SOMERS POINT

CHAPTER 4

Home Care of Common Ailments

MORRIS FISHBEIN, M.D.

In the United States pharmacies are permitted to sell over-the-counter remedies which are safe when taken according to the directions. With advancements in scientific medicine and pharmacy, many remedies are so powerful and so specific in their actions that they can be prescribed only by a doctor. People should not, of course, attempt to treat themselves for any serious condition. However, minor symptoms are often easily cared for.

Before 1900, physicians were most doubtful about anyone attempting to treat himself for anything. The tradition that prevailed then and which has long since disappeared was that remedies were unsafe and should never be taken except when prescribed by a doctor. Doctors in those days might have been adamant against the patient's taking a laxative or cathartic, a tablet for a cold, a syrup for a cough, or anything that might be rubbed on the skin. Nevertheless, before the passing of the food-and-drug laws many people purchased patent medicines of unknown composition and of doubtful efficacy. Scientific pharmacy had not yet developed in those days the antiseptics that destroy germs, the treatments for itching, the drugs that stop congestion in the nose, or any of the other wonderful drugs that can reduce pain or induce sleep that are now available.

When a person takes a remedy or uses one, he should be intelligent enough to know that the medicine is either accomplishing what he hopes or will not do what he thinks it will. However, in the vast majority of instances the efficiency and relatively nontoxic reliever of pain does exactly what it is expected to do. This applies also to laxatives which can hasten a reluctant bowel, to anti-itch remedies that are useful in ivy poisoning, to decongestants that permit breathing, to drugs that can stop headache, and to many other similar preparations. Americans now treat themselves with such remedies knowing that they will be helpful, although occasionally the treatment is experimental.

Among the self-medication products everyone knows about are cough drops, headache remedies, products for the relief of colds, laxatives, vitamins, anti-airsickness and anti-seasickness preparations, and some products said to be helpful for sleeplessness, poison ivy, fever sores, indigestion, or stomach upsets (which used to be called biliousness), and antisepsis.

Long ago the Council on Pharmacy and Chemistry of the American Medical Association recognized the desirability of having so-called "household remedies" which persons could buy in a variety of stores. In the many years that have passed, I know of few instances indeed when such sales had an adverse effect on the purchasers or on medicine generally. In England "household remedies" are available on open shelves in all of the drugstores or chemists shops and on the open shelves of department stores. I know of no laws in England that will prevent their sales in supermarkets in England. In Italy one may purchase anti-sea and -air sickness remedies "over the counter" and in some places on open self-service shelves. Indeed every airplane hostess has available for passengers in need aspirin, Dramamine®, and similar remedies. After traveling more than a million miles I have never seen harm come to any person from such administration of simple remedies by airplane hostesses.

Probably the most frequent of all common ailments is the common cold—for which scientific medicine does not have any specific remedy. (See the article on this subject.) Statistics indicate that the average child has somewhat more than four colds each year and the average adult more than two. The United States Army dispenses millions of doses of relief-giving agents for this condition, in most instances leaving the dispensing to nonmedical officers or even enlisted men. A similar formula to that used by the United States Army is available in many proprietary preparations, including aspirin itself in various forms, and other combinations. The question arises whether either a pharmacist or a physician is needed to dispense these home remedies.

Among the most frequent symptoms from which people suffer are headaches. The headaches may, of course, represent a brain tumor, an encephalitis, accumulations of fluid in the tissues, an aneurysm, or any one of a hundred other conditions, but these are rare; whereas the vast majority of headaches may be due to emotional stresses, slight variations in the circulation of the blood, or, again, hundreds of less serious causes. Relief of headache is easily accomplished with many available proprietary remedies. It would be simply impossible for physicians to see all the people who have headaches at the time when they have headaches. I doubt that any licensed pharmacist is able to determine when the average person with a headache should take the remedy that gives him relief any better than the person who has tried a half dozen remedies and has found one that helps him.

Another common symptom is dizziness—not easily diagnosed by the physician; certainly not diagnosed by the pharmacist, and not likely to be self-treated by the patient. However, dizziness is quite different from the nausea that is related to dietary indiscretions. This may frequently be associated with changes in stomach acidity. About fifteen to twenty per cent of the American people suffer now and then with symptoms of excessive acidity and they are accustomed to treating themselves with baking soda, which is sodium bicarbonate, or with any of several dozen innocuous substances that lessen irritation. Such people should have diagnoses, but once the condition is recognized, little necessity exists for either the physician or pharmacist to prescribe every time a condition like this needs alleviation.

Another frequent symptom is itching. Available over the counter are many remedies for itching conceded to be relatively, if not absolutely, harmless. For the average person who has had bites by insects, association with ivy, occasional sensitivities to food, easy access to quick relief is a merciful arrangement. Persistent symptoms will always lead to consultation with those recognized as capable of giving accurate information.

Our existing laws in most states and under the federal government afford a maximum of protection in this country compared with most other countries where I have traveled. Any substance used to excess may be harmful, including water. Over the years this fact has become apparent. Restrictions have been placed on substances likely to be used in excess. Sale of such substances as aspirin, cough drops, headache remedies, substances for the relief of colds, milk of magnesia and other laxatives without intermediation which would add to the costs of these medicaments is permitted. Restrictions which would make more difficult access to these substances would, I am sure, be opposed by the mass of the people generally.

Among the most frequent users of home remedies and products purchased over the counter are the aged, of whom there are now about eighteen million in the United States. A principal cause for concern is the medical care of the aged and the costs invariably associated with such care. More than a few competent geriatricians, who are the specialists that care for the aged, are convinced that old people need a regular intake of certain vitamins, particularly because, first, they do not eat well; second, they do not absorb well what they eat; and, third, they frequently suffer with symptoms indicating that they need the vitamins whose absence is associated with certain effects. I have in mind particularly the vitamins of the B complex, some of which are said to enhance appetite and indeed to improve alertness and some in the B complex which are related to digestion and a vitamin which is certainly concerned with the production of red blood cells. Old people are particularly unlikely to have sufficient calcium and with it the vitamins concerned with proper absorption and utilization of calcium. Old people suffer inordinately with dizziness, with itching, and with a number of other discomforts which are in most instances easily relieved by certain home remedies. Few physicians would be unwilling that such patients be instructed as to what they should have and what they should purchase regularly in sufficient quantities to meet their needs.

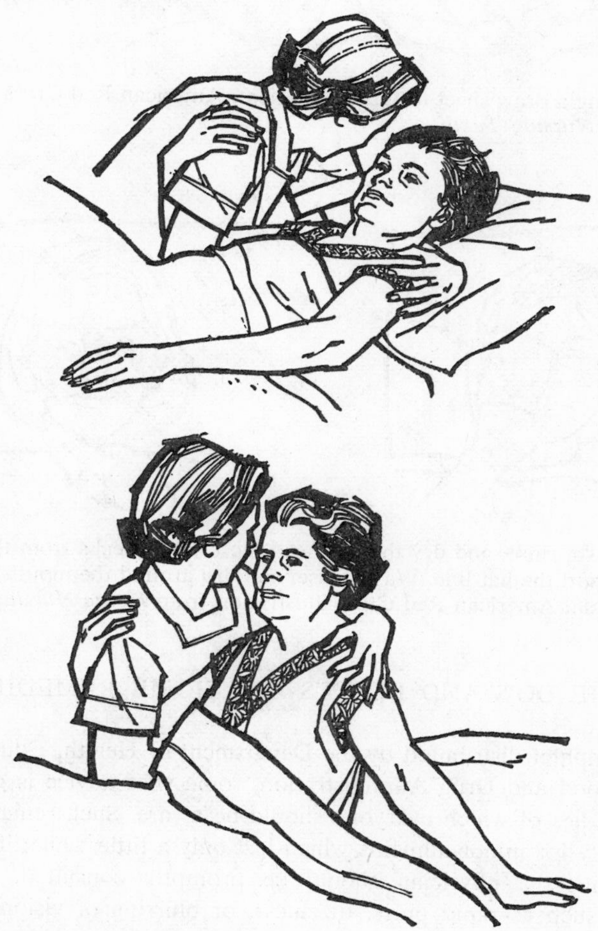

Fig. 7. Helping patient sit up. Lock near arms with patient; support head and shoulders with other arm; on signal, help patient come to sitting position. American Red Cross illustration from *Home Nursing Textbook*.

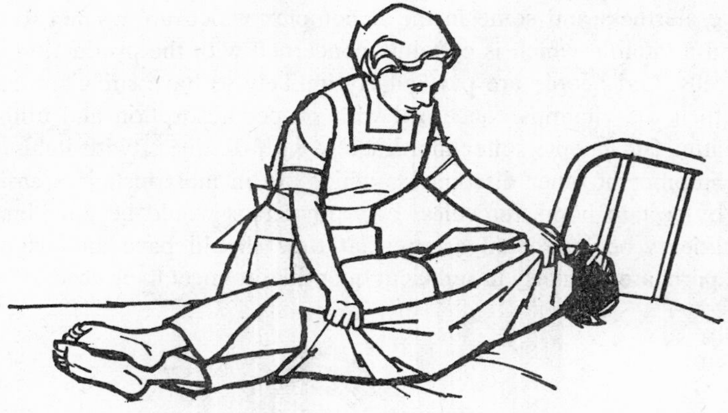

Fig. 8. Using a draw sheet to turn the patient. American Red Cross illustration from *Home Nursing Textbook.*

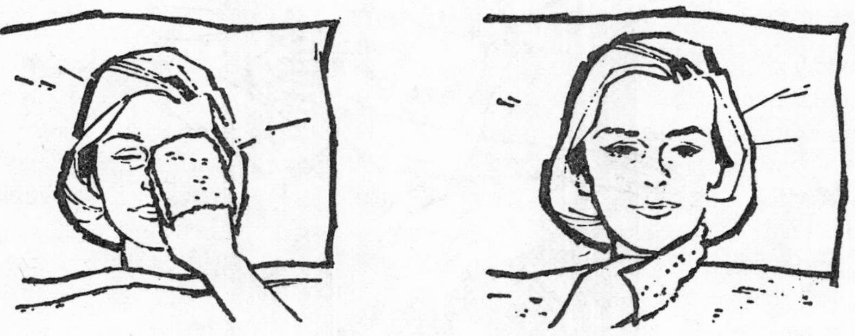

Fig. 9. Wash, rinse, and dry the forehead, nose, and cheeks from the center of the face toward the hairline. Wash, rinse, and dry around the mouth and chin in an "S" motion. American Red Cross illustration from *Home Nursing Textbook.*

THE DO'S AND DON'T'S FOR HOME REMEDIES

In a pamphlet distributed by the Department of Health, Education, and Welfare, Food and Drug Administration, some wise advice is given about home remedies of which everyone should be aware. Such remedies should be used only for minor ailments which last only a little while; if the condition continues, a physician should be promptly consulted. If unusual symptoms such as rapid pulse, dizziness, or blurring of vision occur, the medicine should be discontinued. If pain persists for more than ten days or if there is redness and swelling, a physician should be consulted imdiately.

Here are some simple directions:

1. Date all over-the-counter drugs when you buy them. Prescription drugs will be dated by the pharmacist.
2. Buy medicines and health supplies in realistic quantities. Old drugs deteriorate and may become ineffective or even dangerous.
3. Be sure to store all drugs out of the way of small children, under lock and key if they cannot be protected any other way.
4. Safeguard tablets which are candied, flavored, or colored, since small children eat them like candy.
5. Never give or take medicine from an unlabeled bottle. Transparent tape over the label will protect it.
6. Never give or take medicine in the dark. Be sure the label can be read clearly.
7. Before measuring liquid medicine, always shake the bottle thoroughly.
8. When measuring drugs, give the task full attention.
9. Weed out the leftovers regularly from the home medicine chest—especially any prescription drugs that may have been ordered for a prior illness.
10. When you throw away drugs, flush them down the toilet, and be sure the discarded containers cannot be reached by children or pets.

Many of the most important discoveries in medicine and particularly in the treatment of disease have been made through accidental use by people not medically trained. For instance, the use of sulfur for the treatment of seven-year itch was developed by an old Italian market woman. The use of digitalis for eliminating fluids from the body was discovered by a woman herb doctor in England. The American Indians discovered the use of leaves of wintergreen for rheumatic aches and pains; later scientists found that wintergreen contains methylsalicylate which is used for lowering fevers as well as for rheumatic pains. The Indians also discovered the purgative action of the bark of cascara. The Incas of Peru discovered the fatigue-relieving properties of coca leaves. The natives of the Amazon found curare, which they used for a poison but which is now used as an ingredient of antispasmodic drugs. The Incas also discovered the sweat-producing properties of ipecac and found out that it can cause vomiting. The Moslems discovered the stimulating and awakening powers of coffee which contains caffeine and the fatigue-relieving properties of tea which contains theobromine. Many different peoples found that fruit juices or grain mashes fermented when exposed to warmth and sunlight from which came the innumerable alcoholic drinks also used in medicines. In Peru cinchona bark was found to have value in malaria.

Many home practices have come down from rural people living far away from access to medication. Some of these were without any scientific basis; others, however, had been found to have actual effects on the human body. Knowing that rheumatic pains are often as much psychological as actual, many rural inhabitants have put copper cents in the shoes, worn rings made out of horse-shoe nails, or carried buckeyes in the hip pocket. The American Indians used decoctions of willow bark which contains considerable amounts of salicylates as do also cranberries. For conditions affecting the lungs, many rural people have used inhalations of hot steam and smoke. For asthma a wide variety of smokes has been tried, none of this, however, having any real scientific merit. Hot lemonade has been used for years to ward off colds but without any proof that it really does so. Purgatives of all kinds have been used, including heroic doses of salts. In Arkansas and New Hampshire, rural people treated diarrhea with blackberry root and juice, and in Arkansas smartweed and teas made from sassafras bark and other weeds have been used. For many years bread-and-milk poultices have been used for inflammations and wounds. Many people have connected with this the use of the moulds, such as penicillin, which are antibiotic. In rural America many years ago, spring tonics were regularly employed, consisting usually of any herb, weed, or chemical that would have a bitter taste. These are called tonics or blood medicines.

SELF-MEDICATION

In a recent symposium on self-medication, Dr. Julius Michaelson of Foley, Alabama, noted that out of every 1000 people, 750 will have some symptom of an illness every month. Of these only 250 will consult a physician. Of the 250, only one will need the highly technical services of a physician. The 500 who do not seek professional medical care either go to the drugstore to buy something that they hope will help them, ask a neighbor, or ask the druggist for something that may be helpful. In recent years people have had access to much more information about self-treatment for minor ailments than was ever available previously. This has come through health columns in the newspapers, feature articles in many magazines, and health books.

Over the years legislative safeguards have been developed in the United States to control the sale of home treatments for minor ailments. Drugs sold directly to people over the counter are considered misbranded if their claims for efficacy are shown to be false or misleading. They are also misbranded if they contain inadequate cautions and warnings against misuse or about diseases in which their use may be contraindicated. The dosage must be specified for adults and children.

VARIETIES OF HOME REMEDIES

In 1965 people in the United States spent over $4.5 billion on drug products, about one third of which was for home remedies. Some of these

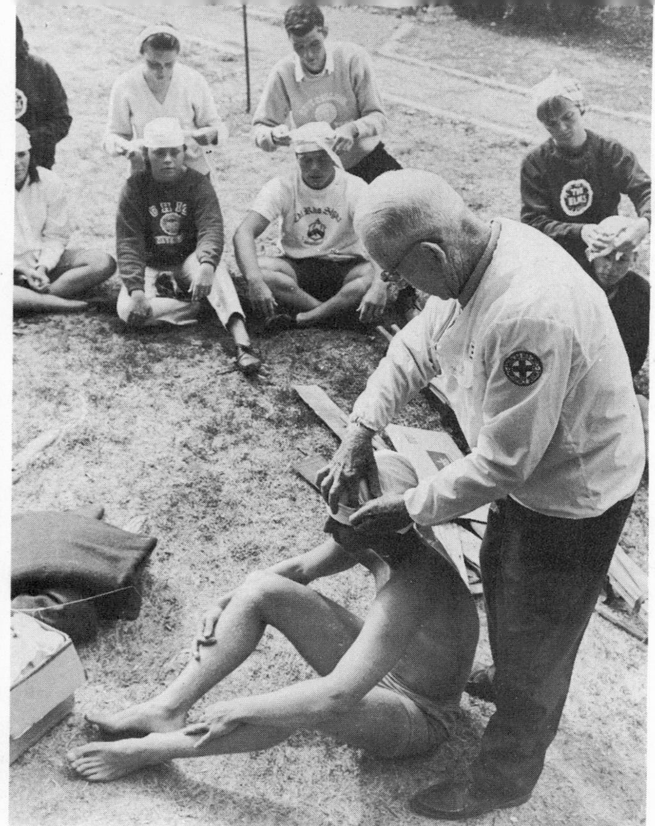

PLATE **16.** Red Cross Youth, formerly Junior Red Cross, conduct leadership training centers sponsored by individual chapters at various sites throughout the country. Here, an advanced first-aid class learns by doing. The proper application of a head bandage requires skill, as demonstrated by Edward M. Davis, first-aid instructor at classes in Hammondsport, New York. *(American Red Cross photo by Rudolph Vetter.)*

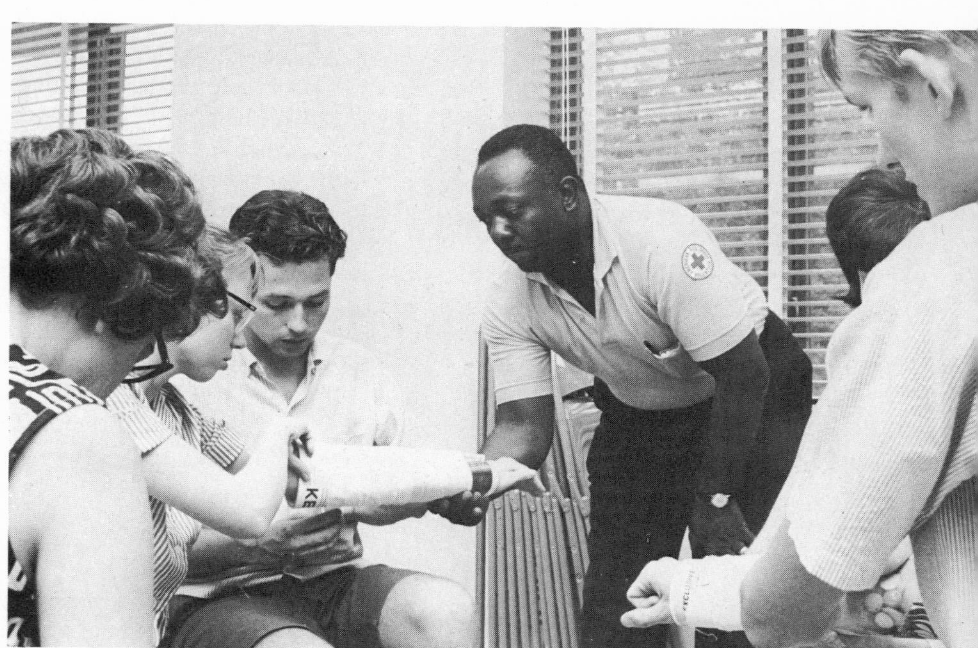

PLATE **17.** Here in Minneapolis, Minnesota, Red Cross first-aid instructor Johnny Walker assists a first-aid class with skills in splinting. *(American Red Cross photo by Frank Fiddler.)*

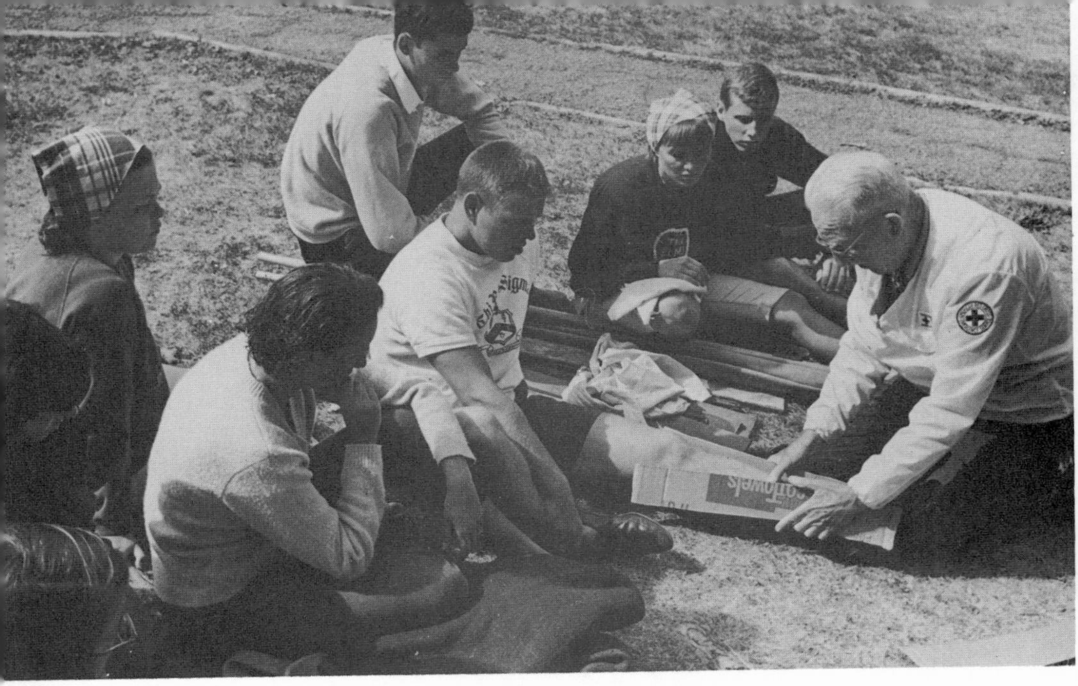

PLATE **18.** "Splint them where they lie," says the American Red Cross first-aid instructor, "and use whatever materials are at hand for splinting broken bones, or suspected fractures." Here at the Aquatic School in Hammondsport, New York, young people learn that cardboard is one good material. *(American Red Cross photo by Rudolph Vetter.)*

PLATE **19.** Students in this Red Cross first-aid course practice carrying a victim with a litter. Proper handling of an accident victim prevents further injury and can save a life until medical help is available. These young people are at the Aquatic School in Hammondsport, New York. *(American Red Cross photo by Rudolph Vetter.)*

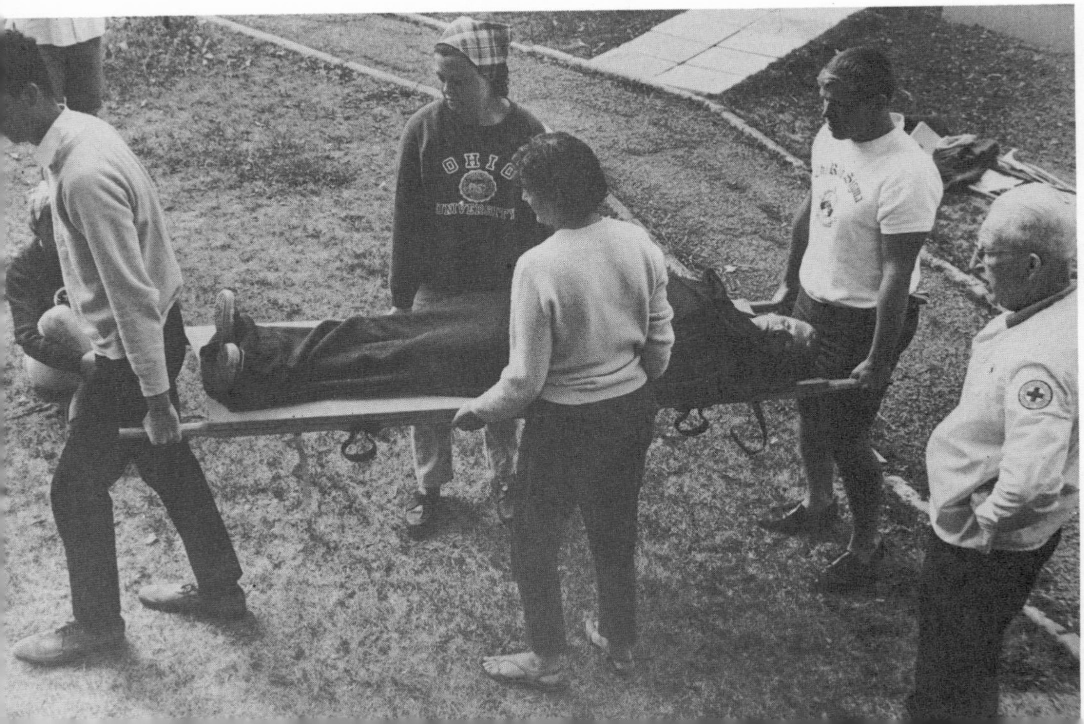

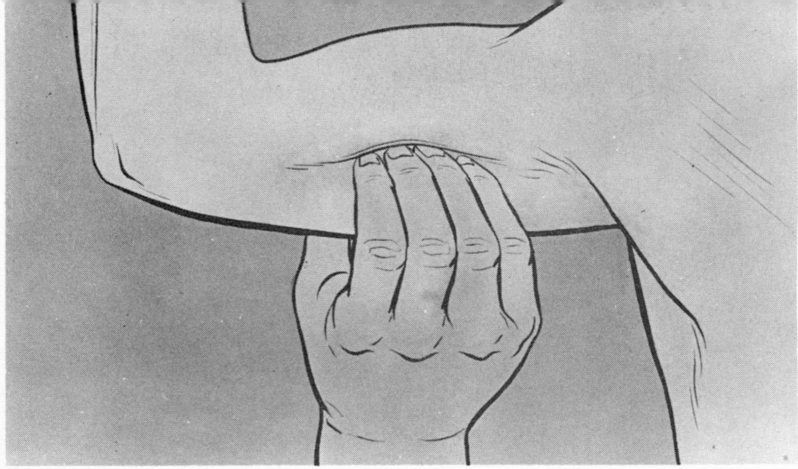

PLATE 20. Pressure on the inner half of the arm, midway between the armpit and elbow, presses the brachial artery against the underlying bone and thus will diminish the flow of blood in the upper extremity below the pressure point.

PLATE 21. Pressure on the front mid-groin area presses the femoral artery against the underlying pelvic bone and thus will diminish bleeding in the lower extremity below the pressure point.

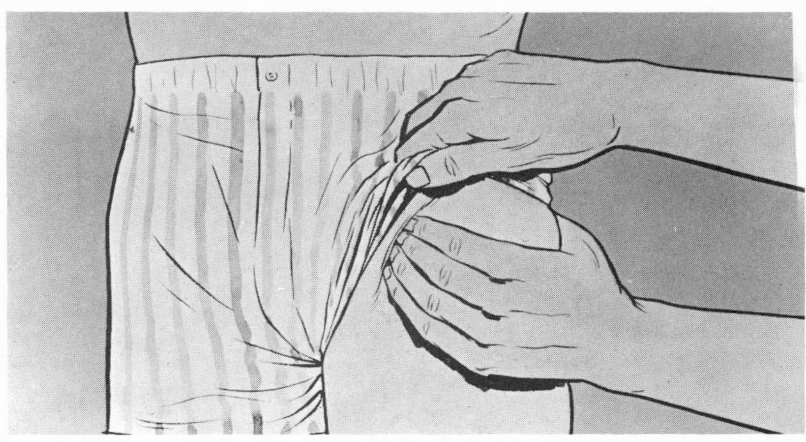

PLATE 22. To stop bleeding, apply dressing or pad directly over the wound and then apply pressure.

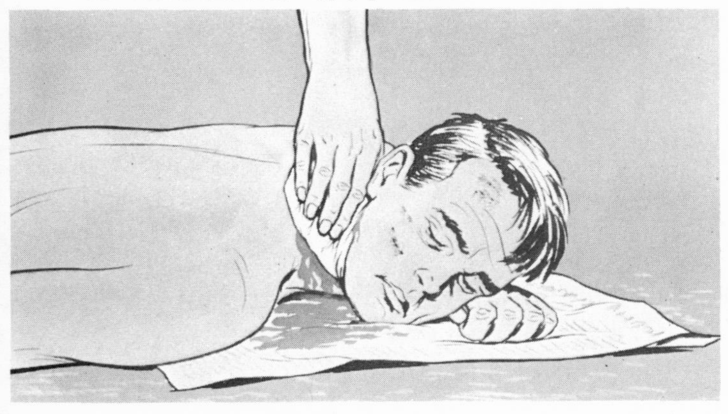

PLATES **20-29** *from "Medical Self-Help Training Program," administered by the Division of Health Mobilization, Public Health Service, U.S. Department of Health, Education and Welfare.*

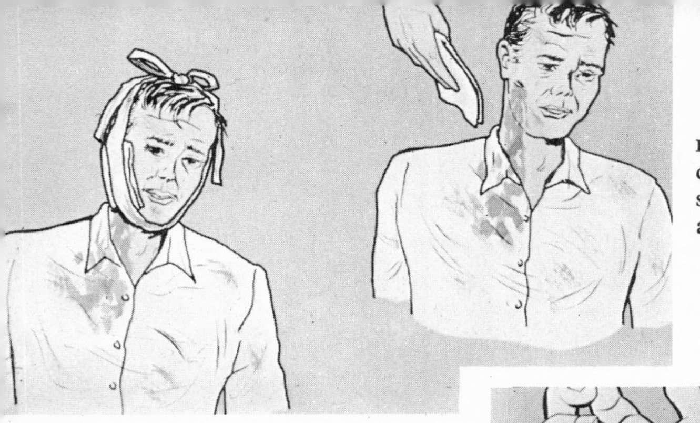

PLATE **23.** After applying dressing directly over the wound, the pressure may be continued by applying a bandage.

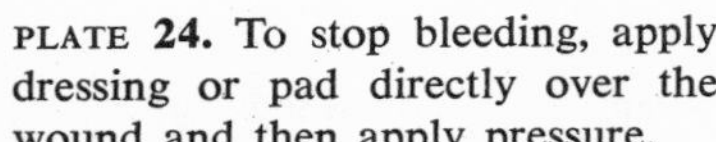

PLATE **24.** To stop bleeding, apply dressing or pad directly over the wound and then apply pressure.

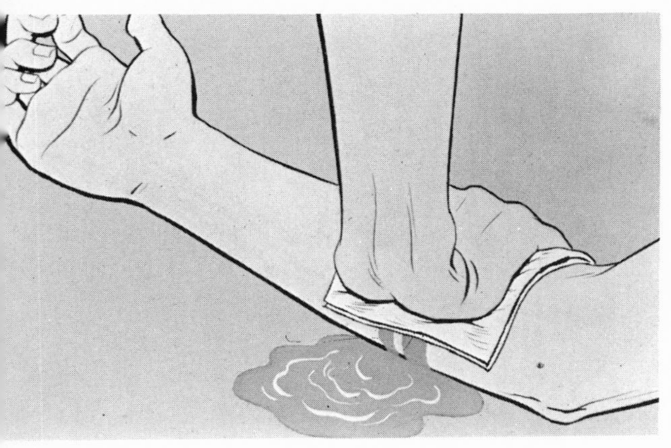

PLATE **25.** Continue the pressure until the bleeding has stopped or slowed to the point where you will be able to apply a bandage. Don't be in a hurry to stop the pressure.

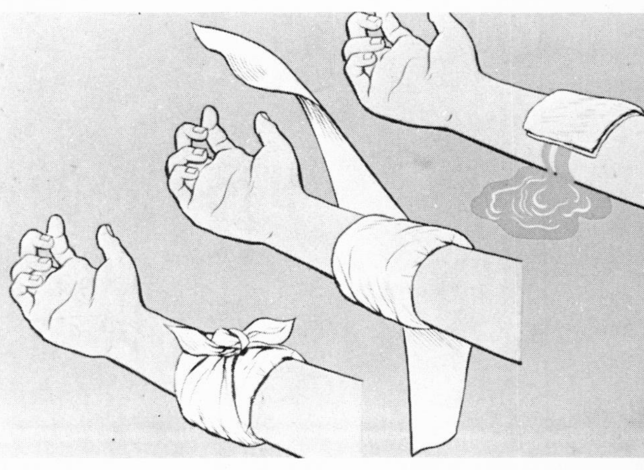

PLATE **26.** Apply the bandage firmly over the dressing to continue pressure and thus continue to stop the bleeding. CAUTION – check the bandage after you have tied the knot to be sure it is not too tight and is not cutting off the circulation.

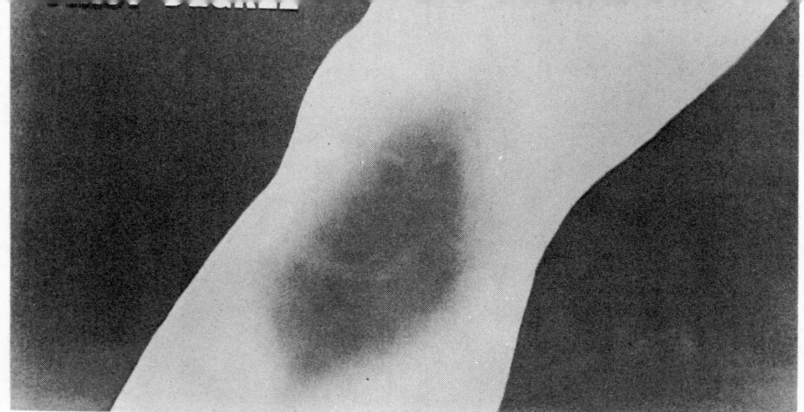

PLATE **27.** A first-degree burn only reddens the skin, and if it does not cover more than 25 per cent of the body, is usually not serious.

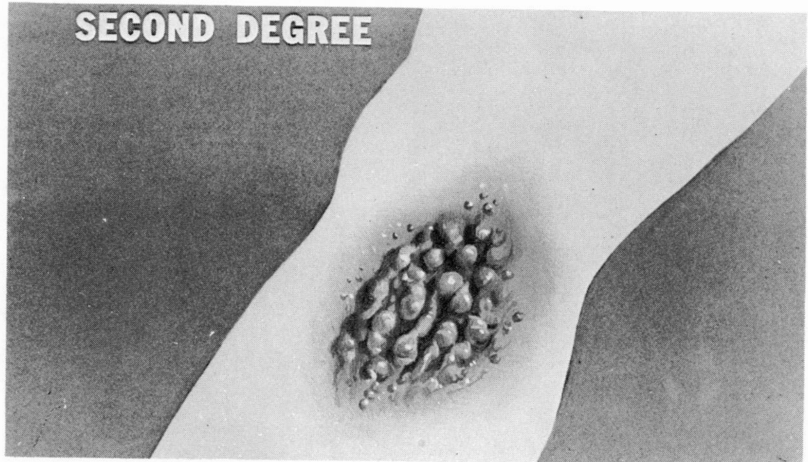

PLATE **28.** In second-degree burns, blisters develop and there is now the very real danger of infection. Extensive second-degree burns will require giving additional fluids to the burned person. Do not apply grease or salve. Cover with sterile or clean dressing.

PLATE **29.** Third-degree burns, even in a relatively small area, are serious. The injury is deep and the underlying tissue has been destroyed. Keep this type of burn clean to avoid infection.

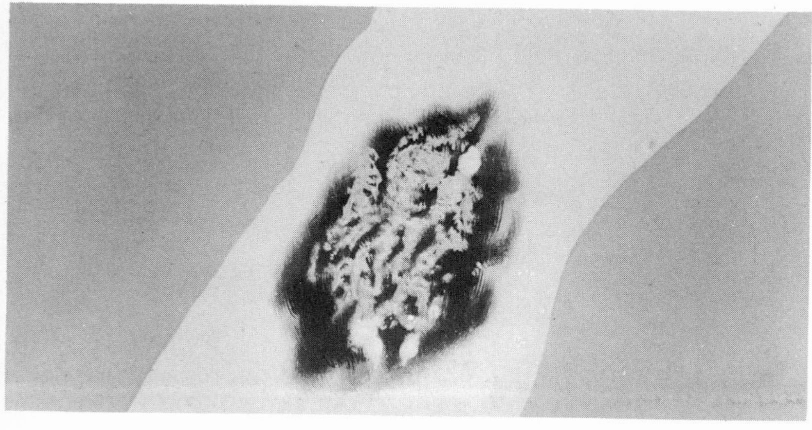

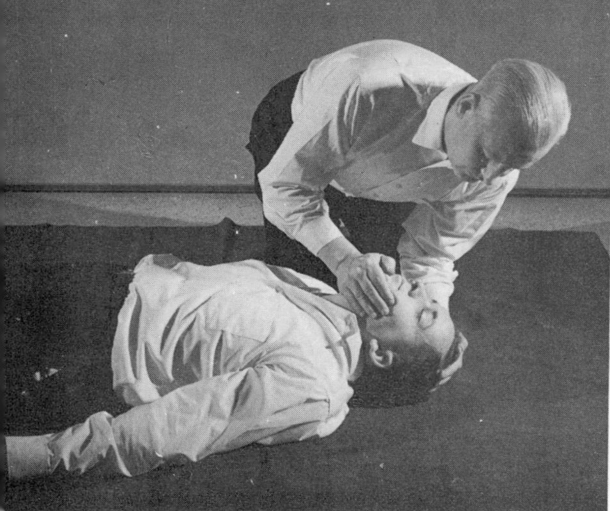

PLATE **30.** Mouth-to-mouth resuscitation. Lift neck and push head down. Pull jaw by holding chin.

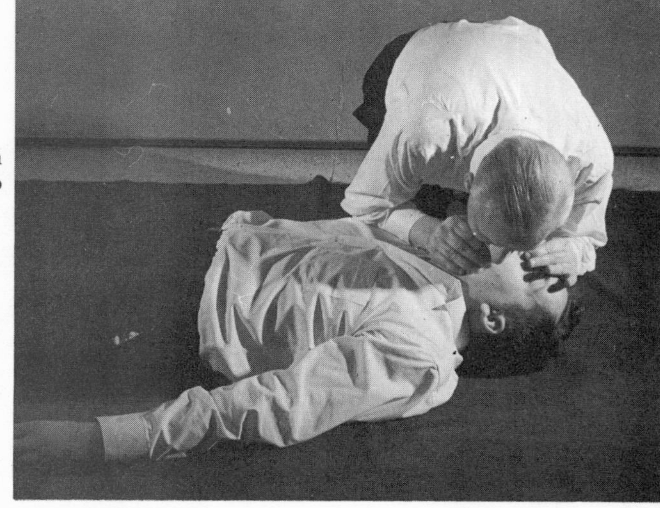

PLATE **31.** Breathe deeply. Put mouth over victim's. Pinch nose and blow into air passage.

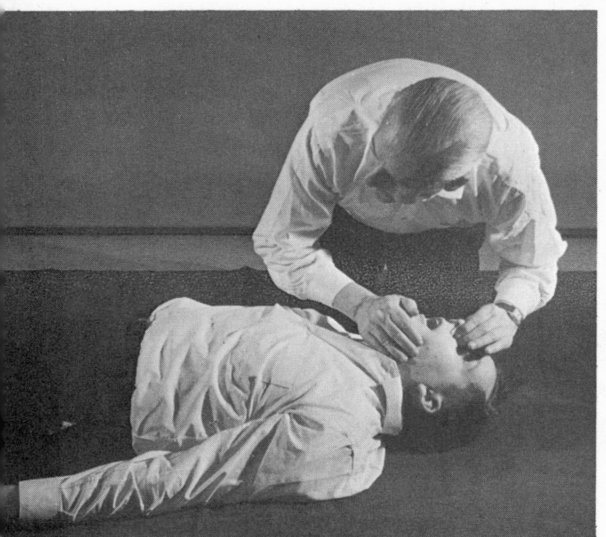

PLATE **32.** Remove mouth, let victim exhale. Inflate lungs again. Repeat twelve times a minute. For a small child, twenty times.

PLATES **30, 31,** *and* **32** *courtesy of Con Edison, New York.*

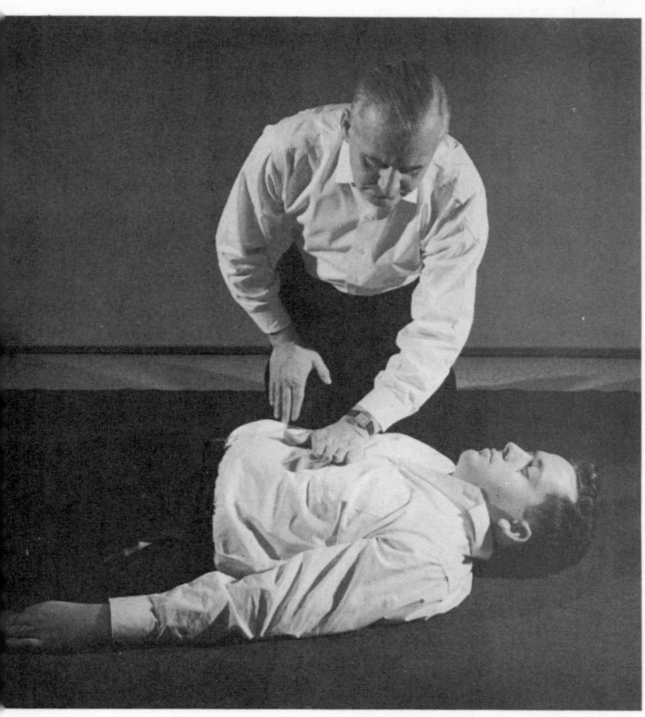

PLATE **33.** Heart resuscitation. Heel of hand on center over lower breastbone. Fingers off chest.

PLATE **34.** Other hand on top. Gently rock forward, exerting pressure down. Heart compresses, pushing blood into lungs, body. Release pressure. Chest expands, heart refills with blood. Repeat 60 times a minute. Use one hand on child, two fingers on infant–80 to 100 times. Two persons can perform these rescue methods at the same time. If you are alone, give victim five or six breaths to begin, then compress heart once a second five times. Continue cycle, one breath to five pressures.

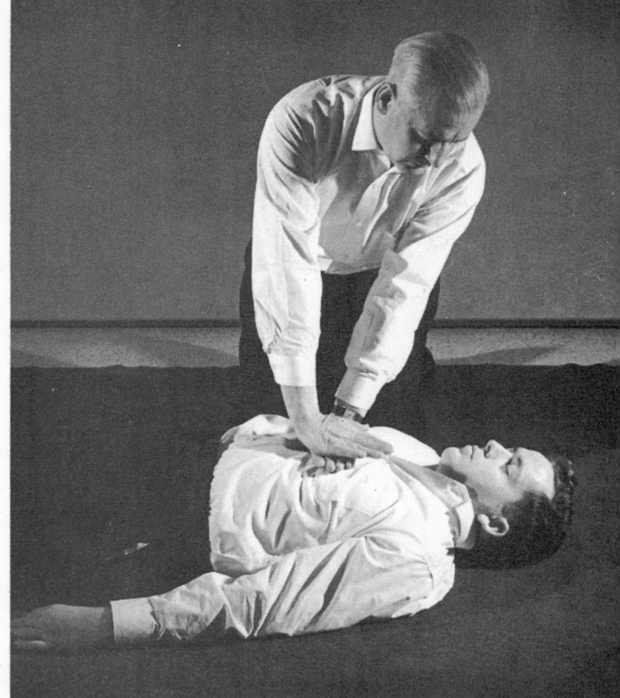

PLATES **33** *and* **34** *courtesy of Con Edison, New York.*

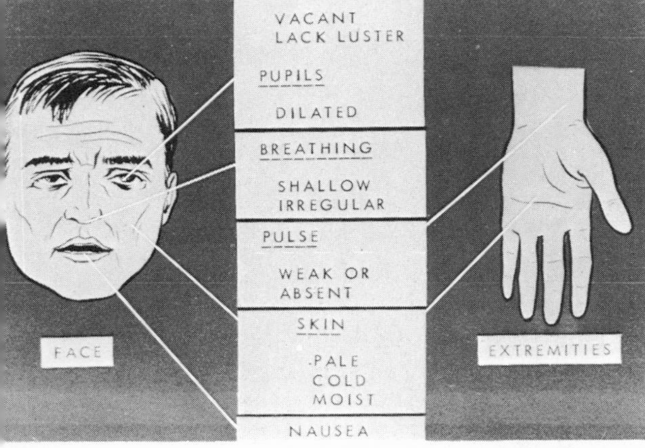

PLATE **35.** Shock is easy to recognize. Shock may cause death if not treated promptly even though the injury which causes it may not itself be enough to cause death. All seriously injured persons should be treated for shock even though all of these symptoms have not appeared and the person seems normal and alert.

PLATE **36.** Encourage fluids by mouth if person is conscious. Use solution of one teaspoon of salt and half a teaspoon of baking soda to one quart of water. Give half a glassful every fifteen minutes. Never attempt to give fluids to unconscious persons.

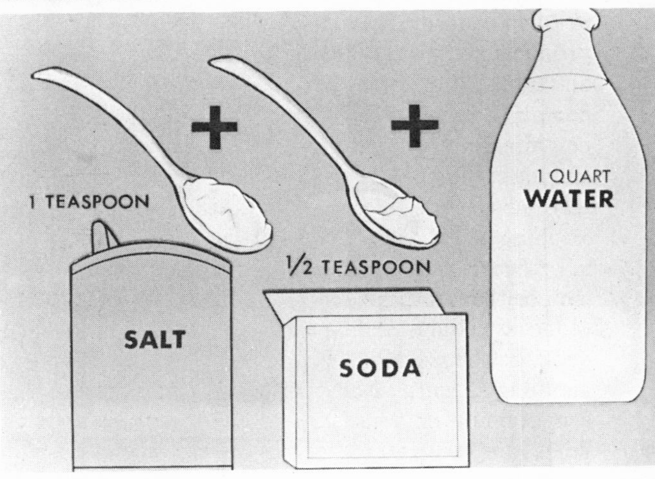

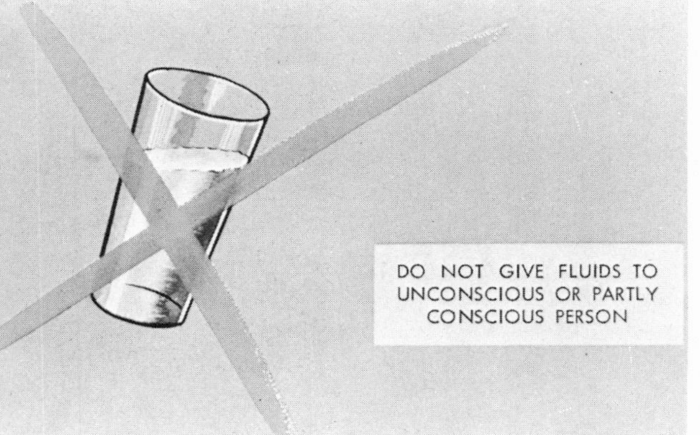

PLATE **37.**

PLATE **38.** If a person does not have a head or chest injury and is in shock, he should be placed in a head-down position. Keep the injured person warm.

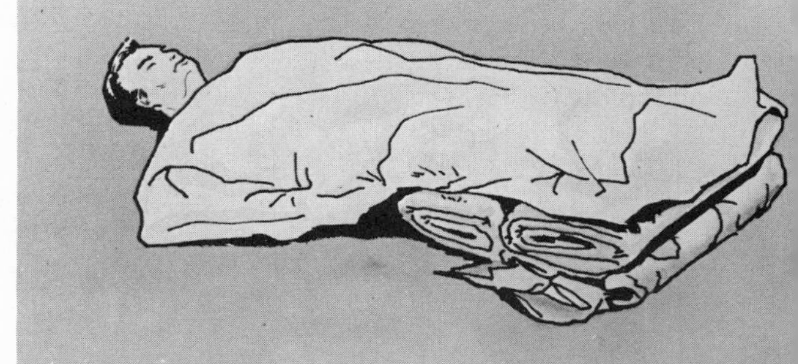

PLATES **35–38** *from: "Medical Self-Help Training Program," administered by the Division of Health Mobilization, Public Health Service, Department of Health, Education and Welfare.*

were classified as health aids; others as toiletries. The chief remedy used was aspirin. About 1000 different preparations containing aspirin are available to the public.

"Cough and cold remedies," according to Dr. H. George Mandel, of the Department of Pharmacology of George Washington University, "include cough drops, expectorants, nose drops and syrups, antihistamines, and decongestants. Expectorants are drugs that help in the removal of exudates from the trachea, bronchi, and lungs. Many of these preparations also contain syrups producing a demulcent or soothing effect on the irritated pharnyx. Laxatives include mineral oil, saline, and bulk-type products as well as glycerine suppositories. External analgesics are the ointments, liniments, and rubbing-alcohol preparations. Tonics frequently contain bitters, which tend to improve appetite, and vitamins. Many also contain iron preparations of value for patients having iron-deficiency anemias. Many diarrhea remedies consist of insoluble bismuth salts, which tend to coat the intestinal walls. Acne aids are largely common antiseptics. Sleeping aids may involve the mild tranquilizer, scopolamine, which is of occasional use in producing sleep in tense individuals. Hemorrhoidal suppositories produce a decongestant effect by their astringent action and reduce swelling, and may provide local anesthetic relief with compounds such as benzocaine. Poison-ivy remedies also contain astringents and soothing agents. Motion-sickness preparations may be constituted of scopolamine or some of the milder antihistaminic agents, and burn remedies are usually ointments with benzocaine-like local anesthetics and menthol, which exert a soothing action."

Eye products include antiseptics and boric acid. Ear preparations are mainly used to soften waxy deposits. There are also products to increase the flow of urine, antibacterial products, and antiringworm products which can be sold over the counter.

In a poll made of 5000 women regarding their purchases of home remedies, practically all used headache remedies. Others, such as antacid preparations, laxatives, or chest rubs were purchased by two out of every three women and one out of three used menstrual pain relievers. Most people buy nonprescription drugs as they need them rather than stocking the family medicine chest. However, headache remedies, mouthwashes, vitamins, items for gastrointestinal complaints, and external pain relievers are usually kept on hand.

Aspirin is probably the most widely used pain reliever and, even with all the deficiencies that have been described, probably the safest. Many different forms of aspirin are available. It may come as plain aspirin, effervescent preparations, mixtures of aspirin and salicylates, and mixtures of aspirin with other drugs. There are also children's preparations which are flavored in various ways.

Dr. Arthur Grollmann of the Department of Experimental Medicine of the University of Texas says also that the analgesics and antipyretics (which reduce fever) are the most widely used of all medications. Pain is the commonest and least tolerated of all symptoms. Aspirin and other pain relievers are used for headache, arthritic pain, and for the general ill-feelings that are associated with most infectious diseases. Aspirin has an anti-inflammatory effect and is, therefore, used also for rheumatic inflammations. One reason why aspirin is used so greatly is that it is absorbed rapidly not only from the stomach but also from the small intestine. Usually within two hours after taking aspirin, it is circulating at its peak in the blood and its clinical effectiveness lasts about three hours; therefore people renew the dose about every three hours.

Many other varieties of salicylic acid are used in pain relievers. The classical formula of aspirin, phenacetin, and caffeine makes a remedy that became widely known during the war as APC. The caffeine was used as a stimulant, and phenacetin is believed to enhance the action of the aspirin so that smaller doses of both may be used when combined.

Among the drugs most used for gastrointestinal conditions are antacids which act against excess acid in the stomach. Most often the acidity of the gastric contents rises after a meal and then declines rapidly. In some conditions, however, the acidity may remain high for many hours, accompanied by pain, cramping and belching. When the excess acid is neutralized, the symptoms are relieved. Many antacids are available and can be purchased over the counter. Baking soda is often used but acts for only a short time. There are also hydroxides, oxides, silicates, carbonates, and phosphates of calcium, magnesium, bismuth, and aluminum. Aluminum hydroxide is also used for diarrheas. Magnesium hydroxide and magnesium trisilicate are palatable and therefore widely used. Manufacturers have developed many products of this kind which are sold under trade names in drugstores.

CONSTIPATION

Constipation is probably the most common complaint of civilized man. It may result from a great variety of causes but is usually due to the failure of the bowel to react properly to the presence of the mass of waste material. When failure to respond to an urge becomes habitual, the condition becomes chronic. The home remedies used for constipation include mineral oil, cascara, and other vegetable preparations, salts, and phenolphthalein. Still widely used are older cathartics such as castor oil, sulphur and senna preparations. Rarely used now is calomel. Some of these preparations act by irritating the bowel, some by causing water to pour into the bowel, and some by stimulating the nerve connections in the bowel. When these drugs are used properly, little harm results. However, continuous use may result in overstimulation of the bowel so that it becomes even more insensitive than it was before.

Other home remedies are used for dyspepsia, indigestion, nausea, lack of appetite, and diarrhea. Still more recently in connection with overweight, preparations are available to decrease the appetite. Some remedies are used to aid digestion. These usually contain enzymes like papain or bile salts and pancreatin. Bile is important in the digestion of fats.

IRON PREPARATIONS

A condition found most frequently in American young people and in very old people is anemia. The anemia is usually a secondary anemia which can be treated effectively with iron. Iron preparations are available in many different forms and are permitted to be sold over the counter.

Although most people take plenty of iron in their usual food, loss of blood may result in iron deficiency. This is particularly the case of women who lose iron during menstruation.

When iron is used for long periods of time, some of it may be deposited in the tissues of the body. Therefore doctors nowadays are careful to watch the use of iron by the patient, allowing intervals so as to permit the body to clear itself of excess.

VITAMINS

Vitamins, which are fully discussed in the chapter on diet and nutrition in this book, are widely used as home remedies to prevent vitamin deficiencies and also to maintain adequate amounts of vitamins in the body. Scientific research has shown that vitamins are essential to maintain the usual chemistry of the body.

Most people who live on complete and well-balanced diets, including the seven basic foods, probably secure enough vitamins. However, the refining of foods and processes like heating, freezing and other methods of packaging may injure to some extent the natural vitamin content. When baking soda is added to green vegetables in order to preserve their color while they are being cooked, some of the thiamine is destroyed. When vegetables are boiled, the water may take out some of the vitamins and minerals that dissolve in water.

As related in the chapter on vitamins, such deficiency diseases as beriberi, pellagra, and scurvy have been practically eliminated in the United States.

Many experts believe that minor deficiencies of vitamins and minerals may unfavorably influence health. When people are on restricted diets, as when they are reducing or if they are diabetic or if a woman is pregnant and loses her appetite, such a person will obviously get an insufficient amount of vitamins. Hence physicians are likely to prescribe vitamins for such people.

WEIGHT CONTROL

Among home products offered people who are reducing are drugs that the doctor prescribes which can interfere with appetite: sometimes thyroid materials when the thyroid supply is deficient, and occasionally products that add bulk in the intestines (of which, among others, are psyllium seeds and cellulose products which draw water from the bowel and make up the bulk).

Many people nowadays buy fixed formula diets of approximately 900 calories a day on which they may reduce without the danger of insufficient vitamins and minerals. Sugar may be lessened and the sense of sweetness satisfied by the use of preparations of saccharin or the cyclamates which are sold as Sucaryl®.

COLD AND COUGH REMEDIES

Among the most frequent of all conditions which people suffer are coughs and colds. As I have already pointed out, the average American has about four colds a year with the usual blocking of the nose, a mild fever, sometimes a cough. Scientists have shown that some eighty different viruses may be associated with the common cold. The preparation of vaccines against such a considerable number of viruses is almost impossible.

Most cold remedies, of which many are now purchasable by anyone at the drugstore, are mixtures of pain relievers like aspirin or phenacetin and decongestant substances which stop the swelling in the nose, expectorant substances which loosen the secretions in the bronchial tubes, and antihistamines, since many people are sensitive to various substances that are inhaled. Some of these mixtures also contain substances that act against a cough. A cough is a reflex response to any irritation in the throat, the trachea, or the bronchial tubes. Such irritations are associated with infections, allergies, the presence of foreign substances like those that may be swallowed and stick in the throat. Coughs may also be associated with inflammations of the nerves in the throat or even with the growth of tumors.

Removal of the cause will stop the cough. However, removal of the cause may require a long time. The discomfort of the cough is reduced by the usual cough remedies. However, any cough that persists for more than a few days should have analysis and treatment by a physician. Whereas most coughs are slight and likely to disappear in a few days, one must always remember that such conditions as tuberculosis, pneumonia, and tumors may produce persistent coughs.

Scientists talk about drugs that are antitussive, which simply means that they are against cough. Many drugs have been proved to be capable of ameliorating conditions associated with coughing.

HAY FEVER AND OTHER ALLERGIES

As described in the chapter on allergy, hay fever and asthma are frequent conditions affecting some millions of people. They represent sensitivities to various pollens that may be inhaled or to such foreign substances as animal hair or chemicals. Allergies may produce skin disturbances such as blisters or wheals associated with the taking of foods to which the person may be sensitive. Generalized itching may be a response. Less serious is stuffiness in the nose and occasional swellings.

Most of the available home remedies are used to prevent the involvement of the sinuses, the sneezing, and the irritation and redness of the eyes that may come with allergies.

The chief constituents of the preparations used are decongestants and antihistamines. These preparations have been found helpful in what are called head colds, in vasomotor rhinitis, sinusitis, hay fever, and even in some cases when the ear reacts with congestion of the eustachian tubes that pass from the throat to the ear.

LOCAL ANTISEPTICS

Among the most commonly used home remedies are mouthwashes and gargles. The old National Formulary contained a preparation called *liquor antisepticus* which was an acid formula and *liquor antisepticus alkalinus* which was an alkaline formula. Such preparations are now available in proprietary products which have the advantage that they are carefully prepared, standardized, and distributed in acceptable packages.

More recently other antiseptic drugs have been discovered, some of them more efficient than those included in the older preparations. Thus the purchaser may have a choice, using the ones which have for him the most pleasant taste and the greatest acceptability.

Among the antiseptic substances recently developed are soaps with antiseptic ingredients, lotions which may contain alcohol that acts as an antiseptic, and all of the common antiseptics such as iodine, mercurochrome, hexylresorcinol, and many others. These efficient antiseptics have taken the place of the old boric acid compounds which were only mildly antiseptic.

For certain special conditions sulphur combinations are available. Our food-and-drug laws also permit the including of certain antibiotic drugs in antiseptic preparations that are applied to the skin for ringworm, burns, barber's itch, acne, impetigo, and other skin conditions.

The law does not permit purchase over the counter of antiseptic lotions to be put into the eye. There are good eyewashes that can help resolve congestion and redness but any more potent drugs are reserved for prescription by the doctor.

TONICS

At the turn of the century many tonic preparations were sold containing iron, quinine, caffeine, and other drugs. Caffeine is a stimulant drug which is found in coffee and which is also included in various headache and similar preparations to counteract drowsiness and fatigue. Iron continues to be a basic constituent of tonics because many people have secondary anemias. Outside of such preparations, the vitamins continue to be the most important tonic preparations. Among the vitamins, thiamine particularly has been shown by scientific study to have stimulating effects.

SEDATIVES AND TRANQUILIZERS

Among the great discoveries of recent years are the sedatives and the tranquilizers which differ from preparations of opium principally used for these purposes in a previous era. The newer drugs are seldom available without a doctor's prescription. However, some preparations of bromides are still available and also derivatives of scopolamine, the dosage being definitely limited to less than toxic doses. Some of these drugs act by producing forgetfulness which may well be an aid to sleep.

MOTION SICKNESS

For seasickness and airsickness, or carsickness, which are forms of motion sickness, new drugs have been introduced which are permitted to be administered by stewardesses on airplanes and which in most countries can be bought without a prescription.

Some of these products have recently been said to be capable of harm in pregnant women who also occasionally suffer from morning sickness or nausea as described in the chapter on that subject. Hence such drugs should not be taken by any pregnant woman unless they have been specifically prescribed by the doctor.

REMEDIES SOLD OVER THE COUNTER

Among the classifications of drugs sold over the counter are, as already mentioned, the vitamins which come in a variety of mixtures designed for adults or for children and containing in some instances additional mineral salts, protein substances, and enzymes. These may be purchased without a physician's prescription but people would do well to ask the doctor if the particular formula chosen is suitable to the patient's condition.

The cough and cold products include tablets, capsules, drops to be put in the nose, liquid preparations, materials to rub on the chest, formulas for coughs, lozenges, mists to be sprayed into the nose and throat, and gargles. For mild conditions these will usually be helpful. If a sore throat is not promptly relieved, study should be made by a doctor. If a cough persists more than a few days, a special examination is needed, as already mentioned. Lozenges have a soothing quality and some of them are slightly anesthetic. In general, they do not kill bacteria. A cough or sore throat can be serious because of the possibility of complications.

The rubs to be put on the chest sometimes contain enough salicylates to have a slightly beneficial effect. They do draw blood to the surface and produce a sense of warmth.

Nasal sprays are decongestant and antihistaminic. Overuse may be harmful.

The headache remedies are mostly based on aspirin with occasionally also phenacetin or modified acetanilid. The claims that they go to any special portion of the nervous system and exert a specific effect are not well substantiated. In general aspirin standardized according to the United States Pharmacopoeia has the same effects whether taken buffered, in capsules, in liquid, or in tablets, although some tablets tend to harden when kept long on the shelves and are not easily absorbed. Other pain-relieving substances are sometimes incorporated, but if in sufficient quantity to be effective, may also be toxic.

Ointment, liniments, and other external medications may relieve burning or itching or inflammation, and occasionally are sufficiently antiseptic to destroy germs.

One should never attempt to treat a skin disturbance of the type of psoriasis without having an examination and prescription by a competent physician who understands diseases of the skin.

Preparations are also available for skins that are extra dry and for those that are extra oily. Similarly many ointments are available for the treatment of burns. In mild burns most of these are helpful. Any severe burn that covers any considerable portion of the body should be cared for preferably in a hospital.

Great numbers of preparations are available for pimples and blackheads but, as described in the article by Dr. Behrman in this book in the chapter on "Diseases of the Skin," proper care of these conditions involves more than just smearing on an ointment.

Preparations for the care of the feet may be sold over the counter directly to people without a physician's prescription. There are corn and callus removers including corn plasters which depend principally on salicylic acid which softens the tissue permitting the corn or callus to be removed. Foot powders will keep the skin dry and prevent spreading of infection and also relieve itching. Some contain specific substances that are antagonistic to ringworm. In severe and continued ringworm infestation, potent products are now available, such as griseofulvin, which can be taken internally and prevent further growth and spread of ringworm.

A considerable number of preparations are listed under the heading "feminine hygiene." These include not only sanitary napkins and tampons but also douche powders and disinfectants which help to keep the organs clean and prevent infection. However, medical science has advanced rapidly so that specific drugs are available for the treatment of infectious organisms. These may be antiseptic or bacteriocidal. Certain infestations by flagellated organisms are now controllable by drugs like metronidazole called Flagyl®. Most of the potent preparations can be prescribed only by a physician but people should realize that such important products are available. The treatment for infestation with the organisms called trichomonas used to require repeated antiseptic douching and sometimes even surgical care whereas nowadays most cases are relieved by use of the tablets of metronidazole.

A great variety of suntan preparations are now available, all of which are safe when used as directed. These contain substances which prevent the burning rays and tanning rays of the sun from acting on the skin.

Many deodorants may be purchased as creams, solutions, powders, sprays, and in other forms. Most of these depend for their effect on limiting the perspiration, being astringent, and also by destroying certain germs which are on the skin. Cleanliness is essential to getting a completely satisfactory result with any deodorant.

CHAPTER 5

Sex Hygiene

MORRIS FISHBEIN, M.D.

INTRODUCTION

Various aspects of sex hygiene affect our lives not only from the physical but also from the mental point of view. The chief contribution of the Freudian psychology has been the emphasis which it has placed on the extent to which the inhibitions of previous generations have operated to establish many neuroses and sexual disorders. Conditions which were formerly thought to be wholly physical in character may have a mental basis, and this mental basis is established by failure to develop proper relationships between the sexes. Much of the background of these disorders is established in childhood and in adolescence.

In previous editions of the *Modern Home Medical Adviser,* Dr. Thurman B. Rice, who died some years ago, discussed "Sex Hygiene." From his chapter I have repeated some of the most significant observations.

The propagation of life is directly dependent on the functioning of the fundamental instincts which bring men and women together in a family or the home. Sex is everywhere about us: in the clothes we wear, in the occupations we serve, and in the sports and games by which we seek relaxation. Short stories, novels, poetry, art, sculpture, music, and the drama constantly remind us of the fact that men and women are different and that they behave as they do largely because of this difference.

THE IDEALS AND PURPOSES OF SEX EDUCATION

Every child and every adult should understand, as well as he may or can, the various complicated functions by which the race reproduces itself and by which the family comes into existence and is held together as a unit.

Sexuality has been confused with sensuality. Sex is supposed to be selfish and seek only its own self-gratification when actually nothing is so unselfish as the love of a mate for a mate or a parent for a child. Sex has ruined many a man or woman, but it has also brought out the best that was in countless millions of others.

Our young people want a positive education. They will not take "don't" as a rule for conduct. When the minds of children–and adults–are loaded high with positive facts and principles based on the assumption that sex is natural, good, beautiful, and entirely proper when in its proper place, there will be little to be feared from the untruths and half truths which may otherwise be so disastrous. We much prefer to have our children turning toward the beauties of virtue rather than fleeing from the ugly face of sin. It is most unfortunate that virtue has so often been made to appear dull and prosaic while dangerous and immoral practices have been made most enticing.

The child should never be frightened when this subject is discussed. The normal child may be told that the benefits of a dental operation are immeasurable, but, just the same, the fact that "it will hurt" when he goes to the dentist outweighs, to him, every conceivable gain. The mother who associates sex with pain and danger is often laying the foundation for an unsatisfactory or even destructive attitude toward life.

Sex throbs with high passion; it lives, and loves, and fights. It is a giant who constructs or destroys, makes or breaks, according to whether it is understood or not. Pink pamphlets for pale people will hardly serve the needs of the robust men and women who make the world go around. As well say "naughty, naughty" to a hurricane as to prescribe certain anemic books as a means of helping young people to control the powerful forces which surge within them. Most publications of this sort have been written by persons who have never known passion or who, having seared themselves in its flame, are now devoutly wishing "to save the young people from what I have gone through."

REPRODUCTION IN THE PLANT AND ANIMAL KINGDOMS

A fairly complete understanding of the reproduction in lower forms of life will give the parent or teacher poise and resourcefulness which will be greatly needed in teaching the subject and in developing a satisfactory philosophy of life.

Obviously each species has some adequate way of reproducing itself, otherwise it would long since have perished from the earth. The continuation of the species is the most fundamental instinct of every plant and every animal species. Most plants begin to die as soon as the seeds are well along toward maturity. All animals except man are ready to die as soon as the end of the reproductive cycle has been reached. Although the self-preservative instinct is supposed to be strongest in man and beast, everyone must have seen men and women risking life, reputation, health, social standing, wealth—everything—in order that they might express themselves sexually or take care of their offspring.

The species may be reproduced by sexual and asexual methods. Animals, except in the very lowest forms, use the sexual method. The same is true of most plants, but there are a considerable number of them which have dispensed with sex as a means of procreation. The bacteria, for example, merely divide in the middle, making two new individuals which are exactly alike and like the parent cell. In a sense the different individuals in a bacterial culture are really different fragments of the original parent germ. Even high in the plant kingdom we see essentially the same thing. A twig from a willow tree becomes itself a willow tree. It is like the parent tree for the good reason that it is a detached part of the parent tree. A number of cultivated species of plants are propagated by tubers, roots, bulbs, cuttings, and grafts, which are all asexual means, though these plants have sexual organs as well. Seed *potatoes* represent a use of the asexual method, while potato *seeds* (occasionally found in small pods where the flowers have been) are of sexual origin. Several of the very low forms of animal life can reproduce themselves merely by dividing or being divided.

Though some forms of life may use the asexual method of reproduction, it is now believed that all have some sort of sex, rudimentary though it may be. Bacteria, until recently, have been considered as being exceptions to this general rule, but many authorities believe that even they manifest an extremely primitive activity which is to be regarded as being essentially sexual. Inasmuch as Nature has used this particular plan in the life of every one of her products, the conclusion is inevitable that there must be some most excellent reason for the phenomenon. Let us suppose that every individual of a given species were free to reproduce himself by asexual means for an unlimited number of generations. A given strain might come rather soon to be quite different from the original species. In this way there would arise an enormous number of varieties, and a condition approaching chaos would result. This is, indeed, exemplified by the fact that those plants which are reproduced by bulbs, cuttings, and tubers commonly have a great number of varieties: roses, dahlias, gladioli, etc. Nature seems, however, to hold the majority of species more constant. Each time the act of reproduction is repeated it is necessary that a given individual fuse his heredity with that of another individual of the same species. In this way each separate drop of living matter is merged with the great ocean of related living matter, and wide deviations from the type species are rendered much less likely to occur.

Sex is fundamental to the continuation of all higher forms of life. Sexual reproduction is the masterpiece of Nature. Into this process she has poured her sweetest perfumes: the flower, for example, is the sex organ of the plant. About it she has drawn her most beautiful patterns. Into it she has dumped her paint pots, as witness the colors of the mating bird, the butterfly, and the flower. On the human level, music and poetry are called upon to adorn it. Sex is motivated by the most precious of all passions, conjugal and parental love. Young girls are as enticing as it is possible to be; young men are handsome and valiant. The young of most species are charming–or, if not that, are at least interesting. Everyone loves the puppy, the colt, the kitten, and most of all, the baby. Who can be so blind as to fail to see in this thing the very essence of life itself?

The insect, in visiting one flower after another, carries the pollen of one plant to the pistil of another. The pollen grains sprout and grow down the entire length of the pistil and carry the tiny cells which unite with the egg cells to form the seeds which are essentially new individuals. The growth of the seeds in the pod–the body of the mother plant–may be easily followed. Essentially the process is the same as is observed in the higher animals, except that the points that are hardest to get across to children are much more simply explained. Most important is the fact that the part of the process which corresponds to the mating of the sexes is the apparently trivial visit of the bee which carries the male element to the female organ of the next flower. In teaching children it is usually this point that puzzles and deters most parents.

Other plants may be used somewhat similarly. The flowers of the members of the melon family–muskmelons, pumpkins, cucumbers–are not all alike. Some have only the female organs, while others have only the male. In this respect they are more like the higher animals. In the case of strawberries and certain fruit trees there are some barren plants which are male. These plants never have fruit, but if they are all pulled out the other plants will be worthless as well.

The fish furnish an excellent example for teaching purposes. The females lay their unfertilized eggs over a clean spot on the bottom of the lake or stream. The male then comes to the nest and pours over the eggs a secretion known as "milt," which consists of millions of the sperm cells. When one of these sperm cells unites with an egg cell a new individual life begins. The young are compelled to get along as best they can after they are hatched, and, as a matter of fact, great numbers of them perish. In consequence, it is necessary that thousands or even millions of eggs be laid. By paddling slowly in a boat about the edge of a lake during the spawning season, the nests of sunfish may easily be found as clean round spots on the gravelly or sandy bottom, over which the parent usually hovers. The parent fish keeps the area clean and will chase away enemies which may come to destroy the eggs.

The mother frog's eggs are put out in a gelatinous material that protects them. Then, too, they are black above and light below, making them harder to see. The dark color absorbs the heat of the sun and hastens the hatching process. The male fertilizes the eggs at about the time they leave the female's body. When the young tadpoles are finally hatched they are usually compelled to get along as best they may and many of them serve as juicy tidbits for birds, fish, and other animals.

The turtle eggs are fertilized before they are laid and are held in the body of the female until a considerable quantity of food has been stored up in them and a firm shell is built about the food and the living portion of the egg. The eggs are then laid in and covered with the sand near the water's edge. There the heat of the sun stimulates growth. They will not be hatched until they are in a rather advanced state of development as compared with the young of the fish and the frog. Far fewer eggs are laid, for the good reason that the few that are laid are better equipped for survival.

The parent birds mate and build a home—a most interesting home, indeed, as may be found by the simple expedient of sitting quietly and watching. The egg is retained in the mother's body until it is large and loaded with food for the young bird. It is then laid in the carefully prepared and concealed nest, where it is faithfully guarded for days by the mother, who hatches it with the heat of her own body. In the meantime, the father bird has protected the nest by driving away enemies, or has attracted attention and danger away from the nest and to himself by flashing his bright colors and brilliant song from a tree safely remote from the nest. When the young are hatched, the parents bring food, the mother keeps the nest clean and picks lice and other vermin off the young. She hovers over them when they are cold or when it is storming; she powders them with dust from the road, thereby discouraging insect pests; she never rests in her untiring efforts to feed and protect them; she teaches them to fly and to find food for themselves.

Higher in the scale the mammal takes even better and longer care of the young. The egg is developed as in the case of the other animals mentioned, but is never entrusted to the dangers of the outside environment—being far too precious—and so the young develop in the body of the mother. When the time comes that they must be delivered, Nature has provided for them a food which is taken from the mother's body and is the perfect food for the growing baby animal. The protective instincts of the mother are easily observed. Here is an example of parental love which is easily recognized even by a young child. The function of the father is often much less inspiring, inasmuch as the male of the most easily studied mammals is generally apparently little interested in his offspring.

The human being is an animal, and as such has many of the ways of an animal. Even a child must learn early that the human being is much more than a mere animal, however, and should conduct himself or herself accordingly. Human children must be given tender care over a long period of time. In this way the child can be made to see the reason for the family as we have it. In this way he comes to appreciate the role of the father and the mother, who have built about him a home that is stable, safe and the core of his existence. The child sees his father working, bringing home food, paying for coal, furnishing a house in which to live, protecting him from injury, giving elemental care, playing and romping with him, planning with him, helping him, and advising him in ways that help tremendously. Every boy and girl should believe that his or her father is far above the level of the father of a puppy. The child sees—or should see—the father and mother exchanging embraces and words of affection. He realizes that sacrifices are being made, and so he comes to thinking that anything that his father does must be quite all right—and as a matter of fact the father's position in the family will be much easier taught when everything that the father does is appreciated.

The male of most of the lower species has little to do that is exemplary in terms of human conduct. Unfortunately, for one reason or another, a considerable number of human fathers also do little that is exemplary by the same standards, and so their purpose is rather hard to explain to the innocent child.

The function of the mother is much more obvious and needs no particular elaboration. The actual deliverance of the child from the body of the mother is usually a considerable ordeal. Children often cannot understand why such a process is necessary. For that matter, it is hard to make adults understand why the bearing of children should be so difficult. A great deal has been done by the medical and nursing professions to relieve that difficulty and danger.

Why must childbirth in the human be so much more difficult and dangerous than in the lower animals? In the first place, there is the erect posture, which has done so much to change the configuration of the pelvis in many women, and particularly in those who may have suffered as children from the disease known as rickets. This disease allows the abnormally soft bones to be excessively distorted by the weight of the body, and, in consequence, the birth canal is made too narrow. Secondly, the nervous development of the human mother makes her much more susceptible to pain than are the lower animals. In the third place, the human child is so precious that Nature strives to hold it as long as possible in the place where it is safest. The newly born human infant is exceedingly helpless even then, and would be dangerously so if it were born any sooner. For this reason the mother must carry the child a relatively long time. Finally, the development of the head, which is made necessary by the large size of the brain, enormously complicates the act of delivery. But that marvelous brain is the one really great characteristic of man, and we must not find fault with that which makes us great among the creatures of Nature.

THE ANATOMY AND PHYSIOLOGY OF THE REPRODUCTIVE SYSTEM

The generative system in either of the two sexes consists of two portions: (1) The sex glands themselves (ovaries in the female, testicles in the male). (2) A system of tubes which carry the sex cells, and later in the female, protect and nourish the developing child.

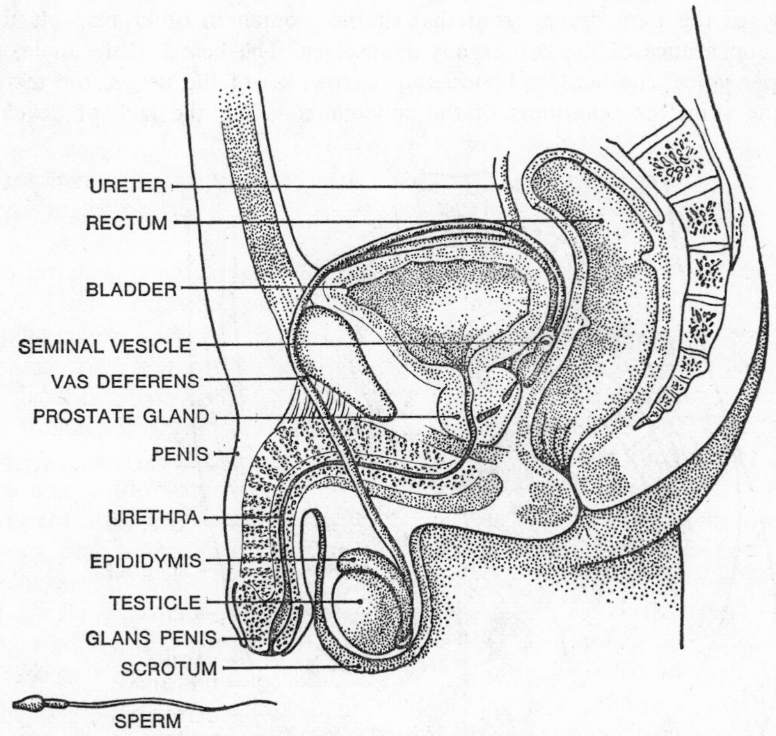

Fig. 10. The male sex organs. At left a greatly enlarged diagram of a sperm cell. Illustration by Lou Barlow.

The sex glands of the male, the testicles, consist of a great number of microscopic tubules which are lined with cells which are constantly undergoing cell division after the individual has attained sexual maturity. These cells become the spermatozoa or sperm cells, which are tiny little living bodies with long slender tails which whip about and in this way propel the sperm in its search for the egg cell. These sperm cells carry the entire inheritance which a given child will or can get from his father. The spermatozoa may live for several days in the tubes of the male, or may even live for a day or two after they have gained access to the female organs. They begin to be produced when the boy reaches puberty (about fourteen years of age), and continue to be formed until senility has been reached. During the period of sexual maturity they are commonly produced at the rate of millions per day.

Another function of the testicles results from certain cells which are called the *interstitial* cells. They secrete a substance which is absorbed by the blood and is responsible for the development of the secondary sex characteristics of the male. Everyone is familiar with the fact that the body of the man differs from that of the woman in other respects than the appearance of the sex organs themselves. The beard of the male, the deeper voice, the heavier bones, the narrowness of the pelvis, the texture of the skin, the scantiness of the subcutaneous fat, the lack of develop-

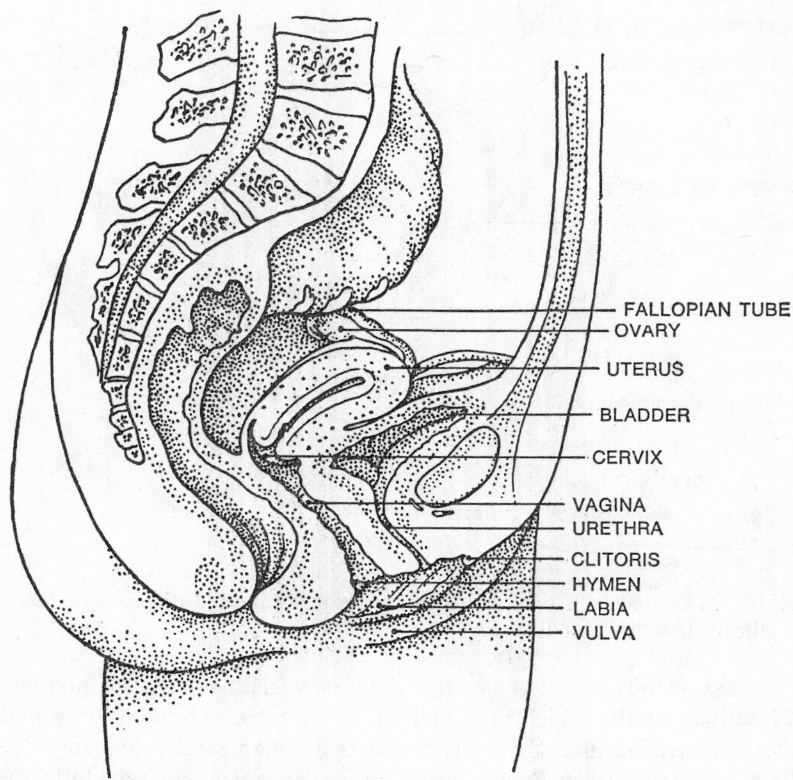

Fig. 11. Female sex organs. Illustration by Lou Barlow.

ment of the breasts are all the results of this secretion. Because of the loss of this substance the castrated male (known as a eunuch) loses the characteristics of a manly man.

The *ovaries* of the female serve a purpose in the female comparable to that of the testicles in the male. The egg cells are already well formed in the ovary at the time of birth, or shortly afterwards. They need to be matured, and stocked with a small supply of food, and then are ready to be extruded from the ovary. At the age of *puberty* (age twelve to thirteen years) the girl begins to produce mature egg cells at the rate of one (occasionally more) per menstrual month (usually twenty-eight days). This is continued until the *menopause* (change of life) is reached. This means that, on the average, less than five hundred egg cells are actually released in a lifetime.

The ovary contains *interstitial* cells which produce a secretion that is responsible for the secondary sex characteristics of the female. The soft skin, the abundant subcutaneous fat, the development of the breasts, the higher pitched voice, the wider pelvis, and a great many other typically feminine attributes are too familiar to need enumeration. Women, because of loss or atrophy of the ovaries, or because of some other glandular disturbance, occasionally lose much of their femininity and may develop a beard or coarse, man-like features.

The *testicles* and the *ovaries* are the essential organs of reproduction. Indeed, many of the simpler animals and plants have hardly any other organs of reproduction than just these. Even in somewhat higher animals, as the fish and the frogs, the eggs are simply turned out into the water, and the spermatic fluid is spread over them there. The accessory organs of reproduction in such a case are exceedingly simple, and sex, as we commonly think of it, can hardly be recognized by examination of the exterior of the body. The episode *coitus* which is considered by the thoughtless person to be the whole of the process becomes a trivial part of the program—merely the spreading of the milt of the male over the eggs laid by the female. In the higher forms of life more and more care is given the fertilized egg. The reptiles and the birds lay large eggs containing abundance of food so that the young may attain considerable size and development before they need to begin to fend for themselves. The mammals give their young even better care, and for weeks and months the female carries the young in her own body, and then, after releasing them, suckles them for another rather long period. Obviously such an arrangement has necessitated an enormous increase in the complexity of the system. The entire body of the female is modified to take care of the fertilized egg, to expel the developed fetus and to nourish the young after it has been born. The body of the male is likewise modified so that it may be able to impregnate the female and protect her and the young during the critical months before and after the birth of the young. Sex as we commonly think of it is highly developed in these animals.

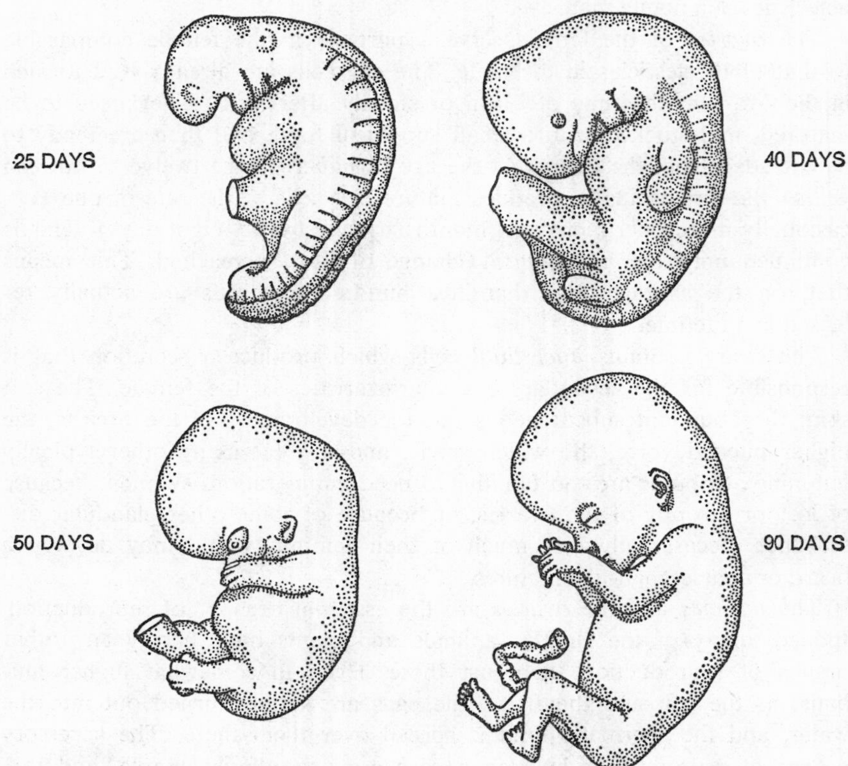

Fig. 12. Fetus in position in mother's body (25 days, 40 days, 50 days, 90 days). Illustration by Lou Barlow.

The human infant has an unusually long period of gestation, infancy, and dependency. This long period of comparative helplessness allows the child to develop countless possibilities which would have been quite out of the question had he been compelled to look after himself from the first. The child needs a highly stable and secure home until he or she is grown, and even longer if the highest interests of the family and race are to be realized.

Anything that tends to hold the father and mother together in a tight union until after the child is born and reared is of tremendous advantage to the individual and the race. This is, then, also a function of the reproductive organs. Fortunate indeed is the child whose parents have learned such functions of the reproductive system that they may derive exquisite pleasure and enjoyment therefrom. That child is safe because he will have behind him a father and mother who love each other and are devoted to him. Such a child will usually go much farther than the one from a broken or loveless home.

The accessory sex organs of the male consist of the scrotum, a baglike sac or pouch, containing the two testicles which produce the spermatozoa or male sex cells; a long tortuous tube from each of the testicles to the corresponding *seminal vesicles* or reservoirs, where the spermatic fluid and the sperm cells are stored until such time as there may be opportunity for extrusion (ejaculation); the *prostate gland,* which secretes a mucus-like fluid which carries the seminal secretion and makes a medium which will permit the spermatozoa to live and reach their objective; and the *penis,* which is an erectile tube capable of depositing the mixture of spermatic and prostatic secretion into the vault of the *vagina* near the mouth of the *womb.*

The accessory organs of the female are necessarily much more complicated for the reason that they must not only protect the egg cells but must provide a home for the developing child for nine long and eventful months. Essentially they consist of two tubes (*Fallopian tubes* or *oviducts*) which are open at the upper end and receive the egg cells when they are extruded from the ovaries. These tubes open into the *womb,* which is a thick-walled, muscular, hollow organ capable of enormous expansion. The womb in turn empties into the *vagina,* which is for the purpose of receiving the seminal secretion, and later of serving as a passageway for the child at the time of birth. The external female organs are called collectively the *vulva.* The breasts nourish the newly born child until it is old enough to eat other food.

The egg cell, after being released by the ovary, passes into the *Fallopian tube,* where it may or may not be fertilized by coming into contact with sperm cells. In case it does not make such a contact it lies there for a few days and then passes down into the womb and finally to the exterior. If it is fertilized it begins at once to divide rapidly and grows apace, utilizing the food that is stored in the egg cell and probably also some food absorbed from the surrounding tissues. It now migrates down into the womb and attaches itself to the inner wall of the womb (*uterus*) much as would a parasite. After a time a *placenta* is formed. This organ is the point of contact between the mother and the child. The bloods of the two individuals remain separate, both the mother and child having a set of closed vessels in the placenta, but fluids and gases can freely pass from the one to the other through the vessel walls by the process of *osmosis.* The mother furnishes food, water, oxygen, and other requirements; the child gives off waste materials of various sorts to the mother. No nerves pass from the one to the other. Various membranes for the protection of the child are also produced. These membranes and the placenta are delivered after the child is born and are collectively known as the "afterbirth." At the time of birth the walls of the womb contract strongly and expel the child and after a time the "afterbirth."

The life of a new individual begins when the living egg cell of the mother is fertilized by the living sperm cell of the father. Really, then, the human child is approximately nine months old when it is born, and more has happened in the development of the individual during that nine months than will take place in the next nine years. There are many who suppose that life begins in the child at about the time that the mother may feel the movements of the child in the womb. Indeed, it is customary to refer to these movements as the "beginning of life." This phenomenon is usually observed at about the middle of the pregnancy. Actually, however, the child is alive from the time of the union of the egg and the sperm, and as a definitive human being has certain recognized human rights.

DETERMINATION OF SEX

As soon as it is known that a baby is expected, parents are usually greatly interested in the speculation as to whether it is a boy or a girl. There is good reason to believe that the sex of the child is unalterably determined at the time of fertilization. To date there is no reliable means of controlling the sex of the offspring, and there is no accurate way of knowing until the child is born whether it is male or female, though the physician may make shrewd guesses which will be correct in a high percentage of cases. According to the most widely accepted theory of sex determination, each cell in the body of the female contains two determiners for sex (*chromosomes*), while each cell in the body of the male has but one such determiner. When the egg cells are produced, each cell contains one of these determiners; when the sperm cells are made, half of them have one sex determiner and the other half have none. If, then, the sperm with one sex chromosome meets an egg cell which always contains one, the fertilized egg cell will have two and is therefore female. If the sperm cell has no sex chromosome, then the fertilized egg cell will have but one—the one from the egg cell—and the sex is then male. If this theory is correct, and there is little doubt about its being correct, it would seem that the control of the sex of the unborn child by any practical means is probably quite outside the range of possibility. Many attempts to control sex have been tried, but none has as yet succeeded.

Even though the sex of the child is determined from the very first, it will be weeks before the differentiation of the organs is such that the sex might be recognized, even if the child could be examined closely. By such careful examination it is possible during the third month of fetal life to determine whether or not the child would have been male or female if it had lived. Previous to this time, the sex organs appear exactly alike, and, even in adult life, it is possible to find in each sex the exact homologue of the organs of the opposite sex. In the early months of fetal life the one or the other set of characteristics begins to be accentuated, and the opposing organs begin to atrophy.

In case a developmental error is made on the part of Nature it may be rather difficult to say without careful examination—an examination which sometimes requires an abdominal operation—whether the full-grown individual is male or female. These unfortunate persons are called *"hermaphrodites."* Usually they are decidedly more like the one sex or the other, though there are some who present considerable difficulty in diagnosis. These individuals are rarely if ever fertile, either as males or females, and never are they actually able to function as both father and mother at the same or different times.

There are three proper functions of the reproductive system in the human species: 1. The production of and the bringing together of the sex cells. 2. The production and the protection of the child, whether it be before, during, or after birth. 3. A means whereby a man and wife may express affection for each other, and on that solid foundation build a home which is, in turn, the foundation of society. All of these functions are absolutely legitimate, proper, and respectable when exercised according to the laws, customs, and ethics of the time and domain.

THE TEACHING OF SEX TO THE YOUNG CHILD

Within the first few days of life the genital organs of the baby should be carefully examined for evidence of defects or abnormalities. In case such defects are found they should be corrected when possible, as such peculiarities are often responsible for irritations or abnormal stimulations which may greatly complicate the sexual life of the child when he or she is older. The tissues of the infant are still highly plastic, and it frequently happens that corrections made early are surprisingly successful for this reason.

The boy baby should be carefully examined to see if he needs circumcision. If the foreskin can be completely and easily retracted most authorities think that circumcision should not be done, but when there is the least doubt about the matter, decision should be made in favor of the operation, which is a trivial one when done within the first week or two of life. When the foreskin is tight or adherent there will accumulate under it secretions which will produce bad odors and cause pain and itching.

Boys should also be examined after six years of age to determine whether or not the testicles have descended into the scrotum. These essential organs of sex are developed in the abdominal cavity, but at the time of birth or rather soon thereafter they should have descended. If they can be felt in the scrotum or can be gently pressed down into the scrotum there is no need for apprehension. If they cannot be found, attention should be given to the matter—without causing too much curiosity on the part of the child—and the advice of a physician obtained. If descent does not take place, an operation to transplant the testicle into the scrotum should be performed before the boy reaches puberty. Undescended testicles commonly atrophy, and if both are in this condition, sterility may result. The proper development of the testicle is important also from the standpoint of the proper secondary sex characteristics.

The girl baby also should be carefully examined for abnormalities. In the washing of the female infant, care must be taken. Sometimes the hymen may be ruptured by rough handling. While it is true that the presence of an intact hymen is by no means proof of virginity, or the absence of it proof of sexual experience, a large percentage of people still believe that such is the case, and so care must be taken to prevent an accident which might later put the baby, grown to womanhood, in an embarrassing position. Washing of the parts should be done in such a way that the friction will not cause erotic stimulation and in this way lead the child to the habit of playing with herself.

Crying babies, male and female, will nearly invariably hush when the genital organs are manipulated. This old, old trick of careless nurses and ignorant mothers, should never be practiced, as it may lead to masturbation. Masturbation is probably far less harmful than has been supposed. The routine care of a child should never be delegated to someone else when it is physically possible for the mother to see to it herself.

During the period when the child is too young to be given definite instruction, much can be done to lay the foundation for sound health and useful habits. The child who learns cleanliness and regularity of body function will be much more likely to respect the purposes of the reproductive system when grown than will a person who as a child was permitted to abuse or neglect the various bodily functions. The strictly normal individual is less likely to develop improper habits or perversions than the one who suffers from various biases or abnormalities. Childhood is the time for health training, and health is the sound base upon which rest normal reactions with regard to sex.

Much of the difficulty in teaching and training children in these matters concerning sex is due to the mistaken idea that children do not manifest interest in such subjects until they are several years old. Sex is far too fundamental to lie dormant for so long a time. The excretory organs are inseparably related to it, and indeed, it has its effect upon the entire body. Regularity in sleep, in eating, and in going to the toilet; pleasant manners and polite speech; love of beauty, truth, and decency; play in the open air; development of a natural attitude toward other children; modesty and respect for one's self are developed in large measure—if they are well developed at all—before the child is four years old. Every one of these traits is of the greatest value in the development of an acceptable sex life.

Great care will be needed in teaching the child that the social conventions are necessary without instilling in him or her the idea that the sexual organs are inherently ugly, unclean, or sinful. The nude baby is proudly exhibited to admiring relatives and friends, the nude child of four is to be seen by the family only, and the boy or girl of eight is expected to be careful about such matters even in the bosom of the family. A fine sense of modesty is of the utmost consequence in the social training of the child. When medical examinations must be made, what has been called modesty is really prudery. The development of poise in these fine qualities is of the utmost consequence. It can be taught only when the child has been led to regard the sexual apparatus with respect rather than shame. The child is made to understand that there are some things that are sacred and for that reason not to be cast before swine; there are some things so fine that they must not be permitted to become common. The child is shown that grown-ups, men and women, cover themselves, and that if he or she would be like them he or she must do so as well.

Many of the difficulties attendant to the teaching of sex are immediately solved when the child is taught the proper, the dignified names for the parts of the body. Hardly better are the baby names and the meaningless terms which are often given them in the vain attempt on the part of the mother to save the child from what she supposes to be vulgarity. The child must acquire a dignified vocabulary if he is to keep the subject clean. Why should it be more embarrassing to the mother to have the child come to her saying that he wishes to go to the toilet than to have him use some of the other expressions which are equally evident in their meaning under the circumstances.

During this impressionable period of life the attitude of the father and mother toward each other will have a profound effect on the character and sexual behavior of the child in later life. The child who sees his father treat his mother with chivalry and respect is much more likely to treat girls and women in the same way. The little girl who sees in her own mother a beautiful character is unconsciously receiving an education in these matters which is infinitely more effective than all the carefully planned precepts which might be memorized from books or articles on sex education.

What shall the mother or the father tell the child when he asks the highly pertinent and searching questions which have perplexed parents for so long? There is but one thing to tell him. It is the *truth*. By this I do not mean that it is necessary to tell a child of four the *entire* truth, or that it is necessary to give him the *detailed* truth. As a matter of fact, that would be impossible for the good reason that not even the wisest man knows the entire or the detailed truth about these matters. When the child asks a question he does not expect the scientifically complete answer, but in later life he will greatly appreciate the fact that he was told the truth in so far as he was able to understand it at the time.

When the child notices the difference between his or her body and that of the opposite sex, explain that there are two sorts of people, and two sorts of everything else that is alive. That is so that each little child and each little baby animal may have a father and a mother to care for him and make a home for him. Birds of certain kinds are different in color and appearance, and there are differences in function which correspond to this difference in appearance. He will have observed that fathers and mothers have different purposes in life, and there are marked differences in dress, in habit, and occupation. The whole process is perfectly natural, and when naturally told to a normal child will give rise to no morbid curiosity whatsoever.

Where did the baby come from? This is a question that every child should have asked by the time he is four or five years old or even sooner if he is interested. What a pity that mothers have seen fit to tell children that babies—they themselves, indeed—are found in garbage pails, in the straw pile back of the barn, under the leaves in the woods, in a hollow log, in the doctor's satchel, and in other monstrous places. Hardly better is the "made in Germany" story of the stork, except that it is somewhat more dignified. The children of Germany love and respect the stork, but the small children of this country know nothing of such a creature.

The question that is most dreaded is, "How did the baby get in the mother's body?" When the father and the mother have loved each other as they should and are legally married, the act that is the expression of that love and the act that enables them to bear beautiful children is not vulgar. The child—bear in mind that this is a young child—can be told that as a result of the love which the parents bear for each other and for the child the baby began to grow in the body of the mother. An older child will need more information, but this is as essentially the truth as the most tediously accurate and scientific account of the union of egg cells and sperms, such as he or she will need at a later stage of development.

The difficulty of explaining the role of the father will fade into nothing at all if the child believes that his father is a great hero who can do no wrong. When the child has seen his father caressing his mother nothing could be more natural—as indeed nothing is more natural—than that they should desire and have children. Many fathers live and treat their families in such a way that the children may learn that their acts are commonly selfish. In the main small children believe that their fathers are great persons, indeed, and that whatever they do is just right. In such case nothing could be easier than proper instruction in these matters. The role of the mother is easily taught. As it is perfectly natural for the child to develop in the mother's body, it is perfectly natural that the child should accept the method as the ancient and honored way of life, and that is all there is to it.

After the child is old enough to understand the simple anatomy of the two sexes, it may be explained that the sperm cells of the male are introduced into the body of the mother and there combine with the egg cells somewhat as the pollen of the male plant fertilizes the female. It should then be explained that such transfer of the male to the female must take place only between married persons, else a child may be born when the parents cannot make a home for it. Even a little child can understand that illegitimacy is a pretty serious thing, in as much as every child needs *both* a father and a mother as he grows up. The process is one that is perfectly proper when the man and woman are married and much in love with each other, and is an act of the utmost intimacy and delicacy.

When the child asks the *details* of birth—as he or she rarely will—care must be taken that he or she is not frightened by morbid details. No small child can understand the forces which come into play in such an event. It is a serious mistake to worry him with the harrowing details. It is enough to know that when the time came, the mother worked hard and was very tired. After such an experience she will need to rest in bed for several days and must be shown every possible deference and affection. She is not *"sick"* in the usual meaning of the word, but is merely *resting* after a tremendously important and vital contribution to the beloved family.

The most important principle in the training of a child in these matters is that the native curiosity of the child should be satisfied. The child must learn that it can depend *absolutely* upon the father and mother as a source of honest and authentic information on this subject, just as he can go to the same source for food, for shelter, and for help of any sort. The child should never be repressed when asking honestly concerning such matters. Once the demand for the truth is filled, the child can then go about his or her normal activities without being bothered with things he or she is too young to understand thoroughly. Questions put by the child should be answered when possible, but they need not be provoked.

The imagination and resourcefulness of the parent will do better than any "canned" information. It is not necessary that every bit of the information be absolutely scientifically up-to-the-minute provided it is earnestly and truthfully set out as the best that the parent knows on the subject. The development of a sound philosophy of life and living is much more needed than are the latest scientific details.

Whatever is done or taught, the idealism of the child must be preserved. The role of the father as hero, provider, and protector; the part of the mother as one who will love and protect whatever may happen, cannot be too strongly emphasized. The child easily understands such teaching and responds eagerly to idealism of this sort.

THE SCHOOL CHILD

The school child is no longer under the eye of his parents. He will hear and learn of sex. The pertinent question is not "Will he learn?" but, rather, "Where and of whom will he learn?" Only a foolish parent would think that a boy or girl in school will remain ignorant of these matters. The child of this age is getting started to school and is beginning to feel that he knows something of life. Quite naturally he wants to understand things as they are. Fortunately he has not yet reached the age of puberty with its many perplexing problems and disturbing urges which will furnish an additional motive for sex interest.

Except that it will be necessary to give these children more information than was given the pre-school child, the problems are not greatly different from those that have just been discussed, for the good reason that the sexual system is still relatively undeveloped, and the child has only a passing interest in such matters. The teaching is still indirect and should consist of principles rather than details. Questions should be answered fully and frankly—in so far as the child is able to understand or is interested—but disturbing questions are not to be raised in the mind of the child.

This is the time when children are so tremendously interested in nature, and they will have observed most of the essential phenomena of sex before they have become involved in the complex social phenomena which so muddle the issue in the human race. The parent who understands the fundamentals of sex and life as they are manifested in plants and animals and has the language to transmit such information will have an enormous advantage in the teaching of his children.

Important during this period is the teaching of a sense of modesty without at the same time teaching shame. Parents all too often shame their children into a state of mind that is mistaken for modesty. Shame, except for some improper act, is an emotion that should never be utilized in teaching. There is nothing about the reproductive organs for which a child need be ashamed. He learns to cover himself because it is the custom to do so, and because the older persons whom he wishes to emulate do so. There is nothing wrong about the genitals, but rather they are so important that they must be protected. They are so intimately one's real self that one must not go about exposing in a cheap and common way that which is so essentially private.

Nearly all normal children have their little love affairs during the first years in school. Since one of the most important tasks in later life is the selection of a worthy mate, even children should be gaining a little proficiency in so vital a matter. Just as the kitten playing with a ball is really learning to catch mice, so these children are practicing the greatest of all arts. Parents or others should not tease children about their love affairs. Such teasing puts the idea into the head of the child that there is something inherently wrong about the whole matter and that he or she has done something that is improper. When, subsequently, a real affair is developing, it will be carefully concealed from the parents. In this way the parent loses his opportunity to be of service in teaching the child how he or she may select the best companions. Furthermore, the curiosity of the child teaches him to seek the evil which he has been led to believe is in the apparently harmless relation which he or she has with another of the opposite sex. With such stimulation he will all too soon find the evil. The truth insofar as he can understand it is far safer than some silly tale which seeks to give a superficial explanation of the facts of life.

Parents who tease their young children about their beaux and seek to deter them from making dangerous alliances should look about them and learn that the best way to insure against these play love affairs going too far is merely to let them run without resistance. Children are far too fickle as a rule to do more than toy with a passion which they are much too young really to understand. Soon it will be forgotten. The parent who attempts to break up such an affair is assuming a grave responsibility. He will be almost sure to intensify it. We naturally tend to protect our friends when they are attacked, and we invariably learn to love those whom we protect. Not only are the children being set into mischief when they are teased, but the parents are accomplishing exactly the opposite result from that which they desire when they indulge in so low a form of correction—or amusement.

The parent who allows his or her children to assume natural relations with other children of the same or opposite sex need rarely fear that mischief will be done. The child, being still undeveloped sexually, gives no thought to the grosser manifestations of the subject unless they are suggested to him by his elders. When the relation is perfectly natural and the parent has abstained from teasing, the child will be free to talk about the matter, and so the parent may keep himself informed concerning the course of events. In case, then, the child gets on dangerous ground, a frank discussion of the matter is possible and will not be resented if skillfully handled. The parent may be able to point out in a kindly manner the good and bad traits in the favored friends, and in this way may be of real service in the important matter of picking the permanent mate a few years later.

Boys and girls will frequently play "father and mother" or "doctor and patient" games. Thus they actually gain experience which may be of great benefit to them in later life. Not unusually children of this age express themselves as to what they will do when they are men or women. For the most part they will do well if they later come up to these expressed ideals. It is also common to hear children say what they will do when they have children of their own, or what their children will or will not do. The wise parent at such a time may well listen and note.

Much worry has been needlessly suffered by devoted parents who have failed to understand children of this age. Boys and girls are curious. They will naturally examine their bodies, or, if the opportunity presents itself, the body of another of the same or opposite sex. The misguided parent thinks that this is exactly the same as if an adult should do so and gets all excited about it. Frankly, we would be inclined to question the mentality of a child who has not done so. The best way to draw the teeth of such a possible menace is to allow the child to satisfy that sense of curiosity which impels him to try to find out how things are made, and, having found out, lets him go on to something else.

Frequently children will get into the habit of playing with or pulling at the genitals. Such children—both boys and girls—may be in need of a thorough examination by a competent physician. Not unlikely circumcision or other special corrective measure is needed. If there is no pathologic basis for the habit, the child should be taught that it is bad manners to behave in such a way and that an ugly habit may be formed. With help, rather than scolding, he may soon correct the ugly practice. Parents should remember that no one can break a bad habit except the person who has it, and that the task is one that sometimes requires patience and perseverance beyond that which a child may be expected to have. Little boys and girls are occasionally found to have developed the practice of masturbation. Normal children of this age will rarely go to excess unless they are being stimulated by some older person. If a child of this age masturbates frequently, a careful watch should be made, not so much of the child as of its older associates. The reason for this is evident, as the child is not often sufficiently developed for the habit to have arisen from within.

Children of this age should be interested in many things, and when they are, one need not worry about their being too much concerned about an instinct which is still far from being mature. All sorts of healthy activities are to be encouraged. Exercise in the open air is far more conducive to good results than excessive poring over books. Regular habits in matters pertaining to health will lay the best possible foundation for a normal sex life in later years. The child should grow in "wisdom and stature" during this time. He or she should develop the body as it was intended to be developed. School interests, play, club work of all sorts, scout exercises, athletic teams, and kindred activities permit little time for those forms of sex activity that might really be dangerous.

The question as to how much direct sex instruction should be given during this period is a rather knotty one. Sex during this period is probably less to the fore than at any time since babyhood, provided the curiosity of the preschool child has been properly satisfied. If the child knows in a general way about these matters, he will let it go at that until the problems of adolescence begin to assert themselves. Matters pertaining to sex in its simpler forms should be frankly discussed by the family in the presence of the child. Questions are answered, and basic principles underlying proper conduct are deeply implanted, and that is about all that is necessary. The subject is far less exciting in the open than when it is concealed.

Girls are being encouraged to be teachers, stenographers, concert pianists, prima donnas, lawyers, doctors, nurses. As a matter of fact, most of them—fortunately—will become housewives and mothers. Why cannot these objectives be held up also as ideals? Then, when they have a home of their own, they will find in the routine a purpose toward their ideal. In case, however, they have been taught that they are to have some glamorous career and then find themselves washing dishes for a family, they are nearly sure to despise their task. There are those who suppose that a career as a mother is a narrow experience as compared with that of typing letters for a concern that sells lumber or vacuum cleaners. Some suppose that a mother needs less education than a teacher who does nothing but teach a single subject in a high school. The mother must be a nurse, a physician, a teacher, a legal adviser, a cook, a dietitian, a financial genius, a diplomat, an authority on child psychology, and a hundred other things—at least, she should be. Why cannot this be made a career toward which girls can be pointed with pride?

Psychologists tell us that the child is half educated before he even starts to school. His mother has taught him—often badly—the mother tongue, his habits, his manners, his attitude toward life, his self-control, his reliability, his respect for truth and right, his religion, his patriotism—and yet the task of a mother is considered too lowly to serve as an ideal! A wife, who has the responsibility of five children, once lamented that she envied a woman of her age who had attained a degree of success in bacteriology. She should be reminded that the other woman grew bacteria in culture tubes, while she was growing men and women in a home. All of this is very important in sex education. The girl who has been brought up to regard her womanhood as a career, the boy who is thoroughly instilled with the principles and practice of manliness, will probably not make great mistakes in their sex lives.

The pre-adolescent age is a period which is immensely important in the orientation of the boy or girl. Orientation is possible at this time for the reason that the strong sex impulses have as yet not taken definite direction because of their relatively immature state of development. A little later they will be so strong that they may take the bit in the mouth and run away. Happy is the adolescent who has been set in such a direction that he or she can permit his or her sex to run away for the good reason that it is running in the direction of the greatest advantage.

THE PERIOD OF ADOLESCENCE

While many sex problems originate before the age of puberty and adolescence, the problems which arise at these times are much more urgent and difficult than those of the earlier years. This is the time when young people really need help and understanding. Powerful and utterly new forces are arising in them. Elated with the new sensation of being comparatively grown up, they may plunge from one extreme to another. They feel that they must do everything possible *to prove that they are grown up.* The boys learn to smoke and to swear great and supposedly manly oaths. They affect deep knowledge of women and girls and tell of their conquests. They rarely, if ever, drive a car slowly. Obviously they are overcompensating for their all too evident inexperience–whistling to prove that they are unafraid.

The girl usually passes through a "boy-struck" period. She giggles and makes herself conspicuous. Unless carefully controlled or endowed with unusual reserve, she is likely to go in for excessively high heels, extremes in dress, and large use of cosmetics. During this period of unrest she is sadly in need of intelligent and *sympathetic* guidance. Such guidance, however, is likely to be extremely distasteful to her. Parents who have neglected the matter of sex education until this time will find it difficult to pick up the reins of control and go serenely forward. Only those children who have been gradually led up to a realization of the forces at work within themselves will be in a position to appreciate the advice that wise parents can give. How may a mother who has told her daughter that babies slid down rainbows now hope to get control of the situation? Long before the time of adolescence the children have learned that their parents *are* sources of accurate information on the subject, or that they *are not* sources of accurate information. They may be expected to behave accordingly.

In continuation of sex education into the period of adolescence the parent or teacher must know that generalities are no longer sufficient. A concrete and detailed instruction in vital matters in which they may be concerned now becomes a necessity. The problems which the boys and girls are likely to meet should be discussed with them in a perfectly natural manner. The instruction should be so natural and so unassumed that the boy or girl is hardly conscious that he has been instructed. Young people of this age should be included in the family conversation about many matters related to the subject of sex. The value of a good example on the part of the parents cannot be overstressed.

Assuming that adolescent boys and girls have had their minds thoroughly satisfied concerning the positive and beautiful phases of the subject, they are then ready to have some of the negative phases mentioned. These young people should know about the possibilities of conception out of wedlock, and that under such circumstances the mother and child are sure to suffer severely from the social stigma which such a birth imposes. They should know something of venereal disease, which is perfectly capable of ruining them, their loved ones, and their careers. They should know of the depreciation of character which invariably follows the promiscuity which seems so enticing. Children of this age should be treated somewhat as men and women, though they are still boys and girls. Young people will appreciate the confidence that is shown when such matters are frankly discussed. They will really be grateful. Discussion between young and old should be as casual as possible. The parent must not be dictatorial and he or she must be able to speak without embarrassment.

In case the young people have not had proper instruction in matters pertaining to sex during their earlier years; if they do not have a dignified vocabulary of terms in which these matters may be discussed; if they see in sex only the possibility of sensuous gratification, it will be difficult indeed—or well-nigh impossible—to correct the omission.

Boys and girls of the age under discussion can become parents of children. The careful parent must explain to his children something of the details of the sexual act. Only those who are willfully blind will pretend that it is possible or desirable to keep young people of the age ignorant of so vital a function. The children should be made to understand that sexual relations are of the utmost consequence to the welfare of the individual, the family, and the race, but that they are only for those who are sufficiently mature to bear and rear children, and are married so that they can do so. Unless this can be done in a way that convinces the young people themselves, it had as well not be done at all. The sexual act must not be made an utterly pleasurable act divorced from all sense of responsibility.

Provided the biology teacher of the high school has an appreciation of the possibilities of his subject, at least one course in this subject should be taken in high school. In a biology class, fundamental matters of sex may be discussed in the most casual manner. When home influences and parental instruction then supplement scientific instruction, little concern need be entertained concerning the welfare of youths and girls who have normal poise and self-control.

Of much importance to the youth of this age is an appreciation of the fundamental reasons for the existence of a stable family life. While it is possible for persons to live in a satisfactory manner without wedlock, marriage is fundamentally necessary. In spite of the fact that many marriages fail, men and women are normally better satisfied and happier in that relation than out of it. Marriage should then be held before young people as a probable goal. All too frequently boys and girls break out into a scarlet rash as soon as marriage is mentioned. Giggling and protesting, they disclaim any such intentions. This behavior is a discredit not so much to these boys and girls as to their parents. It shows clearly they have not frankly discussed such subjects with their offspring.

The sanctity of marriage may well be taught and illustrated at any age of development, but should be increasingly emphasized as the child approaches the age when he or she may be expected to enter into such a contract. Many people cannot understand why marriage should be more than a mere civil contract. The reason is that children will probably result from such a union. Conventional marriage is the foundation on which is built the home, and the home is the basis of every one of the other social institutions—the school, the church, the government, industry, and social relations. A community of good homes invariably has good schools, influential churches, thrifty, industrious, intelligent, educated people, and an acceptable government. A community of bad homes is hopelessly in the mire. Happy marriages and healthy homes are not the products of accident. They are worked out by persons informed in matters pertaining to real human values.

The young people of today develop sexually earlier than they should and would, were it not for the omnipresent sex stimulation which they are constantly receiving. They see moving pictures and television of the most sophisticated sort; they pick up risqué books or hear such books discussed; they hear suggestive songs; they see all sorts of irregularities. At any early age they have been more or less intimately introduced to the urges and passions, but are generally not permitted to marry until they are well into their twenties.

Parents of earlier generations were not let out into society until they were sixteen or seventeen, and were solidly married, frequently, at the age of eighteen or nineteen. In the early months of the period of courtship, they were so awkward and uninformed they could hardly get into serious mischief. If we are going to bring children up to avoid the awkward stage, we are under obligation to help them take care of the passions which are aroused but may not be gratified. The awkwardness of the adolescent boy or girl is a protective device of no mean consequence. Those children who come through this adolescent period slowly and naturally will be better adjusted than those who are hurried through by socially ambitious parents, or who are turned loose on the streets.

For this reason athletics are important for boys and girls of this age. Many suppose that athletics are solely for the purpose of developing the physique. They are of much more consequence when they develop character. Strenuous athletics at this time in life may, and frequently do, actually injure the body when not properly controlled. Play and recreation, rather than highly competitive sports, are needed. The boy who plays tennis, basketball, baseball, or engages in any of the many other wholesome sports, is not in much danger of dreaming too much about the girls. He plays until he is tired enough when he goes to bed to go promptly to sleep.

Girls will usually be somewhat less interested in athletics, though there are many exceptions. The reaction of girls toward athletics is essentially like that of boys, but there are certain differences which should not be entirely forgotten. The pelvis of the girl is broader and more loosely jointed than that of the boy. This is a relation which is necessary, as the pelvis must be built in such a way as to sacrifice strength for the contingencies of future childbirth. Heavy or excessive muscular exercise, or the carrying of heavy weights can for this reason more seriously injure the girl than the boy. Nature insists that the demands of the reproductive system shall come first. For this reason the blood supply of the pregnant or nursing woman is commandeered for the reproductive organs and the breasts. Athletics for girls should be somewhat less strenuous and competitive. Girls do much better with the types of games that are mostly individual endeavor; boys need the highly cooperative games. In later life, men, as a rule, work with others, while a housewife for the most part does her work alone.

Every child of adolescent age should have a hobby. Collections of all sorts are made by interested young people: butterflies, beetles, plants, stamps, match-box covers, marbles, buttons, and a thousand and one other things. The exercises prescribed by the Scout Manual have been of incalculable value in keeping boys and girls in pursuits which permit them to come along without too much attention to the developing forces within them.

Don't call the child in from play to give him his weekly instruction in sex. Sex is life. The teaching must be casual and matter of fact. The best that the adolescent can do is to grow and develop naturally and normally.

Masturbation is likely to be developed during this period. The practice is of little consequence unless the boy or girl worries about it or is degraded by it. Masturbation causes none of the ailments of which it has been accused.

Boys are frequently alarmed by the occurrence of seminal emissions or discharges of prostatic and seminal secretions while asleep. Mothers finding the stained sheets are sometimes greatly disturbed. It means nothing except that the boy is developing properly and is probably not indulging in masturbation or sexual relations. Nature has provided the reproductive organs with a safety valve in the form of seminal emissions. They are perfectly normal, and are indeed an accurate indication of proper and safe development. In the same category are the voluptuous dreams which boys and occasionally girls may experience.

MENSTRUATION

Before she is twelve years old the girl should have menstruation explained to her. Otherwise she is likely to be frightened by it and may be ashamed to say anything about it if she is not accustomed to confide in her mother. Formerly careful mothers put their daughters to bed for a day or two at each menstrual period and stopped all activity and bathing during this time. The girl was taught that she was "sick" and that she might expect for the next thirty years to be an invalid once a month and then to pass through a "change of life." The absurdity of such a method is now recognized. Girls are told to pay no attention except to protect clothing from soilage. Menstruation is a normal process, but sometimes approaches the pathological. Bleeding, for example, is otherwise always associated with pathology of some grade, as also is pain. The uterus of the menstruating woman is congested, and there are changes in the distribution of the blood; the nervous system is often considerably more unstable at such a time, and there are other evidences of altered physiology. Moderate exercise is rarely harmful; exposure to fresh air at such a time will be of no consequence unless there is chilling; bathing in warm water will rarely have a bad effect. Certainly the girl should be taught that the menstrual function is essentially normal and that it should be treated as being such except when there is reason to believe that something is wrong.

LOVE AFFAIRS

Children frequently experience intense love affairs. The adolescent is, of course, considerably more inclined to such attacks of "puppy love." Some young people become so self-conscious in matters pertaining to sex that they go to the opposite extreme. Either reaction is easily understood and may be regarded as normal. Boys who are so delighted with their developing manhood are likely to become rather contemptuous of girls who have not their virile qualities. Girls who are becoming more careful of many little fine points of life are sometimes inclined to regard boys as being hopelessly uncouth. These reactions are also quite natural and do not presage a continuance of such feelings.

All of these manifestations are normal, and strictly the affair of the individual concerned. The boy or girl should be allowed to develop his or her own individuality provided he or she is not taking a route that leads to deviations from what is considered to be a normal reaction.

Adolescence is a period of much dreaming and idealization. Children at this period are frequently dubbed lazy because of their propensity for dreaming and also because nature is protecting their rapidly growing and developing bodies from injury that might be inflicted by too energetic parents wishing to capitalize on the apparent—but more apparent than real—strength. High ideals and religious motives are characteristic also of this period and may be utilized in helping to hold the young people to trends of action that may be considered safe.

THE MATING PERIOD

A time comes in the life of every normal boy and girl when he or she is vastly interested in members of the opposite sex. The urge to mate, first in a process of courting and later in a permanent marriage, becomes the dominant factor in the determination of conduct.

In the United States, particularly, the way of the lover is made easy. Young people may choose their own mates almost without help from their elders. Free choice is the inalienable right of every young person. No one is so unpopular as the stern parent who frowns on the dashing young daredevil who for the moment sends his daughter into a state of ecstasy. In many other countries the young people have little or nothing to say about the matter and must mate according to the wishes or convenience of the parents. This New World freedom imposes a need for responsibility upon the part of the young people themselves; young people must be taught the facts of life as they are related to this subject.

Young people should be taught before the mating period is too urgently upon them that it is important indeed to look their companions over pretty carefully before allowing themselves to get too deeply involved. This is what is meant by "falling in love intelligently." We commonly speak of "falling in love" as if it were a sheer accident against which there was no way of protecting one's self. It is said that "love is blind," but surely this is a time for having the eyes wide open.

How may we hope to teach young people to use more discretion in the vital matter of marriage selection? Who is a suitable mate, anyway? How may one know whether the particular person is going to wear well or not? Certainly the following points are extremely important:

1. The prospective mate should come from a family that is free of serious hereditary defects. The family should be one of intelligence, industry, thrift, and such social standing as will be compatible with the status of the person making the choice.

2. The health of the individual is important. The marrying of an invalid is a mistake that is rarely corrected. Physical attractiveness is of some importance, but exceptional beauty need not be required or particularly desired.

3. Similarity of interests and cultural background should by all means be considered. A vivacious wife and a phlegmatic husband are hardly likely to be happy. Likewise a boob, a boor, a clown, or a gigolo will be badly miscast among "in-laws" of the opposite type. Character, industry, thrift, honor, sobriety, and kindred qualities are by no means to be disregarded.

4. Education should be considered. By education we mean the ability to know what should be done in a given set of circumstances and when and how to do it. We have little respect for mere "book-learning" or diplomas in the present connection. Acceptable manners are a part of education, as are cooking, sewing, and the ability to earn funds and use them wisely.

5. It is well to know how the given individual treats the members of his or her family, and how he or she is regarded by the other members of his or her own and the opposite sex.

6. Each party should understand the attitude of the other toward children, toward sex, and toward sexual morality. When such matters are understood it would be very foolish to disregard such information in making the final decision to marry or not to marry.

7. Misgiving is sometimes expressed when the prospective husband is much larger than his mate. It is feared that she may have difficulty in giving birth to his children. This is much less serious than was formerly the case, for the good reason that obstetrical science is now far more proficient. Cesarean section offers a solution in case trouble should arise. In general, it is better for the couple to be near the same size, but a match need not be called off because of difference of this nature. The small wife of a large man should in all cases see her physician as soon as she finds herself pregnant. If the child appears to be growing too large for safe delivery the physician has several resources which he may use.

8. An accurate inventory of cash on hand, assets, liabilities, the ability to maintain or take care of a home, and a frank understanding of the financial status is essential. By this we do not mean that we would condemn marriage to a person who is financially poor, but we are merely insisting that the situation be understood and soberly considered.

9. It will be much better if the individual has long been known and if the courtship has been long enough and under diverse conditions enough that the wearing qualities have been tested reasonably well before the marriage is actually consummated.

10. In general it will be much better if both of the mates are of the same race and social level. In some instances differences in religion, and even in politics, may cause trouble.

11. Concerning the matter of love for the individual there must be no doubt. One must be willing to make any sacrifice for the loved one, and to prefer him or her above all others. Anything short of a mutual unselfish devotion will almost surely break down in the stress and strain of married life.

Few young people have the discretion soberly to count the debits and credits of the suitor after the love affair has developed, but children who have had such ideals held up to them from an early age will be somewhat less likely to err in so vital a matter when they are older. Young people who understand and appreciate something of the nature of the problems of married life will be much more likely to use judgment. It is too much to expect that children who have had no instruction in sex and character will listen to their elders when they are in the heat of a fervid love affair.

Strangely enough, most parents, when they try to exert an influence upon the choice of mates which their children are making, produce an effect which is just the opposite of that which was desired. An undesirable young man brings daughter home from a function of some sort. The next morning she is questioned, and there is a scene. She is frequently told that he is worthless, good-for-nothing, and altogether impossible. She defends him, of course; we come quickly to love those whom we defend. Nothing will so certainly drive a couple into matrimony as will the idea that the poor dear one is being mistreated and persecuted. An uncouth young man, or a silly girl, can much more easily and certainly be eliminated by inviting him or her into the home and allowing the daughter or son to see him or her in comparison with persons of known value and merit. Many an unhappy marriage has been contracted because the young people have revolted against what they considered an infringement of their sacred right to choose.

Naturally the parent feels that he has some rights in the matter—as indeed he should have, if he has sense to be worthy of the opportunity—and as indeed he does have, if he has made the most of his opportunities in the training of the child. Does not a parent have the right to have some say as to who shall be the other parent of his grandchildren, in whom he will be tremendously interested? Does he not have some rights in saying who shall share the property which he will leave to his child? Does he not have the right to protect his child from what he believes is a disastrous marriage? The answer is that he does have some rights, but that he will have to use all the diplomacy and tact in his possession to get those rights. This is no place for the bungling despot of the home to "lay down the law" or "set his foot down." This is the prerogative of him who has spent two decades or more in preparing a son or daughter for the most important decision that he or she will ever make.

The superior experience of parents *should* make them capable of real aid to the young people. In many cases the judgment of the young may be better. The mother who insists that her son or daughter shall consider social standing above everything else, and the father who demands a fat bank roll, think that they are looking after the welfare of son or daughter, but are really setting up obstacles which will be cleared with difficulty if at all. Loveless, sordid marriages made with an eye on the bank book will rarely be made by the young people themselves. Young people are rather prone to the "love-at-first-sight" sort of infatuation which may lead them into hasty, ill-considered marriages which rarely turn out well.

A difficult matter in modern courtship is that concerning the payment of expenses. Formerly it was possible for a couple to spend evening after evening in the most delightful companionship without the expenditure of a cent. There were no shows to attend, no gasoline to buy, no sodas, no expensive presents, no boxes of candy, no flowers. Now expense is of considerable consequence. As likely as not the girl is earning as much or nearly as much as the man, but the old relic of chivalry demands that the man shall pay the bill and that he shall be ever so generous. Many girls are slipping a coin—or a bill—to the boy-friend sometimes, or are asking him not to spend more than is absolutely necessary, but there are others of the "give-me" type who are bleeding their consorts to the limit and are looking for boys with fat allowances and beautiful cars.

Unfortunately expenses must be considered. Sometimes girls have been led to believe that they are under obligation to repay in ways that are destructive to morals and character. So long as the girl was entertaining in her own home, and furnishing lemonade or home-made fudge, she might bid her suitor begone when he made improper proposals; when, however, she has accepted a theater ticket, a soda, and an automobile ride and finds herself miles away from home in her friend's car, the situation is considerably more complicated. An inexperienced girl who wishes to continue the theater parties, sodas, and rides will sometimes solve the problem in the wrong way. There is also a strong temptation for a sexually aggressive young man to take advantage of the situation. He reasons that he should have something in compensation for the outlay he has made. Being uninstructed in sex ideals, as are most boys, the form of the compensation desired is easily guessed.

Organizations in the large cities give parties and entertainments which throw young people together with the express purpose of making it possible for courtship to progress as naturally as possible. Coeducational colleges serve a most useful purpose in this connection. Various church organizations and societies serve the same end. Rooming houses and girls' dormitories usually have some sort of parlor where a degree of privacy may be had. Private homes should give some thought to the matter of providing a place where the daughter may be the hostess and therefore in control of the situation. A midnight lunch from the family ice box will be deeply appreciated by the young chap who has none too much money to spend. It will also put him under a wholesome obligation to be a gentleman, whereas under a different set of circumstances the girl might feel obliged to repay him for favors received.

Privacy is of some consequence. In this country a young couple expects as their right a degree of privacy which is nearly equal to that which they will enjoy after they are actually married. To deny it would be to drive them to places where they could get privacy under much less favorable circumstances, or to appear to persecute them, which would have the effect of making them tend to wish to abuse whatever opportunities for privacy they might have. The use of a living room from which other members of the family are not entirely and rigidly excluded is a proper medium.

The city mother used to worry when she had reason to believe that her daughter was alone with her friend on country roads. The country mother thought nothing of her daughter driving alone with a young man in the country, but was afraid for them to go to the city. Each mother rather intuitively understood that the young people were most in danger when they were in unfamiliar surroundings.

Some have supposed that the relation of the two sexes can be controlled by the use of chaperons. A chaperon thinks that she is saving the virtue of a girl when she compels a couple to use some restraint in their dancing positions. The couple that wishes to dance in an indecent manner will not be restrained by a chaperon who all too often has been a prim dowager who hasn't the slightest idea what the whole thing is about. We need chaperons, but the chaperons should be built into the character of the young people themselves; otherwise they are simply figureheads who believe that there is no mischief simply because they have seen none. The conventional chaperon serves a useful purpose when she prevents couples who are improper from suggesting such activity to those who otherwise would have had no thought of it.

Love between the two sexes is a pure and fine emotion. For an individual to simulate the expressions of deep affection when such feelings are really not held is to invite an inevitable deterioration of character which will eventually rob that individual of the power of fine and noble emotions of this sort. A girl will soon find herself marked as one who has been pawed over; a boy will soon lose his respect for clean womanhood. Marriage for the sordid purposes of fortune and social position is an unclean thing. He who cheapens so precious an emotion as love will rue it if he has any of the finer sensibilities. He who sincerely and deeply loves another and who has earned the right to legitimate favors is entitled to them, but this presupposes that he would wish to bestow his affection only upon the favored one and has a legal right to do so.

Marriage is of such consequence that it should be carefully considered. The couple expecting to make such a contract should thoroughly discuss every phase of the subject before doing so. All reliable sources of information should be sought, and notes should be compared. Each should frankly tell the other what he or she expects. The desirability or undesirability of having children must be thoroughly threshed out before going ahead. Agreement upon a marriage date that will fit into the menstrual cycle may well be made. Arrangement for the use of contraceptives in the early days of the marriage, and an understanding of such use, is rather important unless the couple is willing to assume the possibility of pregnancy before they are ready for it. If the bride-to-be is anxious that sexual relations not be consummated at once, that point should be understood beforehand—and respected afterward.

THE HONEYMOON

The honeymoon is the period between the marriage ceremony and the time when the young people shall have become more or less settled into the routine of a married couple. It is frequently used to designate a trip that is taken for the purpose of getting away from prying eyes. It is a period of adjustment to the new regimen and may be wisely or unwisely spent. Not a few marriages are utterly wrecked during this time, and a great many others are so strained as to weaken or damage the prospect of future happiness and usefulness. It is a time of high emotional tension and needs to be rather soberly considered. The obvious purpose of the honeymoon is to grant to the newly married lovers an unusual degree of privacy while they are experimenting with the new status in which they find themselves.

Unfortunately many ugly customs have developed about so beautiful a thing as a wedding. Pranks without number are played upon the couple; many of these pranks are in exceedingly bad taste, and not a few are positively indecent, or dangerous.

Wealthy families are inclined to make much of a wedding. There are parties, showers, receptions, and elaborate ceremonies, and finally a long and tiresome honeymoon is planned. A trip to Europe or a tour around the world seems like an ideal wedding present, but may be entirely too long. On such a trip the lovers are thrown entirely too much into each other's company and may utterly exhaust themselves and their interest in each other. The fatigue of travel and of sight-seeing, added to the strain of adjustment and the enervating effects of excessive sexual exercise, is entirely too much.

Families in moderate circumstances often exceed their means in attempting to give their young people a big and elaborate wedding and trip. The worry as to whether the funds will hold out, and the consciousness that the rocketlike celebration is going to end with a thud, make a bad start. Better no honeymoon at all than one that cannot be afforded.

The most important relations of the period, however, are not those which are commonly called the honeymoon. They are those which take place in the very first days and nights of married life. The happiness and even the health of the couple may be seriously crippled by the bungling caresses of one who is not ready for real marriage or is utterly lacking in understanding of the processes involved.

Biologic marriage and conventional marriage have entirely different purposes, but the two are supplementary to each other and are best consummated at approximately the same time. In case the biologic marriage has lagged and one or another of the pair is not ready for the actual union, the process of courtship should continue until the mate—usually the bride—is really ready for sexual relations. Theoretically, legal marriage gives each the right to the body of the other, and many men have been crass enough to insist on those rights as soon as the privacy of the bedroom has been reached. Embarrassed, shocked, frightened, and even sometimes subjected to physical pain, the bride is essentially forced by one who has but a short time before promised to love and cherish her. Under such circumstances she is set against the whole process and, indeed, may never learn to take a normal attitude toward a relation which should be exquisitely pleasurable to both partners. In a short time the husband, being disappointed in the fact that his wife is no longer a lover, may become disgusted and seek mistresses who can take an interest in such things.

Every prospective bridegroom should understand that, unless he has positive and first-hand assurance to the contrary, the bride may probably wish to delay the climax of the ceremony which has just been performed. Brides without previous sexual experience may be reluctant indeed, in spite of the fact that they are intensely in love with their new husbands. In such case there is nothing for the *gentleman* to do but bide his time and divert himself in the gallant and romantic manner which has so far won her approval that she has been willing to take his name, and share her life with him. The rights which the law gives him are as worthless as dust until they have been ratified by her approval. "Women first" is the code of the gentleman. If this fact could be impressed on the consciousness of bridegrooms most of them would be only too glad to wait until the loved one is ready to invite his amorous advances. Young people, when newly married, are in a highly idealistic and romantic state and are more liberal and unselfish probably than at any other time in their lives. But the young man, being intensely stimulated himself and never having been told that the feeling of the bride may be different, supposes that she as well as he is eager to bring about the consummation of their marriage. If she is so, very well! There is not the least reason for formality in cases where courting has progressed to such a stage. When, however, the bride is reluctant, courtship must be continued, and courtship only.

All or most of these difficulties can be avoided by a frank prenuptial understanding. The couple who are so excessively modest that they cannot discuss this subject had better grow up a little, learn something about themselves, and really get in love before going ahead with a wedding. If the girl seems reluctant, her fiancé can make her happy and reassured if he will promise her that he will consider her wishes in these matters as well after marriage as before. She, in turn, should assure him that she understands the purpose and nature of marriage, and that she will do her best to become interested in that which is so vital to happiness and unity.

Sheer clothing, athletic uniforms, and brief bathing suits have accustomed each sex to the general appearance of the body of the other sex. This has helped greatly to prevent excessive embarrassment in the act of disrobing. A couple intensely in love and entering into a relation of significance and beauty will find an exquisite delight in coming frankly and gladly together devoid of covering. The accomplishment of the first act of sexual congress is not without its hazards. In case the male organ is of unusual size care will need to be taken, particularly if the wife is small. After some time adjustment will be made and normal relations may be assumed, but until that time the husband may have to practice restraint. The first union will be facilitated considerably if some lubricant is used. Vaseline will serve in this capacity, but a surgical jelly is better. The hymen of the young wife will occasionally present real difficulty: it is so resistant in some instances that considerable pressure may be required to break it. In rare cases it may even require the aid of a physician to remove this obstruction. Occasionally there will be some pain, and there may be slight bleeding as a result of the first union. When such is the case, the greatest care must be taken, and the wife should by all means be granted the privilege of being the active party. An aggressive husband essentially attacking a sensitive, frightened, and unprepared wife and hurting her may jeopardize the reasonable hope of a full and happy married life.

Concerning the hymen there is need of exact information, else innocent wives may be accused of having had previous sexual experience. At one time the intact hymen was considered an infallible proof of virginity. It is now known that many virgins have lost the hymen as a result of athletic activities, accident, horseback riding, or manipulations incident to bathing. Ignorance of these facts has many times caused the most cruel injustices to be committed.

Many people who should know better suppose that all of these delicate relations can be trusted entirely to the instincts and that for this reason there is no need to discuss them. Nothing could be further from the truth. Nature has furnished us with certain instincts, it is true, but they are the "law of the jungle." These instincts have caused much trouble in times past. Instinct is utterly disregardful of anything except the desire of the male to consummate sexual relations at every possible opportunity, and to bring about fertilization as quickly as possible. Modern marriage is—or should be—on a different basis. In no other species than man is the pleasure or welfare of the female given more consideration than is necessary to gain her physical acquiescence, but man is more than a beast and should behave accordingly.

Because sexual relations as they are practiced by men and women serve another function than merely that of reproduction they cannot be successfully practiced from instinct alone. They are of the nature of an art; they express fine and noble emotions just as do the other arts. Because they constitute an art they must be learned and practiced before a high degree of proficiency may be attained. Even after many years a well-matched couple may still be improving in technique and in appreciation of the legitimate pleasures of conjugal love. Books are available which give the most detailed description of every phase of the copulative function, but one can hardly expect to learn to play the piano by reading about it. If definite difficulties arise, such information may be of service, but otherwise the couple should be somewhat less sophisticated in the early stages of the honeymoon period. Both should remember that *the act is perfectly proper* and that the spirit of love demands that *each shall show the utmost solicitude for the comfort, happiness, and pleasure of the other.*

THE YOUNG MARRIED COUPLE

Much has been said about the advisability of the wife working after marriage. Until the couple can get a start there can certainly be no objection to the wife's holding her former job or getting another one. It will mean extra hours of work and less leisure now that she has the care of a home or an apartment, but it is all for the good of the cause. It would be a poor wife, indeed, who would not put her shoulder to the family wheel and help to make it turn.

Unfortunately, however, there is more to the matter than just that. It will be hard later for her to give up the outside job and devote herself exclusively to homemaking with its comparatively intangible rewards. We need not be surprised that she is loath to give up the independence that comes with a check at the end of the week. There are so many things that are needed and can be had only if the wife as well as the husband earns.

So it is customary to put off, and put off, and put off the real purpose and culmination of marriage—children. If two have trouble making ends meet with two salaries—as two commonly do—how shall three or four or five live on one salary? It is hard to criticize a couple who gradually work their way into this predicament. If the wife works there should be a definite understanding concerning the time when she shall be promoted to the much more important work of real homemaking. Marriages when both parties are poor but in good health and willing to work are frequently the best of marriages. We frequently see the young wife working to help her husband complete his education, and it makes a most inspiring picture.

Likewise, the wife may continue her education after marriage. These are the young people who know what an education is. They will get along.

Health is of the utmost importance to the welfare of the home builders.

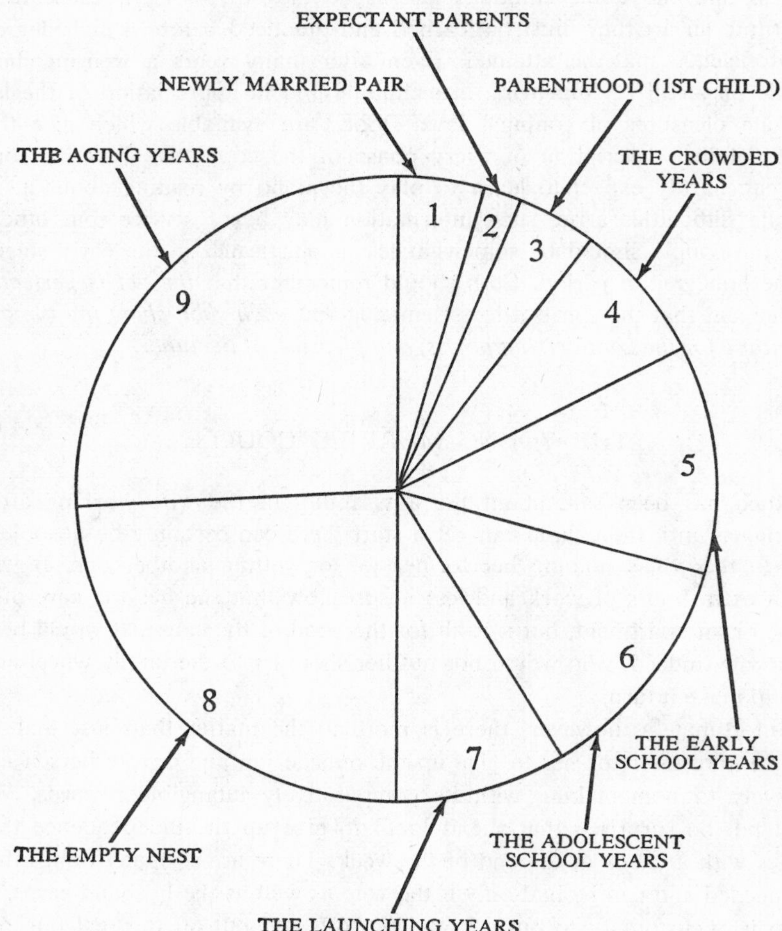

Fig. 13. The family life cycle. At each stage of the family life cycle there are understandings to be sought, adjustments to be made, problems to be solved, crises to be faced, decisions to be acted upon as members of the family seek to meet their personal needs, fill their roles and achieve their goals. This is also true if the family seeks to function effectively as a group. American Social Health Association.

In the first place, only those who have health are fit to marry. It is foolish indeed for a young person to marry an invalid or semi-invalid—immensely romantic in some instances and highly idealistic, but nevertheless foolish.

It is much like marrying a drunkard to reform him. Better reform him first! Besides, it is most selfish for a sick person to fasten himself or herself upon another person and call it love. Marriage is a big job at the best; it is entirely too much for sick people. When sickness comes after marriage, as of course it is probable that it will eventually come, there is nothing that honor can condone except to see it through, but even so it may and often does utterly wreck the family.

Several particular health hazards must be considered by people of this age group. The bearing, nursing, and caring for children undermines occasionally the health of the mother, particularly if the children come too close together. Hard work on the part of both in the years when they are so anxious to get a start, accepting extra jobs, taking few vacations, worrying, and falling for the temptation to avoid the expense of doctors' bills when there is real need for professional attention, all take their toll. Nervous breakdown from overwork, pneumonia, organic heart disease, occupational diseases, and other related conditions are prone to attack this group. Health is a matter of much more than personal concern to these people. It involves the welfare of the entire family and for that reason deserves to be considered seriously in this place. What one of us has not heard our fathers and mothers wondering, "What will become of us if one of us should get sick?"

Life, accident, and health insurance have proved themselves of the greatest possible consequence in solving the problems which inevitably arise when health is impaired. As soon as the family can possibly afford to do so, investment should be made in some form of time-tried insurance. When there are children there is particular need of such protection.

Unless there is a dependable income, unless the housewife and her husband know how to manage so as to keep within that income and have a little to spare for savings, there is trouble ahead. A savings account, a house to live in, a few life insurance policies and other conservative investments, are essential to the welfare of a home.

One of the biggest questions which the young couple must decide is that concerning children. Will there be children? And, if so, how many? There are many excellent reasons why a particular couple should not desire children at a given time, and there are even reasons why they should not have them at all. A couple may not dare to have children because of some hereditary taint or disease. They act wisely in taking precautions which will prevent conception. Unfortunately they did not find out about such matters before marriage and act accordingly. A couple may feel that the health of one or the other is such that the burden of parenthood should not be added. This is a legitimate reason, though many of these persons were ill before marriage, and because of that unfit for marriage. The economic position of the family is often such that children might be endangered by being brought into the home at such a time.

An average of more than three children to the couple is required for a given stratum of society to maintain itself numerically as some die before marriage and others do not marry. Any family of less than four is, then, on the average, falling behind. Unfortunately, those families which should have no children sometimes have many, and those that might be expected to bear and rear superior children too often have few or none.

For those couples who cannot for some reason bear children there are infinite possibilities in adoption. With care the adopted child that has come from a good family has an even chance with the blood descendant of the same age and physical opportunity. Adopted children do not turn out worse than others; they may on the average do better, when they have been carefully selected. A careful physical and mental examination should be made of all children who are being considered for adoption. Couples without children may also satisfy their parental instincts and do a great service by taking up some phase of work which has to do with the welfare of children and young people.

The care of the children after they are born is enormously important. It is discussed in succeeding chapters of this work.

There are many problems which are sexual in the sense that the term is usually used. A husband and wife, a man and woman, in vigorous health and living in the intimacy which is properly granted to a married couple, have many opportunities for expressions of love and affection. Shall we deny them the privileges of sexuality except for purposes of reproduction? Certainly not! They will need to learn well the art of love so that they may know the exquisite pleasures of conjugal love. The stability of the marriage will depend largely on this ability, though, of course, there are other factors serving toward this end.

In most cases where there is dissatisfaction with the conjugal relation at this stage in life the cause is to be found in the fact that women are more slowly aroused and require a longer time for gratification than is the case of the man. Husbands are prone to forget that courtship is as necessary after marriage as before. Quickly aroused and quickly satisfied, they are inclined to forget that the partner in everything else should also have her share in the emotions of sex, else she will become disgusted and intolerant of the whole process. Part of the trouble is also due to the fact that a large percentage of women suppose that sex gratification is not for them and that there is something akin to vulgarity in any manifestation of pleasure or interest in it. With the husband as considerate as he should be and the wife convinced of the propriety of legitimate conjugal relations there should be little difficulty in building a sex life that will bind the family together with hoops of steel.

Considerable effort has been made to determine in an accurate way the limits of safe and proper sexual indulgence. The frequency with which the act may be safely performed without injury to health or vigor is not something that can be reduced to formula. It will vary widely in different couples, and it is impossible for an outsider to set out rules. So long as the act is mutually pleasurable, and both the partners are able to go about the usual day's work without unusual fatigue or lassitude, no harm is being done. In case either partner feels the strain, moderation must be practiced. The average among Americans is probably about two to three times a week. As in the case of everything else, it is better to err on the side of too little than too much. No one would wish to give up the pleasure of eating food, but everyone is disgusted with gluttony. Hardly anything can be so revolting as sexual gluttony. The love embrace is too sacred a thing to be made common.

In practically every family at some time it is considered best that conception should not take place in the immediate future. Improper methods may on one hand fail to control the size of the family, or on the other may cheat the couple of such sexual experience as is essential to health and happiness. The pair that lives in constant fear of pregnancy can hardly be happy and can hardly go about the business and pleasure of living in a way that makes for good family life. There are individuals who by virtue of strong wills, or who by lack of the normal desires, may solve this problem by refraining entirely from intercourse, but the vast majority of couples cannot go along happily on such a regimen. In the chapter on "Hygiene of Women" the details of conception are more fully discussed.

Common opinion takes it for granted that sexual appetite is something that cannot be controlled. It is astonishing how many people suppose that a "red-blooded" individual is utterly at the mercy of any sexual passion that may chance to blow. The attitude of irresponsibility for sexual misconduct is a convenient alibi for those who have not the strength of character to stand by their ideals—if any. Such is not a strong and manly attitude, but is a sign of weakness in those who cannot or will not be strong.

SEX IN MIDDLE AND ADVANCED LIFE

Most men and women are apprehensive as they approach and pass the age of forty. They have learned to look upon "fat and forty" as being the zero hour of romance. Actually, however, a large percentage of people are happier after this age than before. Particularly is this true of those who have lived and loved wisely and well. The person who can adjust his life and thinking to the fact that he is no longer a gay and irresponsible young thing will find many compensations. The woman who can relax a bit at this time and smile indulgently at the mad struggle for beauty and youth has before her many happy days of comparative quiet and serenity.

Of great importance in this process of adjustment is that which has to do with sex. Ordinarily people of forty and above do not bear children. A few children are born of mothers above this age, but it is a rather risky adventure, as some of the children are hardly up to the standard of their brothers and sisters born at a more vigorous period of life. A small percentage of these children may be defective and are called "exhaustion products." Men may continue to be fertile for a long time past the forty mark, but there is some objection to men being fathers after they are much above forty. The possibility that the children will be left orphans in such case is obvious.

Are we to suppose, then, that all of the functions of the reproductive apparatus have been filled? Not at all. Usually there are children to be raised. The family still has a purpose. Couples who have enjoyed the embraces of earlier life will still continue to enjoy them and will not need to consider the possibility of pregnancy and additional children with their many responsibilities. With the children from underfoot it is not unusual to see a couple much more attached to each other than when they were so busy. It is, indeed, not unusual to see them almost like two young lovers, or perhaps more often as Darby and Joan contentedly living a life of placid, uneventful domesticity.

It is difficult for younger people to see in this period anything but a tiresome and monotonous existence, and there are many who find themselves at forty or above in an openly rebellious attitude. They want one more fling at "life" and may do foolish things in the effort to get it. The man who has been circumspect and careful about all such matters may get sympathetic for himself and think he has missed a great deal. Somewhat bored with the faithful but unromantic wife, he is prone to yearn for a younger and more vivacious companion. If some degree of affluence has rewarded his labors, he is in a position to indulge himself—and be an easy mark for gold-diggers who really hold him in contempt. Occasionally a woman of forty retains her youth better than her husband and may be tempted to "step out" a bit with a snappy "gigolo" or a neighbor whose "wife doesn't understand him." She yearns for a lover instead of a tired workhorse who prefers his house slippers and shirt sleeves to a "tux" and a ballroom. Not unlikely this period offers more urgent temptations than does any other. The opportunities for making a fool of one's self during this time are unexcelled.

Likewise the unmarried person of this age is in danger. The unmarried woman who is approaching the end of what would and should have been the reproductive period of her life sees her youth slipping. Until this time she has usually hoped that the opportunity for family life would come, but she now rapidly resigns herself to the prospect of a lonesome and not unlikely bitter old age. She feels cheated. Life is going without ever having really bloomed or borne fruit. Something of the same feeling is experienced by married couples who have not had children. Fortunate indeed are such childless persons who have attained a vicarious parenthood either by adopting children or by interesting themselves in the children of their friends or in young people.

It is not uncommon to hear men say that when they are no longer interested in a pretty face or figure they will be ready to die—life will no longer be worth living. The loss of virility in men is looked on as a calamity of the highest degree. Such an attitude reveals an utter lack of understanding of the real meaning of life.

Loss of virility is Nature's way of insuring against "exhaustion products;" it is her way of making sure that fathers will probably live until the work of rearing the child is accomplished; it is her protection for the weakened and wasted organs of the body which in the wear and tear of life have likely become injured to such an extent that ardent wooing and frequent sexual embraces are exhausting.

The elderly widower gets himself a young wife. How can a young woman be really in love with a man thirty or forty years her senior? For that matter, how can a man of that age who understands things be truly in love with a young woman? Ten years more will find him an old man while she will be just starting. Clashes between the wife and his children —as old as she perhaps—are inevitable. The suspicion that she loves his money rather than him; the fear that she may be stepping out with younger men; the painful effort to entertain her as a young wife deserves to be entertained; the fear that children may be borne at a period in life when children would be a burden; and a dozen other fears real and imaginary, take away every iota of the tranquility that should be the heritage of him who has lived long. Much wiser indeed is he who chooses a companion who is near his own age.

Life to many older women seems to be nothing except a struggle against the onslaughts of age. Hours are spent with hairdressers, skin experts, and beauty doctors of all sorts. For those who are at middle age and are capable of reading it, nothing is so valuable as a little book by Aldred Scott Warthin, for forty years professor of pathology at the University of Michigan. The book is entitled *Old Age* and is the life philosophy of Dr. Warthin written when he was old and wise. Warthin points out that at every age some part of the body is old and worn out and is making way for something else. Even before birth some parts have atrophied and have made way for growing structures. At the time of birth the senile "afterbirth" or placenta is dropped as worn out and no longer needed. It has served its purpose and is cast aside as useless baggage. The thymus of the child is old, or should be when the child is adolescent; the womb and the ovaries are old at forty-five; the prostate and the testicles are commonly old in the sixties; the body as a whole is old at seventy or shortly thereafter.

Senility and death are seen by Dr. Warthin as being perfectly natural processes provided they do not come too soon. Death is, indeed, quite as necessary as birth. If there were no deaths there soon could be no births, because the earth would be full and running over with old people living in the past. The aged must make room for those who are younger and more vigorous. Even death is in this view a part of the reproductive act. We must do our best to get our children ready to do the work of the world, and then we must get out of the way so that they can do it. Unjust? Not at all! As young people, we took the places of those who were older and as old people ourselves we can expect the same inevitable fate. In the relay race that is life, each runner is expected to do his best and then pass the torch to his successor. Having done so, he can perform a last and valuable service by getting out of the way and taking care of himself in such a way as will not divert the attention of the one who is at the time carrying the responsibilities of the race.

Health is frequently said to be more important than anything else. This false philosophy is responsible for the despondency which comes to those who are attaining advanced age. Health is not, or should not be, an end in itself but merely a means to an end. The earnest parent is anxious to remain well, not so much because he or she is afraid to suffer as that he or she wants to be able to take care of the children until they are able to take care of themselves. When a parent dies, the neighbors lament not so much the loss of a friend and neighbor as they look with apprehension upon the fact that he or she left little children. The parent who would not jeopardize his own health or safety for the sake of his child is not a real parent but a miserable imitation. The individual with this outlook will not be buffered against the shock that comes at the age of forty.

THE PURPOSE OF MARRIAGE

The real purpose of marriage is the creation of a home into which children may be born legitimately and reared in decency and self-respect. The fitness of a person to be a father or a mother is ultimately more important than the fitness of the same individual to be merely a husband or wife. The prospective bride or bridegroom should consider the family tree of himself or herself and of the preferred mate. It will be well to consider whether or not a given man is likely to be able to provide for a family, or whether a given girl is of the domestic or maternal type who will enjoy caring for babies. The couple contemplating marriage should frankly discuss the probability of children being born and should come to some agreement in such matters before the ceremony of marriage has been performed. Young people should "fall in love intelligently," a phrase which has been much ridiculed by those who believe that love and marriage should never be considered in any other light than that of the moon. The marriages which have been carefully worked out are more likely to be permanently and solidly "romantic" than those which have been consummated in a fever.

The young of the species desire the company of the members of the opposite sex. The real purpose of such an attraction is that the species may be reproduced. If Nature alone were consulted, there would be no such thing as conventional marriage, and as a result there would be no such thing as the civilized home, and, indeed, no such things as civilization itself. Marriage, by which we mean conventional marriage, has been evolved by man as a means of rising above the chance mating of the animals and as a device for placing about human offspring the care and protection of parents who continue to love each other after the heat of sexual passion has waned.

Since the day of creation, our ancestors have been hardy enough to live to the age of sexual maturity. Each has had the normal instinct to reproduce himself or herself and has been sufficiently comely to be sought and accepted by a member of the opposite sex. In the gigantic relay race that is life, a billion, billion ancestors have passed the torch from one to the next in never-ending sequence until the present generation is reached.

The real, the primary purpose of marriage, then, is children. That two persons should enjoy the constant society of each other is most fortunate but is really of little concern to anyone but themselves, unless there are children. When there are children the setting is established for an ideal home. That two persons should quarrel and fight is again of little importance to anyone except themselves, unless there are children. When there are children in such a distraught home, there is tragedy. The couple without children may separate for some trivial reason, and such marriages are often highly unstable. Judges are much more free in granting divorces to childless couples than to those who have dependent children to consider.

When one considers the importance of the relationship which a person to be married is about to assume, it makes him wonder why society has been so careless in permitting any Tom, Dick, or Mary who can find a willing mate to enter into such a contract. The parent, in addition to his or her duties as a provider or housewife, must furnish the biological inheritance, must serve as nurse, physician, dentist, teacher, preacher, legal adviser, companion, administrator, and adviser to the child. The parent should be an authority on mental hygiene, infant care, dietetics; he or she should speak the mother tongue with accuracy, beauty, and force; he or she should train the child in proper habits, in obedience, thrift, industry, appreciation of truth, beauty, and virtue. The parent, usually without scientific or even practical training in child care and guidance, is responsible for the education of the child before he goes to school and all of the time during school except for about six hours a day, five days a week, and nine months of the year.

Society requires of the applicant for a marriage license less than of the applicant for an automobile driver's license. In most states of the union, or more likely in all of them, almost anyone can get a marriage license if he is persistent and can find a partner. In consideration of the great importance to society and to the individual, the schools should have worked out a method of imparting instruction that would really "help solve the problems of life." Children are taught nearly everything except what might be expected to help them support or care for a home and a family. In recent years girls are being taught domestic science but many such courses are quite impractical. Biology courses can, and occasionally do, give a valuable insight into the problems of life.

The family is the real unit of society; the home is the place where the unit lives, and marriage is the bond which holds the family together until the task is really finished. A community of good homes is one with good schools and churches, flourishing business enterprises, and loyal community interest. The teachers have little trouble at school; and policemen patrol the district only to protect it from outsiders; there are no riots, no antisocial manifestations, no need of the strong arm of the law. A community of vicious or wretched homes, on the contrary, is a constant menace. All the policemen, all the teachers, all the jails, all the hospitals, all the correctional institutions in the world will not be able to undo the ills that are bred in ugly homes.

When the home is inadequate, society is compelled in various ways to try to assume the relations which should have been assumed by the parents. But so often the parents will not, cannot, or at least do not accept their responsibilities, and in such cases organized society can do no less than to attempt to palliate the evil. We go to great expense to stand *in loco parentis* for these children who are obviously unfit for the problems to be met in modern life. There is nothing else to do about it. We have permitted these people to be born, now we must take care of them. It seems that at present they are rather rapidly increasing, and society is assuming more and more responsibility for them.

The ultimate purpose of marriage is superior children. Legal marriage gives these children a name, property rights, citizenship, establishes their legal status, and places the protection of the state about their home where they may be born and reared in security. In addition to these legal bonds there should be other bonds which hold father, mother, and child in a tight and compact unit. Any relation which will strengthen that bond is of the greatest possible consequence, while any relation which endangers the bond is pregnant with dire results for the individual and for society at large.

ABNORMALITIES OF SEXUAL FUNCTION

The individual with normal emotions and sensibilities may regard his (or her) sex as the core of his (or her) personality. Any deviation of sex from normal as seen in others or as experienced in one's own self is sure to make a profound impression and to arouse most unpleasant emotions.

MASTURBATION

Masturbation is admittedly a habit. Millions of people used to believe that it caused insanity, feeble-mindedness, epilepsy, loss of virility, pimples, specks before the eyes, and a dozen other symptoms. It does nothing of the sort. Many wild animals practice some form or another of self-sexual stimulation (auto-eroticism). At some time in life nearly all men and boys have practiced this form of self-gratification, and likewise a great many women and girls. The reason many people vehemently deny ever having practiced masturbation is that they really have done so and are ashamed.

The bad effects of masturbation are the indirect results of the act and of the attempt on the part of the elders to stamp out the practice. Children are shamed, they are whipped, they are spied upon, they are threatened with insanity and all sorts of dire consequences, they are led to believe that they are lower than the dirt, and, as a result of these clumsy attempts at correction, they really are injured. The constant reminder of these awful consequences keeps the child thinking about what it is much better to forget.

When children are taught early that the reproductive organs are clean and wholesome; that sex is something that has a usefulness; that it is something to be kept unspoiled for the future, and that it serves a purpose that is essentially sacred; when children are kept busy with wholesome play, work and planning, and when they are loved and understood in matters such as these, a little masturbation may occur but will be speedily forgotten. Be sure the children are healthily tired when they go to bed. Be sure that there is no need of circumcision, or if there is that it is corrected. Be sure the organs are clean so that they will not be irritated by foul secretions. Be sure that tight underwear does not demand constant pulling at the clothing.

Excessive masturbation is injurious in itself, but is rarely seen except in the mentally defective or in those who are driven too much into themselves.

Persons who are extremely restless because of urgent sexual desire may possibly be more injured by the racking and the loss of sleep than by the act that will permit them to obtain relief. Husbands or wives who make excessive demands on their mates might well practice masturbation rather than wreck their home life by insisting upon their conjugal rights when the partner is sleepy, tired, or for any reason unwilling to cooperate. As the potent male rather regularly has seminal emissions if he has no other sexual outlet, masturbation becomes merely a waking instead of a dreaming activity. Physiologically, its effect, when not in excess, is no greater than emissions, which are merely an overflow. Psychologically, the effect is nil, bad, or extremely bad, according as no, some, or much attention is paid to it.

EXCESSIVE SEXUALITY

A dangerous form of sexual abnormality puts excessive emphasis on the subject. The male of this type is sometimes referred to as being a satyr. The damage which such a person can do is incalculable. He spreads venereal disease, he seduces wives and maids, he becomes the father of illegitimate children, he may commit rape or other crimes of sexual violence. No woman or girl is safe while he is about.

When the female displays excessive sexuality she is known as a nymphomaniac. The nymphomaniac is not to be confused with the normal woman who properly desires a pleasurable relation that is legitimate. Proper sex education of little girls will probably be of aid in preventing cases which are not on a pathologic basis. Dissatisfaction with existing marriage relations may be a cause that can occasionally be corrected.

SEXUAL FRIGIDITY

At the opposite extreme are women, many of them married, who either have no desire for sexual experience, or are even definitely averse to it.

Many causes of this condition are recognized which is commonly called *frigidity*. The instruction which many girls receive from their mothers may produce in them an intense distrust of the male of the species, and repulse any normal instinct with regard to sex. The mother often deliberately teaches the daughter to take this attitude, doubtless thinking that she is protecting the girl from temptation. She does not realize that she may be preparing the daughter for an unhappy marriage. The girl whose father has been crude and repellent may develop unnatural attitudes as a result of the harsh treatment he has shown his wife and children.

The commonest cause of frigidity is lack of preparation for marriage. Awkward bridegrooms have frightened, shocked, shamed, and even injured their brides at a time when the destiny of the marriage was in the balance. With such a start, and with the same act repeated as often as the new husband is able or may wish, the wife is set strongly against the whole program and may develop into a woman who has the most intense disgust for anything of a sexual nature. Wooing should continue until the conventionally married couple are really ready for biological marriage. When this is done and patience is practiced—when the bride is shown the same deference as the fiancée—there will be few women who will fail to develop a strong desire for the conjugal embrace.

Another common cause of frigidity is fear of conception. Wives may have ever so many excellent reasons why they do not desire children at a given time. Frequently most or all of the responsibility for the prevention of conception is placed upon them. They dread the long months of pregnancy. Frequently there have already been born more children than is best for the welfare of the family or the mother. Under such circumstances the wife is under the constant dread of another conception and as a result wishes to avoid every possibility of such a happening. In a similar relation is the woman who has reason to believe that her husband is unfaithful to her.

Sometimes religion, sometimes training, or lack of it, sometimes abnormality of the organs, sometimes a disproportion between the organs of the two mates, sometimes psychological incompatibility between the two may be responsible. Whatever the cause, a couple will be unhappy if the wife is frigid. If there are children, the couple may stay together but furnish the children a decidedly bad environment; if there are no children divorce or separation is nearly inevitable. Not only does a satisfactory relation pay large dividends in personal enjoyment, but it enables couples to form a strong and stable marriage which will insure that their children have a good home until they are old enough to take care of themselves. Body odor, sweaty or dirty skin, untidy garments, beds, and bedclothing may easily cause disgust in a sensitive person; vulgar language, uncouth behavior, or untoward behavior may cause revulsion on the part of a person who is fastidious in such matters.

SEXUAL COMPLEXES

The Oedipus complex is seen when there is an unusual attachment between mother and son. The Electra complex is the relation when a daughter has an excessive love for her father. These excessive attachments may do serious harm to the exemplary young men and women who are so unfortunate as to get caught in their mesh. Parents—particularly parents of a single child—should watch for this trap into which an adoring child may be lured. Particularly if the father lives alone with the daughter or the mother with a son there is danger.

Much has been said concerning repressions of various sorts, and of sexual repressions in particular. Some have even advised that one should not attempt to control or repress the impulses that arise for the reason that terrible complexes may develop if such is done. Society could not exist if everyone simply followed any urge that he might feel. However, spinsters, bachelors, and persons who have been disappointed in love or have strongly loved someone under conditions which made it necessary to conceal the feeling are subject to disturbances which may seriously undermine the health of the body and mind.

Extremely important is suggestion or direct teaching of irregular practices. A child who has wrong ideas can ruin a school or a neighborhood. Children who have evolved a vacuum in their minds regarding sex are easily led into almost any sort of abuse of the sexual apparatus. Children who have had adequate sex instruction will be far less attracted to perverted persons and also much less likely to follow improper suggestions. Disgusting practices are in many instances more directly to be charged to the parents who failed to instruct the child in healthy ways than they are to be held against the unfortunate victim of distorted perspective who has taught the unsophisticated child in these matters.

THE HYGIENE OF THE REPRODUCTIVE SYSTEM

A fine watch does best when it is meddled with least; the same is true of the generative apparatus. When there is reason to believe that something is really wrong, the family physician or a specialist whom he may designate should be consulted at once. The physician should be furnished with a full and frank history of the ailment and its possible causes. Furthermore, he must be permitted to make such examinations and to ask such questions of the parents as he may think necessary.

CLEANLINESS

The first principle in the hygiene of the reproductive system is cleanliness. By this we do not mean to imply that lack of cleanliness will often jeopardize the physical health of the individual. Actually there is more danger that meddlesome methods of attaining cleanliness will cause disease than that lack of cleanliness will cause it. This is particularly true in the case of the woman. The reproductive organs must be clean if they are to be held in high regard; they must be free of odor; they must be wholesome; they must not offend. They are exceedingly important to the welfare of the race, the self-respect of the individual, and the happiness of family.

Odor is a first consideration. The fact that we wear clothing complicates the situation because clothing does not permit the free ventilation that will carry away odors before they become concentrated. Clothing should be as light and as well ventilated as comfort will permit. Great improvement in underwear has been made in recent years. Undergarments should be changed as often as one's finances will permit and should never be worn after they are definitely soiled. Night clothing should entirely replace the underwear that has been worn through the day. This will give opportunity for airing and drying of the various garments which would be most likely to offend.

Washing of the external genitalia is extremely important. The external organs need washing and not the internal. Much harm has been done by the excessive use of antiseptic or even cleansing douches. The normal vagina nearly always contains germs. These germs are not only harmless, but actually beneficial, because they prevent the growth of other germs which can cause trouble. If they are frequently washed away with cleansing douches or inhibited with antiseptics, abnormal conditions may develop in the vagina, and trouble may ensue. Furthermore, strong antiseptics frequently irritate the mucous membrane and make it more susceptible to invasion by other bacteria.

Sometimes, particularly in the male, it is impossible to hold down odors merely by washing the external genitalia. In some men the foreskin is so tight about the end of the penis that it cannot be retracted and the groove beneath it cleaned of the white secretion—known as smegma—which accumulates there. This secretion is of an oily nature and easily becomes rancid, producing exceedingly bad odors and also irritation of the mucous membrane. At the time of birth every male child should be carefully examined to determine whether or not he is in need of circumcision which consists in removing the foreskin. When done in the early days of life the operation is a trivial one. Later it is somewhat more serious, but never dangerous when performed by a competent surgeon. Even those who are not in need of circumcision should retract the foreskin and clean the groove beneath it carefully at least once a day. A child in need of circumcision is often made nervous by the irritation of the rancid secretions and will be constantly twisting, squirming, and pulling at himself. He may also develop the habit of masturbation as a result of the irritation which induces him to handle his penis.

Occasionally discharges of various sorts from the genital organs will complicate the habit of cleanliness. In every case in either sex the cause of any discharge should be ascertained if possible. The family physician or a reliable specialist should be consulted, always.

MENSTRUATION

During menstruation the pelvic organs are considerably congested, and for this reason are more subject to infection and circulatory disturbances. Excessively long hours of standing on the feet, dancing, strenuous athletics, and similar activities are not advisable for many women. Likewise sexual excitement will intensify the effect and may cause trouble. Bathing was formerly interdicted but is now permitted. Local washing is usually

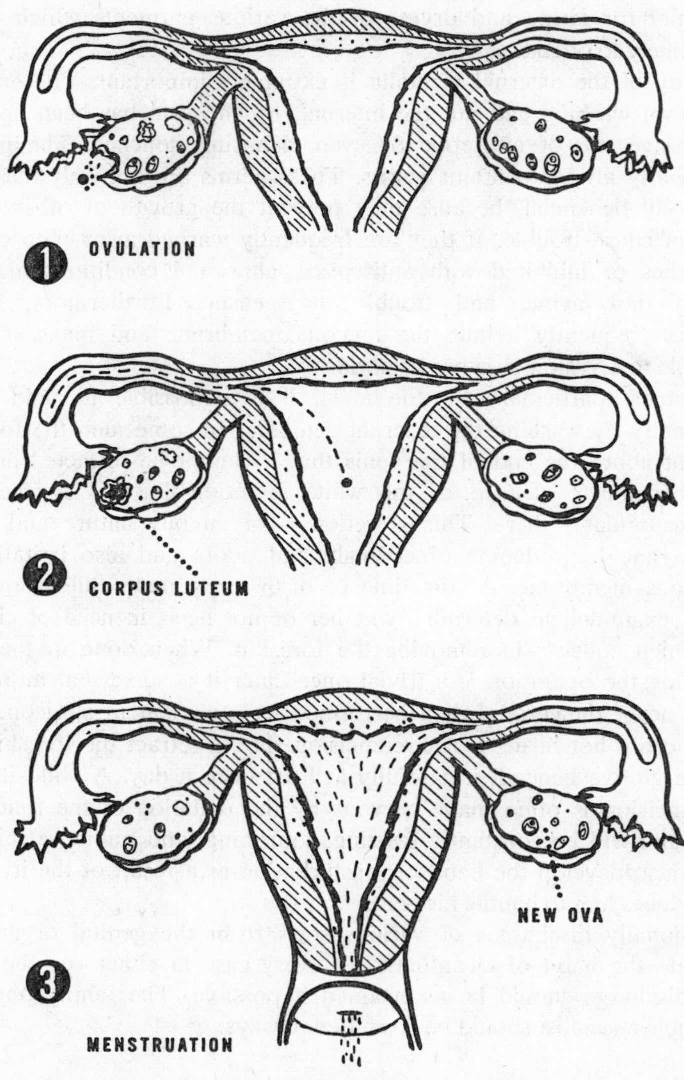

Fig. 14. Menstrual physiology. Technically, there are four phases to the menstrual cycle: (1) period of rest; (2) ovulation; (3) building up of the endometrium; (4) discard, or menstrual flow. The issuing of a ripened ovum from the egg case (follicle) is known as ovulation. After the ripened ovum has been expelled, the follicle turns yellow in color and is then known as the corpus luteum (yellow body). Copyright © 1947–59, Kimberly-Clark Corporation.

safe. Many women and girls can even swim in cold water while menstruating.

In case the menstrual periods should cease in a girl or woman who is probably not pregnant, careful physical examination should be made to determine the cause. Patients with anemia of any sort or those with nervous disturbances are also likely to cease menstruating until they are restored to their normal condition. Of great importance is the mental attitude of the woman toward her menstrual periods, and toward the "change of life," at which time the periods gradually cease from natural causes. In times past, girls were literally taught to make invalids of themselves, and women were led to believe that "the change" was something greatly to be dreaded and a time of danger. Menstruation is a normal process, and the menopause need cause little apprehension if it is approached with understanding and poise. The fact that women are now so much less embarrassed in visiting a physician about such matters has opened a way of escape from many of the dangers and discomforts.

With so much advertising of absorbent pads and other aids to feminine hygiene, it is hardly necessary to describe in detail the means by which women may avoid the soiling of their clothing with the menstrual discharges. Young girls should have these matters explained before they are twelve years of age, or by the time they are ten or eleven if they are somewhat precocious in their development. The girl should be taught so that she will not be frightened by the first appearance but will come to her mother for aid and advice. This is an excellent opportunity for the mother to explain something of the nature and purpose of the genital organs and to impress the girl with the value of the process of which the menstrual cycle is a part.

DISEASE OF THE GENITAL ORGANS

Various serious diseases of the genital organs need to be understood so that they may be detected at the earliest possible moment. The venereal diseases are discussed in a later chapter. Various other chronic inflammations and infections resulting from childbirth or injury usually manifest themselves by symptoms or pain of some sort.

At the present about one woman in eight above the age of forty years is dying of cancer. About one third of these cancers are of the womb, usually the mouth of the womb. Any sort of unnatural bleeding from the privates should be investigated thoroughly. Excessive bleeding, bleeding after the change of life, continuous bleeding, or the passing of clotted blood, constitute "unnatural" bleeding. These signs indicate that there is something wrong, and that a thorough examination is needed. The physician should prove if at all possible that it is not cancer before the investigation is ended. Once the diagnosis of cancer is made, treatment in the hands of a reliable surgeon or radiologist is the only hope. The Papanicolaou test is preventing deaths from cancer of the cervix. A small scraping can be taken and examined under the microscope permitting early detection and removal of anything abnormal.

Another third of all deaths from cancer among women is from cancer of the breast. These growths are always small before they are large, always localized before they are generalized, and always painless before they are painful. The growth usually manifests itself as a lump or nodule in the breast, or sometimes as a thick place in the skin reminding one of a piece of bacon rind. It is usually irregular in shape, attached to the skin and deeper tissues, and solitary in number in the earlier stages at least. As the breast is moved the nodules cause dimpling. If near the nipple, they commonly cause the nipple to be drawn in. The chances for recovery are good if the diagnosis is made early and the appropriate treatment begun at once. If surgical treatment is delayed, the operation is much more severe, and there is less chance of cure. Rarely cancer of the breast is seen in the male.

Cancer of the prostate and bladder are fairly common in the male. The earliest symptom is usually blood in the urine or difficulty in emptying the bladder. These symptoms should call for an immediate examination to determine the cause.

The reproductive system of the female is much more complicated than that of the male and is for this reason more subject to disease and injury. It furthermore is under far greater stress in the performance of its function of reproduction. For this reason care must be taken to avoid as many as possible of the dangers which beset the sexual life. In the first place, women—and men, too, for that matter—should not marry unless they are reasonably sure that they are free from disease and deformity.

The pregnant woman should consult her family physician or the specialist of her choice as soon as she becomes aware of her condition. If the pregnancy is the first, there is additional reason for such professional care. Likewise the women beyond the age usual for childbearing and those who have reason to believe that they may have weak hearts and kidneys should take extra precaution. All pregnant women should have their blood type known. In case the wife is Rh negative while her husband is Rh positive there is particular reason to know.

SEXUAL INTERCOURSE IN PREGNANCY

Many couples wonder if sexual intercourse may be indulged in during the period of pregnancy. This will depend upon several factors. There is good reason from the standpoint of the possibility of infection for refraining during the last few weeks of the pregnancy. In case the wife seems to have been injured by marital relations on previous occasions, or if she is one who is easily aborted, continence is the only safe rule. In those instances—and they are many—in which the wife desires the relation at this time and does not seem to be injured by it there is no real objection. The fear that the child may be injured is quite without foundation except in those women who are easily aborted.

ABORTION

In many instances when contraceptive measures have failed, abortion is practiced. This is always a more or less dangerous procedure. When done under the most careful conditions dangers are minimal. When abortion is done by ignorant persons under urgent necessity of concealing the act and not quite free to call the physician as needed it is exceedingly dangerous and often ends fatally for the mother as well as the child.

SEXUAL STIMULATION

The health of the reproductive system can be injured also by various attempts to stimulate the sexual function. The elderly or weakly man attempts to boost his waning powers. Old men's bodies are not able to stand the strain of highly active glands. Elderly men should not be parents and should be potent only when the psychological mechanism for such a purpose is functional of its own accord. The use of drugs which are supposed to stimulate sexual desire is dangerous. Cantharides (Spanish fly) is particularly dangerous and must never be used for this purpose, as it is an intense kidney irritant. Furthermore, it cannot do what popular tradition claims for it.

Of utmost importance in sexual hygiene is temperance in the exercise of the various functions. The individual who does not permit, or cannot enjoy, the reasonable use of the reproductive system, misses one of the most satisfactory activities in life. The man or woman who has shortcircuited the reproductive act and so has escaped the responsibilities of parenthood has cheated himself. Sex is the foundation of marriage but by no means the whole thing. Properly understood and exercised, the sex life of a married couple is a source of tremendous enjoyment and both physical and mental health.

CHAPTER 6

Adolescence

MORRIS FISHBEIN, M.D.

The word adolescence comes from a Latin word meaning "grow up." Adolescence is the time from puberty, when the sex glands and organs begin to mature, until the body has attained maturity. Puberty usually begins at the ages of nine to twelve, although nine is a little early in most cases.

The changes from puberty to maturity are controlled primarily by glands of the body, including the pituitary gland in the brain, the thyroid gland at the front of the throat, the adrenal glands just above the kidneys, and the sex glands. The sex glands in girls are called ovaries and are inside the girl's body. In boys these glands are contained in the sac that

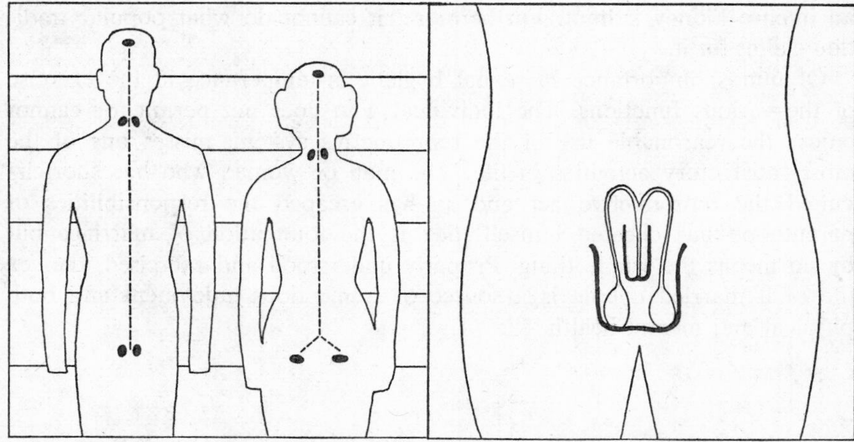

Figs. 15 & 16. During adolescence a small gland near the brain gives off a substance called a "hormone." This hormone, carried by the blood, affects other glands in the body, such as the sex glands, and causes them to give off hormones too. Taken from *The Gift of Life,* © New York State Department of Health, available from Health Education Service, Capitol Station, Albany, New York.

hangs down from the organs that permit urine to pass out of the body. From these glands, which are called testes or testicles, tubes pass upward into little chambers that hold seminal fluid until it is discharged from the body through the male sex organs.

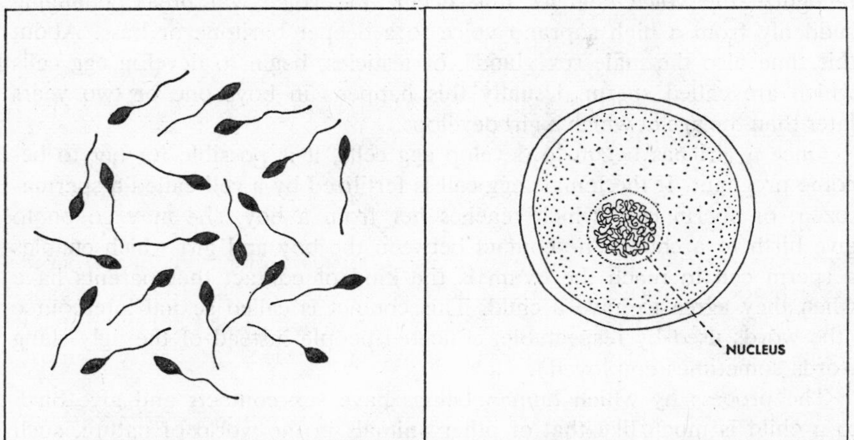

Fig. 17. (LEFT) The sex glands also produce the male and female sex cells. The male sex cells, or sperm, are very small. Enlarged many times, they look like the picture above. Taken from *The Gift of Life,* © New York State Department of Health, available from Health Education Service, Capitol Station, Albany, New York.

Fig. 18. (RIGHT) The female sex cells, or ovum (egg) although a little larger than the male sperm (seed), are no bigger than a pinpoint. Inside . . . both the ovum and the sperm is the substance that makes a child look like his parents. Taken from *The Gift of Life,* © New York State Department of Health, available from Health Education Service, Capitol Station, Albany, New York.

CHANGES IN THE BODY

As a girl reaches puberty, an increase takes place in the width of the area between her hips, and the nipples on her breasts enlarge slightly. Boys change not nearly so much. Girls also may have a slight enlargement of the tissue of the breasts; then hair begins to grow under their arms and above the sex organs. At about twelve or thirteen years of age, girls begin to have a discharge of blood from the sex organs. This is associated with the development in the ovaries of an egg cell, called an ovum. This cell comes out of the ovary into tubes which pass downward into the girl's uterus, or womb. If the egg does not become fertilized by a cell from the male, it simply passes out of the body.

At adolescence the boy may also have a little swelling and pain in his "breasts", but this is not significant. Hormone action in the body is believed to be responsible. Most boys now develop hair under the arms and above the sex organs and, shortly afterwards, the beard begins to grow. The next changes that occur are associated with the voice. Most boys recognize the voice changes that occur; the voice will break, changing suddenly from a high soprano voice to a deeper baritone or bass. About this time also the male sex glands, or testicles, begin to develop egg cells which are called sperm. Usually this happens in boys one or two years later than the age at which a girl develops.

Once a girl has begun to develop egg cells, it is possible for her to become pregnant. If the female egg cell is fertilized by a cell called a spermatozoa, or sperm cell, which reaches her from a boy, she may go on to give birth to a child. The contact between the boy and girl which enables a sperm cell to reach the ovum is the kind of contact that parents have when they agree to have a child. This contact is called sexual intercourse (the words used by respectable, educated people instead of the ugly slang words sometimes employed).

The process by which human beings have sex contacts and give birth to a child is much like that of other animals in the world of nature, such as the hog and sow, the bull and the cow, the stallion and the mare, and the male and female dog or cat. This process developed over thousands of years of differentiation of the lowest forms of life into what is now recognized as the highest form of life . . . human beings.

FAMILY RELATIONSHIPS

In a good American family, the child will have observed early in life that his parents love and respect each other and that they practice kindness and courtesy. Proper education about sex means not only knowledge of how human beings have sex relationships and give birth to children, but also how emotions and social attitudes affect these relationships.

A child begins to be curious anytime after two-and-one-half or three years of age. A child wants to know about why boys are shaped differently from girls. A little boy may wonder why his play leads him much more to playing with boys than with girls. He may actually begin to develop a dislike for girls. Little girls, of course, will react just the opposite. Sometimes, by five or six years of age, a child may ask his mother or father where babies come from. Sometimes, however, he has asked other children with whom he plays; sometimes he has been told by other children even without asking for the information.

Even before going to nursery school, the child may have learned about the physical differences between girls and boys. By the time he reaches elementary school he will already have been associated with other boys and girls. In school, teachers know that they sometimes have to tell children some of the basic facts about the way people grow. When the child studies nature, he learns still more about the differences in sex, and about the way puppies, kittens, rabbits, chickens or guinea pigs are born.

Questions about sex should not be avoided. When a child displays interest, sometimes because of something he has seen in pictures, motion pictures, television or other places, the parents must be prepared to give an answer.

By the time the boy and girl reach high school, they will find that in many schools biology is taught. This deals with the structure of living things, the methods by which they reproduce, their health and growth. Furthermore, courses in social studies are offered that consider education for family life, relations between people, how to make a home, social hygiene, and health. Once such courses were taught separately to boys and girls. Attitudes have now changed, and in most instances, boys and girls are educated together about the kind of relationships they will have in life.

Dr. John Money, associate professor of medical psychology and pediatrics in the school of medicine of Johns Hopkins University, notes that children begin to differentiate about the age of three or four. The girl develops feminine ways and mannerisms in posture, behavior, and talk that are like those of her mother, grandmother, older sister or governess. The boy begins to imitate his father. Little girls become flirtatious around men. A little girl will wheedle and cajole her father in a way quite different from that of her brother. The father will be more stern with the brother. The boy has a special place in his mother's heart. Little boys know that there they can find a soft spot when father gets too strict. The little boy also likes to play the man's part when he goes along with his mother on a shopping trip. Thus one frequently hears little boys and little girls saying that they will marry their mother or their father.

This also is the time when girls begin to play at baby care with dolls, and boys to operate toy trains and trucks. What is important is the choice of items and ways of play. A girl may like to play house, but if a boy joins her, he should join her as the man in the house. The boy who causes some alarm to psychologists is the one who constantly organizes games of house and wants to play a girl's part. Psychologists see a great difference between the four-year-old boy who has a girl doll and plays mother to it, and the boy who has a boy doll to which he plays father.

Dr. Money has also observed that children are bound to pick up sexual knowledge and piece it together; this occurs with any child who is not deaf, dumb, blind, or feeble-minded. Therefore parents should give sexual information to guard against errors of fact, conviction, or emotional attitude. When boys and girls develop behavior opposite to that of their own sex, the origin frequently is something that occurred in childhood.

A three-year-old child who is going to have a baby brother or sister will want information about why the mother is different. Surely at this time the child can be told that the new baby lives and grows within the mother; but certainly he need not at this tender age be given so much factual information as to produce mental indigestion. The child may ask "How does the baby get out?" The answer should be: "The body of the mother is built with a tunnel through which the baby will come when it is born."

The child may also ask about the way in which the baby begins to be born. Psychologists have found that the next installment in instruction should introduce the fact that the father contributes to the mother some 200 million sperm cells which enter into a race to meet the mother's egg cell, which has developed in her body. Only one sperm can win. In telling this story, one may easily use simple diagrams showing how sperms develop in the body of the father and how they swim out of the father and into the "baby tunnel" in the mother.

The time when information is to be given depends, of course, on the amount of curiosity manifested by the child and the judgment of the parent as to when the time is ripe to give information. If a child is observed with other children in play that involves sexual attitudes or practices, certainly the time is right to give adequate information. In a statistical research made by Professor Alfred C. Kinsey, 40 per cent of young children before adolescence had been found to indulge in sex play with children of the opposite sex. Almost all children engage in exhibiting the sexual parts to other children, but 20 per cent stop at this point. About 81 per cent of children have felt with their fingers the organs of a child of the opposite sex. About 55 per cent actually try to imitate sexual play as in the case of adults. (This last type of play is three times more frequent in boys who mature early.) The average age of the first play between sexes is eight to nine years.

In his advice to parents, Dr. Money recommends that parents do not indulge in undue condemnation of the child who is observed in sex play activities. The idea should be to inform the child that this type of activity is not looked upon with favor by most people. Such relationships may be indulged by adults but not by children, exactly as there are many other activities suitable for adults that are not suitable for children. Children respond easily to proper instruction and suggestion. They should not be driven into the belief that all sexual relations and sexual pleasure are abominable. They should not be driven to avoidance of the opposite sex.

All authorities now agree that masturbation is physically and mentally harmless except when condemnation has been so severe as to create worry and a sense of guilt. Practically every child can understand that this is a practice of which his parents do not approve.

The child who has reached the teen ages will or should know the basic essentials of the manner of human reproduction of life and how the body responds in such activities. What the teenager needs is information and guidance about how boys and girls should behave together. The girl especially should be given enough information to create in her a wish to avoid getting pregnant. She should understand the hazards of an emotional stimulus that makes her reduce her guard. Unfortunately some parents are so much handicapped by their own prudery, particularly women who were raised in the prudish atmosphere that prevailed in the early years of the twentieth century, that they find it difficult to concern themselves properly with the sexual problems of their children.

MODESTY

In many families, children have seen their naked bodies and those of other children before they are four years old. The baby will not realize that exhibiting his sexual organs is not to be practiced unless he is so informed. Mothers are always showing naked babies to admiring relatives and friends. However, by the time the child is four years old, exhibition of its body is not usual. A boy or girl eight years old is expected to be careful about running around naked, even in the family home. Modesty is a necessary part of the social training of a child. A child is therefore taught to regard the sexual organs with respect, but not necessarily to be ashamed of them. The child observes that grownups, men and women, cover themselves and do not appear naked.

Customs differ throughout the world. In some European countries, nude bathing is common practice. In the United States, customs have changed greatly from the time when women and girls went into the water wearing dresses that covered the entire body down to the ankles and long stockings that went high above the knees.

Unfortunately, the prudery of the past has led to all sorts of slang names for the sexual organs of the body. Doctors have scientific names for them. The boy has a penis, and associated with it, a scrotum, or sac, in which lie the testicles. Probably all of us would benefit if these scientific words came into common usage, and replaced the slang terms.

Similarly, mothers who are training a child about excretion develop what are commonly called "cute terms" for urination, for emptying the bowels, or even for going to the toilet. The child can easily learn to say "toilet" when it wants to go to the toilet. Similarly, it could learn to use such terms as "I want to urinate" or "I want to empty my bowels."

Many girls and women do not really know the proper names for their sex organs. They use, therefore, the slang terms and, along with these, half a dozen different terms for the act of menstruation. Menstruation is the right word for the bleeding that occurs in the girl periodically after she begins to mature. Since this condition occurs periodically, the use of the

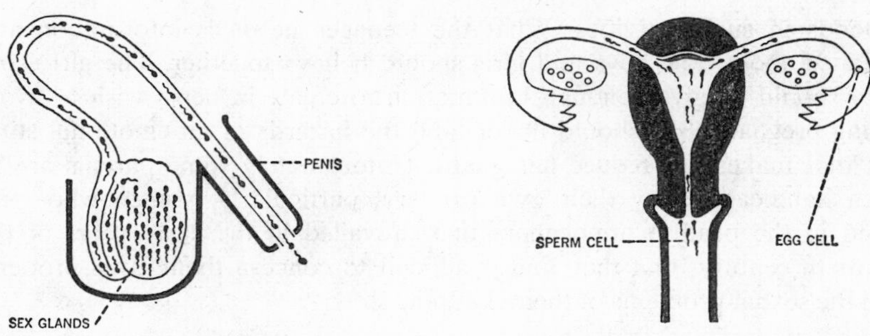

Fig. 19. (LEFT) When a boy is around 14, his sex glands begin to produce sex cells, or sperm. These cells may pass out through the penis during sleep, a natural happening. This also occurs later during mating. Taken from *The Gift of Life*, © New York State Department of Health, available from Health Education Service, Capitol Station, Albany, New York.

Fig. 20. (RIGHT) The male sex cells use their threadlike tails to move into the womb and to seek out the egg cells. If one of the male sperm meets and unites with an egg cell, a new life begins. Taken from *The Gift of Life*, © New York State Department of Health, available from Health Education Service, Capitol Station, Albany, New York.

word period is not considered a slang term. However, the girl in high school or college or the girl who works will probably have picked up from other girls such slang terms as "the curse", "red flag", and similar terms. Properly named, the sex organs of the girl include the outer organ, which is the vulva, and the inner tunnel, which is the vagina. Associated with these organs is the nerve bundle that gives the girl sexual satisfaction. This is called the clitoris.

When the egg cell, or ovum, reaches the uterus and is met there by a sperm cell from the male, which in sex play may have been deposited at the very entrance into the body—that is, the vulva—or higher up, in the vagina, the girl may become pregnant. If she does become pregnant, the two cells joined together begin to grow at once from an infinitesimal amount of material that cannot be seen with the naked eye into a baby, which will at the time of birth, if normal, weigh anywhere from five to nine pounds. During the child's development in the womb or uterus, the mother's abdomen swells to make space for the growing infant After nine months, in the ordinary case, the child's body begins to descend, passing through the vagina, through the vulva, and out. Actually, then, the process is much like the one that occurs in other animals. The male sex organ is adapted to depositing the sperm in the vagina of the girl during sexual intercourse. During this act the organ, by the flow of blood into it, becomes engorged and harder and stiffer so as to be able to penetrate into the vagina.

The sex act must be regarded with respect, not only because it is fundamental to the perpetuation of the life of man on this earth, but also because it constitutes the most intimate personal relationship that can occur between men and women. For this very reason, educators and philosophers since the earliest times have given much thought to the customs and regulations that control such human relationships.

TELLING THE CHILD

Children are invariably interested in babies and, indeed, often ask their mother or father if they can have a baby brother or baby sister. When the child asks such questions, or when he wants to know where a baby comes from, the answer should be truthful and honest within the limits of the child's understanding. During the era of prudery, children were told that babies were brought by the doctor in his medicine bag, or that they were found in a rosebush, or that they were brought by the stork; somehow people delight in perpetuating these fables.

The child who has come near the period of adolescence may be told that the baby grows in the body of the mother. The child may be told that the mother contributes an egg cell and that the father contributes a sperm cell, and that these two join to begin the development of the baby. They may be told that the father and mother's act of joining together to make a baby is a demonstration of their love for each other, of their love for their children, and of their desire to have a family. Actually the child already knows, in most instances, that there must be male and female elements to give birth, as he has observed this among lower animals.

Most important in the education and training of the child in matters related to sex is satisfying the questions that occur in the child's mind that may serve as the basis for more education later. If parents equivocate and fail to give full information, the child will doubt that he can depend upon the mother and father for honesty and authenticity.

Children should not be reprimanded, repressed, or punished for asking honest questions about these matters. However, the child should not be encouraged to dwell upon sex or to make it a major interest of his life. Parents should not be constantly prompting the child to ask for further information. Children who are growing have many other interests which are probably far more pleasurable and important to them than detailed knowledge about sex. Once given authentic information, they will be quite willing to wait for details.

SHAME

Modesty can be taught without making the child ashamed of himself or of his body. Shame is an emotion that should not be utilized in teaching.

The child learns to cover himself because it is the custom to keep the sex organs covered. If the child knows that older persons always keep their sex organs covered, he will want to do the same.

Nearly all normal children have little love affairs during their first years in school. They will come home when they are six or seven years of age and announce that another child is their girlfriend or boyfriend. Nothing need be made of such incidents. Moreover, parents should not tease children about childish love affairs. Teasing may cause the child to believe that there is something inherently wrong about liking, love, or sex, or that these emotions are improper. If the child has been teased, when a real love subsequently develops, the child will carefully conceal all information from the parents.

Without interchange of information, the parent does not have an opportunity to help the child learn how he or she may select the best companions. Furthermore, as was emphasized by Dr. Thurman Rice, a teacher in Indiana University Medical College, the curiosity of the child may lead him to regard as evil an apparently harmless relationship with some member of the opposite sex.

Parents who tease their young children about friends of the opposite sex and seek in that way to prevent them from making dangerous associations should learn that the best way to insure that so-called puppy love will not go too far is merely to treat it as a matter of course. When a parent demands that a child break a friendship, the tendency is for the child at once to protect the friend. This may intensify a friendship that would otherwise not become anything more.

Boys and girls frequently play "father and mother" games. Harm seldom comes from such play unless through some mischance the children think of the sexual relationship as the only relationship between the father and mother. Another type of game in which the children frequently indulge is playing doctor. When a doctor comes he frequently inserts a thermometer in the rectum; when the child sees this done or knows that it is being done he may want to expose the body for the same purpose. Much worry has been suffered needlessly by devoted parents who fail to understand their children. All children are curious. They naturally will examine their bodies, or, if the opportunity presents itself, the body of another child of the same sex or of the opposite sex. Misguided parents may think that this is exactly the same as if adults were to do this. Actually the child may be told that once his curiosity has been satisfied, there is no reason for doing this over and over again. The curiosity has been satisfied, and that is the end of the episode. On the other hand, if the children are severely punished, they will remember that the punishment was for something that should be hidden, and so possibly they will continue the experience whenever there is an opportunity to do so without being caught.

MASTURBATION

The word masturbation, or "self-stimulation," was for many years taboo in any kind of discussion except medical discussion. Children frequently find that playing with the genitals conveys a pleasurable sensation. In other circumstances, itching or burning may be a symptom that causes the child to finger himself repeatedly. If the habit persists, a physician should study the child's condition to make sure that nothing is physically wrong. If a physical condition is not related to the habit, the child should be taught that playing with the organs is simply bad manners and attracts unfavorable attention. Parents should remember that one cannot break a bad habit from the outside. Only the person who has the habit can break it. Patience and perseverance may be required beyond what the average child can be expected to have.

Normal children will seldom practice masturbation to excess unless they are being prompted by some older child or some other person. For this reason their relationship with other children may require study. However, children of young ages have many interests. One need not worry about their being too much concerned about an instinct to play with the body. Healthy activities can be encouraged instead. Exercise and play in the open air are far more conducive to good results than having the child sit alone in a room poring over books and pictures. School interests, play, club work of all sorts, scout exercises, athletic teams and similar activities will permit little time for forms of sex activity that might be harmful.

The attitude toward masturbation has changed greatly with further study and with open discussion of the matter. Normal children, free from psychological attitudes that are wrong, are not likely to practice such play to excess.

If the boy is developing rapidly, he may have, during this changing period of life, emissions from the sex organs while he is asleep or dreaming. When mothers find the sheets stained in this way, they often become unnecessarily alarmed. They should realize that what has occurred is normal. Too much attention paid to the incident will focus the attention of the boy on the sexual organs rather than give him a natural attitude toward the occurrence.

THE TEEN AGES

When children enter the teens, which is at thirteen years of age, they really need help and understanding. At this time powerful and utterly new forces are arising in the body. New impulses bring unfamiliar stimulation.

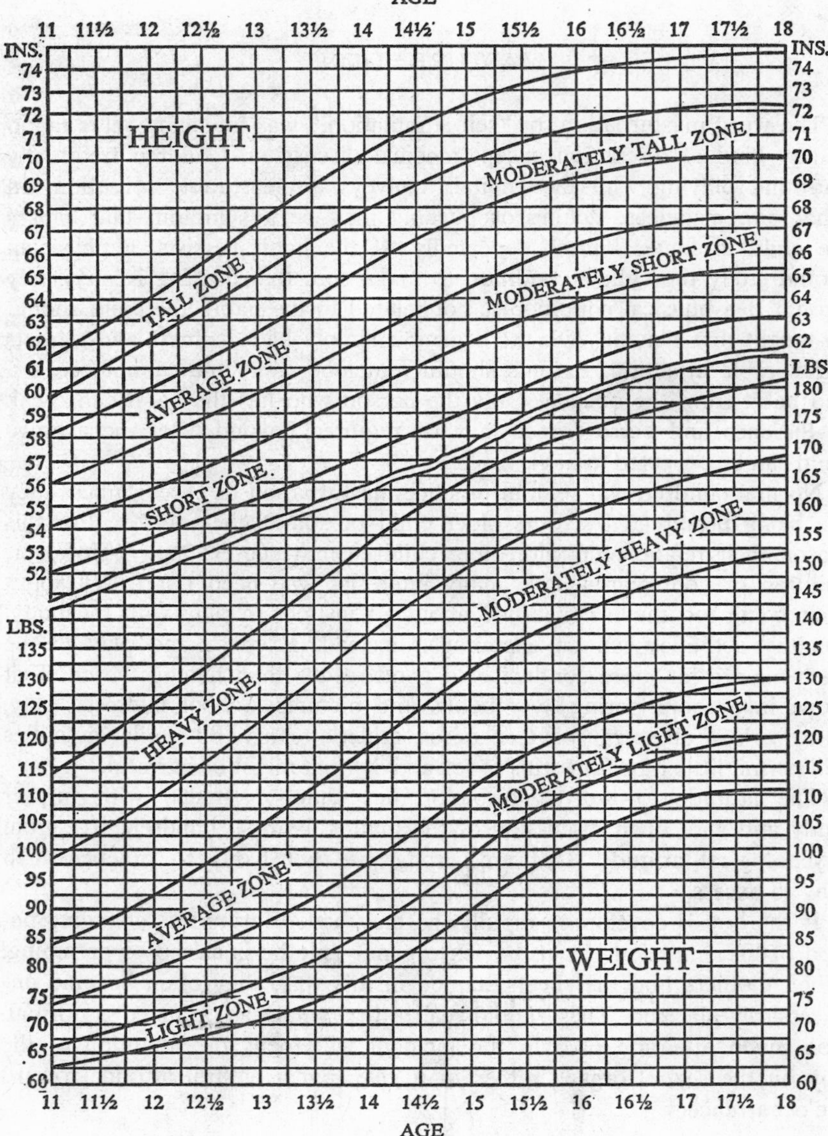

Fig. 21. A physical growth record for boys. The figures on this physical growth record come from scientific studies of many boys as they grew. On the chart, ages are shown in six intervals along the top and bottom. Height is marked in inches along the sides of the upper portion. Weight is marked in pounds along the sides of the lower portion. There are five zones for the heights of boys at each age from 11 to 18. These are labeled "tall," "moderately tall," "average," "moderately short," and "short." There are five zones for the weights of boys

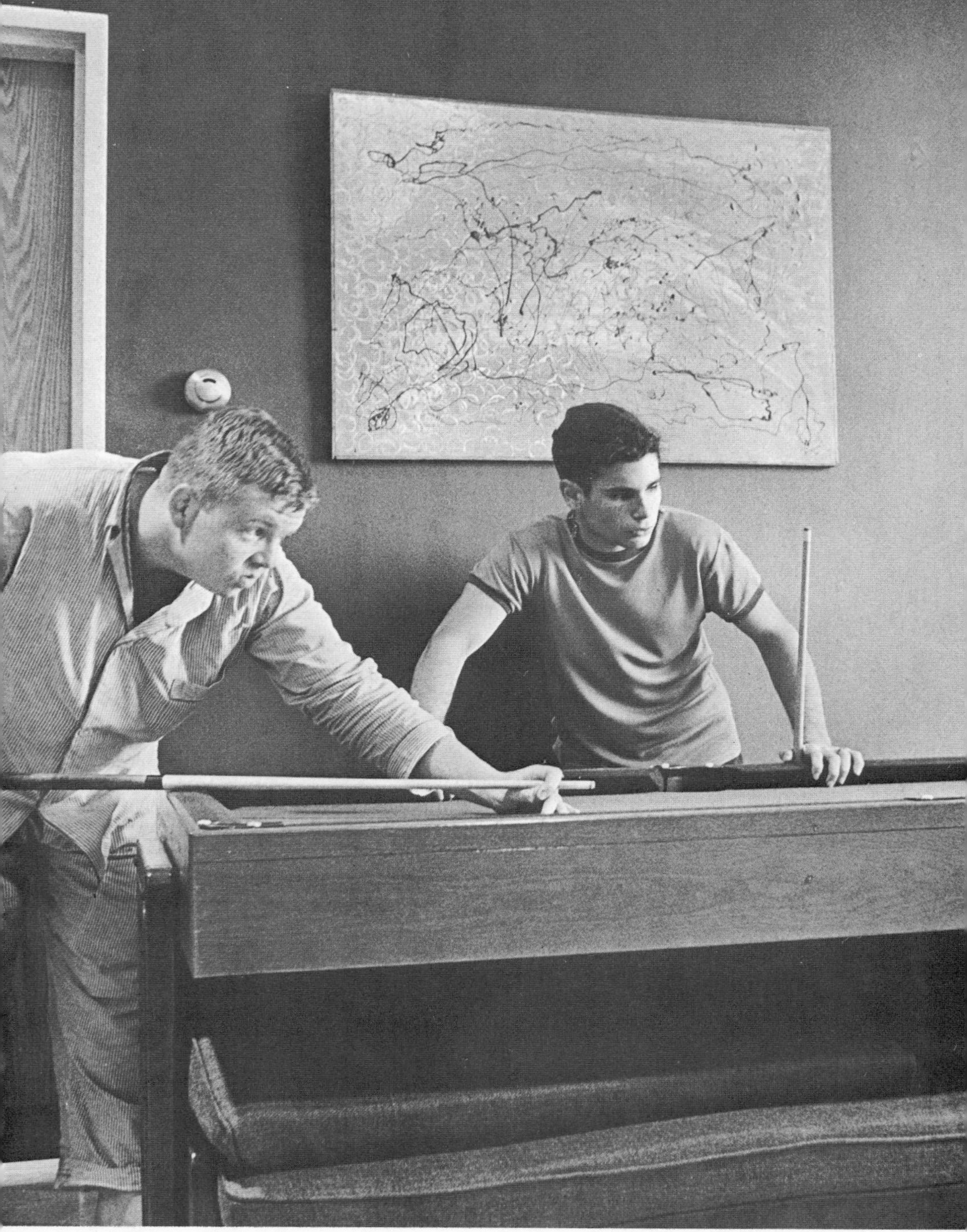

PLATE **39.** Patient in Montefiore's Adolescent Unit shoots a game of pool in the lounge with a teen-age visitor. One of the most recent innovations in hospital planning, the Adolescent Unit is devoted exclusively to patients aged 13 to 18. *(Courtesy of Montefiore Hospital and Medical Center, New York, and Ed Bagwell.)*

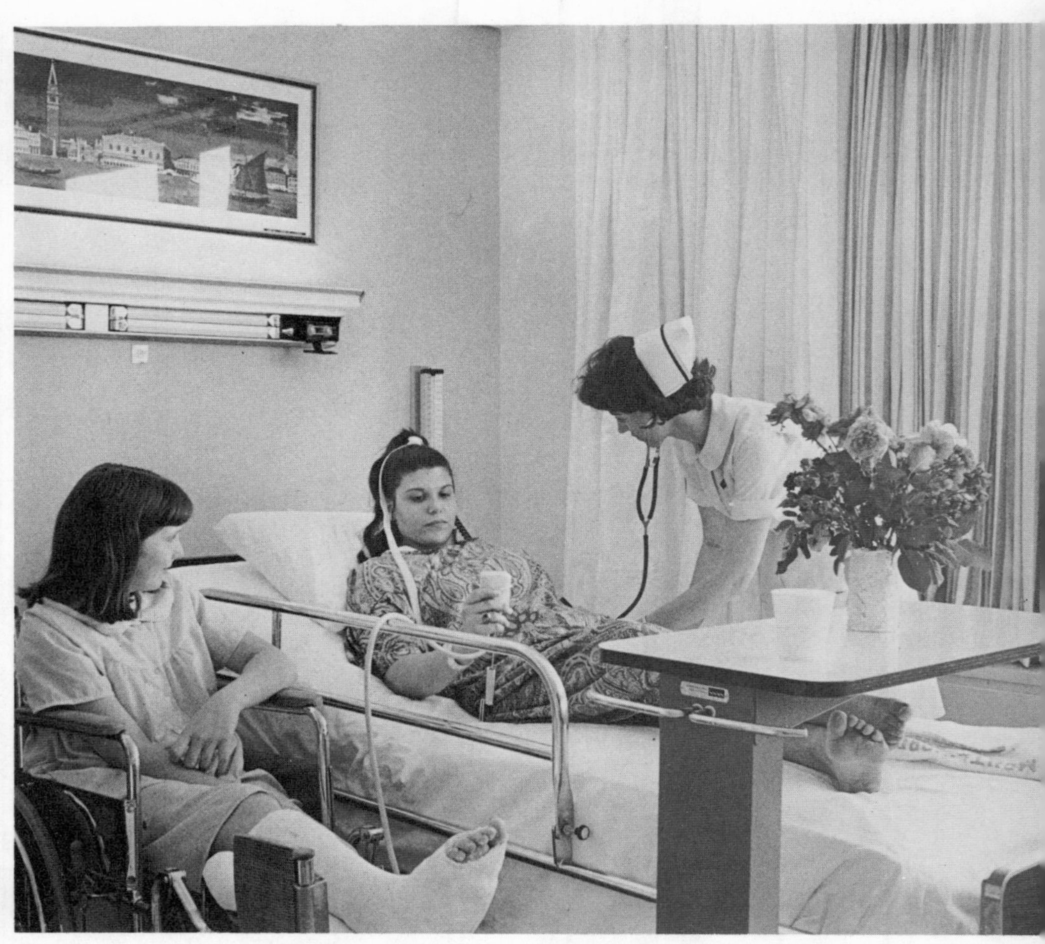

PLATE **40.** Nurse Norma Ellis interrupts a gab fest between two teen-age patients to take a blood pressure reading in Montefiore's Adolescent Unit. *(Courtesy of Montefiore Hospital and Medical Center, New York, and Ed Bagwell.)*

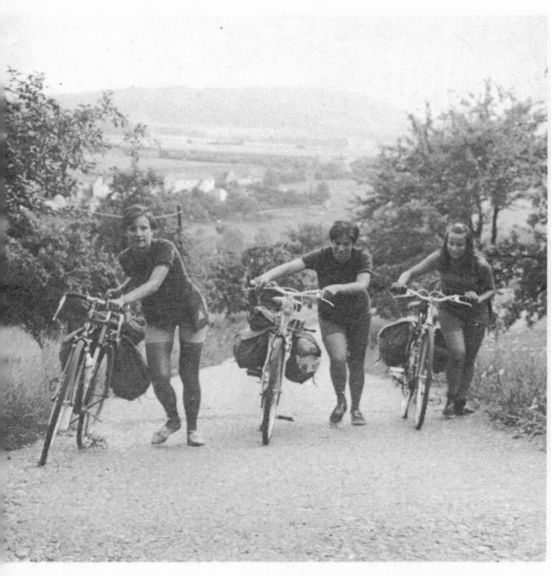

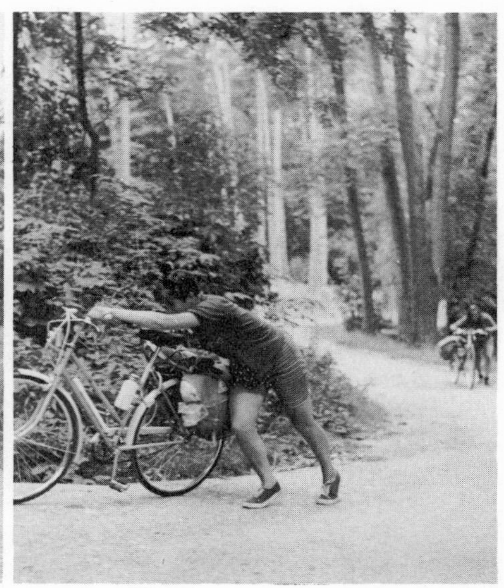

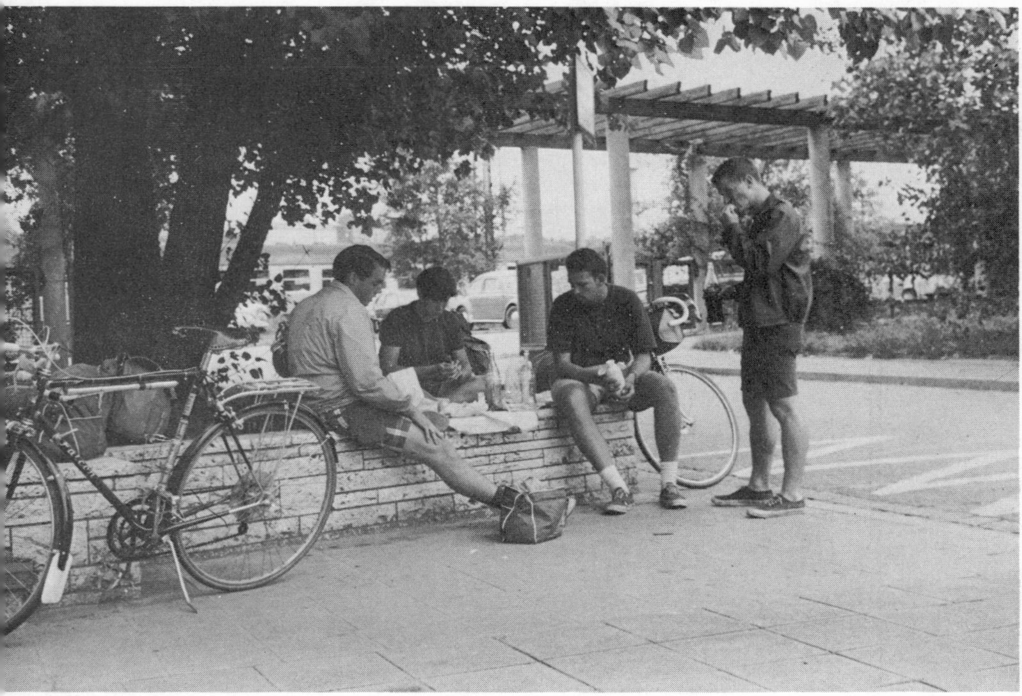

PLATES **41–43.** Exercise in adolescence. Young boys and girls growing into manhood and womanhood face new problems and new situations as their bodies and minds begin changing. During the teen years the body must be cared for and developed. These young people know that physical exercise helps develop one's muscles, stimulates blood circulation, builds up a good appetite, and promotes sound sleep. *(American Youth Hostels, Inc.)*

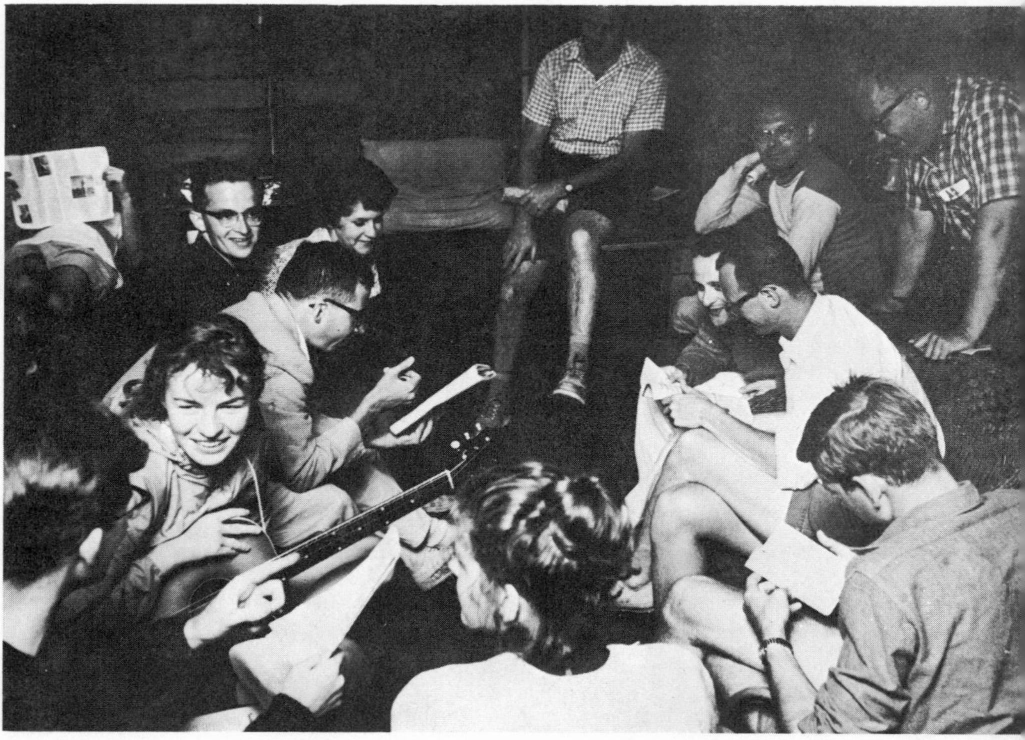

PLATES **44–45.** Group social activities in adolescence. Adolescence is a time for making many friends, taking part in group activities, and winning the attention of members of the opposite sex. These young people are having a good time together, talking, sharing their ideas, and gaining a better understanding of each other. *(American Youth Hostels, Inc.* and *92nd Street Young Men's and Young Women's Hebrew Association, New York City.)*

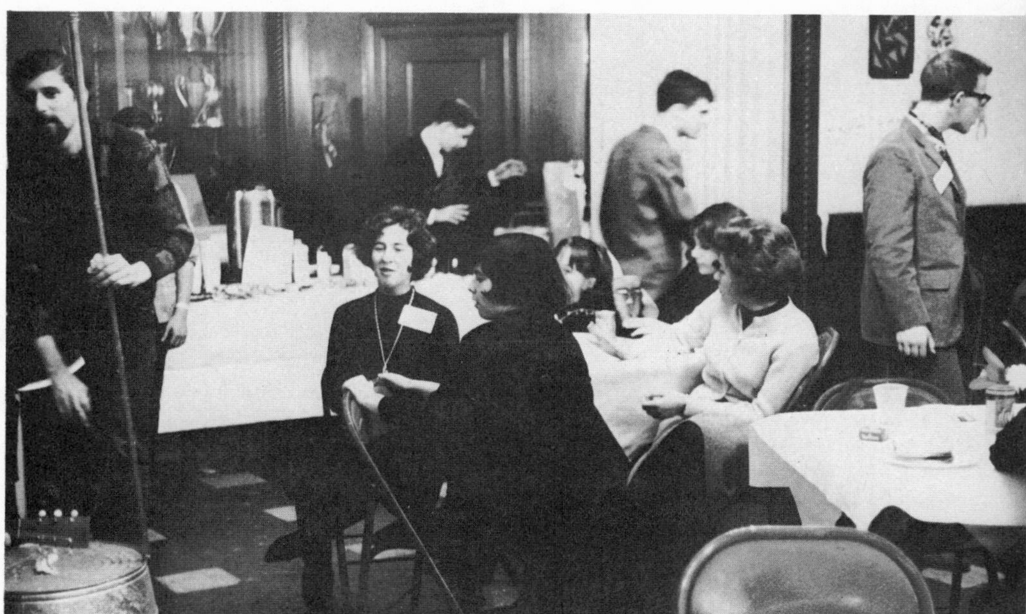

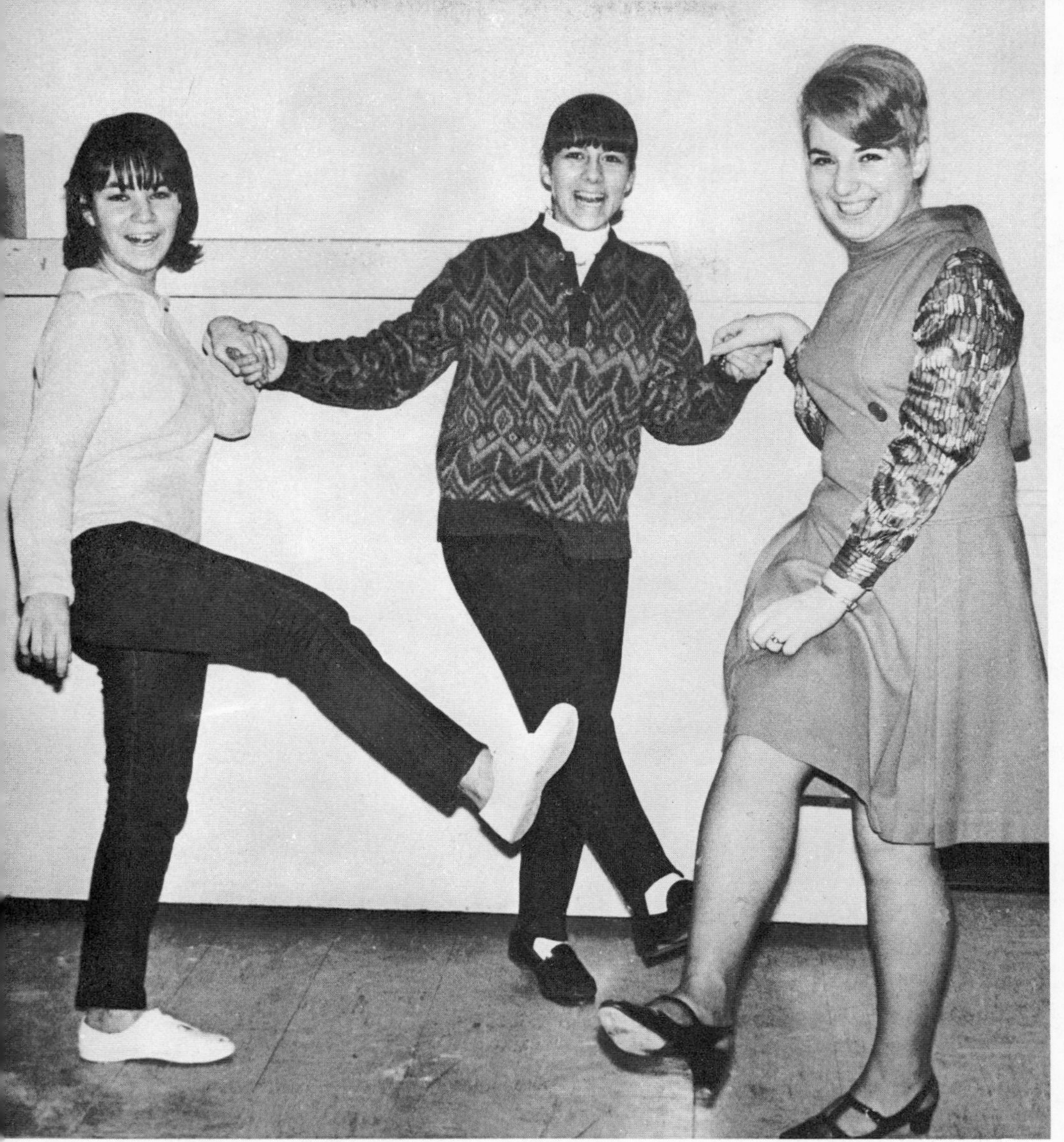

PLATE **46.** These girls are putting on a skit before a group of their friends, obviously aware of the importance in the teen years of developing charm and attractiveness. *(92nd Street Young Men's and Women's Hebrew Association, New York City.)*

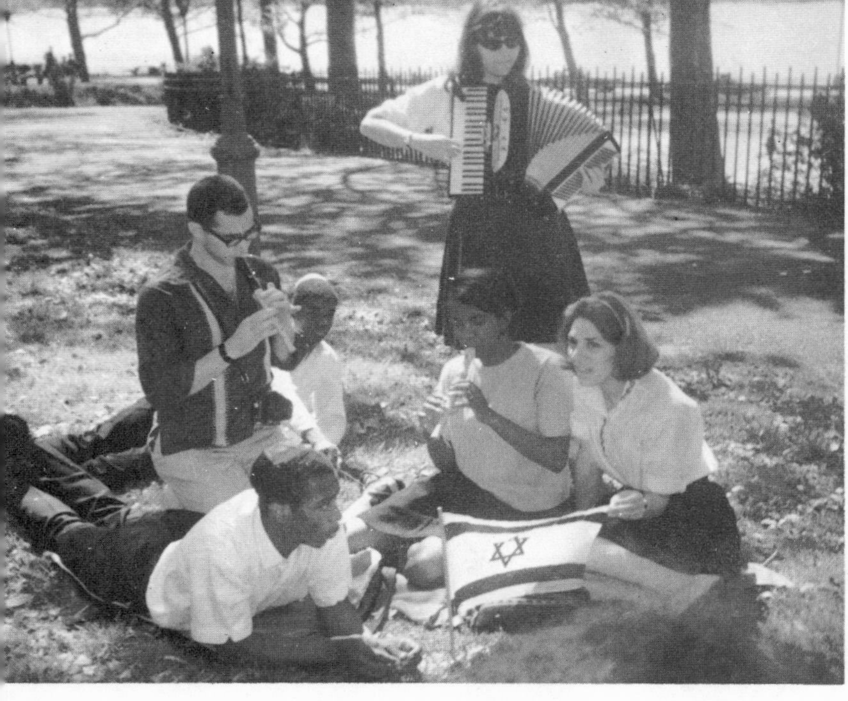

PLATES **47–48.** Taking part in group activities, such as these youngsters are doing, will help them to develop mentally, emotionally, socially, and spiritually. *(Hatzaad Harishon Youth, 92nd Street Young Men's and Young Women's Hebrew Association, New York City.)*

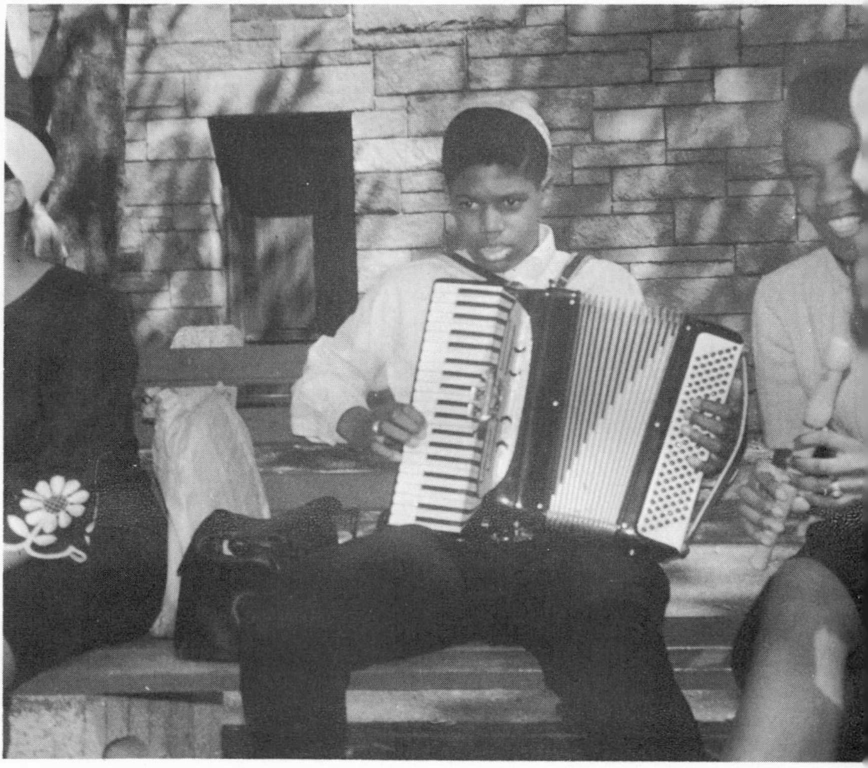

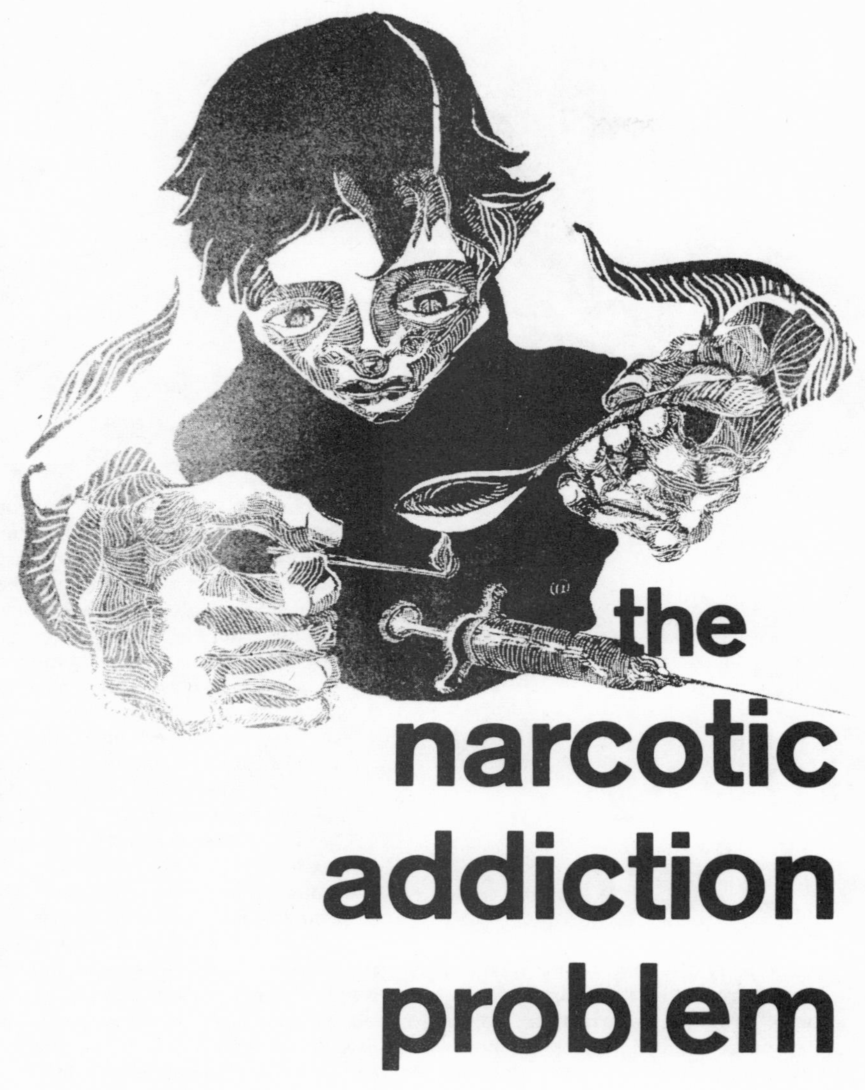

PLATE **49.** The Narcotic Addiction Problem. No one can say with complete certainty how many people are addicted to drugs. It is usually estimated that there are some 60,000 addicts in the United States. Addiction is characterized by three separate but related phenomena: tolerance, habituation, and physical dependence. A substantial number of addicts in large cities begin using narcotic drugs when they are around sixteen years old, the age when adolescents are likely to be confronted by new challenges of maturity. *(From* The Narcotic Addiction Problem *by Dr. Charles Winick, The American Social Health Association.)*

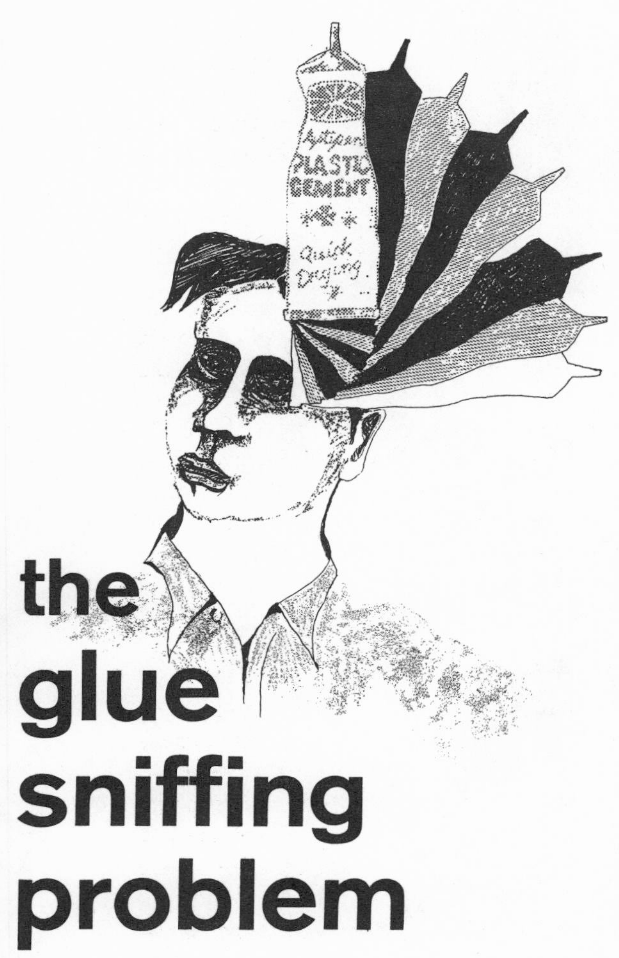

the glue sniffing problem

PLATE **50.** The Glue-Sniffing Problem. The most recent manifestation of modern youth's quest for sensation has been a substantial number of young people who have begun sniffing glue. The current glue-sniffing epidemic is a manifestation of an age-old interest in the gratifications provided by inhalation. According to some estimates, the national figure for the number of children and adolescents who sniff runs into many thousands. As with the effects of alcohol or other drugs, there are substantial individual differences among those who sniff glue. The available findings indicated that glue sniffing is for a passive retreat, and the personality of a sniffer is likely to display many of the characteristics found in alcoholics and drug addicts. At least two basic types of sniffers can be identified and described as the *hard core* (one who is strongly dependent on the practice); and *accidental* (one who engages in glue sniffing under the influence of peer-group contacts but is not strongly involved in the practice and can give it up without too much disappointment). Information disseminated about the dangers of glue sniffing is best presented in a scientific manner, with emphasis on dangers to health. The availability of educational materials, and of experience in the rehabilitation of glue sniffers, all provide opportunities that should enable the communities to mount campaigns that have a reasonable chance of being effective. Parents can help in coping with the problem if they become more aware of its nature and of the symptoms and causes of glue sniffing. *(From* The Glue-Sniffing Problem *by Dr. Charles Winick and Jacob Goldstein, The American Social Health Association.)*

Joyful with the new sensation of being "grown-up," and perhaps even overwhelmed by a feeling of freedom previously unknown, children may go to excess. As long as there is some doubt that the child is really growing up, he may want to prove that he is grown up. Boys learn to smoke and swear. They affect far more knowledge of women and girls than they really have, and they like to tell other boys of their conquests. If they are permitted to drive a car, they like to prove their ability by excess speed. The child of this kind is overcompensating for inexperience–whistling in the dark to prove that he is not afraid.

Adolescence is also a period in which there is much dreaming and fantasy. The child may be called "lazy" because of the desire sometimes to sit and dream. However, the periods are quite normal, and the child should not be injured by being called shiftless or lazy.

At this time, too, the girl usually passes through a "boy-struck" period. She giggles and makes herself conspicuous. She wants to use plenty of cosmetics, wear excessively high heels, put on long dresses for evening visits. At this time, more than ever, she needs sympathetic guidance. If the child has not been previously informed of the nature of sex relationships and of the various functions of the sex organs, this is the time to give the information. The facts should be given in a natural manner when it seems likely that the information is needed.

Assuming that adolescent boys and girls have been thoroughly informed concerning the subject, particularly the positive and beautiful phases, they may at this time be told of some of the negative and doubtful phases. This should not be done with the intention of shocking or alarming the child excessively. However, such young children should know that conception without marriage constitutes a tremendous problem, and that the girl who becomes pregnant before marriage will suffer severely from social condemnation.

Venereal diseases were formerly uncontrollable by most of the methods known to medicine; frequently young people were infected, and their entire lives were often ruined. Since the discovery of antibiotic drugs, the cure of venereal diseases is possible. Of this more will be said later. However, the child should know that contacts of sex organs may lead to infection of such organs, and that the danger lies in concealing the infection and in failing to get medical attention promptly. This is the kind of infor-

---

at each age. Each zone is labeled to correspond to a similar height zone. For example, "moderately heavy" corresponds to "moderately tall." You will see that the zones of weight are wider than the zones of height. This suggests that normally boys of the same age vary more in weight than in height. *A Boy and His Physique,* National Dairy Council. Prepared by the Joint Committee on Health Problems in Education, National Education Association and American Medical Association, using data prepared by Harold V. Meredith, State University of Iowa. The record is produced by courtesy of the Joint Committee.

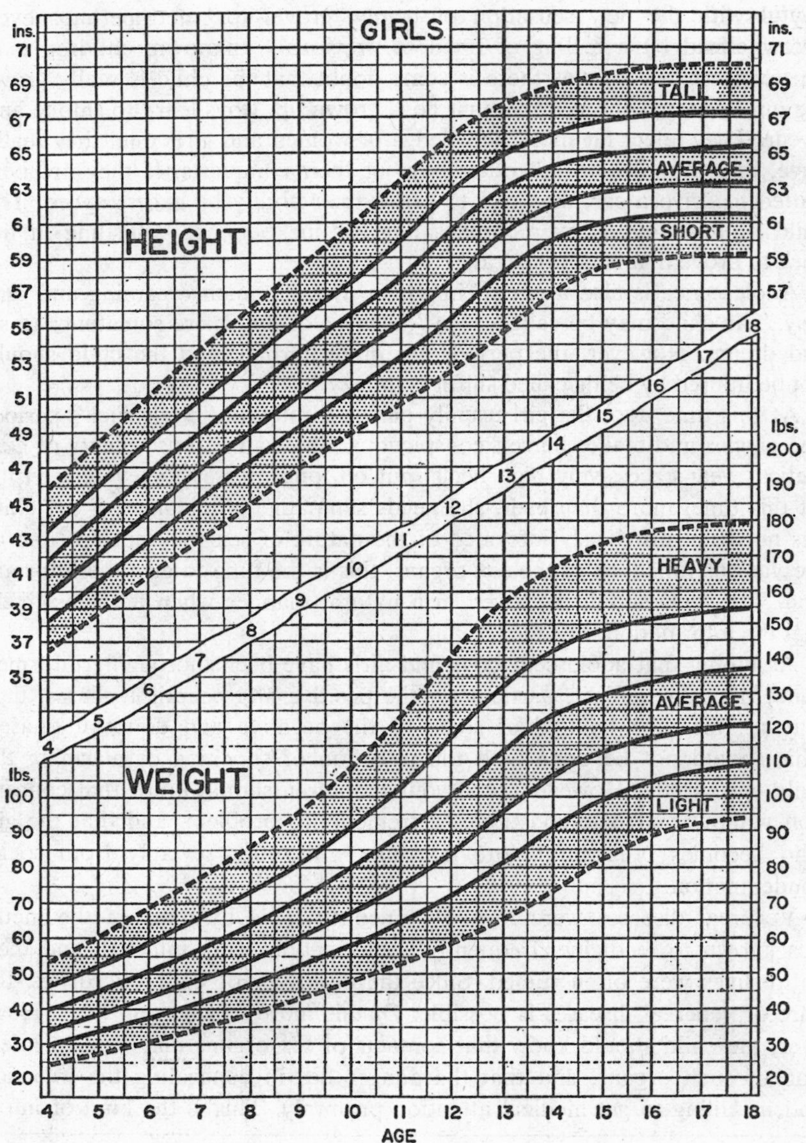

Fig. 22. A Physical Growth Record for Girls: These figures come from scientific studies of many girls as they grew from 14 to 18 years. The record for these years is shown here. Ages are shown in yearly intervals along the middle and bottom. Height is marked in inches along the right and left sides of the upper portion. Weight is marked in pounds along the right and left sides of the lower portion. There are three zones for the heights of girls of each age from 14 to 18. These are labeled "tall," "average," and "short." There are three zones for the

mation that should be given equally to older children or to adults. If the information is given in a factual manner, the child is likely to appreciate the confidence and to realize that the information was supplied for his own protection.

Boys and girls over thirteen years of age have probably already heard much about sexual relationships. The careful parent need not hesitate then to explain to the child something of the details of these relationships. Unfortunately, one of the first steps required may be to get rid of a vast amount of misinformation that has been given by playmates and other children. Moreover, many parents themselves believe many facts that are not really the truth.

This is the time when a child can be made to understand that sexual relations are of the utmost consequence to the welfare of the child himself, to his family, and to his nation. Sexual relationships are for those who are sufficiently mature to have children and to raise them. They should obviously be married in order to do so. Sexual relationships are a great responsibility and should not even be considered without this sense of responsibility.

TEEN-AGE MARRIAGE

Teen-age marriages are becoming more and more frequent. Pregnant teen-age girls are coming more and more frequently to the hospitals. Obviously, a teenager is seldom ready to be married or to have a child. The importance of marriage may be taught at any age of development. However, this knowledge becomes especially important as the child reaches the end of the teen-age period, when he or she might consider marriage.

Marriage is more than just a license for two people to live together and have sexual relationships. Marriage is the foundation on which the home is built and maintained. The home is the basis of the school, the church, the government, industry, and all social relationships. Thurman Rice emphasized, "A community of good homes invariably has good schools, influential churches, thrifty, industrious, intelligent, educated people, and an acceptable government. A community of bad homes cannot survive."

---

weights of girls of each age. Each zone is labeled to correspond to a similar height zone. For example, "heavy" corresponds to "tall," and both are shown in the same shade. You will see that the zones of weight are wider than the zones of height. This suggests that normally girls of the same age vary more in weight than in height. From *A Girl and Her Figure,* National Dairy Council. Prepared by the Joint Committee on Health Problems in Education of the National Education Association and American Medical Association, using data prepared by Harold V. Meredith, State University of Iowa. The record is reproduced by courtesy of the Joint Committee.

These facts should be made plain to young people and, if they are reasonably intelligent, they will adjust themselves accordingly.

Young people today are in a difficult position. They develop sexually early in life and they are constantly stimulated sexually by the society in which they live. They see sophisticated motion pictures, pick up risqué books at any newsstand, hear suggestive songs on the radio and on television, and may actually see all sorts of irregularities whenever they go to a soda fountain or restaurant. Yet, strong social and religious restraints are put upon them to repress this sexual stimulation until they marry.

ATHLETICS

Athletics and sports are important for boys and girls during the teenage period. Not only do they help develop strong muscles, but they also have an important role in the development of character. Tennis, basketball, baseball, and track are further valuable in that they occupy the attention of boys to such an extent that they are much less likely to be concerned with sex relations. When the young athlete gets sufficiently tired, goes to bed and falls promptly to sleep, he is not likely to become involved in sexual fantasies. Moreover, athletic training requires a somewhat abstemious life, and success in athletics is built upon self-discipline.

Girls were formerly little interested in athletics. Modern life has, however, brought many possibilities for young women to engage in such games as basketball, tennis, softball, swimming and various forms of track events. The problem for the girl is whether or not to continue athletic sports at the time of menstruation. Unless the menstruation is excessive or accompanied by unfavorable symptoms, the girl will find herself quite able to continue most of her activities after the first day.

THE CRUSH

From time to time, as girls grow, they develop a deep friendship with some other girl, often with a teacher. Girls usually call this a crush. Such crushes, if not too deep or enduring, are a normal part of growth. Usually this may be the young adult's first experience of really loving someone outside his own family. Often girls with a crush will want to hold and to kiss the person for whom they have this deep feeling. However, the crush should not be allowed to develop to an intimacy which approaches a homosexual level. Marriage must be between people of different sexes. If they want to fulfill their lives as they grow up, they must do what they can to avoid intensifying the feeling and the intimacy of the crush.

RELATIONSHIPS WITH THE OPPOSITE SEX

Dr. Katherine Whiteside Taylor, who has been concerned with such problems in the Baltimore (Md.) public schools, points out that parents must do what they can to enhance interest in the opposite sex. The first step is to provide an opportunity to meet as many attractive members of the opposite sex as possible. The second is to encourage interest at the first sign that the youngster has an interest in someone of the opposite sex. An example of this interest is that a growing boy normally admires pictures of actresses or admires beauty in women.

In a previous generation, children went to parties where kissing games were a tentative attempt at intimacy. There, however, a whole group of other boys and girls and parents were available as protection. Just how far youngsters today are to go with holding hands, necking, and kissing is a problem that concerns everyone interested in adolescent behavior. Some attempt to make contact with the opposite sex is normal. What becomes hazardous is the intensity of necking that involves the handling of portions of the body sensitive to sexual stimulation. One parent said to his son who started off on a date, "You are lucky to have such a nice girl to take out. Try to give her a wonderful time. She probably won't be hurt if you even try to caress her just a little. But you know where to stop, and both her parents and yours can trust you."

Couples begin to pair off; then starts the period called "going steady." In the life of the 1960s, going steady has become far more frequent than was the case in the 1920s. Teachers have observed that going steady begins far too early in many high schools because it is the fashion. Girls like to display their ability to hold a young man. They like to wear a fraternity pin or other symbol of "possession." However, such relationships should not be established before they can have some real meaning for some future sharing of the lives of the two people most concerned.

One of the serious difficulties with going steady is the considerable reaction that may develop if one or the other parties to this relationship suddenly decides that it must be ended. At such times, understanding parents can be helpful. Young women suffer inordinately with what is called "a broken heart" at the ending of such a love affair. The suffering can be about as severe as any in human experience. The suffering is particularly intense for the person who has been rejected. At such times parents and friends and other counselors can help the rejected person understand the reasons for the break-up and can build up the confidence of the rejected person in himself so that he will be able to re-establish his life. Once a person has passed through such an experience he will perhaps on the next occasion have a better realization of the significance of real love as a true partnership.

CHOICE OF A MATE

One of the most important choices to be made in human life is the choice of a mate, certainly more important than the selection of a business, trade or profession. If the choice of a mate is made on the basis of romance associated with reason, the chance is greater of success in the end than if it is made wholly on the basis of sexual attraction. In the United States, young people are supposed to be free to make their own selection of a marriage partner. The parents may indicate their preferences, but they should not arbitrarily interfere. When young people are under age, they must have the consent of their parents to marry. In American social life, the path to marriage commonly passes through five stages: dating, keeping company, going steady, private understanding, and engagement.

DATING

Dating is society's way of giving young people an opportunity to become acquainted with many persons of the opposite sex before they finally choose the one they want to marry. Boys and girls go to parties, dances, plays, or games with different members of the opposite sex, learning in the course of this simple trial-and-error system the ones with whom they are likely to be most compatible. If they find promptly that they have few common interests or few ties as far as concerns family, religion, nationality or other similar factors, the dating can be ended.

KEEPING COMPANY

If a boy and girl find after a date that the time has been enjoyable and that the other person is someone they wish to see more often, they can begin to have more dates with the person who pleases them, but at the same time occasionally having dates with others. This is called "keeping company." When boys and girls keep company, they are expressing a preference for each other. As long as they are teenagers, they should not try to shorten this period too soon.

GOING STEADY

After keeping company, which shows some preference, the boy and the girl may find that they have a really strong attachment for each other.

Hence, they may propose that they go to parties and games just with each other and not with other boys or girls. Going steady is a period in which the couple learn to know much more about each other. During this period they can find out if they are truly in love. They can test their ability to get along with each other. They can determine whether their personalities merge satisfactorily.

PRIVATE UNDERSTANDING

After a couple have been going steady for some time, they may decide between themselves to have a private understanding. This has been characterized as a mutual avowal of love. Usually this understanding is kept secret or shared only with close friends or the immediate family. The young man and young woman may at this time wish to visit each other in their homes and to meet other members of the family and find out to what extent other members of the family, particularly their parents, believe that the choice is a good one. The value of the private understanding is that it permits a final decision to be made before a formal and public engagement. A private understanding may be terminated without the shock and embarrassment that come with a broken engagement.

ENGAGEMENT

The final test before marriage is the engagement. With this must come the determination of how long the engagement is to last before marriage. Some experts insist that at least one year is the minimum time for an engagement in order to determine that the couple is really compatible in personality and temperament. However, the exact time is not as important as is the certainty of the desire to marry. The engagement period may be used by the couple to settle many questions in advance of marriage which may be important to the final adjustment. Such questions may have to do with the nature of the work that is to be done by the couple and how they are to live following their marriage. Many a marriage has been broken and gone into the divorce court because the engagement period was too short to bring solutions to some of the serious questions that should have been decided before the relationship was made permanent.

COMPATIBILITY AND TEMPERAMENT

How are a boy and girl to know anything about the personality of the opposite sex when they have seen each other only over a short period of time and only on their best behavior? The boy and girl who are going on a date are likely to clean and groom themselves carefully. Often this temporary performance gives way to laxity and carelessness once marriage has been achieved. A boy or a girl may not show a fit of anger or an emotional upset when each is trying to do the most to please the other. However, soon after marriage may come a difference of opinion that will end in a temperamental storm quite unbelievable to the person who has never seen such a reaction before.

Professor Ernest Burgess says that a person with an optimistic temperament is more likely to be happy than one with a pessimistic temperament. A person who knows how to yield is more likely to be successful than one who is continually dominating and insisting on a superior position. A considerate and sympathetic person is a better risk in matrimony than one who is critical and inconsiderate. For these reasons, two sympathetic persons are happier in marriage than two who are constantly criticizing others. However, a critical and a sympathetic person would have a better chance to make a successful marriage than would two critical persons.

MATURITY

Marriages made at too early an age have a high record of divorce. The average age of marriage is, as has been said, becoming lower. From the point of view of the most chance of success in a marriage, the optimum age is from 22 to 30 years. Much depends, however, on the extent to which the person has really matured, regardless of his age in years. Of the greatest importance is sufficient maturity so that the partner in the marriage is no longer emotionally dependent on the father or on the mother, but is quite able to adjust to another adult, to make his own decisions, and to be responsible for his own obligations.

INFATUATION

When people fall in love, the attraction may be romantic and of such depth as to be infatuation. An infatuated person is completely dependent on the whim or the will of the one with whom he or she is infatuated. Here the emphasis is on physical attraction and is often called "love at first sight." When people are infatuated they do not wish to be with other people, and they are indifferent or hostile to the advice of parents and friends. However, infatuation is never a reasonable basis for marriage. Infatuation is often likely to end in an elopement or hasty marriage, followed in turn by disillusionment and divorce.

LOVE AND SEX

Much better is the love that is based on friendship associated with affection and admiration. The chief gain to be obtained from marriage is companionship and the sharing of mutual interests and desires. People are more likely to be well-adjusted and happy in their marriage if they have received some sex instruction before marriage, if they have been properly informed and their curiosity satisfied. They will be unhappy if they have disgust or aversion toward sex. The best marriages are those in which sexual desires are of about equal strength, and those between persons who have not been too sexually promiscuous before marriage.

SEX RELATIONSHIPS BEFORE MARRIAGE

During early adolescence, boys and girls often prefer to go around in groups rather than to have dates with just one person. The moment the relationship becomes more intimate, a question arises as to how far the couple will indulge in sexual relationships.

The word petting is understood by all young adolescents. While the word means "to fondle or to caress," many modifications have developed referring to the manner of the fondling and the extent of the caressing. One psychologist has defined petting as "physical contact for pleasure which is an end in itself." It arises from sexual desire in one or both parties but stops short of actual sexual intercourse. It does, however, stir up sexual emotions and develops increased tension which can be relieved only by sexual intercourse or by some substitute for it. If the sexual tension is not relieved it tends to persist and may become an annoying problem. Heavy petting usually means caressing the breasts and the thighs; often it may stimulate the sexual organs so strongly that a climax or orgasm occurs. The more intimate petting becomes, therefore, the more dangerous it can become to the couple who cannot go on because of social inhibitions to the complete sex act.

Dr. Anna O. Stevens has stated this problem clearly. She says: "Many adolescent girls begin to practice petting at the request of their boyfriends because they believe that that is the only way to be sure of getting another date, or of proving that they are grown up enough to continue dating, or because they have been led to believe that they owe it to the boy who has given them a pleasant evening. Only after the practice is well established do they learn its real physiological significance. Then it is difficult to establish a new pattern of behavior unless both the environment and the boyfriend are also new. The young boy may begin petting because he thinks girls expect it of him or that they will be impressed with his maturity. In many instances he recognizes the sex urge before he begins to pet, or at least much earlier than the girl does. Believing that the girl shares his sexual stimulation, he assumes that her reasons for continuing are the same as his. As petting becomes more intimate, the girl may be bewildered by his ardor and insistence, while he is confused by her resistance or her surprise at his intentions. The result is often unhappy for both of them. Certainly young people should be fully informed as to the significance of petting and as to its possible harmful results."

CONDUCT WHEN DATING

We all have friends about whom we think much that is good, others about whom we have our doubts. Often in high school or college, children are thrown with persons who come from different social atmospheres. These persons may be of different color, race, religion, nationality, and economic status. Marriages are made often between persons of different status, but experience has shown that people are more likely to have long-lasting marriages when they marry people of similar background rather than those of an entirely different background. After all, marriage is a family affair. Brothers, sisters, fathers, mothers, aunts, uncles, and cousins become involved, and all of these may have some influence on the permanence of a marriage.

People who are dating before marriage have to make many decisions which should be given thought and not made hastily. Dr. Ernest Burgess suggests that each young person should inquire of himself as to where he stands on the matter of chastity, and each girl as to the question of maintaining her virginity. They must think about what constitutes an ideal marriage. They must determine in advance whether they will persist in maintaining their standards of conduct or yield to pressure for premarital sex relations. There comes a question as to whether one wishes to break up a friendship or maintain standards against pressure from a friend. When the decisions are made, the boy or girl who is convinced in his own mind as to the ideals he holds, and the price he is willing to pay to maintain those ideals, is in a better position than one who has never previously considered the possibilities.

When it comes to courtship, the decisions are even more important because the temptations are greater. Without question, physical contacts on an intimate basis increase the temptation. Here, then, physical intimacy needs to be held within certain limits, for pressure for early marriage is likely to result in hasty or ill-considered marriage. Excess petting, which is a constant stimulus to sex desire, can lead to premature marriage. If, however, the courtship is associated with planning for the future, with consideration of work, and with recreation, sports, and other social activities, the pressures are likely to be much less.

ALCOHOL

Another important aspect of modern life is the part that alcohol plays in our social gatherings. Nowadays cocktail parties among teenagers are not unusual. Wild drinking parties are sometimes reported in the press. The chief effect of alcohol on the human body is to suppress inhibitions, to make people depart from their standards when otherwise they would not. Even one drink may affect judgment, especially if the person is emotionally aroused. The best rule is: Do not drink if you can possibly avoid it. This applies especially to boys and girls in social gatherings.

BLIND DATES

Among the special considerations is the question of blind dating. One of the interesting aspects of social life is the desire of a boy or girl who has an intimate friend to bring along that intimate friend on his date. This means that the girl or boy must provide a partner for the "blind date." Often a blind date turns out to be a bore, someone dull or stupid or someone intent primarily on a sexual relationship. If the two couples have little in the way of common interests, the situation may deteriorate into a petting party. The petting party is particularly serious when it involves a person about whom the one of the opposite sex knows little or nothing. These considerations apply especially to the case of girls going out with strange men. If a girl will insist that the other girl in a foursome be someone whom she knows, and someone who shares her own ideals and standards of conduct, she will not be put in the difficult position of being the only dissenter at an intimate party. Two girls who stick together in opposing conduct of which they do not approve will usually win. Two girls who incline to relaxation of standards will relax more easily than would one girl alone.

CHANGES IN SEXUAL ATTITUDES

Today teenagers begin dating much earlier than they did in the first twenty years of this century, indeed sometimes as young as eleven or twelve years old. Going steady, with the exchange of pins or rings as tokens, may begin as early as fourteen or fifteen years of age.

Times have changed in relation to new methods of communication, prolonged schooling, increased delays in going to work, the threat to life that constantly exists with modern methods of warfare, and finally the sexual freedom of girls from the prudery of previous generations. Moreover, the hazard of pregnancy has been reduced by widespread knowledge of methods of preventing conception, including not only various devices but also the new hormone pills which can prevent the passing of the egg cell in the girl's body.

Thus new scientific discoveries related to pregnancy and marriage have served to bring about changes in sexual attitudes. An investigation among college girls indicated that some of them would permit intercourse before marriage but never with a boy whom they contemplated as a partner in marriage. A new approach that is gaining acceptance as a part of the teen-age code will permit sexual intercourse before marriage, but only with the one to whom the person is engaged to marry.

Variations in the teen-age code depend on the locality in which the boy or girl lives, his status in his own society, and the extent to which his group, either family or community, is identified with or segregated from the whole community. Investigators have found that teenagers subdivide into groups with different standards of sexual morality. One small group may be called the "hot-rodders," or the "rock-and-roll" set, and are obviously more likely to be involved in delinquency and sexual promiscuity. The opposite group are frequently those who are academically serious and ambitious. These people are more reserved in dating, and particularly in going steady. Usually an in-between group is known in the community. They have no special name, but sometimes they suffer from their isolation and have problems in identifying themselves with the group.

THE IMPORTANCE OF KNOWLEDGE

The way to know is to ask. Parents should teach their children that the way to find out is to ask, to read, and to study what others have written about these matters. Every public library contains books which young people can read to find out everything that they really want to know. Parents should always be willing to tell a child anything he needs to know, and if they are unable to inform him, they should refer the child to a doctor or a counselor who can give the kind of information that the child should have.

Every young person must be concerned with many aspects of his sex life in order to conserve what nature has given him. Sexual knowledge is also necessary in order to get full enjoyment out of sex—because in sex life there is pleasure—without any of the great hazards and distresses that may be associated with misuse of sex or with lack of knowledge of the meaning of sex. Knowledge is extremely important to inform young people and their parents of what a great treasure we have within our bodies, and why we should treat this treasure with such definite care.

CHAPTER 7

Hygiene of Women

MORRIS FISHBEIN, M.D.

The boy and girl, until the age of twelve, may be reared in much the same manner. Their health problems are approximately the same. Thereafter, however, the problems of the girl are distinctive. At this period in her life her organs begin to differentiate to prepare her for her functions as a mother. The mother should prepare the daughter suitably for recognition of the changes that are to come. In the majority of girls these changes take place so gradually that they are not noticed.

The startling change which appears is the development of the menstrual flow. In far too many instances, notwithstanding the advance in health education that has been made in the last quarter century, girls still come to this phenomenon without any knowledge, and some of them sustain mental shocks which mark their lives thereafter. Until menstruation appears, the girl is not likely to bear children; with the coming of menstruation, the organs develop and the possibility exists.

Before that time, the body configuration of most girls has been much like that of the boy. After puberty, which is the time when the menstrual flow appears, the breasts, the pelvis and neck enlarge, hair develops in the armpits and over the sexual area, and the voice changes.

The onset of the menstrual flow is not always an abrupt and complete development. The first flow may be brief; it may disappear and not appear again for weeks or months; it may, at first, be irregular and then later regular. Just as soon as the flow appears regularly at a definite interval for several months, menstruation is established.

Associated with this physical change are also mental changes. Many of these changes are associated with interests in the male sex, in more mature occupations, in a different type of reading, and in many new interests.

Our views have greatly changed in the last quarter century. Girls used to be sick in every sense of the word during the menstrual period. Nowadays they are likely to go through without the slightest alteration in their habits. There are instances in which the function is accompanied with severe pain or with physical disturbance. When these occur, they should have the attention of a physician.

The adolescent girl is undergoing rapid development. For this reason her posture must be carefully watched. If she grows too rapidly and is somewhat tall, there may be an inclination to slump the shoulders forward, the abdomen out and the chest in. Such posture is bound to lead to a poor figure later in life. Exercises, described in the article on posture in this book, will help to develop a proper position when standing and when sitting. The chin and abdomen should be kept in and the chest forward. Many young girls worry about the development of the breasts and, not understanding the changes that occur, attempt to hide them. Poor posture may result from holding the shoulders in such a manner as to draw in the chest.

The girl, at this period of life, needs plenty of sleep; ten or eleven hours in twenty-four is not too much. Extra relaxation in the form of a nap in the middle of the day, such as is given to smaller children, may be exceedingly useful in maintaining her body tone. There need be no special attention to the diet other than the certainty that it contains the necessary proteins, carbohydrates and fats, mineral salts and vitamins that are necessary in any well-balanced diet.

Many girls passing from adolescence into adult age feel that it is necessary for them to adopt sophisticated habits. Whereas they have formerly avoided tea and coffee in favor of milk, they want to partake of these and even of alcoholic beverages as giving them somewhat more of an adult status in the family. Smoking cigarettes is not necessary, and again may be considered as a habit to be controlled until a later date when it can be used with intelligence and restraint.

Some girls at this age put on so much weight that they are seriously disturbed. The weight may increase so rapidly that the skin of the abdomen stretches and red marks appear along the curves of the hips. These should not cause worry because they will fade when the weight of the body is more definitely adjusted. For the control of the tendency to overweight, a suitable diet with a lowered amount of carbohydrates is desirable. Nowadays most people have learned enough about calories and carbohydrates in relationship to overweight to exercise a certain amount of control over this danger.

Special attention should also be given at this period to the condition of the thyroid gland. In some children a tendency to overactivity of the gland develops, which is marked also by rapid heart, nervousness, perspiration, and similar symptoms. If any sign appears of overactivity of the thyroid gland, the basal metabolism should be determined by a competent doctor and the condition of the thyroid gland controlled in relationship to the results. If there is overweight or underweight, the basal metabolism test should also be made to determine whether or not the activity of the thyroid gland is related in any way to this unusual development.

In the Great Lakes area and in the Northwest, the water and the soil lack iodine, hence there is a tendency among young children to develop simple enlargement of the thyroid gland that is known as simple goiter. There is a special chapter on this condition elsewhere in this book. Any tendency of the thyroid gland toward enlargement should, of course, be studied by the family doctor. In most cases, however, intelligent parents nowadays give small doses of iodine regularly each week to supply the iodine deficiency and thus effectively prevent the appearance of simple goiter.

DISORDERS OF MENSTRUATION

Menstruation may be occasionally irregular during the first year without causing any anxiety. Certainly, by the end of the first year it should be regular, in the majority of women, occurring every twenty-eight days. Menstruation occurring regularly anywhere from twenty-one days to five-week intervals may be considered within normal limits.

Sometimes, in connection with the first appearance of menstruation, the usual signs of adolescence appear, including pimples and blackheads on the face, back, and chest, soreness and swelling of the breasts, and headache. These may appear as the result of the changes in the glands that occur at this time.

Ordinarily menstruation should cause no more pain than any of the other functions of the body. When the pain occurs, it is usually associated with a disturbance of the circulation or of the glands. Sometimes failure of the bowels to act properly is a complication, which may be easily corrected by establishment of regular habits, sufficient rest, drinking of plenty of water, and the other measures suggested in the section on digestion.

Doctors now recognize a period of a few days before menstruation when symptoms of distress, irritability, anxiety, flushing, nausea and such, make what is called premenstrual tension. Control may involve study of the glandular condition and prescription of suitable treatment.

EXERCISES

Various exercises have been described for use by growing girls at this time. Some of these simple exercises involve not only the usual bending and standing, which are good for posture, but also kneeling in the knee-chest position, walking on the hands and feet as the monkey or cat walks, and other postures which help to develop the ligaments which hold the organs of the pelvis in position. Since menstruation is a normal function of women and involves several different organs, its control must involve study of the organs concerned.

Emotional shocks and nerve shocks may tend to be associated with pain at this time. A change in the altitude, extraordinary changes in the diet, over- and under-exercise, and many similar factors may yield difficult symptoms. For this reason, the routine of the girl's life during the menstrual period should be disturbed as little as possible.

She may take her baths daily as always, preferably a warm bath; but if she is in the habit of taking cold baths, she may take these also. There is no good reason why most women should not take a bath during the menstrual period. If the flow of blood is profuse, strenuous swimming may make it excessive; also a very hot tub bath may increase the amount of blood lost. A very cold bath taken just before or at the beginning of menstruation may occasionally stop the bleeding. The danger of infection from the water is very slight.

Indulgence in competitive games during the menstrual period should be carefully controlled. Such games involve emotional stress and high tension. They place a considerable burden upon the heart. They bring about shocks and jolts to the internal organs for which these organs are not competent. Every girl who participates in athletic sports should have a physical examination in relationship to her feminine constitution.

PAINFUL MENSTRUATION

A tremendous number of remedies have been suggested for painful menstruation. Sufficient rest and sleep, proper hygiene and treatment for anemia, if that is present, are especially important. Some patients get immediate help from rest in bed and the use of an enema for emptying the bowels. Others are relieved by placing a hot-water bag over the painful area. Aspirin and similar drugs which relieve pain are used by many girls and are not harmful, if taken in small doses and preferably under the direction of a physician.

Sometimes it is necessary for the doctor to make certain modifications of the glandular mechanism of the patient. The administration of suitable glandular substances which are known to have control over the menstrual functions sometimes yields successful results in eliminating pain.

In the process of menstruation several organs are involved: the pituitary gland, adrenals, ovaries, and the uterus. Regular bleeding from the uterus, called menstruation, is nearly always dependent on proper functioning of the ovaries. These, in turn, are controlled by a portion of the pituitary gland in the brain. The pituitary gland has been called the motor of the ovaries. When there are unusual symptoms during the menstrual period, such as flushing, numbness of the fingertips, fainting spells, and crying, the glands and their secretions are ordinarily responsible, related in turn to various mental influences.

Because of the tendency to bleed at this period, some women bruise more easily during the menstrual time; others suffer with nosebleeds. These symptoms usually disappear when the menstruation ends.

When menstruation is exceedingly scanty, the state of the blood should be studied as to whether or not there is anemia. There should also be an investigation of the basal metabolism and the general nutrition.

During menstruation the vast majority of women wear a simple cotton pad, such as is now commercially available in many different forms. Vaginal tampons are also used satisfactorily and safely. Where there are unusual odors of any kind, a careful investigation should be made by a competent doctor to determine the presence or absence of infection. In most cases, annoying odors are a sign of infection, and they cannot be corrected by application of deodorants or powders of any kind.

The tampons do not seem to be quite dependable for women who have a profuse flow. This applies also to various types of rubber cups that have been devised for controlling the menstrual flow. For persons in the theatrical profession, for acrobats, and women who indulge in sports of various kinds, such devices may be especially desirable.

The medical profession has not settled definitely the question of the advisability of using douches before and after the menstrual period or at any other time. About an equal number of specialists in diseases of women are arrayed on each side of this question. Women who are not infected in any manner and who do not have excessive discharges of mucus and other material from the genital tract need not employ douches regularly. Ordinary bathing will suffice for the purpose. However, in cases in which there are excessive discharges, or in which, as has been mentioned, an odor is present, a physician should be consulted in order to determine the presence and nature of the infection. The infection should be treated by the means that the physician will recommend. This recommendation will in most instances involve the use of suitable cleansing and antiseptic agents used in the form of douches and in similar ways.

ABSENCE OF MENSTRUATION

Most people know that menstruation disappears when a woman becomes pregnant and is to have a child. It disappears also at a period known as the climacteric, which is also an important epoch in the life of women. This period is also called the menopause, as an indication of the fact that the menstruation disappears at this time.

There are, of course, other factors which occasionally produce a change in menstruation and in some instances even a temporary absence. A change of geographical location, which involves chiefly a change of climate and perhaps of altitude, not infrequently produces alterations in menstruation. Usually the flow may stop, but in some cases the amount of blood lost is excessive. Because the process of menstruation is controlled by glandular action, disorders of menstruation, including stopping for no apparent reason, are generally assumed to be due to some glandular difficulty.

Women who do not menstruate are not in any way inferior to those who do. They rarely show any abnormal symptoms, and their sex life is about the same. The whole difficulty lies in the minds of such women. They feel they are subnormal; they may become exceedingly disturbed mentally worrying over the condition. Frequently a physician can bring about menstruation in such patients by the experimental use of various glandular preparations.

MENOPAUSE

The discontinuance of menstruation at the menopause is, of course, a different matter. The average duration of menstruation in women is from 30 to 32 years. The average age for the beginning of the climacteric or menopause in the temperate zone is about 47 years. However, there is an enormous variation in the ages at which the symptoms of climacteric may arise. Cases are known in which the change of life occurred as early as 27 years of age and as late as 59 years. Usually in the United States the discontinuance of menstruation occurs between 45 and 50 years of age in 50 per cent of women; between 40 and 45 in 25 per cent; between 35 and 40 in 12½ per cent, and between 50 and 55 years in 12½ per cent.

In most instances there is a definite association between the onset of puberty, or the beginning of menstruation, and the time of the appearance of the menopause. In general, the earlier the menstrual function begins, the longer it will continue. Girls who have an early puberty will have a long, potential, reproductive career and a late menopause. A physician named Gallant published a chart of approximate ages as to when the menopause would appear, based on the age of the onset of puberty. The table, which is for healthy women, follows:

Year in Which Menstruation Appears	*Menopause Should Occur*
10	Between 50 and 52 years
11	Between 48 and 50 years
12	Between 46 and 48 years
13	Between 44 and 46 years

14	Between 42 and 44 years
15	Between 40 and 42 years
16	Between 38 and 40 years
17	Between 36 and 38 years
18	Between 34 and 36 years
19	Between 32 and 34 years
20	Between 30 and 32 years

Exactly as parts of the body change at the onset of puberty, so also do similar changes occur at the menopause. Usually the spleen and lymphatic glands decrease in size. There is an increased tendency to constipation, because of changes in the wall of the intestine. Most women have some physical discomfort and some mild mental or nervous changes, but some women cease menstruating with slight inconvenience. As a rule, the woman may miss one or two or more periods, then will have menstrual periods that seem almost normal; then she will miss other periods, and finally the periodic flow will cease altogether. This variability is due to the fact that the glandular changes which are occurring take place gradually.

There may be, during this period, slight inflammation and swelling of the sexual parts. These are, however, of little significance. The most difficult symptom which may develop at this time is excessive bleeding. Whenever excessive bleeding occurs, however, either at the menopause or at any other time, a physician should be consulted immediately so that he may make a study of the condition and determine its cause. It is well established that the appearance of blood is sometimes associated with the appearance of cancer. The only way to make certain is to have a direct examination of the tissue to guard against such a possibility.

Occasionally there is a good deal of itching, particularly after bathing. In such cases the use of an ointment, such as 12 per cent boric acid in an ointment of rose water, is helpful. If such mild treatment does not secure a good result, a physician should be consulted for the prescribing of something more powerful.

While it is true that states of mental depression and other abnormal mental states occur somewhat frequently at or about the age of menopause, it must be remembered that these are not really important abnormalities, and that they occur also in men around the age of fifty. Unless they are extreme, there is nothing to do in the way of treatment.

Since many different forms of mental disorder may occur at this period, it is always advisable to have a scientific diagnosis as to the character of the disturbance that occurs. In some women there seems to be increased sexual desire at this period. In such cases also the treatment is good hygiene, including also the avoidance of any unnecessary stimulants. The avoidance of coffee, and a good deal of outdoor exercise, may be helpful. In other cases there is a gradual loss of sexual desire. This also may be quite temporary. Many women continue to be sexually active for considerable periods after the menopause. Not infrequently there is a mild degree of overactivity of the thyroid gland, and, associated with this, increased excitability. There may also be a slight elevation of the blood pressure.

All of these symptoms, however, are associated with the gradual change in the glandular mechanism and, unless severe, need not be considered seriously. New substitutes for missing glandular substances may be prescribed by the doctor to overcome symptoms.

The changes associated with this period demand slight modification of the general hygiene of the body. Usually older people will want less food. Because of the difficulties of digestion, foods rich in carbohydrates, including sugars, cake, candy, preserves, and jelly, should be taken with moderation, as also foods that are known to cause indigestion in many cases; for example, foods fried in a good deal of grease, hot breads, pastry, cheese, and similar substances.

Since there is a considerable amount of congestion in the abdomen, the care of the bowels should be a special problem. A daily, free evacuation of the bowels is essential to health. The use of mild laxatives may bring a good deal of relief. The kidneys must be especially watched for the onset of any degenerative changes.

It is necessary to keep the skin in good condition by bathing—sometimes alternate hot and cold baths. Massage is helpful in toning up the nervous system and the circulation. Exercise daily in the open air is helpful in steadying the nerves and stimulating the body generally.

From the point of view of the mind, it is particularly necessary at this time of life that some pleasant occupation be followed. Usually by this time children will have passed the age when they need constant supervision, and the mother must take relaxation from her home cares. Many women at this time of life become expert bridge players or golfers, although previously they may have taken but little interest in such diversions. Any mental occupation that will take the woman into a new interest is the best possible safeguard against the slight mental difficulty which develops in some women at this period.

The estrogenic hormones including the natural and the synthetic, stilbestrol, will aid in overcoming headache, hot flashes, and melancholia, which are so distressing at this time. These substances should never be taken except when prescribed by the doctor. Physicians also prescribe some androgen or male sex hormone particularly when there is depression or fear of loss of sex-life.

THE RHYTHM OF MENSTRUATION AND THE SAFE PERIOD FOR PREVENTION OF CONCEPTION

A definite relationship exists between the time a woman menstruates and the time when an egg cell or ovum passes from the ovary into the uterus. If a woman menstruates regularly every twenty-eight days, it is usually impossible for her to conceive between the first and tenth day of her menstrual cycle, the first day being the one on which the menstrual flow begins. She can conceive on the eleventh day and up to and including the seventeenth day, but she will not be able to conceive from the seventeenth day on. Therefore, the days on which conception is most likely are the days from the fourteenth to the sixteenth day after the first day of menstruation. This is the period in which the mother cell or egg cell is produced by the ovary. In a woman who menstruates every twenty-eight days, the egg cell comes from the ovary on the fourteenth day.

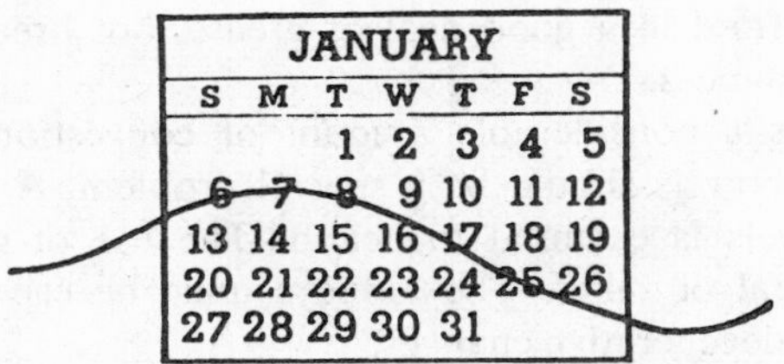

Fig. 23. The rhythm method is based upon a "safe period" each month. A doctor can help the woman figure out her safe period. From *To Be a Mother, To Be a Father,* Planned Parenthood Federation of America, Inc.

The period of nine days, referred to as the period when conception is most likely, includes three days for the production and discharge of the egg cell, one day allowed for variability, and two to three days for the survival of the fertilizing power of the male cell. It has been definitely shown that the male cell will not survive much over three days, unless it meets the egg cell of the female and brings about conception. The extra three days added to these seven are in the interests of safety against any irregularities.

Records have now been kept of many thousands of cases in which women have observed this safe period, and failures, when absolute observance prevailed, are exceedingly few. Of course, the matter is complicated when the menstrual cycle in the woman is more or less than twenty-eight days. For the majority of women, therefore, it will be necessary to determine the exact dates and variations of the menstrual cycle. This is done by keeping an accurate record for several months of the exact dates on which menstruation begins, how many days it continues, and the number of days from the first day of menstruation to the first day of the next menstruation. All sorts of calendars and devices have now been developed for keeping records of this kind.

It is known that a good many women have occasional variations in their menstrual cycle. Thus one authority said, "The only regular thing about menstruation is its own irregularity." Just as soon as the cycle is definitely established, it becomes possible for the woman to calculate the periods when she is likely to conceive, or the fertile period, and the period when she is not likely to conceive, or the sterile period.

THE TEMPERATURE CONTROL METHOD

Many people think there is a chance for conception whenever the male sperm cell is deposited in the woman's genital tract. Actually, the sperm cannot fertilize an egg cell or ovum unless the ovum is there when the sperm reaches the Fallopian tube. Only one ovum, smaller than a pin point in size, is released by the ovary during the woman's periodic cycle. This takes place about 14 days before the beginning of the next cycle. If pregnancy is to occur, intercourse must take place within 24 hours of ovulation, since the life of the ovum is not more than 24 hours, and the sperm cells have fertilizing power for only 24 to 36 hours. Hence, if a woman can determine the exact time of ovulation, she can increase her chances of conception by having intercourse then.

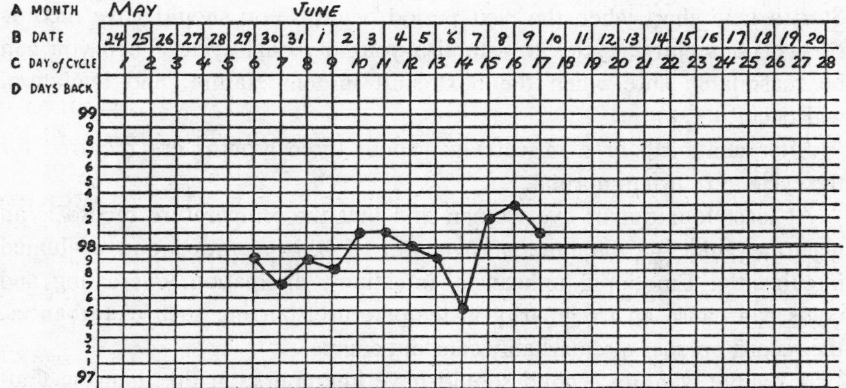

Fig. 24. Typical temperature chart. Another method of finding the time of ovulation is by taking and recording the temperature each morning when one wakes up. The temperature varies from day to day during the course of the menstrual cycle, and when it is recorded it normally follows a pattern like the one in this sample record. From *The Safe Period,* Planned Parenthood Federation of America, Inc.

The most practical method of achieving this is to keep a careful record of body temperature on arising each morning. Whereas a man's temperature follows a regular pattern day after day, the temperature of a woman is altered by the normal functioning of the ovaries. For several years thousands of women have kept daily temperature records, which physicians have studied and interpreted. We now know that the release of the ovum raises the level of a woman's temperature during the latter half of the menstrual cycle.

Your doctor can help you get charts especially designed for daily temperature records and show you how to use them.

Take your temperature immediately after waking up in the morning. Do not get up to go to the bathroom first, or drink water or smoke a cigarette. Just reach over, get the thermometer, put it under your tongue, lie back and remain quiet for five minutes. Then record the temperature on your chart. If it differs from those recorded before, and particularly if it is lower, shake the thermometer down, put it back under your tongue and hold it for another five minutes to verify the reading.

Temperature drops 24 to 36 hours before the onset of the menstrual flow, reaching a low point during the first day or two after the flow begins. This low level continues until the middle of the interval between two menstruations. This is the time when ovulation usually occurs in the woman who has a 27- to 31-day cycle. A sharp drop often takes place just before the rise that indicates the ovulation is occurring. During the next 24 to 36 hours, the temperature goes up abruptly. It stays at the higher level until one to two days before the beginning of the next flow. Start a new chart when the next period begins. You should have records of two consecutive cycles to establish your personal cycle. Then you can be reasonably sure when the next shift in temperature, and ovulation, will occur.

After childbirth or a miscarriage, about three months are required for the cycle to return to normal.

At least four out of five women find that the temperature record is an accurate guide to the time of ovulation if it is recorded and evaluated intelligently. Emotional upheavals, infections, dissipation, overeating and colds can cause an irregularity in temperature; barring such disturbances, the record pursues a remarkably constant course.

A couple wanting a child should have intercourse at the time the temperature falls, just before the rise that precedes ovulation. Intercourse should be continued daily during the rise of the temperature and when it has reached its peak after ovulation; however, too frequent intercourse causes a decrease in the number of sperm cells and lessens a man's fertility.

A carefully kept temperature record will also indicate the beginning of pregnancy. If the elevated temperature that develops after ovulation does not drop in its customary fashion, the woman is pregnant. Failure of the temperature to drop during the first week of the missed menstrual period is reliable evidence.

This natural method of child-planning is within the normal range of human functions, and it does not require procedures that might cause objections for religious or esthetic reasons. An intelligent young couple can plan to have their babies when they want them. When a baby is born, the mother can be given full opportunity to recover from the stress of that birth before undertaking another pregnancy. This will mean healthier mothers, healthier babies, happier families.

PREVENTION OF CONCEPTION

There are many different reasons to be considered when a woman wishes to avoid pregnancy. These reasons may be related to a possible illness of the prospective mother or father. The physician who is fully familiar with the physical condition of the prospective parent will be able to advise whether or not any of the available methods for the avoidance of pregnancy is to be tried. Frequently childbirth may be difficult so that the mother's health needs to be fully restored before another pregnancy. If she is nursing a baby that is still small and dependent on her, it may be harmful for both mother and child as well as for the prospective child to have another pregnancy too soon. Sometimes after a difficult childbirth the tissues of the mother will be injured and surgical repair may be necessary before she is to become pregnant again. When the health and even the life of the prospective mother may be threatened by another pregnancy, most specialists in the care of women do not consider it wise to depend on the so-called "safe period." In such instances they are likely to advise the use of some of the techniques which are much more certain to prevent the contact between the sperm cell of the male and the egg cell of the female that is necessary to begin a pregnancy.

The method to be used must be practically certain to succeed and it must be free from harmful psychic as well as physical effects. Many marriages are endangered by the use of methods for the control of births that do not meet with all of the objections that arise from both psychic and physical considerations.

Whenever any method of birth control is used that conflicts with the religious beliefs of either of the partners to a marriage, serious conflicts may arise in the minds of those concerned. Indeed, marital discord as a result of such conflicts is not unusual. Any method that interferes greatly with the normal conduct of sex contact may be distasteful to the married partners and may even be physically harmful. Almost every physician condemns techniques which involve separation of the partners before culmination. Moreover, several widely observed religions are definitely opposed to this practice. Finally, the method is not at all dependable because it is difficult to practice and the percentage of failures is very high. Physically it may leave the tissues congested and the nervous system in a state of unrest.

Those methods which involve materials placed over the male organ of sex called condoms are not always successful because of the possible breakage or faulty character of the device. Even when such devices are ample in size and properly lubricated, they are difficult to use artistically, and their obvious character sometimes sets up resistances and deters the emotional response in the female partner. Frequently the male partner will complain that such material interferes with the feeling of release and gratification.

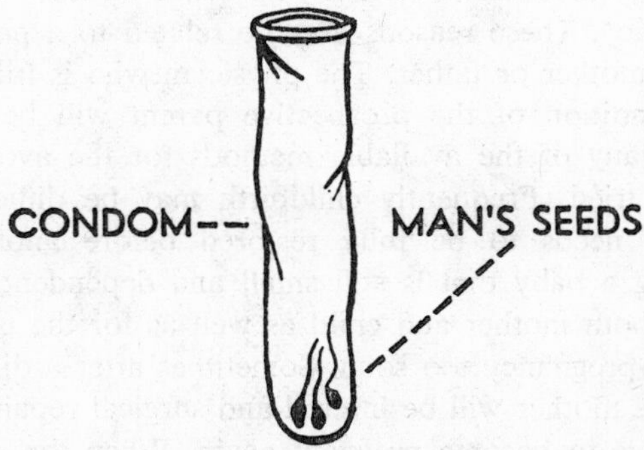

Fig. 25. No prescription needed. Another way is using a condom (rubber). The condom is placed over the man's sex organ (penis) before sex relations. The man's seeds then cannot reach the egg. From *To Be a Mother, To Be a Father,* Planned Parenthood Federation of America, Inc.

The use of various chemicals and washes and pastes should be attempted only with the advice of the family physician because many such materials are harmful and even more are quite without dependability. After the male egg cell has once entered the uterus no such material can reach it. The American Medical Association has accepted a number of products as suitable for safe use when prescribed by the doctor. The list includes "Contra-Creme," "Laktikal Creme," "Lorophyn Jelly," "Koromex Cream," "Lanteen Jelly," "Lygel Cream," "Lygel Jelly," "Ortho-Creme," "Ortho-Gynol Vaginal Jelly," "Ramses Vaginal Jelly," "Marvasan Creme," "Veritas Kreme," "Cooper Creme," and also "Lorophyn Suppositories" and "Pernox Vaginal Capsules."

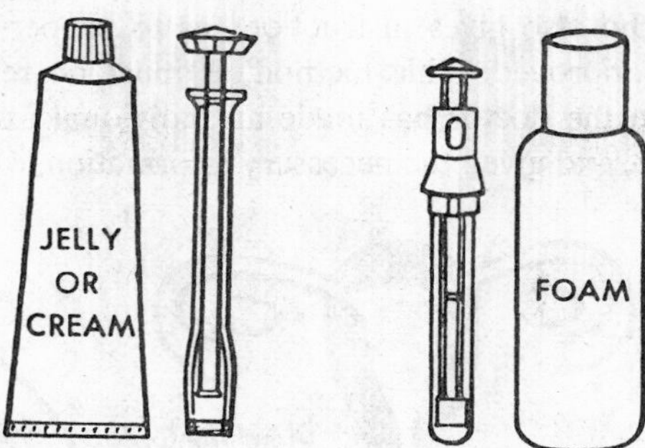

Fig. 26. No prescription needed. Contraceptive foams, creams, jellies, vaginal tablets, and suppositories can be put into the birth canal before sex relations to kill the man's seeds. These can be bought at any drugstore. From *To Be a Mother, To Be a Father,* Planned Parenthood Federation of America, Inc.

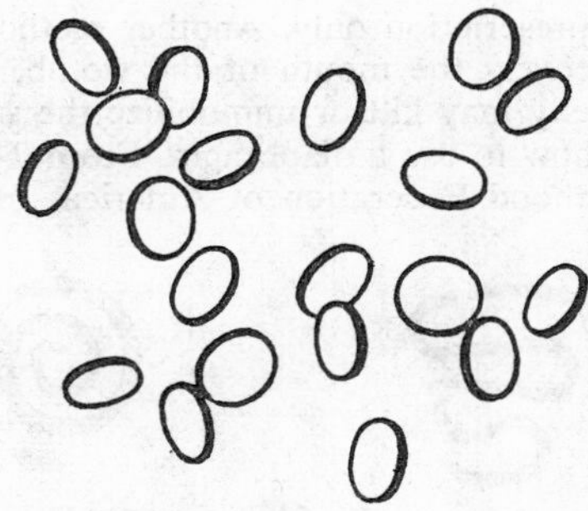

Fig. 27. By doctor's prescription only. Birth control pills taken by mouth according to directions stop the ovary from forming eggs. If there is no egg, pregnancy cannot occur. From *To Be a Mother, To Be a Father,* Planned Parenthood Federation of America, Inc.

Many women have the superstition that pregnancy is not possible unless the female receives complete sex gratification during the sexual act. This is a superstition without the slightest scientific basis.

Glandular materials can be taken in pill form as prescribed by the doctor. When taken from the fifth to the twenty-fifth day of the cycle, ovulation is prevented and the woman cannot become pregnant. When the pill is stopped, the cycle promptly returns. Among the pills most frequently used in the United States are Enovid®, Ortho-Novum®, Provess, and others.

Even women in some of the savage tribes of Africa and South America have attempted to prevent the entrance of the male sperm cell by obstructive devices made of wool, sponge, metal, or rubber. Such devices are frequently prescribed by physicians when they are necessary for reasons of health. The diaphragms which are prescribed and carefully fitted by the doctor who also gives instructions as to proper use is a technique now frequently approved. This method, it must be remembered, is only dependable when the doctor has made an individual examination, selected the proper device, and given the necessary information.

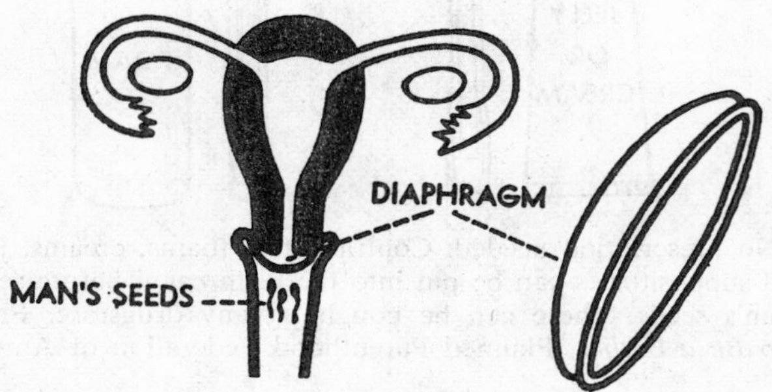

Fig. 28. By doctor's prescription only. Another method is the diaphragm and jelly. The diaphragm covers the mouth of the womb, keeping the sperm out. Special contraceptive jelly may kill or immobilize the sperm. A doctor must fit and teach the woman how to use a diaphragm. From *To Be a Mother, To Be a Father,* Planned Parenthood Federation of America, Inc.

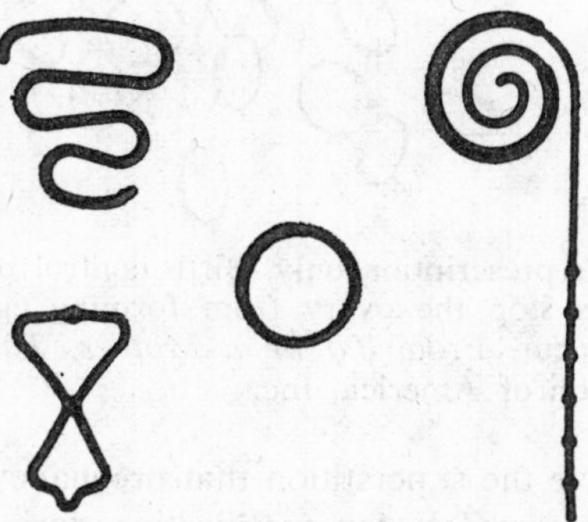

Fig. 29. By doctor's prescription only. Small plastic or stainless steel contraceptives—called intra-uterine devices (IUD)—are placed in the womb by a doctor. Once in place, this birth control method requires little further attention. From *To Be a Mother, To Be a Father,* Planned Parenthood Federation of America, Inc.

Spring devices, made of wire or plastic to be inserted in the cervix or opening of the uterus are available. Many doctors recommend these new devices, insert them, and teach women how to use them safely.

A successful marriage depends on the presence of children. Methods for the prevention of conception should be used only when they are definitely indicated, and most marriages are far more likely to be permanent and happy if children come soon to complete the marriage bond.

CHAPTER 8

Care of Mothers before and after Childbirth

J. P. GREENHILL, M.D.

INTRODUCTION

Women used to keep secret, even from their husbands, and as long as possible that they were going to have a baby. As the time approached when the child was to be born, the prospective mother would notify the physician. In many instances, however, the doctor was called posthaste at the moment of childbirth. Then, in the home, with the aid of a neighbor or a relative, the child would be brought into the community.

The advances of scientific medicine have greatly changed our points of view in relationship to what is proper in childbirth. Nowadays the intelligent woman may consult her physician even before trying to have a child. She finds out whether or not her health is such as to permit her to have a child without seriously injuring herself and without danger to the prospective child. When the physician's examination has revealed that her condition is satisfactory she may proceed.

The intelligent woman consults her physician as soon as she realizes that she is pregnant. He then examines her again to make certain of the diagnosis. This he confirms by various tests in the laboratory as well as by physical examination of the patient herself. During this period her life must be regulated according to her condition. Her diet, her exercise, her rest, her work, and every other factor of her existence are controlled. Examinations are regularly made of her excretions in order to determine whether or not the organs are functioning satisfactorily.

Such prenatal care in childbirth is of the utmost importance for lowering the death rates associated with this condition, and also for bringing into the world healthy and normal children.

M. F.

Because of ignorance, negligence, territorial inaccessibility, financial distress, or other reasons, many women in this country fail to be examined by a physician while they are pregnant. These women do not call in expert aid until the child is actually ready to be born. Since most of the mishaps from childbirth may be prevented by proper care before the baby arrives and by skillful management of confinement, every woman who is to have a baby should visit a doctor long before the expected date of confinement. Not only will the lives of hundreds of mothers be saved, but countless other women will be spared temporary or permanent invalidism. Furthermore many thousand babies will be born alive who would certainly perish in the absence of proper supervision. The care which a woman receives before the baby arrives is known as antepartum care. In contradistinction to this is the care after the child is born, and this is spoken of as postpartum (or postnatal) care.

A confinement case begins at the time of conception. Hence the woman should consult a physician as soon as she believes she is going to have a baby. The ideal arrangement would be for a woman to have a thorough examination before she decides to have a child, because not infrequently abnormalities are found which, unless corrected, may make childbearing a hazardous undertaking. Occasionally a medical disturbance is found such as serious heart, kidney, or lung trouble, which absolutely precludes pregnancy. A woman should know this before she conceives. She should seek a physician who has a sympathetic nature and one in whom she can have utmost confidence. Faith in the doctor is important to allay the fears which young prospective mothers have. Advice should be sought from the physician and not from well-meaning but misinformed friends and relatives, many of whom instill fear rather than dispel it.

If a woman cannot afford the services of a specialist in obstetrics or an experienced general practitioner, she should visit one of the numerous maternity clinics to be found in every large city and in many small ones.

SIGNS OF PREGNANCY

A woman may suspect she is to become a mother in a number of ways. The most important sign is absence of the monthly flow, especially in a young woman who has usually had regular monthly periods. A second significant sign is morning sickness or nausea and vomiting. Frequently the breasts feel full, they are tender to the touch, and they have peculiar sensations such as tingling or throbbing. The skin around the nipples becomes darker in color, especially in brunettes. Another sign is a desire to pass urine at frequent intervals. Not one of these symptoms by itself indicates pregnancy, but a combination of two or more is presumptive evidence that a baby may be expected. A physician can nearly always detect a pregnancy as early as six weeks after the last monthly flow. If he is in doubt he can have biologic or other tests performed which correctly indicate the presence of a pregnancy in at least 96 per cent of all cases. A woman does not usually feel the baby move around until the sixteenth or eighteenth week of the baby's development. At this time the abdomen is usually enlarged sufficiently to verify the suspicion of a pregnancy, and a physician can feel the baby and hear its heart beat. After the fifth month a baby or at least parts of it may be shown on X-ray pictures. A new device known as ultrasonics can detect a living baby much earlier than the baby's heart can be heard by the physician.

VISIT TO PHYSICIAN

When an expectant mother visits the doctor the first time, he will take a history and make a thorough examination. This includes external and internal investigation of the organs directly associated with childbearing; also an examination of the teeth, thyroid, breasts, nipples, and other organs. The blood pressure and temperature will be taken, the urine examined, the weight recorded, the blood studied for anemia, syphilis, the Rh factor and the blood type. This knowledge is important in case a blood transfusion is necessary and also because a very small percentage of babies suffer when there is a difference in the Rh factor in the husband and wife.

A woman should visit her doctor at least once every three weeks during the first seven months of pregnancy and once every two weeks thereafter. If abnormalities exist, the patient may have to see her physician more often. At each visit she should bring to the physician a three- or four-ounce bottle of urine. The bottle should be carefully washed before it is used, because its former contents may be the cause of false tests. Once a week it is advisable to measure the amount of urine passed in twenty-four hours. If there is a considerable reduction in the amount usually passed and the patient has been drinking the customary amount of fluids, this fact should be reported to the physician. It may indicate a disturbance of the kidneys. A label should be attached to the bottle giving the patient's name, the date the specimen is collected, and in certain instances the amount of urine passed in twenty-four hours.

SERIOUS SYMPTOMS DURING PREGNANCY

During each visit the doctor will ask the patient certain questions and listen to any questions or complaints. He will usually inquire about the following symptoms: nausea, vomiting, swelling of the hands, feet, or face, headaches, constipation, dizziness, pain in the abdomen or legs, spots before the eyes or other visual disturbances, bleeding from the vagina, movements of the baby, shortness of breath, nervousness, and other symptoms.

He will observe the patient's blood pressure, the pulse rate, abnormal swellings, excessive gain or loss in weight, and the results of the examination of the urine. It is not necessary to be examined internally at each visit, but at least one examination should be made in addition to the first one, and this preferably about four weeks before the expected date of confinement.

ESTIMATING THE DATE OF BIRTH

It is impossible to predict accurately the day when a baby is to arrive. However, the approximate date can be estimated in a number of ways.

1. Add seven days to the first day of the last monthly flow and subtract three months. Thus if the last menstrual period began July 10th, add seven days, giving July 17th, and subtract three months, which gives April 17th as the approximate day labor may be expected. In most cases the confinement will take place within a few days before or after this calculated date.
2. A woman having her first baby may add twenty-two weeks to the day she first feels the baby move. A woman who has already borne children should add twenty-four weeks because she usually recognizes movements of the baby about two weeks earlier than women pregnant for the first time.
3. If the exact day of conception is known, 266 days added to this will give the approximate date of confinement.
4. By repeated internal examinations, a physician can often tell within a few days when a baby will be born.

THE DIET

The child in the womb depends on its mother for its supply of food. The nourishment is not given to the child directly, because there is no direct connection between the mother and her child. The latter lies in a sac filled with fluid which permits the child to move about freely. In one part of this sac is an organ known as the placenta or afterbirth. This is made up of myriads of small projections known as villi, in each of which is a small blood vessel. These villi dip into a collection of the mother's blood, and it is the coverings of these villi which extract from the mother's blood the constituents which the child requires. The nourishment which the villi take up is transported from the small blood vessels in the villi to large blood vessels which pass through a tube connecting the afterbirth with the child. This tube is known as the umbilical cord, and it usually contains one vein and two arteries. The vein carries fresh blood containing nourishment to the child, whereas the arteries carry blood containing waste products from the baby to the afterbirth. This impure blood is transmitted from the afterbirth to the mother's blood, and the mother purifies this blood in the same way she cleanses her own blood, namely, by eliminating the waste products through her bowels, kidneys, lungs, and skin.

Since the connection between the mother and the child is as intimate as just mentioned, it is obvious that the child's development depends to a large extent upon the mother's nutrition. The child's growth is not entirely dependent on the mother's food intake, because if the diet is lacking in certain substances which the child requires, these substances in many instances will be extracted from the mother's tissues, usually to her detriment. Hence it is important that the mother's diet contain both the proper quantity and quality of food each day to supply all the demands of the fetus.

Not only is the mother's nutrition important for the baby, but it is important also for her own benefit. In order to avoid trouble there should be certain additions and restrictions to the diet the expectant mother has usually followed. As a general rule it may be said that the expectant mother should eat a well-rounded diet, just as she eats in the non-pregnant state, except that she should drink plenty of milk, eat more fresh fruits and vegetables, and less condiments. A woman should not make the serious mistake of overeating because she believes she must eat for two individuals. The excess food is not transferred to the baby but is stored in the mother. This may lead to serious consequences. However, women should not starve themselves in an attempt to keep down the weight of the baby, because the weight of a newborn baby is not dependent entirely or even in great part on the amount of food its mother eats. Heredity is a much more important factor than diet.

A proper diet during pregnancy, which should contain about 1800–2000 calories, will result in a total weight gain of about 20–25 pounds above a desirable nonpregnancy weight. Such a diet contains the following:

1. *Water,* which serves many functions. About eight or ten glasses of liquids a day in one form or another should be taken.
2. *Proteins,* which build and repair the tissues of the body. These are found chiefly in meat, eggs, milk and milk products, and such vegetables as peas and beans.
3. *Fats,* which furnish fuel for heat and energy. These are found in cream, butter, cheese, oils, and fat meats.
4. *Carbohydrates* or *starches,* which also supply fuel. They are found chiefly in sweets, sugar, bread, potatoes, cereals, milk, and rice.
5. *Minerals,* which are the most important substances for the growth of the bones and teeth. They are found especially in milk, certain fruits, and most vegetables. If vegetables are cooked, the water should not be thrown away but should be used for soup. The chief minerals necessary during pregnancy are calcium, phosphorus and iron. Every pregnant woman should take iron in one form or another daily throughout her pregnancy.

6. *Vitamins,* which regulate the growth of the body. They are found in milk, eggs, meat, whole wheat, fruits, vegetables, and cod-liver oil.

7. *Iodine* in certain regions of the country is necessary to prevent the development of a goiter in the mother and the child. It is found chiefly in such sea food as oysters and salmon. Iodized salt or iodine tablets may be used, but only under the direction of a physician.

It will be observed that milk is the ideal food because it contains water, proteins, fat (in the cream), sugar, minerals, and vitamins. It is easily digested in all its forms (regular, skimmed, or buttermilk). At least a quart of milk should therefore be taken every day not only throughout pregnancy but also after the baby comes as long as the baby is nursed at the breast.

Some pregnant women have a strong desire for unusual foods out of season or odd things. Chief among these are pickles, highly seasoned foods, and chalk (calcium). This perversion of appetite is known as "pica," and unless these foods disagree with the mother, they may be indulged in.

A definite relationship exists between the diet of the mother and the condition of the baby at birth and for a few weeks after. A proper diet produces a healthy child. Premature, stillborn, and abnormal babies are born usually to mothers who have had an inadequate diet in pregnancy.

SPECIAL DIETS

During the first three months of pregnancy at least 50 per cent of all women suffer from nausea or vomiting or both. These women should not attempt to eat the usual three meals a day but should take small amounts of solid food, especially starches and sweets, every two or two and a half hours. If part or all of the food is vomited, more solid food should be eaten immediately. Water should not be taken with these meals but between them. The following diet may prove useful:

Before getting out of bed:

Crackers or dry toast.

One half-hour later breakfast consisting of the following:

Orange, grapefruit, stewed prunes or apricots.
Cereal with cream and sugar.
One soft-boiled egg.
Thin buttered toast.
Milk, cocoa, weak tea or coffee with sugar.

10:00 a.m.:

Glass of milk with low-salt crackers.

Lunch:

Cup of cream of celery, asparagus, spinach or potato soup.
Soup crackers.

Salad of lettuce, tomato, endive, etc., with sugar and a small amount of lemon juice.
Whole-wheat bread, or toast, buttered.
Ice cream, water ice, or custard.

4:00 p.m.:
Milk, cocoa, chocolate or weak tea.
Small piece of cake, low-salt crackers, or wafers.

Dinner:
Cup of bouillon or vegetable soup, especially tomato.
Soup crackers.
Small lamb chop, broiled steak, or veal chop, well done.
Baked potato, mashed potatoes, or carrots.
Thin bread, or toast, buttered.
Lettuce or tomato salad.
Ice cream or water ice.

At bedtime:
Glass of hot milk, chocolate or malted milk.
Graham or oatmeal crackers.

The nausea and vomiting usually cease spontaneously after the fourth month, and from this time on the following diet is recommended:

Breakfast:
Fruit, such as orange, grapefruit, stewed prunes, or baked apple.
Cereal with cream and sugar.
One boiled or poached egg.
Two slices of crisp bacon.
Buttered toast, roll, or corn muffin.
Cup of cocoa, chocolate, weak tea, or coffee, with sugar and cream.

10:00 a.m.:
Glass of milk.
Fresh fruit or fruit juice.

Lunch:
Cream of celery, tomato, or asparagus soup.
Low-salt crackers or wafers.
Baked potato with butter.
Lettuce or tomato salad with sugar and small amount of lemon juice.
Ice cream.

4:00 p.m.:
American or cream cheese sandwich.
Glass of milk.

Dinner:
Celery, pea, spinach, or corn soup.
Salt wafers.
Small lamb chop, steak, or equivalent in fish.

Mashed or baked potato, carrots, peas, beet tops, or spinach.
Lettuce, tomato, endive salad with sugar and lemon.
Cheese and crackers or toast; nuts.
Ice cream, jelly roll, plain cake or fruit.
Cup of weak tea or coffee with cream and sugar.

At bedtime:
Glass of hot milk.
Low-salt or sweet crackers.

If a woman finds that certain foods disagree with her, she should eliminate them from her diet for a while. If the distressing symptoms reappear when she resumes eating them, these foods should not be eaten for the remainder of the pregnancy. In general it is advisable to avoid highly seasoned, spiced, greasy, fried, or fatty foods, rich pies, pastries, and other desserts, too many sweets, strong condiments, and strong coffee and tea. A woman who is underweight when she becomes pregnant may eat more than one who is overweight.

When the blood pressure rises and there is excessive gain in weight and swelling of the legs, hands, or face, the physician will ask the patient to avoid table salt as much as possible. The following foods should not be eaten:

DIETARY SUBSTANCES GENERALLY TO BE AVOIDED IN SODIUM RESTRICTION[1]

1. Smoked or cured meats and fish, such as ham, bacon, corned beef, cold cuts, frankfurters, sausage, tongue, salt pork, chipped beef, and anchovies.
2. Meat extracts, bouillon cubes, and meat sauces.
3. Salted foods, such as potato chips, nuts, and popcorn.
4. Prepared condiments, relishes, Worcestershire sauce, catsup, pickles, and olives.
5. Vegetable salts and flakes, such as onion, garlic, or celery salt; celery and parsley flakes.
6. Sodium in any other form, such as sodium benzoate as a preservative and monosodium glutamate as a flavoring aid.
7. Bread or bakery products unless prepared without salt and other sources of sodium.
8. Frozen fish fillets and shellfish, except oysters.
9. Prepared flours, flour mixes, baking powder and baking soda.
10. Frozen peas and lima beans.
11. All canned meat and vegetable products, unless prepared without salt (dietetic pack).
12. Canned pears, figs, and applesauce, unless prepared without salt (dietetic pack).
13. Butter, cheese, and peanut butter, unless prepared without salt.

[1] From Marie V. Krause in J. P. Greenhill's OBSTETRICS, 13th Edition, W. B. Saunders, 1964.

Most of the water should be taken on arising in the morning, between meals, and before retiring at night. On the day the twenty-four-hour specimen of urine is measured, the amount of water taken should also be recorded, and both of these figures should be given to the doctor.

CARE OF THE BOWELS

A pregnant woman should have a bowel movement every day, in order to eliminate not only her own waste products but also those of the baby in the womb. As a general rule, women have a strong tendency to be constipated while carrying a baby. Constipation is still more likely to occur in women who do not drink enough fluids and do not eat the proper kinds of food, and in those whose bowels did not move regularly before pregnancy supervened.

In order to prevent constipation as much as possible and also to overcome it when present, the following rules should be observed:

1. An abundance of water should be taken upon arising, during the day, and before going to bed.
2. Every day an attempt should be made to have a bowel movement at exactly the same hour. The best time for this is after breakfast, and one should have patience. However, there should not be too much straining. A glycerine suppository inserted into the rectum may stimulate the bowels to move.
3. The diet should contain a large amount of fresh fruits and vegetables. The fruits should include apples, apricots, cherries, figs, grapes, ripe olives, oranges, peaches, pears, pineapple, plums and prunes, raspberries and strawberries. The vegetables should include asparagus, beans, cabbage, carrots, celery, corn, lettuce, onions, peas, spinach, tomatoes, and watercress. Other foods which may help are bran, cereals, and bread. Tea should be avoided if there is marked constipation.
4. In some cases it may be necessary to inject four to six ounces of warm olive oil into the rectum before retiring. This is to remain overnight, and its purpose is to soften the stool, protect the lining of the rectum, and prevent or remove a spasm of the bowel.
5. If the above measures do not prevent or relieve constipation, drugs must be used. In nearly every case such simple substances as metamucil (every other night), or milk of magnesia (one tablespoon every night), usually suffice. In more stubborn cases it may be necessary to take a teaspoonful of fluid extract of cascara sagrada each night. An enema should be the last resort, and the fewer that are taken throughout pregnancy the better. The simplest enemas consist of weak salt solution or a very weak soapsuds solution. A simple and convenient enema is Fleet's, all prepared in a plastic container.

CARE OF THE KIDNEYS IN PREGNANCY

The kidneys have an extra amount of work to do during pregnancy, and they sometimes give rise to serious disturbances. If a woman knows she has or has had kidney trouble she should visit a physician before she plans to have a baby and let him tell her whether it is safe for her to bear a child. Women who have serious kidney disturbances, such as chronic nephritis, should not attempt to have children, because the kidney trouble will nearly always be aggravated, and the baby in many instances will not be born alive. However, if a woman has only a mild degree of nephritis she may go through a pregnancy without complications provided she is carefully watched by a competent physician.

Women with normal kidneys should have a specimen of urine examined at least once every three weeks, and more frequent examinations toward the end of pregnancy. However, women with kidney disturbances should have their urine examined at least once a week, and they should measure their urinary output every day. At least three pints of urine should be passed daily, and if the amount decreases the doctor should be informed.

If swelling of the feet, ankles, hands, or face is noticed, the doctor should be notified. Frequently these swellings indicate some abnormality in the function of the kidneys.

Chronic nephritis is not the only kind of kidney trouble which occurs during pregnancy. There may be a condition known as pyelonephritis, in which part of the kidney is inflamed and the urine contains pus and bacteria. Examination of the urine will also reveal whether diabetes or a tendency to diabetes is present.

CLOTHING IN PREGNANCY

The manner in which an expectant mother dresses herself is important. Comfort should not be sacrificed for the sake of appearances. In cold weather sufficient clothing should be worn to keep warm, whereas during the hot months the clothing should be light. In some regions it is important to be prepared for sudden changes in the weather in order to avoid chilling. Most of the clothing should be simple and should be washed frequently. None of it should hinder free movements of breathing or of the arms and legs. There must be no circular constrictions anywhere; hence it is important to give up using round garters, belts, tight corsets, or tight skirt bands. Side elastics attached to a maternity corset are the proper type of garter.

Underclothing should always be worn, the kind and amount depending upon the weather. It may consist of one or two pieces, but it is best that the drawers be closed. The under-garments should be changed every day or as often as possible, because they absorb the waste matter eliminated by the skin. All clothing should be well aired at night.

Women who have a flabby abdominal wall must wear a proper maternity corset, or they will have a good deal of discomfort, especially backache. On the other hand, most women carrying their first baby are comfortable throughout pregnancy without a corset.

Most women must wear a support for the breasts, or the latter will be painful. This support should not be tightly applied, but should elevate the breasts.

Proper shoes are essential. Shoes with narrow, high heels not only cause pain but theoretically cause harm. During the latter months of pregnancy the feet spread and enlarge somewhat, hence slightly larger shoes may have to be worn. Furthermore, as the abdomen continues to grow, there is a tendency to pull the body forward. To overcome this, the woman instinctively throws her shoulders back. If the woman wears high heels, the body is pushed still farther forward, and to save herself from falling she must throw her head and shoulders much farther backward. This causes a good deal of backache, discomfort in the lower part of the abdomen, and fatigue. The proper shoe for a pregnant woman with this problem is one which is sufficiently wide and has low broad heels somewhat on the style of the Cuban heel, or one still lower and wider. Rubber heels lessen the amount of jarring while walking.

It is natural for women to want to prevent the ungainly shape which some of them have after giving birth to a child. Most of this is due to relaxation of the skin and the rest of the abdominal wall and to markings on the skin known as striæ gravidarum. Massaging the abdominal wall with mineral oil or olive oil every day during pregnancy is said to diminish these conditions but their effectiveness is doubtful. In women with an inherited predisposition to flabbiness, little can be done to prevent relaxation of the abdominal muscles or striæ gravidarum.

EXERCISE IN PREGNANCY

A woman who expects a baby should take a certain amount of exercise daily. The benefits derived from exercise are improvement in the circulation of the blood, better appetite and digestion of food, better elimination of waste products of the body, more restful sleep, and an opportunity to divert the mind from household responsibilities.

The amount and kind of exercise for an expectant mother depend to a certain extent on the individual woman. One thing is certain, however: the expectant mother should never exercise to the point of fatigue. She should stop as soon as she begins to feel tired. The nearer the day of confinement, the more readily does fatigue set in. Women who are accustomed to participate in strenuous sports can tolerate more than women who lead an indoor and sedentary life. Women who have many household duties to perform do not need as much exercise as women who do not have such duties.

WALKING

Practically the only active exercise available for expectant mothers is walking and this should be outdoors, except during inclement weather. For this purpose, broad, low-heeled shoes with wide toes should be used, because high-heeled shoes may cause backache and missteps. It is best to walk during the hours of sunlight, because the sun's rays are beneficial. However, during the summer months the expectant mother should be cautious about taking a walk in the hot sun. While walking, it is advisable to proceed leisurely and to avoid crowds. Long tramps may be too strenuous for most women. About two or three miles is a fair average daily walk.

If even a short walk produces a tired feeling, the expectant mother should not walk much but should rest in the open air. While resting, the mind may be occupied with reading, knitting, or chatting. At least two hours each day should be spent outdoors. This time is best divided into two periods, one in the morning and the other in the afternoon. When the weather is unusually bad, a walk should be taken at home, either on an open porch or in a room with all the windows wide open. In winter, warm clothes should be worn for this, just as if one were on the street. It is needless to emphasize that the home should be well aired at all times, night as well as day.

VIOLENT EXERCISE

Violent exercise in any form should be avoided. This includes running, tennis, golf, swimming, cycling, skating, and horseback riding. Dancing should be indulged in only occasionally and for short periods of time; but the prospective mother should not dance in a crowded room.

TRAVEL

Driving an automobile should be given up during the last two months of pregnancy. However, most women may safely undertake long journeys by train, automobile, ship or airplane without mishap. The chief drawback is that should trouble arise during the journey or at the destination, skilled obstetric care may not be available.

Women who have lost babies before full term should avoid traveling whenever possible and should undertake a journey only after consultation with a physician. When railroad travel is imperative for a woman who has had miscarriages, the smoothest road and the most comfortable accommodations should be chosen and she should recline as much as possible during the journey.

HOUSEWORK

A certain amount of housework is not only permissible but is desirable. Here also the expectant mother should never proceed to the point of fatigue. Only light work should be done. If there is a young child at home, the expectant mother should not lift and carry him around any more than is absolutely necessary. By observing these precautions many backaches and much fatigue will be avoided.

An expectant mother who has much housework to do and who tires quickly from the additional walking outdoors should take only a short walk and spend most of the outdoor allotment of time sitting and resting, especially when the sun is shining. This will insure not only physical but also mental relaxation.

REST AND RECREATION

The prospective mother should learn to rest frequently, especially if she does housework. Most women, and more particularly those who tire easily, will find an afternoon nap of an hour or more of great help. Even if one does not actually sleep, complete relaxation in a reclining position will prove refreshing. To obtain the full benefit of such relaxation, it is essential to undress and go to bed. Where there are young children in the home, the mother may take her siesta when the children take theirs. If exercise is taken during the day, there need be no fear that an afternoon nap will prevent sleeping at night.

Places of amusement may be visited, but those that are poorly ventilated or overheated should be avoided.

Massage during pregnancy is rarely necessary but women who must remain in bed for a few weeks during pregnancy need massage.

BATHING

The skin should be kept clean at all times, but more especially during pregnancy, because the activity of the skin is greater than usual at this time. This is due to the increased elimination and excretion of the body during pregnancy, and the skin constitutes an important organ for these purposes. The expectant mother must eliminate not only her own waste products but also those of the child within the womb.

The skin contains myriads of openings called pores, which lead to sweat glands. By means of these pores certain excretory products of the body are eliminated. If these pores become clogged, proper elimination is prevented, and the expectant mother suffers in consequence.

The water and waste products that cannot be thrown off by the sweat glands remain in the blood until the kidneys, the bowels, and the lungs do the work. An unpleasant odor usually develops. To keep the pores open, to remove the accumulation of degenerated skin, dirt, grease, and dried perspiration, and to keep the skin functioning, it is necessary to wash the entire body with soap and water, and this must be done daily. One may take a shower, sponge, or tub bath, but the water should be neither too hot nor too cold. Very hot baths cause fatigue. The water should preferably be at a temperature between 85 and 90 degrees F. Even the woman who is accustomed to a cold bath each morning should increase the temperature of the water during pregnancy; for while a cold bath is stimulating, it is not as efficacious as a warm bath for actually cleansing the skin. However, women who are accustomed to a cold shower or tub bath may take such a cold bath in the morning and leave the cleansing bath for the evening.

Since the object of a bath is not only to cleanse the skin but also to stimulate the circulation, it is advisable to rub the whole body with a rough towel fairly vigorously. It does not matter much whether the daily warm bath is taken in the morning or in the evening before retiring. However, for women who do not sleep well, it is best to take the warm bath at night, because it is soothing and will promote sleep. If the warm bath is taken in the morning or during the day, at least an hour should elapse before one goes outdoors. If the bath is taken in the afternoon, at least two hours should have passed after the midday meal.

Shower or tub baths may be taken up to the time of actual confinement. When taking tub baths, women should be especially cautious to avoid slipping or falling while getting in and out of the tub.

The following types of bathing should be avoided by most women: cold tub baths, cold plunges, cold showers (except for those who are accustomed to such baths), and ocean bathing. Sweat baths should also be shunned, because they usually prove to be too exhausting and rarely do any good.

CARE OF THE BREASTS

Special attention should be paid to cleansing the breasts and nipples. Care must be exercised to avoid compression of and injury to the breasts;

this holds true not only during pregnancy but also during the entire life of the woman, from early infancy.

During pregnancy a breast supporter should be used, especially if the breasts are large. The skin of the breasts should be washed with soap and water daily just as the rest of the body. Special precautions should be taken to remove the scales that frequently cover the nipples. These scales are due to drying of the discharge which normally exudes from the nipples during pregnancy. If the prospective mother is to nurse her baby, the nipples may be anointed daily with cocoa butter, cold cream, or lanolin. Astringents, such as alcohol, should not be used because they harden the nipples, thereby favoring the formation of cracks, which may become avenues of infection.

If the nipples are flat, they may be drawn out for a few minutes each day during the last few weeks of pregnancy; but this must be done with the utmost gentleness and after demonstration by a physician or nurse.

CARE OF THE GENITAL ORGANS

The genital organs may require attention. During pregnancy there is increased secretion, but this does not require removal. If, however, the discharge is profuse or has a disagreeable odor, or there is an itch at the opening of the vagina, the doctor should be told about it. Douches should never be taken.

SEXUAL INTERCOURSE

Sexual intercourse need not be restricted during pregnancy unless it is painful or disagreeable. However it should be discontinued no later than three weeks before the baby is expected, because of the danger of rupturing the bag of waters and of serious infection. Women who have a tendency to abort, who have bled during the pregnancy or who have had premature labors should indulge in as little intercourse as possible throughout the entire pregnancy.

CARE OF THE HAIR

The hair should be washed once a week. The scalp should be massaged and the hair brushed daily. If the hair is dry or there is dandruff, olive oil should be rubbed into the hair and scalp. There is no harm in having a permanent wave but this should not be done in the last four weeks of pregnancy.

SMOKING

It is best for the expectant mother who smokes to limit the number of cigarettes to ten a day. There appears to be a relationship between excessive smoking and prematurity. It is best to give up smoking entirely.

CARE OF THE TEETH

It is important for every expectant mother to have her teeth examined and cleaned at least twice during her pregnancy. If the dentist finds defects which he can remedy, it is perfectly safe for him to correct the abnormalities. But he should not do more than is absolutely necessary. He may fill, clean, and pull teeth, but not attempt work which requires a long time and causes a good deal of pain unless it cannot be postponed until after delivery.

The teeth should, of course, be carefully brushed at least once a day and dental floss, stimudents, or water under pressure used to remove particles of food lodged between the teeth. If the gums have a tendency to bleed they should be vigorously massaged with the fingers two or three times a day.

THE MIND

The expectant mother should try to lead a quiet, cheerful life and avoid mental as well as physical upheavals. There is usually nothing to fear about pregnancy and labor, and the best proof of this is that millions of women constantly go through these physiologic processes without harm, all over the world. It is best to avoid contact with friends or relatives who relate tales about difficult obstetric cases they know. If a woman has any fears she should speak to her doctor about them. He will usually be able to prove there is no basis for them, and if there is good cause for the fears the physician will be able to correct or overcome the cause. Reading cheerful books helps a great deal.

SIGNS OF TROUBLE

There are certain signs and symptoms which arise during pregnancy and which may be forerunners of trouble unless attention is paid to them. The following is a list of them, and when any of them are present they should be called to the attention of the physician without delay:

1. Persistent vomiting of most of the food eaten in the first three months of pregnancy and any vomiting after the fifth month.
2. Stubborn constipation.
3. Frequent or persistent headaches, especially if associated with dizziness and marked constipation.
4. Swelling of the feet, ankles, hands, eyelids, or face.
5. Rapid gain in weight.
6. Diminished output of urine.
7. Blurred or double vision, or spots before the eyes.
8. Shortness of breath or inability to sleep unless the head is elevated on a few pillows.
9. Frequent fainting spells.
10. Any infection or fever.
11. Failure to feel the baby after it has been definitely felt for a while.
12. Cramps or pain in the abdomen.
13. Escape of bloody or watery discharge from the vagina with or without cramps in the lower part of the abdomen. During the early months of pregnancy these are symptoms of a threatened or beginning miscarriage or abortion. Should they occur, someone should notify the doctor and the patient should get into bed. She should not become excited, because nothing serious can happen during the first few hours, and a doctor can surely reach her during this time. It may happen that the fetus and afterbirth are expelled spontaneously. All tissue, including blood clots, which is passed, should be saved in a towel or in a jar so the doctor may see whether all the parts came away. This is important, because if part or all of the afterbirth is left in the womb, it will have to be removed with instruments.

MINOR AILMENTS DURING PREGNANCY

HEARTBURN AND BELCHING

Many women are greatly disturbed by frequent attacks of heartburn or belching or both. In spite of its name, heartburn has nothing to do with the heart. It is a peculiar burning sensation in the chest and throat, accompanied by the presence of a bitter fluid which escapes from the stomach into the throat. Sometimes heartburn may be prevented by drinking a glass of milk and cream mixture a few minutes before meal time. The fat in the cream and milk prevents the secretion of acid in the stomach. However, when heartburn is actually present, fats will not help. In fact, they may even aggravate the condition. The best remedies for heartburn are a half-teaspoonful of baking soda (sodium bicarbonate) in a half-glass of water, a teaspoonful of milk of magnesia, or two or three soda-mint tablets. These substances neutralize the acid which causes the heartburn. However, the amount of sodium bicarbonate and other alkalis taken during pregnancy should be strictly limited.

FAINTING AND DIZZINESS

It is not uncommon for pregnant women, especially those who are anemic, to have attacks of fainting or dizziness. The condition is not serious; hence, there is no cause for alarm or worry. If a woman feels faint she should immediately lie down on a couch or bed. If she is in a place where there is no bed or couch, she should gently slip down to the floor and lie flat. The faintness will pass away in a few minutes. If the attacks are frequent, it is a good thing to keep spirits of ammonia or smelling salts in the house within easy reach or in the purse. If a woman becomes dizzy she should sit down and lower her head to her knees in order to permit more blood to reach the brain. This symptom should be reported to the physician.

VARICOSE VEINS

Varicose veins are much more common in women who have had children and there is a large hereditary factor in most of these women. Women who have varicose veins on the legs and thighs should keep the legs up on a chair or a stool while they are sitting. They can read, sew, or fulfill most sedentary occupations with their legs elevated. This relieves the distended veins of the extra load of blood they must carry when the patient is standing or sitting with her feet lowered in the usual position. Care must be exercised not to injure varicose veins, because they may bleed or become infected. In cases where the veins are unusually large, supportive stockings or elastic bandages must be worn. This should be long enough to extend above the highest visible varicose vein and should be put on the leg in the morning before the woman gets out of bed. Occasionally an operation is necessary during pregnancy. The results of this type of surgery are good.

HEMORRHOIDS OR PILES

Many pregnant women are troubled by piles. The usual symptom is bleeding from the rectum while having a bowel movement or pain may be present. They are much more common in women who have had children than in those who are pregnant for the first time. It is important to eat the proper kinds of food and to go to the toilet at the same time every day because hemorrhoids are always aggravated by constipation and straining during bowel movements. In addition, a tablespoonful of metamucil should be taken by mouth morning and evening. If the piles are much swollen, ice or witch hazel compresses will help. If the hemorrhoids do not readily go back into the rectum, they should be pushed back with a lubricated finger, because there is danger of obstruction and infection of these veins. If they cannot be pushed back or if they bleed frequently the doctor should be notified.

CRAMPS IN THE LEGS

Cramps or muscular contractions occur rather frequently, especially in the second half of pregnancy, and particularly during the night. They may be relieved by changing position, by rubbing the cramped part, by applying heat or cold, by bending the foot at the ankle, and by standing on a cold slab such as the floor of the bathroom. Leg cramps may be prevented or relieved considerably by (1) reducing the intake of milk temporarily, (2) the use of calcium salts free from phosphorus or (3) adding small quantities of aluminum hydroxide gel to the diet in order to remove some of the dietary phosphorus from the intestines. If the cramps are severe the physician will prescribe specific medication.

PREVENTION OF GOITER

In pregnancy the function of the thyroid gland is increased, and, because of this, slightly more iodine is needed than otherwise. If insufficient iodine is eaten, the thyroid gland of both mother and baby may enlarge. In most parts of the country there is ample iodine in the drinking water and in the vegetables and grain grown in these regions. However, in certain localities like the Great Lakes region there is a lack of iodine, and the expectant mothers in these places must take iodine in some form such as iodine tablets, iodized salt, or Lugol's solution. However, none of these should ever be taken without orders and strict supervision by a physician, because harm may result.

PREPARATIONS FOR CONFINEMENT

Nearly all women have their babies in a hospital because of the numerous advantages gained thereby. The doctor or the patient may make the necessary arrangements. Since premature delivery is not uncommon, it is a good plan to have certain articles packed in a suitcase a few weeks before the expected date of confinement. These articles should consist of two nightgowns, a bathrobe, two pairs of stockings, a pair of slippers, a few handkerchiefs, a toothbrush and toothpaste or powder, and a comb and brush. In most hospitals the baby's clothes are supplied by the hospital until the child is ready to leave. Hence the day before the patient expects to depart from the hospital, the husband or someone else should take to the hospital for the baby a shirt, a nightgown or robe, safety pins, a few diapers, a sweater, a cap, and two blankets. Of course these are only a few of the things which the expectant mother should have bought a few weeks before the baby arrives. Since newborn babies quickly outgrow the clothes, not much is needed at the time of birth. Nowadays clothes for the baby are made to be comfortable for the child and easy to put on and take off. They should be of light texture, particularly, because in steam-heated apartments babies are generally burdened with too many clothes.

The following is a list of clothes necessary for a baby:

Shirts. Four shirts are usually sufficient. They should be infant size No. 2 for they will soon be outgrown. For summer, cotton mesh should be used and for winter, cotton and wool. The shirts should have long sleeves and high necks, they should open in the front and they should reach down below the hips.

Dresses. Two dresses are ample because they are worn only occasionally. They should open all the way down the back.

Kimonos. Four kimonos should be purchased because they are used more than dresses. They should consist of cotton and wool, flannelette or cashmere.

Nightgowns. Six nightgowns are usually necessary. They should be made of soft flannel or stockinet. Most of the nightgowns have drawstrings in the sleeves and at the bottom in order to keep the baby warm should it become uncovered during the night.

Diapers. At least four dozen diapers should be obtained. They should be soft, absorbent, and of loosely woven material such as bird's eye, stockinet, or cotton flannel. Many diapers are made to throw away after they are used once. In large cities there are laundries which for a fee deliver clean, sterilized diapers every day and take back the soiled ones. The laundries provide diaper containers.

Bootees. Two pairs of bootees are sufficient. They should be long enough to extend over the knee. Stockings are not to be used.

Sweaters. Two sweaters either knitted or made of cashmere are necessary. They should be open down the front, so there will not be any need to slip them on over the baby's head.

Cap. One cap will suffice.

In addition to the foregoing list of clothes for the baby, other articles may be secured. For the baby's nursery the following will be necessary:

1. A bed or large basket with a suitable mattress.
2. Four sheets made of cotton knit.
3. Two large rubber sheets to be placed between the mattress and cotton sheet.
4. Six pads made of Turkish toweling each about 20 by 20 inches.

5. One rubberized pad, about 20 by 20 inches, to be placed under the Turkish toweling pads.

6. Two woolen blankets.

7. A bath table for bathing and dressing the baby. Most of these are collapsible.

8. Scales which may be purchased or rented. They should be of the balance or beam type and not of the spring type.

9. A clothes horse for hanging and drying the baby's clothes.

10. A baby's toilet tray on which should be placed a rectal thermometer, a bath thermometer, nursing bottles, safety pins, and covered jars containing rubber nipples, bottle caps, cotton balls, toothpick swabs, a bottle brush, albolene and soap.

11. Towels and wash cloths.

WHEN TO CALL THE DOCTOR FOR CONFINEMENT

Labor is the term applied to the process of giving birth, and there are usually three signs by which the beginning of labor may be known:

1. Rhythmic contractions of the womb which the woman experiences as abdominal cramps. These may be felt by placing the hand on the abdomen, because the latter becomes hard during a contraction and relaxes when the cramp subsides. At first these cramps or labor pains are irregular in frequency and intensity, and they begin in the back and radiate to the front. Later they become more frequent, more regular, stronger, and located in the abdomen. "False pains" are weak contractions which occur a few days or a few weeks before actual confinement. They may be distinguished from true labor pains by the fact that they do not increase in frequency, intensity, or duration, and they subside after a while.

2. The escape from the vagina of water which is not urine. This is due to rupture of the bag of waters in which the baby lies. Labor pains usually do not begin for a few hours after this starts, but it is advisable for the patient to go to the hospital after notifying the doctor.

3. A thick, mucous, bloody discharge from the vagina, known as the "show."

Only one of these signs is usually present at first, and it is sufficient to warrant notifying the doctor. Then the hospital should be informed that the patient is on the way. Abnormal symptoms may sometimes arise just about the time of confinement, and the doctor must be told about them without delay. These symptoms include bleeding from the vagina, a sudden fainting attack, severe persistent cramps in the abdomen, vomiting, disturbances in vision, and muscular twitchings. It is a good thing to keep the telephone numbers of the doctor, his assistant if he has one, and the hospital, in a place where they can be obtained without delay.

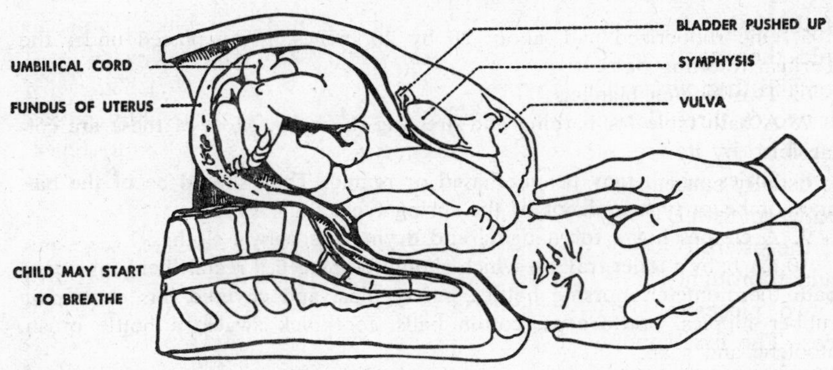

Fig. 30. Birth of a baby. After the baby's head emerges, it turns as the shoulders are rotated. The head is gently and firmly supported by the attendant. As contractions continue, the head is guided over the receding and thickening perineum and the rest of the baby's body slides out. From *A Baby Is Born,* Maternity Center Association.

WHAT TO DO IF THE BABY IS BORN AT HOME BEFORE THE PATIENT CAN GO TO THE HOSPITAL

The average duration of the first labor is about thirteen hours, and the length of labor after the first one is about eight hours. Hence there is no need to be panic-stricken when labor begins. With few exceptions there is always ample time to get to the hospital. Occasionally, however, for one reason or another, especially in the case of a woman who has had a few quick labors, the entire duration of labor may be so short that the baby is born at home. When it is obvious that the child will be born in the home, the patient's physician should be informed of what is happening. If he cannot be reached, his assistant or another physician should be called to act in the emergency. A kettle of water should be placed on a stove to boil, and a small pair of scissors and two pieces of tape or string dropped into the water.

The cleanest room should be chosen for the patient, and there should be sufficient warmth, especially for the sake of the baby. The expectant mother should, of course, remain in bed. If a baby can be born in such a short time, the process is nearly always normal and easy. As soon as the baby is born, if it cries spontaneously, nothing need be done except to wrap a warm, clean towel around its body to keep it warm. There is usually no harm in leaving the child in bed just as it is, provided it is breathing normally and its color is pink. If the doctor is informed of what happened at home he will usually be able to arrive in time to clean his hands properly to tie the cord and see that the afterbirth is delivered.

If the baby does not breathe or cry immediately after birth, someone should thoroughly wash his or her hands and fore-arms with soap and water and then with alcohol and should rub the baby's back up and down with two or three fingers. If this does not produce crying, the baby should be held up by its feet, and its buttocks gently spanked a number of times. This usually causes the baby to cry. Then it should be kept covered with a clean warm towel.

If the afterbirth should be expelled before the doctor arrives, someone should thoroughly scrub his or her hands with soap and water, and with the two pieces of boiled tape or string, tie the umbilical cord in two places. The first should be about one inch from the baby's body and the other about one inch farther away. Before tying the two tapes, iodine or other antiseptic on a cotton applicator should be applied on the part of the cord where the strings are to be tied, and the strings should be

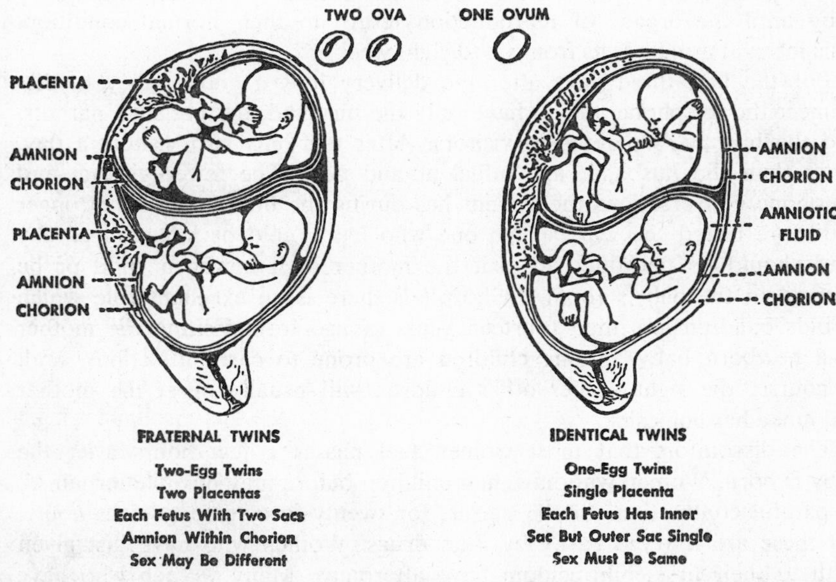

Fig. 31. The two babies in the left of the picture are fraternal twins. This means that they developed from two separate ova and were fertilized by two separate sperm. Each twin has its own double membrane, sac, and placenta. They may or may not be the same sex. Fraternal twins are frequently no more alike than any other brother and sister. The two babies in the right of the picture are identical twins. They were developed from one ovum, fertilized by one sperm. If you look closely you will see that there is one chorion (outer membrane) shared by both babies. Each baby has its own amnion (inner membrane). They share the same placenta. Identical twins are always the same sex and each is the mirror image of the other. From *A Baby Is Born,* Maternity Center Association.

saturated with iodine. The cord should then be cut between the two pieces of string with the scissors which is in the kettle of boiling water. More iodine or other antiseptic should be applied to the cut edge of the cord which is attached to the baby. It is important to be sure there is no bleeding from this end of the cord. If there is bleeding, another piece of string should be applied tightly.

The afterbirth and the sac should not be thrown away but should be saved for the doctor to see. It is important to know whether all of the afterbirth and the sac came away intact. If a piece is left behind, it usually causes hemorrhage and frequently infection unless it is removed immediately.

THE PUERPERIUM

The puerperium is the time interval that extends from the birth of the baby until the organs of reproduction return to their normal condition. This interval usually lasts from six to eight weeks.

For the first three days after the delivery it is a good policy to disconnect the telephone and to have only the husband, the patient's parents, and the husband's parents as visitors. After this only two visitors a day, other than the husband, are sufficient and best. The fewer visitors and telephone conversations the patient has during the first week, the stronger and more rested she will be. No one who has a cold or infection of any kind should be permitted to visit the mother of a newborn child or be allowed in the baby's room. In hospitals there is an excellent rule which forbids children less than fourteen years of age from visiting the mother of a newborn baby. Young children are prone to carry infections, and, of course, the sight of her other children will usually upset the mother and make her homesick.

The discomfort that most women feel passes a few hours after the baby is born. Women who have had children before may have "afterpains," or painful contractions of the uterus, for twenty-four to forty-eight hours, but these are relieved easily by mild drugs. Women who have just given birth to their first child seldom have afterpains. Many women who have stitches on the outside of the vagina suffer a good deal of pain. In addition to the use of medicines for the relief of the pain, a helpful procedure is to sit in a hot tub once or twice a day. For generations tub baths within the first few days or even weeks have been taboo, but there is no harm in indulging in them and they afford great relief from pain.

On the third or fourth day most women complain of pain and swelling of the breasts. This is caused by the onset of the flow of milk. The discomfort is seldom troublesome and generally disappears after twenty-four to forty-eight hours when the baby, by its sucking action, has regulated the amount of milk in the breasts. Babies are generally put to the breast only twice during the first twenty-four hours, and after this they nurse every four hours, except during the night. Breast nursing is beneficial to the mother as well as to the newborn baby. The genital organs return to normal more quickly in women who nurse their babies.

Today patients are permitted much more freedom than was the custom in previous years. We generally permit our patients to get out of bed and even walk the day the baby is born, but surely the next day unless there is a strong reason against this activity. Most mothers may safely return to their homes when the baby is four or five days old.

If the patient had some disturbance during pregnancy, she will need special aftercare. Thus, if a woman had high blood pressure, she will have to have repeated blood-pressure readings. If she had a kidney infection, her urine will have to be examined every day. These women must be watched not only during their hospital stay but for months and perhaps years afterward. Such follow-up care is important for the patient's future health and certainly for a decision about having more children.

POSTPARTUM CARE

Postpartum means after delivery. When a patient leaves the hospital she may walk the steps leading to her apartment but she should walk up slowly. Since there is considerable excitement incident to dressing the baby, packing suitcases, saying good-bye to the nurses, riding home, meeting neighbors, and so on, in the process of getting home, it is advisable that the patient lie down on a couch or bed for about thirty minutes. Once in the home, the patient should not go into the street until the baby is more than two weeks old.

Probably the most important factor necessary to safeguard a happy household with a newborn baby is a mentally calm and unperturbed mother. This is determined to the largest extent by the health of the baby. As was previously said, the day of departure from the hospital is one of excitement. As a result the baby not infrequently loses weight on that day. After the first day at home the mother must learn to be more or less callous to disturbing influences. Certainly petty inconveniences should not be permitted to interfere with her peace of mind. If there is a nurse at home, she, of course, assumes much of the responsibility in the care of the child. Tranquillity of mind and regularity in feeding the infant will usually guarantee a thriving baby.

During the puerperium the mother should have an abundance of sleep and, in addition, should rest in a reclining position for definite periods of time in the morning and in the afternoon.

During the first week at home visitors should be restricted to two a day besides the immediate family. Tact is necessary to avoid talkative visitors or to limit their stay. Likewise, telephone calls should be limited in number and length, especially if at the other end of the wire there is a garrulous individual or one who wants to impart information concerning dreadful occurrences. Visitors who have colds or infections should not be seen and definitely must not be admitted to the baby's room.

If the mother herself has a cold, she should cover her mouth and nose with a handkerchief or a mouthpiece when nursing or bathing the baby. No medicine should be taken by the mother or given to the baby without the sanction of a physician. Many drugs reach the baby through the breast milk.

If there are three- or four-year-old children in the home, the development of jealousy in them should be looked for and averted. Sometimes they resent the attention showered on a new arrival. Showing the baby off before relatives and friends may aggravate such a tendency.

When nursing the baby one may sit up or recline. An extremely important thing to avoid is constant observation of the baby while it is at the breast; for this not only strains the mother's eyes and produces headaches, but strains the muscles of the neck and back, which likewise become the seat of pain.

For the woman with a lax abdominal wall a supporting garment is most helpful. Showers or tub baths should be taken daily during this time. Exercise, especially walking, is advisable after the second week; but strenuous exercise, such as playing golf or tennis, swimming, skating, or even driving a car, should be avoided during the first four weeks. Social functions during these weeks should likewise be reduced to a minimum.

RETURN OF MENSTRUATION

The return of menstruation varies in different individuals. In those who do not nurse their babies the flow usually returns at the end of six weeks, while in those who do breast-feed their babies the first menstrual period appears sometime after the third month. In a few, however, the menses do not return until the baby is weaned. The first period is usually profuse, sometimes enough to cause alarm. At the time of the first period it is best for the woman to keep off her feet as much as possible; but if the flow is too profuse, the advice of a physician should be sought. In fact, if the mother has any doubt concerning herself or the baby she should consult her physician rather than take the advice offered by well-meaning but often misinformed friends and relatives. Cracked or bleeding nipples or painful breasts particularly call for immediate notification of the physician.

It is customary for a patient to return to her physician at the end of the puerperal period; namely, six to eight weeks after the birth of the baby. At this time the physician will determine, by an examination of the breasts and an abdominal and vaginal examination, whether the reproductive organs have returned to their normal state. Generally this checkup is designated as the "final" examination. This is unfortunate, because the patient regards it as the final contact with her physician until a new pregnancy begins or some disturbance arises. It is advisable for women to see their obstetricians when the baby is six months old, and again when it is a year old. All women should be examined once a year, preferably twice, even if they feel entirely well. This is most important to keep women healthy but especially to prevent or detect cancer of the breast and uterus early. Every female should have a yearly smear (Papanicolaou) test. Such tests have already resulted in a decrease in cancer of the uterus. On the other hand cancer of the breast is increasing frighteningly and as yet we do not know how to prevent this except by frequent examinations by both patients and physicians.

WEANING THE BABY

The time when a baby is to be weaned varies considerably. Women who have an abundant supply of breast milk should nurse their baby for four to six months. However, few women have a supply of milk which will last as long as this. Women with ample breast milk should not wean the baby during the first few months without an urgent reason. A doctor's advice should be sought before a woman with a good supply of milk decides to discontinue breast feedings.

SUPERSTITIONS AND MISCONCEPTIONS ABOUT CHILDBIRTH

From the dawn of history there have been innumerable superstitions associated with childbirth. The ancients held such peculiar notions about reproduction that we consider them ludicrous. However, the vast majority of the laity who today scoff at the credulity of the uncivilized and the semicivilized peoples hold fast to enough erroneous beliefs about childbirth to make physicians laugh at them in turn.

There is an almost universal belief among the laity in so-called maternal impressions. This expression signifies that a child in the womb may be marked in some obscure way by what the mother thinks, feels, or sees during pregnancy, especially if the experience is disagreeable or shocking. This belief is one of the oldest in history. Not only was it prevalent among the uncivilized peoples, but many of our most prominent literary celebrities used it as a theme for their writings. Among the latter may be mentioned Goethe, Scott, Dickens, and O. W. Holmes. When a child is born with a birthmark, those who believe in maternal impressions make an effort to detect a special form in the birthmark and link it up with some frightful occurrence which the mother experienced during the last few months of pregnancy. However, there is absolutely no support for the belief in maternal impressions. In the first place birthmarks and other defects are usually accidental aberrations in the growth of the child. These abnormalities begin to manifest themselves when the fetus has been in the uterus only a few weeks, because the fetus is almost completely formed by the time it reaches its tenth week of development. Hence nothing which happens to the mother in the latter part of gestation can possibly affect the child in the womb. Secondly, there is no direct contact between the mother and the baby in the womb, by way of either the nerves or the blood. The nerves connect the mother with the womb but not with the baby; hence the worst thing which can occur is stimulation of the uterus, with subsequent interruption of pregnancy. Even this occurrence is uncommon. The baby receives nourishment from the mother, but only because the afterbirth extracts the necessary ingredients from the mother's blood. Thirdly, in most instances, where the child presents defects, the mother was never frightened or upset in any way. In spite of the horrors to which women abroad were subjected during World Wars I and II, there were no more "marked" babies than are usually born.

Another common belief is that a baby born during the seventh month of its intrauterine existence can live, whereas one delivered during the eighth month cannot. This is incorrect. The truth is that the longer a baby remains in the womb, which is by far the best incubator, before it is born, the more advanced is its development, and hence the greater its chances for survival. The few exceptions do not disprove this rule.

There are many misconceptions concerning the determination of the sex of a child before birth. It is commonly held that if a baby's heart tones are more than 140 per minute the baby is a girl, whereas if the heart rate is less than 140 the child is a boy. This belief is based on the fact that large babies usually have slower heart rates than smaller ones, and since boys are generally larger than girls it is assumed that slow heartbeats indicate boys. The truthful physician will tell his patients that he guesses the sex of babies incorrectly almost as often as he guesses it correctly. Normally about 105 boys are born to every 100 girls, and this ratio holds true regardless of seasonal variations and geographical divisions. Hence, if a physician guesses boys more often than girls, over a long period of time, his correct guesses will be slightly greater than his incorrect ones. Among premature babies the proportion of males is higher than 105 to 100, and among fetuses which are expelled during the early months of pregnancy the males are still more predominant. There is as yet no satisfactory explanation for this phenomenon.

Some people believe that the sex of a baby depends on the time in the menstrual cycle when conception takes place. This is wrong. In human beings the sex is determined at the time the female egg is fertilized by the male spermatozoön or sex cell. It is the latter which determines whether a child is to be a male or a female. There are two types of spermatozoa, one of which produces males and one of which is responsible for females.

Some individuals believe that a woman who has only one ovary is capable of having only male or only female children. This belief is not true, because women with only one ovary may give birth to babies of either sex. Likewise these women have a menstrual flow every month, and not every second month. In other words, women with one ovary are just as capable from a reproductive point of view as women with two ovaries.

There is an almost unanimous belief that a woman who has a Cesarean section must have all her subsequent babies delivered in the same way. This is erroneous, because many women have babies through the natural passages after having had a Cesarean section. Of course, if the first operation was performed because a woman has small pelvic bones, the operation will have to be repeated for each baby unless the babies are unusually small. On the other hand, if abdominal delivery was resorted to because of such complications as hemorrhage, convulsions, etc., and this complication is absent during subsequent pregnancies, delivery may often be accomplished in the natural way. However, if natural delivery is awaited after the old type of Cesarean section, there is a distinct risk of rupture of the uterus. This hazard is slight after the new type of abdominal delivery.

Another misbelief is that a Cesarean section cannot be performed until a woman is in actual labor. However, this operation may be done at any time during pregnancy, even weeks and months before the time of the calculated confinement. Likewise it may be performed at any time during labor, but the longer a woman is permitted to have labor pains before the operation is resorted to, especially if the bag of waters has ruptured, the greater the risk of infection.

Some individuals are of the opinion that a woman can have only two Cesarean sections. The truth is that there is no limit to the number of these operations a woman may have. In fact, there is a case on record of a woman who had thirteen babies by Cesarean operation. Fortunately this is a unique case. Because every abdominal operation carries with it some risk, usually a physician will sterilize a woman after her third Cesarean operation if she so desires. Sterilization as performed today does not prolong a Cesarean operation greatly and does not increase the risk of the operation. Even if the womb is removed after delivery of the child, there is no increased hazard. The womb is seldom removed unless it is diseased. In rare instances however, it is taken out at the time of a Cesarean section as a means of preventing conception.

Contrary to a common notion, sterilization as now performed has absolutely no deleterious effect on a woman afterward. If she were not told that she can no longer have babies she would not know she was sterilized. All her normal functions, including menstruation, continue except the ability to conceive. It is only when the uterus is removed by operation or its function is destroyed by radium or the X rays that the menstrual flow ceases. If for some reason the ovaries are also removed at the time of Cesarean section (and this is extremely rare) the symptoms of the change of life may set in. This is not a calamity because we possess inexpensive hormone tablets which women may take to prevent or overcome the symptoms of the menopause.

A fairly common misconception is that which maintains a woman is incapable of becoming pregnant as long as she nurses a baby. Many women have had an opportunity to learn otherwise. Conception is possible at this time regardless of whether a woman menstruates or not. Most women begin to menstruate within a few months after their babies are born. Those who do not nurse their babies usually have the first flow at the end of about six weeks, whereas those who nurse do not begin to menstruate until a few months later. Strange as it may seem, pregnancy is possible not only during the period of nursing but also before a young girl of twelve or thirteen years begins to menstruate, and also at the end of the reproductive career for a year or more after a woman ceases to menstruate because of the change of life. In other words, even though there is no monthly flow, the ovaries may produce and expel ova or eggs which are capable of being fertilized.

A common belief not only among the public but also among some physicians is that the size of the baby at birth is dependent for the most part upon the amount of food the mother eats during gestation. While this appears to be logical, it has not been proved. There is no constant ratio between the gain in weight in the mother and the size of the baby. The size of babies depends chiefly on heredity but also in some cases upon abnormal conditions in the mother. For example, women with kidney trouble usually have puny babies, and mothers with diabetes frequently have abnormally large offspring. Physicians carefully control the weight of obstetric patients because an excessive gain is primarily deleterious for the mother and only secondarily for the baby.

Since the baby is in reality a parasite, it takes all the nourishment it needs from its mother's blood. If the mother's food does not contain all the ingredients a baby requires, the child will obtain these substances at the expense of the mother's tissues. Hence it is important for a pregnant woman to take not only the proper amount of food but also the right kinds of food, minerals, vitamins, etc.

Of lesser extent is the belief that one can tell the sex of a baby from the shape of the mother's abdomen. Thus a high prominence is said to indicate a boy, whereas a more even distribution to the sides and to the back is said to be indicative of a girl. These notions have absolutely no truth in them. Likewise there is no basis for the belief that if a woman extends her arms upward to reach for objects the baby will be born with a loop or cord around its neck. In the first place, stretching cannot result in lassoing the child around the neck because the baby moves about freely in a spacious sac of fluid. Secondly the finding of one or more loops of cord around a baby's neck at birth is fairly frequent and usually has no significance at all. Only rarely does a loop of cord wound around a child's neck produce trouble.

A way is known of definitely telling the sex of a baby while it is still in the uterus. This consists of obtaining some of the fluid which surrounds the fetus and examining the cells in the fluid for sex chromosomes. However, this can be dangerous; and unless there is a special reason to carry out this procedure, it should not be tried.

Many women and physicians believe that a tight binder applied to the woman's abdomen after childbirth will result in the restoration of a normal figure. Unfortunately this is not true. No matter how snug a binder or bandage is applied, it cannot restore tonicity of weak abdominal muscles. On the other hand a tightly applied abdominal binder may result in harm. A loosely applied binder helps to steady the enlarged uterus when the patient moves around in bed, it relieves the feeling of emptiness in the abdomen, and it allays the minds of those women who believe that the binder will restore their anteconceptional figure.

CHAPTER 9

Care and Feeding of the Child

ALWIN C. RAMBAR, M.D.

INTRODUCTION

Children and adults in 1968 are taller than they were some years ago; since 1885 progressive average increase in both height and weight has occurred. Among the reasons are improved economic conditions allowing for better diets and advances in medical care.

DEVELOPMENT OF THE INFANT

There are extreme variations within normal limits of the infant in its first year of life. In this time usually the question arises of whether the baby is developing normally. Mothers often use their own knowledge of previous siblings or neighbors' children as their standards for comparison. To evaluate progress properly, some fundamental knowledge of the limits of how a baby grows and develops is necessary. The average newborn infant weighs about 7 pounds at birth, the male usually being slightly larger than the female. However, weight from 6 to 9 pounds at birth may be considered normal. The American Academy of Pediatrics has set the standard of prematurity at 5½ pounds or less. Under certain circumstances a full term baby may weigh less than 5½ pounds at birth and perhaps should be considered an immature baby. Infants born of diabetic or pre-diabetic mothers may weigh over 9 pounds at birth; this is an indication for investigation of possible diabetes in the mother.

In the first few days of life, some loss of weight appears which is mainly a loss of water from the baby's tissues; this is a normal balancing process. Unless the loss is more than ten per cent of the birth weight, it should not cause concern. After the fifth day, usually a gradual gain in weight ensues if the feedings are satisfactory. This continues at different rates throughout the growth span of the child's life. The average newborn doubles its birth weight at four to five months, and approximately triples it at one year. Thus the growth rate is faster during the first few months than in the latter months of the first year. The appetite of the infant is concurrent with the rate of growth and it is normal for it to eat more vigorously during the early period when growth is more rapid. This is also particularly noticeable during the growth spurt periods in later childhood when parents feel that they cannot "fill him up."

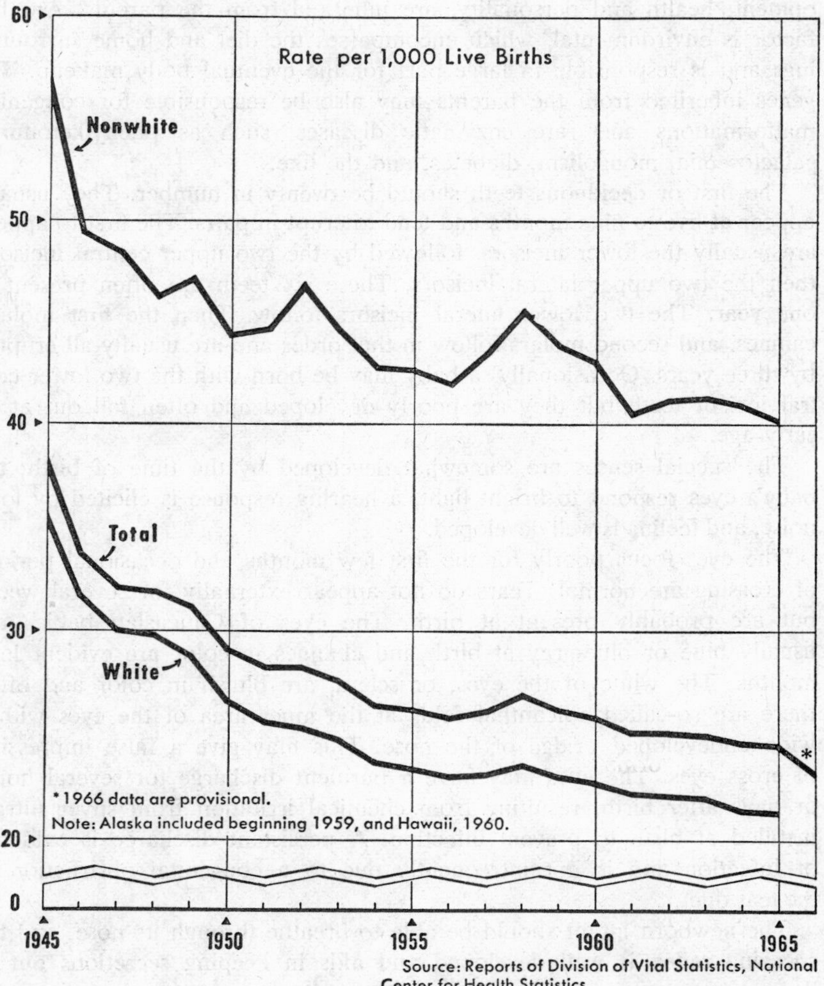

Fig. 32. Trend in Infant Mortality, United States 1945–66. *Statistical Bulletin*, Metropolitan Life Insurance Company.

One of the easily recognized signs of an infant's progress is its gain in weight. This is continuous from year to year as a result of constant growth, and the expected rate of gain changes from one age period to another. These age periods can be divided into the pre-natal period, from fertilization of the ovum until delivery of the fetus; neo-natal, the first month of life; infancy, the first two years; preschool, 2 to 6; childhood proper, six to ten for girls, six to twelve for boys; adolescence, ten to eighteen for girls, and twelve to twenty for boys.

Genetic factors which are responsible for the size, build, rate of development, health and personality, are inherited from the parents. Another factor is environmental, which encompasses the diet and home surroundings and is responsible in large part for the eventual body makeup. The genes inherited from the parents may also be responsible for congenital malformations and rare enzymatic diseases, such as phenylketonuria, galactosemia, mongolism, diabetes, and the like.

The first or deciduous teeth should be twenty in number. They usually appear at five to nine months and tend to erupt in pairs. The first to appear are usually the lower incisors, followed by the two upper central incisors, then the two upper lateral incisors. These six teeth are often present at one year. The two lower lateral incisors follow. Then the first molars, canines, and second molars follow in that order and are usually all erupted by three years. Occasionally, a baby may be born with the two lower central incisor teeth but they are poorly developed and often fall out at an early age.

The special senses are somewhat developed by the time of birth; the baby's eyes respond to bright light, a hearing response is elicited by loud noise, and feeling is well developed.

The eyes focus poorly for the first few months and occasional periods of crossing are normal. Tears do not appear externally for several weeks but are probably present at birth. The eyes of Caucasian babies are usually blue or blue-gray at birth and changes in color are evident in 3 months. The white of the eyes, or sclera, are bluish in color and often there are so-called epicanthal folds at the inner area of the eyes with a wide undeveloped bridge of the nose. This may give a false impression of cross eyes. The eyes may have a purulent discharge for several hours or days after birth, resulting from chemical irritation from silver nitrate instilled at birth to prevent infection. A persistent discharge is evidence of infection and is not infrequently due to a congenital obstruction of the tear duct.

The newborn infant should be able to breathe through its nose, and the sneezing reflex is well developed and aids in keeping secretions out of the nasal passages.

There is a great variety in the hair on the scalp of newborns. In some it is sparse and stays so for a few years. In others it is profuse, extending down the back of the neck, over the forehead, and with long sideburns. Some babies also have fine hair on their shoulders and back. Much of this excess hair disappears in the first few years.

Other normal characteristics of the newborn are a tendency for slight trembling of the chin and extremities. Breathing may be somewhat irregular in depth and rhythm. The skin at birth is covered with a cheesy material called vernix, which is usually cleaned off in the nursery. Often the palms of the hands and the soles of the feet are bluish in color (acrocyanosis) which disappears in the first day or two. The skin may normally be slightly jaundiced after the first twenty-four hours and this should disappear within a week or so. Some scaliness of the skin may be present. A pink area is often seen on the inner aspects of the upper eyelids, the middle of the forehead, and especially on the nape of the neck, all of which tend to disappear by the end of the first year. A birthmark called a hemangioma may be present at birth or develop during the first few months. These are characteristically small tumors composed mainly of blood vessels and are popularly known as "strawberry marks." They can appear on any part of the body. Unless they are extremely large, they tend to disappear within the first few years and should receive no treatment to speed the resolution process. The flat purplish port-wine stain type of birthmark, on the other hand, extends deep under the skin and tends to remain throughout life.

The head may be misshapen with a protrusion of the part that was presenting at the outlet. This is called a caput and it quickly disappears. The sutures of the head may be overriding at first, and there are openings at the top of the skull called fontanelles. The anterior one, which may be large or small, allows for growth of the head and it closes at from 1 to 2 years of age. Actually, a pin-point opening at least, remains until about 2 years. The posterior fontanelle is always relatively smaller and closes by one month.

The infant's breasts often secrete milk for the first week or two due to the maternal hormones present in the baby's blood. The breasts may be engorged and slightly reddened during this time. Severe redness and swelling may be evidence of infection.

The umbilical cord which is tied at birth rapidly becomes dark brown or black and dries up. It normally falls off by about 2 weeks, although the practice of painting the cord with dyes to prevent infection, tends to keep the cord on longer. After it has fallen off, occasionally the umbilical area may protrude, due to the failure of the muscles beneath to grow together. This is never due to improper cutting or tying of the cord in the labor room. This so-called umbilical hernia can remain for several years and only in rare instances is surgical repair necessary. Taping of the protruding navel probably does little or no good, but it does hide the condition and makes the parents feel that something is being done for it.

If the baby is a male and has not been circumcised, the foreskin should be gently retracted and cleansed beneath. Several months may pass before this retraction can be completely accomplished and force should never be used. It is easier to care for the penis of a newborn who has been circumcised, but even then, the small amount of foreskin left should also be retracted and the edge of the glans, or head of the penis, cleaned daily.

The female genitalia may be swollen at birth and some mucus be present for a few days. Occasionally some transient bloody discharge is visible and this is normal, but any continuation requires investigation. Gentle cleaning of the labia is advisable.

The normal newborn has a distinct type of body build. The chest is round, as is the abdomen. The trunk is relatively long and the extremities relatively short. By the end of the first year, the chest is more flattened and the extremities are approaching a longer relationship to the trunk.

One of the causes for retardation of growth is faulty nutrition. Thus an insufficient amount of certain vitamins results in specific diseases, such as rickets or scurvy. An insufficient amount of protein may be the cause of defective over-all growth, while overeating produces obesity. Chronic diseases and insufficient oxygen in the blood from certain congenital heart defects may result in over-all malnutrition, just as interference of proper blood supply to a portion of the body inhibits growth in that part.

As a result of insufficient rest and sleep, chronic fatigue also produces poor growth. Diseases and injuries which interfere with activity and appetite have a direct influence on the progress of growth and development.

The effect of emotional factors must not be underestimated. Parental love and care have as great an influence on the physical development of the child as any of the nutritive factors. Proper diet and rest are closely associated with the emotional climate. Unhappiness can induce poorly balanced meals and overeating, leading to obesity. One extreme example may be seen in the neglected infant who will not eat any solids and eventually fails to respond to external stimuli. Another extreme is the child denied the normal responses to his appetite, who has food forced on him at every meal until there is a complete distaste for the normal pleasure of eating. Emotional problems may affect the digestion of foods with such diseases as peptic ulcers and ulcerative colitis, just as occur in the adult. The emotions also have an effect on the child's social life, his learning capacity, his exercise, and his progress in school.

Perceptual handicaps must be recognized in any child who fails to develop normally in any specific field of learning. Proper examination of the eyes and the neurologic makeup are necessary to differentiate these children, and appropriate teaching methods instituted early to allow normal learning.

Since the mental development of the infant is judged by its physical development and accomplishments, any deviation from normal should demand evaluation. If a child has had good food, loving care, and no severe illness, mental retardation should be suspected when purposeful motor behavior of all types is abnormally delayed, or when the infant is inattentive to familiar sights and sounds.

PHYSICAL CARE AND HYGIENE

The baby should always have his own bed. Whenever possible he should have a room exclusively for his own use. The room which he occupies should be well ventilated or the air changed frequently. During his waking or play hours the temperature should be in the neighborhood of seventy degrees Fahrenheit. During sleep time the temperature can be ten or more degrees lower than this, depending upon the age, size, and vigor of the baby. When the room is kept cold for sleep, a warm room should be available to which he can be taken when necessary. When properly supervised and protected, a baby can spend much of his time out of doors after two weeks of age in summer, or after three months, in winter. Common sense must be used in putting the baby out of doors, particularly in winter. One criterion for the winter is the baby's reaction to cold; if his face becomes pale and blue and his hands and feet cold, he should not be left outside. The baby must be provided steady warmth and fresh air; if this cannot be done out of doors, the baby must be kept indoors. In the summer babies are placed out of doors in the shade. Extreme care must be used in exposing them to the direct sun. The amount of sun necessary to produce a deep tan may be harmful and sun bathing must be carefully supervised. Sunstroke from excessive heat is possible. The eyes should be protected from direct sunlight. The first exposure should be no more than 5 minutes and only to a small area, gradually increasing the amount and area of exposure. Occasionally, a sunburn is so severe that second-degree burns with blisters appear.

THE BABY'S BATH

After the navel and the circumcision are healed, the baby should be bathed daily. Usually the bath is given before feeding but convenience may necessitate any other time. The bath should be a pleasant time for both the baby and mother and is only unpleasant to the baby if some unfortunate experience such as soap in its eyes, or too hot or too cold water have at some time frightened him. The bathroom should be about 75 degrees Fahrenheit, with the bath water moderately warm, as determined by dipping the elbow into it. Any mild soap is appropriate. Absolute rules need not be followed for the bath procedure and each mother should follow the most comfortable method. In general, the face is washed first, with or without soap, as desired. The eyelids may be cleansed but never the eyes. The ears should be washed with a finger in the washcloth and the ear canals should be let alone. The edges of the nostrils may be cleansed gently with a washcloth, and the mouth need not be touched. The scalp can be washed each day if desired. If a yellowish scaly material collects on the scalp, "cradle cap," the head may be washed with a soap called Fostex® (Westwood) which helps to dissolve this material. The remainder of the body should be washed well with soap and water, especially the diaper area. Clean carefully behind the ears and the creases of the neck, arms, and legs.

Any of the various baby oils or lotions may be applied to the skin and small quantities of talcum powder, if desired. The fingernails and toenails should be trimmed periodically.

When the 8 incisor teeth have all erupted, they may be brushed with an infant's toothbrush and mild toothpaste. Toothpowder should never be used as it may be inhaled into the baby's lungs.

CLOTHING

The clothing needed for babies varies with the climate and the geographical area. Selection of clothing should be guided by needs and common sense for the baby's health. Since the fetus has been tightly confined in the uterus, there is some justification in wrapping the newborn snugly in blankets during its first few days. After this, loose clothing allowing freedom of movements is advisable. Since babies grow so rapidly during the first months, clothes are quickly outgrown. Care should be taken that neck openings are large enough. Long-sleeve shirts are rarely needed and belly bands are archaic and never necessary. A list of clothing for the newborn should include several dozen diapers, 6 shirts and 3 nightgowns, sweaters, and cotton blankets. Bonnets are not needed in warm weather and unless it is very cold, baby's ears do not need to be covered. More babies are overdressed than underdressed, and excessive clothing results in perspiration and prickly heat.

EXERCISE

While exercise is necessary for good muscular development, a great amount of pressure from some popular authors overemphasizes this phase of infant care. When the infant is very young, it moves its arms and legs in an uncoordinated manner and is relatively helpless. Its exercise comes from being picked up, held, and walked about by its mother.

As muscular development progresses, the baby gets sufficient exercise by kicking and other movements and while lying unrestricted in its bed. Later, he sits, plays, crawls, and eventually walks. Formal exercises are not necessary for normal development of the muscles.

TRAINING AND DISCIPLINE

The practice of pediatrics encompasses the "whole child." Besides the care of the growth and physical development and diseases of childhood, the mental and psychologic care must be given equal consideration. The home is the most important influence on the child's future character and mental health. At first the mother is all-important and her love and attention provides a security essential to proper maturity. A continuous uphill progress proceeds from a helpless baby to independence. The child needs a calm home with patience and understanding from his parents. Parents must learn not to expect more than his abilities enable him to produce and should not show disappointment at his failures. Undoubtedly, most of the problems that children have are due to unskilled handling, starting with the simple tasks of feeding, weaning, toilet training, sibling relationships, and school attitude.

Aldrich stated, as long ago as 1938, the basic emotional needs of children. He said that physical and mental progress are so merged in the plan of growth that they cannot be considered separately. Since mental growth in infancy is measured by physical accomplishment, mental hygiene cannot be separated from physical hygiene. Thus competent physical care for the baby is good mental care. By giving the warmth, comfort, and cuddling that he needs in addition to the basic physical needs, the mother is laying the groundwork for a healthy mental attitude. Encouraging new accomplishments adds to the baby's progress.

The parent must make plans for discipline. As the baby grows older, a definite schedule for eating and sleeping should be established. Overpermissiveness is as harmful as overdiscipline. The child should learn the importance of the word "no," which should be used sparingly and only for necessary discipline.

Training in safety is important, for after the age of one year, accidents are the major cause of death in childhood. All drugs, detergents, cleaning agents, pesticides, etc., must be kept in a safe place and never left available even for a minute. The natural curiosity of childhood encourages the eating of anything that can be placed in the mouth.

Some infants can be bowel trained at an early age. If the baby sits well and has bowel movements at a regular time, he may be placed on the toilet for a few minutes at advantageous times. A floor seat is better than one that can be attached to a regular toilet. By the time 30 to 36 months is reached, regular training procedures should be established. The parent must be patient and encouraging.

When the baby remains dry for an hour or longer, urine training may be started.

When a mother has doubts as to the proper course in caring for emotional problems, she should discuss them promptly with her doctor in order to avoid the possibly serious consequences that may result from indecision.

THUMB SUCKING

Thumb sucking is a normal form of gratification and should not cause concern to the parents. Regardless of the amount of sucking during nursing, some infants apparently need more. This may be accomplished by the use of a pacifier, but if this device is used, it should be discontinued by 8 months of age. Thumb sucking does not do harm, although displacement of the deciduous teeth, and a callous of the thumb may result. The habit is undesirable if it is practiced to excess, or after 5 or 6 years of age. If it occurs only at bedtime, it may be disregarded. All mechanical devices, scolding, or shaming should be avoided. If the habit continues, treatment should be directed toward the probable cause.

NUTRITION OF THE INFANT

Nutrition deals with the food we eat and the structures which the body makes of it. A diet which is adequate to maintain the body in good nutritional health must include the essential food materials. These essentials are protein, carbohydrate, fat, mineral salts, and water.

The body needs all these various food materials at all ages of life, although the amount and the form in which they may be offered vary according to the age. The infant, the child, and the adult need exactly the same essential food elements. The foods chosen to supply them must be adapted to the digestive capacity and the relative need of the individual. Many foods as prepared for the adult are not in a suitable state for digestion by the infant. Because milk is so easily digested by the infant and because it is so nearly a perfect food, it is commonly the basis on which the infant's diet is constructed.

In the life processes of the body, certain materials are constantly being broken down to simpler ones; the process is comparable in some respects to the burning of fuel in a furnace. This combustion takes place even when the body is in complete repose, and it is increased by activity in proportion to the degree of muscular exertion. In the process of combustion, heat is liberated. This keeps the body warm. Heat produced in this manner can be measured. The measurements are made in heat units or calories. A known amount of food will give rise to a definite amount of heat, which can be calculated. Thus food is often measured in terms of calories. If insufficient food were furnished, the body would consume itself to the point where life would be impossible. It is necessary therefore to supply energy (food capable of producing energy) to the body for the purpose of maintaining life. In order that the infant may grow and develop properly, energy must be supplied in addition to that which will only maintain life. Growth takes place only when food is supplied in excess of the amount needed to replace that which is burned to maintain the body. The infant's need for energy is relatively (per unit of body weight) far greater than that of the older child or adult and the effects of an inadequate supply show themselves more quickly. Between 85 and 90 per cent of the infant's energy needs are supplied by fats and carbohydrates, this being the chief function of these two food materials. The remainder of the energy is derived from protein.

Protein is an essential part of all cells; without it, life would be impossible. Plants can form protein from substances which they are able to obtain from the soil and the air. Man and animals cannot do this but must have the constituents of protein supplied to them either from plants or from other animals. For existence a certain amount of protein must be supplied in the diet, and for body growth an increased amount is necessary. Since no other food material can replace it, protein is an essential part of the diet. A sufficient amount may readily be supplied by the milk of the infant's diet, provided the amount of milk offered is adequate. A moderate deficiency of protein causes slow growth and feeble musculature. Gross deficiencies will eventually lead to death. A disease called Kwashiorkor, due to deficiency of protein, is found in many underdeveloped countries. Proteins from different sources differ in their chemical structure. When a protein has all the components necessary to build the kind of protein needed by the body, it is called a "complete" protein. Milk protein is considered complete. The vegetable proteins are not complete and as a consequence are not as adequate for producing good growth as are the proteins from animal sources.

The food materials that have been discussed (fat, carbohydrate, and protein) are present in our food in relatively large amounts. Other food essentials are present only in small or even minute amounts. The latter group includes both the minerals and the vitamins that are necessary for growth and the maintenance of health. The materials that have been grouped under the general term of vitamins differ widely from one another, yet some similarity exists in that all are organic substances similar to enzymes and hormones. Formerly they were designated exclusively by letters of the alphabet, but as their structure becomes known, their chemical names are used.

VITAMINS

Vitamin D is essential to the body for the proper absorption of calcium from the intestinal tract into the blood stream and for its proper utilization along with phosphorus in the formation of bone and teeth. A deficiency of this vitamin in infancy leads to rickets, a condition in which the bones become soft and often crooked.

Vitamin D is present in fish oils and is commercially available in the form of multivitamins which should be administered to all babies. Vitamin D is also supplied by the presence of cholesterol in the skin which is changed to Vitamin D by the ultraviolet rays of the sun. Since one cannot determine the exact amount produced in this manner, it is necessary to augment this with a measured additional dose. Most milk, especially evaporated milk, and commercial formulas are fortified with the equivalent of 400 units of Vitamin D to the quart. This is the average amount needed daily for the maintenance of good nutrition for healthy infants and children. The usual practice in infant feeding is to start a supplemental amount of Vitamin D at 2 weeks of age or earlier in the amount of 0.3 cc. or 0.6 cc. of a vitamin preparation such as Trivisol® (Mead Johnson) containing Vitamins A, C, and D. This and similar preparations contain 400 international units of Vitamin D, 60 milligrams of ascorbic acid or Vitamin C, and 3000 international units of Vitamin A in each 0.6 cc. A larger amount should not normally be given, as an excess of Vitamin D may lead to digestive disturbances, weight loss, and undesirable calcification of some of the organs of the body.

Vitamin A is necessary for growth, for normal state of the skin and the various mucous membranes, for ability to see in a dim light, and for certain other normal functions. Vitamin A is found in variable amounts in milk fat, egg yolk, and glandular organs, such as liver. All yellow and green plants contain the precursor of this vitamin in pigments, the commonest of which is carotene, so-called because it was first prepared from carrots. By chemical action in the body, carotene is converted into Vitamin A. Lack of Vitamin A lowers resistance to infections, causes night blindness, and maldevelopment of the teeth. Overdosage of Vitamin A with large amounts given over a long period of time, may cause serious damage to health, resulting in loss of appetite, drying of the skin, enlargement of the liver and spleen, and pain in the long bones.

Vitamin C or ascorbic acid is found commonly in fruits and vegetables. It is however a fragile vitamin and tends to be destroyed in cooking. Deficiency of Vitamin C in the diet leads to the disease called scurvy, with symptoms of debility, spongy bleeding gums, hemorrhage into the body tissues, and even death. The most available form of Vitamin C is present in orange or tomato juice. Orange juice may be started at 3 months of age in small amounts and gradually increased to 2 to 4 ounces a day. Giving orange juice at an earlier age is believed by some pediatricians to precipitate allergic reactions. If a nursing mother receives adequate Vitamin C in her diet, there is an ample supply in the breast milk. Cow's milk, however, contains much less Vitamin C and this is partially destroyed in pasteurization. The present recommendation is to add Vitamin C as in Trivisol® or other multivitamin preparations at the time artificial feedings are started.

The Vitamin B complex is composed of a group of vitamins which tend to occur together, although the relative proportions of each vary in the different foods. Deficiencies of a single member of the group are thus improbable, although deficiencies of one vitamin may predominate. Thus, beriberi is chiefly a thiamine deficiency disease, pellagra results from a shortage of niacin, and a shortage of riboflavin causes sores about the corners of the mouth and disturbances of twilight vision. The B complex occurs in the embryos of seeds, in meat, milk, eggs, fruits, and vegetables.

The amount of the B vitamins in human milk depends in large measure upon the amount in the diet of the mother. The diet of many mothers is so incomplete that the B in the milk is often dangerously low. For this as well as other reasons, the diet of the infant is advantageously supplemented at an early age with B-containing foods. Although a deficiency of Vitamin B leads to a loss of appetite, not all babies have their appetites improved by an addition to the diet of Vitamin B preparations, because there are many other causes for poor appetite. If fruits, vegetables, and egg yolk are included in the infant's diet at an early age, it is rarely necessary to give special Vitamin B preparations.

Vitamin K is occasionally given to mothers in labor or to newborn babies to prevent hemorrhagic disease of the newborn, a condition in which bleeding occurs because of a disturbance of the clotting mechanism. Vitamin K is distributed in nature especially in green leafy vegetables and in pork liver. If used, it is administered in very small dosage to the newborn by hypodermic injection. Overdosage has been known to cause damage to premature infants.

Vitamin E, a fat-soluble vitamin, is apparently necessary since deficiency may result in faulty absorption of fats and may cause deteriorative effects on muscles and degenerative changes in nerves. However, this vitamin is present in so many foods that deficiencies seldom occur.

Under usual circumstances all the necessary mineral salts of the body, with the exception of iron, are supplied early by the milk in the infant's diet. Normally a baby is born with a store of iron which will serve his needs for several months. However, the small amount of iron in milk is supplemented by the early addition of solid foods containing iron enrichment. Infant cereals are especially prepared with iron that amply supply the baby's needs. Thus, cereal should be the first solid food added and it is customary to start feeding this at 2 to 3 months, or earlier if so desired. Occasionally an infant 8 or 9 months old who is very well nourished, but deathly pale with only ⅕ or ⅙ of the needed iron in its blood is seen, and it is discovered that this baby has been entirely fed on cow's milk. Such lack of iron produces nutritional or iron deficiency anemia with pallor, irritability, lack of appetite, and decrease in normal activity.

Iron is also found in egg yolk, meat, vegetables, and fruit, so that an average good diet contains the amount needed. Premature babies are born with a lower initial supply of iron and require an additional amount to keep pace with their rapid growth. This may be given at 3 to 4 weeks of age in special formulas such as Similac with Iron® (Ross Laboratories) or the iron may be administered in prescribed medicinal form.

Calcium and phosphorus are essential minerals needed for growth and are found abundantly in formulas, in cow's milk, and in cereals. Rarely is any additional amount needed.

Water is essential for the storage and combustion of foods, the excretion of waste products and for many other life processes. The baby's needs for water are relatively much greater than those of the adult, and he shows the harmful effect of deprivation or loss much more quickly and more seriously. Many babies, however, do not need or will not take an additional quantity over that in the formula, since milk is in large proportion water. The normal amount and extent of wetness of the diapers is an indication of proper hydration.

In certain illnesses such as diarrhea, with severe water loss in the stools and from vomiting, with the consequent failure of water retention, a baby may become so dehydrated that its life is threatened. Under these circumstances, the administration of fluids intravenously is often essential. Additional water may be needed in hot weather or in case of excessive sweating from any cause. Because of the difficulty of determining when a baby is thirsty, water can be offered regularly at suitable intervals as a routine measure.

FLUORIDE REQUIREMENT

More than thirty years of useful objective evaluation of fluoridation have substantiated its tremendous value in reducing tooth decay. To obtain its greatest effect, it should be available from birth on, until at least 8 to 10 years of age. Since the tooth buds form at the sixth week of prenatal life, fluoride supplementation should be given to the pregnant woman. The best way to provide an adequate amount is to add fluorine to the public water supply in those areas that are deficient. It may be given in tablets or as a vitamin addition such as Tri-Vi-Fluor® (Mead Johnson) in deficient areas. The Council on Dental Therapeutics of the American Dental Association recommends a supplementation of 0.5 mg. of fluoride ion per day for children from two to three years and 1.0 mg. per day beyond three, continuing until eight or ten years of age.

DIGESTION

The digestive capacity of the infant is limited. Many foods served to adults would cause digestive disturbances if fed to an infant. The basic food of an infant's diet is milk. The stomach of the newborn baby seems to have acid and digestive juices adequate to digest human milk without difficulty. Unmodified cow's milk may tend to cause more or less digestive difficulty in the early months of infancy. The common modification of cow's milk, such as boiling, acidification, or dilution, makes it better adapted to the digestive capacity of the infant.

Babies who are fed cereals or other starches in the early weeks usually do not have difficulty from them, but an undigested part of starch may pass through as a harmless foreign body. Only occasionally are fermentative processes set up with their consequent distress.

Other foods commonly offered to infants (fruit juices, fruits, sieved vegetables, vitamins) usually do not cause digestive difficulties, although sometimes the coarser parts of some of these foods are not digested and are passed in the stools.

The emptying time of the infant's stomach is of some importance. The stomach usually is empty in from two to three hours after a feeding of human milk; and two and one half to three and one half hours are required for cow's milk in the usual modifications. Babies should not be fed at such short intervals that the stomach still contains some food from the last feeding. Too frequent feeding leads to digestive disturbances. Illness from any cause tends to delay the emptying of the stomach, and to affect the digestive capacity sufficiently to cause digestive symptoms. If vomiting or diarrhea are prominent symptoms and the responsible illness somewhat obscure, the illness may be attributed erroneously to the digestive tract.

STOOLS

The first material that is passed from the infant's intestinal tract is a dark green or blackish sticky substance called meconium. After food is started, the character of the bowel movement changes and takes on the type influenced by the food eaten. By the fifth day the typical stools of infancy appear. If the baby is breast-fed, the stools are canary yellow, soft, and from 2 to 5 a day, with a slightly sour non-objectionable odor. The stools of a cow's-milk-fed baby are less frequent, 1 to 3 daily, more solid and with a stronger odor. The total quantity passed is in direct relationship to the amount of food ingested. Usually, the last movements in the day are looser. As the baby becomes older, the stools change in appearance and odor with the addition of new foods. Cereal gives a more grainy and solid appearance, vegetables produce a darker color and often show evidence of passing unchanged in small quantities through the intestinal tract. As the child grows older a definite bowel pattern evolves. Even before training, when defecation is purely an involuntary reflex affair, the number of movements can be as few as one a day. After training, there may be from 1 to 3 movements a day. Some children do not have a bowel movement every day and have no untoward symptoms or difficulties resulting.

In infancy the passage of the digestive material through the intestinal tract may be unusually rapid and the bowel movement does not have time to turn from the normal green (due to bile pigments) to a yellow color, and thus the stool is green. In a well and happy baby this green color has no significance. In cow's-milk-fed babies especially, there may be curds in the feces. These curds are composed of soaps which are derived from the fat in the milk, and in moderate quantity are without significance. Mucus may appear in the stool when the intestinal tract is irritated for any reason.

BREAST FEEDING

Breast milk is the natural food for the new infant and nursing is preferable for those mothers who are able and desirous of doing so.

The mother who desires to breast feed should be heartily encouraged. Recent research has definitely shown appreciable amounts of antibodies to certain diseases in human milk, and thus the baby derives benefits greater than from the food value alone. The fixing of the baby's mouth on the mother's nipple, together with the firm holding of its body by the mother, and the clawing touch of its hands on her breasts have a psychologic benefit that both initiates the mothering instinct and the feeling of security in the infant.

Despite the fact that human milk is such an excellent food, the milk varies in quality with the diet and habits of the mother. For example, the various vitamins cannot be present in the milk unless they have been taken in adequate quantities by the mother. In order that her milk be at its best and serve well its intended purpose, the mother must observe the common rules of good hygiene and diet. These rules are fully as necessary for her own health as for that of the baby. Mothers frequently develop cavities in their teeth during lactation, because they secrete more calcium in the milk than they ingest. The mother should have sufficient sleep and moderate exercise but never to the point of fatigue. Worry and other nervous states often have a harmful effect which may be reflected in the quality of the milk.

The diet of the mother may be varied, and any food is permissible unless it causes digestive disturbance. The avoidance of acid foods is a fallacy. Examples of a well-balanced diet for the pregnant and nursing mother are given in another chapter.

Sometimes the mother is unable to secrete adequate quantities of milk. If her diet already is good, the milk supply cannot be increased by increasing the diet, although her milk may be increased by improving the diet when this has not been satisfactory. The best stimulus to maintaining or increasing the milk is regular and thorough emptying of the breast. When milk accumulates in the breast because of incomplete emptying, parts of the breast tend to become hard and painful from the pressure of the retained milk.

To give the tired mother some rest, or occasional time off for shopping or relaxation, all babies should be given an occasional bottle. So too, if the mother becomes ill and cannot nurse temporarily, the infant will have had some experience with a bottle and will more readily accept it as a substitute.

There are some reasons for the mother not to nurse her baby. She should not nurse if she has tuberculosis or a serious chronic illness. Nursing should be suspended temporarily during a severe illness. Menstruation is not a good reason for weaning, even though the baby may be uncomfortable for the first day or two. Should the mother become pregnant the baby should be weaned gradually to avoid overtaxing the mother. Medication taken by the mother need not constitute a reason for weaning, for it is doubtful if any drugs given in customary doses are secreted in the milk in harmful amounts.

In extremely rare instances, mother's milk may be the cause of severe jaundice in the newborn. A few mothers apparently produce a hormone that interferes with the metabolism of bilirubin (a bile pigment) which normally is present in the first few days of life. This excessive pigment may produce kernicterus (staining of the basal nuclei of the brain) with associated degenerative changes and mental retardation. A history of previously jaundiced babies is found in these mothers. If breast feeding is stopped and a formula substituted, the jaundice clears rapidly.

TECHNIQUE OF NURSING

When a baby is first brought to the breast, it should nurse no more than 5 minutes on each side, gradually increasing to 10 or 15 minutes. Feeding on both breasts is preferable as frequent emptying and stimulation increase the milk supply. If there is a great deal of milk, nursing on alternate sides is advisable. The baby gets most of the milk in the first 5 minutes and if sucking continues for a long time, there is usually insufficient milk. Most mothers have more milk during the early feedings and less later in the day. Successful breast feeding is obvious. The infant is satisfied, need not be fed too frequently, and appears to be thriving. Breast-fed infants may have to be fed rather frequently at first, perhaps as often as every 2 or 3 hours until the milk supply is established. These babies often cry late in the day regardless of the amount of milk that they obtain from their mothers, and this is not a sign of unsuccessful nursing.

All babies swallow some air with the milk. This may cause vomiting or discomfort. It is desirable therefore to hold the baby upright after each nursing and to pat him gently on the back until eructation of the air occurs.

The care of the mother's nipples is important. They should be bathed before and after each feeding. A fissuring of the nipples may occur. This is always painful and sometimes leads to breast abscess. Fissuring of the nipples has the same cause as chapped hands, and can be prevented in the same manner, viz., keep them as dry as possible as far as the milk is concerned, and if necessary keep them greased with some simple nipple ointment, such as vaseline or cold cream.

WEANING

The baby may usually be weaned from the breast at the age of 6 to 9 months. This may be done gradually by substituting an increasing number of bottle or cup feedings. If the baby has reached the weaning age without being accustomed to a bottle or cup, he may refuse it as long as he can get the breast. Thus abrupt weaning is necessary at times. In the case of abrupt weaning, when the baby is unaccustomed to cow's milk, it is usually preferable to have the formula slightly weaker for a few days than it would be normally for the baby's age. Weaning in the summer is still feared by many mothers. There need be no such fear if the milk formula and other foods are appropriate for the baby, and are properly prepared. Occasionally medication is necessary to dry up the breasts and relieve the pain of engorgement.

ARTIFICIAL FEEDING

Human and cow's milk are similar in many respects. They have the same constituents, but the proportions are different. Chiefly because of these differences in proportion, digestive difficulties occur when unmodified cow's milk is fed to young infants. The milk of all cows is the same except for the quantity of fat. For infant feeding, milk of medium or low fat content, such as is found in dairy milks conforming to local legal limits is generally advisable.

Milk is easily contaminated in the milking and handling and is an excellent medium for the growth of bacteria. All harmful bacteria and most of the others are killed by pasteurization. Boiling milk for several minutes also kills the bacteria and in addition alters the milk in such a way that the casein forms a finer curd and is thereby more easily digested by the infant.

Evaporated milk is ordinary fresh cow's milk which has been concentrated to slightly less than half of its volume by the evaporation of the water, then sealed in cans and sterilized. It has been shown to be an excellent, safe, and convenient food for the artificial feeding of infants. For use it may be diluted back to its original volume with water and used in the same manner as fresh milk. The sweetened varieties of evaporated milk (condensed milk) are not suitable for the routine feeding of infants, as the protein content of such milk is so low that it does not permit proper growth of muscle tissue.

Dried milk is milk which has had practically all of its water removed. It is useful in infant feeding, although usually more expensive than fresh or evaporated milk. Some dried milks are prepared from skimmed milk instead of from whole milk. Dried milk is used frequently in communities and foreign countries that cannot obtain fresh milk, and also for other special reasons. To obtain a product similar to whole milk it is necessary to add one tablespoon of the dried whole milk to 2 ounces of water.

SUGARS AND CARBOHYDRATES

Milk alone may not be a suitably balanced food in early infancy without the addition of sugar, and when the milk has been modified by dilution, sugar is necessary to satisfy the energy requirements of the infant. Thus some variety of sugar is usually used in the milk formula. Sugars that are used are lactose (milk sugar), cane sugar (table sugar), and derivatives of starch (dextrin, maltose, dextrose, and mixtures of these). These serve the baby equally well after they have been absorbed from the intestinal tract. The choice of sugar is based upon its cost and upon its behavior in the intestinal tract of the infant. Certain sugars are more laxative than others. For example, lactose is absorbed relatively slowly and usually passes far down the intestinal tract before complete absorption. This long presence in the tract has a laxative effect. At the other extreme is dextrose, which is absorbed quickly and consequently is a good sugar to use in cases of diarrhea. Corn syrup is a mixture of dextrin, maltose, and dextrose, and has found favor because it is inexpensive, as well as useful, although it is less convenient to handle than the dry sugars. Dry dextrin-maltose mixtures are the most commonly used.

DILUENTS

One of the chief aims in the modification of cow's milk to make it more suitable for young infants is to alter the casein in such a manner that it forms a fine curd in the stomach. This object is commonly achieved by dilution with water.

FORMULAS FOR WELL BABIES

Milk satisfies the need of the infant for most of the nutritional essentials when at least 1½ to 2 ounces for each pound of weight is given each twenty-four hours. By the time the baby is taking a quart of milk a day, other foods should be added to supplement the diet in such a way that more milk is unnecessary.

The amount of sugar added to meet the total food requirement is usually one ounce daily during the first two months and one and a half ounces during the succeeding four months. More or less than this may be indicated under special circumstances.

The amount of diluent (water) used should be sufficient to bring the total volume to that which the baby will take conveniently in twenty-four hours. A young baby should take at a single feeding two to three ounces more than his age in months. More than 8 ounces should rarely be given at a feeding at any age, for by the time the baby is receiving 8 ounces he is taking foods other than milk.

During the first one or two weeks after birth, the milk dilution usually should be a little greater than that which has been specified, until the baby becomes accustomed to the cow's-milk feeding. The original mixture should never be less than half milk, and this should be used for only a few days. Customarily one starts with two thirds milk and one third water.

A feeding schedule which will be found suitable for the majority of well babies is as follows:

Age Months	*Average Pounds*	*Milk Ounces*	*Water Ounces*	*Sugar Ounces*	*Feedings Number*	*Feedings Ounces*
½	7	11	7	1	6–7	2½–3
1	8–9	16	8	1	5–6	4
2	10	20	8	1¼	5–6	5–6
3	12	24	8	1½	4–5	5–6
4	14	28	6	1¾	3	7–8
6	16–17	Whole	0	0	3	7–8

Sugar Equivalents
1 ounce by weight of cane sugar = 2 level tablespoons.
1 ounce by weight of lactose = 4 level tablespoons.
1 ounce by weight dextri-maltose = 4 level tablespoons.
1 ounce by volume of corn syrup = 2 level tablespoons and contains 1 ounce of sugar.

The formulas and schedules given are calculated for the average baby, and adjustments frequently will be necessary for the individual baby. A baby who is hungry, not gaining as he should, and who is not having digestive difficulties should have more food than is indicated in the schedule. Often minor adjustments in the quantity or type of sugar will make the difference between constipation and loose stools. For these and many other reasons the infant's feeding should be under the supervision of one who is expert in such matters.

Preparation of Formulas

The milk, sugar, and water should be mixed and then boiled from one to three minutes with constant stirring. It should be poured immediately into boiled nursing bottles, stoppered and cooled rapidly, and placed on ice until ready for use. This is known as the aseptic method.

An easier means of sterilization is to use the terminal method. The bottles and nipples are washed carefully and the formula mixed in a clean pan, and then poured equally into the number of bottles desired. The caps are placed on the bottles loosely, and then the bottles are set in a rack in a receptacle partly filled with water, and then placed on the stove. This water should be kept boiling lightly for 30 minutes. After cooling, the bottles are removed from the rack, the caps screwed on tightly, and then they are placed in the refrigerator.

Ready-Mixed Formulas

A number of preparations are available that are excellent formulas. In alphabetical order, Bremil® (Borden), Enfamil® (Mead Johnson), Similac® (Ross Laboratories), SMA® (Wyeth) are the most popularly used. In the first week a dilution of ten ounces of the liquid preparation mixed with fourteen ounces of water is advisable. After the first week or two, equal parts of the milk and water are easily digested by the baby. These preparations may also be obtained in a powder form, and in the first one or two weeks, 10 tablespoons (or measures which are enclosed in the can) should be mixed with 24 ounces of water. After this, the full strength formula should contain 12 tablespoons of the powder to 24 ounces of water. While these formulas are designed to have 4 ounces in each bottle, this is more than newborns usually take, and not enough for older babies. The average young infant takes about 1½ to 3 ounces at a feeding; occasionally a hungry baby will take more. It is advisable to have more formula in a bottle than the baby needs and allow him to decide how much to eat. Mothers should always realize that the baby knows its own needs and should never encourage or force him to take more than he is enthusiastic for.

There are also ready-mixed formulas in cans or bottles with special nipples, which may be immediately used. These are of special benefit for use in travel.

SOLID FOODS

Until the 1930s solid foods were not routinely introduced into the infant's diet until late in the first year. At times since then, the pendulum has swung to the extreme of giving almost any solids in the first few days of life. The Committee on Nutrition of the American Medical Association states that no one today should doubt the nutritional inadequacy of a diet exclusively of milk throughout the first year. Proof is lacking that feeding of solid foods at ages earlier than four months is nutritionally or psychologically essential, or on the other hand, actually harmful. However, giving milk alone to a baby for six to fifteen months produces severe deficiency symptoms, especially anemia. While the weight of such babies may appear to be adequate, they may become pale and waterlogged and have chemical imbalances. These symptoms are not seen in infants receiving an adequately varied diet. Long experience has shown that giving babies cereals, such as pablum, which contain adequate iron, can be started at one to two months. The addition of fruits, including fresh ripe banana, at two to three months and strained vegetables and strained meats at three to four months will supply the needed nutritional requirements. To decrease the possibility of allergic reactions new foods should be introduced one at a time. Start all new foods slowly with one or two teaspoons and increase daily until a satisfactory amount is given. One-half cup of cereal with milk added and one-half jar of other food is usually sufficient at a feeding.

Babies occasionally have to learn to swallow solid foods, and those who do have difficulty are perhaps not ready for them. Urging or forcing should never be attempted, for when the baby is ready, he will stop resisting. The easy acceptance of solid foods corresponds to the time of his nutritional needs.

At seven to eight months tastes of table foods should be offered, and at eight months or later coarser foods may be started. Many babies choke or even vomit when given lumpy foods, and obviously are not ready for this change. Teeth are not necessary for chewing, as babies will gum soft foods without difficulty. Certain foods should be avoided, namely, those that are so crisp and hard that they will not soften in the mouth. These include nuts, raw carrots, or cucumbers, for if the baby chokes with any of these in the mouth, particles may be aspirated into the lungs.

TIMING OF FEEDING

Most newborns need to be fed at about three-hour intervals during the first week and at three to four hour intervals thereafter for the next couple of months. In the average hospital nursery, babies are fed at four-hour intervals from the beginning, but this is due to the necessity of nursery routine and dependence on the amount of help that is available. In hospitals with rooming-in, babies are fed when they are hungry. Whether the baby is breast or bottle fed, he will make his feeding needs known to the mother. After the infant leaves the hospital, he should be fed when hungry, the so-called self-demand or self-regulatory method. The mother soon learns the cry of hunger as opposed to the fretful cry of an uncomfortable baby. Self-demand does not mean that the baby should be nursed or given a bottle every time it cries. Some babies may want to take small quantities every hour or two, day and night; this is obviously an impossible situation. Do not feed an infant at less than approximately 3 hour intervals and allow it to sleep almost any length of time between feedings. After 2 to 3 months, a fairly routine schedule should be established.

TECHNIQUE OF FEEDING

In the hospital bed mothers may at first be uncomfortable holding the baby for nursing or for its bottle. As soon as possible, the mother should sit in a chair and assume a comfortable position. When she goes home, a rocking chair is of great comfort to both the mother and infant. A young baby should always be held while it is being fed, both for safety and the benefits obtained from the holding, fondling, and love that it needs. A bottle should never be propped and left with the baby lying in bed.

For feeding, the milk should be warmed to body temperature by placing the bottle in a vessel of hot water. The size of the hole in the nipple should be such that when the bottle is inverted, the milk drops out rapidly but does not flow in a steady stream. The baby should be fed in a position in which the shoulders are higher than the buttocks. Any milk refused should be discarded.

Burp or bring up the air bubble in a baby's stomach usually only in the middle of a feeding, and at the end. The infant is frustrated by burping him more frequently. Some babies like to play with the bottle in their mouths and stretch out the feeding for an inordinate length of time. Thirty minutes is long enough for the feeding, for by that time the baby will have taken all of the milk that he needs. If more sucking is needed, a pacifier may be used.

FEEDING PROBLEMS: FAILURE TO GAIN

Every baby gains in its own fashion and the heaviest baby is not necessarily the healthiest one. If he is happy and gaining only a small amount, nothing is usually wrong. This is especially true at certain periods in breast-fed infants. If this extends over too long a period a formula should be substituted. In bottle-fed babies the formula should be strengthened, but not beyond full normal strength; rather this is an indication for the early addition of solid foods. If failure to gain continues despite proper feeding, the infant should be examined thoroughly by the doctor.

CARE OF THE SICK INFANT

The illnesses of an infant are usually of an acute rather than of a chronic nature, and the general care is similar for all illnesses. The infant should be allowed to lie quietly in bed, and the feedings, treatments, or other attention should be spaced at as long intervals as possible. There is often a tendency to keep doing things to the patient, with the result that little of the much-needed rest is obtained, and the baby becomes exhausted. Excitement should be avoided and unnecessary entertainment reduced to a minimum.

An effort should be made to have the air of the sickroom fresh at all times, but this does not mean that it need be raw, cold winter air. No illness of infancy requires any special type of clothing. The clothing should be that to which the infant is accustomed during sleep in health. Except in the case of premature and delicate infants, the patient should have a cleansing bath daily. There is no acute illness in which bathing is harmful, except perhaps eczema. The feeding of the sick infant is discussed elsewhere.

A common and effective method of reducing high temperature is by thoroughly sponging the entire body with one-half rubbing alcohol and one-half tepid water.

EXCESSIVE CRYING

Nothing is so disturbing for a family as a baby that cries a lot. Changes in the social life of a family are associated with the advent of a new baby. The young family has become accustomed to a certain way of life, without demands other than those needed for husband and wife alone. There is ample time for the housework, cooking, social life, and the love and attention of husband and wife for each other. The arrival of a new individual in the family produces changes that perhaps neither parent expected. Each must get used to the presence of the baby, whose needs must be constantly fulfilled, and each must be prepared to give up much of the attention that was previously available. The father should help the mother with the care of the baby. Most babies cry a little in the evening and apparently especially at the time when the father has returned from a hard day's work. Even though the father is tired, he must realize that his wife is also tired. Babies respond to tenseness in the home by becoming tense and unhappy themselves. A certain amount of crying, however, is normal but this varies greatly in different infants. Thus the initial cries after birth help to expand and ventilate the lungs. Crying in the newborn normally occurs when the baby is hungry, wet, or otherwise uncomfortable, or because it is lonely and needs to be picked up and comforted. Some babies cry while feeding, at sudden noises, or from sudden changes of position. Mothers occasionally are unable to leave a happily sleeping infant alone. They find it necessary to fuss with the baby, with the baby responding in the only way it can, by showing its displeasure. Mothers often say that they wish they could have had their second baby born first, since it is so good in contrast to the first one. They recognize that they are now relaxed and were unable to accomplish this with their first baby.

From the ages of five to eleven months, strange faces, voices, or places may produce fear and crying. As the child grows older, frustrations, such as inability to reach a toy, may cause crying. Important is recognition of the baby's needs, especially for love, comfort, feeding, and opportunities to develop normal skills. Do not hesitate to pick up a young infant who is crying and do not worry about spoiling him.

COLIC

The definition of this poorly understood condition is excessive crying. Although the so-called colic infant is not uncommon, a specific condition has not been found to be the cause. These infants cry or scream a lot; they are often not comforted by holding, and seem to need an excessive amount of food which, by itself, may contribute to the discomfort. They are often distended, pass a large amount of gas, and have an increased number of loose stools. Changes in formula are occasionally successful. If an allergy to cow's milk is suspected, one of the soybean preparations such as Mull Soy® (Borden's), So Bee® (Mead Johnson), Isomil® (Ross), or Soyalac® (Loma Linda) may be used. Every colicky baby should be thoroughly examined by the doctor to ascertain that all is normal, and this should include a rectal examination.

The colicky baby needs to be held, rocked, and comforted. A pacifier should be tried and certain medications that relax the intestinal tract should be used. Colic usually ends by the time the baby is six months old, but the intervening time is trying.

VOMITING

Sometimes the newborn infant vomits its gastric contents shortly after birth, and occasionally some spitting or vomiting of mucus or fluid occurs in the first few days. Not infrequently, the first few feedings are regurgitated. At this time, the baby must be observed to ascertain that it has passed meconium to exclude the possibility of some congenital malformation, with intestinal obstruction. Diagnostic signs of obstruction include distension of the abdomen, and visible peristaltic waves. The area of the obstruction can sometimes be anticipated by the character of the vomited material. If it is watery or mucousy, the obstruction is probably high, while if it is bile stained, it is below the stomach.

As the infant grows older, vomiting may occur from many causes. The first necessity is to differentiate spitting from vomiting. Until the baby stands, its stomach is relatively high in the abdomen. After it is able to stand, the weight of the food causes the stomach to drop lower and eventually become fish-hook shaped. When the stomach is high, it is easy to regurgitate food because the distance to the mouth is relatively short.

Too large feedings, or feeding at too short intervals when the stomach is only partially emptied, may result in vomiting. Also the stomach may be distended by a large amount of swallowed air in addition to the usual feedings.

Illness is a common cause of vomiting. Almost any acute infection will produce this. Vomiting is largely the result of irritation of the stomach by the fermentation of foods, which remain there unusually long due to the impaired emptying power of the stomach in illness. Common causes, also, are the eating of spoiled or inappropriate foods. Certain viruses which affect the intestinal tract specifically are frequently responsible, as in epidemic vomiting. Administration of medicines may also result in immediate vomiting.

A few babies vomit merely because of an apparent desire to do so. Rarely, they may repeatedly regurgitate small amounts of food shortly after eating and then swallow it again, much as cattle do. This is probably due to some abnormal psychologic factor in the mother-child relationship, and proper advice for the mother should be sought.

An occasional cause of obstruction is pyloric stenosis. This is due to an enlargement of the muscle at the pylorus, the area at the outlet of the stomach. The pyloric valve may become elongated and thickened to twice its normal size and appear much like a large olive. This condition occurs much more often in first-born males, but girls are also affected. Rarely, it recurs repeatedly in families. The symptoms usually start gradually after the first week of life, often in the second or third week, when forceful (projectile) vomiting, loss of weight, scanty stools with constipation, dehydration, and visible peristaltic waves in the abdomen appear. Palpation of the enlarged pyloric mass confirms the diagnosis. Occasionally an X-ray examination is necessary. The treatment is to correct the dehydration, and then surgical repair should be accomplished.

Occasionally these same symptoms, but to a lesser degree, may occur when the pylorus is in a state of spasm (pylorospasm). In this, the same type of projectile vomiting and visible peristaltic waves are present, but this rarely leads to dehydration. A mass is not felt and X ray shows little or no real obstruction. The treatment is to use milk feedings thickened with cereal, and the administration of antispasmodic drugs such as atropine and phenobarbital. Some commercial preparations, such as Bentyl with Phenobarbital®, or Pamine with Phenobarbital®, are also useful.

This is not a complete enumeration of the causes of vomiting but the discussion does include the most common ones seen. Treatment must always be adopted to the probable cause.

DIARRHEA

Diarrhea is usually the result of irritation or abnormal stimulation of the intestinal tract. Because of the unusual stimulus, the intestinal movements are increased in intensity, and food material is passed along at a rapid rate. During this passage some of the food and much of the water are not absorbed; as a consequence, the stools are fluid and often contain an unusual proportion of undigested food.

The increased stimulus may be caused by infection and inflammation of the intestinal tract. In this group belong bacillary and amebic dysentery, and typhoid and paratyphoid (salmonella) infections. With better hygiene and improved care of milk and other food, some of these infections are much less common than formerly. In each of these the stools show evidence of the disease. In dysentery, pus and often blood are present. In all these infections, the cause can be determined by bacteriologic examination and appropriate treatment given by testing the germ against the various antibiotics. Bacillary dysentery is usually controlled promptly by sulfonamides and other antibiotics, although salmonella infections are often resistant. Typhoid infections respond to Chloromycetin® or Ampicillin® properly prescribed. There are very useful remedies for amebic dysentery.

A rare type of diarrhea, difficult to manage, is one that occurs epidemically among newborn babies. Many of these, if not all, are the result of a virus infection for which a specific remedy is not yet available. Most of the babies recover if expert medical and nursing care is given. Some epidemic diarrhea in infants is due to a pathogenic colibacteria.

Diarrhea, often accompanied by vomiting, may occur as a complication of infection elsewhere than in the intestinal tract, such as an inflammation in the ears. In these instances the diarrhea responds to treatment of the infection and to appropriate changes in the diet.

Diarrhea may also occur as the result of taking improper food, or food that has been contaminated by bacteria which produce toxic products in their growth. Even perfectly proper foods may be a cause of diarrhea if they are given in excess of the infant's ability to digest and absorb them. In many instances the cause cannot be determined, although many are due to allergy to food, especially cow's milk.

Other causes may be cystic fibrosis of the pancreas, congenital megacolon (Hirschsprung's disease), deficiencies of sugar-splitting enzymes, malabsorption syndromes (celiac disease) with inability to digest and absorb glutens (wheat and rye flours), metabolic disorders such as hyperthyroidism, and in older children, emotional excitement and even fatigue may cause diarrhea.

Some food loss occurs in diarrhea but the most serious effect is water loss. In the usual mild diarrhea, the baby is not particularly ill and the water loss seldom becomes apparent. However, when diarrhea is severe and prolonged, serious, and even fatal dehydration may occur. Important at that time is determination of the mineral content of the baby's blood and replacement of those minerals that are lost with proper fluids given intravenously. This is often a life-saving measure.

Even though diarrhea may not be primarily dependent upon the diet, certain alterations are desirable for treatment. During a brief period food should be withheld, but water, tea sweetened with sugar, or apple juice, may be administered as tolerated. This fasting period need not be more than a few hours in mild diarrhea. In severe diarrhea, fasting may have to continue for several days, but the baby's fluid and mineral contents must be maintained. The first food after the fast may advantageously be one which is high in protein and low in sugar and fat. Boiled skimmed milk is a customary means for fulfilling these requirements. As the diarrhea improves, other foods are gradually replaced in the diet.

CONSTIPATION

Constipation usually refers to difficulty in evacuating the feces, or at least to an unusual retention and delay in emptying the intestinal tract. Parents often refer their own bowel pattern to their infants; thus many babies are believed to be constipated simply because the number of the baby's stools is less than their own.

The causes of constipation may be dietary due to underfeeding, vomiting, or a result of faulty diet. There may be an overabundance of cow's milk, starches, or protein, too finely purėed food, or even a lack of adequate water. In hot weather infants frequently lose an excess of water through perspiration, and may not have a sufficient amount of fluids to liquify the intestinal contents, with the result that the stool becomes dry and hard. Occasionally, a small anal fissure or crack which is painful may cause the infant to hold back the stool. In illness an insufficient food intake and lack of exercise may also produce constipation.

Organic diseases, especially congenital abnormalities, may however be the cause. At birth, the anus may be imperforate due to a membrane in the lower intestinal tract, which has to be surgically removed. Other rare abnormalities, such as intestinal atresia or stenosis, malrotation, constriction of the intestines by other organs, cysts, etc., are occasionally present. Rarely, there is an absence of nerve cells in the lower intestinal tract above the anus, causing a functional obstruction known as Hirschsprung's disease. In this condition the stools are often dry and pea-like, sometimes ribbony with occasional periods of diarrhea. Examination usually reveals an empty rectum, although masses of feces may be felt in the abdomen. Diagnosis is proved by X ray and rectal biopsy. After the condition is proven, surgical correction is necessary.

Treatment is not needed for mild constipation, but if there is discomfort an infant glycerin suppository may be inserted. It may be necessary to add or change the type of sugar in the formula; or adding prunes to the diet may easily solve the problem. Rarely, stretching of the rectal muscles is indicated. In general, one should avoid the use of laxatives, suppositories, or enemas as much as possible and give attention to changes in the diet.

EXAMINATION OF THE NEWBORN

The first examination of the newborn is of great importance and should be performed as soon after birth as practical, certainly within the first twenty-four hours. It is necessary to know the history of the pregnancy, and the type of labor and anesthetic used. The blood type of the mother should be noted, and the length of pregnancy should be estimated and compared with the expected date of delivery. The information about the fetal heart rate, the time and extent of the first cry and any difficulty in initial respiration should be available. After this, a complete physical examination, with the general appearance, the baby's color, the presence of any unusual amount of mucus in the nose or mouth, the type of breathing, and the cry should be noted. Normally, the color is pink. There should only be a small amount of mucus in the mouth, the respirations may be irregular normally, and the baby lies quietly. The skin is examined for birth marks and rashes and for any abnormalities at the base of the spine, neck, and ears. The head may be misshapen depending upon the length and type of labor. The eyes should be examined for abnormalities such as cataracts or tumors; malformed or low-set ears call attention to possible abnormalities of the kidneys. Abnormalities of the nose, mouth, jaw, or neck are occasionally found at the initial examination. The shape of the chest and the use of the stethoscope may show signs diagnostic of diaphragmatic hernia, or lung cysts which may demand immediate surgery. Auscultation and examination of the heart may reveal abnormalities which also may require ultimate surgical correction. The shape and size of the abdomen may suggest tumors, intestinal obstructions, or diaphragmatic hernia. The doctor will scrutinize the umbilical stump for abnormalities or infection. The anus should be inspected and a rectal thermometer inserted to ascertain that it is open. The genitalia must be examined for abnormal openings or failure of normal descent of the testes, or hydrocele. The spinal area must be looked over for abnormal openings or bulgings. The extremities are inspected for normal motion, shape, and possible dislocation of the hips. A good examiner feels the femoral pulses to make sure that no obstruction to the circulation of the legs is present. Besides this, the baby's urine and blood should be examined for inborn errors of metabolism, notably phenylketonuria, and occasionally routine blood counts, urine examinations and cultures are indicated.

The baby will also be carefully examined before it goes home, as many minor difficulties, such as skin infections may be found and treatment begun.

THE PREMATURE INFANT

The standard of prematurity is weight of 5 pounds 8 ounces or less, a length not exceeding 18½ inches, and a head circumference of less than 13 inches. Undoubtedly some full-term babies have statistics that fall in this category, while some prematures born of diabetic mothers may weigh much more. The figures should be revised for offspring of Negro parents as they often weigh less than their white counterparts. About 7 to 8 per cent of all babies in the United States are prematurely born. The cause for this in the majority of instances is unknown, but certain factors are known to predispose for premature birth. There are more female prematures than males, probably because the average female weighs about 4 ounces less than the male. Multiple pregnancy, twins or triplets, account for 17 per cent. Fetal malformations and maternal infections, hemolytic disease of the newborn (so-called erythroblastosis or Rh disease) or other blood incompatibilities, race, maternal age, illegitimacy, economic factors, dietary deficiency of protein, complications of pregnancy, diabetes, heart disease or size of the maternal heart, the amount of hard work done by the mother, are all known causes of prematurity.

Since all premature births occur before forty weeks of gestation, the maturity of the various organs depends on the length of the pregnancy. Under twenty-eight weeks the fetal organs are too poorly developed to permit life. After this, the premature must be treated with particular reference to the immaturity of his temperature control, his inadequately developed lungs which tend to produce hyaline membrane disease, his inadequately developed digestive system associated with difficulty in digesting fats, and his poorly developed kidneys. He is more susceptible to infections and his blood vessels are fragile with a greater tendency to birth injuries and severe hemorrhage. Severe jaundice due to liver immaturity is also more common in prematures. All these factors must be taken into consideration in the proper care of the premature, and incubators with regulation of temperature and humidity, special formulas or breast milk, and nurses trained in the techniques of feeding such small infants are essential. Unless complications occur, the undersized premature grows rapidly and catches up with the full-term infant in one to two years. Special attention must be given to the emotional needs of the premature. If the baby is small it may have been in an incubator for many weeks and needs a great deal of holding and loving, for it has been deprived of the normal mother-baby relationship. Mothers are often afraid of an exceedingly small baby and should be reassured that it will be as sturdy as any other infant. Spock has remarked that the anxiety of the mother may be inversely proportional to the size of the infant.

UNEXPLAINED SUDDEN DEATH

In infrequent instances, so-called "crib deaths" occur in apparently healthy infants between the age of two and eight months. Adequate post-mortem examinations may reveal sudden overwhelming pneumonia, or meningitis, or some undiagnosed congenital defect such as congenital heart disease, agammaglobulinemia, or a foreign body aspirated into the larynx. In general, however, these deaths occur in apparently well babies who, at the most, may have had signs of a mild cold. Since babies most often sleep on their stomachs, suffocation by bedclothes is often attributed as the cause, but this is rarely true. Formerly, an enlarged thymus gland was often diagnosed. Parents of these babies may feel that they have been guilty of neglect, but they should be assured that they are in no way to blame. In the majority of cases, a definite cause for death cannot be found.

CONGENITAL STRIDOR

Noisy breathing in infants is rather commonly observed, usually noticed in the first month or shortly after. Parents often think that the baby has a cold. The common variety of this condition has a noisy sound on inspiring air that becomes worse on activity or change of position, and is rarely heard when the baby is asleep. The voice, cry, and color of the baby are normal. This is important in differentiating a more serious condition. While there are many causes of noisy breathing, congenital stridor is usually considered as being due to a "soft larynx" which flutters during inspiring air. This condition normally corrects itself by one year. X rays and examination of the larynx may be necessary to be certain that no real abnormality exists.

INTUSSUSCEPTION

Intussusception is the telescoping of a portion of the intestinal tract into an adjacent segment. This, together with incarcerated inguinal hernias, or ruptures, are the most common acquired causes of intestinal obstruction in early childhood, and are among the most frequent surgical emergencies in this age group. Intussusception is rare in early infancy; over one half of all cases occur in male babies between six and eighteen months of age, with most occurring between the fourth and tenth month. Some belief prevails that this condition is caused by the change of a diet of milk alone to a more solid type, with a resulting alteration of the peristaltic movements of the intestinal tract. Since early feeding of solids is now usual and since there has been no increase in intussusceptions, there is considerable doubt as to this being true. Other causes may be abnormalities of the intestinal tract, peritoneum and mesentery, constipation, strong laxatives, diarrhea, foreign bodies, allergy, polyps, and swelling of the lymphatic areas of the intestinal tract due to a virus infection.

The symptoms are typical in most instances. A sudden onset with severe colicky pain is frequently associated with vomiting. The infant becomes pale with each attack of pain. Bloody stools occur in 85 per cent of cases, but often not before twelve to eighteen hours have elapsed. The typical stools are described as being like "currant jelly." The abdomen is soft at first but later becomes distended and hard. A sausagelike mass may be felt by the doctor, and a rectal examination or a small enema may reveal the presence of blood in the stool. Intussusception is often overlooked because it usually occurs in well-nourished, healthy babies. Not until the obstruction has lasted for several hours does the baby show the picture of severe illness with attendant pallor, sunken eyes, dehydration, rapid pulse, fever, and severe prostration.

The early treatment is the use of hydrostatic pressure to reduce the obstruction, by a barium enema given under fluoroscopic attention. By this procedure the diagnosis may be accurately assessed and the obstruction may be reduced at the same time. If more than a few hours have elapsed an emergency operation may be necessary to reduce the obstruction. The danger is the complication of gangrene of the obstructed intestine. While occasionally an intussusception may reduce by itself, untreated cases are usually fatal. The mortality rate is very low if reduction is accomplished in the first twenty-four hours, but becomes progressively greater with the passage of time. A small percentage of treated cases tend to recur.

CELIAC SYNDROME

The Celiac Syndrome, or celiac disease, is one of a number of conditions described under the title of Intestinal Malabsorbtion Syndrome. This term embodies those conditions in which there is an inefficient passage of digested nutritional components from the intestinal tract into the body tissues. Celiac disease comprises a set of symptoms that are rather typical. The fully developed case has a history of repeated severe diarrhea, starting between six to eighteen months of age, with foul, large, offensive, greasy-looking stools, abdominal distension, wasting of the body tissues especially noted in the buttocks, stunting of growth, and loss of appetite. There are a number of causes of this disease, but it is mainly caused by an intolerance to wheat glutens or lactose in cow's milk. It is a genetic disease caused by a specific enzyme deficiency. Treatment consists of withholding wheat in any form such as bread, cereal, or baby foods containing wheat, or in the case of milk sensitivity, withholding cow's milk. In treating this, care must be exercised to read carefully the label on all cans or jars to determine the contents. These children do well with proper treatment.

CYSTIC FIBROSIS

Cystic fibrosis of the pancreas is also a congenital defect inherited as a recessive trait with symptoms resembling Celiac disease, combined however, with recurrent pulmonary disease, and disturbances of the sweat mechanism. In a few cases, symptoms of intestinal obstruction appear at birth due to mechanical blockage of the bowel with hardened meconium. These infants do not gain weight, although their appetites are usually large. The abdomen becomes distended and the typical large foul-smelling stools are apparent. The treatment is to reduce the amount of fat, since this also reduces the number and size of the stools, and to add pancreatic enzyme (Viokase®, one-quarter to one-half teaspoon at each meal). Larger amounts of vitamins than normal are needed, and also extra salt to replace the large amount lost in perspiration. The chest complications may be improved with the early and continuous use of some broad-spectrum antibiotics. The presence of a rectal prolapse should alert the physician to the possibility of cystic fibrosis. The pulmonary complications are the most severe aspect of this disease and are often associated with progressive debility. The diagnosis of this disease should be based on the following criteria: 1) increase in salt in the sweat, 2) absence of pancreatic enzymes, 3) chronic lung disease, and 4) family history.

ERYTHROBLASTOSIS (RH DISEASE)

Erythroblastosis, or hemolytic disease of the newborn due to Rh incompatibility, is the most common cause of severe jaundice in the newborn. Physiologic jaundice is present in some degree in every newborn infant. This incompatibility exists in some infants where the mother's blood is Rh negative and the father's is Rh positive. Genetically, it is possible to predict which infants may be affected by whether the mother and father are monozygotic or heterozygotic. Approximately 85 per cent of all white persons are Rh positive, and 15 per cent are Rh negative. Statistically then, one in eight marriages bring together an Rh negative female with an Rh positive male. Not all of these incompatible matings result in a baby that develops hemolytic disease, but about 1 in 200 pregnancies produce an affected baby. The sensitization process starts with the first pregnancy but never results in a baby with the disease, unless the mother has had a previous transfusion with Rh positive blood. The first pregnancy paves the way for the sensitization and the disease may show itself in the recurrent pregnancies. Often this sensitization increases with each subsequent pregnancy.

The disease is caused by the passage of incompatible blood from the fetal to the maternal blood circulation, by way of the placenta. This incompatible substance causes the mother's blood to produce antibodies against it, which then pass back into the baby's circulation and set up the hemolytic process which destroys the fetal red blood cells. In some instances, the disease is so severe as to result in a stillborn, or edematous baby. More often there is a gradual hemolysis with jaundice and anemia in the first twenty-four to forty-eight hours. If the jaundice is severe it may stain the basal nuclei of the brain and cause kernicterus. Kernicterus produces neurologic symptoms with either death or severely brain damaged infants having athetosis, deafness and mental deficiency. For this reason erythroblastosis must be treated early. The blood of the parents should be examined early in pregnancy and preparations may then be made for the proper treatment of the baby. Mild cases do not require treatment, but more severe ones may need repeated exchange transfusions with Rh negative blood. An exchange transfusion consists of removing the infant's damaged blood, and as nearly as possible, replacing it with fresh blood of the same type as the mother. Gradually increasing jaundice with certain positive laboratory tests, such as a positive Coombs test, the presence of unusual numbers of normocytes, and an increasing amount of bilirubin may necessitate the exchange transfusion.

Hemolytic disease of the newborn may also occur when the mother and father have an incompatibility of blood group (ABO system). ABO disease is probably as common as Rh but it is usually less severe. However, this disease may be present in the first born. This incompatibility may also require exchange transfusions.

Most hospitals are well equipped for exchange transfusions and while there are some dangers associated, they are less than the sequellae of kernicterus. It is now possible to prevent this disease by the use of a new drug called Rhogam (Ortho). This is a specially prepared gamma globulin, containing Rh antibodies. These antibodies provide protection against Rh positive red blood cells that may enter the mother's blood after the delivery. The intramuscular injection of one dose of Rhogam will prevent the mother's blood from producing antibodies which become permanent. Rhogam should be given to Rh negative mothers, who have an Rh positive baby, and who have not already produced antibodies from either this, or a preceding pregnancy, or blood transfusion. Rhogam should be given within seventy-two hours after the delivery of an Rh positive baby, or after a miscarriage, and must be repeated after every similar delivery or miscarriage.

THRUSH

Thrush is a mild infection that may be seen in the mouths of the newborn, characterized by the formation of white milk-curdlike lesions caused by a fungus, Candidia (monilia) Albicans. Most cases are due to vaginal infections of the mother and may be anticipated by the obstetrician and prevented by prophylactic treatment of the baby's mouth in the nursery. Other cases occur from improper sterilization of bottles and nipples, from the mother's breasts, or from infected attendants. The lesions respond well to treatment, such as daily painting of the mouth with 1 per cent gentian violet, or the use of a specific antibiotic, Nystatin®, given by mouth. This fungus also may produce skin manifestations particularly in the diaper area, and Nystatin® ointment will usually result in a cure after about a week's use.

CONVULSIONS

Convulsions may be due to a variety of causes, such as low blood calcium or low blood sugar in the newborn. Convulsions sometimes occur as a result of brain damage or brain hemorrhage occurring in very difficult deliveries, or as a result of disease in the mother. The most common cause in the child over six months, is fever from infections, especially of the throat or ears. Usually the fever is high (over 103°), but some infants may have convulsions with a low fever (101°).

It is always important to ascertain that the convulsion is not due to an infection of the central nervous system, such as meningitis or encephalitis, and a spinal fluid examination may be needed.

Repeated convulsions in apparently well children may be caused by epilepsy and this can be correctly ascertained by neurologic examinations, including an electroencephalogram.

The treatment for febrile convulsions is to sponge the child over his entire body with one-half rubbing alcohol and one-half tepid water, or by placing the child in a lukewarm bath. Medicines as recommended by your doctor should be used to prevent further convulsions, or be given at the onset of the fever if the possibility of a convulsion is suspected. There are many specific drugs used in the control of convulsions caused by epilepsy.

HERNIA (RUPTURE)

Ninety per cent of inguinal hernias, those found in the groin, appear in the male. In the fetus the testicle develops high in the posterior wall of the abdomen and gradually descends to its resting place in the scrotum. The testicle descends along the inguinal canal together with the peritoneal lining of the abdomen and enters the scrotum still retaining a communication with the general peritoneal cavity. This communication normally closes, but if it fails to do so, a hernia results with the intestines free to project down into the open inguinal canal and scrotum. Since the right testicle descends at a later period than the left, and its inguinal canal closes later, this probably accounts for the greater frequency of right-sided hernias. In the female, the embryonic development is similar to the male and they likewise are susceptible to hernias although to a lesser degree. Occasionally an ovary may be found in a hernia in a girl.

Inguinal hernias are frequently discovered in the newborn, and actually most are seen in the first few years of life. Crying, straining, severe coughing, or standing, may force the intestines down into the open canal at which time the hernia becomes visible as an unusual bulge in the groin, or as an enlarged scrotum. One must differentiate this from a hydrocele, which is a collection of fluid in the scrotum, from a hernia. Occasionally, however, hydroceles are associated with hernias, especially in the young infant. A hernia may be without symptoms unless it becomes obstructed or incarcerated; then pain, fretfulness, constipation, and poor appetite may result.

About 60 per cent of inguinal hernias are on the right side; 10 to 25 per cent on the left side, and the remainder bilateral. The recommended treatment is surgical repair. A truss is inadvisable because it only postpones the inevitable, and may produce damage by pressure upon the underlying spermatic cord, and is unsanitary. There is no contraindication to surgery in the newborn.

INFECTIONS

The newborn has some immunity to disease in the first few months of life, probably inherited from the mother. However if she has not developed immunity to certain diseases she cannot transmit what she does not have. Since the average mother has had the common communicable childhood diseases, her infant is immune to them during the early months. Therefore measles, mumps, or chicken pox rarely occur in the newborn. A few cases of chicken pox and mumps, however, have been seen during this period in the offspring of mothers who have not had these diseases. Newborns can catch colds if they are exposed to them. Immunity may be transmitted to the infant by mothers who had vaccines or serums for their own immunization, such as diphtheria, tetanus, or poliomyelitis. Immunity to poliomyelitis has been positively demonstrated in breast milk. Babies are extremely susceptible to tuberculosis and must be immediately separated from any contact with this disease. In certain circumstances, it is wise to inoculate a high risk (fairly certain of exposure) baby with BCG vaccine, which should produce immunity to this very serious disease. Influenza, fungus infections such as histoplasmosis, protozoal infections such as toxoplasmosis, may occur infrequently in the newborn.

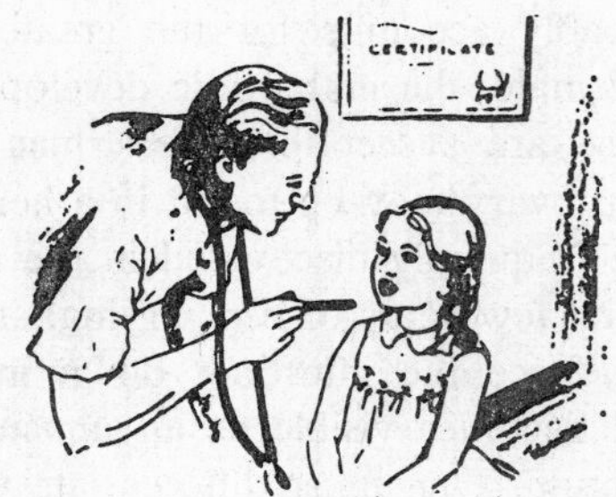

Fig. 33. Health exam is important. School boards in some communities require a health exam for beginning students. The AMA recommends a thorough health examination for 5 and 6 year olds who are starting school for the first time. Most doctors feel that four or five thorough examinations during the school years are sufficient for healthy youngsters. These usually are spaced at the start of the first school year, about the fourth grade, about the seventh grade, at the ninth or tenth grade, and upon graduation. From *Health and Safety Tips,* American Medical Association.

The most common infections during the newborn period are caused by the staphylococcus, especially involving the skin. This germ may be present on the mother's skin or in her nose and throat causing impetigo, pustules, or boils in the baby. The germ is occasionally found in nurseries, or in the nose and throat of hospital personnel, and all hospitals are alert in the prevention of the dissemination of the staphylococcus.

Impetigo in the newborn usually manifests itself by one or more thin, clear, or yellowish blisters on the skin, most frequently in the diaper area. These are usually seen at any time during the first month of life. These blisters break easily and leave a red, shiny, round, open area. Impetigo spreads rapidly if untreated. Babies with impetigo should be bathed with a soap containing hexachlorophene (Phisohex, Winthrop), with special care to cleanse the area about the navel, and an antibiotic ointment used on the infected areas. If the disease is severe, antibiotics should be given either by mouth or injection.

Boils should be opened and drained and appropriate antibiotics used. All rashes are not infectious, but aside from simple diaper rashes, or blemishes of the face, prickly heat, etc., it is advisable for a rash to be seen by the doctor and properly treated.

Pneumonia is one of the more frequent complications of the newborn. It may result from aspiration, either of maternal fecal material or infected vaginal secretions during delivery. It may also be blood-borne as a result of maternal infections, or it may be from air-borne or contacted infections. Occasionally pneumonia ensues from aspiration of foods or gastric contents. The disease may be mild with few symptoms and with complete recovery, or it may be severe enough to produce marked respiratory distress and death. Treatment with oxygen, humidity, fluids, and antibiotics is indicated.

HYALINE MEMBRANE DISEASE

Hyaline membrane disease is a serious condition of the lungs whose cause is unknown, occurring mainly in premature infants, the offspring of diabetic mothers, or in babies born by complicated Cesarean section. The symptoms of difficulty in breathing, cyanosis, with increasing respiratory distress, occur within the first few hours and may prove fatal to at least half of the babies so affected. The treatment also includes oxygen, high humidity, antibiotic drugs, and the intravenous use of soda bicarbonate and glucose. A respirator (Bennet) designed for infant use may also be of great value.

RETROLENTAL FIBROPLASIA

Retrolental fibroplasia is fortunately now a rare condition. Formerly this was a major cause of blindness in small premature infants, but was found by Patz to be due to the concentration of a high percentage of oxygen, together with the length of time spent in such an atmosphere. Since this discovery, prematures who need oxygen as a life-saving procedure, are kept in oxygen at the lowest possible percentage necessary, and for the shortest possible time.

BIRTH ABNORMALITIES

In Dr. Fishbein's book *Birth Defects,* Dr. Gilbert W. Mellin reported that approximately 3 per cent of infants have malformations discovered at birth, and after one year from 4 to 7.4 per cent are found to have abnormalities. These defects vary from race to race. Thus, malformations of the brain occur more often in whites than Negroes. Spina bifida, a malformation at the base of the spine, is found twice as often in whites as Negroes and twelve times as often in whites as Japanese. Extra fingers, as an example, occur seven times as often in Negroes as in whites.

While the cause of many abnormalities is unknown, careful investigation has revealed a vast material of information regarding the causes of certain birth defects. Much is known of certain genetic causes, that is, where the genes of one or both parents carry the defect. An example is mongolism (Down's Syndrome) which is found especially in the offspring of mothers of advancing age (over 45). Radiation to the reproductive organs may affect the future baby and radiation to the fetus itself may produce damage. Certain virus diseases carry a risk to the newborn. The best known of these is German measles or rubella. If a mother is infected by this disease during her first three months of pregnancy, the infant may be born with eye, ear, heart, and brain defects. There is no definite evidence that other viruses produce developmental defects in the human.

Certain drugs or chemical agents are known to cause abnormalities. The tragic results from the use of thalidomide in early pregnancy are well known, causing abnormalities or absence of the extremities, and associated heart defects. Certain drugs used in the treatment of cancer or leukemia can produce abnormalities. Possibly other drugs rarely may be a cause of birth defects and women in the child-bearing age should refrain from taking even common medicines without the specific advice of the doctor.

Inborn errors of metabolism, an inherited dysfunction of certain necessary enzymes, is a rare cause of abnormality. Phenylketonuria is perhaps the best known, since there is a popular test, the PKU urine and blood test, to determine its presence. With this rare disease the child is normal at birth but in a short time develops mental retardation. The urine possesses a rather strange odor and the early recognition of the disease necessitates the use of a special diet to help prevent the ravages of the abnormal chemicals (phenylalanine) resulting from the absence of the enzyme.

Hemophilia is one of the oldest hereditary diseases known to mankind. Severe bleeding from minor causes occurs in childhood, and is due to a rare gene usually carried by the female with the disease transmitted to the male. The blood of patients with hemophilia lacks a factor essential to the normal clotting.

Agammaglobulinemia is a genetic disease which interferes with the development of gamma globulin in the blood, a substance that carries the immune property of the individual. This disease occurs only in males who may have recurrent attacks of such common diseases as pneumonia, chicken pox and others. They may be treated with regular repeated injections of gamma globulin in order to protect them from infections.

THE ALLERGIC CHILD

The term allergy is used to indicate an altered reactivity to a foreign substance known as an antigen which causes the production in the body of a new substance called an antibody. Probably allergic symptoms and disease result from this antigen antibody union, which results in the liberation of certain chemicals, such as histamine. There is apparently an inherited capacity to become sensitized to foreign substance. If there is allergy in both parents, about 70 per cent of their offspring may show symptoms at some time. If only one parent is sensitive, about 50 per cent of the children may show allergic symptoms. The foreign substances most commonly encountered are pollens of trees, grasses, and weeds; spores of molds; dust, certain foods and drugs. These may enter the body by inhalation (pollens), ingestion of foods, injections of drugs, or by direct contact with the skin (poison ivy). The more commonly encountered allergic conditions in children are asthma, hay fever, eczema, and drug reactions.

In infancy, the principal evidence is gastrointestinal, which may show itself in colic, vomiting, or diarrhea. Eczema is a common skin manifestation of allergy and this is often due to cow's milk, egg, or possible orange juice. Respiratory allergies may also appear in infancy with running nose, sneezing, and coughing. This is difficult to diagnose at this period of life. Wheezing, not unlike asthma, often accompanies respiratory infections, and is known as asthmatic bronchitis.

In older children the symptoms of allergy usually involve the respiratory system resulting in sneezing, stuffy nose, coughing, and wheezing.

The diagnosis of an allergic condition requires a careful and detailed record of growth, physical examination, certain blood tests, nasal smears, and allergy tests. There are several methods of allergy testing, but the most commonly used are the scratch and intradermal types. The principle of skin testing is to introduce the suspected antigen or foreign substance into the patient's skin by a scratch or by injection with a small needle. If a specific reaction occurs, the patient may be considered allergic to that particular substance. However, the results of skin testing are not infallible and require interpretation along with results of the other studies.

Emotional causes also undoubtedly play a great part in the symptoms of allergy. Certainly, asthma may result from unusual tension, and consideration of this must be included in the allergic study.

The treatment of the allergic child requires knowledge of the positive factors, frequency, severity, and type of allergy. In some instances the symptoms may be mild and insignificant and require no treatment other than simple avoidance or elimination of the offending agent, or the use of antihistaminic drugs. In other instances such as asthma, more intensive measures may be necessary, which include the injection of the offending agent over a period of time to produce desensitization. Environmental manipulation, such as removal of animals, strict avoidance of dust, and the use of antibiotics and vaccines to reduce infections, are also helpful. Other general measures include adequate diet and nutrition, rest, and the elimination of any psychologic and disturbing factors, and also general medical supervision.

CONGENITAL HEART DISEASE

Congenital heart disease is defined as a structural abnormality of the heart present from birth. This condition has replaced rheumatic fever as the commonest cause of heart disease in children. Since the fetal heart is intact by eight weeks after conception, the stimulus that produces the defect must act before this time. For instance, one cause of abnormalities of the heart, along with other abnormalities, is German measles (rubella), occurring in the mother during the first 8 to 10 weeks of pregnancy. In the overwhelming majority of children with congenital heart disease, a cause cannot be determined. While congenital heart disease is not truly hereditary, a slightly increased frequency of occurrence is noted in families in which it has previously appeared.

The incidence of congenital heart disease is about 1 per 3000 live births and diminishes to 1 per 10,000 population by ten years of age, due to its high mortality rate.

Over 100 different types of malformations may occur, and in many cases more than one defect is present in the same heart. The defects most frequently involve malformations in the septum or wall which normally divides the right and left sides of the heart, or narrowing of the valves leading from the heart to the great arteries which conduct the blood to the lungs and the rest of the body. Other defects that commonly occur may be outside the heart and involve abnormalities of the arteries leading away from the heart. The malformations may be so severe that death in the first few days of life is inevitable. On the other hand, the defects may be so slight that they add no burden to the heart and there is no discernible effect on the child, even though the physical signs of the defect may be detected by a physician. In other words, he may hear a distinctive type of murmur on listening to the heart with his stethoscope. The majority of defects, however, do shorten the life span to some extent even though they may permit normal growth and activity.

A small number of types of defects constitute over 90 per cent of the cases. These are ventricular septal defect, tetralogy of Fallot or "Blue Baby," atrial septal defect, patent ductus arteriosus, coarctation of the aorta, pulmonary stenosis, and aortic stenosis. These defects produce various changes in the function of the heart and alter the cycle of blood through it, such as leakage of blood between the right and left sides, obstruction of flow through the valves, and delivery of unoxygenated blood (dark blue) back to the tissues without passing through the lungs. This altered function produces overwork for the heart muscle which may eventually fail and cause death.

In the developing fetus, the lungs do not function and oxygen is obtained by the baby through the placenta from the maternal blood. In the fetal heart, blood bypasses the unexpanded lungs and is shunted from the right to the left side of the heart through two temporary openings which should normally close after birth, when the child has started breathing and using its lungs. Occasionally the blood vessel that connects the pulmonary artery to the aorta stays open after birth and this constitutes one of the common types of congenital defect, patent ductus arteriosus. After birth the signs and symptoms of congenital heart disease appear at varying intervals depending on the type and severity of the defect. The most characteristic sign is a heart murmur produced by blood passing through an abnormal opening. It should be pointed out, however, that innocent or functional murmurs which have no significance can be heard in up to 75 per cent of all children. The differentiation of an innocent murmur from one originating in a cardiac defect should be left to an experienced physician.

Recurrent bronchitis, pneumonia, and shortness of breath are frequently found in children with congenital heart disease. Retarded growth also occasionally results. The majority, however, manifest normal growth and have no exercise limitations. Pain is not a symptom of congenital heart disease.

If possible, those defects that overburden the heart must eventually be corrected by surgery. The first successful repair of congenital heart defect was a patent ductus arteriosus in 1938. Since that time, great advances in diagnostic and surgical techniques have occurred culminating in the successful use of a heart-lung machine in 1956 which permitted direct repair of defects inside of the heart.

Consideration for surgery requires a prior precise structural and functional diagnosis. Although the clinical examination aided by an X ray and electrocardiogram supply much information, cardiac catheterization is necessary. In this procedure a hollow tube or catheter is introduced into a vein and advanced under fluoroscopic control until it reaches the heart, and various measurements are then taken.

The results of surgery on congenital heart disease today constitute one of the amazing stories of advancement of scientific knowledge. The mortality rate for many of the more common defects now is practically zero. However, in very poor risks, such as small infants and very complicated defects, the mortality rate may be as high as 50 per cent. With further experience and refinement of techniques in the relatively new field of open-heart surgery, results will continue to improve.

IMMUNIZATIONS

Preventive pediatrics, which in its most usual aspects, is to protect against the common communicable diseases, has completely changed the incidence of disease in the infant and young child. At one time, whooping cough was one of the most common causes of death in infants less than one year old, and measles, in children under five years. Now it is no longer necessary for a child to have these serious contagious diseases.

Active immunization; that is, the administration of a vaccine or a toxoid which calls upon the body's immune apparatus to produce protective antibodies against a specific disease, should be started in the first year of life. Routinely today all infants are immunized against diphtheria, whooping cough (pertussis), tetanus, poliomyelitis, smallpox, and measles, during their first years, and given booster inoculations at appropriate times thereafter.

Since there are varying opinions as to the best time and methods of immunizations, the recommendations of the Committee on the Control of Infectious Diseases of the American Academy of Pediatrics are followed here with certain modifications.

The Committee recommends that all infants be inoculated against diphtheria, whooping cough, and tetanus with a course of combined antigens (triple) started at 2 months of age. The initial course should consist of three injections at approximately one month intervals, and a fourth injection about 12 months later.

There are two acceptable vaccines against poliomyelitis (infantile paralysis), both of which have great merit. The inactivated or Salk vaccine is given by injection and may be started as early as 2 months at the same time as the triple antigen, in monthly injections at the second, third and fourth month, with a booster at 15 months of age and at intervals thereafter.

The oral (Sabin) vaccine is now used by more doctors than the Salk vaccine, as its effects are more permanent. It is customary to administer it directly into the baby's mouth in drops, starting at two months of age, and giving three doses at two month intervals. Further doses may be given at eighteen months, and on entering school.

If the Salk vaccine has already been given, it is all right to give the Sabin vaccine at a later date.

RECOMMENDED SCHEDULE FOR ACTIVE IMMUNIZATION AND TUBERCULIN TESTING OF NORMAL INFANTS AND CHILDREN* (1)

2–3 months	DTP–Type 1 OPV or Trivalent OPV[2]
3–4 months	DTP–Type 3 OPV or Trivalent OPV
4–5 months	DTP–Type 2 OPV or Trivalent OPV
9–11 months	Tuberculin Test
12 months	Measles Vaccine
15–18 months	DTP–Trivalent OPV–Smallpox Vaccine[3]
2 years	Tuberculin Test
3 years	DTP–Tuberculin Test
4 years	Tuberculin Test
6 years	TD–Smallpox Vaccine–Tuberculin Test[4] Trivalent OPV
8 years	Tuberculin Test[4]
10 years	Tuberculin Test[4]
12 years	TD–Smallpox Vaccine–Tuberculin Test[4,5]
14 years	Tuberculin Test[4]
16 years	Tuberculin Test[4]

ABBREVIATIONS—DTP (Diphtheria and Tetanus Toxoids and Pertussis Vaccine combined)
OPV (Oral Poliovaccine—if trivalent OPV used—interval should be 6 weeks or longer)
TD (Tetanus and Diphtheria Toxoids, Adult Type)

* Report of the Committee on the Control of Infectious Diseases, 15th edition, 1966, American Academy of Pediatrics.

1 See separate disease sections for more detailed discussion of recommendations, contraindications, and precautions.

2 Immunization may be started at any age. The immune response is limited in a proportion of young infants and the recommended booster doses are designed to ensure or maintain immunity. Protection of infants against pertussis should start early. The best protection of newborn infants against pertussis is avoidance of household contacts by adequate immunization of older siblings. This schedule is intended as a flexible guide which may be modified within certain limits to fit individual situations.

3 Initial smallpox vaccine may be given at any time between twelve and twenty-four months of age.

4 Frequency of repeated tuberculin tests dependent on risk of exposure of children under care and the prevalence of tuberculosis in the population group.

5 After age 12 follow procedures recommended for adults: i.e., smallpox vaccine every five years and tetanus toxoid booster every ten years as TD.

Smallpox vaccination is recommended after the first year and should be repeated every 5 years. For travel abroad, a revaccination is needed every 3 years. Measles vaccine should be administered to all children who have not had the disease, providing that they are at least one year old, or older. The immunity provided by the vaccine then will probably be lifetime. While there are two kinds of vaccine, one made from live virus, and one made from killed virus) only the live virus vaccine should be used.

Dear Parents,

Now is the time for your new baby to be receiving protective vaccine against Diphtheria, Whooping Cough, Tetanus, Smallpox and Polio.

To let us know about your baby, please fill in the following information and mail this card today. NO STAMP IS NEEDED.

Please check (✓) one box only:

☐ My baby is already getting protective vaccines
☐ My baby will be getting protective vaccines soon

Name of Doctor or Clinic

Your Name

IF NAME OR ADDRESS IS
INCORRECT, PLEASE CHANGE

140M-DP 518125-526139 (67)

Estimados Padres,

Ahora es el tiempo para que su nuevo bebé esté recibiendo las vacunas para la protección contra la difteria, tos ferina, tetano, viruela y polio.

Para nosotros saber de su bebé por favor llené la planilla a continuación y ponga la tarjeta en el correo hoy mismo. NO NECESITA SELLOS.

Marque asi (✓) en sólo uno de los cuadritos:

☐ Mi bebé ya comenzó a recibir vacunas de protección
☐ Mi bebé va a recibir vacunas de protección, pronto

Nombre del Médico o Clínica infantil

Su nombre

CORRIJA SU NOMBRE Y DIRECCÍON
SI ESTÁ EQUIVOCADO

Fig. 34. This reminder card is used in approximately 75 large metropolitan areas across the country. In New York City, the system was initiated in January of 1967. Names of newborn babies are recorded in the Department of Health. This card is sent to parents of all babies born in the five boroughs of New York, 90 days after the baby is born. Bureau of Public Health Education, Department of Health, City of New York.

In my experience, vaccine made from the Schwarz strain causes fewer reactions, and produces as good immunity as vaccine made from another (Edmonston) strain. As far as is known, if the vaccine is given at one year or later, no booster injections will ever be needed.

There are certain contraindications to these injections. Unless immunization is urgently needed because of community-wide epidemic, any child with an acute respiratory disease should have the procedure deferred until recovery.

Any infant with cerebral damage should have the DPT injections modified in dosage and postponed until after one year of age.

A baby with eczema, impetigo, or any form of dermatitis, should not be vaccinated against smallpox until the rash has completely cleared. Actually no one person should be vaccinated against smallpox if anyone in the home has eczema, because of the danger of crossinfection. The eczematous areas may become infected from the vaccination resulting in a serious disease called eczema vaccinatum. If vaccination is necessary under these circumstances, it is possible to obtain a special attenuated vaccine that is safe.

In the future an effective vaccine against German measles will become available. Then all girls and women in the child-bearing ages should be immunized. Since accuracy in making this diagnosis is so difficult, it is hard to know who is really immune.

Routinely all children who have been immunized against diphtheria, tetanus, and whooping cough need an occasional booster. Older children should not be given the vaccine containing whooping cough, as reactions may be severe.

Tetanus boosters are necessary in puncture wounds, animal bites, burns, or any dirty type of injury, especially those around barnyards, if it is over one year since immunizations or boosters have been given. In any case, the physician should be consulted as to the advisability of a tetanus booster. If a child has not been immunized against tetanus, human tetanus antiserum is available and effective. Antiserums made in animals are also available for human use but are more likely to produce reactions.

Under certain circumstances influenza vaccine should be administered and boosters given each year. Children with rheumatic heart disease or other heart ailments, and those with chronic pulmonary diseases, such as asthma, cystic fibrosis, chronic bronchitis, bronchiectasis, etc., or any debilitated or chronically ill child, should receive this vaccine.

An effective live virus mumps vaccine is now available. There have been some questions raised as to the proper age at which it should be given. Some authorities recommend its use only in older children, or adults who have not had the disease. This is based on the fact that the length of immunity is not certain, and protection is of greater importance in the adolescent and adult. Mumps, however, is not an innocuous disease, as all pediatricians can attest, since deafness (usually in one ear) occasionally results. It is my present recommendation that this vaccine (which rarely produces any reaction) be given in the second year of life to all children who have not had mumps. It is possible that a booster may be necessary, at some later time.

Rabies vaccine must be used after exposure by bites of a rabid animal. If licking of a mucous surface (mouth) by a rabid animal has occurred, the vaccine is necessary. In severe bites, or bites of the head and neck, rabies serum should be used first and the determination of giving the vaccine also, is up to the physician. Bites by unknown animals require immunization, unless the physician advises against this. Bites by skunks, foxes, and bats are especially dangerous.

BCG vaccine is advised by the committee, for all children who live in or plan extensive travel to areas in the world where tuberculosis is prevalent, and also to those who are likely to be exposed to adults with active or recently arrested cases of this disease.

Typhoid vaccine should be given when travel outside the continental United States or Canada is anticipated.

PASSIVE IMMUNIZATION

If a child has not had previous immunizations and is exposed to certain diseases, temporary protection may be conferred by the use of gamma globulin, convalescent serum, or other materials.

Infectious hepatitis. Exposed individuals, especially household contacts, should be given gamma globulin.

Measles. Gamma globulin should be used for prevention in all unimmunized infants under two years, and modified (made lighter) in older unimmunized children.

Mumps. An exposed male over the age of puberty with a positive skin test for mumps may be given a hyperimmune globulin to help protect him.

Whooping cough. Intimately exposed, unimmunized children under the age of three, should be given hyperimmune globulin.

German measles (rubella). There is no reason to attempt to protect children against this disease. Gamma globulin may be given to susceptible women in the first three months of pregnancy, but the protective effect is uncertain.

Smallpox. Convalescent serum or vaccinia immune globulin will prevent or modify smallpox if given within twenty-four hours following a known exposure. This material must be obtained through the American Red Cross Volunteer Consultants for the Distribution of Vaccinia Immune Globulin.

Other immunizations. There are special requirements for those contemplating travel in foreign countries. The United States Public Health Service will give advice regarding specific problems in any area in the world, especially in regard to cholera, typhus, plague, and yellow fever.

THE TUBERCULIN TEST

A tuberculin test should be performed annually, starting at 9 to 12 months of age. There are several methods of testing, the most practical of which is the Mantoux or intradermal test, using a specific material PPD, in proper dilution. The Tine test is also a very useful test. The test is read in 2 to 3 days and if induration and sufficient redness are present at that time, the test is considered positive. A positive test means that the child has been exposed to someone, probably an adult, with active tuberculosis, and has inhaled some tuberculosis germs. These germs have produced a primary tuberculous infection, probably of a mild nature. Most of these infections show no sign of illness and heal by themselves. The degree of reaction, however, is some indication of the severity of the infection and also the degree of activity of the infection. If tests are done each year, it is possible to tell at what age the child has had the contact. Any child under the age of 5 with a positive tuberculin test should be given appropriate antibiotic treatment to prevent possible consequences. A child who has changed from a previously negative to a positive test within the past year who is under the age of puberty, or possibly even older, should also receive this treatment. Isoniazid by mouth is used either alone or in combination with other drugs, given daily, for at least 12 to 18 months.

These children should have an X ray of the chest when the positive tuberculin test is noted, and an occasional X ray during the treatment period, and once a year thereafter. These children should be watched carefully during puberty and the adolescent years.

CHAPTER 10

The Prevention and Treatment of Infectious Disease

MORRIS FISHBEIN, M.D.

About one hundred years have passed since it was first shown that germs actually cause disease. In the intervening period thousands of germs have been identified definitely as associated with certain diseases that attack human beings. In 1880 the germ associated with typhoid was isolated. Since that time such important diseases as tuberculosis, diphtheria, glanders, pneumonia, cholera, lockjaw, undulant fever, meningitis, dysentery, plague, syphilis, whooping cough, gonorrhea, leprosy, and many other specific infections, have been definitely related to invasion of the human body by specific germs or viruses or other living organisms.

ABOUT GERMS

Few people really know what a germ looks like or how it invades the human body. Germs are so small that it takes three hundred billions of an average germ to weigh a pound. They multiply rapidly under favorable conditions. One germ can produce two new ones in twenty minutes. Anyone who has tried to estimate how much money he would have by beginning with a penny and doubling his fortune every hour can realize how rapidly germs multiply. If a germ divided and made two new ones every hour it would, at the end of a day, have sixteen and a half million descendants.

Doctors identify the germs that cause disease in various ways. First they take some of the material from the infected saliva or from the discharges or from the blood of the person who is infected. They examine this under a microscope. The germs are seen as little round dots, or as rod-shaped organisms, or even as long, slender filaments when they are greatly magnified under the microscope. Like human beings, the germs tend to live preferably in certain forms, sometimes two together, sometimes a group of many, sometimes a chain. Some germs are surrounded by capsules, usually a sort of fatty envelope that enables the germ to resist attacks in the body or in the blood of the animal it invades. Other germs have little tails like fins which enable them to move about.

Some people talk about the germ theory. Germs are no more a theory than are plants, birds, and other living things that live and reproduce. The power of most germs to cause disease can be tested on animals. When the germs are injected into animals they produce changes in the tissues of the animal which are specific for the germs concerned.

A pneumococcus in the lung of a man produces pneumonia; first a consolidation of the lung due to invasion by red blood cells and other material and later a softening of this mass and a clearing up of the lung if the patient lives.

When the typhoid germ gets into the human body it produces ulcers in the intestines, and germs are found in the ulcers. When the meningococcus gets into the linings of the spinal cord and brain it sets up an inflammation of these linings, which are called meninges; then the person has meningitis, an inflammation of the meninges. When the spinal fluid is examined the germs can be found in the fluid.

These tests which were developed by the great Robert Koch, with Louis Pasteur, a founder of modern bacteriology, constitute the acid tests for determining with certainty that any germ is associated with the production of a certain disease. If the germ can be found in the infected tissues, if the germ can be artificially grown outside the human body, if the germ can then be injected into an animal like the monkey and produce in that animal a condition like that in the human being from whom the germ was originally taken, it is the cause of that particular disease. Anyone with a reasoning mind should be willing to grant that the germ actually causes the disease.

INCUBATION PERIODS

The common contagious diseases include measles, scarlet fever, diphtheria, whooping cough, mumps, chicken pox, and German measles. The best way to avoid these diseases is to keep away from people who have them. However, many parents do not feel their responsibilities greatly and do not see to it that their children, when ill, are kept away from other children. The chief responsibility rests on the parents of the sick child for the prevention of infectious diseases rather than on the parents of the well child.

Most of the common infectious diseases are caused by organisms which get into the body and then begin their action. A certain amount of time elapses between the period when the germ first gets in and when its visible manifestations appear. This is known as the incubation period; and it varies with different diseases. For instance, in meningitis it is from two to four days, in erysipelas from one half to three days, in measles from ten days to two weeks, in German measles from five days to twenty-one days, in scarlet fever from a few hours to a week, in smallpox from ten days to two weeks, in typhoid fever from six days to twenty-five days, and in chicken pox from four days to sixteen days.

In most of these diseases an eruption occurs in the surface of the body. These eruptions have characteristic distribution on the skin, so the physician asks particularly as to whether the redness first began on the face, the neck, the hands and feet, the abdomen, or the chest. The eruptions also differ greatly in their appearance: from tiny red spots to large red patches, from tiny pimples to crops of blisters.

Practically all of these conditions are likely to begin with a mild cold. In some of them the sore throat is severe; in most of them fever, slight headache, dizziness, nausea or vomiting ensue. Do not disregard any of these symptoms, particularly when they appear in a child.

The excretions which carry disease include the material that is coughed from the throat, that is spread by spitting, by sneezing, or that may pass from the body in the form of discharges of one kind or another. Therefore, mothers should guard particularly against contact of a well child with one that is coughing, sneezing, spitting, or that manifests any of the other signs of infectious disease that have been mentioned.

RESISTANCE TO INFECTIOUS DISEASE

Four factors are chiefly responsible for infection of the human body: First, the presence of a germ with sufficient virulence to grow in the body; second, a sufficient number of these germs to overcome attacks by the body against the germ; third, some special condition in the body that makes it possible for the germ to live and grow; and fourth, some method of getting the germ into the body.

Were it not for the fact that human beings develop within their bodies conditions which make it difficult for germs to live and grow, the human race would long since have been destroyed by the bacteria. However, the resistance which the human being has is not absolute. The constitution of the human body changes from time to time. Resistance is decreased when the body is greatly undernourished, when a person is exceedingly fatigued, when he has been exposed to sudden severe changes of temperature, or in several other ways.

The line of defense varies in its intensity from time to time. When the enemy is sufficiently numerous, or sufficiently strong, a breakthrough occurs. For this reason, even in the most severe epidemics, some people escape, although there are conditions in which practically everyone attacked is unable to resist. Such conditions occur, for example, when a population among whom a disease has never previously appeared suddenly comes in contact with it. This occurred in the Faroe Islands when measles was brought by a ship carrying white men; at that time more than half the population of the islands died of that disease.

Sometimes the resistance of the body to one disease is broken down by a mild attack of another previous disease. For instance, a person who has had influenza, diabetes, tuberculosis, or some other chronic disorder, may thereafter develop pneumonia, typhoid fever, rheumatic fever, or tuberculosis much more easily than he would have previously.

CARRIERS OF DISEASE

Frequently people who are healthy carry about in their bodies germs which do not attack them but which have sufficient virulence, toxicity, strength, or poison to invade the body of another person and in that person to cause disease. A person who carries the germs about is called a "carrier." Should the carrier suddenly have his own resistance lowered by any of the factors that have been mentioned he might suddenly be invaded by these germs, although previously they had not been able to set up infection in his body.

All of us are constantly being invaded by germs in contaminated food and water, in breathing, in touching infected items with our hands, which are then conveyed to the mouth and nose. Germs occur on money, in clothing, and on various other objects. However, the dosage of germs received through such contacts, or the virulence of the germs, may not be sufficient to bring about disease. The exposure of the germ to fresh air and sunlight, and the fact that it is trying to live on a substance not suitable to it as a habitation, may prevent its multiplying and may cause the germ itself to lose its strength.

Under other circumstances, germs multiply in tremendous numbers, so that the human being who comes in contact with them sustains a massive assault. For instance, an infected fruit peddler may use saliva to polish the fruit, and the germs might grow well on the fruit thus polished. Germs may be deposited with sewage in running water and multiply tremendously in the sewage. When the water from the contaminated stream is drunk by a human being he gets in enough germs to cause prompt infection.

Sometimes an infected food handler is employed to mix a potato salad, to bake a custard, or to make a pie which is then kept under insanitary conditions before being eaten, so that the germs multiply profusely. When this occurs anybody who eats the infected food may become seriously infected, as occurred recently at a picnic when eight hundred people became sick from eating infected potato salad.

PATHS BY WHICH GERMS INVADE

Germs can get into the body in all sorts of ways: with food and water, by inhaling, through open wounds on the skin, by the bite of an insect, as occurs with mosquitoes in malaria and yellow fever, ticks in Texas fever, fleas in plague, and tsetse flies in African sleeping sickness.

When the means by which the germs get into the body are understood, scientific medicine develops methods for keeping them out.

Often the germs produce disease by developing a poison which is then absorbed by the body. After absorption, the poison acts on the nerves or the muscles or the blood vessels. Sometimes the germs themselves gradually break up, and the products of their disintegration are poisonous. Again clumps of germs float around in the blood and cause death by developing in overwhelming numbers in the blood. On other occasions the germs may attack certain organs of the body and so injure these organs that death ensues.

The germs like to pick out certain places in which to live under the conditions which suit them best. This happens, for instance, with a germ called the pneumococcus which settles in the lungs and produces pneumonia, but which also may infect the eye or the spine. The germs of meningitis practically always settle on the coverings of the spinal cord and of the brain, the typhoid germ settles in the intestines, the germs of lockjaw, of hydrophobia, and of epidemic encephalitis attack the nervous system. Some germs, like those of tuberculosis or syphilis, may affect any tissue in the human body although preferably entering by way of the lungs or mucous membrane. Tuberculosis of bones, of joints, of the eye, and of the nervous system is recognized. The organism that causes syphilis actually attacks every organ and tissue in the human body.

RESPONSE OF THE BODY TO GERM INVASION

When germs get into the body and release their poisons the tissues react usually in definite ways. One of the reactions of the body is fever which is apparently due to the effects of the poisons of the germs on the nervous mechanism of the body which controls the body temperature.

Associated with the fever the chemical changes that go on in the body are speeded so that there may be perspiration and, as a result of the increased activity, a loss of weight. For this reason it has become customary to feed fevers rather than to starve them.

Associated with the disturbance of the nervous system there may be dizziness and loss of appetite, also vomiting and an increased activity of the motion of the bowels. This helps to cause loss of material from the body. Due to accumulations of fluid or swelling of tissue aches and pains in the joints and in the muscles may appear. The interference with the action of the kidney may cause fluid to be retained in the body. The blood usually responds by an increase in the number of the white blood cells, but in some conditions the number is decreased, notably influenza and typhoid fever.

Because the fever is considered to be one of the mechanisms of the body in defense against the attack of germs, scientific medicine does not always attempt to reduce the fever too suddenly or too rapidly by the use of drugs. A fever that is not exceedingly high or prolonged for any length of time is not especially harmful to the body, particularly if the amount of fluid in the body is watched and enough of the right type of food is put into the body to prevent too great a wastage of the tissues.

A normal temperature is 98.6 degrees F. A great many investigations indicate that temperatures over 100 degrees F. are unfavorable to the growth of bacteria and may inhibit the action of some of the poison developed by the bacteria. Much better is prevention of infections rather than to endeavor to treat them after they have been established.

STAMPING OUT DISEASE

By scientific methods applied since the nature of the germs and their methods of attack on the body have been discovered, certain diseases are now practically eliminated as of exceeding danger to mankind. Yellow fever occurs now in only a few isolated spots throughout the world. In the United States the number of cases of typhoid fever has been so greatly reduced that many young physicians never see a case even in the hospitals where they take their training. Cholera and plague are limited to the remoter areas of China and India and are seldom if ever seen in the United States.

Mankind has undergone progressive changes from the beginning of time; the diseases of man, particularly such as are caused by living organisms, likewise undergo such changes. True, some diseases have been overcome and eliminated, but new diseases constantly appear and demand consideration. The development of new methods of transportation and conveyance, such as the airplane and the ease of intercommunication between various portions of the earth, have brought into the temperate zone the diseases of the tropics which were formerly limited to such areas.

Many a great civilization has fallen because of the development, endemically or epidemically, of diseases that were previously under control, or because of the introduction of some new disease that had previously been considered a rarity. The great civilizations of Greece and Rome fell because of epidemics of malaria. In the United States today certain forms of infections of the glands, certain forms of infestation by tapeworms, and similar disorders, are seen with comparative frequency, whereas formerly they were practically unknown.

The time will never come when man will be free entirely from the fear of disease. The battle is unending, but more and more mankind can celebrate the fruits of victory. As diseases change and as new diseases appear, scientists observe them in their earliest stages, determine their causes and their modes of transmission, and prevent their development.

PREVENTION OF INFECTION

The prevention of disease must be related to our knowledge of the way in which infectious disease gains entrance into the body. Everything possible must be done to see that the germs in the person who is infected do not get into contact with other people. If this could be done in every case, many infectious diseases would probably disappear.

If everything possible is to be done, all of the sheets, pillow cases, clothing, handkerchiefs, and, in fact, everything touched by a person who is infected, will have to be sterilized by boiling or by steam under pressure before being permitted in contact with other people. All of the excretions from the body of the infected person must be disinfected by proper antiseptics or by burning. The person with a discharge from the nose, such as occurs in the common cold, might at all times wear a face mask. To carry out completely these procedures would mean such an obstruction and hampering of the usual routine of existence that it is not likely to be generally adopted.

The next step is to do everything possible to prevent infected material from being passed from one person to another. This means complete control of food, drink, and air, also the earliest possible detection of human beings, animals, or insects which carry disease, the control of such carriers and their possible elimination.

A human being who is carrying typhoid cannot be eliminated but must be controlled. Since there are millions of persons who carry disease constantly, it is not likely that this source of infection will ever be brought completely under control. Moreover, there are some diseases of which the cause is not definitely known, and it is unlikely that healthy carriers of such diseases will ever be controlled until the cause of the disease is known.

PERSONAL HYGIENE

The best step that the average person can take to prevent infectious disease is to raise his individual resistance by practicing the best possible personal hygiene. This means the eating of a suitable diet, the securing of sufficient exercise and sunlight, and enough rest to give the tissues of the body opportunity to recuperate from fatigue.

Moreover, it is possible to aid resistance to certain infectious diseases by injecting the human being either with blood that has resistance, such as the blood from a person who has recovered from the disease, or by injecting serums from an animal which has been infected with the disease and which has in its serum substances opposed to the disease. A considerable number of such specific preventive serums and vaccines will be discussed under each of the infectious diseases as it is considered.

INCIDENCE OF INFECTIOUS DISEASE

The number of cases of the various infectious diseases varies from time to time. There have been great epidemics of influenza such as the epidemic of 1918, in which tremendous numbers of people were involved, whereas there have been minor epidemics in which relatively few people were concerned. Cases of influenza are difficult to differentiate from the common cold.

The death rates for such conditions as measles, chicken pox, scarlet fever, mumps, and whooping cough have dropped to figures under 0.5 per 100,000 population since new discoveries of antibiotics, preventive vaccines, and serums. The rate of incidence of tuberculosis has dropped greatly. The number of deaths from this disease has dropped from 275 per hundred thousand people in the United States to rates as low as 5.0 in more than ten states of the United States.

Notwithstanding that typhoid fever can be completely controlled by proper measures, some cases of typhoid fever still occur annually in the United States. Notwithstanding that we have in vaccination and in isolation certain methods of controlling smallpox, a few cases and deaths from this disease are still reported.

CLEANLINESS AND INFECTION

If infectious disease is to be prevented and brought under control, people must learn to know the nature of disease, the method of its spread, and the methods of prevention. They must do everything possible to keep themselves in such fit condition that infectious disease will not readily attack them.

Much infectious disease can be prevented by keeping as clean as possible, including frequent bathing with plenty of soap and water. Thorough washing of the hands with plenty of soap, particularly before eating, will destroy millions of germs which may otherwise infect human bodies. Vaccination against smallpox is important for everybody. Children should be protected against diphtheria by the use of diphtheria toxoid or toxin-antitoxin. When there are epidemics of typhoid or of other infectious diseases, physicians should be consulted as to the desirability of using other specific vaccines, serums, or antitoxins. Remember that most infectious diseases are spread by contact with persons who have the disease or who may be recovering.

TREATMENT OF INFECTIOUS DISEASES

In the treatment of most of the common infectious diseases, rest in bed is absolutely necessary. The diet should invariably be mild and bland, depending largely on milk, but supplemented with well-macerated vegetables and occasionally with enough thoroughly macerated liver or lamb's kidney to supply the necessary iron and vitamins that are needed in the diet.

For many of the specific infectious diseases there are now specific methods of treatment. For example, there are serums, vaccines, antitoxins, and antibiotic drugs available against scarlet fever, measles, diphtheria, whooping cough, tetanus, meningitis, erysipelas, and undulant fever.

Typical of the treatment of most of the infectious diseases is the usual method of handling measles. Every child with this disease should be put to bed and kept there, with light covers, as long as it has any fever and for a few days thereafter. If the eyes are irritated, they may be treated with iced cloths soaked in a cold solution of boric acid. The doctor may prescribe the application of an ointment which will keep the lids from getting sticky. The itching and burning of the skin which frequently occurs in the infectious diseases is often relieved by bathing with a simple solution of bicarbonate of soda or a calamine lotion.

The doctor will treat the cough, if it is distressing, by small doses of sedative drugs. The restlessness, headache, and general discomfort may also be relieved by small doses of aspirin or similar remedies, as the doctor prescribes. When, however, any patient develops serious complications or symptoms, such as dullness, stupor, or convulsions, whenever he breathes rapidly or turns blue, it is well to have the physician in immediate attendance. Under such circumstances, the application of a bath, a pack, or a proper remedy may mean a turning between the tendency toward recovery or the tendency toward a more serious condition leading to death.

The details of the treatment of infectious diseases are discussed much more fully in the chapters dealing with individual diseases. The sulfonamide drugs and the antibiotics have revolutionized the treatment of infectious diseases. Penicillin, aureomycin, and terramycin are most widely used with chloramphenicol or chloromycetin in typhoid. Thus far specific substances are not available for chicken pox and measles. The forms of sulfonamides most widely used are sulfadiazine, gantrisin, and gantanol.

CHAPTER 11

Infectious Diseases of Childhood

MORRIS FISHBEIN, M.D.

DIPHTHERIA

In a novel, *The Marriage of Simon Harper,* by Neil Bell, appears an account of a diphtheria epidemic in a small town in England in the period just preceding the discovery of diphtheria antitoxin. The author depicts graphically the child who is severely infected by this disease. Tchekhov also depicts the horror of this deadly disease in an earlier day. Its conquest has been as dramatic as any struggle known to man.

The condition begins with a sore throat and with repeated attempts to expel, by spitting, the membrane that forms in the throat. If the disease continues, severe paralyses prevent swallowing and injure the heart. There comes a period when breathing becomes impossible, and finally, death. No one who has read such a description or who has actually seen a child with this condition, and who has then seen the marvelous effects of a suitable dose of antitoxin given early in the disease, can fail to appreciate what a great blessing this conquest has been for mankind.

In an earlier day, the physician would frequently be called in the middle of the night to the bedside of a gasping child. Then he would either suck the membrane from the throat by mouth-to-mouth suction or through a tube, if one was available. In severe cases he sometimes opened the windpipe with a knife to permit the child to breathe through the throat beneath the membrane.

Then came the great discovery by the German, Von Behring, and by Roux, a pupil of Pasteur, that an antitoxin could be prepared which would overcome the poisons of this disease. Since that time, there have been developed preparations called toxin-antitoxin and toxoid which can be injected into children early in life and which will give them immunity, or protection, against being infected with diphtheria.

In 1883, shortly after Pasteur had announced his discovery of the germ causation of disease, Klebs and Löffler isolated the germs that cause diphtheria. These germs are known as diphtheria bacilli. They are found in the membrane which appears in the throat of a person infected with diphtheria.

In order to determine whether or not infection is present the physician takes a smear from the throat and sends it to the health department, which then studies the germs to see if they are the germs of diphtheria. By taking a smear one means merely the introduction into the throat of

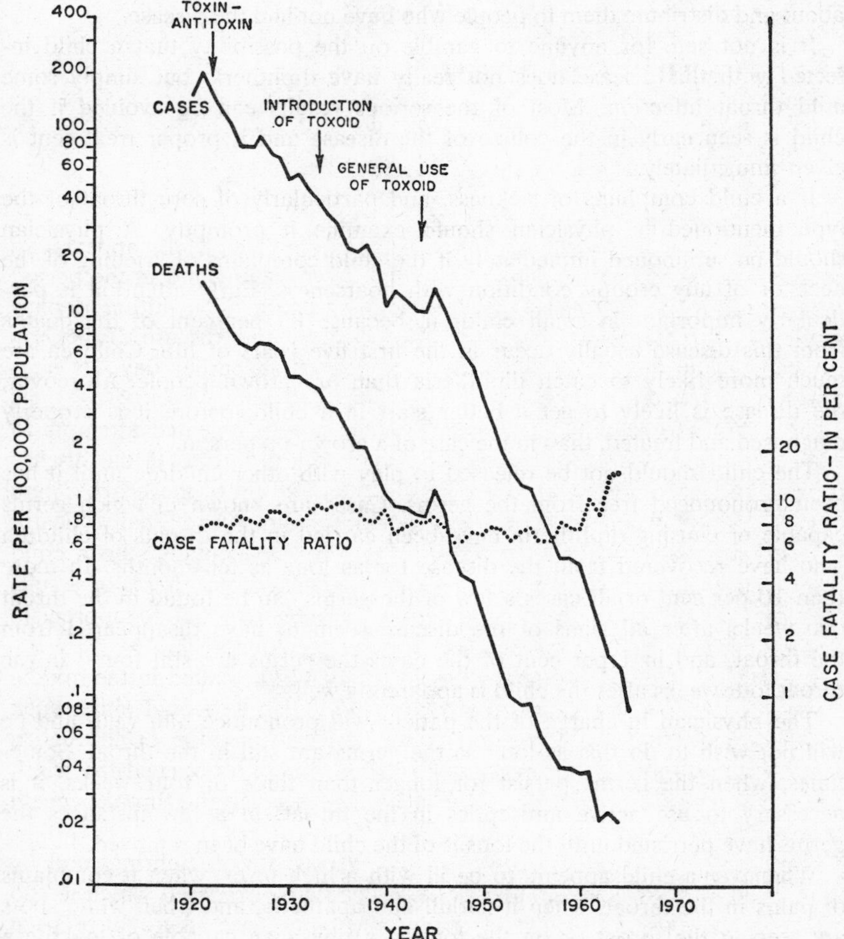

Fig. 35. Diphtheria–Reported Annual Case and Death Rates, and Case-Fatality Ratio–United States, 1920–65. From *Disease Status Report,* October 1966, National Communicable Disease Center, Atlanta, Georgia.

some cotton on the end of a stick, which collects a small portion of the infected material. This is deposited on a preparation which permits the germs to remain alive until they can be studied.

There are various ways in which diphtheria may be spread from an infected person to a well one. The germs have been found on the bedclothing, on handkerchiefs, candy, shoes, hair, pencils, and drinking cups used by infected children. They are, of course, found in any discharges coming from the noses or throats of children who have the disease or who are recovering from it. There are, moreover, healthful carriers of diphtheria who, although they have recovered from the disease, still carry the germs about and distribute them to people who have not had the disease.

It is not safe for anyone to gamble on the possibility that a child infected with this disease does not really have diphtheria but simply some mild throat infection. Most of the serious results can be avoided if the child is seen early in the course of the disease and if proper treatment is given immediately.

If a child complains of sickness, and particularly of sore throat of the type mentioned, a physician should examine it promptly. A physician should be summoned immediately if the child complains of swelling of the neck or of any croupy condition with hoarseness. Early attention is particularly important in small children, because 85 per cent of the deaths from this disease usually occur in the first five years of life. Children are much more likely to catch diphtheria than are grown people. Moreover, the disease is likely to get a better start in a child, before it is properly diagnosed and treated, than in the case of a grown-up person.

The child should not be released to play with other children until it has been pronounced free from the germs. Cases are known in which germs capable of causing diphtheria have been carried in the throats of children who have recovered from the disease for as long as ten months. In more than 10 per cent of all cases a few of the germs can be found in the throat two weeks after all signs of the disease seem to have disappeared from the throat, and in 1 per cent of the cases the germs are still found in the throat four weeks after the child is apparently well.

The physician in charge of the patient will pronounce him well, and he will not wish to do this as long as the germs are still in the throat. Sometimes, when the germs persist for longer than three or four weeks, it is necessary to use active antiseptics in the throat; in a few instances the germs have persisted until the tonsils of the child have been removed.

Whenever a child appears to be ill with a high fever, when it complains of pains in the throat, when it is dull and apathetic, and when white spots are seen in the throat or on the tonsils, a physician capable of making a diagnosis should see the throat and should have immediate charge of the child's care. The more the throat is involved, the greater the spread of the membrane in which the germs are found. The longer the time that the poisons developed by the germs are permitted to get into the system, the more danger there is of death or of serious complications. Hence it is urged that such cases be diagnosed as early as possible, and that when diagnosed large amounts of antitoxin, to be determined by the doctor in charge, be given promptly.

It used to be thought that from 3,000 to 5,000 units of antitoxin were sufficient for a first dose, in the vast majority of cases. Most physicians now prefer to give 10,000 units of antitoxin immediately, and in severe cases 20,000 to 30,000 units of antitoxin as a first injection. The danger of death, or of various forms of paralysis, or of serious complications is far more likely from the disease than from any excess amount of antitoxin. Most strains of the diphtheria germ are sensitive to penicillin and this is beginning to be given routinely in treatment. Throat cultures become negative earlier in patients who receive penicillin.

The child will be immediately put to bed and it will have prolonged rest in bed in order to prevent serious complications. The development of such complications demands particularly the constant care of a physician.

Years ago, a physician named O'Dwyer developed a method for permitting persons with diphtheria to breathe when the membrane had developed to such a point that it obstructed the throat. This method includes the use of gold tubes, called intubation tubes, which an expert can pass through the throat and from the throat into the larynx, or breathing tube, thus permitting the child to breathe. The use of such tubes requires expert knowledge; they are a most valuable method in certain types of cases.

As the condition improves under the use of suitable doses of antitoxin, the membrane disappears, and the child usually coughs up the tube and gets rid of it. In other instances the physician easily removes the tube when it is no longer needed.

During the first few days of diphtheria the child should have a liquid diet as nourishing as possible, including plenty of milk and eggnog and cereals. Thereafter its diet may be gradually improved, particularly with substances that will aid the rebuilding of blood which may have been injured by the infection.

In the prevention of diphtheria in recent years chief reliance has been placed on the use of the Schick test, on toxin-antitoxin and on toxoid. The Schick test is simply a method of injecting a very small amount of the toxin of diphtheria into the skin. Those people who have in their blood antitoxin against the diphtheria poison will have a negative test. On the other hand, those who do not have antitoxin or who cannot develop it will have a positive Schick test.

In a positive Schick test the spot at which the toxin was injected becomes red and slightly raised within twenty-four to forty-eight hours. The application of Schick tests in thousands of cases has shown that about 8 per cent of newly born and young infants are susceptible to diphtheria, which means that they are likely to become infected if exposed to the disease. The remainder are not likely to have the disease at this early age because they have from their mothers a certain amount of resistance to the disease. This is gradually lost, however, so that from 30 to 40 per cent of children will be susceptible at one year of age, and about 65 per cent at five years of age. Apparently, through mild infections, this susceptibility then begins to decrease so that approximately 30 per cent are susceptible at ten years, and 18 per cent at fifteen years.

In the presence of an epidemic it is, of course, desirable that Schick tests be performed on all of the children exposed so as to know which ones are to be especially watched and which ones are to be immediately immunized against the disease by the use of toxin-antitoxin or toxoid. Millions of children have been given toxin-antitoxin and toxoid without the slightest harmful reactions, so that it has become customary in most large cities where there are competent health departments to recommend immunization of all children against diphtheria. Your family doctor will inoculate all the children against diphtheria. You should have this done as soon as possible.

Few people understand the difference between toxin, antitoxin, and toxin-antitoxin. When a horse is injected with the poison which diphtheria germs develop, he develops in his blood a substance which opposes the poison of the diphtheria germ. The poison is called toxin.

The material in the blood which opposes the poison of diphtheria is antitoxin. If a child does not have enough of this antitoxin in its blood to overcome diphtheria infection, the physician gives it antitoxin to help it. If a child has been exposed to diphtheria, and it is necessary promptly to give it something to help it ward off the disease, antitoxin may be injected.

However, this antitoxin does not protect for a long time; its effects wear off in about three weeks. If a person has diphtheria, the antitoxin, when injected, helps to overcome the disease, and when the person recovers he has developed in his own body his own antitoxin, which is one reason why no one seems to have this disease twice.

If one is injected with small doses of toxin or poison, he builds up resistance to diphtheria in his own body. If it is desirable to stimulate his resistance-building factor still more, it is necessary to give him larger doses of toxin. However, such a procedure would be unsafe. Therefore, it is customary to add antitoxin to the toxin, which prevents it from working harm but does not prevent the body from responding to the injection of the toxin by building up more resistance. Toxoid is merely toxin detoxified by the addition of formaldehyde.

Few people realize the background of the way in which the body opposes disease. The process is called immunization. The terms vaccination, inoculation, injection, and similar terms refer to the fact that the substance is being put into the body in order that the body build the materials to oppose it.

The preparation called toxoid has been developed for use in protecting children against diphtheria. Toxoid does not contain any horse serum, but is merely toxin detoxified by the addition of formaldehyde. It is used in the same way that toxin-antitoxin is used and serves to stimulate the development of immunity, or of resistance to diphtheria.

Some people react unfavorably to injections of antitoxin because they are sensitive to horse serum. Hypersensitivity of this kind is the same type of hypersensitivity that produces asthma, or hay fever, or eruptions of blisters, or similar manifestations. When there is a possibility that a child is going to be especially sensitive to antitoxin, the physician can find out by injecting under the skin a small amount—one or two drops—of the antitoxin and then waiting for an hour to see if there is going to be a reaction. Whenever a reaction appears it can be combated by giving suitable preparations of drugs which serve to control the reaction.

TREATMENT OF DIPHTHERIA

In the treatment of diphtheria, the antitoxin, as has already been mentioned, has been of the utmost importance. A delay of two, three, or four days in giving antitoxin may mean damage to vital organs in such manner that they can never recover completely. Moreover, the first dose of antitoxin that is given should be large enough to control the disease. This antitoxin is usually injected by the doctor in the back below the shoulder blade, but sometimes into the thigh or under the breast. In very severe cases the antitoxin is injected directly into a vein; in less severe cases, into the muscles, and in the milder cases, under the skin.

In the vast majority of cases a striking improvement is seen shortly after the antitoxin is injected. The improvement is demonstrated by a fall in the fever and a favorable change in the general condition of the patient. Usually within twenty-four hours after a sufficient dose has been injected, the membrane in the throat stops spreading, becomes softened and loosens up, and the swelling goes down.

There are patients with diphtheria who come to treatment so late that the antitoxin seems to be of little help, but even in these cases it exercises a tremendously beneficial influence in comparison with the effects when antitoxin is not given. In an occasional case of diphtheria there is sensitivity to the antitoxin, so that the patient may have a severe eruption or a reaction. These are exceedingly rare, developing perhaps in one out of every one thousand people. Death from severe reaction to the serum occurs in only one in about seventy thousand people. These reactions occur more often in people who have had severe asthma or who have developed sensitivity to horse serum following a previous injection.

The heart is usually subjected to a severe strain in diphtheria, so that the patient should always be at rest in bed. Moreover, the heart must be watched carefully for several weeks after the patient recovers to make certain that it has not been damaged in any way.

There was a time when it was customary to wash the nose and throat of a patient with diphtheria with all sorts of gargles and sprays, usually of some alkaline solution. Nowadays it is customary to leave the nose and throat alone. In most instances when there is a foul odor in the throat, a mild wash or gargle may be desirable.

Antitoxin is supplemented with penicillin in cases of diphtheria to control secondary infections and because it helps to prevent formation of diphtheria toxin.

In the most severe cases of diphtheria, when the patient seems to be strangling because of lack of air, it may be necessary, as previously mentioned, to pass an O'Dwyer tube into the larynx so as to permit breathing. In the still more severe cases, an emergency operation is sometimes done, the physician opening the tube that leads to the lungs so that the patient is able to breathe. These cases are, however, exceedingly rare, since a powerful diphtheria antitoxin has been introduced, and since the vast majority of doctors give a large dose of antitoxin immediately, as soon as the patient has been examined and the diagnosis has been made.

Most patients stop showing germs of diphtheria in the throat after three or four weeks. Others continue even after several courses of treatment with penicillin. The virulence of the germs should be determined by the state laboratory before the doctor relinquishes control of the patient.

In many communities where almost the entire population of children has been immunized against diphtheria, the disease has been practically eliminated. The prevention of this disease by application of the various methods that have been described represents one of the greatest contributions of modern medical science to the welfare of humanity. Recent tests show that 80 per cent of the children who have been immunized by the use of toxin-antitoxin or of toxoid remain immune for at least ten years after the injections. Diphtheria is no longer a prominent menace to any child.

MEASLES

Measles is one of the oldest diseases known to modern medicine. It may have existed in the early Christian Era. It is even described in the writings of physicians of the seventh and ninth centuries. However, it was for a long time confused with scarlet fever, and it was not until the seventeenth century that it was clearly distinguished from scarlet fever. Moreover, it was occasionally confused with smallpox, and it was not definitely distinguished from smallpox until the eighteenth century.

Two of the greatest names in English medicine are associated with these two observations. Thomas Sydenham distinguished measles from scarlet fever, and William Withering, who introduced the use of digitalis, distinguished measles clearly from smallpox. The English word measles resembles a word in Sanskrit, *masura,* and the German word is *masern.*

For a long time it was generally believed that every child had to have measles. In fact, mothers used to expose their children to the disease with the idea of getting it over. Now it is known that the disease is definitely transmitted from one person to another, and that it is possible, by exercising precautions, to avoid the disease in most instances.

Measles is essentially a disease of childhood. More than half the cases occur in children under five years of age, and more than 90 per cent occur in children under ten years of age. There are occasional epidemics of measles in which considerable numbers of people are affected, even people of advanced years. In such cases it is usually found that the people concerned have come from rural areas and that they have not previously been exposed. For example, there were severe outbreaks of measles among the soldiers in the training camps in 1917 and 1918, because large numbers of recruits came from farms, ranches, and remote districts and had never had measles before.

Measles among a people who do not have anything resembling resistance through heredity may be a most serious and fatal disease. A terrific epidemic of measles occurred in the Faroe Islands in 1846. There were 7,800 people on the Islands and 6,000 of them had the disease in a few months. There was also a great epidemic in the Fiji Islands in 1875. A British ship carrying measles brought the disease to the Islands. Out of a population of 150,000 there were 40,000 deaths in a few months. Part of this was due to the great virulence with which the disease attacked a community without resistance. Much of the fatality is ascribed to the fact that so many people were sick at the same time that there were not enough well people left to take care of the sick. Some people died of starvation, and many died from lack of care.

As with diphtheria, measles is spread mostly through direct contact with those who have the disease. Apparently, the virus or poison that causes the disease is present in the secretions of the nose and throat. Hence it is spread by coughing and sneezing. Fortunately, the virus which carries the disease is injured by exposure to air and sunlight, so that it is seldom likely that measles is carried from one person to another through the medium of a third person or an animal. For this reason it is safe for doctors and nurses who see cases of measles to go in the open air to visit other patients.

However, those who take care of patients with measles should observe all the precautions that are associated with the care of infectious disease generally. This means thorough washing of the hands after visiting a patient, the wearing of a clean gown on entering the room, and removal of the gown on leaving. Moreover, the dishes, bedding, and other materials associated with the child sick with measles must be boiled before they are used again.

From the time when the child first comes in contact with a case of measles, and thereby develops the likelihood of catching the disease, until the disease appears, is usually twelve to nineteen days. This is known as the incubation period. During this period the patient does not have symptoms. However, he does develop early three definite signs which permit a physician to diagnose the disease in its earliest stages. These signs include fever, running nose and watering of the eyes, and an eruption on the mucous membranes lining the mouth. Measles is particularly infective during the stage before the rash appears when the nose is running and the child is coughing and sneezing.

The inflammation of the eyes differentiates measles from other infectious diseases, in which this symptom is not common. The child avoids the light and, as has been mentioned, the eyes are moist and full of tears. Particularly interesting are the little spots which appear on the sides of the mouth and on the palate and which resemble the rash that is later to appear on the skin. These little bluish white spots, surrounded with an area of red inflammation, were described by a New York physician named Koplik and are commonly called Koplik's spots. A Dutch physician on an isolated island described them earlier, but his report did not circulate; hence Koplik's name goes with the spots.

Three or four days after the running nose and the slight fever appear comes the rash. The child breaks out on the face, the mouth and chin, and then over the trunk, arms, thighs, and legs with red spots which enlarge and join together. The color is purplish red. During this period the child is likely to be sicker than at any other time in the course of the disease. He may have lack of appetite, a coated tongue, even looseness of the bowels; there may be a slight cough and other disturbances related to the lungs.

The child with measles should be placed in a room alone and not permitted to come in contact with other children. Particular attention must be given to the prevention of chilling, because this is especially harmful in measles. The secondary complications affecting the lungs are far more serious than the disease itself. The room should be well ventilated, but care must be taken to avoid drafts by placing screens properly before open windows. This does not mean that the room is to be kept stuffy or hot. It is the draft that should be avoided.

For years it was customary to keep darkened the room used by a child with measles because of the trouble with the eyes. Now it is realized that strong sunlight should be excluded because glare will cause pain in the eyes. The child should not be permitted to read nor should there be a brilliant artificial light. If the child complains particularly of the light, colored glasses may be worn. If the eyelids tend to stick because of the slight inflammation they may be bathed with boric acid solution or with plain warm water, which removes the crusts and prevents pain and irritation.

During the period of restlessness the child will sleep better if it is given a warm sponge bath just before going to sleep. This serves to cool the child and to bring down the fever slightly. It also avoids chilling. After the sponge bath the skin may be powdered with any light, clean talcum. This helps to avoid irritation.

It is not necessary to cover the child with heavy woolen blankets or to use flannel sleeping garments. The child should be kept warm but not made uncomfortable.

The food to be taken by the child with measles should be chiefly light and fluid as long as there is any fever. Just as soon as the fever disappears and the child begins to convalesce, plenty of nutritious food should be supplied, particularly foods containing iron and vitamins, as these will help to build up the depleted blood. Laxatives and cathartics should be given only on the order of a physician. It is much better to keep the bowels regular by the use of proper foods. It is also well in these conditions to give plenty of fluids, including drinks tending toward alkalinity, such as orange juice and lemon juice.

When a person has an infectious disease he builds up in his blood materials for opposing the disease. When he recovers, the material remains. For this reason the person who has measles, scarlet fever, or another infectious disease, usually has the disease only once. For this reason also it has been found helpful, in the presence of severe epidemics of measles, to inject into those who are exposed small amounts of the blood of those who are getting over the disease. This procedure has been found to be safe. It seems to minimize the severity of the disturbance if it does not prevent it. In addition to serum from convalescents, ordinary adult serum and placental preparations have been used.

It is the contagious material from the patient with measles that spreads the disease. This contagious material is found chiefly in the excretions from the nose and throat. Every possible step must be taken to prevent other children from coming in contact with these excretions. Occasionally also there are infections of the ear with discharges. The discharges from the ear may also contain the infectious substances, although quite frequently the ear is infected secondarily with other germs, such as the streptococci, which are always present in the throat.

When the resistance of the body is broken down by any one disease a human being becomes susceptible to infections from others. Measles is particularly important in this regard. It has been noticed that epidemics of measles are frequently followed by invasion of other contagious diseases, such as whooping cough, chicken pox, diphtheria, and scarlet fever. Measles is noted also for lowering resistance to tuberculosis so that children who have quiescent infections from tuberculosis in the glands, the bones, the joints, or the lungs may develop activity in these foci when they become infected with measles.

Dr. John Enders developed in 1966 a vaccine against measles using living attenuated virus grown in cultures outside the body. Several preparations of virus vaccine are now available for prevention of measles.

In measles, antibiotics and sulfonamide drugs are of immense importance for preventing and controlling secondary complications such as may affect the eyes, nose, sinuses, throat, ears, lungs, heart or kidneys. The streptococcus, pneumococcus, meningococcus and the organism of tuberculosis are most frequent secondary invaders.

Whenever a case appears in a school, the parents of other children should be warned that a case has occurred and that they should be on the lookout for symptoms of infection in their own children. Parents should be warned particularly to keep their children who have measles, or who are just recovering, away from other children who may not have had the disease.

When a child with measles is put to bed promptly and given satisfactory care of the type that has previously been mentioned, it tends to get well. The prevention of the complications in measles is largely due to the kind of attention that is given. Careful management, skillful nursing, and early control of complications by competent medical attention make all the difference between prompt recovery and the possibility of permanent complications or death.

GERMAN MEASLES

German measles brings on one of the reddest eruptions of any disease that affects mankind. Its scientific name is *rubella,* and in German it is called *Rötheln.* Because of its red eruption it is frequently confused with scarlet fever or with measles. Fortunately, it is not nearly so severe a disease, although it is highly contagious.

From fourteen to twenty-three days after a child comes in contact with another who has had German measles it will begin to feel ill and break out with the eruption, which occurs first on the chest and face and then gradually spreads over the body. There is not much fever in most cases. However, the lymph glands, particularly those at the back of the neck, swell up and get hard, a condition that seldom occurs in other infectious diseases. Associated with this swelling and hardness of the glands at the back of the neck there will be tenderness and even stiffness.

The physician must be sure about the cause of such tenderness or such stiffness of the neck because many of the conditions of infection which concern the nervous system, such as meningitis, brain fever, and infantile paralysis, also develop stiffness and pain on motion of the neck. Conditions occur in which lymph glands are infected in which the glands later soften and develop pus which has to be released by an opening. In German measles, however, the glands gradually soften and disappear without developing pus or matter.

The doctor tells the difference between German measles and ordinary measles by the absence of the spots in the mouth and by the slightness of the condition, by the nature of the eruption and by the absence in measles, in most cases, of the hard spots at the back of the neck.

Few, if any, people die of German measles. The disease usually proceeds toward prompt recovery. The chief trouble with it is that it causes loss of time from school. Seldom is anything required in its treatment except good care, a mild diet, cleansing of the throat by proper gargles, and the early care of any secondary complications.

Since the chief danger from measles has been the secondary complications, early use of penicillin and sulfonamides has lessened complications and made mortality minimal. At the earliest sign of infection of ears or chest the antibiotics are administered.

German measles and other virus infections are especially serious for pregnant women, since such infections during early months of pregnancy are now definitely related to deformities in the newborn child. Gamma globulin from serum of persons recovering from German measles is given to pregnant women not less than eight days after contact or exposure to a case of German measles, as a method of protection.

SCARLET FEVER

No doubt scarlet fever was known to the ancients, but only within the last ten years has its nature actually been thoroughly elucidated. It is an acute infectious disease that comes on suddenly, with a red rash which disappears gradually and is followed by peeling of the skin.

For many years it was known that a germ called the streptococcus was associated with scarlet fever. Only recently has the definite relationship of this germ to the cause of the disease been established. The germ can be found in the throat, the blood, and other tissues of people who have the disease; the disease can be produced in human beings by putting the germs into their bodies; and there is a reaction in the skin of a human being who does not have the disease when the toxin or poison taken from the germs is inoculated into the skin.

Scarlet fever usually comes on in epidemics that are worst in the winter or fall. The chief factor necessary is contact, usually of a child, with someone who has the disease. Most of the cases develop in children between five and twelve years of age. Probably something that the child gets in its blood from the mother in most cases prevents children below one year of age from catching the disease.

Scarlet fever does not spread nearly as rapidly as measles; apparently only about one in ten people who come in contact with cases of the disease later develop it. Possibly people are infected with mild attacks of scarlet fever which are overlooked, and as a result they are later protected against the disease. Scarlet fever is one of those diseases which happen once in a person's lifetime and then are not likely to happen again. In other words, one attack of the disease protects.

Occasionally scarlet fever is spread through milk or through the excretions or secretions of persons who are infected, but the spread through food is far less frequent than the spread directly from person to person. Most people are interested to know whether or not the scales or the skin that peels off after scarlet fever will transmit the disease. Apparently the scales will not spread scarlet fever unless contaminated with the secretions of the nose and throat.

From two to four days after a person has been in contact with someone who has had scarlet fever he will have a chill and complain of severe sore throat. If the person affected is a child, he is likely to be nauseated and vomit. Promptly the pulse becomes rapid as the fever goes up. The fever may rise as high as 102 to 104 degrees. There is severe headache. Then bright red spots about the size of a pin point appear, usually first on the neck and chest, then rapidly spreading over the rest of the body. The face is flushed because of the fever, but the eruption on the face is seldom severe.

After two or three days the rash or eruption begins to fade, and in about a week the skin appears to be normal in color. Then ten days to two weeks after the disease first appears the skin begins to peel. Great patches of skin may come off the hands and feet, but over the rest of the body the skin comes off in small scales. Occasionally the teeth, the hair, and the fingernails also are affected by the destructive process. An interesting symptom of scarlet fever is the appearance of the tongue. Because of its bright red appearance and because the tissues of the surface of the tongue swell so as to show tiny pits, the tongue of scarlet fever is called a strawberry tongue.

Scarlet fever in many instances is a fairly mild disease. When, however, it is complicated by certain forms of invasion of the kidneys, the ears, the glands or the joints, it may be most serious and destructive.

Scarlet fever varies in its severity from time to time, from epidemic to epidemic. In the presence of a severe epidemic with numerous serious complications, it is advisable to give the specific drugs that prevent the growth of the streptococcus.

Because of the danger to other children from a child or an adult who has scarlet fever, the patient should be promptly put to bed and kept separate from other people for about six weeks. If there are discharges from the nose and throat or from the ears the patient should be isolated until all discharges have ceased. These discharges are extremely dangerous in spreading the disease.

Beyond this placing of the patient in a separate room, attention must be given to protecting the kidneys and the heart from the special strains associated with activity at a time when they are exposed to the actions of the poisons that come from the germs. Therefore, every patient with scarlet fever should remain in bed for at least three weeks. It is customary to give a light, soft diet consisting mostly of liquids until the fever has disappeared, and then gradually to add cereals and similar soft foods until the peeling has begun. Then it becomes necessary to build up the tissues and the blood again. This can be done by feeding plenty of milk, fresh vegetables, foods rich in vitamins, mineral salts like calcium and iron, and more protein than is allowed in the active stages of the disease.

It is important to avoid exposure to cold. Therefore, the patient should be bathed with sponges of lukewarm water. Sometimes the skin may be oiled, which aids the peeling and prevents irritation.

In most cases the throat can be let alone because the initial soreness and swelling soon disappear. If, however, there is severe pain from the sore throat, the usual mild gargles may be used. It is well, however, that only persons who have already had the disease should be in contact with the patient and help him with these procedures.

There is no certain method of preventing the complications that affect the kidneys in so many cases of scarlet fever. All that one can do is to make sure that the patient is quiet and that the diet does not throw an undue burden on the kidneys. For this reason it is customary, during at least the first two or three weeks, to eliminate meat and eggs from the diet.

In treating scarlet fever doctors usually prescribe remedies that will prevent headache and pain, giving small doses to avoid irritation of the kidneys. If earache occurs, the ears are closely watched so that the eardrum may be punctured and the infectious material allowed to escape before there is danger to the internal ear from pressure of the poison and danger of mastoiditis. If the infection is virulent, these complications may develop in spite of every precaution.

The discovery of the sulfonamides and of penicillin has revolutionized the prevention and treatment of scarlet fever. Penicillin, aureomycin, terramycin or sulfadiazine will suppress streptococci in the pharynx. Penicillin and erythromycin have been proved effective in treating scarlet fever. Most patients recover with few complications when properly treated with these drugs, and the incidence of complications is much less. These drugs are apparently specific against the streptococcus that is associated with scarlet fever. So efficient is penicillin against the scarlet fever streptococcus that routine administration has also been proposed for prevention of infection when there are epidemics. However, antibiotics for the ordinary use are not recommended although they are used prophylactically during epidemics. Penicillin also eliminates the streptococcus from carriers.

WHOOPING COUGH

At least four hundred years ago diseases were described which resemble what is called whooping cough today. It was known in Scotland as the "Kink" which meant a fit or paroxysm. This condition is one of the most difficult with which health officials and physicians have to deal. A few cases appearing in any group of children spread rapidly to include all who have not had the disease previously.

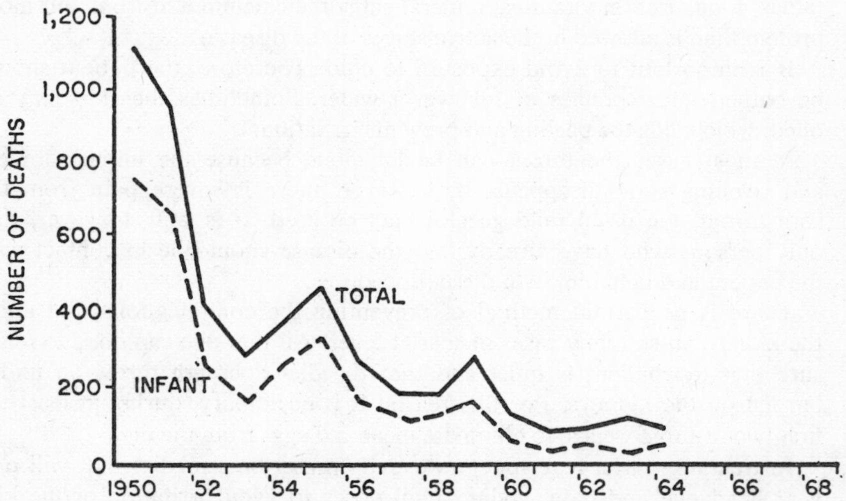

Fig. 36. Pertussis reported deaths, United States, 1950–64. From *Disease Status Report,* October 1966, National Communicable Disease Center, Atlanta, Georgia.

Whooping cough causes more deaths than do most of the other infectious diseases of childhood. It is fatal chiefly to the young, and the immediate cause of death is nearly always some secondary infection. In older children whooping cough may be followed by pneumonia or tuberculosis and is especially menacing from the point of view of these complications.

A germ was found in connection with the disease in 1906, by two Belgian investigators, Bordet and Gengou. The germ is called Bordetulla pertussis.

The chief epidemics of this disease occur in winter. Whooping cough is transmitted, of course, by the material coughed out from the lungs. It has been shown that the explosive cough which occurs in this condition can throw droplets of infected saliva six feet or farther. Far too frequently parents permit children to begin playing with other children just as soon as they are without fever. Yet these children, if they continue to cough, may be active in spreading the disease to children who have not had it. Moreover, there is evidence that whooping cough is infectious in its earliest stages, so that children who are not put to bed and kept isolated until after they have been coughing for some time may also actively spread the disease.

It is the duty of parents not only to their own children, but also to others, to put a coughing child to bed as soon as possible. Moreover, they ought to keep him in bed until a physician says that it is safe for him to be up and around.

What is called the incubation period in whooping cough is the period from two to fourteen days before the patient begins coughing. During this period the child is infected but not sick. Therefore, the child exposed to whooping cough must be watched carefully for at least ten days after its contact for the signs of whooping cough. During this period there may be symptoms resembling those of a common cold. After the characteristic whoop and the paroxysm of coughing appear, the child is likely to be able to spread the disease for at least three weeks longer. Therefore, doctors advise that children be kept alone as long as the cough continues and for two weeks after it ends.

The doctor diagnoses whooping cough not only by the typical coughing spells, which are usually accompanied with redness of the face and the development of a thick, sticky mucus in the mouth, but also by changes which occur in the blood in this disease. Not only do the white blood cells increase in number, but a particular form of the white blood cells, known as the lymphocytes, mononuclear or single nucleus cells, increases even more than do the others.

As has been said, the chief danger from whooping cough is not from the disease itself, but from the secondary pneumonia and changes which may affect the heart and lungs.

The total period of quarantine may be as long as six weeks. In attempting to control whooping cough all sorts of methods of prevention have been tried, including inoculation of the blood from people who are recovering from the disease, the injection of germs that have been killed, with the idea that these injections will stimulate the body to form antisubstances against the germs of the disease, and many similar measures. The use of the vaccines, which means a mixture of killed germs, is established as valuable in preventing whooping cough in children who are exposed, and also in diminishing the severity of the symptoms. Several specific vaccines have been developed and the use of such preparations for prevention is now generally recommended. Preventive inoculations begin as early as six months of age. Booster doses of vaccine are given at four year intervals.

As soon as the child who has had whooping cough is free from fever and any other serious symptoms, it is customary to permit him to be about, particularly where there are sunlight, warmth, and fresh air, but the child should not be exposed to air that is too cold.

Because the coughing spells are frequently accompanied by vomiting, such children sometimes lose weight and may suffer from a lack of water in the body. Hence, the parents must aid the physician in seeing to it that the child has sufficient water and also that it eats between meals, if necessary, or in fact whenever it can retain food, so as to keep up its nutrition.

Because coughing may bring undue pressure into the abdominal cavity and thereby cause rupture or hernia by pushing the abdominal contents through the wall, it is advisable in some cases to put an abdominal binder on the child, which helps to support the abdominal wall and, at the same time, gives the child comfort during severe coughing.

Although the use of various drugs does not cure whooping cough, sedatives which a physician can prescribe lessen the severity of the coughing. Streptomycin, chlortetracycline and polymyxin are new antibiotics successful in whooping cough. Other antibiotics to be tried include chloramphenicol and oxytetracycline. The whooping cough vaccines now available are more efficient in preventing the disease and lessening its severity.

One of the simplest methods of relieving a cough is to inhale warm steam perhaps medicated with a little tincture of benzoin. Fill a cup with boiling water, drop in a teaspoonful of the tincture of benzoin, and inhale the hot steam for five or ten minutes. Such medication is more useful for an ordinary cough than for whooping cough, however. In this condition, frequently, the only way to get relief is by taking sedative remedies that are so strong they can be taken only with a doctor's prescription.

As in other types of infectious disease, all drops from the nose and throat should be disinfected, and all articles contaminated by such discharges should be disinfected or burned.

In keeping up the nutrition of the child, it is well to rely primarily on milk and the use of vegetables containing plenty of vitamins and mineral salts.

In preventing the spread of whooping cough everyone must cooperate. If parents know of other children in the neighborhood who have whooping cough and who are permitted to play outdoors with children who have not had the disease, the health department should be notified. In most communities the parents who have children with whooping cough are permitted themselves to go to work and to go outdoors, although the children are kept under isolation.

CHICKEN POX

All sorts of names have been applied to chicken pox, not only by the public, but also by physicians. In some parts of the country it is known as water pock, glass pock, sheep pock, and crystal pock. These names obviously are related either to some resemblance of the blisters to similar conditions occurring in animals, or, in fact, to the resemblance of the blisters to water or crystal. Scientifically, the condition is called *varicella,* but it was also called *variola spuria,* or spurious smallpox, because it was so frequently mistaken for smallpox.

The cause of chicken pox is a virus. The viruses of chicken pox and herpes zoster or shingles resemble each other. Chicken pox in children may induce shingles in adults. Shingles, whether in children or adults, may be followed by epidemics of chicken pox. The condition occurs most often in children and, because it is so highly contagious, spreads rapidly. Usually a person who has had the disease once does not develop it again. The infectious agent is present in the blisters. The blisters appear early and break almost as soon as they appear. Probably the disease may be spread before the eruption is visible in the form of blisters. About two weeks after a child has been in contact with children who have chicken pox, it will probably come down with this disease.

The blisters on the skin appear in groups, usually first on the back, the chest, and the face, but most profusely on those parts of the skin that are covered by clothing.

As has been mentioned, the condition may be spread not only from contact with infectious material that is in the blisters, but far more frequently through some infection that may be inhaled.

A physician's daughter, sixteen years old, developed a slight sore throat and was immediately isolated in a room in the upper story of her home. On the following day she was found to have the eruption of chicken pox. An eight-year-old brother who was with her on the previous day was kept in a distant part of the house, but sixteen days later he also came down with chicken pox. His only possible contact with the disease was through his sister.

Nobody knows how long a person who has chicken pox remains infectious for others, but it is safe to keep the person who is recovering away from other people until the skin is entirely free of the original crusts.

Chicken pox is not a particularly serious disease, since it is seldom associated with high fever or with much depression. Usually the fever disappears in from one to three days, although it may last four or five days. With the exception of German measles, chicken pox is probably the mildest of all the infectious diseases that attack children.

Usually all that is necessary in such cases is to make certain that the child does not scratch the spots with the likelihood of secondary infection. The fingernails of children should be closely trimmed to prevent such scratching.

Ordinarily, the blisters, if let alone, will last a few hours, break, dry up, and form a crust. This crust disappears in from two to four days.

The diet is mild and soft. Mild, warm baths are used, and it may be desirable for the physician to prescribe powder to prevent itching, or ointments and antiseptic solutions to prevent secondary infection.

Chicken pox seldom concerns older people. Most children have had it by the time they grow up. If, however, they have not had it, they may get the disease later. Chicken pox can be exceedingly inconvenient for a grown-up person, but the most important step for a grown-up person is to make certain that he really has chicken pox and not smallpox.

After a patient recovers, it is merely necessary to wash the bedding thoroughly with hot water and soap and to clean and air the room in which the patient has been while sick.

It is also well for everyone who is in contact with the child to wash the hands thoroughly after leaving the room and preferably to wear a gown or covering while in the room.

The giving of sulfonamides or penicillin and the application of tyrothricin to the blisters prevent secondary infections. The lesions of shingles may require sedative ointments. Reports indicate the possibility that ultraviolet irradiation of air or glycol vaporization may help to prevent spread of chicken pox in schools.

MUMPS

Of all the annoying diseases that afflict the child, and which also occasionally attack the adult, mumps is the one most likely to arouse the risibilities of those in the vicinity. Swelling at the sides of the face gives the person who is infected a distinctly comical appearance. Superstition holds that the person with the disease cannot eat pickles and that anything sour will pucker up his face like the phenomena that follow the eating of a green persimmon.

The condition is infectious, because it spreads rapidly wherever it gets a start among a group of young people. Cases have been described as long ago as one hundred fifty years. In 1934 the cause of mumps was definitely established to be a filterable virus.

Most often mumps appear in a child from five to fifteen years of age from 14 to 21 days after exposure to infection. Because the glands most commonly concerned are the parotid glands, just in front of the ear, the disease is called scientifically parotitis. The Germans fondly call it *Ziegenpeter,* which perhaps has some reference to a goat.

In most cases, mumps is a mild condition. It occurs usually during the cold season of the year. Out of 150 epidemics, only 21 occurred in the warm months. The mouth becomes dry and there is pain on chewing or swallowing.

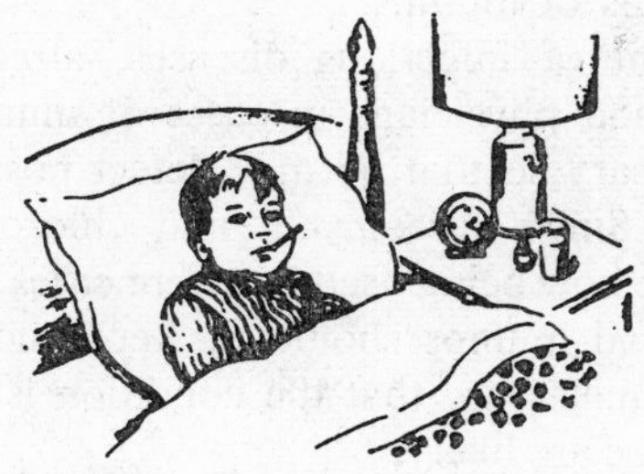

Fig. 37. Mumps is a virus infection of the parotid gland, one of the salivary glands, immediately below the ear lobe and behind the angle of the jaw, says *Today's Health,* the magazine of the American Medical Association. Mumps is not excessively contagious and almost direct contact with the afflicted—such as drinking from the same cup or being sneezed at—is required to contract the disease. Mumps cannot be prevented at present, but recent research promises a vaccine soon. *Health and Safety Tips,* American Medical Association.

Mumps is primarily a disease of adolescence, but cases have been observed in a woman eighty-four years of age, and in a man ninety-nine years of age—possibly both in their second childhood.

Mumps is probably spread from one person to another by the saliva. Occasionally a third person may become contaminated with this infectious saliva and, although himself not infected by the disease, carry it from a sick person to a healthy one. Study of the disease shows that it is most contagious during the early days, and that once convalescence begins it is not nearly so dangerous. For this reason it is not customary to quarantine or isolate cases with mumps for more than two weeks.

Beyond the stiffness of the jaw and the pain on opening the mouth, which are associated with the swelling of the glands, the person with mumps usually has little trouble. There are, however, cases in which the mumps seem to spread particularly to the glands of sex. When this occurs, it is a serious complication. There are instances in which the ability to have children has been irreparably damaged by this secondary complication. Incidentally, the complication is more likely to occur in grown people than in children. With a complication of this character there may be fever that is fairly high.

Not much can be done about mumps, except to make certain that the person is absolutely quiet and that there is no secondary complication in the form of pus infection. When this occurs either in the glands in front of the ear or in the sex glands, a competent physician can be of much service. Gamma globulin from cases of convalescent mumps is used in treatment. Cortisone or ACTH has been reported helpful in controlling the inflammation. In the majority of cases the condition gets well without any complications. Usually it is mild. Aureomycin has been helpful in the secondary complications of mumps.

The usual treatment of infectious diseases, already described, is ordinarily applied by good physicians in cases of mumps. The attention of the physician is necessary so that he may detect possible complications at the earliest moment. Since aureomycin and chloromycetin are effective against viruses they are now being used in severe cases of mumps.

People who have had mumps should be kept under observation for at least three weeks, to make sure that the condition is fully healed and that no further complications are likely.

INFANTILE PARALYSIS

Of all the diseases that strike dread to mankind, none was more feared by mothers than acute poliomyelitis, or, as it is more commonly known, infantile paralysis. This is an acute infection in which the inflammation attacks the tissues in the front part of the spinal cord. Possibly it has occurred throughout the centuries, but it was first widely recognized as an epidemic disorder around 1887, since Medin described the epidemic of that year in Stockholm in a paper published in 1891. No

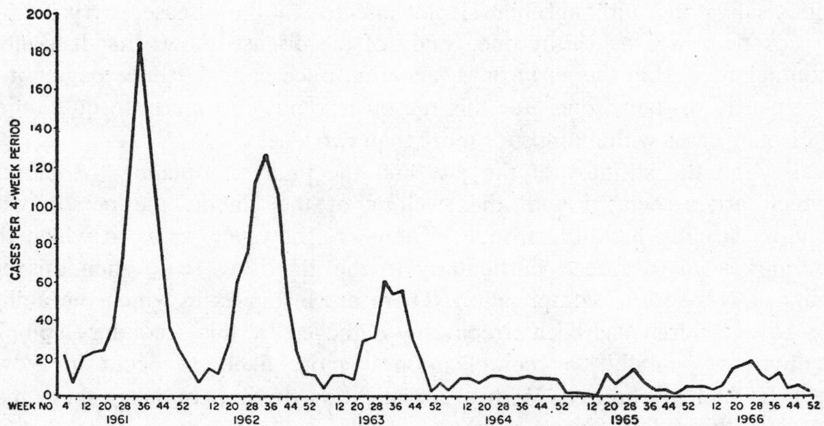

Fig. 38. Paralytic poliomyelitis, 1961–66, cases by date of onset. *Annual poliomyelitis Summary, 1966,* National Communicable Disease Center, Bureau of Disease Prevention and Environmental Control.

doubt, previous to that time, cases of this disease were confused with meningitis and paralysis due to other disorders.

The majority of cases of this condition occur in young children, afflicting boys and girls in about equal proportions. There are, however, numerous cases in which the condition attacks older persons, among the most conspicuous examples being Franklin D. Roosevelt, who was infected late in life.

A virus of several types, an infectious agent too small to be seen with the microscope, is recognized as the cause of this disease. The virus can be cultivated outside the body on living tissue. Several different types of poliomyelitis virus have been isolated. Its infectious character is certainly established through transmission from one animal to another. The disease is spread through contamination, possibly by direct contact with those having the disease, and possibly also by healthy carriers of the infection. The virus is found regularly in material excreted by the bowel and this may also be a source of infection. The appearance of the paralysis usually follows three or four days of fever and disturbances of digestion. In some cases the preliminary symptoms are so slight that the paralysis is the first symptom noted. In other cases, the paralysis may be so slight that the condition is unrecognized except for the fact that the child happens to be sick at a time when infantile paralysis is prevalent in the community. The disease usually appears 7 to 14 days after exposure and the incubation period may be from 5 to 35 days.

The condition occurs usually in warm weather, but is not especially a disease of tropical countries. It is most frequent in the temperate zone.

The disease attacks rich and poor alike and appears equally in good and bad sanitary situations. Whereas 95 per cent of those attacked are children, the condition seldom occurs during the first year of life. This may be due to the fact that the infant, during this period, is separated from the community generally. It is also due, however, in some part, to the fact that the mother transmits to the infant at birth a certain amount of resistance against this as well as other infectious diseases, and that perhaps a year is required for the immunity of this character to wear off.

In any event, when infantile paralysis is present in a community, any child with the slightest symptoms of a cold or a fever should be given most careful study by a physician.

Those who have been exposed to infantile paralysis should have temperatures taken regularly for a period of at least three weeks so as to detect the onset of fever and symptoms at the earliest possible moment. During times when there are epidemics in the community, children should not be allowed to mingle with crowds, and travel should be discouraged. The occurrence of fever, headache with vomiting, drowsiness, and irritability when disturbed, flushing, congestion of the throat, and notable sweating during a period when infantile paralysis is prevalent in a community should be looked on with suspicion. Any evidence on the part of the child of stiffness of the back and resistance to movement of the neck is to be considered as a suspicious symptom, demanding the most careful medical investigation.

Careful epidemiologic studies indicate that a community has 200 abortive or non-paralytic cases for every one paralytic case of poliomyelitis.

Since 1952 inoculation against infantile paralysis has been practiced. Enders grew the virus types in pure culture outside the body on monkey kidney tissue. Salk combined the three chief viruses in a vaccine. Doses are given two weeks apart; then after a lapse of seven to ten months a booster dose is given. By adoption of vaccination, principally oral, with booster doses, poliomyelitis has been practically eliminated as a threat. In 1967 less than fifty cases of paralytic poliomyelitis occurred in the United States. Albert Sabin developed vaccination with living attenuated virus vaccines taken by mouth.

The secretions and excretions from the patient with infantile paralysis should be handled exactly as we handle the material from the patient with typhoid. Particularly dangerous is hand-to-mouth infection. Everyone associated in the care of a patient with infantile paralysis in its early stages should make certain to wash his hands with soap and water each time he is near the patient.

EARLY DIAGNOSIS OF INFANTILE PARALYSIS

As soon as infantile paralysis is well established it becomes important to have a careful examination of the muscles in order to find out which are permanently involved so that plans may be outlined for treatment leading to recovery of the power of motion.

Among the remedies used in the treatment of infantile paralysis it is necessary to mention first absolute rest in bed. This is important in avoiding any unnecessary irritation to the affected tissues. Research has shown the significance of fatigue and exhaustion in extending and making paralysis more severe.

Among the most important factors in giving relief from serious pain and depression in this condition, good nursing is especially to be emphasized. Good nursing in infantile paralysis must be exceedingly gentle. It must minimize as much as possible any movement of the patient and avoid any unnecessary output of energy. The physician can prescribe various drugs which tend to keep such patients quiet. The nurse may aid in giving warm baths which help in bringing about relief.

Once the active disease has passed, a complete examination of all the muscles is necessary to find out which have become weakened and which have lost their functions entirely; then the weakened muscles may be benefited. In cases in which some functions have been lost entirely, re-education of the muscles may be used to enable children to walk and to carry on other activities. Throughout all treatments it is necessary to guard against too much fatigue. Children should not be encouraged to walk too soon. They should never be allowed to stand in a deformed position. If the legs are too weak, splints may be applied, and corsets, jackets, and braces may be worn in order to aid in supporting the weakened tissues.

Exercise in water has developed a great vogue, particularly through endorsement of the Georgia Warm Springs Foundation by former President Roosevelt. The chief advantages of the use of the swimming-pool method are the aid derived from supporting the limbs by the buoyancy of the water. Even under the best of conditions, however, the swimming pool itself is not a cure for paralyzed muscles. It is the training given in the swimming pool by competent teachers that brings about restoration.

Of the greatest importance in the care of such patients is the proper handling of all their normal functions. They should be moved sufficiently often to prevent the occurrence of bed sores. There is danger of pneumonia. The patient should not be allowed to lie continually on the back. If he cannot swallow the mucus and saliva which develop in the mouth, he must be turned so that these will be drained out. More recently the development of mechanical devices to aid normal breathing during the period when the lungs are paralyzed has saved many lives.

The majority of children who have had infantile paralysis still retain the ability to perform certain movements but lack the power to make other movements. For this reason general exercises which are good for normal people are not suited to the unequal movements of these patients.

A physician selects exercises which are graded according to the amount of the deficiency of the muscle, and gradually increases the scope of the exercise to be performed as the weakened muscles strengthen. No exercises of any kind are recommended for use during periods of active inflammation in this disease.

As an example of how a handicapped person can overcome his disability of this type, it is well to recall the story of Sir Walter Scott, who lived one hundred years ago. He was one of twelve children, the first six of whom all died in infancy. In the period in which he lived deaths among babies were frequent. Indeed, the infant mortality rate was in many places as high as four hundred per thousand, which means that two out of every five infants that were born died before they were one year of age. Today the rates vary from fifty to one hundred per thousand.

In fact, Scott himself almost succumbed because his parents employed for him a nurse who was tuberculous and who concealed this fact. Fortunately the famous professor of chemistry, Dr. Black, discovered it and notified the parents, who then dismissed the nurse. Even at that time the risk to the child of being nursed by a tuberculous woman was understood.

When Sir Walter Scott was eighteen months old his first serious illness overtook him. Apparently he suffered with the cutting of teeth and a fever. On the fourth day thereafter he was found to have lost the power of his right leg. His parents consulted every possible type of medical practitioner, both scientific and unscientific, and, all of this being without success, he was finally sent to the country to recuperate. This was, of course, an attack of infantile paralysis, not sufficient to cause death but sufficient to produce permanent crippling, for Sir Walter Scott was thereafter lame for the rest of his life. It was probably excellent advice to send the young boy to the country to recuperate.

As Scott himself said, "The impatience of a child soon inclined me to struggle with my infirmity, and I began by degrees to stand, to walk, and to run. Although the limb affected was much shrunk and contracted, my general health, which was of more importance, was much strengthened by being frequently in the open air, and, in a word, I who had probably been condemned to hopeless and helpless decrepitude, was now a healthy, high-spirited, and my lameness apart, sturdy child."

CHAPTER 12

Transmissible Diseases

MORRIS FISHBEIN, M.D.

TYPHOID FEVER

If the case rates and death rates for typhoid fever that existed in 1890 prevailed now, the city of Chicago would have in one year 60,000 cases of typhoid fever and approximately 6000 deaths. Instead, the city of Chicago has seldom had any cases in recent years.

In an earlier day, the family doctor claimed that he could smell typhoid fever. His guess was likely to be accurate, since one out of five seriously sick people whom he saw was likely to have typhoid fever. In the United States typhoid fever is a rare disease, but in many countries as yet undeveloped the disease still prevails.

Typhoid fever is an acute infection caused by a germ which used to be known as the typhoid bacillus and which is now called *Salmonella typhosa.* The germ can be found in the blood of a person seriously sick with the disease, and in 80 per cent of the cases is found in the stools or excretions of the sick. The germ is spread from the sick person to those who are well by means of the excretions, by soiled food and clothing, particularly by contaminated water and milk, and to a large extent by people who carry the disease; that is to say, they themselves have been sick and have recovered, but they still have in their bodies germs which reside frequently in the intestinal tract and also in the gall bladder, and which may get out of those places and infect other people.

There was a time when cases of typhoid fever occurred from the use of ice made from water in polluted streams. Today the vast majority of ice used in this country is made artificially from clean water, and there is no danger of typhoid. Milk used to be a common source of typhoid germs; and milk products such as ice cream, butter, buttermilk, and cheese were also known on occasion to carry the germs. Once the eating of infected oysters was a prominent cause, because the oysters were developed in contaminated water. In fact, the best fattening grounds for oysters were known to be in and around sewers. Now the control of oyster breeding in uncontaminated water, and suitable methods of storage and transmission for oysters, have largely eliminated the shellfish as a source of contagion. Cases have been reported due to the eating of raw vegetables which had been fertilized with contaminated materials or watered with contaminated water.

It was thought for a while that flies were more responsible for spreading typhoid fever than any other cause, but today it is not believed that transmission by flies is important. However, the fly does feed filthily and may transmit any condition associated with the filth on which it feeds.

Typhoid fever used to follow a long and serious course once a person became infected with it. After a person gets the germs in his body, from three to twenty-one days elapse, known as the incubation period, during which the germs develop and liberate their poisons. The average length of time is ten and a half days. The condition begins with the usual symptoms of infection, such as headache, pains in the body generally, a feeling of exhaustion and loss of appetite. Sometimes there are chills. Quite frequently there is nosebleed, and almost invariably there is disturbance of the action of the bowels in the form of constipation or diarrhea. With the coming of modern methods of treatment using chloromycetin the duration of the disease has been shortened and its severity diminished. The fever is brought under control in a few days.

In addition to the loss of appetite, there is a tendency to the formation of gas with bloating of the body; and sometimes, because of the ulcers in the bowels and the bloating, sudden severe hemorrhages from the bowel. Sometimes the infection and the poisoning affect the nervous system so that there is delirium and even the appearance of mental disturbance during the course of the disease.

The physician who examines a patient with typhoid fever makes his diagnosis from the history of the case and from the appearance of the symptoms, and also by careful studies of the blood. It is possible to examine specimens of the blood and to determine by the use of a test, called the Widal test, after the Frenchman who discovered it, whether or not the condition is quite certainly typhoid fever. Any serious complications such as hemorrhage, perforation of the bowel, and changes in the heart action and in the nervous system, demand prompt and careful attention by a competent physician.

A person who has typhoid fever must be kept alone and preferably cared for by an experienced nurse. The room should be screened if the condition occurs during the summer, when flies are a common pest. Because the person with typhoid may remain long in bed in severe cases he should have a bed with a firm mattress, and arrangements must be made to change the bed linen any time it is soiled. The patient must be bathed

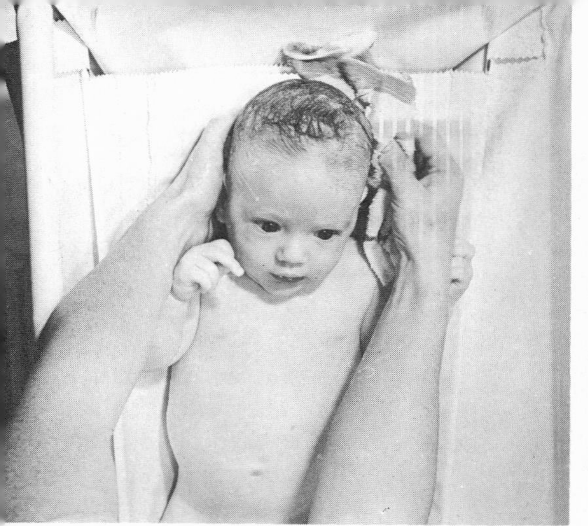

PLATES **51–52–53.** Bathing of the baby should be done not just to keep the baby clean and his skin in good condition, but as a social experience for the baby—one that he should enjoy. Wash the baby's neck, giving particular attention to the folds of skin in which moisture, lint, and dust may accumulate. Rinse and dry. Wash his head with a gentle rotary motion, using the hand or a washcloth. Rinse and dry. Beginning at the baby's chest and arms and using firm, continuous strokes, soap his entire body. Rinse the front of his body. Lean him forward against the wrist and rinse his back. While the baby is young, hair and scalp should be washed daily at the time of the bath. This is done with soap and water as for the remainder of the body. *(Children's Bureau photographs by Philip Bonn, Department of Health, Education and Welfare.)*

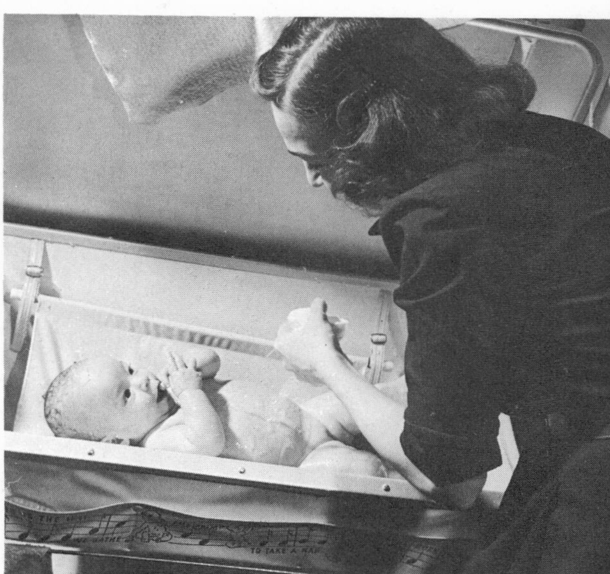

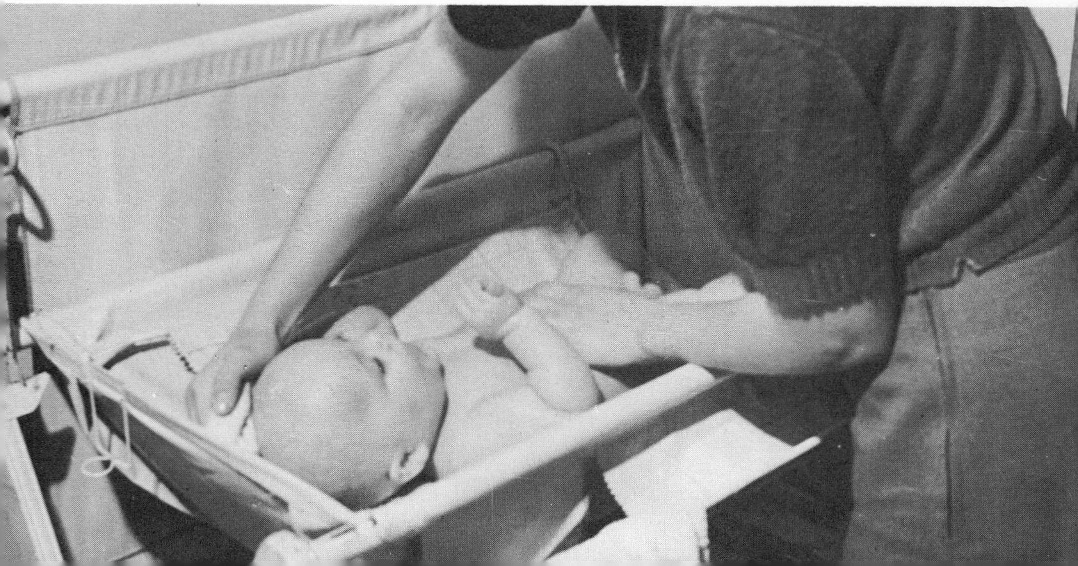

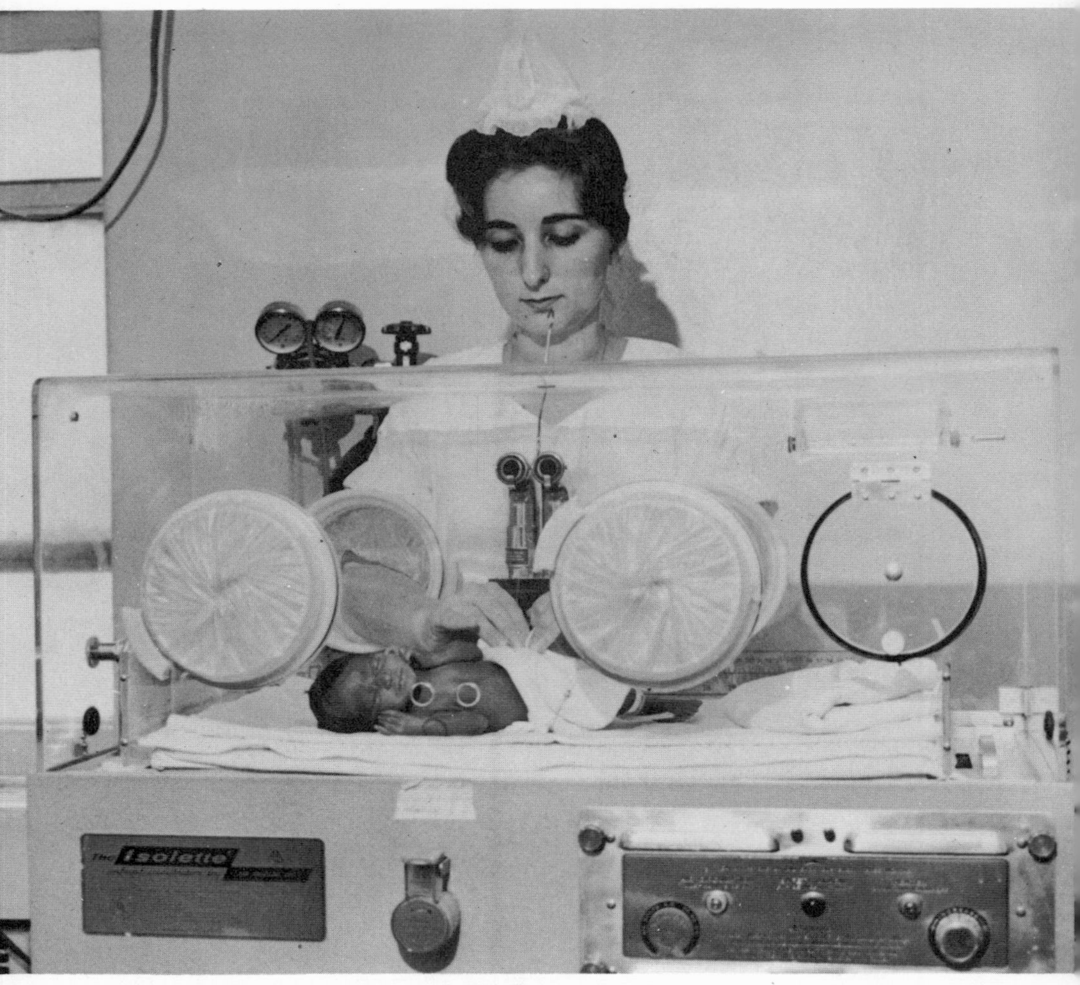

PLATE 54. Miss Sharonanne Paul, RN, supervises a newborn in an Isolett, an infant incubator, in the nursery of the Long Island College Hospital. *(Long Island College Hospital/ United Hospital Fund of New York.)*

PLATE 55. *(facing page)* From 10,000 to 15,000 babies between the ages of two weeks and six months die suddenly and unexpectedly in the United States each year from causes completely unknown. The infants are in apparent good health when last seen alive. Death occurs almost instantaneously causing no suffering; it is completely unpredictable and, therefore, not preventable. It may be said with certainty, however, that death is not caused by the baby smothering. Potentially dangerous communicable disease is discovered very early at autopsy so that there is usually no danger of infection to the family. Statistics indicate that roughly one in five hundred live-born infants will die from the Sudden Death Syndrome, but it is not a hereditary disease and the chances of more than one such death occurring in the same family are extremely small. *(National Foundation for Sudden Infant Death.)*

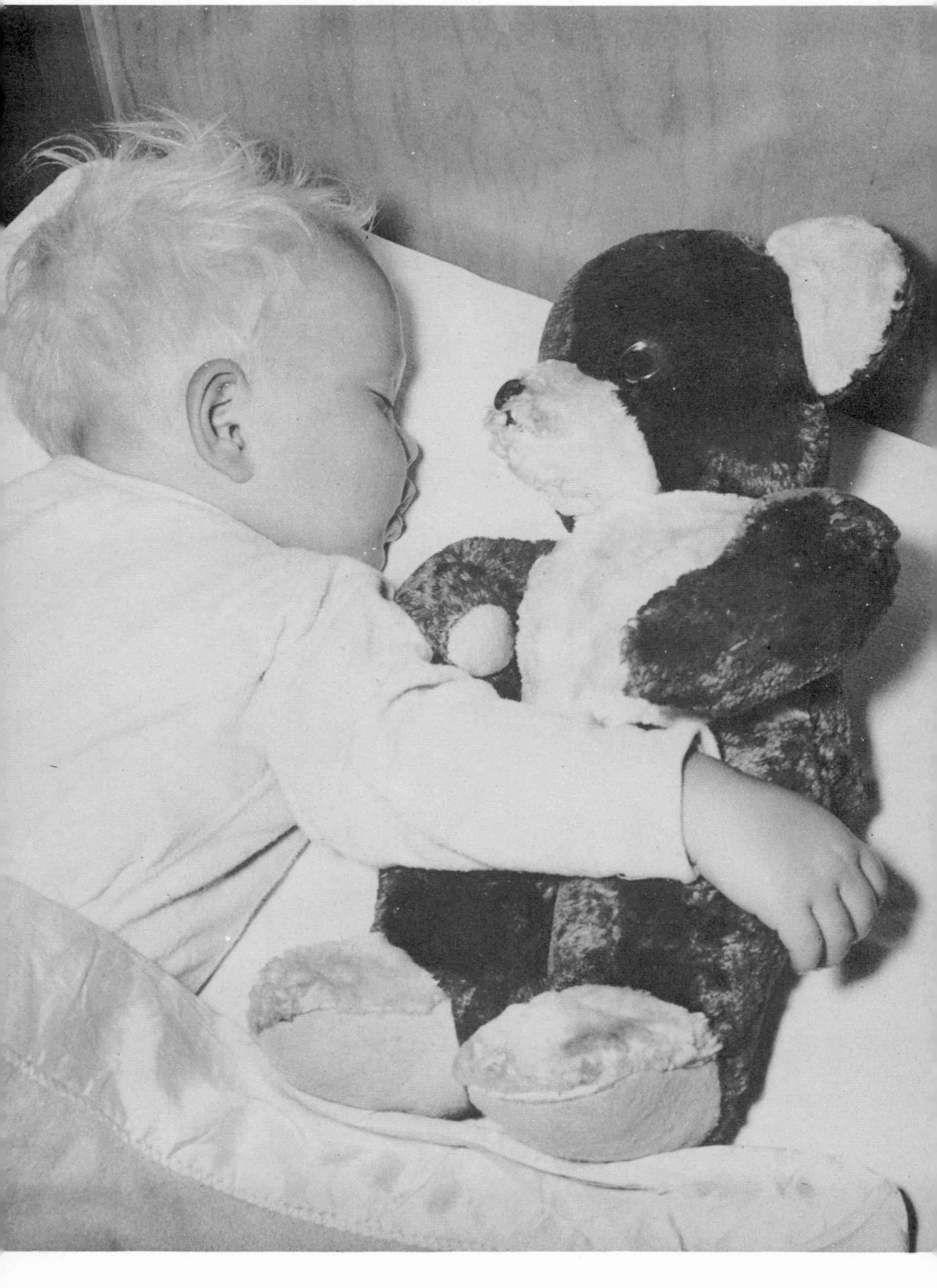

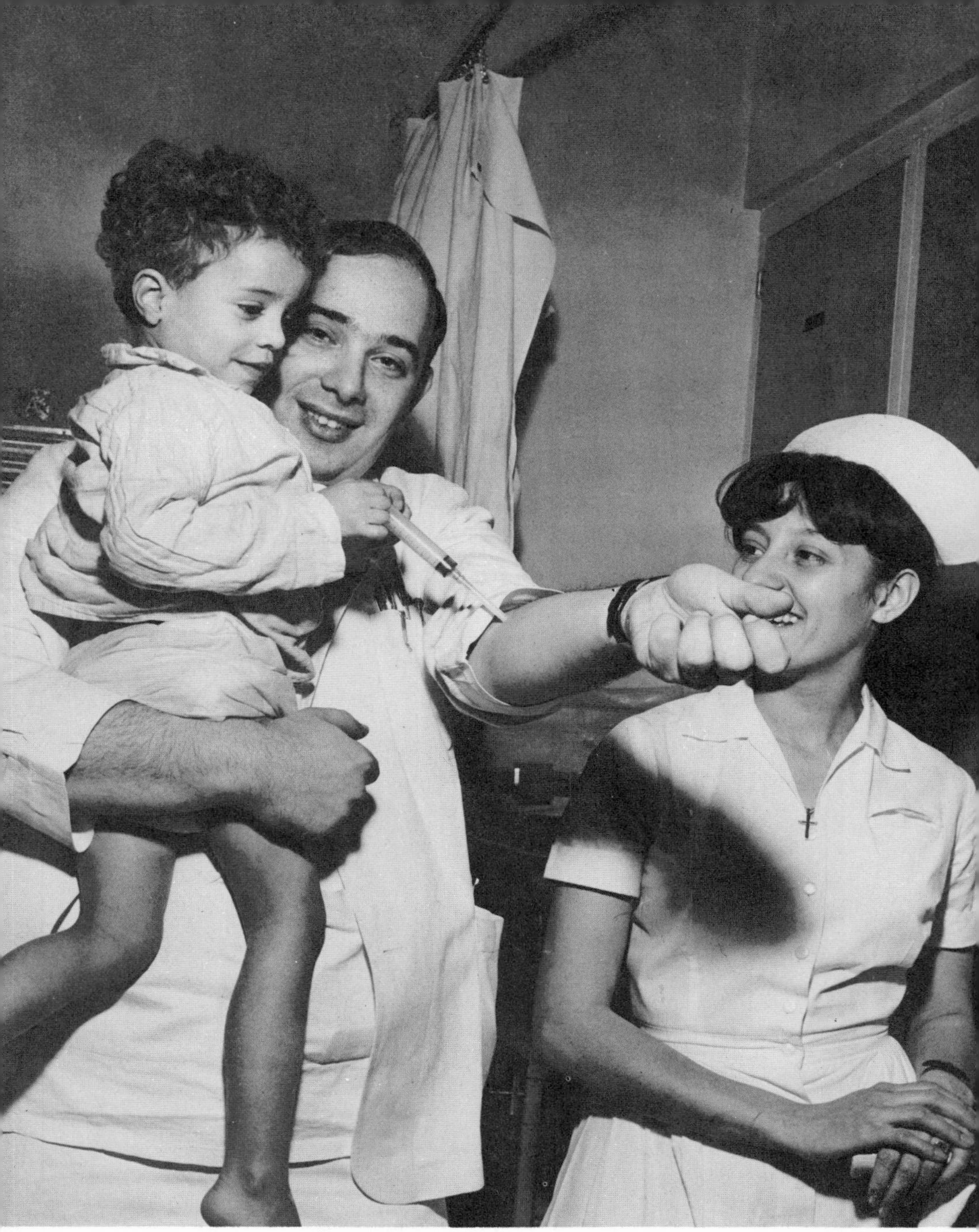

PLATE **56.** Dr. Steven Witover gives a young patient a chance to get even as Nurse Carmen Nieves looks on. Fortunately for Dr. Witover, there is no needle in the syringe. *(Courtesy of Montefiore Hospital and Medical Center, New York, and Wagner International Photos.)*

Just one shot protects your child. Local Child Health Stations give the vaccine free
to pre-school children. Call DI 9-2255 and ask where. Or see your doctor.
MEASLES BITES THE DUST!
New York City Department of Health

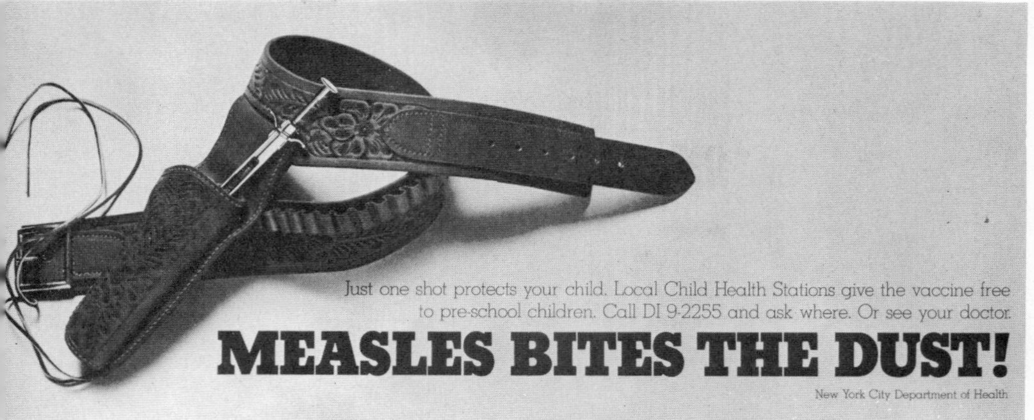

PLATE **57.** An example of the type of campaign poster used for encouraging free vaccinations against measles to pre-school children. *(Bureau of Public Health Education, Department of Health, City of New York.)*

PLATE **58.** Measles Immunization Campaign, Measles Bites the Dust. Bess Hart, Mrs. Hart, and Dr. Howard Shapiro, M.D. *(Bureau of Public Health Education, Department of Health, City of New York.)*

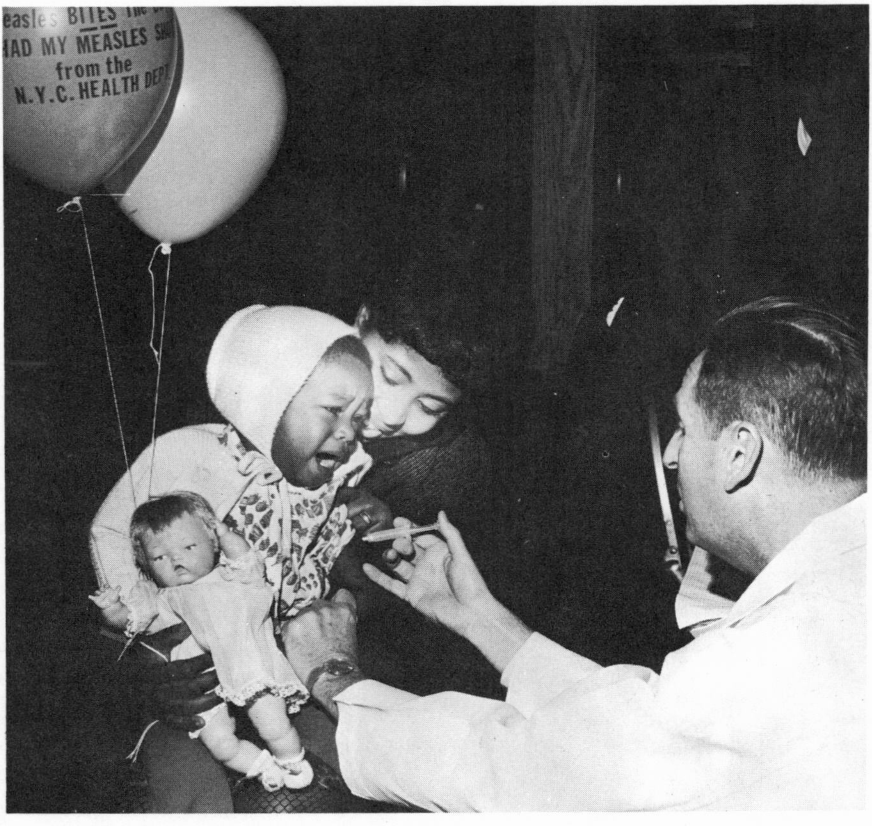

1
2
KA-
3
KA-
4
KA-
CHOO
5
COVER
YOUR COUGHS
AND SNEEZES

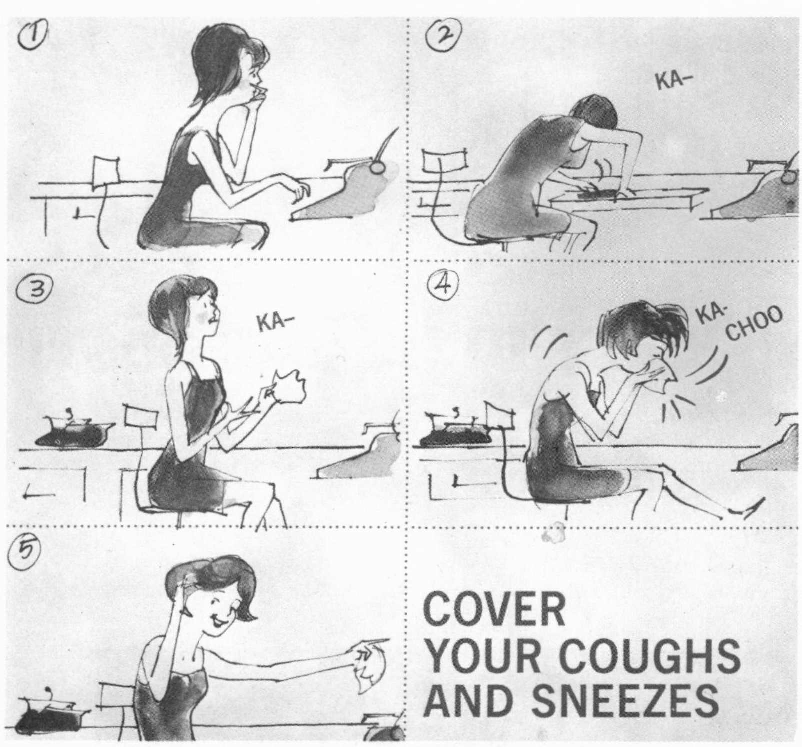

PLATES **59-60.** *(National Tuberculosis Association.)*

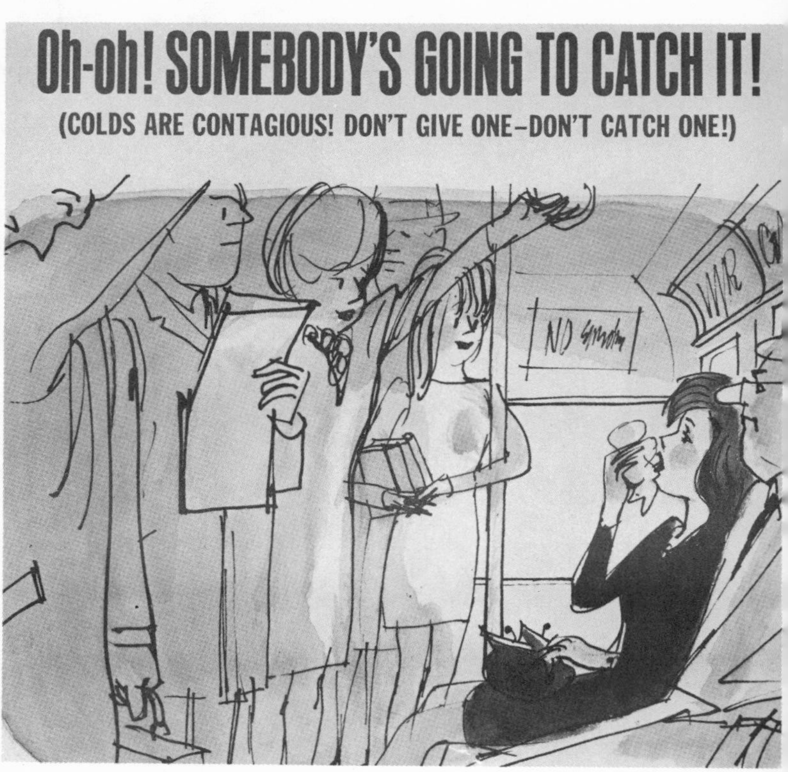

Oh-oh! SOMEBODY'S GOING TO CATCH IT!
(COLDS ARE CONTAGIOUS! DON'T GIVE ONE–DON'T CATCH ONE!)

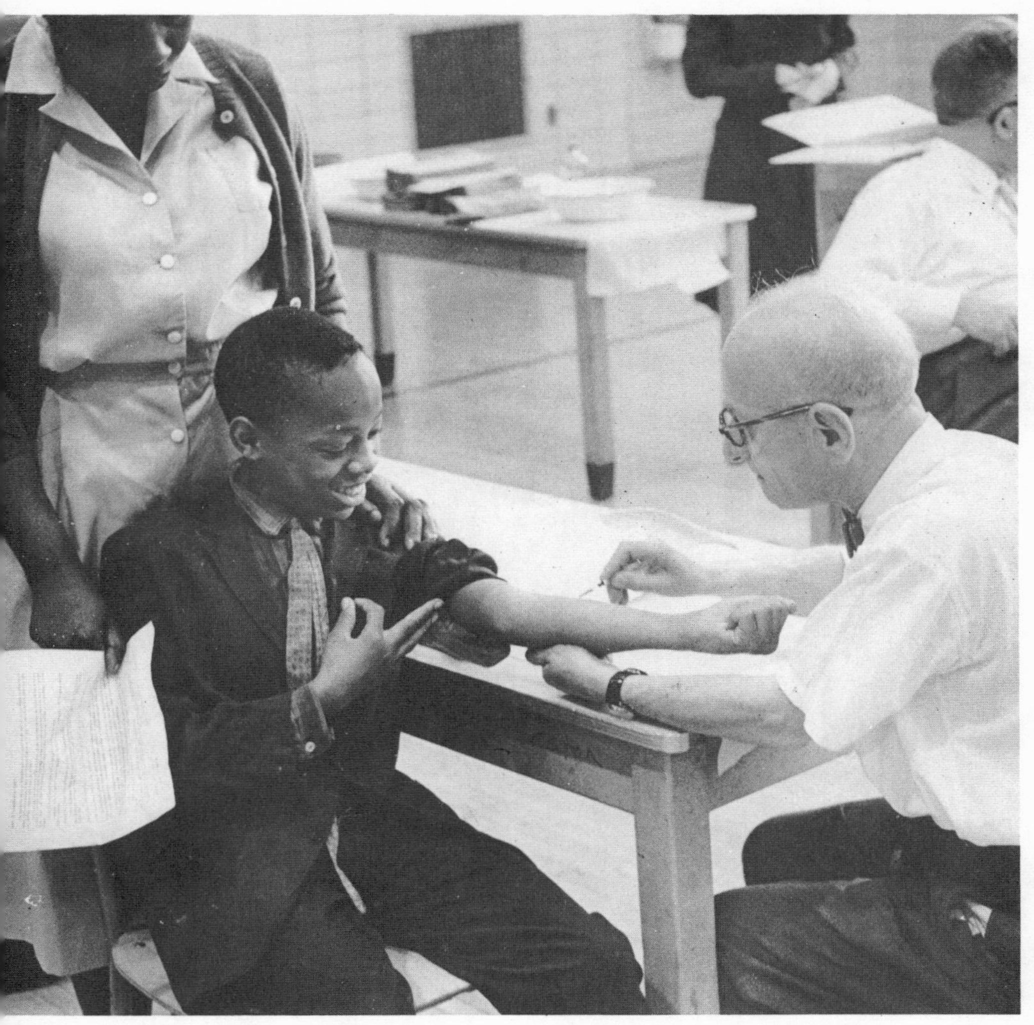

PLATE **61.** Tuberculin testing in Brooklyn schools, spring 1964. *(Brooklyn Tuberculosis and Health Association, National Tuberculosis Association.)*

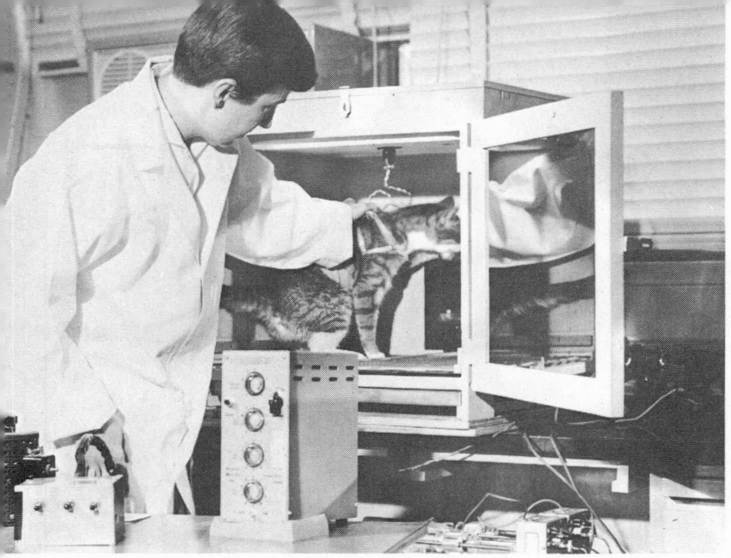

PLATES **62–63.** Cats are used in research study by Dr. Bernice Wenzel and Dr. Robert Tschirgi, of University of California, who are exploring the relationship between learning capacity and the central nervous system. This cat has learned how to press a lever which turns on the light. *(The National Association for Mental Health, Inc.)*

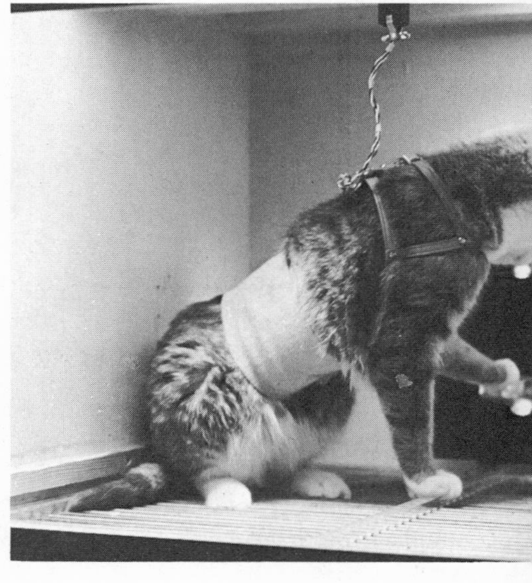

PLATE **64.** Records of electrical, spontaneous responses to stimulation at various points from the brain are mounted on cards for analysis and measurement. What the records signify as to how the brain operates under conditions of the experiment performed are not always easily interpreted. Here are Margaret Clare, M.A., Research Assistant, and Dr. George H. Bishop, Professor of Neurophysiology, Division of Neurology, Department of Psychiatry and Neurology, Washington University Medical School, St. Louis. *(The National Association for Mental Health, Inc.)*

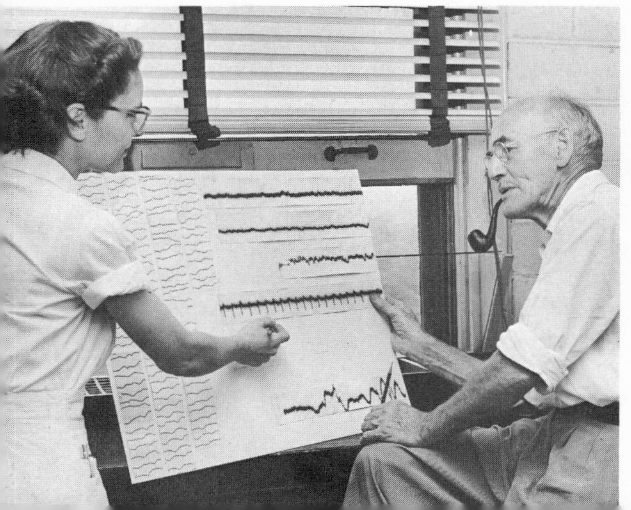

at least once a day and the back and buttocks kept clean in order to prevent secondary infections. It is also important to see that the mouth is kept clean and rinsed each time after food is taken.

There was a time when it was thought advisable to starve patients with typhoid fever. The condition interferes with the nutrition of the patient, so that present methods involve the giving of a diet of from 3,000 to 3,500 calories. Then the patient will not lose weight during the course of the illness.

A vaccine made of the killed germs of typhoid fever is of value in preventing the disease. This was quite certainly proved during World War II. Anyone who is likely to be exposed to the taking of contaminated food or water ought to be vaccinated against typhoid fever. In the entire American army during World War II there were only slightly over one thousand cases of typhoid fever among something like five million enrolled troops. If the rate for typhoid which prevailed during the Spanish-American War had existed, there would have been approximately a million cases.

It is customary to give three injections of the vaccine against typhoid fever at ten-day intervals, although the intervals between injections may be shortened in time of necessity. Obviously, the giving of such vaccines is the work of a physician or of a trained nurse, since the average person cannot inject himself and does not understand the technique of preparation. Only rarely indeed are there reactions of a serious character following the injection of ordinary doses of antityphoid vaccine.

Persistent attention to water supplies and disposal of sewage, pasteurization of milk, education of the public in hygiene, and the control of typhoid carriers will eventually eliminate typhoid fever entirely throughout the civilized world. Means are now available in most states for proper control of carriers when they are discovered, but the discovery of a carrier demands expert bacteriological investigation.

The rates for typhoid fever have been falling steadily. With antibiotic drugs complications are controlled and chloromycetin, also called chloramphenicol, has proved especially valuable in this condition. Some research has shown even more rapid improvement with combined use of cortisone and chloromycetin.

ERYSIPELAS

The condition called St. Anthony's fire is an acute inflammation of the skin caused by the streptococcus, an organism of the same type as that which causes scarlet fever and many other infections. Apparently, the condition was known in the time of the ancient Greeks and Romans. In fact, the greatest writers of those days, Hippocrates, Galen, and Celsus, all described this condition and credited it to living under unhygienic conditions. Finally, in 1882, a German investigator proved the specific character of the disease by isolating the germs.

Erysipelas starts most often in a wound, abrasion, or rubbed place on the skin, and particularly in those places where the mucous membranes, such as those which line the nose and the mouth, join the outer skin. In hospitals, in the past, there were frequently epidemics of erysipelas because the infection was carried from one patient to another by attendants. Nowadays the great danger of erysipelas in a surgical ward has been recognized, and a person with erysipelas is promptly put in a room by himself and attended by a nurse who is not attending other people. In cases which occur in homes under ordinary conditions it is necessary to make certain that the other people in the family do not come in too close contact with the patient. The spread of this disease is almost always by the hands of the person who is taking care of the patient.

Erysipelas usually begins with a severe fever and a chill and associated with this all of the usual symptoms of an acute poisoning of the body such as headache, loss of appetite, vomiting, and, in the case of a high fever, perhaps some delirium.

The disease usually lasts from five to ten days, the average being eight days. When the erysipelas affects large areas of the body it may continue for as long as fifteen days.

Usually erysipelas begins on the face and extends from day to day, so that it eventually covers the entire side of the face, including the eyelids, which become enormously swollen and filled with fluid. Sometimes the swelling is sufficient to close the eye completely. Then the disease spreads onto the ear, which thickens tremendously, and finally reaches the line of the hair, where it stops abruptly. In other cases it may spread down the back. In many instances the condition begins on the bridge of the nose and spreads rapidly to each side so that it forms what is called a "butterfly" pattern.

Often any natural boundary such as the hairline, the nape of the neck, and places where the skin is tight over the cheekbones, will stop the spread of the disease.

When the inflammation of the skin stops, the fever begins to drop. Sometimes the skin peels where it has been greatly swollen. If the disease occurs again and again, almost a permanent thickening may develop, which is, of course, exceedingly unsightly.

The doctor is able to diagnose erysipelas certainly by studying its general character and also by examining the blood in which the white cells are found to have been increased tremendously.

The most serious complication in erysipelas is a secondary infection. Under such circumstances the swelling changes to abscess. In the vast majority of cases erysipelas is not a fatal disease. In young infants and in old and sickly people it may be exceedingly serious, but in general it causes a death rate per year of about three people for each hundred thousand in the community.

Numerous remedies have been developed for the treatment of erysipelas. Doctors used to attempt to control the disease by painting on iodine, silver nitrate, and similar preparations. Modern authorities feel that these accomplish little, and besides may so hide the spread of the disease as to interfere with its control. If the eyelids are involved, it is customary to drop some mild antiseptic solution, which the doctor will supply, directly into the eyes.

Since erysipelas is caused by a streptococcus, the condition is now controllable by the use of the antibiotics, particularly penicillin, aureomycin and terramycin and by the use of sulfadiazine. The manifestations on the skin are treated with direct application of specific remedies. Since erysipelas arises in most instances from a small beginning, early and prompt treatment of scratches and minor infections has greatly reduced the total number of cases of erysipelas. Cold compresses are often soothing and some physicians recommend moistening the compresses in a mild solution of aluminum acetate (Burow's solution, 1:1000).

Because erysipelas, like other infectious diseases, tends to break down the blood and weaken the patients generally, it is well to give people who are sick with erysipelas plenty of fluids, actually forcing them to drink not less than ten and as many as sixteen glasses of water daily. It is also well to have the food easy to digest and nourishing, in fact, what is ordinarily called a nutritious soft diet.

TETANUS OR LOCKJAW

The ancient Greeks knew about lockjaw. Indeed, the father of modern medicine, Hippocrates, described it and made some statements about the likelihood of recovery which are still good. Not until 1865 was it thought to be infectious. The germ was not described until 1886. Today it is possible to isolate the germ, to grow it artificially, and to produce lockjaw in animals by injecting the germs into their bodies. The germ is called *Clostridium tetani*.

The poison produced by these germs is one of the most powerful poisons known. Most people used to think that tetanus, or lockjaw, was always caused by scratching the skin with a rusty nail. Today it is known that the rusty nail produces the disease because it is contaminated with material containing the germ of tetanus.

When this germ gets into the body by any means whatever, it sets up inflammation of nerve tissue. Because these germs have a special predilection for certain nerves, the condition called lockjaw is produced.

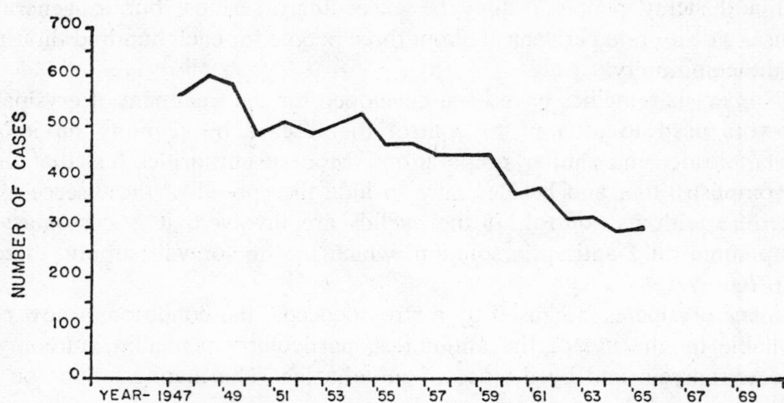

Fig. 39. Report of Tetanus in the United States, 1947–65. From *Disease Status Report,* October 1966, National Communicable Disease Center, Atlanta, Georgia.

Certain types of wounds are more likely to cause tetanus than others. Most important are wounds which are deep, penetrating, lacerating, or crushing and which, because of that fact, permit particles of foreign matter containing the germs of tetanus to go deeply into the tissues and to remain there. This germ lives much better in the absence of oxygen. When it is pushed deep into a wound it is without oxygen and therefore is under the best possible conditions for its growth. The effects are produced more by the poisons produced by the germs than by the germs themselves. The poison, or toxin, is transported by the lymphatics and in this way it reaches the nerve tissues.

The germs of tetanus seem to live preferably in the intestinal tracts of cattle, horses, and man. Because the germs are fairly widespread it is remarkable that the disease is not more common. Apparently, however, it is necessary for the germs to get deep into the tissue through a wound in order to multiply and produce the disease.

In the United States around one thousand to thirteen hundred deaths occur each year from tetanus. The number is less now than formerly because of the disappearance of horses and manure from city streets, because of the diminution of Fourth of July accidents associated with explosives, and because of the use of new methods of prevention which were not formerly generally available.

Tetanus usually begins about seven days after the wound which permits the germs to get into the tissues. It may, however, come on somewhat later or, rather rarely, earlier. The first signs are a sense of drawing pain in a wound with the twitching of muscles near by; also the usual signs of infection such as irritability, headache, chilliness, and fever. Then comes the stiffness of the muscles of the jaw and neck which gives the disease its name.

It becomes more and more difficult to open the mouth, and finally the jaws may be clamped shut and the neck rigid. Attempts to open the mouth intensify the spasm. Due to the fact that the muscles of the face are contracted, the corners of the mouth are drawn back and the eyebrows raised. This gives the person a typical grinning appearance which is described by the scientists as *risus sardonicus*—in other words, a sardonic expression.

Eventually, of course, other muscles and nerves are involved so that there are serious spasms and convulsions. In fact, there may be from three to forty spasms in an hour. The whole body may be involved, including even the muscles of the bowels and of the bladder. Of course, when the heart and the breathing muscles are involved, the condition is fatal.

Even under the best of treatment, patients with lockjaw may die because of the potency of this poison. Much depends on the time at which the antitoxin is given and on the amount. Of greatest importance is the prevention of lockjaw through the proper treatment of people who have been wounded, at the earliest possible moment. It should be taken for granted that a wound acquired in localities where the soil is likely to be contaminated, such as wounds acquired in fields, stables, and farmyards, or such as gunshot and powder wounds, are infected.

A physician who treats such a case will probably open the wound widely, removing any clothing, soil, or other visible contamination that may be present, and then treat the wound with proper antiseptics such as tincture of iodine or hydrogen peroxide to destroy the germs that can be reached. The opening of the wound is especially important, because this germ multiplies in the absence of air. Opening of the wound permits air to be present. It also permits removal of contamination, and it allows the antiseptics to reach the infectious material.

It is also important at this time to inject under the skin the specific antitoxin against tetanus, and perhaps to give another injection one week later.

If the disease develops in spite of preventive treatment, the patient should be placed in a quiet room, preferably in a hospital. The room must be kept darkened, and all noises or vibrations prevented, because they may serve to stimulate spasms. It may be necessary even to use an anesthetic to prevent these spasms. In order to feed the patient it is sometimes necessary to pass a narrow tube through the nose and down into the stomach, because the jaws may be so tightly clamped as to make it impossible to get food into the body otherwise. Someone must be constantly with the patient to prevent injury from convulsions and to guard against sudden death from paralysis of the breathing.

Several reports have appeared on beneficial effects of combined treatment using antibiotics such as penicillin or terramycin with antitoxin.

In no condition is the constant and immediate attention of a competent physician, and at the same time good nursing, so important. This makes the difference frequently between life and death. The antitoxin which opposes the poison must be given early in the disease and in large doses. Because of the great irritability of the patient it is sometimes necessary to put him to sleep in order that the antitoxin may be given. Under the best of treatment it is possible to save the lives of from one half to two thirds of the people who are infected. By the use of oxygen under pressure, in a special hyperbaric chamber in some hospitals, many lives are saved that would formerly have been lost.

RABIES OR HYDROPHOBIA

The word *"rabies"* is Latin for madness or rage. "Hydrophobia" means fear of water and thus defines what seemed to be the most significant symptom of the disease. It is one of the oldest of the diseases definitely classified by man. Around 100 A.D., Celsus recommended cauterization of wounds produced by mad dogs. As early as 1804, long before the nature of the disease was discovered by Pasteur, it was known that the saliva of a person or of a dog that had the disease would transmit it. Since, however, no means was known for preventing its spread, sufferers at that time were sometimes put to death by strangulation or smothering because people so greatly feared the disease. Until the time when Pasteur made the great discovery which freed mankind from fear of hydrophobia it was customary, as a means of treatment, to burn with a redhot iron the flesh of a person who had been bitten by any mad animal.

Some strange superstitions about hydrophobia still remain. One is that it commonly occurs in the "dog days." It has been believed that the danger from mad dogs was greater at that time than at any other. There is no evidence to support this view, because the bites of mad dogs occur at any time. They are likely to be more frequent from April to September than from October to March because dogs run loose more often and more generally in the spring and summer than they do in winter.

When a mad dog bites another animal or a human being the disease is transmitted by the saliva, which contains the poisonous virus. It is called a virus because it is so small that it will pass through the pores of a clay filter. The time when the disease attacks is from fourteen days on. There are wide variations in the period of incubation, in fact from ten days to twelve months, but in the vast majority of cases the onset follows the bite in from twenty to ninety days. It is rarely less than 15 days or more than 5 months.

During this period of incubation the person may show only signs of restlessness and apprehension, sometimes of irritation or tingling and pain at the site of the bite. However, when the disease begins, the horrible symptoms which give it its name reach their peak. A slight huskiness of the voice and a sense of choking are followed by severe spasms of the muscles of swallowing and breathing. There is shortness of breath. So severe are the symptoms following any attempt to swallow that the affected person will refuse to take water. This, of course, gave rise to the name hydrophobia, or fear of water. Eventually the convulsions and spasms may affect almost the whole body, and the nervous system is so sensitive that the slamming of a door or a sudden draft of wind will bring on an attack. Finally, the spine may stiffen and bend and death results from paralysis of the apparatus of breathing.

Because the affected person or animal is unable to swallow, thick saliva accumulates and drips from the mouth. Because of the paralysis of the muscles of breathing the breath comes in harsh gasps. The person who is infected does not necessarily foam at the mouth or bark like a dog, but the nature of the symptoms is such as to give people this impression.

Because of the great danger associated with this disease, everything possible should be done to prevent its spread. At times when hydrophobia, or rabies, is prevalent in any community the lives of both dogs and children may be freed from menace by protecting them from exposure to the bite of a mad animal. Homeless animals should be picked up and disposed of by the usual methods. A failure to enforce the laws regulating the control of homeless animals represents nothing in the way of friendship for the animal and exposes innumerable human beings to the danger of one of the most serious of diseases.

The dog that is kept in a good home is usually watched carefully, kept from contact with savage dogs, and is not so likely to be involved as the one that runs free. However, any dog may suddenly bite a human being, under provocation or sometimes without provocation. Because of the terrible possibilities of rabies, there is only one course to follow after a dog bite. The animal should be penned up or kept secured for at least ten days, during which time it will either die or develop the symptoms of hydrophobia, if it has that disease.

Far too often, when police are called to kill a dog suspected of hydrophobia, the dog is shot in the head or the head crushed with a club. This should not be done, because it is difficult for a laboratory to examine the brain of the dog when it is too severely injured.

The diagnosis of hydrophobia is made by examination of the brain of the animal under the microscope. When this disease is present the brain contains certain substances known as Negri bodies, which can be seen by the investigator. If there is the slightest suspicion that the dog which has bitten a person was mad, the Pasteur treatment for the prevention of hydrophobia should be begun immediately. If there are bites on the face or even on the hands it is wise to commence immediate treatment because of the increased hazard when bites occur in these places. Otherwise it may be safe to delay for a few days to make sure that the animal was rabid or mad.

The wounds should be immediately cauterized with carbolic or fuming nitric acid. The Pasteur treatment is administered by any private or state laboratory. Moreover, it is available to physicians in any village or town through material that can be supplied by pharmaceutical houses. In the Pasteur treatment a special vaccine is used which is prepared from the brains of rabbits that have been injected with the disease. In these tissues the virus has been attenuated by passage through many animals and by other treatment, such as drying. There are no contra-indications to the use of this treatment.

The success of the Pasteur treatment for preventing hydrophobia is almost certain. Failures occur in less than one half of one per cent of the cases in which it is used. Notwithstanding the fact that information concerning this disease has been widespread for many years, there are still more than one hundred deaths annually from the disease in the United States. These are preventable deaths. Once the disease has developed, the physician can do much to relieve suffering and should be in constant attendance for this purpose.

Control of rabies includes measures which prevent dogs from biting, licensing of dogs, seizure and destruction of stray dogs, quarantine or muzzling of dogs during outbreaks of rabies and subjection of all imported dogs to six months quarantine. These measures eliminated rabies from England and Canada. Vaccination of dogs against rabies is recommended where quarantine cannot be enforced or where the disease prevails among wild animals.

VINCENT'S ANGINA

In 1898 a French physician named Vincent described an infection of the mouth and throat due to a peculiar spiral organism called *Treponema vincentii* and *Borrelia vincentii.* Apparently the disease occurred only in man, was accompanied by slight general disturbances with but a small increase in temperature, but there was pain on swallowing, enlargement of the glands, and a yellowish gray membrane in the mouth and throat. Because of this membrane, the disease was often mistaken for diphtheria until the differences were clearly established.

Sometimes the germs responsible for Vincent's angina were found in mouths that were not infected, but which were in bad condition. Occasionally also the disease appeared to be especially favored by fatigue, chill, exposure, improper food, or the excessive use of alcohol or tobacco.

During World War I the disease spread widely among the soldiers and was given the common name of trench mouth, a name which has persisted. Many infections of the mouth result from the herpes virus, others by candida albicans or monilia.

In this common infection penicillin has already been established as especially helpful in combating infections. With good dental care and suitable application of such remedies the condition is controllable.

When the disease is once established, it may be treated by the repeated use of solutions of hydrogen peroxide or by the application of a paste of sodium perborate, as the physician or dentist may advise. In severe cases treatment includes injections with sulfanilamide or neoarsphenamine and also local application of drugs. For prevention it is also advisable to have the teeth clean and smooth and to discontinue tobacco as long as any evidence of the disease remains.

UNDULANT FEVER OR BRUCELLOSIS

Years ago, British soldiers quartered on the island of Malta developed a disease in epidemic form which was called Malta fever. Later, as the disease spread about the world it became known as Mediterranean fever. Finally, it was called undulant fever because of its intermittent character; that is, the fever went up and down in waves. Three types of organisms are now known as causative including *Brucella melitensis, Brucella abortus* and *Brucella suis*. The condition is related to contagious abortion of cattle.

The menace of undulant fever is not the menace of epidemics of yellow fever or even of influenza. The disease insidiously creeps into a population and gradually affects increasing numbers of people. Fortunately, it is likely to spread slowly, if at all, in American communities, because milk is the most important medium in transmitting the disease. Since 1900, milk supplies in the United States have been controlled through suitable public health laws and measures. Milk is made safe for human consumption by pasteurization, in which the milk is heated for a sufficient length of time to destroy dangerous germs.

Before 1927, undulant fever was regarded as a curiosity when it occurred in a human being in the United States. Since that time cases have appeared in practically every state of the union. In the great majority of cases the taking of raw milk containing the germ, which is identified also as the one which causes contagious abortion of cattle, was demonstrated to be the source of the infection. Apparently the condition is more likely to be spread by goat's milk than by that from cattle, particularly since the goat's milk is not usually as well controlled in its assembling and distribution as is the milk of cows. Moreover, the infection is more generalized among goats than among cattle.

From ten to thirty days after the person becomes infected with this disease he has the usual symptoms associated with an infectious disorder—weakness, tiredness, chilliness, loss of appetite, general aching, chills and fever. The condition develops slowly, so that frequently weeks may pass before the person who is infected considers himself sick enough to call a physician. He is inclined to believe that he has something like a persistent cold or rheumatic condition and that it is hard to break up.

Eventually, the symptoms of a person who has contracted undulant fever develop with sufficient fullness and persistence to make him realize that he is subject to a serious complaint. The physician who examines the blood of a patient with this disease finds that changes have taken place in the blood, and it is possible for a laboratory to make the kind of test that is made on the blood in typhoid fever and to determine with certainty that the patient is infected with undulant fever.

The disease resembles many other infectious diseases, such as typhoid, tuberculosis, malaria, or almost any other infectious disorder. In a few instances, perhaps two out of every one hundred cases, death may occur as a result of the seriousness of the infection or from secondary complications.

The way to avoid undulant fever is to avoid milk that has not been properly pasteurized. Men who work in packing houses where they come constantly in contact with infected animals should, of course, take the necessary precautions in their work. Men with wounds or abrasions on their hands should be certain to wear gloves and perhaps to clean their hands thoroughly at frequent intervals.

The real control of this disease will rest on the ability of government bureaus and of the veterinary industry to eliminate the condition from domestic animals.

The patient who has undulant fever must be handled in much the same way as one who has had typhoid. He must be put into a separate room; the health authorities must be notified; all of the excretions and secretions must be sterilized before they are disposed of in any way. This means either burning, boiling, or the use of proper antiseptic solutions. The patient, of course, must remain in bed and be properly fed to overcome the loss of weight, the anemia, and the weakness that are due to constant chills and fever. The wearing effects of such conditions on the body are extremely serious in producing changes in the nature of degeneration of important organs.

A treatment with sulfadiazine and streptomycin or with aureomycin or chloromycetin or terramycin or tetracyclines has been found most effective in treating undulant fever. The drugs are administered by the doctor. Sometimes corticosteroids help to make the toxic manifestations less.

AMEBIASIS AND DYSENTERY

Since the outbreak of amebic dysentery, from a source in two Chicago hotels during 1933, the world has become increasingly aware of the menace of this disorder, which was formerly considered a tropical disease. Instead of being caused by an ordinary germ, this condition is caused by a large type of organism known as the *entameba histolytica.* This organism gets into the large bowel, and once there sets up symptoms that are exceedingly serious. Moreover, the organism may spread to the liver particularly, or to other organs of the body, and there set up secondary places of infection which are also a menace to health and life. Although this condition was formerly unheard of in the northern portions of the United States, more recent evidence indicates that from five to ten per cent of all the people of this country are infected.

The organism which causes this disease multiplies in the bowel and gives off daughter cysts. These cysts are passed out of the body with the excretions, and if they reach food or drink in any way are naturally swallowed. They pass through the stomach and small intestines and then get into the upper portions of the large intestines. Here they divide and multiply organisms which invade the walls of the bowels.

Ordinarily, the entameba histolytica which infects mankind comes in food or drink that has been contaminated in the manner suggested. After a person has had the disease and recovered, he may carry the organisms in his bowel for long periods of time, and as a carrier of the disease is constantly able to transmit it to other people. These carriers, who apparently are healthy or who have mild symptoms of the infection, are the ones most concerned in transmitting the disease.

Occasionally, however, the disease is transmitted by impure water supply. It has been shown that the cysts of the entameba histolytica may live for days and several weeks in water, depending on the temperature of the water and the number of bacteria in the water. It was thought in the past that these methods of transmission were of comparatively little importance in this country, except in the rural districts where people deposit their excretions on the soil, and where wells and springs are the chief sources of the water supply.

More recently, it has been found that any severe contamination of the water supply in a large building may result in the spread of amebic dysentery.

In China and Japan human excretions are frequently used as fertilizing material for vegetables. This is a serious menace to health, because it has been shown that the cysts of this parasite will remain alive in the moist excretions for as long as two weeks, and when they contaminate the vegetables, they may in this way transmit the disease.

It has also been shown that it is possible for the fly, which feeds on excretions, to carry the organism and deposit it on food. The most common method of transmission of this disease, however, is through the contamination of food and drink by food handlers who happen to be carriers of the entameba histolytica. The food handlers concerned may be waiters, cooks, dish washers, or any other kitchen personnel in a family or in a large hotel.

As the organism may live in the intestines for months or years without producing serious symptoms, it is not possible to say just how long a time is required for infection to develop. However, there is some good evidence that the swallowing of the cysts of entameba histolytica is followed in from ten to ninety-five days, with an average period of 64.8 days, by the beginning of the symptoms which are characteristic in this disease. Usually the disease comes on suddenly, but often it begins with mild diarrhea which gradually becomes worse. When the disease begins suddenly, there is severe abdominal pain with nausea and vomiting and a chilly sensation. The irritation of the bowel becomes acute, and the patient tries to evacuate the bowels repeatedly. This irritation may be so constant that the number of actions of the bowels will vary from six to eight in twenty-four hours to as many as thirty to forty actions of the bowels in twenty-four hours in severe cases.

As a result, the patient becomes exhausted, complains of aching in the back and great weakness in the legs, and is likely to be mentally depressed. There may be little or no fever; even in severe cases the temperature reaches at most from 100 to 102 degrees, but in very severe cases may go higher.

As a result of the extensive action of the bowels, such patients have tenderness in the abdomen, the skin appears sallow and jaundiced, and the patient loses weight rapidly. The doctor will want to examine the blood to find out how much the red cells of the blood have been injured and also whether or not there is any significant rise in the number of white blood cells. Frequently the distinction between this condition, appendicitis, and peritonitis will depend on a careful examination of the blood.

In times when amebic dysentery is prevalent and physicians are naturally on the lookout for it, they are likely to check up the cases. However, in the past physicians have not been particularly aware of this disease; certainly not in the northern parts of the United States. Since the diagnosis is made with certainty only after the excretions have been examined under the microscope in order to determine whether or not entameba histolytica is present, it is not safe to make a diagnosis until such a microscopic study has been made. At the same time, the man who makes the laboratory study must make certain that the ameba is the real entameba histolytica and not a form of the other amebas that live in the bowels without causing symptoms. He must also distinguish between the dysentery that is caused by the ameba and the dysentery which follows infection with some bacteria.

There are certain ways in which the community may protect itself against amebiasis. Much depends on having a properly guarded water supply, on the proper disposal of sewage, the protection of food from flies, and on suitable examinations and treatment of waiters, cooks, dish washers, and other food handlers in public eating places.

Chlorination of water will sterilize it so far as bacteria are concerned, but it takes one hundred times as much chlorine to kill the cysts of the entameba histolytica as it does to kill bacteria in water. In fact, the addition of this amount of chlorine to water would make the water unfit for drinking. Therefore, whenever water is heavily contaminated with entameba histolytica, the only way to make it safe is to boil it: obviously a difficult matter for any city water supply.

In controlling food handlers, it is necessary that they be examined at fairly frequent intervals, and that their excretions be examined in the laboratory to rule out the presence of the organism.

Fortunately, there are now available several methods of treatment which have been established as useful in controlling amebic dysentery. All of the remedies concerned are potent. Since they are powerful remedies, they are dangerous if taken in excessive dosage and should never be taken except under the advice and control of a physician. Among the remedies most commonly used today, and proved to be valuable, are chiniofon, carbarsone, and vioform, also milibis and various combinations. The drug called emetin, which is much used in this condition, is especially valuable in controlling the symptoms of the disease and is usually given early in order to bring about prompt recovery of the patient.

Aureomycin, chloramphenicol and terramycin have all been used successfully. Amebiasis is difficult to cure and relapses are frequent.

TULAREMIA

For the last fifty years, market men have known about a condition called "rabbit fever." About 1911 cases were described under the name of deer fly fever. Finally, in 1912, investigators of the United States Public Health Service found a plague-like disease among the squirrels in one of the counties of California and discovered that this disease was caused by a germ which they named in honor of Tulare County, Calif., the *bacterium tularense* now called *Pasteurella tularensis.* Then, Francis, another investigator from the United States Public Health Service, found in 1919 that this germ which caused both the plague-like disease of rodents and deer fly fever could infect human beings with a condition which was named tularemia. Francis later examined the livers of a thousand rabbits offered for sale in the markets of Washington, D. C., and found at least one hundred seventy of these rabbits infected with the same germ.

While the disease caused by the bacterium tularense is not an especially serious disease, seventeen out of four hundred twenty people who had it died. The human being who becomes infected with this germ usually does so in the handling or dressing of rabbits sick with the disease. The rabbit sick with tularemia is not likely to be active. Health authorities warn particularly against eating rabbits that can be knocked over with a stick. If the rabbit gives a good chase and has to be shot with a gun it is probably not a sick rabbit.

The person who has tularemia develops swellings of the skin with the formation of abscesses, swelling of the lymph glands and nodules, and small spots of infection in the internal organs. The typical history of such a case is that the man in question or the woman in question dressed wild rabbits, that he or she had at the time a sore on the finger, and that shortly thereafter the sore developed into an ulcer; then the glands became involved, and finally other organs of the body.

Rabbit meat, even from rabbits infected with this condition, is harmless as a food if it is thoroughly cooked, since a temperature of 133 degrees F. will kill the germ. It is safer, however, for everyone who is dressing rabbits for use as food to wear rubber gloves during the process.

This condition can be transmitted from one animal to another, including the human being, by means of deer flies, wood ticks, rabbit ticks, and lice; and such creatures as the sheep, the coyote, the cat, the quail, and the grouse may be infected, as well as rabbits and squirrels. However, as far as is known, the horse, cattle, dogs, and chickens have not been infected with this disease. In the Eastern states it is most likely to occur during November, December, and January.

Most people who become infected with tularemia have to go to bed for ten days to three weeks, and sometimes recovery is slow. There is no specific serum. The discovery of streptomycin provided a new specific treatment for tularemia that is quite effective. Aureomycin, chloramphenicol and terramycin are also effective.

Sometimes it is necessary to put hot packs on the spots of infection and then to open the abscesses in order to relieve the pressure of the broken-down material. In this infectious condition, as in every other, it is wise to convalesce slowly, since any disease with considerable fever and infection throws a strain on the heart and the circulation.

MALARIA

Authorities in medicine have attributed the fall of the Roman and Greek civilizations to the development of malaria among the population. Certainly, malaria can devitalize any person.

Any community that is willing to spend sufficient money to stamp out the disease can do so. Malaria is becoming less prevalent in the United States each year. Nevertheless, a million people in the United States constantly suffer from malaria. Possibly one third of the people in the world are infected. Malaria has been called the greatest single destroyer of the human race.

The physician diagnoses malaria by the characteristic symptoms, which include regularly recurring attacks of chills and fever, the presence of an enlarged spleen, and the presence of the malarial parasite in the blood of the sick person. He must not only diagnose malaria but also the special form that is present.

The plasmodium, as the organism which causes malaria is called, was discovered by the famous scientist Laveran, who received the Nobel Prize for this discovery. Ross and Grassi, a British and an Italian investigator, proved that the organism of malaria is transmitted from one human being to another through the bite of the anopheles mosquito.

Although malaria has practically disappeared as one of the great medical problems in large cities, the disease is still to be found in many rural communities, particularly in the southern portions of the United States.

In river valleys and creek bottoms malaria has been found to be highly endemic, averaging fifteen cases for every one hundred persons. The worst infection is always found in the immediate vicinity of some lake, pond, or marsh which could be the natural habitat of the malaria mosquito. The district extends about a mile in every direction from the pond, which marks the range of flight of the mosquitoes. Country-club ponds must be watched particularly, as these artificial pools have been found frequently to be excellent breeding places for the mosquito.

The malaria mosquito bites most frequently at dusk. If it has fed on a sick person and then bites a well one, the latter is likely to be supplied with some malarial infection. In summer resorts where the population is mixed, including people coming from all sorts of localities, the chance of infection is greater.

One of the means used to destroy the mosquitoes that carry the malaria organisms is to stock all lakes, ponds, and sluggish streams with the variety of fish that lives on the larvæ of the mosquito. The routine for mosquito control should include the clearing of the edges of the ponds of willows, cattails, water grasses, and floatage. Thus the bank of the pond is left sharp and clean, so that the fish can swim close to the bank and feed on the mosquito wiggletails.

The fish that has been found to be most active in feeding on the mosquito larvæ is the little top minnow *Gambusia affinis,* also called the potbellied minnow. This little fish swims in the most shallow waters.

The drainage of small ponds or marshes and the use of oil sprays are methods suitable to areas where it is not necessary to preserve the pond for decorative or for amusement purposes. Adult mosquitoes can be destroyed by DDT.

As long as the adult parasites are present in the blood of the individual in sufficient quantities to infect the mosquito that bites the individual, the person is a possible conveyor of malaria. Since the parasites remain in the blood for months, providing that the individual is not properly treated, anyone who is not undergoing regular treatment is a menace to those around him.

Children suffer more severely with the disease than do adults. Negroes apparently are less affected than are the white people. Malaria has been practically stamped out of northern communities, and cases are rarely seen even in large charity hospitals in the northern part of the United States.

In the more serious types of malaria not properly treated, anywhere from 10 to 30 per cent of the people die. The milder forms of the disease become chronic, and the fatality rate may be less than 5 per cent.

In controlling malaria, patients who are sick with the disease are protected from the bites of the mosquito. It has been established that the regular use of sufficient doses of quinine will control the condition. Many varieties of antimalarial drugs are now available. Quinine and atabrine are best known. Primaquine and pyrimethamine are newest. Paludrine and Camoquin can arrest the full blown development of the disease. Chloroquine or Aralen is used both for suppression and treatment.

RAT-BITE FEVER

When human beings are bitten by animals of the rodent type, including incidentally not only the rat but the weasel and the pig and occasionally, as will be seen later, even the cat, they are sometimes infected with a peculiar organism called a *Spirillum* which produces a disease of the whole body. This disease is characterized by short attacks of fever alternating with periods without the fever, and also an eruption on the skin. Such cases have been known in the United States for a century, and medical journals have reported approximately one hundred.

The usual course of such a case is as follows: After the person has been bitten, the wound heals promptly unless a secondary infection occurs. From one to three weeks after the date on which the patient was bitten, the spot of the bite becomes red and swollen, and the person who is infected develops the usual symptoms of infections in general: namely, headache, general pains and fever, sometimes a chill and a general feeling of sickness. Finally an eruption appears, at first most prominent in the region of the wound, but later spreading over the body.

From this time on, attacks of fever will occur every five or six days, sometimes less frequently. Gradually the person loses weight and may become exceedingly sick due to the loss of nutrition and general health. Somewhere between 6 and 7 per cent of the people who are infected eventually die of the disorder, but the tendency is for the majority to recover.

There have been instances reported in medical periodicals of children who have been bitten by rats when left alone by their parents, particularly when they live in basement homes or poverty-stricken tenements. Of course, a cat may become contaminated through its hunting of the rats.

The doctor makes his diagnosis of this condition not only by the symptoms that have been mentioned, but also by finding the germ which causes the disease in the wound, and sometimes in material taken directly from lymph glands near the wound. There are also cases in which people have been bitten by rats and become infected, not with this organism but with the usual germs that cause infection, such as the staphylococcus and streptococcus.

Formerly this condition was treated like syphilis, with salvarsan or arsphenamine or, as it was more popularly known, "606." Now penicillin seems to be fully effective in rat-bite fever, as in syphilis.

ROCKY MOUNTAIN SPOTTED FEVER

As was shown years ago in investigations made by Dr. Theobald Smith, many diseases of man are transmitted by the bite of a tick. Among the most serious of these is the condition called Rocky Mountain spotted fever, an infectious disease seen frequently in eastern Idaho and the Bitter Root Valley of Montana, but also occurring in most western states and occasionally in eastern portions of the United States. This condition occurs most commonly in men because of their occupations as surveyors, foresters, hunters, fishermen, sheep herders, or cowboys. These occupations expose them to the bite of the tick. If bitten, women and children are just as likely to become affected.

The tick is found on the rodents in the areas mentioned, and from these rodents picks up the organisms which it then transfers to man when it bites. From four to seven days after he is bitten, the man comes down with the disease. At first there are loss of appetite, general aches and pains, and slight fever. Then suddenly there is a chill followed by a high fever. This may reach 104 or 105 degrees. At first there are severe headache and backache with pains in the muscles. Even the skin may be tender. Eventually the nervous system may be involved, with restlessness and lack of sleep and even disturbance of the action of the bowels.

About the third to the seventh day, the infected person breaks out with tiny pinkish spots which generally appear first on the wrists and ankles, and which give the disease its name—spotted fever. In serious cases the spots run together. Since they are due to blood, they gradually turn purple. The fever remains high for a week to ten days and, if recovery occurs, falls gradually. In the fatal cases death occurs from the seventh to the tenth day, with high fever.

The physician is able to make his diagnosis certain by examining the blood, in which he finds not only changes in the blood cells but also specific reactions which are certain evidence of the presence of the disease. This condition resembles the old typhus fever, or jail fever, as it was called when jails were almost universally unsanitary, which is transmitted by the bite of a louse.

The use of paraminobenzoic acid has been recommended and also aureomycin, terramycin and chloromycetin. The diet should be nutritious and high in carbohydrate. Plentiful liquids are given. Most serious complication is pneumonia.

The obvious method of preventing this disease is to avoid the bite of the tick which causes it. This has been attempted in some places through eliminating rodents and through dipping cattle. As a method of prevention this has not, however, been extremely successful.

Investigators of the United States Public Health Service have developed a vaccine made of the ground-up bodies of the ticks. This is found to be a protection against infection with this disorder and can minimize severity.

GLANDERS

Most farmers think of glanders as a disease affecting horses and mules, but occasionally it attacks human beings. It has been reported also in cats, rabbits, sheep, mice, and various wild animals of the cat tribe.

Because the disease is commonly transmitted by horses and affects horses more frequently than any other animal, it is now rarely seen in large cities, from which horses have practically disappeared.

In the first twenty years of the present century there were seven cases of glanders in the wards of the Bellevue Hospital, New York City, but since then, not a single case has been seen.

Glanders is caused by a germ known as the bacillus of glanders. From three to five days after the germ gets into the body, the symptoms first appear. There are the usual symptoms of infection, such as nausea, headache, vomiting, chills, and some fever. Quite soon, however, nodules appear on the skin, associated with inflammation of the lymphatic ducts and glands near the places where the abscesses are located. Sometimes a hard nodule develops which ulcerates and breaks down, discharging a profuse, sticky substance. If the disease attacks the lungs it gives symptoms like those of pneumonia.

Nowadays, a diagnosis of glanders is hardly likely to be made unless the condition described happens to occur in someone who is constantly working around horses. The acute infection is very serious in the human being, and most of the patients die.

In the control of a disease like glanders, everything depends on stamping out the source of the infection in the animal which transmits it. Hence, it is recommended that practically every animal with glanders should be promptly destroyed and the stables thoroughly disinfected, including all harness and watering buckets. All animals that have been exposed should be examined for the infection and kept under observation until well past the time when there is any likelihood that the infection may develop in them.

A doctor who takes charge of such cases treats them usually by the surgical method of opening the abscesses and draining away the infectious material.

PSITTACOSIS OR PARROT DISEASE

In 1904, three cases of psittacosis or "parrot disease" were reported in Boston. In the fall of 1929 an outbreak of this disease was reported in Buenos Aires, and more outbreaks have since been reported in the United States. In Hamburg, Germany, twenty-eight cases, with five deaths, occurred in the fall of 1929. In the epidemic of psittacosis which occurred in Paris in 1892 there were forty-nine cases and sixteen deaths, and it was reported that the infection had been caused by parrots brought from South America.

When psittacosis occurs it begins with a chill and fever, with a good deal of weakness and depression, and usually some inflammation of the lungs.

"Parrot disease" is essentially a medical curiosity and need occasion little alarm among the people of the United States. The symptoms resemble those of other infectious diseases, and one should be certain that the disease is actually psittacosis and not pneumonia or other infection of the lungs.

Obviously, the first step is to get the suspected parrot and to find out whether or not it contains the germs which are responsible. In addition to parrots many other bird pets occasionally become infected, including love birds, cockatoos and parakeets.

The occurrence of this condition is another demonstration of the fact that we are likely to contract diseases from all sorts of contacts and that it is not safe to demonstrate too much fondness for our animal neighbors.

Psittacosis has been known for a long time as a disease of parrots, but the first cases of pneumonic infection traced directly from parrots to man were described in 1879 in Germany.

The proof of the fact that human infection has come from the parrot depends on isolation of the germ from both the parrot and the affected human being.

In parrots, psittacosis is highly fatal, killing from 50 to 95 per cent of the infected birds. The disease can be transmitted from one parrot to another by infected feathers, food, water, dishes, or the soiled hands of attendants. Mice or insects may carry the infection from one cage to another. When a parrot becomes infected it gets weak, loses its appetite, has diarrhea, and is likely to die in a few days. Then the germs will be found in practically all of its organs.

As might be expected, a disease that can pass from parrot to man may also infect chickens, rabbits, mice, and guinea pigs. It is interesting that this disease which chiefly infects the intestinal tracts of birds strikes the lungs in man. In many instances the infection is due to the fact that the parrot is fed by the mouth-to-mouth method. Not infrequently, however, it occurs merely from handling the sick birds, and not infrequently the person in a family who becomes sick passes the disease on with infected hands to other members of the family.

Fortunately, this disease is rare in civilized communities, probably because parrots are not nearly so frequent as pets as are other animals and birds, and probably also because the disease kills the parrots so rapidly that the likelihood of infection is lessened.

The occurrence of cases of psittacosis in the United States is new evidence of the fact that methods of transportation, exchange of products among various nations, and the complete abolishing of boundary lines between peoples make it impossible any longer for a nation to be isolated. The disease of one people will sooner or later appear among others.

The sulfonamide drugs help to stop the growth of the virus. Aureomycin and terramycin are also effective in checking the disease.

EPIDEMIC ENCEPHALITIS

No one knows when the first epidemic of lethargy associated with fever and destruction of brain tissue first afflicted mankind, but several observers have pointed out that Hippocrates, the famous father of modern scientific medicine, himself described an epidemic of this character which appeared in the spring and continued on into the autumn, at which time it was more fatal. It was suggested that there were similar epidemics in the sixteenth century in various parts of Europe. At the end of 1890, such an epidemic occurred in southern Europe and was described under the name of *nona*.

The modern condition called epidemic encephalitis was described in Vienna in 1917, during World War I, and was given the name *encephalitis lethargica* because it is an inflammation of the brain associated with drowsiness and somnolence. The disease spread to England and to the United States and Canada; it seems possible, however, that there were individual cases in the United States before 1915.

Encephalitis means inflammation of the brain. Now many different causes of such inflammations are recognized. Transmitted by insects are St. Louis encephalitis, Japanese B, Australian X, Western equine, Venezuelan equine and Russian tick borne encephalitis. These are distinct from the condition called *nona* or epidemic lethargic encephalitis.

Epidemic encephalitis occurs most frequently in February and March but may occur at any time of the year. The condition is caused by a virus and at least seven different types of virus more or less closely related to each other have been distinguished. Principal varieties include the so-called eastern type and western or St. Louis type. The disease seems to have been more common in the United States and in Europe than on other continents. It is quite mildly contagious, but outbreaks have been reported in schools, asylums, and barracks in which large numbers of people are housed.

There has been much research in an attempt to find a preventive serum based on the discovery of virus. The virus may be transmitted to humans from lower animals like birds, rats, horses or domestic pets. Such conditions as the louping ill of sheep, X disease of Australia, "B" virus disease in monkeys, and other virus diseases are believed to be related in a group.

In most cases of encephalitis the disease occurs in three stages: first, the beginning, which is sudden; second, a milder condition following the first acute condition; and, finally, a sort of chronic condition in those who recover. In the acute stage there are the usual symptoms of infection, such as fever, weakness, headache, and running of the nose, but in addition in these cases there are quite frequently double vision and emotional disturbances indicating that the brain has been affected. Most of the patients become lethargic or sleepy at the beginning of the disease and remain in this condition until the recovery from the acute stage has taken place. There are, however, other cases which actually have insomnia, and there are some who are lethargic in the daytime and awake at night.

While these patients seem to be completely unconscious, there are recorded instances in which the patient who apparently slept was aware of everything that went on in the room. The brain was affected in such a manner that the patient could not speak or let other people know that he heard what was being said. In association with the somnolence or lethargy in many of these cases there is a delirium in which the patient may have emotional outbursts, delusions, or periods of depression. An exceedingly interesting phenomenon is the development of what is called occupational delirium, in which the person who is affected dwells constantly on the occupation; the orator continually makes speeches, the teacher lectures, the accountant adds figures.

In association with the primary symptoms that have been mentioned are many other symptoms indicating that the nervous system has been involved, such as paralyses, convulsions, tremors, and similar disorders.

After the patient has recovered from the first stage, which may have been slight—in fact, so slight as hardly to have had medical attention—comes the second stage of this disease, in which the patients are weak and say that they have been sick since an attack of influenza. They remember that they were drowsy, but they never feel well, and they are likely to be called neurasthenic or hysterical or simply plain lazy by their families. However, the condition is likely to go on to the time when anyone can realize that these patients are seriously sick, since they begin to develop symptoms like those of Parkinson's disease, or the shaking palsy. In this condition the face is mask-like, the arms and legs are held rigid, the movements are slow, the speech monotonous, and the thumb and forefinger move rather constantly in a pill-rolling movement.

In association with this there may be an apparent oversupply of saliva with some drooling from the mouth because of the changes in the muscles of the face.

There develop frequently in the later stages difficulties of behavior in children who tend to become moral imbeciles. These children are cruel, disobedient, destructive, abusive, rather filthy in their habits, and may actually become a menace from the point of view of their lack of sanity. Without a recognition of the disease which is involved such children are frequently brought before the courts and treated as criminals rather than as invalids. In the same way adults occasionally develop strange mental conditions following encephalitis and constitute a problem for those responsible for their care.

None of these patients are actually sleeping over months or years, but the mentality is seriously disturbed, and the rhythm of sleep may be changed.

Unfortunately, scientific medicine has not yet developed any specific method of treatment that will prevent this disease or arrest its progress. It does, however, attempt to aid these patients by what is called symptomatic treatment, treating each of the symptoms as it develops by well established methods. A number of serums and vaccines have been tried.

These patients have been injected with non-specific proteins in the form of typhoid vaccine; malaria germs have been injected to produce shock and artificial fever; and artificial heat has been tried, but thus far the results are quite inconclusive, and no one can say definitely that any of these methods of treatment actually stops the progress of this disorder.

During 1938 outbreaks of a form of brain inflammation or unconsciousness called encephalitis broke out in North Dakota, Minnesota, Vermont and Massachusetts. In the same area at the same time there were numerous cases of a form of inflammation of the brain among horses called equine encephalomyelitis. The investigators proved that both conditions were caused by a virus of a certain type and that this virus is also to be found in a disease that affects the field mouse and other rodents, as well as partridges and pigeons. With an understanding of the nature of the disease which has thus been made available it only remains to find the chain of communication from the animals to man. Then it will be possible to prevent the further appearance of the disease among human beings.

These conditions are diagnosed by doctors through laboratory studies which demonstrate neutralizing or complement fixing antibodies in a patient's serum two weeks or more after infection. Both types of antibody persist for two years at least. After death the conditions found in the brain are not specific, but a diagnosis can be made by the demonstration of virus through intracerebral inoculation of mice with brain tissue. The virus is virulent for mice, monkeys, rabbits, guinea pigs, rats, and sheep.

CHAPTER 13

The Respiratory Diseases

MORRIS FISHBEIN, M.D.

THE COMMON COLD

When William Osler wrote his *Principles and Practice of Medicine,* the most popular textbook of medicine ever published, he began with typhoid fever, probably because typhoid was one of the most serious and incapacitating diseases affecting a vast number of people. Students learned to study diseases according to the way in which William Osler systematized knowledge of typhoid. Typhoid is definitely under control and disturbs but few people.

The most widely used textbooks of medicine began in 1965 with the common cold—and rightly. Infections of the nose, throat, and sinuses are responsible for more than one half the time lost by wage earners due to sickness. Everybody knows how to cure a cold, and, even if he does not, will tell *you.* You can put your feet in a mustard bath, drink several glasses of hot lemonade, carry a buckeye in your right rear pocket, wear an iron ring, indulge freely in many of the widely advertised remedies, and even take some of the beverages that once required a doctor's prescription and about which the government expressed considerable doubt as to curative value—and at the end of three days you will probably begin to get well almost regardless of the treatment.

The common cold is essentially a self-limited disease. Unfortunately, however, it does not, like an attack of measles or scarlet fever, induce in the person who has it a resistance or immunity which will prevent him from having a cold soon again. People who have colds seem to have them often. Those who are easily susceptible constitute about 23 per cent; they have colds four or more times a year. Sixty per cent of people have colds two or three times a year and 17 per cent once a year or not at all.

The common cold is not like the epidemic influenza that devastated the world in 1918. That was a definite infectious disease, highly contagious, affecting vast numbers of people and causing a terrific number of deaths. The history of medicine shows that at least eight great pandemics of influenza had previously swept the world, beginning with one in 1580, the seventh occurring in 1889–1892. The common cold is something quite different.

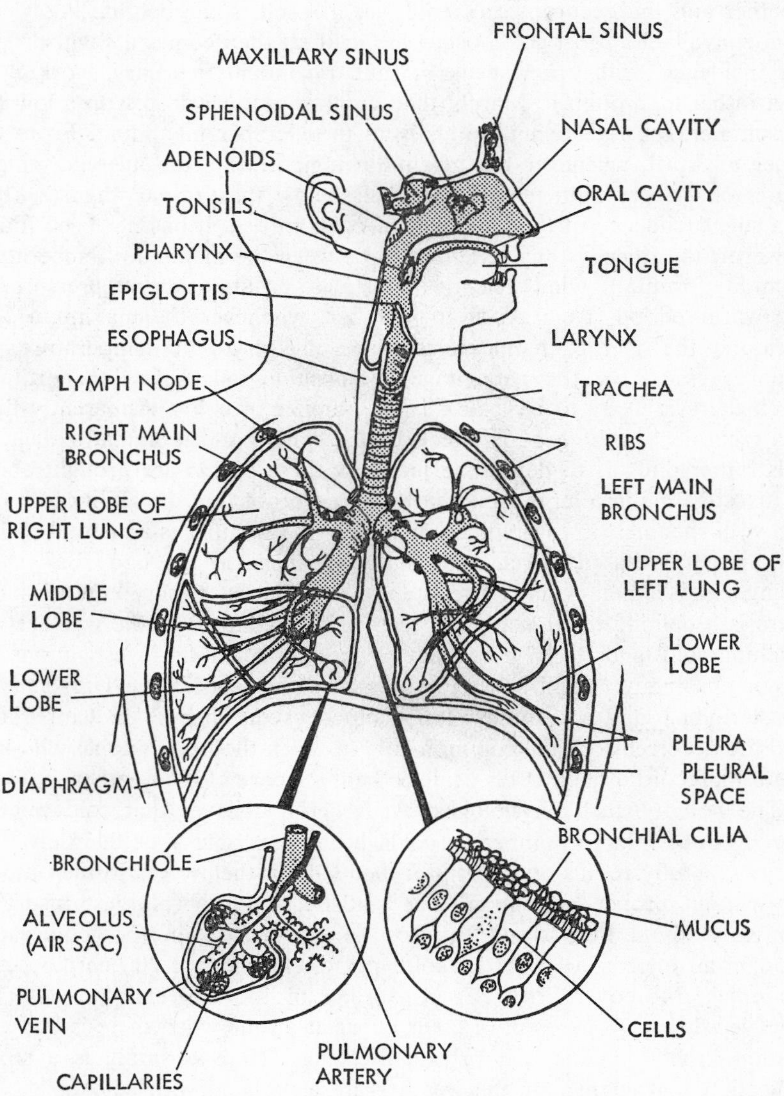

Fig. 40. The Respiratory System. National Tuberculosis Association.

CAUSES OF COLDS

Changes in the weather have been incriminated as a cause of colds from the time of Hippocrates. Geologists, geographists, physiographers, and biometricians have tried to find certain relationships between changes in the weather and the occurrence of colds; as a result, some definite knowledge is now available. Most colds occur in October; then comes a slight drop in the incidence, with a new peak in January and in February, working up to a rather high point in March; then another gradual drop with a low rate in summer, the rate rising gradually to the October maximum. From October to April, whenever the maximum temperature, the average temperature, or the dry bulb temperature falls below the ordinary figures, there is a slight tendency of the incidence of colds to rise. It has not been found, however, that there is any relationship between the maximum temperature, humidity, rainfall, wind velocity, sunshine, or atmospheric pressure. In the warm period, from April to October, whenever the maximum temperature, the average temperature range, the dry bulb temperature, the vapor pressure, or the percentage of sunshine falls below the ordinary level, there is likely to be a rise in the number of colds. Apparently there is a great deal in the general effect of atmosphere on the human being, but it is rather difficult to determine just how these effects are brought about.

Investigators in a large clinic have offered proof that the ability of a person with rheumatism to predict a change in the weather is an actual ability, and that it is based on changes that take place in the body before the change in weather occurs. The opinion of at least twenty centuries that there is a definite relationship between sudden changes in the weather and catching cold tends to be borne out by modern scientific investigations but is not absolutely established. A professor of hygiene in the University of Amsterdam found a definite relationship between changes in temperature and the occurrence of the common cold in seven thousand people who kept a careful record of their colds while he kept a record of the weather.

The noted British physiologist, A. V. Hill, believes that cold weather brings about a large number of colds because people shut themselves up in warm, stuffy rooms and perspire; then submit themselves to the outdoor air without proper protection. The statistician for our largest insurance company found that a sudden drop of 10 degrees in the temperature brought an increase of eighteen colds per week among 6,700 employees in his office. Moreover, Prof. E. O. Jordan of the University of Chicago discovered that 90 per cent of colds occur at a time when there is less ventilation in both public and private dwellings. Here certainly is a strong indication that changes in the weather are associated with colds.

Everybody has experienced the development of a cold following a night in a sleeping car, a swim in the pool, or a shower bath immediately after being overheated by exercise. Investigators are convinced that the overheated and dehydrated air in the homes and in offices in the United States lowers the resistance of the membranes of the nose; then germs or viruses, which are almost constantly present among human beings, begin their work of infection.

Extreme cold does not cause colds. Eskimos seldom have colds. A group of explorers found on visiting one Eskimo settlement that there was not one cold among the Eskimos from the tiniest infant to the most ancient patriarch of the tribe. Seventy-two hours after the expedition, which included several people who had colds, arrived in the settlement, practically every one of the Eskimos developed the characteristic symptoms. That ought to be sufficient proof that there is some transmissible agent which produces the infection. It correlates with the fact that germs do well on new soil.

Many investigators have been searching for a specific virus as a cause of the common cold. The evidence suggests that several different viruses may be involved. When the cause is isolated, specific measures of prevention may follow.

Granted that the cold is caused by an infectious organism, there must apparently be other factors or all of us would have colds all the time. These factors constitute what are called predisposing causes. Tobacco, dust, gas, the amount of sleep, sitting in a draft, constipation, perspiration, and footwear have all been suggested as possible predisposing elements. A research made by investigators at Cornell University failed to incriminate definitely any one of them. Changes in the weight and quality of underwear that is worn have been suggested. Enough evidence is available to indicate that the wearing of woolen underwear is not a panacea; besides, it itches!

Experts in diseases of the nose and throat feel that obstruction in the nose and enlarged tonsils are important in relationship to the number of colds. Numerous studies recently made failed to prove that either one of them is a certain factor. Obstructions in the nose ought to be taken care of because they interfere with breathing and perhaps bring about congestion. Enlarged and infected tonsils are a menace to health and should be removed. But the person concerned may have just as many colds, if not more, after these factors are attended to than he had previously.

Our modern methods of living may be largely responsible for the increased incidence of colds. We are crowded together in offices, in motion-picture houses, at football and basketball games. We are packed into elevators and subway cars. We breathe constantly, cough frequently, and sneeze unexpectedly in one another's faces. Moreover, our hands are constantly in contact with door knobs, pencils, dishes, and other utensils, also handled by other people. We carry our hands to our mouths and to our noses and thus transmit by what is called hand-to-mouth infection.

SYMPTOMS OF COLDS

Because of its symptoms and its rather poorly understood character in relationship to other diseases, the common cold is variously called by a number of high-sounding scientific titles, in most instances related to the part of the body particularly affected. What is known as a head cold is called coryza. Because of the increase in the temperature and the outpouring of fluid from the nose, the cold has been called acute catarrhal fever. Because the running is principally from the nose, it has been called acute catarrhal rhinitis. If the throat is hoarse, the portion affected may give the title to the disease so that it becomes acute pharyngitis, acute laryngitis, or acute tracheitis.

These anatomical designations nevertheless hardly convey the stuffiness, the chills, the irritability, the loss of appetite, and the other symptoms that are commonly associated with this disorder. The chief changes in the tissues involved are those which affect the mucous membranes of the nose and throat. The lining of the nose is red and swollen, and from it pours continuously the fluid that causes much sniffling and blowing. With the sniffling and blowing comes irritation of the skin around the nose and mouth, and, if the trouble extends down far enough, there is coughing without much discharge from the throat. The mouth is held open during sleep so that the tongue becomes thick and coated.

PREVENTION OF COLDS

What everyone wants to know is how to prevent a cold, how to stop a cold, and how to cure one. In every infection of the human body three factors are concerned: First, contact with the infecting substance; second, sufficient virulence in the infecting germ to overcome the resistance of the body, and third, sufficient resistance in the body to overcome the infecting germ.

The human family, particularly in large cities, is so crowded that it is practically impossible to avoid contact with those who have respiratory infections. Our modern apartment dwellings are simply great barracks into which families are packed, and dwellings are like cans into which the individual members of the family are crowded closely together.

If a germ or virus is responsible for the common cold, it may vary in virulence from time to time exactly as diphtheria, scarlet fever, and similar infections vary in their potency. However, what is called a variation in virulence may really be the reflection of lessening of resistance or the development of a new generation that has not the resistance of a previous generation. One conception of epidemic influenza emphasizes that it occurs in cycles of some thirty years which permit the development of new generations of human beings not capable of resisting the infection. Since the germs are living organisms, conceivably they may vary in their power from one occasion to another exactly as human beings vary.

Germs may be affected exactly as human beings are affected by the atmosphere in which they live, the soil on which they rest, the diet on which they thrive. The organism of the common cold may die readily on the surface of the skin but grow happily on a mucous membrane. It may die readily on a normal mucous membrane, but multiply exceedingly on a mucous membrane that has been vitiated by the continuous residence of its possessor in a hot, dry, stuffy, dusty room. Here then comes the question of a proper supply of clean air as a factor in the onset and in the prevention of the common cold.

The most serious problem is the question of proper heating and the provision of sufficient moisture in the air. Private homes should be heated to 68 or 70 degrees, and large halls to 60 or 65 degrees F. The large halls require less heat because human beings will provide from their own bodies enough extra heat to make up the deficiency. Equally important with heat is moisture. A sufficient amount of humidity prevents chilling. Moisture can be obtained either by special devices built into furnaces which are now widely advertised and which have been proved to be efficient, or by special electric devices which have been developed for moistening the air.

The common impression that chilling, dampness, and fatigue are predisposing factors in catching cold is, as has been shown, supported by much good scientific evidence. The theory is that chilling and dampness induce a cold through disturbing the heat-regulating mechanism of the body by sudden evaporation of moisture from the surface of the body. For example, one who is quite well may sit in front of an electric fan and get up after fifteen minutes with the nose congested and with all of the beginning symptoms of a cold. The draft from the electric fan brings about chilling of the surface of the body and disturbs the circulation of the blood in the mucous membranes of the nose.

Conditioning against colds has behind it the acceptance of many hygienic authorities. The technique of conditioning involves the building of resistance through proper hygiene and a few special measures directed specifically against the predisposing causes. One of these techniques is the cold-bath technique. A cold shower is all right for anyone who wants it, provided he rubs himself thoroughly thereafter with towels so as to restore a brisk circulation to the congealed surface. The majority of people probably do better with a lukewarm bath taken primarily for purposes of cleanliness and only secondarily with the idea of benefiting resistance to disease.

There is also the conception that children may have their resistance increased by wrapping their throats and chests with towels wrung out of cold water. There is no good evidence in favor of this notion. Then there are the mothers who believe that they help the health of the child by baring to the wintry blasts the portion of the leg from the calf to the upper third of the thigh. It remains to be shown that any child had its resistance to colds increased by this exposure.

Certainly the biometricians have not credited such statistics as are available in favor of conditioning to cold by subjecting one's self unnecessarily to it. The reasoning in favor of the procedure is only symbolical, like the suggestion that the proper treatment of smallpox is to put the patient in a room with red velour hangings.

Germs in general succumb to sunlight. For human beings sunlight is pleasant. Hence the argument early advanced that exposure to the rays of the sun or to the rays of ultraviolet from the artificial sun lamp, using either the carbon arc or the quartz mercury vapor burner, would aid in building resistance to colds. The Council on Physical Therapy of the American Medical Association, after examining all of the evidence that could be offered in support of such measures, has withdrawn its approval from sources of ultraviolet that are advertised as beneficial in the prevention of colds. Perhaps the ultraviolet does enhance the power of the body in some generally beneficial way, but certainly it has not been proved that its effects are specific against respiratory diseases. Indeed, the exact words of the council are, "As far as normal persons are concerned, the claim that exposure to ultraviolet rays increases or improves the tone of the tissues or of the body as a whole, stimulates metabolism, or tends to prevent colds, has not been conclusively substantiated."

Vaccines Against Colds

Another measure of which much is heard in these advanced times, when people are beginning to understand medical progress and medical methods, is the use of the vaccine for the prevention of colds. The hoi-polloi refer to the use of vaccines or of any other substances administered by injection as "shots." Physicians build resistance against typhoid fever by injecting the patient with vaccine made of killed typhoid and paratyphoid germs. The injection of these killed germs stirs up the tissues of the body to resistance against the constituents of the typhoid organism. Some physicians inject mixtures of the killed bodies of germs frequently found in the noses and throats of people with colds, with the idea of building resistance to infection by these germs. There are two reasons, however, why many scientists do not approve the use of the "shots" in the cases of people with frequent colds. First, none of these germs are specifically the cause of or definitely related to the colds; second, it has not been shown that the injection of these germs will stimulate resistance. Two viruses known as influenza A and B are associated with symptoms like those of a cold and vaccines against these are available. Another cold or influenza virus is called virus X. Most colds are mixed infections. The United States Public Health Service has recommended inoculations against influenza for older people and women in early pregnancy.

TREATMENT OF COLDS

First, everybody who knows advises rest in bed until the temperature is normal, with head of the bed elevated in order to make breathing easier. Actually, only hygienists or people who are quite serious in medical affairs go to bed when they have a cold.

The skin is usually so uncomfortable that a sponge bath with water of a temperature about 98 degrees F. is desirable, and the skin may be fairly well rubbed with a rough towel after the bath. If the bowels are inactive, it is advisable to clear them of their digested and undigested contents. The clearing may be accomplished either by washing out from below or by the usual laxatives administered above.

Fever burns tissue. Hence the diet during a cold should consist of nourishing food. Since appetite is lost in most instances anyway, food should be appetizing and enjoyable. A child should not be forced to eat what is repulsive, particularly in the presence of disturbed appetite. Let the child have what it wants. Many physicians administer sugar and fruit juices with a view to providing calories and to preventing the acid reaction which is believed to be favorable to the persistence of the cold.

The common home remedies, such as bathing the feet in mustard baths, perspiring freely under hot blankets, drinking quantities of hot lemonade and orange juice, are time-tried helps to comfort. Of a similar character are the home remedies employed to lower fever and to diminish pain. Of this type is aspirin, a widely used home remedy. Any good aspirin will do, and fifteen or twenty different pharmaceutical houses now make it available. Aspirin, like every other remedy, is a two-edged sword, capable of damage when employed improperly as well as of good when given in proper dosage at the right time.

Diets for Colds

Then there is the specific diet. Rats which have had in their food an insufficient amount of vitamin A begin to develop a breakdown of the mucous membranes of the nose and throat. Rats that are fed sufficient amounts of vitamin A do not develop such changes. From this it has been argued that human beings who eat proper amounts of vitamin A or even excess amounts should be able to preserve the integrity of their mucous membranes and thereby avoid colds. Such experiments as have been done over short periods of time not only on chimpanzees but also on human beings do not support the idea strongly. A well balanced, nutritious diet will supply sufficient vitamin A. If doubts exist about the diet the well-recognized vitamin tablets will take care of the need.

Nose Sprays for Colds

A man with an eruption wants something to put on it. A man or woman with a running nose wants something to put in it. Hence the development of innumerable antiseptics, sprays, ointments, and lotions for administration in the common cold. There are drugs which dry up the secretions, but apparently that is not the road to cure. There are other drugs which increase the secretions, but the duration of the cold still seems to average three or four days. The experts in diseases of the nose and throat feel that the discomfort when too great should be relieved by one of the sprays which diminish secretions, and which include either the old adrenalin or the modern ephedrine. For years camphor-menthol solutions and preparations of oil, camphor, menthol, and eucalyptus have been used to give relief in nasal irritation. The actual worth of such preparations in curing the cold is doubtful. Their value in securing comfort is considerable.

Most recent in the control of colds are the antihistaminic drugs, used alone or combined with aspirin or phenacetin or sprayed in the nose with camphor or menthol. Such preparations are useful in colds which begin as a running nose due to allergy and these constitute a large percentage of all colds.

General Treatment

When the cough is relieved, the discomfort in the chest usually becomes less. Many remedies are used to loosen the cough, most of them being what are called expectorant remedies, containing ammonium chloride. The dose of ammonium chloride usually prescribed is eight grains to each teaspoonful. This is given every two hours. The ammonium chloride is put up with some pleasant syrup. Sometimes sodium citrate, taken in ten-grain tablets mixed with lemonade or warm water, will help to loosen the cough.

Most important in this condition is taking plenty of water. A person with a cold should take a half tumblerful every hour while awake. The water can be as is, or as lemonade or orangeade. If a more alkaline drink is desired, a little baking soda or sodium bicarbonate—usually about 10 grains—may be added to the lemonade.

Lots of people think they want a cathartic every time they have a cold, to clean out the system. Really the cathartic, when the cold begins, does not seem to make a great deal of difference. Sometimes it is so irritating as to induce a condition much more discomforting and worse than the cold itself.

SUMMER COLDS

Beyond the common cold there comes with the beginning of spring another type—the allergic cold, rose cold, summer cold, or hay fever. The spring or rose cold is due to sensitivity to various protein substances derived in the spring primarily from the dandelion, the daisy, maple, and poplar, and also from various other pollens of weeds and grasses. The season and the nature of the sensitizing agent depend on the location in which the person lives and the kinds of grasses and flowers in his vicinity. The symptoms of onset are much the same as those of the common cold, but with most of the emphasis on the redness of the eyes and on the sneezing. That type of cold is a special condition prevented and treated by proper diagnosis and attempts at desensitization. See the chapter on Allergy in this book.

If you must blow your nose, be careful not to blow it so hard as to force the infected secretions from the nose through the eustachian tube into the ears. Always keep one nostril open as a safety valve. Be careful to protect yourself so as not to develop the secondary complications of bronchitis and pneumonia. The cold itself is not a fatal disorder. The complications of colds in the form of infected ears, bronchitis, pneumonia, cause long maladies and many fatalities. Try going to bed for a day, give yourself a fair chance, and get well soon!

PNEUMONIA

At the seasons, with increasing cold and exposure, when epidemics of influenza strike in various parts of the country, the number of cases of pneumonia increases rapidly and also the number of deaths. The number of deaths varies from year to year, apparently related to the severity of the climatic conditions and also perhaps to changes in the nature of the germ that causes the disease.

This germ is known as the pneumococcus, a round germ which passes with the discharges from the mouth and nose of the infected person to others, and which may occasionally be carried by a healthful person who is not himself infected, and thus is distributed to others. The germs causing pneumonia are of many types. The overcrowding and the innumerable human contacts associated with modern life aid in the dissemination particularly of diseases of the mouth, nose, throat, and lungs.

Since normal persons may have the germs in their breathing tracts without having the disease, factors related to the person himself may be involved with the question of whether or not he will develop the disease.

Any factor which will break down the resistance of a person will tend to cause him to become more easily infected.

A direct injury to the tissue of the lung, such as might occur from inhaling a poison gas, or such as might occur from inhaling some foreign body which would cause an irritation, will open the way for infection by the germ of pneumonia.

The disease occurs in people of all ages but is rather rare during the first year of life. It is much more serious during the earlier and later years of life than it is during the middle period. The rate of incidence and death is high during infancy, decreasing up to the age of ten, and then gradually increasing up to the age of forty, when it again begins to become exceedingly high.

Pneumonia, as shown by statistics, is much more serious in the colored race than in the white. It also follows frequently after such conditions as measles, smallpox, scarlet fever, and even after typhoid. Exposure to severe fatigue, to bad weather, and to malnutrition gives the germs of pneumonia greater opportunity to attack. Hard drinkers have been believed more likely to suffer with pneumonia than others, but this has also been related to the fact that hard drinkers occasionally lie out in the open and are exposed to rain and freezing temperatures for long periods of time.

Crowding is an important factor in the occurrence of pneumonia. The disease is more frequently found in the city than in the country and is probably more fatal in the city than in the country. The chance for infection from one person to another is much greater where people are crowded together. In trains, street cars, theaters, motion-picture houses, in tenements and under similar conditions, human beings come into contacts that are intimate for fairly long periods of time. Under such conditions germs pass directly from the mouth, nose, and throat of one to another.

When the germs of pneumonia attack the lung it becomes filled with blood, so that quite soon the person begins coughing and spitting material which contains the red streaks showing the presence of blood in the lung. This lung is, however, rather solid because of the presence of the material in it. The physician, therefore, fails to hear the air passing because of the obstruction in the air spaces. Moreover, when he thumps the chest over the lungs it gives forth the dull sound of a solid object rather than the resonant reverberation of one which is full of air.

After a time, depending on the severity of the condition, the lung begins to clear up, the breathing takes place with less difficulty. At the same time the fever goes down.

Pneumonia sometimes begins suddenly with a chill, pain in the chest, vomiting and coughing and difficulty in breathing. In other cases there may be fainting and weakness. In the serious stages of pneumonia the fever may vary from 104 to 106 degrees. Because of the difficulty in getting the blood through the lung there is great stress on the heart. Furthermore, the obstruction to the circulation causes the patient to develop a blue color which indicates that the blood passing through the lung is not receiving enough oxygen. Especially valuable is the use of X ray to make certain of the diagnosis in pneumonia and to differentiate between lobar and virus pneumonia.

Most people know that the usual case of uncomplicated pneumonia used to last from a week to ten days and that then it cleared up by what is called a crisis; or more slowly by what physicians call lysis, or a gradual dissolving of the disease. In those cases that clear up by crisis the patient suddenly begins to get better and within a few hours is without high fever. He feels much better, his pulse is better, his breathing is slower, and in every way he is improved. In most instances the recovery is gradual. Recovery is due to the fact that the blood of the patient has developed the power to overcome the germ of the disease.

In preventing pneumonia remember that contact with those who are infected is the chief source of its spread. Certainly, a baby should not be taken into a room in which someone is suffering from pneumonia. Mothers must do everything possible to prevent their children from coming in contact with other children who have running noses, coughs, colds, and sore throats. It is especially important to protect children against sharp falls in temperatures which, through centuries of experience, have been associated with the onset of fall and winter colds.

In some cities people with pneumonia are isolated, as with other serious infectious diseases. This has not yet been done on sufficiently large a scale to permit accurate estimation of the worth of the procedure, but there is reason to believe that its effect may be definitely for good.

The person attending a patient with pneumonia should wear a clean gown which is changed before contact with other people. The hands should be thoroughly cleaned with soap and water after attending the patient. The room of the patient should be kept as clean as possible and thoroughly aired, washed, and sunned after the patient's recovery.

When a person is isolated for an infectious disease the utensils, bedclothing, personal clothing, handkerchiefs, and other material in close contact with him should be sterilized. They should be kept separate from similar materials used by other members of the family.

Most important in the care of the patient with pneumonia is to keep him as quiet as possible, both mentally and physically, and to give him the best possible nursing care. The difference between good and bad nursing may mean the difference between life and death.

Because of the importance of proper care and nursing in such a case, most physicians feel that a patient with pneumonia is better off in a hospital than at home. Moreover, it is better to get the patient under good care early and not to wait until he has reached a critical stage before transferring him to a hospital.

The patient with pneumonia should have a large, well-ventilated room with plenty of access to good fresh air. This does not mean that a patient with pneumonia is to be exposed to storm and stress. In inclement weather it is much better to prevent such additional exposure. The patient himself is frequently the best judge as to when he is breathing with most ease and least distress.

The number of visitors must be kept to a minimum. The patient should not have to worry about troubles in the family or business affairs and must be kept flat on his back for at least a week after recovery has begun. Only gradually is he allowed to assume a sitting posture.

The diet in this condition, as in any serious infection, must be chiefly liquids such as soups, gruels, milk, and soft-boiled eggs. Occasionally it is well to add milk sugar to keep up the energy. Rest and quiet are more important even than nourishment in the serious stages of pneumonia. When recovery has begun, feeding is gradually extended so as to aid the improvement of the blood and the broken-down tissues.

It is well for patients with pneumonia to have plenty of water. This does not mean, however, much more than two to three quarts a day. The patient will not drink unless the water is given to him when he is quite sick. Under such circumstances it is perhaps best to give water with a teaspoon, giving small amounts frequently, or to have the patient suck small pieces of ice.

Of greatest importance in the treatment of pneumonia is care directed by a competent physician. He himself must direct the nursing and determine its value. He himself must administer proper remedies at the proper time in order to support the extra work of the heart, in order to relieve stress from the circulation, in order to permit the patient to sleep, and in order to control the actions of the bowels, the skin, and of all the other organs. There is no substitute of any kind for the type of care that a well-trained physician can give in this disease.

The use of oxygen in the treatment of pneumonia is exceedingly valuable. Tents have been developed which may be placed over the patients as they lie in bed, and many large hospitals have oxygen rooms into which the entire bed may be moved and in which the nurse may remain and attend the patient. Oxygen is not to be considered an emergency measure to be applied when the patient is at the point of death, but instead one which is to be used promptly when the physician feels that it is required.

While any of the sulfonamide drugs are useful in the treatment of pneumonia, most frequently used nowadays is sulfadiazine, which is less toxic. Penicillin, chlortetracycline and oxytetracycline as well as newer antibiotics are valuable in the attack on the pneumonia germ. Large amounts of penicillin can be given by injection into the muscles and a sufficiently high level of penicillin maintained in the blood to bring about prompt control of the infection.

The former fatality rate of 25 to 30 per cent in pneumonia has now dropped to 5 per cent.

VIRUS PNEUMONIA

The pneumonia that is caused by the pneumococcus is now recognized as distinct from virus pneumonia. Fortunately virus pneumonia is not as serious a disease as lobar pneumonia. Deaths from virus pneumonia are exceedingly rare. Various antibiotics are recommended for this condition to control possible secondary infections.

TUBERCULOSIS

The protection of mankind against tuberculosis is based on two principles which were formulated by the famous Pasteur and Robert Koch. The first is to preserve the child against infection with the germ of tuberculosis by removing it from contaminated surroundings; the second is the isolation of the sick and the education of the well in the prevention of the disease.

Tuberculosis is a social disease in the sense that it affects groups of mankind as well as individuals. Second, it is involved with the economic status of those who are infected. For example, in Vienna in 1913 deaths from tuberculosis were five times higher in the poorer quarters than in the better class quarters.

Tuberculosis attacks all races, all ages of mankind, and indeed all classes of human society, but it is largely a disease of poverty and malnutrition. The number of deaths from tuberculosis per hundred thousand of population is steadily decreasing throughout the world.

The death rate drops among people who have had tuberculosis for many decades. The death rate rises when tuberculosis comes into a country area or into a district in which the population has previously been relatively free from tuberculosis. The coming of the industrial era with crowding and long hours of labor produced a higher death rate for this disease. Then came the protection of labor, particularly of child labor, social hygiene, improved nutrition and improved housing, with a lowering of the rates for tuberculosis.

With the truly extensive knowledge of tuberculosis which we have, its complete prevention ultimately should be a possibility. However, perfect success in a problem of this kind is not likely in a day, a month, or even a generation.

The path to prevention seems to be clear. Young children must not be exposed to infection, or, in any event, the possibility of infection in young children must be reduced to a minimum.

Let us consider what this means in our modern civilization. Human contacts have been multiplied enormously. Today the home has largely disappeared in our great cities; instead, we have the apartment house, housing from three to fifty families. Obviously under such circumstances children are exposed not only to their own parents and relatives, but to vast numbers of other children and other families.

The child of an earlier day played in its own backyard at least until the age of six. Today it goes early to nursery school and thereafter to kindergarten. Moreover, human beings now assemble in crowds of thousands in motion-picture houses and of tens and hundreds of thousands at baseball and football games.

It is easy enough to suggest that young children be not admitted to the presence of known consumptives. It is far more difficult to establish the principle that they be kept out of all gatherings where they may be exposed to infection from unknown sources.

There are, of course, still some differences of opinion as to the proper procedure for eliminating tuberculosis. We are not at this time prepared to isolate all carriers of the germs of this disease or to exterminate them. The fact is emphasized when it is realized that practically everyone has had the disease by the time he is fifteen. Were this not the case, the mortality among adults would be terrific. The earlier infection establishes a resistance against the severe infection of later years.

The Negroes in the crowded districts in northern cities have the highest tuberculosis rate of any group in the community. The Mexican population of Chicago has eleven times the average rate of the rest of the population.

The attack on tuberculosis has been thus far an economic attack. Realizing that it is primarily a disease associated with bad hygiene, great importance has been placed on physical well being.

The treatment consisted largely of good diet, sufficient rest and fresh air. Special attention was paid to housing and types of employment, to the prices of food and wages, since it has been shown that a drop in wages is usually related to an increase in tuberculosis.

In the United States the number of beds available for patients with this disease increased from 10,000 in 1904 to more than 100,000 in recent years. Moreover, there has been a tremendous growth in open-air schools, preventoriums, clinics, and dispensaries.

With the development of new methods of diagnosis and treatment of tuberculosis the demand for sanitarium beds is decreasing. In 1954 and 1955 many sanitariums for tuberculosis were closed, including the famous Trudeau Sanitarium at Saranac Lake, N. Y. More and more patients are being treated while ambulatory with the newer drugs including streptomycin, para-aminosalicylic acid (PAS), and isoniazid.

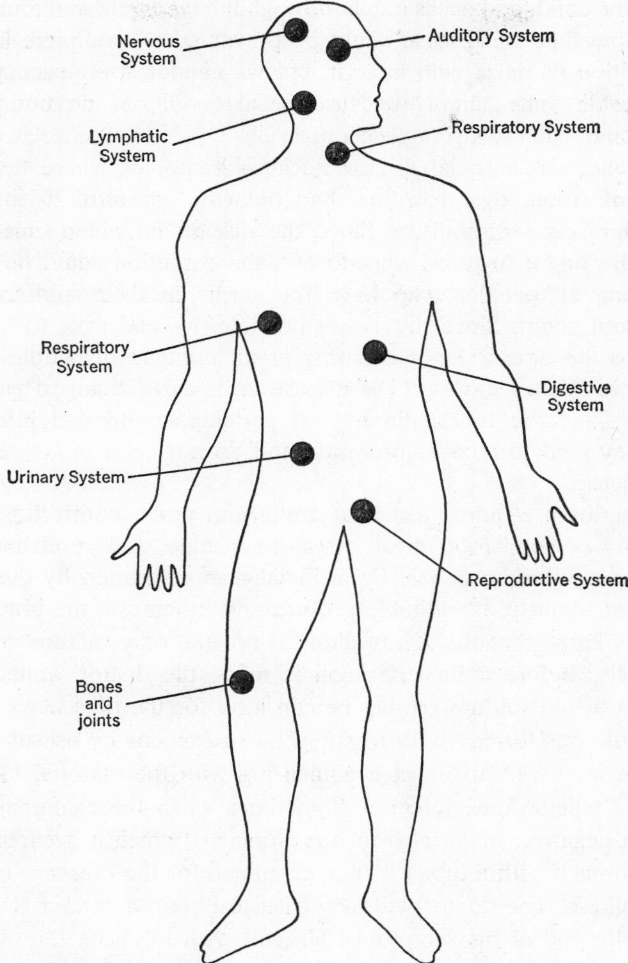

Fig. 41. TB's Other Targets. Tuberculosis most commonly attacks the lungs, yet it may be found in other parts of the body. TB germs, which are usually breathed in the air and lodge at first in the lungs, may invade other organs of the body in either of two ways: sputum containing TB germs is coughed up from the lungs into the throat and mouth; the other route which TB germs travel is through the blood and lymph systems. Among other parts of the body which may become tuberculous are: the digestive system (intestines or rectum); respiratory system (bronchial tubes); auditory system; lymphatic system; bones and joints; urinary system; reproductive system (the Fallopian or uterine tubes in the female and the prostate gland in the male); and the nervous system. National Tuberculosis Association.

In tuberculosis, we know the cause of the disease: namely, the germ of bacillus of tuberculosis. We know the method of transmission, which is from the patient with the disease to the person who does not have it, particularly the child, and occasionally through infected milk and food.

We know that the disease could be prevented by complete isolation or extermination of those who have it, but we cannot apply such procedures on a suitable scale, simply because social conditions do not permit the application of such stringent procedures.

Tuberculosis is a social disease because it spreads where there is poverty, malnutrition, overcrowding, bad housing, exposure to the elements and similar social disabilities. Since the disease is spread chiefly from a person who has it to those who do not, the condition could be controlled by isolating all persons who have the germs in their sputum and who spread them about. Since this is not possible, we endeavor to increase resistance to the disease by inoculating great numbers of people with BCG vaccination. We try to detect the disease in its earliest stages by the use of the X ray and the tuberculin test. If patients are treated in such early stages, they tend to recover promptly and do not become active spreaders of the disease.

The condition requires rest in a sanitarium under controlled conditions with plenty of good food, fresh air and sunshine, and good hygiene. The ailing lung can be put at rest by artificial pneumothorax, by the operation called thoracoplasty, by suitable posture and by cutting the phrenic nerve.

Doctors know that the X ray alone is not the only method of detecting tuberculosis. Before a final decision is made the doctor wants to obtain specimens of the sputum so that he can look for the presence of the germ of tuberculosis. He may wish to study the specimens by use of the microscope. He may wish to inject a guinea pig with the material to see if the guinea pig will become infected. Sometimes when the examination of the sputum is negative, material from the stomach (which is secured by washing the stomach with a tube) is then examined for the presence of the germ of tuberculosis. The doctor will also wish to obtain a careful record of the person's life and of his symptoms. He will wish to check the observations by studies of the chest, by percussion or thumping or by listening with the stethoscope.

The following hints for good hygiene in tuberculosis come from the National Tuberculosis Association:

"Babies and little children must stay out of your room. You must insist on this, because they are very likely to catch your germs. The best plan is to send them somewhere else to live while you are sick.

"Do not allow pets in your room.

"Never allow anyone or any animal to eat the food or drink that has been in your room. Left-over food should be burned; if liquid, poured into the toilet.

"Do not let visitors come close to you, shake hands with you, handle your things, or put their coats, hats, gloves, etc., on your bed.

"Never kiss or allow anyone to kiss you! This is a hard rule to obey—probably the hardest for most families. You will have to be the one to insist on it, since if you forbid kissing and remind the family of the danger, they will be less likely to think you want to be kissed, or are feeling hurt at their neglect. Kissing is a very easy way to spread your germs. Show your real affection for your family by refusing to kiss or be kissed.

"Your doctor or nurse will teach your family what to do with your dishes, linen, and other soiled articles, but the most essential thing for you to remember is this: *Protect others from your sputum!*

"Your sputum (spit or phlegm) is dangerous because there are tuberculosis germs in it. Everything your sputum soils is dangerous to others. Therefore you must catch your sputum when it comes as spit or spray from your mouth and nose in sneezing, coughing or spitting. You do this by covering your nose and mouth with paper tissues or soft old rags and burning them after use. Your supply of tissues should be placed beside your pillow or on the bedside table where you can reach them without stretching. Then do as follows:

"1. Take one or two and hold them in your cupped hand, protecting your hand and fingers. You may need two thicknesses of material.

"2. Cover both your nose and mouth.

"3. After use, drop the tissue into a paper bag (grocery bag, or one made of newspaper) pinned to the side of your bed or bedside table, where you can reach it without stretching and without missing.

"When the bag of soiled tissues is about three-quarters full, it should be taken out by your family helper and burned. Do not fill the bag so full that anyone has to touch the soiled tissues in unpinning and holding the bag.

"Never cough, sneeze or spit without using the paper tissue or rags in this way. Always turn your head away from anyone when you cough or sneeze. Later, when you are up, the doctor may let you use a sputum cup (a metal container with a paper filler), but tissues are safer.

"Try to remember that everything soiled or sprayed by the moisture from your nose and mouth is dangerous to others. Be careful! Have your set of toilet articles, toothbrush, towels, shaving kit, and, if allowed, smoking supplies. You can save your family helper many steps and much trouble by being careful about this rule of separate belongings. Your linen and dishes must be boiled before being used by other members of the family."

DIET IN TUBERCULOSIS

The diet is important in the treatment of tuberculosis. Some people simply do not get enough food. Many people are badly fed because they do not know how to select the right foods and to make the best use of what food they have. There seems to be not the slightest question but that malnutrition has an extremely unfavorable effect on the death rate from tuberculosis.

The charts of deaths from tuberculosis show a high peak in earliest infancy, then a definite drop in the rate during later infancy and school age, and a rise at the beginning of adolescence. This points definitely to the periods when children must be most closely watched for the development of symptoms and when everything possible must be done to keep up their nutrition and to see to it that they have plenty of rest and good hygiene.

CONTROL OF TUBERCULOUS CATTLE

Of special importance in the prevention of tuberculosis is the control of tuberculous cattle. The germ of tuberculosis of the type which lives in cattle is rather rare as a cause of tuberculosis of the abdomen, the glands, the bones, and the joints. There are certain methods for controlling tuberculosis in cattle which are now subject to legislation in this country.

In the first place, milk for children, unless coming from cattle free from tuberculosis, must invariably be pasteurized, and in fact it is probably better to pasteurize all milk for children—at least there is more certainty of safety. Second, it is desirable to stamp out tuberculosis among cattle. This is commonly done by testing cattle for the presence of the disease and then destroying all that are infected, at the same time compensating the owners for the loss of the animals.

CLIMATE AND TUBERCULOSIS

Dr. James Alexander Miller tabulated certain conclusions which should be borne in mind by every person with tuberculosis who may contemplate a change of climate.

Here they are:

1. The regimen of regulated rest and exercise, proper food and open-air life, is the fundamental essential in the treatment of tuberculosis. Suitable climatic environment makes this open-air life more easy, enjoyable, and beneficial.

2. When these essentials are assured, a change of climate is of definite value in a considerable number, probably the majority, of cases, but with the proper regimen many cases will do well in any climate.

3. Any change of climate involving the fatigue of travel is contraindicated in acute cases with fever or hemorrhage, or in very far advanced and markedly debilitated cases. Absolute bed rest is the one essential here.

4. No patient should be sent away in search of climate who cannot afford to stay the reasonably expected time and to have the necessary food, lodging and care.

5. Competent medical advice and supervision are essential.

6. One of the most valuable assets of change is the education of the patient. This may, of course, be obtained in a suitable environment without reference to climate, as in a sanitarium near home.

7. Selection of a suitable locality is an individual problem for every patient, depending upon his temperament, tastes, and individual reaction to environment, as well as the character of his disease. The advising physician should have an appreciation of these as well as a knowledge of the particular environment to which the patient is being sent. Contentment and reasonable comfort are essential.

8. There is no universally ideal climate. For each patient there may well be a most favorable environment, if we are wise enough to find it.

9. There is a reasonable amount of evidence that certain medical types of cases are more favorably influenced by certain conditions of climate, everything else being equal. For example, reasonably cold, dry, variable climate, such as is found in the mountains, for young or vigorous constitutions which will react well. Dry, sunny climates for laryngeal cases and those with marked catarrhal secretions. Equable mild climates at low altitudes for the elderly and those of nervous temperaments, as well as for those with arteriosclerosis, weak hearts, or marked tendency to dyspnœa.

10. Successful selection of climate and environment for cases of tuberculosis requires wide knowledge of human nature, of places, and of the disease. This can only be acquired by patience, skill, and experience.

SKIN TESTS FOR TUBERCULOSIS

Many years ago it was proved that almost every human being has tuberculosis before he dies.

Indeed, the vast majority of people become infected with the disease in childhood and recover. However, a considerable number do not recover, and these represent the constant mortality from this disease. The death rate from tuberculosis has been cut tremendously through the advancement of modern medical science and modern hygiene.

In order to detect cases as early as possible and to apply as soon as possible suitable methods leading toward recovery, several systems have been established. The first is to examine all school children physically and by means of the X ray and to give all of them the tuberculin test. The tuberculin test is a simple skin test, less painful than a pin scratch and much less dangerous.

One of the advantages of such a procedure is the fact that during the physical examination for tuberculosis, it is also possible to detect any other disease which may happen to be attacking the child.

Another method is to select from among school children those who seem particularly likely to have tuberculosis and to limit the examination to them. When a child is found to be positive to the tuberculin test, a thorough study is made of its physical conditions, then the X-ray examination is made. The X ray reveals even small changes which may have taken place in the lungs.

If a child is found to be susceptible to tuberculosis or in a very early stage it can be put under a course of hygiene which will aid its prompt recovery in the vast majority of cases.

One of the modern developments in the care of tuberculosis is the establishment of the preventorium to which children are taken who have very mild degrees of tuberculosis or who come of families in which tuberculosis is prevalent. There they have opportunity to recover under the best conditions.

REST IN TUBERCULOSIS

Since rest is the most important single measure in aiding recovery from minimal tuberculosis in its early stages, the provision of adequate facilities in a sanitarium is fundamental to the control of tuberculosis in any community. Some states already have more beds than they need because of lowered number of cases.

Rest, fresh air, and food, it has been repeatedly emphasized, are the important trilogy by which the person with tuberculosis must regulate his life. The sanitarium teaches the person how to follow this trilogy automatically and as an everyday procedure.

The person with active symptoms must have absolute rest. As symptoms quiet down the competent physician is able to tell the patient how much exercise is to be taken along with the rest to secure the best results. To most people fresh air means a lusty breeze pouring through a window or below-zero weather on an outdoor sleeping porch. It is important to realize that fresh air does not demand physical discomfort. Windows may be kept open, but the temperature should be equable, and drafts are unnecessary.

One of the chief values of the sanitarium is to teach the patient the routine facts regarding such matters as rest, exercise, diet, and fresh air. It will teach him also how to prevent the contamination of clothing, dishes, and other human beings with the organisms that are in his body. It will teach him his limitations in work and help to find work that he can do.

Thus will it have fulfilled a most useful function and when he is improved sufficiently to be on his way, the place he occupied will be filled by another pupil, and he will go out to help educate the public.

TREATMENT OF TUBERCULOSIS

For many years all sorts of specific remedies have been tried on the tuberculous, and millions of dollars have been mulcted from the people for patent medicines.

The first drug proved to be specific against the germ of tuberculosis is streptomycin. It seems to have established value in tuberculous meningitis, in miliary tuberculosis (which spreads rapidly throughout the lung) and in very severe cases of tuberculosis when there is secondary infection with pus in the chest cavity. The drug is also of value in tuberculosis of the kidney, the peritoneum and of the intestines. At present physicians do not believe that streptomycin should be used in the mild, early cases of tuberculosis because these cases are best cured by older techniques which establish suitable resistance in the patient. The use of streptomycin in tuberculosis, combined with para-aminosalicylic acid (PAS), and the combination of streptomycin with drugs like promin or diasone or tibione, which are sulfonamide derivatives, may bring about even more satisfactory improvement. The drugs are not a cure for tuberculosis; they supplement bed rest and specific methods of resting the lung.

Newest among drugs in tuberculosis are preparations of hydrazides of isonicotinic acid called isoniazid including remiofon, marsalid and pyrazidin. They bring about improvement, aid appetite and give a feeling of well-being.

People with tuberculosis suffer frequently with fever and sweating at night. When these symptoms become oppressive, the doctor can prescribe drugs which will control them. An alcohol rub at bedtime or a sponge bath with lukewarm water containing about one gram of alum to the ounce is also helpful.

One of the most severe symptoms that may occur in a patient with tuberculosis is bleeding from the lungs. The appearance of this symptom is a danger signal which should cause the patient to lie down immediately and to get medical attention at once.

In the sanitarium in which the patients are treated for tuberculosis, one of the most useful remedies thus far developed is artificial pneumothorax. This involves the injection of air into the chest cavity, which serves to put the lung at rest. The same effect is also brought about by cutting the nerve which leads to the diaphragm, or by performing surgical operation on the ribs.

Tuberculosis could probably be completely controlled if every case with germs in the sputum could be isolated until freed of germs.

MENTAL ASPECTS IN TUBERCULOSIS

One of the most important factors in the care of the tuberculous is the cooperation of the patient in the handling of his disease.

In a thesis prepared in the University of Minnesota, Blanche Peterson insists that the most important single factor in the cure of tuberculosis is an intelligent attitude of the patient.

Doctors, nurses, and social workers endeavor, therefore, in every possible way to influence the patient to assume an intelligent and constructive outlook.

A questionnaire sent to a score of leading physicians who have specialized in this subject resulted in the almost universal response that reasonable and courageous attitudes are highly constructive. The worst states are those of fear, anxiety, and depression.

The patient with tuberculosis who becomes discouraged, hopeless, pessimistic, or rebellious is difficult to treat and aids in his downfall.

When a person first learns that he has this disease, he is likely to be upset and depressed. Knowing nothing of modern care, he is likely to feel that the disease will be promptly fatal.

If, however, the physician who makes the diagnosis will tell the patient that help is possible, that the disease is curable if treated sufficiently early and sufficiently long; that dozens of persons have achieved world-wide fame even though suffering from this disease, he is likely to have a different attitude and to cooperate fully in treatment.

Courage and reasonableness can come only with complete understanding of the situation. For this reason the health education of the tuberculous has come to be one of the most important factors in the control of this condition, and a vast literature has been developed for the purpose.

Practically every tuberculosis sanitarium and tuberculosis society now publishes books and pamphlets which are helpful in informing the tuberculous of the important facts relative to their condition.

The National Tuberculosis Association, 1790 Broadway, New York City, publishes much material that is useful. Such books as the guides and calendars for the tuberculous, edited by Lawrason Brown, are exceedingly helpful.[1]

Above all, the persons living with and surrounding the tuberculous must realize that it is their duty to keep the patient in a hopeful frame of mind and not treat him as a helpless invalid from the moment the diagnosis is made.

[1] *Laws for Recovery from Pulmonary Tuberculosis.* Lawrason Brown, Saranac Lake, N. Y.

HEALTH HINTS FOR THE TUBERCULOUS

Here are some hints for people with tuberculosis. Many of these hints constitute excellent advice regarding hygiene for everyone who is slightly run down, whether tuberculous or not.

1. Never exercise to the point of fatigue. If you find yourself tired, you have done yourself harm.
2. Rest comes before exercise. By resting a surplus of strength and energy is built up and stored in the body.
3. Aim to spend as much of each day outdoors or in absolutely fresh air as possible. The air, to be fresh, need not necessarily be cold.
4. Ideal food should be appetizing, nutritious, and not too bulky. If appetizing and not nutritious, it will not nourish you; if nutritious and not appetizing, you will not eat it; if too bulky, however appetizing, it upsets your stomach.
5. Eat up to the limit of your digestion. It is the food which is digested and absorbed, and not what is put into your mouth, which will do you good. A glass of milk with each meal is advisable. Raw eggs are not as digestible as cooked eggs.
6. If your digestion is poor, tell your doctor.
7. Eat your meals at regular hours. Do not take reading matter to the table.
8. Approach and leave each meal in a rested condition. Never eat when tired. Never exercise immediately after eating.
9. In winter, wear warm, light, or medium wool underwear; in summer, ordinary summer cotton underwear.
10. Never wear heavy underclothing or chest protectors.
11. Let your shoes be stout and warm in winter and wear warm woolen socks, by all means. Woolen socks at night are often a great comfort. In winter, a flannel shirt is much more comfortable than anything else. When sitting out in winter, have an extra wrap near by.
12. If you get overheated and perspire, change your clothing and rub dry.
13. A healthy condition of the skin is most important. A warm bath once or twice a week if ordered by your physician is advisable, and a cool sponge bath or a tub bath in the morning if your doctor permits it. The water should be cool but not ice cold. If you do not have a proper reaction after your bath, if you feel chilly or are blue, the water is too cold. Ask your doctor about it. See that your room or bathroom or wherever you take your bath is warm.

ULTRAVIOLET RAY IN TUBERCULOSIS OF THE LARYNX

Tuberculosis of the larynx has been considered, until recent years, one of the most dangerous forms of the disease, leading usually to fatality.

The drugs such as streptomycin and isoniazid are used. Tuberculosis in any part of the body demands careful treatment with the methods that are used for tuberculosis of the lungs and special methods designed for kidneys, skin, larynx or other part that may be involved.

With the discovery of the apparatus which yielded ultraviolet rays, in the form of the carbon arc and the quartz mercury vapor lamps, it became possible to apply concentrated sun's rays directly to the larynx. In order to get the rays directly to the laryngeal cords, various systems of mirrors have been devised, and also quartz stems along which the ultraviolet rays pass.

It has been found that people who are very frail, those with advanced tuberculosis of the lung, and those who have very severe lesions in the throat are treated better by means of the mirror reflection than by other methods.

A steel mirror will reflect about 44 per cent of the valuable rays into the larynx whereas ordinary glass mirrors absorb these rays and reflect only about 9 per cent. It has been found that practically all of the patients treated by direct sunlight to the cords tend to heal.

CONCLUSIONS

Particularly of importance in controlling the spread of tuberculosis is the use of dispensaries in which the disease can be diagnosed in its earliest stages and properly controlled. Experimentation with the method of vaccination against tuberculosis by Calmette has not yet gone sufficiently far to warrant its general adoption in this country.

The most powerful social factors in controlling the disease are housing, nutrition, and education. In educating people, it is desirable to educate them not only in general hygiene but also especially as regards the prevention of tuberculosis. The regular examination of school children and teachers, studies of the nutrition of the school child, and education of those who are infected in methods of preventing the spread of the disease are significant factors.

The preventive institutions against tuberculosis today include holiday camps, open-air schools, preventoriums for children who are perhaps not certainly infected with tuberculosis but in such poor state of nutrition and general health that they offer easy prey to the disease, and certainly removal of children as soon as possible from contact with adults who are infected.

CHAPTER 14

Stress and Disease

RAYMOND D. ADAMS, M.D.*

The idea of a possible relationship between psychological disturbance and disease dates far back into the antiquity of medicine. But only in the past two or three decades has it been subjected to more precise observations and scientific scrutiny. The influence of psychosocial factors in illness has now become so widely accepted that almost every person tends to ascribe his many ails to the situation in which he finds himself. This allows of the possibility of error in two directions: one, the false attribution of disease to nervousness, fatigue, and worry when in fact the causation is of quite different nature; the other, the false attribution of a nervous state to some more strictly organic, pathological process in the visceral organs when in fact the functional derangement is due to anger, fear, or despondency.

The word "stress" in itself is not apt, for it has many other meanings in our language; some refer to the effects of physical force, others refer to accent or emphasis. In medicine stress has still another meaning: the sum total of unfavorable environmental agencies which cause either normal or maladaptive processes within the human body. These processes may take the form of a temporary disturbance of function without any apparent physical basis, or lead to a demonstrable lesion, i.e., a gross or microscopic change in the tissues themselves. The former of these might be roughly classified as a normal but distressing reaction, often mistaken for illness; the latter is generally accepted as a disease per se. The distinction between these two conditions is not easy. Disease defined as a state in which there is a lesion or demonstrable change in an organ is too restrictive and must be broadened to include those states in which an anatomic abnormality may be inferred because of a consistent physical or biochemical disturbance. In many established diseases such as delirium tremens, coma due to kidney disease (uremia) or sugar diabetes, and mongolian idiocy, even the most meticulous postmortem examination of the brain tissues fails to show a consistent structural change under the microscope.

* This chapter has been modified and re-edited from the original chapter written by Dr. Harold G. Wolff for an earlier edition.

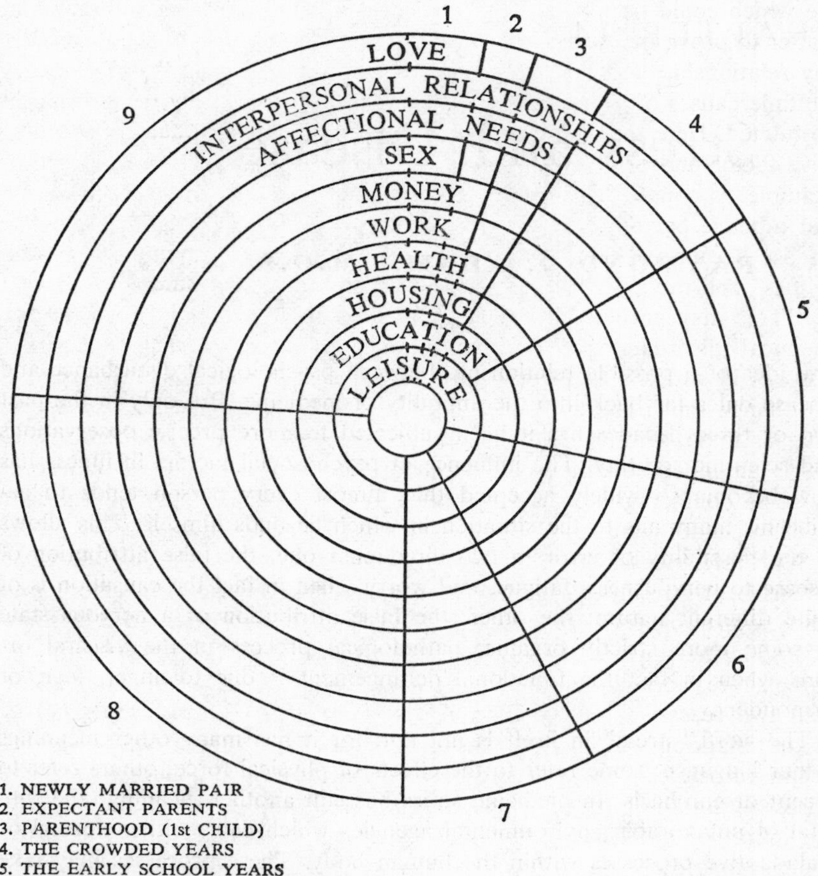

Fig. 42. Family life concerns. This chart identifies ten concerns. Each concern assumes varying degrees of importance at various life cycle stages. Not only are these and other concerns of interest throughout the life cycle, but also they are interrelated. Their interrelationships are complex. Further, the relationships between these concerns shifts as the individual of the family progresses through the stages of the cycle. American Social Health Association.

In theorizing about the causes of many obscure diseases the medical profession has tended to rationalize the problem in one of two ways; the first is to invoke in all abstruse illness a psychological or environmental stress, presumably unknown to the patient; the second is to invoke for any mysterious disorder multiple causation. With a little probing every patient will be found to have worries and unresolved difficulties in his daily life which could be related to a medical complaint. But it is quite another matter to prove their relevance to an illness. Neurotic persons tend to deny any relationship between worry and disease. In declaring the existence of multiple causes of a disease, when one is not known, many factors may be postulated. Here the difficulty is one of evaluating the primacy of the causative factor and of giving weight to the different factors. Tuberculosis, for example, is caused by a bacterium entering the lungs through inhalation. But tubercle bacteria are inhaled by many people who do not develop the disease because of their general state of health, racial immunity, or other factors. The tubercle bacillus is the primary cause; the others are secondary. This may be illustrated even more strikingly in certain inherited biochemical disorders due to abnormalities of germ plasm, i.e., genetic diseases in which a faulty gene or chromosome may result in a biochemical change that never expresses itself unless the person receives a certain drug or toxin which he cannot metabolize. Many believe that schizophrenia is an inherited disease in which the symptoms are often occasioned by some conflictual situation occurring in the patient's personal life, again an example of the operation of primary and secondary causes.

With reference to the appearance of genetic diseases, the concept is not exclusive of stress, since the latter may evoke symptoms in an organism made vulnerable by heredity. Parenthetically, such diseases need not have existed in the parents or have been present at birth. In recessive traits the parents are normal and only when they mate, thus producing children with two recessive traits, will a disease arise. Then a predictable portion of the offspring will have the disease, according to well established Mendelian principles. The causative factor is endogenous, that is to say, it arises within the body. Unless it blights early development before birth, the infant or child may be normal for years until finally some chemical change caused by the defective gene begins to damage the organism. If recognized early, before tissue injury has occurred, the biochemical change may be controlled and thus its effects or progress prevented.

If one uses the word "stress" to apply to all environmental factors, such as psychological threat, inadequate or unbalanced diet, the ingestion of substances that may prove toxic, then stress may figure in the creation of disease in many ways. However, as medical thought has evolved, the concept of stress has been restricted more and more to psychological and social influences, with a tendency to ignore the effects of undernutrition and the physical climatic and geographic conditions in which man lives. The reason for this emphasis is that the social factors in man's environment are amongst the most ubiquitous, the most complex and difficult to analyze. Modern man is a gregarious creature. He seldom stays alone for any period of time, preferring to be a member of some type of group, whether it be family, community, or nation. Growth, maturation, and education involve fundamentally a broad series of adjustments between man's private impulses for survival, personal need, sexual gratification, or other goals, and those rival influences of self-discipline, continence, and altruism demanded by society. People seem to be the most poignant source of human emotional disturbance; man is above all creatures the most susceptible to "crowd diseases." The degree of stress felt by anyone is in a sense inversely proportional to the success of his ability to adjust to the social forces which surround him.

MAINTAINING THE STABILITY OF THE BODY (HOMEOSTASIS)

The health and survival of the human organism as it moves around in its varied physical and social environment depends on the maintenance of a stable fluid and chemical balance in all the vital organs of the body. The precision of the physiological mechanics in the maintenance of this stability is almost incredible. Man's fluid needs are maintained by thirst, which is adjusted to losses of fluid through the kidneys, respired air, and sweat. A regulating mechanism in the center of the brain indicates the slightest deviation from a particular standard and adjusts the fluid intake to the fluid loss within fine limits. Similarly man's appetite for food is adjusted precisely to his energy requirements so that the average person rarely changes weight more than a few ounces in a year's time. Temperature regulation, sleep, oxygenation of the blood, the levels of sodium, potassium, calcium, magnesium, and all the essential chemical substances that maintain the activity of cell membranes are also finely adjusted. The regulation of all of these complex systems is through the vegetative nervous system, the central control of which is in the hypothalamus, a series of groups of nerve cells in the center of the brain just above the pituitary gland, which controls the entire endocrine-hormonal system (thyroid, parathyroid, ovaries, testes, adrenal cortex, and medulla). At every level in this neurovegetative-hormonal system a change at one point results in compensation at another with constant feedback control.

The adjustments in the autonomic or sympathetic nervous system and endocrine system provide not only for the homeostasis or stability of the internal organs but are the basis of all instinctual and emotional reactions. These latter are unlearned and unconscious, being to a large extent built into the form and structure of the organism. Nature has thought it prudent to place these functions outside "the control of an ignorant will" as was shrewdly remarked by the great French physiologist Claude Bernard.

The conditions of the external environment are prevented from exerting prolonged and significant changes in the internal environment of the body by adjustments effected by the nerve-controlled and glandular mechanism. Some of the most extreme of these effects necessarily require effective action on the part of the whole organism, as when it is threatened by violence or provoked to intense anger or to powerful amiable feelings. Each of these emotional states is associated with alterations in the autonomic or vegetative nervous system and the endocrine system, preparing the human for flight, fight, or approach. Man's awareness of the danger and of his own organ changes constitutes the experiences which we recognize as emotional.

Peculiar to the human organism, however, is the degree to which minor degrees of environmental stress can be differentiated and future ones anticipated. This is largely a matter of education and training (learning). Indeed, man may be aroused to an emotional state when only a word symbol such as a description of the effective stimulus is presented. The differentiation of these situations or the meaningful symbols thereof involves the action of many parts of the cerebrum that are not to be found in the nervous system of the largest primates such as the gorilla or orangutan. Thus one might conceive of man's nervous system as a great nervous and muscle apparatus whereby information about the environment is transmitted through the sensory system to evoke movement of the organism and effect vegetative adjustment. And human instinctual and emotional reactions, then, can always be viewed as having an unconscious (visceral) and conscious aspect.

Persistent stimulation of the autonomic or vegetative systems by stressful situations may tax the organism's capacity to adjust and give rise to functional disorders that simulate disease.

THE RELATION OF ANXIETY AND MOOD DEPRESSION TO THE PRIMARY EMOTIONAL STATES

In everyday life man is subjected to rather few life-threatening situations or highly charged emotional circumstances. Instead, he is more likely to be involved in conditions that give rise to milder and more protracted states of emotion expressed as anxiety, worry, discouragement, and depression or their opposites. These latter may be viewed as milder forms of the stronger emotions. Unlike the strong primary emotional states, however, anxiety and depression may be evoked by either a recognizable stimulus or environmental situation of which the person himself is aware, or they may occur without the subject knowing their cause. These latter are believed to be unconscious emotional reactions and are often aroused by only the symbols of dangerous situations. The relation between these symbols and their attendant emotion may only be elicited after a series of interviews which explore the pattern of the person's behavior through free association (psychoanalysis). Once the patient sees the connection, the effects of the emotion on the organs of the body lose their mysterious quality, being now but the normal emotional reaction of a healthy person. The evocative stimulus then is dealt with in realistic fashion.

Some of the control mechanisms of the nervous system whereby irrelevant stimuli are suppressed or the reactions to stimuli inhibited may be deranged by body chemicals may suffer internal derangements as part of an innate disease. The patient is plunged into a state of dejection or apprehension which bears no relationship to real or fancied environmental stimulus. Indeed, the patient while in the throes of his disturbed emotional state may in fact alter his environment or single out only those stimuli which are compatible with his mood. *Thus worry or concern about particular situations may be the effect rather than the cause of his condition.* These two almost antithetical possibilities of human reaction have been the source of grave confusion in medicine and have led to two almost diametrically opposed hypotheses about mental illness and disease. Neither concept seems universally applicable to all medical problems and each has its place. But the first hypothesis—that many of the serious derangements of the human organism are consequent to real or fancied environmental stresses—shall be examined more critically here.

WAYS IN WHICH THE BODILY FUNCTIONS OF MAN MAY BE DISTURBED BY CHRONIC EMOTION

The fact that strong emotion may disturb the functions of various organs in the body is widely known. Our language contains phrases indicating that men have long been aware of the relationship between their feelings and bodily changes. We hear, for example, "that he was pale with rage"; "it took one's breath away"; "he was in a cold sweat"; "it makes me sick"; "it turns my stomach"; "I had a lump in my throat"; "he got a weight off his chest"; "he trembled with fear"; "he shook with rage"; "he had cold feet." The frequency with which the heart and circulation are engaged in these emotional states has led to the common belief that they must stem from the heart. In the index of Bartlett's Familiar Quotations one can find nine columns of phrases including the word "heart." Also, in the index of Roget's Thesaurus the word "heart" appears more than any other word. Indeed, the heart has come to stand as the symbol of the human spirit, hence the words hardhearted, warmhearted, coldhearted, steelhearted. But even a moment's reflection will bring to mind other organ or tissue effects which man has come to identify with his feelings and mood; he speaks of them as though they were the sources of the emotion. How important these changes are to ill health and how they disturb a man's effectiveness or even jeopardize his life will be next discussed.

SKIN

The skin undergoes some of the most dramatic changes during stress. For example, the state of the minute vessels of man's skin, called for convenience *capillary tone,* if tested as regards the ability to retain blood is readily modifiable. If the left arm be forcibly struck, immediately a red area appears which begins to swell, indicating a deterioration of the capillary tone. But curious as it may seem, the skin of the right arm sometimes behaves in the same way even though it is not struck. Then the left arm gradually returns to its former state, whereas the right arm recovers a little sooner. If the experiment is repeated but instead of actually striking the arm the blow does not make contact with it, being brought up just short of the arm, the skin of the left arm behaves just as if it had been struck. The skin of the right arm does not respond. Gradually the left arm returns to its former state. In other words, the subject, through his skin, reacts not only to an actual blow but also to the symbol of the blow by releasing histamine into his tissues, thus causing dilatation of the blood vessels and the escape of a certain amount of blood plasma. This seems to represent not only a reaction to tissue injury but also a means of protecting it against serious damage. The whole procedure may be repeated, except that this time the subject is warned of what will happen. Now the expected sham blow fails to evoke bodily change.

When man's skin is stroked vigorously, chemical poisons (histamine and pilocarpine) are released. Normally the skin is insensitive to these substances. If such a person is required to discuss his family troubles, at the height of his emotional reaction his skin turns red and then blanches along the line of stroking. The same mechanical and chemical stimuli that failed previously to produce an effect now cause a definite one. In other words, the patient's emotional state has rendered him vulnerable to the mechanical and chemical stimuli. With reassurance he soon returns to his original condition.

Some of these skin reactions are important sources of aggravation of skin diseases such as eczema and allergic dermatoses. This is embodied in the term *neurodermatitis*.

STOMACH

The entire gastrointestinal tract is highly susceptible to emotional disturbances. Everyone knows this from personal experience, but the phenomena can be easily reproduced and measured in the physiology laboratory.

One of Dr. Harold Wolff's experiments was to present appetizing food to a man who was somewhat hungry and to measure the blood flow in the lining of his stomach. It was found to be increased. A mechanical record of the stomach showed that it was churning and contracting and also that the digestive juices were being secreted in increased amount. This meant that the stomach was preparing for the act of digestion even though the man was only looking at the food and had not yet placed a single morsel of it in his mouth. When the food was removed, the blood flow and contractions gradually returned to their initial level. When other food was offered which was not at all appealing, the man's appetite was not stimulated and there was no change noted in the gastric function.

The next step in the experiment was to remove the food from view and instead of introducing something that the man could see or smell, food that he liked was discussed. Immediately the stomach again prepared for digestive activity. Words symbolic of food rather than food itself were the stimuli.

A topic which was extremely unpleasant to the man was then introduced. It referred to an underhanded business deal carried out by a business partner during the time when the patient was ill. As the man discussed his partner's activities, he became exceedingly angry but, surprisingly, his stomach and upper gastrointestinal tract acted as though they were preparing to digest food. Thus an inappropriate response of an organ was evoked by an emotional stimulus.

In one of the classic physiological experiments on a man named Tom who had a window in his stomach, due to a previous injury, Dr. Wolff was able to make many observations on the effect of emotion on gastric function. Actually the hole had been made in the stomach because the esophagus leading to it had been damaged by swallowing a scalding liquid and after recovery he was required to feed himself by putting food directly into the stomach. The patient had gone through adolescence and adult life under this great handicap, becoming a good citizen, father, and worker. He was shy, taciturn, with strong feelings about respectability and his role in the community. At the time Dr. Wolff experimented on him, he was employed as a helper in the New York Hospital. Each day he was persuaded to come into the laboratory and the blood flow in the stomach lining was measured. The redder the stomach lining appeared, the greater the blood flow, as one would expect, and when pallid the blood flow was reduced. The secretion of gastric juices and the churning activity of the stomach were also measured. At the same time notes were made concerning the patient's current fears, hopes, wishes, frustrations, and satisfactions.

On one occasion when the patient was in the laboratory, a physician entered saying that a certain important protocol, the safekeeping of which had been charged to the patient, was missing. The patient grew pale in the face and his stomach was also pale. The irritated doctor opened and closed drawers, muttering imprecations. He finally found the protocol and left.

The patient said, "I was scared that I had lost my job." This statement has to be seen in symbolic terms. The man was in terror that he had lost his position not only as a worker but also that he had lost face as one who had been entrusted with responsibility. His stomach was pale, hypoactive, and non-functioning. It was "out of condition," distended, and the digestion was slow. He complained of air in the bowel. Food remained in his stomach for a long time. He experienced gaseous eructations or belching and felt nauseated. Under comparable circumstances at other times he vomited through the opening in his stomach. This may serve as an example of an organ failing to function properly under conditions of stress.

In contrast, another emotional state resulted in a quite different reaction. One day while Tom was again reclining on the observation table, he was told that a particular job of dusting and cleaning which he had been assigned was improperly done. As he was being told about his inadequacy, he became red in the face and red in the stomach; the acid in his stomach increased in amount; his stomach began to churn. Finally he was told that he was "fired"; by then his stomach was exceedingly red. His accuser then left, whereupon Tom muttered, "I'd like to wring his neck." Along with this expression of anger he felt abused.

Such changes in the stomach may last for weeks. The acid secretion and the color of the stomach before, during, and after a period of crisis were exemplified in the following situation: Receiving a small salary, the patient, Tom, was obliged to accept the contributions of a benefactor who meddled in his personal affairs. This threatened his independence, and he repeatedly made efforts to throw off his benefactor. Finally during a two-week period the meddling was particularly irksome, and his stomach exhibited a high acid secretion and a deep red color. A slight raise in salary enabled him to be rid of his benefactor and his stomach returned to its former state.

This case is not unique. Dr. Wolff studied another man who had had a similar abdominal opening through which his stomach could be viewed. When the man was tranquil, the lining of the stomach had a natural pink color, but when the name of a certain doctor was mentioned, a man whom he hated because it was believed that he had failed to diagnose his illness correctly, he became exceedingly angry. He sputtered and was profane, and his stomach mucosa became dark red. Thus as part of his reactions to a topic involving his hates and fears, nerve impulses went down the vagus nerve, which converted the mucous membrane of the stomach from a resting state to one of readiness for eating and one which, if sustained, could conceivably lead to irritation and illness. Finally it became necessary to cut the major nerve to the patient's stomach, that is, the vagus. After surgery, discussion of this same doctor was associated with every outward show of anger, but no change was observed within the stomach. Presumably prolonged discussion would have diminished his reaction to the thought of this doctor, but by then the stomach was so overly sensitized that it was stimulated by even less strong emotional states.

Because of these remarkable observations in which the experimenter has witnessed some of the same alterations in the gastric mucosa and the acid secreting cells as are found in peptic ulcer or gastritis, many physicians and surgeons have come to believe that these latter diseases are due entirely to psychological problems, i.e., are psychogenic. The proof of this hypothesis has not been forthcoming, however. A view more consistent with available medical facts is that these are diseases of unknown cause and that the symptoms of them may be enhanced by anger, fear, or anxiety, which happen to act on the same structures. Helping the patient understand and control his emotional states may aid in the treatment of the peptic ulcer but does not eradicate its cause, again an instance of a disease with a large psychosomatic component.

BOWEL

The effect of strong emotion on bowel function is perhaps less obvious to most people. Again Dr. Harold Wolff and his colleagues obtained information concerning this relationship in four persons with abdominal apertures allowing views of the lining of the large bowel (colon). As an experiment he put a thumbscrew arrangement on top of the head of one subject. The patient willingly volunteered to have this done although it would hurt. Painfully squeezing the head caused the bowel to become red and to begin to contract. It was learned then that although the subject appeared placid, he was in fact quite apprehensive. A second man, despite the fact that he wished to participate and knew what was going to happen, became angry and showed it. Indeed, he would not permit the experiment to continue. This second man had, in reaction to exactly the same stimulus under the same circumstances, precisely the opposite bodily reaction as did the first man. His bowel became pale and contractile activity stopped.

A general principle was thus exemplified: Here were two people exposed to the same assault, yet because of a difference in constitution or possibly in the interpretation of the meaning of the procedure, they experienced opposite reactions.

In a similar study another person's bowel, when he was in a state of relative tranquility, was observed to be pink in color. During a period featured by dejection or sadness, it became pale and relaxed. During a period of anger, it contracted and became dark red; a balloon inserted inside the bowel showed it to be irritable and excessively motile. About twenty minutes after eating, the colon was again observed to be red and hypermotile even while he was tranquil. This is the so-called gastrocolic reflex and is the basis of the urge to empty the bowel shortly after meals. It normally serves a good purpose; but what was pathological was the tendency for this condition to persist after anger had subsided. The same man was observed on another day, after lunch, apparently under the same circumstances, but showing none of this reaction. It was then discovered that he was dejected because of an unfortunate and humiliating incident involving a neighbor which had occurred just a few hours before. The subject under these circumstances had no urge to evacuate the bowel and indeed considered himself constipated.

Mucous colitis and ulcerative colitis are diseases in which the bowel is overactive for long periods of time with resulting diarrhea. In the second of these diseases there is chronic infection, hemorrhage, and sometimes perforation; and death may occur if the condition continues untreated. The effects of emotional disorder are prominent in part because of the disagreeable nature of the illness and the disability it creates. These conditions are not psychogenic. Psychotherapy has been useful in some cases, but the usual treatment continues to be dietary control in the first and cortisone or some related compound or surgery in the latter.

THE NASAL PASSAGES AND RESPIRATORY SYSTEM

Man's respiratory system is also remarkably sensitive to his emotional state. This may be demonstrated by mere inspection of the color of the nasal mucous membranes. In some persons they are the same color day after day. In others they may be red one day and pale the next, or red in one nostril and pale in the other. When a normal person is exposed to smelling salts, he suddenly gasps and the mucous membrane of the nose becomes dark red and swollen. A watery secretion pours out and hardly any air will pass through the nose. He may be unable to speak, and his chest seems held in a vise. This is a reaction to neutralize, wash away, and shut out a noxious element in the environment.

An allergic person suffering from hay fever or allergic inflammation in the nose, when exposed to rose pollen, develops many of the same symptoms. Again this appears to be an attempt to shut out, wash away and neutralize an agent which to him has become noxious. This is one of the proper uses of the nose.

But consider a woman with a long history of trouble with her nose resulting in several operations. She is no longer able to breathe freely and her nose seems stopped up much of the time, particularly at night and especially when her husband is in the room smoking. When her physician suggested after an interview that perhaps some of her trouble might be related to her attitude toward personal problems and particularly toward her husband, she violently rejected the suggestion but burst into tears. The mucous membrane on the inside of her nose became dark red and there was much secretion and swelling. A little while later it appeared pale, boggy, and solidly occluded. This woman acted as though she were shutting out, neutralizing, and washing away some noxious agent.

Changes of this type may last for minutes or days, as exhibited by an ambitious young physician who was much concerned with his career and was obliged to work intimately with a professional partner in his hospital, some years his senior but his junior in experience and wisdom. He resented working with this colleague and feared that his future was jeopardized by the inadequate performance of his associate. Their relationship deteriorated rapidly. During a two-week period while his conflicts with his colleague were most severe, he exhibited red and swollen mucous membranes with quantities of fluid pouring out and scarcely any space for the passage of air. Moreover he developed headache which he called sinus headache and had red eyes, tender, swollen, flushed cheeks, and tender forehead. His nasal mucous membranes were exceedingly sensitive to touch. During an interview the mucous membranes swelled further, additional secretion pouring out; and increased quantities of pus cells were then seen in the secretion. These men were separated and soon thereafter the patient became symptom-free and his nasal mucous membranes became paler and much less swollen, with little secretion and no obstruction.

A combined or summative effect is evident when one kind of noxious stimulus, to which the patient is allergic, has superimposed upon it another occasioned by an emotional state or the repeated use of irritating drugs. Such a patient was brought into a room containing a constant amount of circulating pollen in the air. She had hay fever in the pollen season and was sensitive to this pollen. And as she sat in this room, her mucous membranes began to redden and swell slightly. Then in addition to the irritating pollen, a topic concerning her troubles and her quarrels with her father was introduced. Immediately her symptoms were greatly augmented and her airways became obstructed. She was then reassured by the words of her physician and despite the fact that she remained in the room laden with pollen, the membranes were restored even to their initial state, akin to that noted before she entered the pollen-laden room. In this instance, then, her relationship to her father rather than the pollen seemed the more potent stimulus, although both were operating.

An anatomical defect in the nose, present since birth, can under certain circumstances take on importance in middle life or later. For example, a deviated septum which has been present for a lifetime may become important when one's relations to others become of such a nature as to call forth the protective reaction of shutting out, washing away, and neutralizing. A man may then need to have his septum removed to allow more air to pass through his nose.

The asthmatic person is closely akin in his pattern of reaction to the one who has trouble with his nose. Indeed, an asthmatic reaction seldom occurs without nasal involvement. The basic disorder is one of allergy, usually genetically caused; but it may become evident by direct inspection that threatening topics, which by themselves may cause sensations of air hunger, tightness in the chest, and butterflies in the stomach, may combine with the asthma to cause the mucous membranes of the bronchi to become redder and wetter and the lumen to become smaller. During a series of observations, topics calling forth feelings of bitterness, regret, and failure also may precipitate asthmatic attacks. Some of the tight, unpleasant feelings of pressure in the middle of the chest during strong anxiety may be mistaken for pains originating in the heart. Also, a benign spasm may occur in the diaphragm, the sheet of muscle separating the lungs and the heart from the contents of the abdomen. When an X-ray picture of the diaphragm of a person in a relaxed and tranquil state is compared with that of his diaphragm when he is anxious, the latter shows a contracted state which would make it difficult to take in more air. A fluttering sensation may be experienced and sometimes spasms may be seen in it under the fluoroscope.

CIRCULATORY SYSTEM

So far patterns of disturbed function involving portals of entry, the mouth and airways, and portals of exit, the bowel and rectum have been considered. Under certain circumstances the organism may act as though it were mobilized for action when in fact there is no call for it. Here the most noticeable reaction is in the heart and blood vessels. If a man runs up stairs or exercises vigorously, he increases the output of blood from his heart with each beat. His heart rate is increased, his blood pressure rises and the amount of resistance offered to the flow of blood by the minute vessels in the tissues of the body is decreased. These physiological changes are necessary in order to assure a good supply of blood to the muscles, thus making action more effective.

Often during an interview with a patient, in which he becomes frankly anxious or frightened, his circulatory system may act as though he were running up stairs or preparing for battle. One such example might be cited: A patient came to his physician in a tense anxious state complaining of pounding of his heart and breathlessness. Climbing a certain number of steps caused his already augmented cardiac stroke-volume (the amount of blood ejected by the heart per beat) to be further increased. The heart rate also was increased. As the patient's general life adjustment improved, his circulation gradually was restored to a more normal state so that ten months later the same physical effort produced only a minimal increase in circulation.

A more complex situation is one in which a patient ostensibly loved his mother but actually hated many of the things that she did, never admitting this to himself. He presented a bland exterior during an interview, but his blood pressure rose and the resistance offered to the passage of blood by blood vessels in many of his organs mounted. His blood became much more viscous and coagulated more readily. During an interview concerning his relations with his mother, his blood pressure went up sharply and as a part of his general increased resistance to the flow of blood, the amount of blood that went through his kidneys was much decreased. These regulatory devices serve presumably to help the animal stop bleeding during mortal combat, but when they are used every time a person comes in contact with his mother, it follows that they serve no useful purpose—another instance of a device that may protect or prolong life being called into action so inappropriately as to derange normal body function.

PAINS IN BACK AND HEAD

General nervous tension and mobilization of the skeletal muscles for action may give rise to backache or headache. The intensity of an individual's muscle tension is indicated by the firmness of the muscle when it is felt. And it can also be shown by a record of the electrical impulses in the muscle, which roughly parallel in amount the magnitude of contraction.

An example of this phenomenon was a man deliberately exposed to a discussion aimed to bring into focus feelings of hostility and anxiety. Contractions of the large muscles of his back and legs increased, presumably in readiness for action for fight or flight. Being thus contracted for long periods but not actually associated with movement (which usually is followed by relaxation), they began to hurt. When topics that interested him and brought him esteem and satisfaction were discussed, the muscle activity was reduced. But with a reconsideration of the threatening matters, the muscle contraction was again increased and again he had backache.

Similar painful contractions occur in the muscles of the head and neck. Headaches can persist for days, weeks, or months due to sustained contraction of the sheet of muscle on top of the head and neck when a person is exposed to an environment which calls forth the need to be on the alert against assaults that threaten but never come. Electrical records of patients with such headaches have been recorded. After anxiety and fear subside consequent to being able to discuss their causes freely, the sheet of muscle is no longer contracted and the headache ends.

Vascular headaches such as migraine constitute a most important source of discomfort. A person subject to this hereditary disease may develop, during an attack, large swollen vessels on the side of his head. Anxiety or simple nervousness, although not causal to this condition, may increase the frequency of these headaches or prolong them, and the assuaging of anxiety may bring about some measure of relief.

REACTIONS TO STRESS

Some of the ways in which certain environmental and particularly psychosocial stimuli may act on the neurohumoral mechanisms of the body have been presented. A number of the visceral responses have been described which, if not understood by the patient, may be mistaken for disease. Further, some of the diseases which utilize these same anatomical structures and are therefore modifiable by stress and emotion have been mentioned. Any person, for reasons not entirely clear, is more likely to respond to emotional upset by a disturbance in one of his organs than in another. Some persons have their "weak spot," their Achilles heel, in their gastrointestinal system, and throughout their lives every emotionally charged symptom adumbrates through their stomach or bowel. Others may be plagued with respiratory symptoms and in still a third group the skin may most accurately reflect the state of emotional equilibrium. Moreover, in any given situation these adaptive and protective reactions may not involve the totality of one of the aforementioned organs or organ systems. Instead of the whole respiratory system becoming involved, for example, only the nose may react.

One of the current hypotheses concerning the type of reaction which one may manifest during periods of stress is that of acquired "organ inferiority." Implied in this formulation is the notion that an organ or organ system becomes unusually susceptible to all autonomic discharges because of disease in prenatal or postnatal life or improper training in early life. Strong emotion may still create in such a person all of the standard reactions that are appropriate to apprehension, fear, and anger, but the milder emotional states may be reflected only in skin changes, deranged gastrointestinal function, respiratory difficulty, nervous tension with pressure headache, trembling, and sweating. Another variant of this hypothesis is that inherited weakness or abnormal vulnerability in a given organ renders it liable to derangement by autonomic nervous activity. For example, shortness of breath, poor tolerance to physical exertion, rapid heart action, concern about health, represent patterns of reaction which run through certain families. However, one cannot decide from existing evidence whether this is an example of child imitating parent or the manifestation of a more basic abnormality that has been genetically determined, though the evocative stimulus in each instance may be environmental.

What makes this whole problem so difficult to study is its inherent complexity. One may overlook the fundamental abnormality in such a person and attach undue importance to some secondary symptom. Thus the fact that a patient has an inherited allergic tendency may be disregarded while his undue responsiveness to annoying social situations, which seems to activate or prolong his asthma, may be emphasized.

Even more confusing is the observation that some individuals lose their older, fixed, ingrained patterns of reaction under extreme stress. For example, a distinguished physician in Holland studied, during the worst years of Holland's occupation by the Germans, a number of patients with stomach ulcers. He had attended their medical needs before the Germans came and also after they had been put in concentration camps because of their religion. Before the war they had been healthy, comfortable, and successful merchants. They suffered a good deal from dyspepsia and other gastric symptoms. In the concentration camps their plight was horrible. Life was intensely unpredictable and full of threats. They never knew in the morning whether they would survive that day. Yet these people lost all manifestations of their peptic ulceration. The ironic aspect of it was that many of them again developed their peptic ulcers when they returned to their homes after the war. The specific type of stress which occurred under these conditions was ineffective in aggravating ulceration in the stomach.

In a similar vein one may cite the medical anecdote of a group of missionaries in Japan who were subject to intense and frequent headaches. During the good times of their missionary activity, they suffered considerably, even though they were esteemed by the people with whom they were working and were presumably effective and satisfied with their work. When these people were put in Japanese concentration camps, with all the deprivations that this entailed, they lost their headaches. When they were freed at the end of the war, the headaches returned. These examples are difficult to explain. Possibly it means that danger has to have a specific meaning to a person in order to produce specific changes.

Regardless of these inconsistencies, however, the function of all the organs of the body which are under autonomic control are subject to derangement during intense emotion, a derangement which initially serves to preserve the biological status of the individual over short periods of time but which, if prolonged as in protracted anxiety and incompletely understood by the patient, becomes a source of complaint and difficulty.

Why do we not all have bodily reactions during stress? Why are we different in these respects? Why do we look at the same assault or threat differently? The complete answer to this latter question cannot be given. Here we must recognize individual differences between every two people. Obviously what is recognized as a threat by one person may have a different meaning to another. Nor do two people deal with a problem in the same way. Do we run toward it? Do we run away from it? Do we try to avoid it? Do we try to act as though it didn't exist? Do we wish to fight but dare not? All of these patterns of reaction can be observed. Perhaps we raise the same issue when we ask why dogs of certain breeds more easily learn to retrieve birds or fight fiercely or follow scents; or why beavers construct dams and squirrels hoard nuts. The implication is that it is easier for a bird dog to learn to be a bird dog.

From this it does not follow that such manifest proclivities of certain organs to respond to emotional upset lead to disease in that organ. There is no proof that this is so. In fact, one might even challenge the statement that repeated or prolonged participation of a given organ or system of organs in a protective pattern constitutes evidence of biologic inferiority of that organ. The individual may be weak or vulnerable, but the organ can hardly be declared weak. Indeed, it may be especially well developed and strong for long periods before its function is seriously disturbed.

THE IMPORTANCE OF ATTITUDES

In these numerous reaction patterns, it has been evident that the evocative stimulus may be either a situation to which a given emotional reaction is entirely appropriate or it may consist of a mere symbol of the threatening situation. This, as was said already, is one of the most unique features of man, that he is able to react to verbal stimuli which stand in symbolic relationship to the initial event or some fragment of the initial stimulus; further he may react to a symbol without even recalling its relationship to the original stimulus. It may be difficult at first to recapture this connection and to see that the symbol is but a fraction of a larger pattern of stimuli which formerly were effective in the life of that person. But an opposite danger lurks for the unwary—that of assuming a relevance of a highly charged topic to some obscure disease when none in fact exists. The experienced physician learns that any given topic may be merely representative of many which pose as threats to the patient and to which he reacts in a similar way. Achieving an understanding of such a topic only temporarily results in amelioration of symptoms.

The effects of an emotionally potent stimulus on the later behavior of the individual is more than a mere stimulus-response situation. Once an organism has reacted to such a stimulus, it is never the same as it was before. The experience of reacting affectively alters a person; he becomes expectant in anticipation of the approach of the stimulus again. This learning process has given him a new perceptive set. The stimulus now has acquired a new significance. An attitude has been created that will modify all future reactions. When analyzed, the first component of this attitude seems to concern the meaning any new experience has for the individual; the second, what he must do about it. These matters may be dealt with at an automatic, instinctive, relatively unconscious level, as when one rids himself of something by vomiting because it is disgusting or unattractive, thus expressing a characteristic attitude. Or it may result in a careful, premeditated plan of action.

Much has been said concerning the conscious versus the unconscious; a careful appraisal of affective or emotional experience usually shows that there are elements of both. The conscious parts are often the least distressing to a balanced personality, for the problems can be resolved in a realistic manner. The unconscious, the less accessible, cause the most trouble, and the individual may suffer from its effects for long periods of time without knowing what is wrong. In this whole class of medical disorders relating to stress, emotional states and prolonged fatigue, both the conscious and unconscious reactions to a stimulus and the fixed attitudes to which they are related figure most importantly.

PSYCHOSOMATIC MEDICINE

From this background of experimental physiological data and medical observation, we may now examine the concept of psychosomatic medicine. This topic, as all informed people realize, has become popular. One hears it discussed freely at cocktail parties and reads about it in daily newspapers. What are psychosomatic diseases and how may they be defined? Psychosomatic diseases include migraine, hay fever, asthma, urticaria, mild forms of dermatitis, peptic ulcer of stomach and duodenum, ulcerative colitis, mucous colitis, dysmenorrhea, and high blood pressure. Common to all are the following characteristics: First, their cause has never been defined; secondly, many of them tend to run in families but do not necessarily have a genetic basis; thirdly, in the majority of instances the symptoms are based on derangements of function, many of which are reversible though in most instances some definite pathologic change, that is to say a lesion, has developed. Hence they are characterized as diseases and not merely as somatic or emotional reactions. They do not have a higher incidence in neurotic individuals. Finally, more than in most diseases, an unusually close relationship exists between the emotional state of the person and attacks of the disease. This latter criterion is often stated, though exact data on this point are difficult to obtain.

For a time it was hoped that by deep exploration of the mind through the techniques of psychoanalysis a particular personality type would be found to go with each of these diseases. This would have affirmed their psychogenesis. Unfortunately this hypothesis has not been supported, and even more troublesome is that many people with a personality structure not unlike that seen in a patient with peptic ulcer or high blood pressure do not seem to have any of these diseases.

The basic assumption has been that these diseases are caused by psychological problems and by social maladjustment because of the close relationship between the protracted emotional states and their visceral counterparts and the disease in question—that is to say, they are psychogenic. Perhaps the most persuasive evidence of this theory has come from the work of Dr. Harold Wolff who found that when the patient, Tom, with an aperture in his stomach was subjected to intense emotion, some hemorrhage and even a slight ulceration of the stomach lining might occur. He conjectured that he had witnessed the formation of a peptic ulcer. The lesion was not that of the usual peptic ulcer. Clear evidence has not yet been adduced that frank gastric ulceration of the type called *peptic ulcer* can be caused simply by emotional disturbance. A sounder view, from present evidence, would be that each of these psychosomatic diseases has its own causation and that prolonged emotional disorders merely add to the disease in a summative fashion or become interdigitated with it.

A tendency prevails to ascribe every obscure complaint to fatigue, overwork, emotional upset. The medical profession has itself been responsible to some extent for this attitude. Common is the statement that in two-thirds of patients coming to a doctor with a complaint, a serious underlying disease will not be found. The implication may be, therefore, that the symptoms are all in the patient's mind or that if there is some evident functional change, it is psychogenic. As medicine progresses, the untenability of this notion becomes increasingly evident. Many minor difficulties which do not lead to any serious structural change in organs may be related to minor inherited biochemical changes or structural peculiarities with which the patient goes through life. Such symptoms may be enhanced by psychological difficulties in times of psychological stress, but the latter is only a contributory factor. And of course the patient's reaction to these disorders and the degree to which he complains or seeks medical attention are matters of culture, education, or mood.

CULTURE AND STRESS

The medical problems created by emotional disorder and psychosomatic diseases are largely products of Occidental culture. Little information has been recorded as to whether any of these diseases occur in the undeveloped parts of the world. In a primitive society, where everyone must fend for himself, little or no time is available for leisure or self-observation. Perhaps man may have this type of disorder but is too preoccupied with other more pressing problems to register complaint about it; and if he did, his relationship to his social group might be threatened. Tolerance to psychosomatic disease could conceivably be a manifestation of an affluent, leisure society.

Similarly, culture may be related in another manner to diseases of stress. In complex social groups, which are necessary when populations become large, man may be subjected to a maximum degree of stress as here defined. This follows from the previously stated fact that the most disturbing agents in man's life are human beings. And organized society offers the greatest number and variety of conditions which conflict with the natural impulses of man and are difficult to cope with directly. It is not as though there were an opponent who threatens and from whom one can flee or launch an attack, but instead a circumstance where the source of threat is uncertain and escape impossible. Man may succumb to illness under such circumstances even though he can rise to the challenge of overt danger and engage effectively in actual physical combat.

Effects of cultural environment are also becoming ever more pressing in contemporary life and they are shown not only in this field of psychosomatic medicine but in all the social institutions. Universal education and liberalized social standards permit one to move from one stratum of society to another. A farm laborer's son goes to college and becomes a judge or bank president and marries a woman from a family of the upper class. He is compelled to forsake the rules of conduct which guided his parents and accept new customs, habits, rules, and traditions which are difficult for him to evaluate. One reaction is to become skeptical and to question all moral and ethical values and repudiate all social rules. Attitudes toward property and possessions, toward woman's place in the economic and political world, one's responsibility to one's employer, church, community, etc., all these and more are open to critical reappraisal. New symbols of success, prestige, and achievement are adopted. These derived cultural influences are of lesser importance than the basic principles of conduct such as those underlying marriage and family, parental responsibility, etc., which may come to be disregarded. As a consequence, conscious or unconscious conflicts arise. These are some of the larger problems which occur in cultural adjustment and which may ultimately have medical implications by causing disturbances of visceral function.

The medical profession has a key role in treating the psychosomatic disorders. Two persons out of three exhibiting stress manifestations can be significantly helped. The thoughtful doctor can do much to indicate which things must come first and give support while a troubled patient reorients himself. As a person of authority, he can help the sufferer regain his self-esteem and acquire new attitudes that may help restore more normal patterns of functioning.

Not all stress and emotional disorder are evil. They are one of man's sources of motivation; they stimulate curiosity and investigation. But the patient must learn that when he pursues a goal, he must pay a price. Once he knows what the price is, he must then ascertain whether the goal is worth the cost. Certainly there are aims in life more important than comfort and occasionally even more important than health. These are matters everyone must decide for himself.

CHAPTER 15

Arthritis, Rheumatism, and Gout

HOWARD F. POLLEY, M.D.

Arthritis, rheumatism, and gout are among the oldest diseases known to affect human beings. Hippocrates, a Greek physician called the "Father of Medicine," described these conditions graphically many centuries ago. Evidence of the occurrence of these diseases even before his time has been found in mummies and excavations from other ancient civilizations. The widespread occurrence of these diseases in the United States at present is indicated by the presence of some form of rheumatic disease in more than 16,500,000 people in this country.

The terms "arthritis" and "rheumatism" have been used synonymously at times, but as a result of advances in our medical knowledge, physicians have been able to recognize almost a hundred different kinds of arthritis and almost another hundred kinds of rheumatism. Arthritic diseases are those that affect singly or in various combinations the tissues of the joint: (1) the *cartilage,* (2) the adjacent *bone,* and (3) the *synovial* (*lining*) *membrane*. Rheumatism, by contrast, affects tissues *outside* the joint, sometimes spoken of as "the soft tissues." These tissues include the fibrous tissue which forms a capsule immediately surrounding the joint and also lines or envelops bundles of muscles and sheaths of nerves, ligaments, tendons, and bursae. Terms such as "fibrositis," "tendinitis," "bursitis," "myositis," or "myalgia," depending on which structure is affected, or the term "periarthritis," meaning around but not in the joint itself, may be used in describing the location of the rheumatism. Rheumatism may affect a person who also has arthritis, but rheumatism can and often does occur without arthritis.

There are both acute and chronic types of rheumatism and arthritis. Persons of any age and either sex may have practically any of the various types of arthritis and rheumatism. The most common type of arthritis is known as degenerative joint disease or *osteoarthritis,* which can be found to some extent in almost all persons past middle age. Hence this type of arthritis is often attributed to the results of "wear and tear" of use of joints of the body over a long time. Fortunately, though most persons may acquire some evidence of osteoarthritis, symptoms from the presence of the osteoarthritis occur only infrequently. Hence the presence of osteoarthritis is not necessarily evidence that a person's "rheumatic" or "arthritic" symptoms are the result of this type of arthritis.

Another type of arthritis of particular significance is *rheumatoid arthritis.* Physicians find that about one out of three patients who have symptoms of arthritis have this type of arthritis. It can affect persons of any age but tends to occur more commonly in the young adult years. Women are affected by rheumatoid arthritis two or three times as frequently as are men.

The most common types of rheumatism include *bursitis, fibrositis, tendinitis,* or *periarthritis* in the various parts of the body in which these tissues are particularly subject to rheumatic involvement. Another kind of rheumatism that is common is that which results from muscular and nervous tension and emotional fatigue. This is sometimes called *neuromuscular* or *psychosomatic rheumatism.*

Gout is a special type of metabolic disorder of the bodily functions which may be manifested by the occurrence at various times of either arthritis or rheumatism. Gouty arthritis (or bursitis or rheumatism) is related to the body's overproduction of or inability to dispose properly of chemicals, known as purines, eaten in certain foods or accumulating (as urates or uric acid) as a result of certain metabolic processes within the body itself. Gout usually affects men past middle age, although occasionally it occurs earlier than this. Gout affects women only infrequently (about one case in fifty), and then usually late in life. Gouty involvement occurs in the region of the "bunion joint" of the great toe, other joints of the feet, the ankles, and occasionally the knees, hands, wrists, or elbows. Usually only one joint or tendon or bursa is affected at a time. Attacks of gouty arthritis develop rapidly, and the affected area becomes red, warm, and extremely painful. The acute episode may last for a few days or perhaps weeks before it completely subsides. Even after the acute attack is gone, however, the basic derangement of bodily metabolism continues to exist and may require treatment. If the disease continues uncontrolled, multiple joints or articular areas may be affected and there may be gouty deposits in the bone and joints or bursae or ligaments which may be affected. This ultimately can result in a change from an acute to a chronic gouty arthritis. Similar gouty deposits are sometimes found on the ears, about the involved joints, and also in the kidneys. Patients with gout often have increased amounts of uric acid (as urates) in their blood, but such increases occur under a number of other circumstances. A test that shows an elevated concentration of uric acid in blood, of itself, therefore, does not necessarily indicate the presence of gout. Treatment for gout may include a special diet and drugs. This is discussed under the heading "Treatment of Arthritis, Rheumatism, and Gout."

CAUSES OF ARTHRITIS AND RHEUMATISM

Arthritis and rheumatism, like diseases of other organs of the body, can result from a number of causes, some known and others as yet unknown. These include (1) injury, (2) heredity, (3) infections, (4) allergies, (5) tumors, (6) metabolic disorders, and (7) fatigue, emotional upsets, or other factors.

INJURY

Injury to joints or related soft tissues may be either acute such as might be encountered in a fall, an automobile accident, or in the course of strenuous sports, or chronic injury such as that which might result from less severe but repeated daily injuries, such as those resulting from certain occupations or from other disadvantageous use over and over again of a certain joint or related musculoskeletal tissues.

HEREDITY

Arthritis and rheumatism can be produced by hereditary influences. The occurrence of a peculiar but common type of osteoarthritis in end joints of the fingers, called "Heberden's nodes," is an example of hereditary or familial development of osteoarthritis. The arthritis of the hemophiliac or "bleeder" is another example; this is more serious but fortunately is not common.

INFECTIONS

Arthritis and rheumatism can result from a number of different types of infections, including streptococcal and staphylococcal infections, pneumonia, meningitis, tuberculosis, venereal diseases, typhoid fever, undulant fever, and many others. Because of the infections which occur predominantly in children, certain types of infectious arthritis and rheumatism occur more frequently in younger than in older persons. Despite intensive investigations and long search, no germ or virus has been found to be the cause of osteoarthritis or rheumatoid arthritis.

ALLERGIES

Allergic reactions, or perhaps more properly reactions of hypersensitivity, may affect tissues involved by rheumatism or arthritis. Unusual sensitivity to drugs or proteins "foreign" to the human body, for example, may result in arthritis or rheumatism. When this type of arthritis or rheumatism occurs, it can be described as an inflammation without an infection.

TUMORS

Like other organs of the body, the joints may be affected by new growths or tumors, but fortunately these are rarely encountered in persons who have arthritic and rheumatic diseases.

METABOLIC DISORDERS

Changes in metabolism or the way in which the body performs its work may affect the joints and related skeletal tissues, thus resulting in arthritis or rheumatism. A severe deficiency of vitamin C, for example, may result in a disease called "scurvy" in which there may be rheumatic complications. A disorder in the body's ability to handle the purine (a type of protein) substances formed during certain metabolic processes or contained in certain foods results in the condition known as gout, which has been described. Ochronosis, a peculiar type of degenerative joint disease, occurs in some persons in whom pigmented chemical deposits develop in cartilage as a result of a particular abnormality of the body's enzymes. Similarly, a disturbance or upset of the balance between the various hormones of the body may affect the condition of joints or result in certain types of rheumatism or arthritis.

OTHER FACTORS CAUSING ARTHRITIS AND RHEUMATISM

Some physicians have suspected from time to time that arthritis and rheumatism may result from disturbances of circulation or disturbances of function of the nervous system. Lowered physical resistance, emotional upset, stress, shock, fatigue, and the like are other factors which might be of considerable importance to the development of certain types of arthritis and rheumatism.

In general, climate is neither a cause of nor a cure of arthritis or rheumatism. A few specific types of arthritis and rheumatism may be related to certain climates or geographical areas, but people in all parts of the world can and do have many of the common types of arthritis and rheumatism.

SYMPTOMS OF ARTHRITIS AND RHEUMATISM

Persons with arthritis and rheumatism often have a background of acute or chronic stress or strain. This may be of either a physical or mental nature or both and may be an important indication which will permit early recognition of the symptoms of articular or rheumatic diseases. Sometimes the first symptom is not directly related to the joints, but is more in the form of tiredness or exhaustion or generalized aching and stiffness. There may be loss of weight, appetite, and strength. The sensation of swelling of joints or muscles may be recognized by the person affected even though it may not be detected by careful examination of the affected areas. As would be readily recognized, these symptoms of a more or less general nature are not always indicative of arthritis or rheumatism. A person with such symptoms should rely on the advice and judgment of his physician in evaluation of these symptoms.

The main symptoms of arthritis or rheumatism are pain, stiffness, limitation of motion, and swelling of affected areas. Pain from arthritis and rheumatism varies from dull to sharp in severity, or may be described as "like a toothache" or "knifelike." In some types of rheumatism burning sensations and feelings of "pins and needles" and numbness may occur in affected areas. The pain may be fleeting or constant and may vary from one location to another or may occur only in an isolated area. The affected area may be warm or hot to touch, and there may or may not be some degree of redness or discoloration of the overlying skin. Pain of arthritis and rheumatism is often characterized by its "ups and downs," but may disappear without returning or may progress either slowly or fairly rapidly.

Patients with rheumatism and arthritis often complain of "stiffness." When rheumatic stiffness is aggravated by rest, it is often relieved by mild exercise and easy movements of the affected areas. When the stiffness is more directly related to fatigue, it may be relieved by rest and inactivity.

Limitation of motion of an affected area may result from pain on motion and consequent avoidance of that painful motion or may be related to muscular weakness or imbalance in muscular function. Sometimes limited motion also is attributed to fatigue. In other instances roughening of the smooth, shiny, cartilaginous surfaces of the joint may be the basis for limitation of motion. Creaking noises or crepitation on motion may also result from such changes in the joint surfaces, but the creaking sounds may be produced just as readily by friction in tissues outside the joint. Hence such sounds do not necessarily indicate that a joint is damaged or even diseased.

Swelling may occur either outside the joint or inside the joint. Swelling outside the joint often can be attributed to generalized fatigue or disturbances in the balance of function in small blood vessels which become "sluggish" in their capacity to remove or circulate the body fluids. Swelling of this type may produce the sensation of rings becoming temporarily tight on fingers or shoes tight on the feet. This type of swelling may occur either after periods of rest and inactivity or in parts of the body that are dependent or hang down during much of the time that a person is not resting.

Swelling that occurs inside the joint results from the collection of fluid in the joint in an amount in excess of that normally produced by the lining (synovial) membrane for lubrication of the joint. This may occur with certain types of inflammation, infection, injury, or other disorders. Local heat or warmth outside the joint often accompanies the collection of excess fluid, although when excess fluid has been present for some time there may not be apparent local heat, warmth, or redness of the covering tissues.

TREATMENT OF ARTHRITIS, RHEUMATISM, AND GOUT

As is to be expected, the treatment of arthritis or rheumatism depends on the type of involvement present. To determine this a careful medical examination is usually needed. When a cause of arthritis or rheumatism such as infection, allergy, tumors, or metabolic deficiencies is found and can be corrected, the arthritis or rheumatism subsides.

When a removable cause of the arthritis or rheumatism cannot be found, treatment is generally directed toward helping the patient (1) improve the ability of his natural bodily functions to cope with the arthritis or rheumatism, and (2) (when needed) maintain as nearly normal joint function as is possible. Thus in the treatment of arthritis and rheumatism both the daily activities and the periods of rest need to be considered carefully; neither should the former be excessive nor the latter be minimized or slighted. Adequate rest and sound sleep, a mind free of worry and daily activities free of anxiety and tension go a long way toward improving the body's ability to cope with the presence of extra inflammation, infection, or other factors requiring special effort by the bodily functions. *How* well this is accomplished is generally more important than *where* it is done. The position of joints during resting hours should be favorable to use of the joints when rest is not needed. This is discussed in the following section on "Physical Therapy." An occupation that protects affected joints and muscles, minimizes fatigue and loss of bodily energy and resistance may be another means of improving the natural bodily resistance against arthritis or rheumatism.

It is sometimes advisable for persons who have arthritis or rheumatism to sleep in a warm room, wear warm socks, mittens, or a head covering, in addition to the bedclothes, or use an electric blanket. Whether any exposure to the sun is desirable is determined by the type of arthritis or rheumatism present. Such persons must rely on the advice of their physician regarding this matter as well as for advice concerning the amount of exposure to sun that is desired.

Extra care to protect against exposure to infections is usually desirable, especially when resistance is low or when fatigue is present. Attention to dental and other bodily hygiene also constitutes an important aspect of the general bodily care of the arthritic or rheumatic patient.

A well-balanced diet, including meat, vegetables, fruit, and dairy products, is usually advisable. The details of a normal diet have been presented in another chapter in this book. The physician can decide when dietary supplements (such as vitamins and iron) are indicated. Many dietary fads have appeared from time to time, but, in general, the arthritic or rheumatic person does best to eat the type of food which would be best for him if he were not troubled by arthritis or rheumatism. It is generally advisable for rheumatic and arthritic patients to avoid being overweight in order to provide additional protection to weight-bearing joints.

The diet for patients with gout and gouty arthritis may require restricted use of foods containing significant amounts of purine substances. Wild game and fowl, and meats derived from animal organs, such as liver, kidneys, sweetbreads, brains, and so on, contain large amounts of purine and are especially to be avoided. Certain other meats and meat extracts used in soups and gravies may be allowed in the diet, but amounts are generally restricted. Alcoholic beverages may be excluded from the diet, but coffee, tea, cocoa, milk, and fruit juices can be permitted. A person with gout can best determine his particular dietary requirements by detailed consideration of his individual needs with his physician or a dietitian instructed by the physician.

PHYSICAL THERAPY

Since efforts to improve a person's general physical condition may involve spending extra time in bed each day, special attention may need to be given to the maintenance of joint function that will be as useful as possible when the patient does not require rest. Pillows under knees or hands, and arms folded over the chest, for example, are positions usually to be avoided during resting hours. Judicious use of splints, sandbags, lightweight plaster or plastic casts, a board under the mattress of the bed, and other supportive measures, however, can be helpful in maintaining a desirable position. During the waking hours and when a person is up and about, strains or pressure on affected joints and soft tissues should be avoided. The additional support of various types of corsets, braces, properly supporting shoes, and other similar devices also can give some assistance. Even when joints have already been affected and *normal* function is not to be anticipated, it still may be possible to obtain some degree of *useful* function. This can be the difference between the person's being self-dependent, that is, in his being able to earn a living or care for a family, and not being able to do these things. Various types of physical therapy are available and can be used to help an arthritic or rheumatic person improve his condition as much as possible.

Heat and Massage

Heat in almost all forms is one of the helpful measures of physical therapy which most arthritic and rheumatic patients can use to good advantage. Occasionally, however, heat will not be indicated or will need to be used limitedly. Applications of heat increase the circulation and induce rest and relaxation in a painful muscle, joint, or other skeletal tissues. Many devices are available for the application of heat in the patient's home, including ordinary electric light bulbs, heat lamps and pads, warm tub baths, applications of warm or hot towels, woolen or flannel materials. Applications of paraffin and use of hot and cold contrast baths, when properly carried out, are other effective methods of utilizing heat. Care must be taken to avoid burns and overheating. It is advisable to consult a physician regarding the details of such treatment.

The application of heat is sometimes followed by massage performed under the direction of a physician or by either a trained physical therapist or a member of the patient's family who has been properly instructed in such treatment. The use of mechanical devices for massage may be hazardous and hence is not advised. The duration and type of massage vary with the type of rheumatism or arthritis, and specific instructions are also required for proper use.

Heat and massage, besides being of value in relieving symptoms of arthritis or rheumatism, also serve as a good preliminary to therapeutic exercise.

Therapeutic Exercise

The use of exercise as well as the type of such treatment which may be advisable is determined by the type of arthritis or rheumatism which may be present. "Therapeutic exercise" is designed to maintain or obtain as nearly normal strength, endurance, and range of motion in affected joints and muscles as it is possible to obtain. A person's ordinary daily activities rarely serve as a suitable substitute for therapeutic exercise, but when properly undertaken, therapeutic exercise, including postural and deep-breathing exercises, can be especially beneficial and should be performed daily. The conscientious application of the appropriate therapeutic exercises for whatever period of time they are needed constitutes one of the best approaches to the problem of how useful articular function may be regained or maintained in many types of arthritis and rheumatism. Therapeutic exercise should be undertaken only on the advice of a physician and when specific instructions regarding such treatment are made available. A physician may instruct a patient to use a pamphlet such as that prepared by The Arthritis Foundation, 1212 Avenue of the Americas, New York, New York 10036, or other supplements to supply additional information for effectively carrying out a program of home physical therapy.

TREATMENT WITH DRUGS AND OTHER MEASURES

Simple analgesics such as aspirin (acetylsalicylic acid) or closely related chemicals of the salicylate family are often of aid in giving relief from the pain of arthritis, rheumatism, or gout. Many highly advertised and ofttimes expensive patent remedies have utilized this beneficial effect by having the inexpensive salicylates as their principal effective ingredient. When a physician advises the use of aspirin or other salicylates, there should be no hesitancy on the part of the patient to use such treatment to best advantage. Of course, these drugs like many others are not to be used indiscriminately, but a popular opinion that such drugs are "bad for the heart," stomach, kidneys, or other organs is exaggerated, if not erroneous. Aspirin and other salicylate drugs can relieve painful spasm as well as counteract inflammation and are not "dope" or habit-forming drugs. However, for nearly all types of arthritis and rheumatism, narcotic drugs which can be habit-forming should be avoided. This is especially true when treatment for arthritis or rheumatism is likely to be prolonged.

For some severe inflammatory reactions other anti-inflammatory and immunosuppressive drugs which need to be used with appropriate medical supervision have become available.

For the special type of arthritis which patients with gout have periodically, a drug known as colchicine is of particular value. This time-tested remedy has been used successfully for more than a hundred years for acute gouty arthritis, but it usually is not of benefit to other types of arthritis or rheumatism. Drugs which either accelerate the elimination of excess uric acid from the body or interrupt internally its formation also often are needed to control gout.

Although it is not yet known just how the benefit is mediated, gold salts given by injection are sometimes helpful for persons with rheumatoid arthritis. Use of X rays, exposure to various radioactive materials, specially prepared or processed foods, blood transfusions, vaccines, or tonics has now been largely replaced by other types of treatment which are more likely to be of benefit. Operations to repair or reconstruct affected joints may reduce disability from certain types of arthritis. With new or better techniques, the results of such operations are continually being improved.

The limitations of such treatment, however, add a further impetus to efforts to prevent whenever possible the development of disability which might require such operative treatment.

TREATMENT WITH HORMONES

Nearly all the hormones of the body which have been isolated have been tested for their value in the treatment of various types of arthritis and rheumatism. The most effective to date have been certain of the hormones of the adrenal gland, known as cortisone and hydrocortisone, and the hormone of the pituitary gland, corticotropin or ACTH, which stimulates the cortex or outer layer of the adrenal gland to produce these adrenal steroid hormones. Prednisone, prednisolone and a number of other synthetic "chemical relatives" of cortisone and hydrocortisone have been produced in recent years. The various chemical modifications which are available and the improvements in techniques of administration of all adrenal hormonal preparations have permitted more patients to tolerate and benefit from such treatment than was the case in the early years of this relatively new type of treatment. However, adrenal hormone therapy generally is restricted to those persons with rheumatoid arthritis, or certain closely related types of arthritis, which are not adequately controlled by other indicated treatments. Thus, treatment with an adrenal steroid hormonal preparation usually will *supplement* rather than be a substitute for other treatments which already have been discussed. To obtain the optimal and sustained advantages of hormonal treatment of rheumatoid arthritis, dosage needs to be highly individualized. This requires careful medical supervision of such treatment. However, when use of these hormones is advised by a physician familiar with them, a person may proceed with the same confidence and consideration he would have in accepting other types of treatment.

Treatment with adrenal steroid hormones may be carried out by using certain preparations that can be injected into the affected joint or joints or inflamed extra-articular tissues, but treatment with adrenal hormones is not advised for many types of arthritis and rheumatism, including the rheumatism from fatigue or nervous and emotional upsets, the arthritis of injuries, or the arthritis and rheumatism resulting from specific types of infections by germs. Injections of suitable steroid preparations may be made into the joints or extra-articular tissues of certain patients with degenerative joint disease or osteoarthritis, but adrenal steroids usually are not given systemically for this condition. Arthritic and rheumatic persons may reasonably anticipate that the further efforts of medical and chemical scientists will improve the physician's ability to affect the course of the various types of arthritis and rheumatism and gout.

RESULTS OF TREATMENT

Use of currently available methods of determining the type of arthritis or rheumatism and adequate application of currently available treatment will provide most patients with considerable comfort and useful joints. Success in treatment is a co-operative venture on the part of the patient and physician. Rarely can the physician facilitate the accomplishment of the objectives of treatment without the expenditure of much time and effort by the person affected.

Most arthritic or rheumatic patients can anticipate a long and useful life, especially when the desire and effort for this are sustained. Improvement sometimes comes when least expected. Though at times the ailment seems to run its course despite effort to control it, in most instances and especially when appropriate precautions are taken to protect affected muscles and joints, some degree of useful function can result. The course of many types of arthritis and rheumatism, fortunately, is generally favorable. Recent surveys of arthritic and rheumatic patients have shown that, while these conditions can be and often are painful and distressing, 90 per cent of such patients did not require assistance either in or outside of their living quarters and three out of four persons could continue the type of work they had been doing. Disabilities may increase with age in all categories, but this is not necessarily so. The arthritic or rheumatic person who with the help of his physician utilizes to the fullest every advantage indicated to improve his condition can be well repaid for his efforts.

CHAPTER 16

Diseases of the Heart and Circulation

OGLESBY PAUL, M.D.

INTRODUCTION

From the earliest times the heart has aroused the curiosity and interest of man to an extent not equaled by any other organ in the human body except the brain. Most people who get sick are inclined to refer unusual symptoms to the heart. This organ has often been associated with the idea of courage, as in the phrase "faint heart," and the average man is likely to speak of the other person as either "weakhearted" or "stronghearted." Once people thought that the heart was the seat of the soul. The heart is still referred to as the seat of one of life's most interesting emotions.

The heart is in fact a muscular pump which circulates the blood throughout the body and moves more than one thousand five hundred gallons of blood a day. During a lifetime it beats two and a half billion times and pumps a total of about thirty-five million gallons. The heart begins working before a child is born and is never quiet until death. The only rest it gets is when its beat is slowed or decreased somewhat in its force. The heart never gets a complete rest.

The heart of a child at birth weighs less than an ounce; that of an adult, a half pound. The energy which causes the heart to contract develops in nervous tissue called the pacemaker of the heart. Apparently its energy is the equivalent of a thousandth of a volt. The heart beats one hundred times a minute or more in a small child, and on an average of 72 times a minute in an adult.

More than seven hundred thousand people died in the United States in 1963 from heart disease. Over fifty per cent of all deaths are due to heart and blood vessel diseases, with about seven per cent of the deaths under the age of 5 years being in this category as contrasted with more than 60 per cent over the age of 65.

The importance of heart disease in relation to the cause of death is paramount; it leads all other causes. Estimates indicate that there are at any time nearly ten million people in the United States suffering from heart and blood vessel diseases.

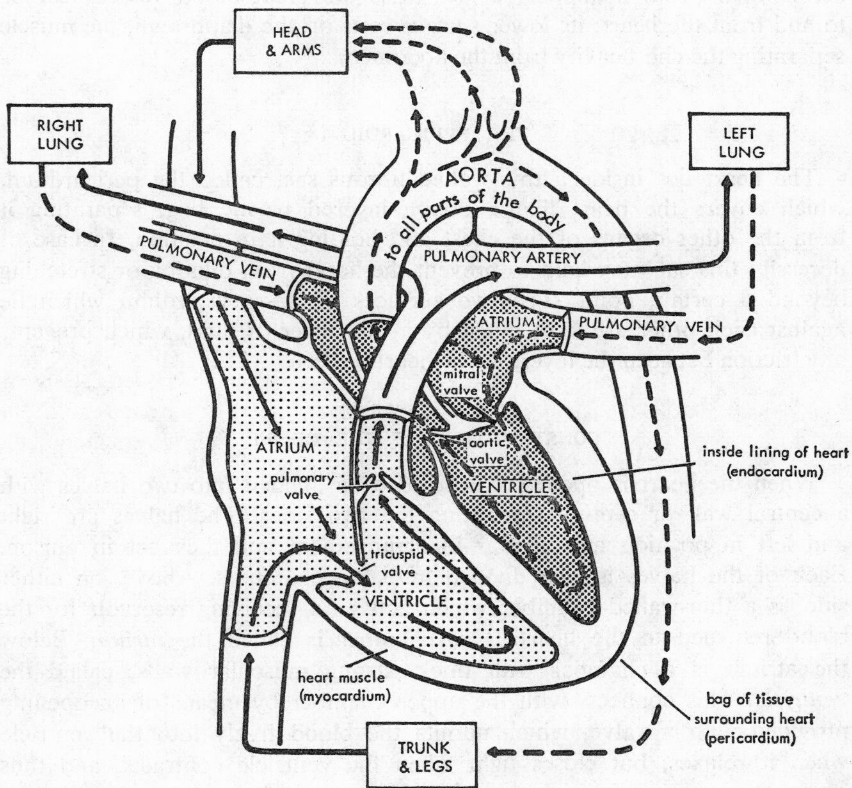

Fig. 43. Your heart weighs well under a pound and is only a little larger than your fist, but it is a powerful, long-working, hard-working organ. Its job is to pump blood to the lungs and to all the body tissues. It is a hollow organ whose tough, muscular wall (myocardium) is surrounded by a fiberlike bag (pericardium) and which is lined by a thin, strong membrane (endocardium). A wall (septum) divides the heart cavity down the middle into a "right heart" and a "left heart." Each side of the heart is divided into an upper chamber (called an atrium or auricle) and a lower chamber (ventricle). Valves regulate the flow of blood through the heart and to the pulmonary artery and the aorta. American Heart Association.

THE ANATOMY OF THE HEART

The heart is the great central pump which pumps blood through the blood vessels to every part of the body. It is a hollow organ with strong muscular walls and its size is about that of the clenched fist of its owner. The heart lies just beneath and to the left of the lower two thirds of the breastbone. From its upper surface arise the great blood vessels leading to and from the heart; its lower surface rests on the diaphragm, the muscle separating the chest cavity from the abdomen.

THE PERICARDIUM

The heart lies inside a thin-walled fibrous sac, called the pericardium, which covers the heart like a double-layered plastic bag, separating it from the other organs of the chest and holding it in position. In case of necessity this sac may help to prevent the heart from dilating or stretching beyond a certain point. The two surfaces of the pericardium which lie against each other are kept moist by a thin layer of fluid, which prevents any friction between the layers as the heart beats.

CONSTRUCTION OF THE HEART

When the heart is opened it is seen to be divided into two halves with a central wall or septum separating the two sides. The halves are right and left in position and similar in arrangement and they act in unison. Each of the halves is also divided into two chambers. Above, on either side, is a thin-walled chamber which acts as a receiving reservoir for the blood returned to the heart. This chamber is called the *atrium*. Below the atrium is a chamber with thick, strong muscular walls, called the *ventricle*. This connects with the upper chamber by means of an opening provided with a valve, which admits the blood freely into the ventricle when it relaxes, but closes tight when the ventricle contracts, and thus prevents the return flow of blood back into the atrium during the contraction of the ventricle. The only essential difference between the right and left sides of the heart is that the muscle walls on the left side are thicker; for the left side must propel the blood through the entire body except for the lungs while the right side needs to pump the blood through the lungs only. Leading from each ventricle is a large blood vessel (artery) which carries away the blood forced out of the ventricle when it contracts. At the point where the blood leaves each ventricle and enters the artery is a valve to prevent the flow of blood back into the ventricle, when its muscular walls relax again after contraction. Thus, *each side of the heart has two chambers, an atrium and a ventricle, and each side also has two valves* (tricuspid and pulmonic on the right side, mitral and aortic on the left side).

THE HEART WALL

The muscular wall of the heart is called the myocardium. Lining it in the hollow interior of the heart is a thin smooth membrane, the endocardium. This is continuous with a similar membrane lining the arteries and veins. From these terms come the names of diseases in which these tissues are inflamed, such as myocarditis and endocarditis.

THE CIRCULATORY SYSTEM

The circulatory system includes the heart and the various blood vessels leading from and to it—the arteries, veins, the tiny capillaries, and the lymphatics. This transportation system for the body carries to the cells, of which every organ and tissue of the body is built, essential materials for construction, and reconstruction of growing tissues and replacement of tissues broken down by wear and tear. The blood carries food stuffs as fuel, and oxygen to burn the fuel, so the necessary energy for repair and rebuilding may be obtained; each cell is thus enabled to perform its special function. Many other products, for instance the secretions of certain glands, must be carried to the cells by this system. The waste products from the cells must also be carried away and taken to organs whose duty is to excrete the waste; or the waste may be utilized elsewhere and made over for certain needs of the body. This circulatory system acts perfectly under normal conditions and takes care of the changing needs of each part of the body. When an organ or tissue is doing active work, that part receives an increased flow of blood, while parts at rest may receive a reduced amount.

The *arteries* are the blood vessels through which blood fully saturated with oxygen flows from the heart to the small *capillaries,* through the walls of which in turn the oxygen and other substances diffuse out of the blood and are delivered to nourish the tissues. The *veins* are the blood vessels through which the blood which has delivered its oxygen and fuel supply to the tissues and picked up waste products is returned to the heart.

The heart muscle itself is supplied with a system of blood vessels, arteries and veins, for its own fuel and repair requirements. This is called the coronary system. The coronary arteries open from the interior of the aorta (the large artery leading off from the left side of the heart). They arise just above the valve which separates the aorta from the ventricle.

THE FUNCTION OF THE HEART

The blood returning from every part of the body is brought back to the right atrium by two large veins, one coming from the upper and the other from the lower part of the body. These two veins are called respectively the superior and inferior vena cava. From the right atrium, the blood enters the right ventricle, which pumps the blood through the lungs. There it gives up its carbon dioxide, carried from all parts of the body, and takes on a fresh supply of oxygen. The blood returning thus from the circuit through the lungs is returned to the left atrium by the pulmonary veins, then passes into the left ventricle, and is finally pumped out into the arteries to supply the tissues.

When the walls of the ventricles relax in their turn, after each contraction, the blood from the distended atria flows into the ventricles. Just before the end of the ventricular diastole or period of relaxation of the walls of the ventricles, the muscle walls of the atria contract, further emptying the atria and more completely filling the ventricles. A fraction of a second later, the ventricles begin to contract. As the walls of the chambers contract and draw together, the pressure of the contained blood increases; the valves leading back into the atria are closed and held firmly shut by the blood in the ventricles pushing against them. When the pressure in the contracting ventricles becomes greater than the pressure in the arteries, the valves leading into the arteries are opened and the contents of the ventricles forced into the arteries. At the end of the ventricular contraction or *systole,* the ventricles in turn relax. As they do so the valves leading back into the ventricles are closed by the pressure of the blood in the arteries, thus preventing a reflow of blood back into the ventricles. During the period of ventricular systole the relaxed atria have again been filling with blood, whereupon the now relaxed ventricles are again filled. This cycle is repeated, many times a minute, hour after hour, and year after year during life. The heart works constantly but the amount and speed of its work varies with the demands imposed by exercise, eating, emotion, or even dreams.

The heart and the blood and lymph vessels which make up the circulatory system of the body constitute a mechanism equipped to meet every need of the body under normal conditions. This mechanism automatically adjusts itself to changing and varying needs in every part of the body. Provision has been made for almost every contingency that may arise. In addition, nature has given this mechanism a wide margin of safety so that it may still continue to do its work, even after a considerable amount of damage to the heart has been sustained.

Frequently our attention is called to the heart by symptoms which we

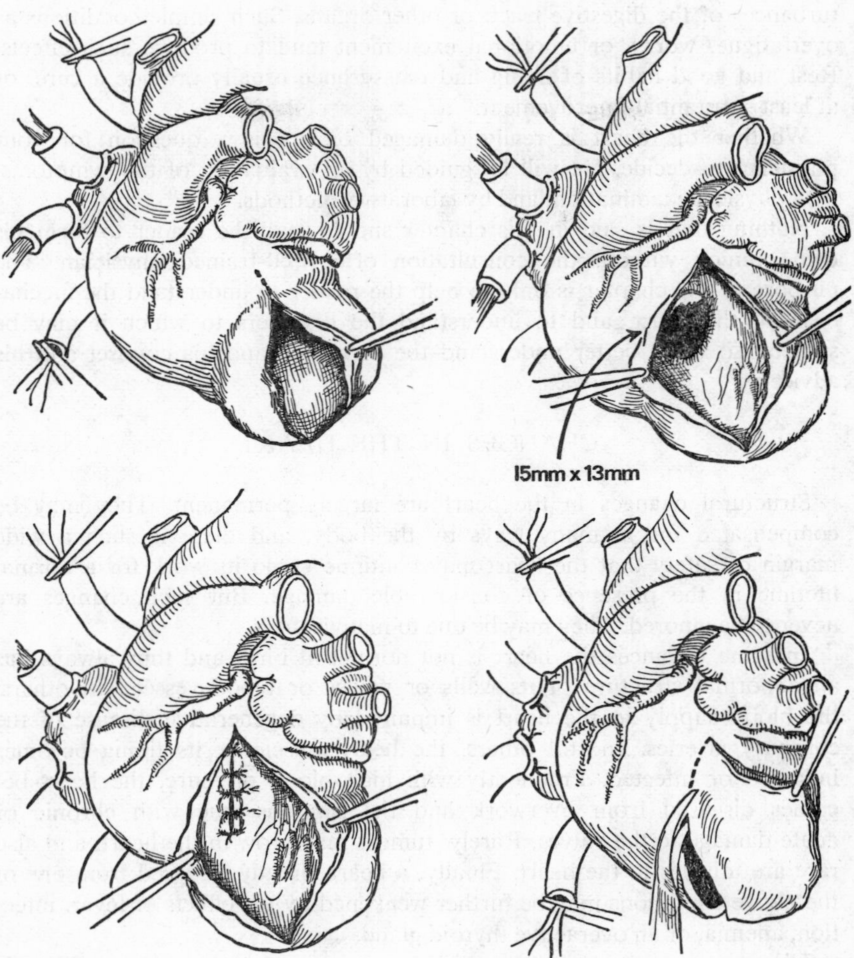

Fig. 44. In the 1950s, with the development of the heart-lung machine—a mechanical device which substitutes temporarily for the heart and lungs—the procedure known as open-heart surgery became feasible. Details of one operation are shown in the accompanying diagrams. Initially, surgeons opened the heart at an aneurysm (ballooning out) of the outer wall. This reveals an opening, or defect, in the inner wall of the heart. The opening is sewn. The damaged tissue of the aneurysm is removed. The heart is reconstructed. Drawings by Lawrence A. Krames, M.D.

interpret as symptoms of heart disease, but which are not due to any disease of the heart or to disease of any organ. Sometimes such symptoms may be troublesome. Usually they are due to an instability of the nervous mechanism which regulates the rate at which the heart beats, or to disturbances of the digestive tract, or other organs. Such simple conditions as overfatigue, worry, or emotional excitement tend to produce such effects. Rest and good habits of living and reassurance usually provide a cure, or at least substantial improvement.

Whether the heart is really damaged or not is a question for your physician to decide. He will be guided by an evaluation of the symptoms, by a physical examination, and by laboratory methods.

Nothing that is said in this chapter should lead the reader to form his own opinion without the consultation of a well-trained physician. The purpose of the chapter is only to help the reader to understand the mechanism of the heart, and to understand the disorders to which it may be subject, so as to better understand the physician and his counsel and his advice.

CHANGES IN THE HEART

Structural changes in the heart are largely permanent. They may be compensated for in many ways by the body, and there is such a wide margin of safety that the heart may continue to do its work for a normal lifetime in the presence of considerable damage. But such changes are never to be ignored. They may be due to many causes.

In some instances the heart is not normal at birth and thus always has an abnormal structure of its walls or valves or blood vessels. In others, the blood supply to the heart is impaired by degenerative disease of the coronary arteries. In still others, the heart muscle or its lining becomes inflamed or infected. Frequently with high blood pressure, the heart becomes diseased from overwork and the same is true with chronic or acute damage to the valves. Rarely, tumors may grow in the heart, and also rare are injuries to the heart. Finally, a heart already diseased from one of the above conditions may be further weakened by the effects of fever, infection, anemia, or an overactive thyroid gland.

Vigorous exertion does not injure a normal heart. Uncomfortable symptoms, or if these are not heeded, unconsciousness, stop overexertion long before the heart is damaged. But overexertion can cause difficulty in a heart in which an active inflammation is present or in a heart previously damaged.

CONGENITALLY DEFECTIVE HEARTS

A small number of children are born with hearts which are structurally defective. This defect may occur as a defect or "hole" somewhere in the central wall or septum, as faulty formation of the valves, or as improper positioning of the large blood vessels as they enter and leave the heart. In some cases, a blood vessel which usually closes at birth remains open and diverts extra blood into the lungs. Frequently, two or more of these defects are present in the same heart. Such congenital defects may be so serious that the child dies at birth or soon after. In other cases, in which the defect is less serious or in which its presence is compensated for by some other abnormal condition, the child may survive for varying periods, with some disability, or may lead a normal life, with the heart doing its work in spite of its handicap.

In some of the children in whom the only evidence of a congenital defect is perhaps limited to an unusual sound or murmur over the heart area and who are normal in growth and development, the physician may well advise that it is safe to disregard the condition if symptoms do not appear on exertion. These children should be allowed to live the life of normal children with the usual attention to health and hygiene but under careful observation. They do not usually require any medicine for the heart.

The problem is more significant if the child does have symptoms. Such symptoms include shortness of breath on exertion, or occasional fainting spells, or a lack of growth and development for the age. In some, the skin, lips, and nail beds may have a bluish cast, and the fingers may be "clubbed," that is, the ends may be broader and flatter than normal. Formerly such children did not survive, or were invalids or semi-invalids. Now surgical procedures can do much to restore such children to normal. The risk of doing such an operation is often small compared with the risk to future health and life if it is not done. The decision is a matter for the careful judgment of your physician, as is also the choice of a surgeon with special training who is skilled in such work.

Fortunately, today, the vast majority of children who have congenital heart disease and who survive the first few months of life can look forward to good futures. The milder cases may lead normal lives without treatment; the more severe cases may often be cured or greatly relieved by surgery.

RHEUMATIC FEVER

The illness responsible for most of the heart disease of childhood and early life, is known variously as rheumatic fever, acute rheumatic fever, or inflammatory rheumatism. Chorea, or St. Vitus' dance, is a manifestation of rheumatic fever.

The name "rheumatic fever" is not always apt. The name "rheumatism" calls to mind symptoms of disease of the bones and joints, and rheumatic fever may exist and cause severe damage to the heart without any such symptoms or with symptoms so slight that they do not attract attention. Fever, while it is doubtless present in some degree at times during the acute phase of the disease, may be minor or may remain undiscovered. However, the name "rheumatic fever" has been in general use for so long that it would be confusing to attempt to change it.

As far as is known, rheumatic fever always follows an infection caused by a small bacteria called the beta hemolytic streptococcus. This is the bacteria which causes scarlet fever and often causes sore throats and tonsillitis. Only a small per cent of people who have an infection due to this streptococcus develop rheumatic fever (less than 3 per cent). Just why some children and young adults develop rheumatic fever after such an infection and others do not is not yet understood. What is clear is that no other bacteria has ever been shown to produce an infection followed by rheumatic fever except this streptococcus. It is thus essential to recognize that rheumatic fever may be a sequel to a streptococcal sore throat or to scarlet fever. However, rheumatic fever is not itself an actual infection by the streptococcus—the streptococcal infection *precedes* the rheumatic fever, and in some way creates a state of sensitivity or allergy which results in symptoms and disease in the joints, heart, and elsewhere which we have come to identify as an inflammation called rheumatic fever.

While rheumatic fever is thought of as a disease of the joints and of the heart, it is really a generalized disease. Its effects are not evenly distributed and it may affect some organs greatly, such as the joints and the heart, while other organs may be only slightly affected, or not at all. The joints may escape and the heart may be involved, without any joint symptoms, but characteristic changes in the smaller arteries may appear anywhere, from the brain down. There may never be any acute symptoms. Often rheumatic fever is a chronic disease and its course in one form or another may cover a period of months or even years. One does not acquire an immunity as the result of one attack, but the whole process may recur following another streptococcal infection. While the joints are often involved at the outset, the important permanent damage is done not to them but to the heart.

Most of the damage done to the heart occurs during the acute stages, but damage may also be going on slowly, though none the less certainly, during the periods when the disease is apparently inactive. Indeed, rheumatic fever may exist and cause structural damage to the heart without any recognizable symptoms. Frequently unquestionable evidence of heart damage due to rheumatic disease is found in patients whose record, after the closest questioning, furnishes no clue to the time when the damage might have occurred.

The milder manifestations of rheumatic fever, unless accompanied by some more definite sign, such as rheumatic nodules, are difficult to differentiate from symptoms occurring in other conditions.

The child may only appear to be below what would be considered the normal health level. Colds and sore throats may appear with more than usual frequency. The weight may be below the normal average, or a loss of weight may occur rather conspicuously and suddenly. Fatigue is present out of all proportion to the play or exertion which brought it on. There may be loss of appetite, symptoms of stomach or intestinal disturbance, headache, nervous instability, or many other symptoms which are not characteristic of rheumatic fever particularly, but which are indicative of mild illness. There may be a pallor, and a blood examination may reveal mild anemia, although sometimes the pallor is out of proportion to the anemia actually present. Blood examination may also show evidences of a previous beta hemolytic streptococcal infection and elevation of the sedimentation rate or other tests for active inflammation. Unfortunately, there is no simple test absolutely diagnostic of rheumatic fever. The pulse may be more rapid than normal. Careful and repeated trials may indicate the presence of fever. An electrocardiogram may show signs of an active process in the heart.

There is nothing characteristic of any one disease in the symptoms described. These cases do, however, demand careful examination and reexamination by the doctor. Particularly important is consideration of rheumatic fever when such vague symptoms follow scarlet fever or a sore throat; have a throat culture to look for a beta hemolytic streptococcal infection.

"Growing pains" may be a complaint and difficult to evaluate. Many such indefinite pains are not significant, but there should always be careful questioning to determine their true nature. If there is any doubt, careful and repeated physical examination by the physician is most important. The growing pains are rather indefinite nagging muscle or joint pains, occurring anywhere, but most often in the legs, in front of the thighs, or behind the knees, or in the so-called "hamstring muscles." Sometimes the child complains of neck pains. Such pains may occur from many causes and are usually not important. However, they may be difficult to distinguish from a true rheumatism, with real involvement of the joints (redness, increased heat, swelling, and pain on motion or touch) representing a manifestation of rheumatic fever. The watchful mother should listen to the child's story so that the true nature of the pains may be determined.

Another manifestation which occurs with variable frequency is the "rheumatic nodule." It is a small round lump or nodule, visible under the skin and movable. It is not tender. The size varies with the location, but on the average is about the size of a small pea. These nodules are most easily found where the tendons join the muscles with the bones, as close to the elbows or wrists, the knees, or the nape of the neck, or over the shoulder or hips, and less frequently over the shoulder blade or the collarbone. The presence of these nodules may be presumed to indicate rheumatic fever, although they have been observed in apparently healthy children, in cases in which rheumatic fever could not be definitely proved.

More frequently the actual onset of rheumatic fever occurs abruptly, most often about two weeks after a sore throat or scarlet fever. It begins with the immediate appearance of joint symptoms or sometimes heart symptoms. There may be a short premonitory stage of fever. In more than half the cases, the attacks begin with an inflammation of one or more joints, particularly the large joints such as the knees, ankles, wrists, and elbows. There is pain in the joint, which is swollen, tender, reddened, and feels hot to the touch. The symptoms may be severe or mild. The joints may be tender with little or no swelling, or slightly swollen with little or no tenderness. Characteristically the symptoms may migrate from joint to joint, with a duration of one to eight days or more for each joint. At a given time, one or several joints may be involved. Fever is present from the start during these stages, and its height varies with each case. Its severity or lack of severity must never be taken as an index of the involvement of the heart.

Pleurisy or inflammation of the membrane lining the chest cavity may be the first symptom of the onset of rheumatic fever. Severe pain on breathing may occur suddenly, without any previous warning, or may follow after a few days of what is apparently only a "cold." The symptom of pain may disappear, and the pleura, or lining membrane of the chest, escape further trouble. Sometimes the pain may be followed by a collection of fluid in the chest cavity. Occasionally the fluid may appear silently without any preceding pain. A form of pneumonia, peculiar to rheumatic fever, may appear at the onset, but is more likely to occur later in the disease.

CHOREA

Chorea, or St. Vitus' dance, is another manifestation of rheumatic fever, occurring rather more frequently in girls, and is limited usually to the early school age. Most cases occur between the ages of five and ten, and most frequently independently of the joint symptoms. The child who has had choreic twitchings will probably have chorea when rheumatic fever recurs, just as the one with symptoms affecting the joints most frequently has joint symptoms when there is a recurrence. In a part of the cases chorea and joint symptoms are present at the same time, or the child may show chorea at one time and joint symptoms at another.

Chorea is often mild, and does not always attract the attention it should. Occasionally it occurs without being noticed. Sometimes there are only minor symptoms, such as fidgeting, restlessness, or lack of attention and concentration. The lack of concentration may be noticed only at school, or the nervousness may show in the handwriting. There may be loss of appetite, headache, and general nervous instability. The child may be forgetful, irritable, emotional, and may have crying spells. In the less mild cases the nervousness is more evident. There are spasmodic involuntary movements of the face and hands. The child may drop things that he is carrying and be unable to sit still. The more severe cases cannot escape attention. The spasmodic movements are more extreme and pronounced; the face is distorted, and there are uncontrollable grimaces. The tongue may be involuntarily thrust out; the speech may be interfered with. Choreic manifestations are always worse during excitement or when attention is attracted to them. The choreic movements disappear during sleep.

Heart disease may ensue in the children with choreic manifestations but not as frequently as it follows with other signs and symptoms. It does not always follow so promptly, either. Children with the joint symptoms usually develop the heart disease while they are still under observation because of the acute attack, or shortly after, although the appearance of heart disease is often delayed in them also. In chorea the heart disease frequently appears later, after the symptoms of chorea have subsided, or even after a period of years.

A child with chorea requires rest and quiet surroundings. Chorea should be considered as active rheumatic fever and treated as such. (*See* later.)

RHEUMATIC INFLAMMATION OF THE HEART

Inflammation of the heart and its consequences are as much a manifestation of rheumatic fever as are the joint symptoms or the nodules. It is not to be regarded as a complication or as an aftermath of rheumatic fever, but as an essential part. Rheumatic fever is a generalized inflammatory condition having an effect on similar tissues in many parts of the body. However, while many tissues in the body may be involved in the initial acute stage, it is the inflammation and subsequent scarring in the heart which may be serious. Thus, while the joints never show any permanent damage, the heart frequently does.

The inflammation may seem to expend all of its energy on the heart, and the effects of rheumatic fever on the heart may appear without evidence of rheumatic fever elsewhere. Occasionally when a child is examined because of an acute attack of rheumatic fever with joint symptoms, or other manifestations, the heart is found to have been already involved at some previous time. In such cases the probability is that minor manifestations of rheumatic fever had occurred and were unobserved. Such cases are not the common rule; more frequently involvement of the heart is associated with or follows one or more of the other manifestations of rheumatic fever. However, as has been noted, the inflammation of the heart may not be noticed at the onset and for a long period give no indication of its presence.

Rheumatic fever may affect the outer sac covering the heart producing pericarditis; it may affect the heart muscle causing myocarditis, or it may involve the inner lining of the heart causing endocarditis. Often, and indeed usually, all three of these occur together.

Pericarditis is an inflammation of the walls of the sac in which the heart is enclosed. As these inflamed walls rub past each other with each beat of the heart, they may cause pain in the front of the chest. In some cases the pain is absent. Frequently fluid appears between the two walls of the pericardium, separating them, and sometimes causing distention of the pericardial sac, even to the point of interfering with the work of the heart. This is called pericarditis with effusion. Pericarditis may be the first manifestation of rheumatic fever and may come on suddenly. More frequently it occurs in the course of the disease and in the presence of other manifestations. It always means that an inflammation of the heart is present.

Because of the frequent inflammation of the lining of the heart or endocardium (*endocarditis*), deformities of the valves which are covered with endocardium develop so that they cannot open or close properly. This may affect any of the valves, but most frequently the mitral valve between the left auricle and ventricle, and the aortic valve at the outlet of the left ventricle are involved. Less frequently the tricuspid valve, between the right auricle and ventricle is affected. The earliest damage to a valve results in inability of the valve leaflets to close properly, and thus the valve allows blood to "leak" back through the valve at the time when the valve is supposed to be closed tight. After months and years, with the lessening of active inflammation and the formation of scar tissue, the valve may no longer open widely enough, a condition called stenosis. Such damaged valves give rise to murmurs—sounds the physician may hear with his stethoscope.

If the heart is affected, the heart muscle is invariably involved in the inflammation to some degree, perhaps slightly, or perhaps to a degree which interferes with its efficiency. The minor involvement by this *myocarditis* may only be evident if a record of the electrical activity of the heart is made—an electrocardiogram. More severe myocarditis results in enlargement of the heart, dilatation of the heart chambers, and loss of pumping power by the heart muscle. It may produce fatigue, shortness of breath, cough, and swelling of the abdomen and legs.

A heart that has been severely damaged is almost always enlarged and in rheumatic fever may become greatly enlarged. When the heart enlarges in order to compensate for the additional work which it must do, the muscle fibers become longer or thicker, or both. The bulk of the muscle is increased. But as the heart muscle increases in size, it cannot grow any new blood vessels, so that the enlarged muscle must be nourished by the same number of blood vessels that supplied it before it became enlarged. The blood vessels per unit of size are fewer in number, in spite of the increased needs. The body may compensate for this in part by increasing the blood flow through the vessels which are present. However a decreased blood flow with increased blood needs may eventually cause serious changes in the heart muscle and the person with an enlarged heart should not leave the entire burden of care to nature, however kindly nature may be. Some restriction of physical activity may be needed, and he should consult with his physician regarding appropriate exercise and the limits of physical strain.

MANAGEMENT OF RHEUMATIC FEVER

The management of rheumatic fever requires first that the diagnosis be properly established by the physician. This involves a careful history of the illness, a complete physical examination, and usually blood tests for evidence of a beta hemolytic streptococcal infection and for signs of active inflammation. Usually, an electrocardiogram is needed and often a chest X ray. Because the disease may be subtle in its manifestations, the physician may find necessary observation of the patient for several days or even weeks, usually at home but at times in the hospital, before a firm diagnosis can be established.

The care of rheumatic fever includes measures to assure general good nutrition and adequate rest, measures to eliminate any active infection with the beta hemolytic streptococcus, the use of drugs to alter and reduce active inflammation, and in some instances specific treatment to help the heart.

The general measures useful are not specific for rheumatic fever and are those suitable for any illness. The child or adult should have sufficient physical and mental rest to permit recovery of strength, avoidance of undue fatigue, and freedom from symptoms. In general, rest is obligatory during periods of fever, rapid pulse, and symptoms such as joint pain, shortness of breath or tiredness. The duration of such rest can only be determined by periodic appraisal by a physician. It customarily necessitates rest for several weeks and frequently for several months. The diet should be a normal balanced one, often light during the first period of symptoms.

In view of the relation of rheumatic fever to a previous infection with a beta hemolytic streptococcus, the physician will usually wish to take a throat and/or nose culture for this organism. If this is found to be present in the nose or throat, a course of treatment with an antibiotic such as penicillin which is known to kill the streptococcus is advisable.

Two types of drugs are helpful in alleviating the signs of active inflammation in the joints, heart, and elsewhere. Many years have passed since aspirin and other members of the aspirin family were observed to have a remarkably helpful influence in lowering fever, in relieving joint pain and signs of joint involvement, and in quieting the discomfort of pericarditis. More recently, substances such as cortisone have been widely used with similar benefit. Thus both types of agent can help to give comfort to the patient. Further, there is some evidence that the early use of substances such as cortisone may lessen the extent of permanent damage. Since these drugs have certain undesirable as well as desirable effects, the decision as to their use is always carefully reviewed by the physician.

Should the heart be severely affected, the physician may wish to administer drugs to strengthen the heart muscle and to help dispose of extra water and salt through the kidneys. Oxygen occasionally is useful for a time. In the milder or moderate cases, such measures are usually not needed. Later, with recovery from the acute illness, many long-term considerations arise. Thus, the child or adult may always attempt to lead a healthy life, avoiding excessive fatigue, and maintaining proper but not excessive nutrition. Most patients who have recovered from the acute phase are able to lead lives of normal activity; for a minority some restriction of strenuous physical activity is needed. Neither a history of rheumatic fever or the presence of a murmur due to rheumatic heart disease necessitate in themselves a limitation of sports and other physical activity. Only those persons with signs of severe damage must be restricted. Any person with a rheumatic history should take especial precautions with respiratory infections and should seek medical advice for any illness associated with fever and a sore throat. Rheumatic fever can recur, such recurrences being due to a repetition of streptococcal infection, and one attack does not convey immunity. While the disease is commonest between the ages of five and twenty, initial attacks and recurrences may occur earlier or later than this, and the possibility of a recurrence must always be considered at any age in a person who has had rheumatic fever once. If there is a history of frequent sore throats, and the tonsils appear chronically diseased, it may be wise to have them removed. However, a history of rheumatic fever is not by itself any reason for such an operation.

Signs of the development of difficulty from rheumatic heart disease may occur during the acute stage, but often do not arise for many years. In those patients with minimal disease, symptoms may never occur despite one or more murmurs and slight or moderate enlargement of the heart. In those with more severe damage, development of some shortness of breath is common, quite often palpitation due to irregular heart action, and perhaps swelling of the abdomen or lower limbs. In certain cases, chest pain or discomfort or fainting spells are seen. Much can be done to help such persons with diet and drugs and advice as to a proper pace of living.

One of the signal and dramatic chapters in medicine has been the availability of surgical operations to help some patients with chronic and disabling disease of the heart valves. In some instances, the surgeon may open valves which have become fused partly closed. In other cases totally new valves may be inserted and the patient's old valve removed. Such surgery may be useful in lessening the effects of the rheumatic damage on the valves, but unfortunately does nothing to attack directly any weakness of the heart muscle resulting from the previous myocarditis. Thus, heart operations are not as yet a perfectly satisfactory answer to the problem.

PREVENTION

Rheumatic fever recurrences can be prevented. With adequate antibiotic treatment of beta hemolytic streptococcal infections, first attacks of rheumatic fever might never occur. Thus, to prevent rheumatic fever in a primary sense, patients and physicians must be alert to detect a sore throat due to the beta hemolytic streptococcus, or to detect scarlet fever. A throat culture is the best means of identification, and once diagnosed, prompt adequate antibiotic treatment almost invariably prevents rheumatic fever from following. For those people who have once had rheumatic fever, particularly children and young adults, the *regular* use of sulfadiazine or penicillin is nearly one hundred per cent effective in preventing further infections with the beta hemolytic streptococcus and thus in preventing more attacks of rheumatic fever. Since each attack tends to produce further damage to the heart, such a program of prevention is vitally important.

BACTERIAL ENDOCARDITIS

Valves damaged by rheumatic fever, or by other processes, or deformed at birth, appear to have a predisposition to infection with certain bacteria. Sometimes after extraction of a tooth, or a respiratory or other infection, bacteria will gain access to the blood stream, be carried to the damaged valve, and lodge there and multiply. This condition is called bacterial endocarditis. Since it may produce further damage to the heart and send out infection to other parts of the body, it is a most important although fortunately not very common condition. It may occur at any age. Less often, an acute bacterial endocarditis may arise on a normal valve usually complicating an acute infection such as pneumonia.

The symptoms of this acute endocarditis are those of a severe acute infection with high fever, chills, and prostration. Prompt treatment with the proper antibiotic is needed if recovery is to take place.

The milder, subacute form is more common. In the subacute form about 85 per cent are due to one type of streptococcus, the S. viridans. As in the acute form, the infection is practically confined to the endocardium, especially to the valves, where it results in a productive inflammation, causing growths called vegetations upon the valves, with underlying ulceration of the tissue. The symptoms may be mild indeed at the onset, so mild as to attract little or no attention for a long time. The condition is frequently similar to mild, incipient tuberculosis. There may be only fatigue on slight effort, weakness, feeling of malaise, or slight digestive disturbance, or loss of weight and strength. There may be some pallor, and an actual anemia is often present.

Fever is present, although there may be periods of days when it is absent. It varies from a rise of only a fraction of a degree in the milder cases to higher temperatures in the more sharp types. In the cases associated with the higher temperatures, chills may occur. The pulse rate is usually faster than normal.

At some time during the disease what are known as petechiae or an outbreak on the skin may occur due to the release from the heart of small blood clots called emboli. They are small round red dots, not appreciably raised, and differing in size, rarely larger than a pinhead in diameter, and do not disappear on pressure. They are frequently seen in the white of the eye, in the mouth, and in the nail beds. The spleen is sometimes enlarged, and the symptoms of the pre-existing heart disease may be accentuated.

Still another sign of the disease is the occurrence of emboli in various other parts of the body. These small fragments which have become detached from the growths on the valves of the heart are carried by the blood stream through the arteries to lodge in some distant part. The symptoms and signs will vary with the site of the artery which is occluded by the embolus. Occasionally the lodgment of such an embolus in the brain, with consequent paralysis, or in the spleen, with intense pain, or in the kidney with pain and the appearance of blood in the urine, or in one of the arteries of the extremity, is the first symptom which brings the disease to the attention of the patient and his physician.

The sooner this infection is recognized, the better. The outlook, with penicillin and the other antibiotics, is immeasurably brighter than formerly. In these days most cases recover, instead of just a few, but it is still an extremely serious disease. To help to prevent it, patients with known valvular heart disease should receive antibiotics before and after dental extractions and other operative procedures.

NON-RHEUMATIC MYOCARDITIS

Syphilis of the heart and aorta, the large blood vessel leaving the left side of the heart is becoming rare. It can be prevented by adequate treatment in the primary or secondary phase of the disease. It may exist silently until extensive or irreparable damage has been done. For this reason blood examinations, like Wassermann or Kahn tests, should be made on those in whom there is any reason to suspect the disease to have occurred. When syphilitic disease of the heart and aorta is known to be present, treatment cannot be curative.

While myocarditis due to rheumatic fever is well known, it is by no means the only type of heart muscle inflammation which is seen. Many types of infection can be accompanied or followed by involvement of the heart muscle by infection. Usually this is mild and unimportant. Rather rarely, the infection in the heart may be severe, the heart may enlarge, and develop signs of weakness as shown by rapid pulse, congestion in the lungs and liver, and engorgement of the veins in the neck. Influenza and various forms of pneumonia may be accompanied by this complication. The outlook is usually favorable, but if the heart becomes quite large, serious difficulties can arise. The heart should be carefully watched, and the observations checked by X-ray examination.

HEART CHANGES IN TOXIC THYROID

In the cases known as toxic thyroid, there is an oversecretion of the hormone of the thyroid gland. In these cases almost invariably one symptom is referable to the heart: the rapid pulse rate. Occasionally there may be an abnormal rhythm, called atrial fibrillation, or some shortness of breath. The presence of a definite increase in the metabolic rate will confirm the diagnosis as will blood tests and a radioactive iodine uptake test.

Such symptoms subside when the abnormal condition of the gland is remedied, by use of drugs like propylthiouracil, or use of radioactive iodine or surgery.

CORONARY HEART DISEASE

The heart muscle is supplied with the blood necessary for its activity by means of coronary arteries, blood vessels which run through the heart itself, dividing and subdividing finally into small capillaries in close contact with each muscle fiber. They bring to the heart muscle material for repair, fuel to furnish energy, and oxygen to burn the fuel. They carry away the waste and the results of combustion. They are essential for the life and the activity of the heart muscle.

These arteries have their origin in the aorta, the large vessel leading from the heart, at its beginning, just as it leaves the left ventricle or left chamber of the heart, and just above the valve which separates the aorta from the ventricle. Hence the flow into these arteries will depend in part upon the pressure in the aorta.

Come from a family with a history of coronary artery disease

risk up 1.7 to 1

Smoke a package or more of cigarettes a day

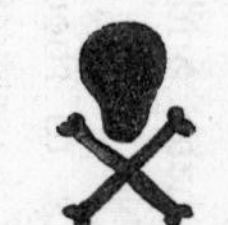

risk up 3 to 1

Get fat

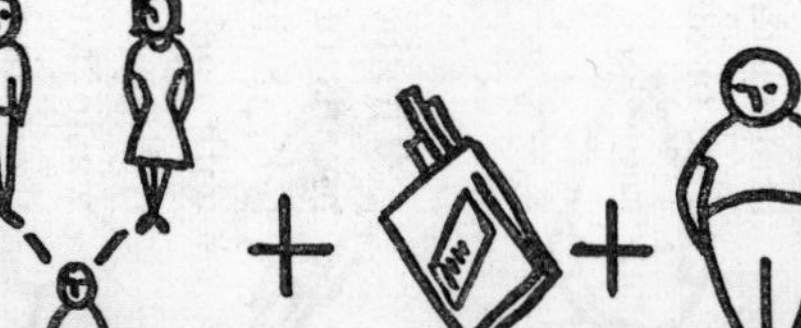

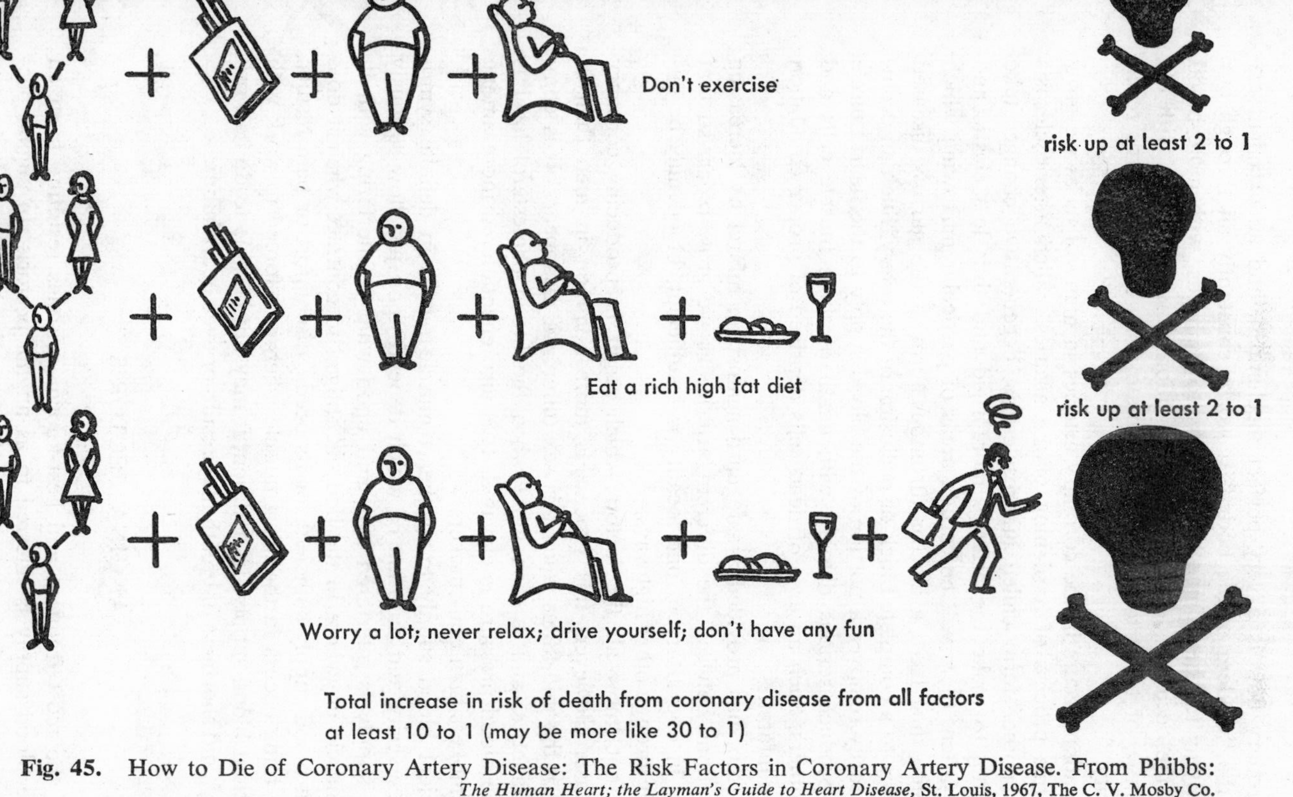

Fig. 45. How to Die of Coronary Artery Disease: The Risk Factors in Coronary Artery Disease. From Phibbs: *The Human Heart; the Layman's Guide to Heart Disease*, St. Louis, 1967, The C. V. Mosby Co.

The coronary flow is a very perfect mechanism, and an excellent example of the "wisdom of the body." It works constantly all through our lives, supplying the heart muscle according to its needs, with more blood or less, as the occasion demands. Any condition which interferes with the coronary flow, or tends to make it inadequate, may shorten life or result in incapacity.

Deterioration occurs in the coronary arteries in many of us as we grow older. In this process of hardening of the arteries, called arteriosclerosis and also another form called atherosclerosis, degenerative changes take place tending to make the arteries more rigid and thus less elastic and narrower. Often, there will be certain areas of particular narrowing which may at some time have a clot or thrombus form at the narrow diseased point leading to a complete block or occlusion of the artery. Such an occlusion necessarily removes a portion of the blood supply to the heart muscle and may produce serious damage with death of some muscle cells and injury to others. Such an area of dead cells deprived of proper circulation is called an infarct.

Nature, too, has provided a safeguard against an infarct by increasing the connections between the different arteries as we grow older, so that if the flow in one artery in one locality is insufficient, blood may be detoured to it through other highways.

We do not know all the factors which result in producing coronary heart disease. However, this process is more common in men than in women until the mid-fifties when this sex difference disappears. It is common in diabetics, and is seen more when the blood cholesterol level is high or the blood pressure is elevated. It is also encountered more among cigarette smokers than non-smokers.

A deficient blood supply to the heart muscle results in definite symptoms, the severity and duration of which depend upon just how seriously the blood supply is interfered with and upon what is interfering with it. When a muscle anywhere in the body is obliged to contract when it does not have a blood supply sufficient for its needs, discomfort or pain results. The same thing occurs in the heart muscle when it is forced to work with an insufficient blood supply. In addition, it may not be able to do its work adequately, and shortness of breath may result, or even heart failure.

ANGINA PECTORIS

One of the most frequent and best-known episodes resulting from an inadequate blood supply is referred to as angina pectoris. In angina pectoris symptoms are of short duration, because the blood supply is only temporarily insufficient for the work of the heart just at that time, when some extra demand is made on the heart. This is encountered essentially when the coronary arteries carrying the blood to nourish the heart muscle become narrowed with atherosclerosis, and thus are unable to carry enough blood to feed the heart properly when an increase in oxygen and other substances is required—as with exercise. This transient inadequacy of the blood supply to the heart causes the symptoms.

Discomfort in the chest is the most important symptom in angina pectoris. The discomfort is usually dull, oppressive, or constricting, and not sharp like a knife. It is usually noted under the breastbone, and more frequently under the upper portion of the breastbone, or across the front of the chest. It may remain in that region, or it may radiate to the left shoulder, or down the left arm, perhaps only as far as the elbow, or the wrist, or it may extend to the tips of the fingers. Occasionally it may radiate to the right shoulder and down the right arm, or it may radiate to both shoulders, and down both arms. In other persons it may radiate to the front of the neck or be referred to the lower teeth. At times, the distress may never be felt in the chest at all, and be felt only at the points to which it may radiate, as the left shoulder, the elbow, or the little and the ring finger, or the lower jaw, or the pit of the stomach.

Except for these symptoms, associated or appearing singly, there is nothing which characterizes an attack, except that it is of short duration, a matter of thirty to sixty seconds or several minutes. Attacks lasting hours, or with other symptoms, are not typical angina pectoris.

There are no certain signs which enable the physician to recognize the presence of an attack or to judge of the probability of the occurrence of such an attack. Nothing characteristic can be found by examination of the heart, or the pulse or blood pressure, or by laboratory methods except that the electrocardiogram is of limited help. The physician must be guided altogether by the story of the attack and such characteristics as the patient tells him.

Attacks are most frequently brought on by exertion or emotion. In some persons they are brought on by moderate exertion at any time; in others by moderate exertion only under certain conditions; and in others the attacks may accompany only unusual exertion. Attacks are especially apt to accompany exertion soon after a meal. With an empty stomach, a man may be able to walk briskly for a long distance without distress and yet find himself unable to walk a hundred feet after a meal without symptoms of pain. In some, the attacks may follow exertion after any meal, or may follow especially some one meal, as in the evening or in the morning. Attacks are likely to follow a meal which is too full.

For these reasons, it is best for the person with angina not to eat heavily at any time. It is well to avoid rich and heavy foods, and to avoid effort soon after eating. Too low a blood sugar may also rarely cause typical anginal pain. This condition may occur with a poorly proportioned diet, or too much insulin, etc. It is a matter of careful consideration by your physician.

Excitement is also well known as a factor which increases the work of the heart and may bring on angina. Thus, some patients learn to avoid going to a football game or watching sports on television.

Angina may also be related to reflex impulses arising from various sources. One very frequent such reflex is that resulting from breathing cold air through the nose or walking against a cold wind. This can be obviated by holding a muffler over the nose and thus breathing warm air through the mouth or nose. Other sources of such possible reflex effects are gallstones or stomach disorders, duodenal ulcers, or a hiatus hernia where the stomach pushes up through the opening through which the esophagus descends to the stomach. Just too full a stomach, or an indigestible meal, may be a cause.

In some with more severe difficulty, an attack may come when sitting quietly, especially after a meal. An attack may occur in the early morning hours in the midst of a normal sleep.

Angina pectoris is by no means the hopeless disease which is often pictured. It may be serious, but it is possible in most cases for patients to go on for many years with recurring but not disabling attacks, or the attacks may cease to occur and the patient lead a normal life. Important are avoidance of overweight, the maintenance of a routine of regular physical exercise as advised by the physician, and the use of the drug nitroglycerin. Patients with angina pectoris usually know about how far they can go without bringing on an attack, and they should conduct their lives accordingly. They should keep in touch with their physician and report at regular intervals. Possibly, also, the physician may wish occasional electrocardiographic tracings made to confirm his observations. If an attack occurs which is different from those usually experienced, which is more painful, or lasts longer, the patient should call his physician.

CORONARY OCCLUSION

In occlusion of one of the branches of the coronary artery, as well as what is referred to as acute coronary insufficiency, the discomfort or pain is identical with that of angina pectoris only it is usually more severe and instead of lasting not more than five or ten minutes may last up to several hours. In angina pectoris there is only a temporary disproportion between the blood supply to the heart muscle and its needs for blood. The pain usually quickly passes away, and no damage to the heart muscle results from the isolated attack. In coronary occlusion one of the coronary arteries is occluded by a clot. The area of muscle supplied by that particular branch is deprived of blood for a length of time sufficient to do serious damage to the muscular wall of the heart. The zone of muscle involved is called an infarct. Muscle cells die, and must be replaced by scar tissue which requires several weeks.

Thus a patient who has suffered a coronary occlusion with an infarct must have a period of several weeks of rest, often requires oxygen and narcotics for the initial relief of his discomfort, and subsequent to the first complete rest must only gradually resume normal activity.

Fortunately, although this condition is a serious one, the body is able to achieve a highly satisfactory repair of the areas affected in a majority of cases. Collateral channels open up to bring blood to the muscle cells formerly provided by the coronary artery branch which has been closed off. Thus, an eventual return to a full normal life is possible for most persons with this sort of an attack. However, particular care should be employed to avoid excessive fatigue and overweight, and to have regular proper exercise. Most physicians advise the complete omission of cigarettes.

A patient with coronary occlusion or coronary insufficiency is usually best cared for in a hospital, where laboratory methods are available to confirm the diagnosis and to check on progress toward recovery. Electrocardiographic tracings are almost always diagnostic, but a lack of characteristic findings in them should not outweigh the other clinical evidence.

FUNCTIONAL SYMPTOMS

In a large group of cases, symptoms appear often regarded as due to the heart and variously referred to as neurocirculatory asthenia, effort syndrome, or anxiety state. In these cases the heart and the circulatory system are normal structurally. However, the person often complains of shortness of breath, a desire to take deep breaths and get air into his lungs, sighing, various chest pains usually unrelated to effort, and palpitation and fatigue. Frequently, the patient believes he or she is suffering from heart disease.

A careful appraisal by a physician in such cases will not reveal evidences of heart trouble. The history points to the nature of the difficulty—a condition not due to any structural disease, and indeed of unknown origin. Called by various names as noted, it is without effect on longevity and never develops into true heart disease. It is annoying but not serious, and may come and go over years.

Often reassurance and explanation are sufficient to relieve the anxiety of the patient and to lessen greatly the discomfort. In severe prolonged cases, the advice of a psychiatrist may be required.

VARIATIONS IN THE PULSE

Some irregularities of the pulse beat are quite normal; others may be significant of conditions which demand the physician's advice. In youth, and at times in later life, there is a slowing of the pulse in breathing out, and a quickening in breathing in, which is normal. Sometimes the alternating change in rate may be noticeable. It is never of any significance.

In many people an irregularity which may frequently attract attention is really an extra beat of the heart coming before the anticipated time, but the long pause following the beat makes it appear as though a beat has been dropped. It is usually described by the patient as a feeling of the "heart flopping over." It is more noticeable with fatigue, or with indigestion, or after too hearty a meal. It often appears with worry or apprehension. The irregularity tends to disappear on exertion and then is more noticeable during the rest which follows exertion. This irregularity is usually of no significance in itself, but its importance, if any, is a matter for the physician to decide.

Attacks of rapid regular heart action coming on instantly, and stopping just as suddenly, occur in some people. They commonly last only a few seconds or minutes, but they may persist for longer periods. They may begin at any time, even in early life. They are inconvenient and troublesome, but not serious. Such paroxysmal attacks occurring with structural heart disease, especially later in life, may be of significance, and a physician should be consulted.

A form of irregularity called atrial fibrillation occurs, especially in those who have had a rheumatic infection of the heart, but may accompany other conditions, such as toxic thyroid. This may also occur in persons who appear to have no structural heart disease. In this, the pulse is absolutely irregular in both rate and volume. This condition with its usually rapid heart rate can be controlled by digitalis and may be adequately moderated for an indefinite period of time. It can often be terminated or prevented by use of the drug quinidine. In selected cases, an electric shock may also be employed to end the irregularity.

CHAPTER 17

Digestion and Digestive Diseases

JOSEPH B. KIRSNER, M.D., Ph.D.

Digestive diseases are among the most common of all ailments and are one of the major causes of chronic and of fatal illness. This chapter is divided into four parts: the structure and function of the gastrointestinal system; tests for digestive disorders; a description of important gastrointestinal diseases; and a discussion of common digestive complaints.

STRUCTURE AND FUNCTION

The main purpose of the digestive tract is to facilitate the utilization of food as sources of energy for the many bodily functions, and to supply the constituents necessary for the growth and the replacement of tissues. Since food is a combination of many substances, including sugars and starches, proteins, fats, minerals, and vitamins, the digestive tract must possess various mechanisms for dealing with these multiple constituents.

The mouth plays an important initial role, in that food must be chewed thoroughly to divide the large, tough portions into smaller pieces for easier swallowing and digestion. The first step in the digestion of starches, such as potatoes and bread, takes place in the mouth, through the action of a specific substance (ptyalin) in the saliva, which digests starches. Substances disintegrating large particles into small ones are called enzymes. The digestive tract has many different enzymes, each with the capacity to subdivide sugars or starches, proteins or fats, into their simple components for easier utilization. Digestion, in the strict scientific sense, therefore, signifies the breaking up of complex food substances into simple chemicals, so that the body may absorb them more readily; enzymes play a major role in this process.

Once the food has been chewed, the act of swallowing forces it into the esophagus, a simple muscular tube connecting the mouth to the stomach. The sole purpose of the esophagus is to propel food by muscular activity into the stomach.

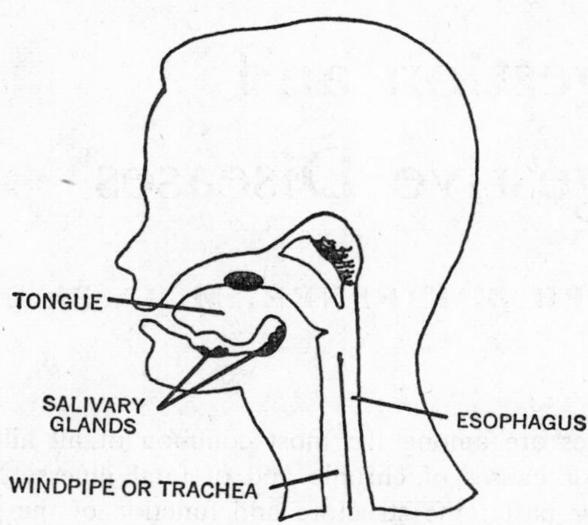

Fig. 46. Carbohydrates begin to change in the mouth. As you swallow, the food passes into a long tube. A series of ringlike muscles squeeze food along until it reaches the stomach. From *How Your Body Uses Food,* by Dr. Albert Piltz, National Dairy Council.

Food entering the stomach is acted upon by powerful muscular action so that the material is further subdivided into smaller particles and also is diluted with water and stomach content. The several types of cells in the lining of the stomach produce stomach juice. These are the parietal or acid-secreting cells; the chief or pepsin-secreting cells, and the mucous cells. Pepsin, an enzyme, helps to digest proteins, as in meat, fish, and eggs. The stomach also produces hydrochloric acid by a complex process, including stimulation of the acid-secreting cells via the central nervous system and the hormone, gastrin, produced within the stomach. At the smell, taste, sight, or thought of food, nerve impulses from the brain are transmitted along the vagus nerves to the salivary glands and to the stomach, initiating the process of digestion. An excess of acid is important in the development of peptic ulcer of the duodenum. Acid also is important in the evolution of stomach ulcers but, because of the lowered tissue resistance of the stomach wall, less acid is required than for duodenal ulcers. Various means of controlling stomach acidity have been devised in the treatment of peptic ulcers, such as neutralization by antacids or suppression of the secretion of acid with antisecretory drugs; this subject is discussed more fully later. Although an excess of acid may be harmful, a deficiency or absence of acid does not impair the digestion of food in any way. The stomach also produces a substance which enables the body to absorb vitamin B_{12}, necessary to prevent pernicious anemia. Except for alcohol, little absorption takes place in the stomach; so that the partially digested food passes into the first portion of the small intestine, the duodenum.

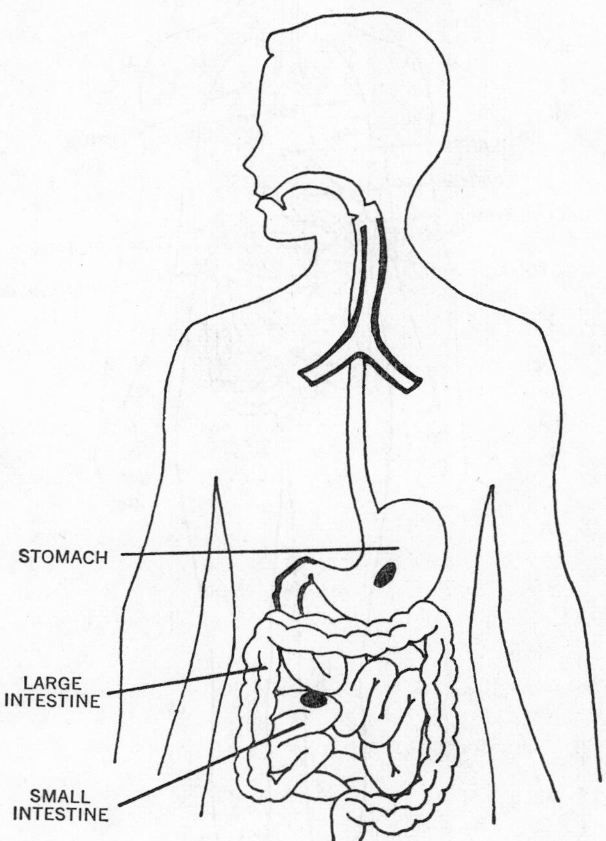

Fig. 47. Proteins are digested in the stomach and in the small intestine. From *How Your Body Uses Food,* by Dr. Albert Piltz, National Dairy Council.

The duodenum receives not only food from the stomach, but also the important secretions produced by the liver and the pancreas. The liver is the largest organ in the body; it manufactures bile which aids the digestion of food, in addition to its many functions essential to nutrition and the health of the entire body. Bile produced in the liver flows into the gallbladder where it is concentrated; it then flows from the gallbladder into the duodenum through a channel, the common bile duct. Bile contains a

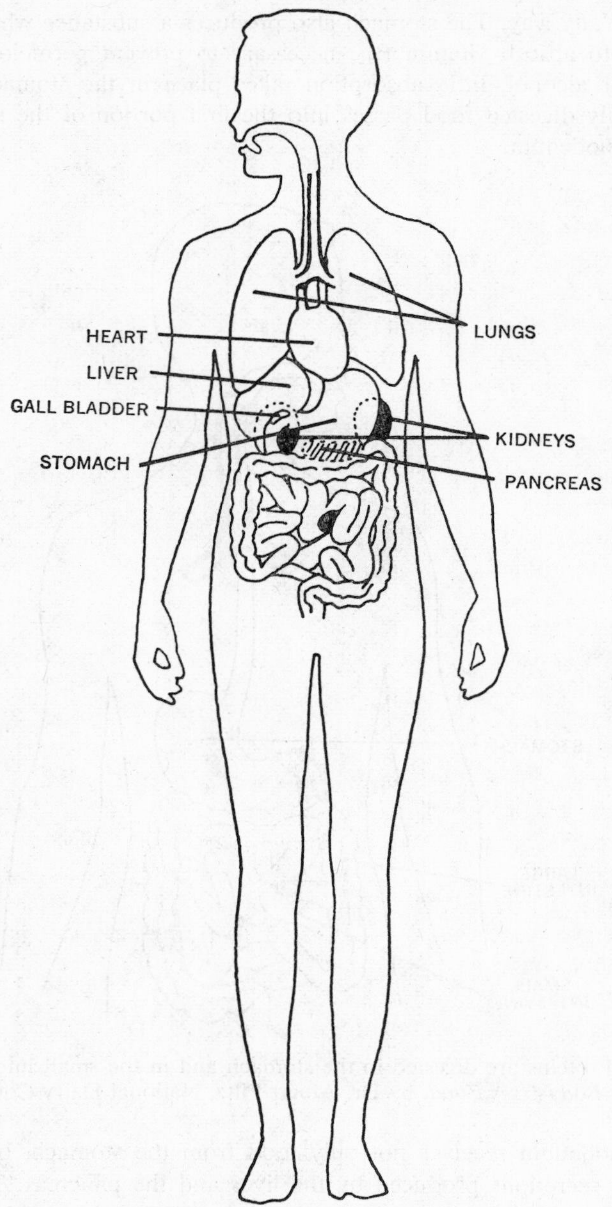

Fig. 48. Fats are digested in the small intestine as digestion of carbohydrates and protein is completed. Notice in the diagram that two organs are connected to the upper part of the small intestine. The larger one is the pancreas, and the other is the gall bladder which is connected with the liver. These organs and other glands in the walls of the small intestine supply juices and enzymes to com-

yellow-green substance, bilirubin, which produces the characteristic brown color to the stools, scientifically called feces, the material that passes out through the rectum, when acted upon by bacteria in the large intestine. The pancreas plays a vital role in digestion since it produces a large quantity of powerful digestive enzymes which digest starches, fats and proteins. The pancreas also manufactures bicarbonate of soda to neutralize the acid entering the intestine from the stomach. The lining of the duodenum and the small bowel elaborate other digestive enzymes, aiding in the subdivision of complex sugars into simple compounds (the disaccharidases).

Once food has been divided into smaller, simple chemicals by the process of digestion, it then must pass through the lining of the bowel for utilization in various parts of the body; this process of absorption takes place chiefly in the duodenum and small intestine. Food absorbed from the small intestine is transported to the liver, which stores sugar and manufactures proteins, fats, and other substances for general use.

As the nutrient substances are removed by the body, the remaining liquid content of the small intestine, now largely composed of waste products (chyme), flows into the large intestine (colon). Huge numbers of bacteria reside in the colon and are responsible for the further breakdown of food that has escaped digestion thus far. The bacteria also contribute to the odor of the stool, and indirectly, to its color. A major function of the colon is removal of water from the intestinal contents by absorption into the tissues and concentrating the liquid bowel content into dry, formed, easily evacuated stools. The stool collects in the last portion of the digestive tract, the rectum, until it has accumulated sufficient bulk to distend its wall; thereby stimulating the rectal muscles and initiating the sensation for a bowel movement. Subsequent contraction of the rectal muscles and relaxation of the anal orifice results in the evacuation of the bowel movement.

The stool is the end product of the ingested food, after the nutritious substances have been absorbed. Thus, stool consists largely of undigested wastes, such as vegetable fibers. Roughly one-third of the stool weight consists of bacteria. The brown color of the stool is due to the presence of urobilinogens, produced by the action of intestinal bacteria upon bilirubin in the bile. Bacteria also supply the odor of stool by their putrefactive properties.

TESTS

Gastric analysis refers to measurement of the volume and concentration of hydrochloric acid in the stomach. Usually, a soft rubber tube is passed

plete the digestion of your food. From *How Your Body Uses Food,* by Dr. Albert Piltz, National Dairy Council.

into the stomach through the nose or mouth, and the stomach content is removed and tested for volume and amount of acid. This test is invaluable in patients with pernicious anemia, where small amounts of juice without hydrochloric acid are produced; or in patients with duodenal ulcer, who often secrete excessive quantities of acid. A qualitative method of establishing the presence or absence of stomach acid involves the "tubeless gastric analysis," requiring only testing the color of the urine after the administration of a special dye compound by mouth; however, this test does not indicate the quantity of acid produced.

Gastric cytology is a method of examining cells from the lining of the stomach after vigorous washing with salt solution. The cellular material is stained with a special procedure and examined under a microscope. This technique is especially valuable in the earlier recognition of stomach cancer and other tumors.

Gastroscopy is a technique for looking directly at the lining of the stomach by means of a unique flexible tube, fitted with a series of tiny lenses fixed on a coiled wire or by a more flexible tube containing glass fibers (fiberscope) which also is capable of taking color photographs of the interior of the stomach. The gastroscope or fiberscope often demonstrates tiny ulcers, small tumors, or inflammation of the stomach too small to be seen by X rays. The lining of the esophagus can be examined similarly by a lighted tube (esophagoscope), permitting direct inspection of the surface.

Stomach X rays involve drinking a solution of barium, which cannot be penetrated by the X rays, and, therefore, casts a shadow of the shape of the stomach and intestines on the X-ray film or the fluoroscopy screen. These X rays must be used by a doctor trained in the science of radiology. The barium delineates an ulcer crater or stomach tumor and thus facilitates prompt recognition of these conditions.

Gallbladder X rays are obtained by eating a fat-free meal and taking tablets of a special dye which is concentrated in the gallbladder and outlines stones or other abnormalities. If the gallbladder is not seen, this indicates the gallbladder is diseased sufficiently not to concentrate the dye.

Small bowel biopsy is the removal of a tiny amount of tissue lining the small intestine, for analysis under the microscope. The tissue is obtained by passing a tube through the mouth into the stomach and from the stomach into the small bowel, where a small opening traps and removes a small piece of intestinal tissue for examination. The procedure is simple and well tolerated, and provides significant information.

Colon X rays are obtained by administering barium as an enema into the rectum and large intestine. The barium outlines the bowel and thus can demonstrate changes in the lining outpouchings (diverticula), polyps growing from the surface of the bowel, or tumors.

Proctoscopy involves directly inspecting the lining surface of the rectum and lower colon by means of a straight metal tube with a light on the end (proctoscope). Usually an enema is given to clean the bowel wall and thus provide a better view. Proctoscopy is relatively simple and facilitates the recognition of tiny polyps and tumors, and other disorders of the rectum and lower bowel (sigmoid).

Stools or the bowel movement can be examined in several ways. One of the most important tests is the analysis for hidden (occult) blood. A test positive for blood may be the first indication of a cancer in the bowel or other digestive diseases and the procedure, therefore, should be a routine test, together with blood counts and urine analyses. The more sensitive and more useful methods require that red meat not be given for several days in advance of the test since the meat may give a spuriously positive reaction. In addition, the stool often is cultured for disease-producing bacteria, which means that they are grown outside the body in a laboratory; this is useful in the diagnosis of various types of dysentery, for example. When worms or other infectious agents inhabit the digestive tract, they or their eggs can be detected by examining a fresh stool under a microscope. Finally, when digestion or absorption of food is abnormal, one clue to the diagnosis may be the presence of excessive fat in the stool. For this purpose, all bowel movements are collected for several days (72 hours) and are analyzed for fat content.

Liver biopsy refers to the removal of a tiny piece of liver tissue with a special needle; a procedure that is useful in detecting the cause of yellow jaundice and other diseases of the liver, including cirrhosis. This test can be done simply in the patient's bed, using medication to numb the skin. The tissue is examined under the microscope for inflammation and scarring.

PEPTIC ULCER

Peptic ulcer is among the more common ailments of man and occurs in approximately fifteen per cent of the population. The condition is found in all people in all parts of the world. Ulcers are more common in the duodenum than the stomach and are much more common in men than women. An ulcer is a circumscribed defect of varying depth in the lining of the stomach or duodenum. If deep enough, it may extend through the wall of the digestive tract and perforate, causing peritonitis; or it may erode into a blood vessel, producing bleeding. The cause of peptic ulcer is not known completely, but hydrochloric acid plays an important role in its development. Hydrochloric acid also is important in the production of ulcer pain; and the continuous neutralization of acid promotes the healing of ulcers. The term "peptic" ulcer relates to the enzyme pepsin which, together with the hydrochloric acid, contributes to the digestive action of the stomach content upon the surface of the stomach or duodenum, presumably impairing the integrity of localized areas and thus leading to the formation of peptic ulcer.

The most common complaint of ulcer patients is a characteristic burning or gnawing pain in a localized area of the abdomen, below the breast bone and above the navel, called the epigastrium. The pain usually occurs one to two hours after meals and commonly awakens the patient from a sound sleep between 1 and 3 A.M. The pain is relieved almost immediately by drinking milk, eating food, taking an antacid medicine, or by vomiting. Ulcer pain often will occur for several days or weeks, then completely disappear for weeks or months, only to return again. In some patients there appears to be a tendency for peptic ulcer to recur in the spring and fall.

Complicated ulcers produce additional problems. Often the appearance of a complication may be the first indication of the presence of an ulcer. The first sign of a bleeding ulcer may be the passage of tarry black stools, indicating blood that has been changed by the digestive secretions; or by the vomiting of bright red blood or coffee-ground-like material. The bleeding may be severe enough to cause shock due to loss of blood. If the ulcer extends through the wall of the stomach or duodenum, it has "perforated," and the leakage of intestinal contents into the abdominal cavity produces severe pain and a generalized inflammation, peritonitis. Finally, an ulcer, by inflammation and scarring, may block the outlet of the stomach or passage through the duodenum and not allow food or liquids to pass readily along the small intestine, producing an obstruction.

An ulcer may be strongly suspected by a physician who carefully notes the pattern of symptoms; but the only certain diagnosis is to demonstrate the ulcer by X-ray examination. This procedure involves swallowing a barium mixture which coats the lining of the stomach and duodenum. The barium will flow into the ulcer crater and reveal it as a dense, circumscribed shadow on the X-ray film. Additional information is provided in measurements of the output of stomach acid, by placing a rubber tube in the stomach and withdrawing the content for one or two hours. Persons with ulcers, particularly in the duodenum, produce more acid than normal people. Ulcers in the stomach may be examined directly, just as a sore in the inside of the mouth can be visualized, by the gastroscope, which is passed down the esophagus into the stomach. Finally, if there is doubt that a stomach ulcer actually may be an ulcerated tumor, washings of the cells from the stomach lining can be obtained and examined under the microscope for the presence or absence of tumor (exfoliative cytology).

Peptic ulcers often are treated by a bland diet (*see* page 409), omitting strong spices and other potential irritants. In recent years, diet therapy has been less emphasized than in the past, but it remains a worthwhile method in preventing the discomfort of ulcer pain. The excess use of alcohol and tobacco, especially cigarettes, will prevent proper healing of peptic ulcers or will promote recurrences. Neutralization of hydrochloric acid, as with milk and cream, food or antacid medications in either powder, liquid, or tablet form, remains the basis of ulcer treatment. The most effective program requires the presence of food or antacid medication in the stomach at all times to neutralize and buffer the acid content. At first, and often in the hospital, either milk, food or an antacid medication is taken at least once an hour; after the ulcer heals, these may be taken every two or three hours. Antisecretory medication may be prescribed to reduce the flow of acid from the stomach. These compounds act by blocking the effects of the vagus nerves upon the acid-secreting (parietal) cells of the stomach. Identification and adjustment of the emotional problems so often present in patients with peptic ulcer also is extremely helpful.

Surgery for peptic ulcer usually is reserved for the complications—perforation, bleeding, obstruction—or for lack of healing after careful medical treatment in the hospital. The most popular operation is vagotomy, in which the vagus nerves are cut at the level of the esophagus, thereby decreasing the stimulation of acid production by this route. Another surgical technique is to remove a portion of the stomach (partial gastrectomy) in order to remove the cells secreting hydrochloric acid. Since the latter operation decreases the size of the stomach, mechanical difficulties may arise subsequently, especially when food is eaten, the so-called dumping syndrome, characterized by symptoms of faintness, weakness, and perspiration. An intermediate surgical method is removal of the lower portion of the stomach, the antrum, which usually comprises about 40 per cent of the stomach, together with vagotomy.

GASTRITIS

Gastritis signifies inflammation of the stomach. It occurs at all ages, but seems to be more common among older people. The term often is used loosely as a catch-all for almost any digestive complaint, particularly heartburn, belching, "sour stomach," and bloating, symptoms that more often reflect irritability rather than inflammation of the stomach. Actually no correlation exists between the presence or severity of gastritis and the presence or absence of symptoms (discussed more fully under "Indigestion"). Some doctors believe that the usual forms of gastritis do not cause any symptoms.

Occasionally, acute gastritis may occur after the heavy intake of alcoholic beverages. In these instances, the lining of the stomach may be reddened, swollen, and bleed more easily. This condition may be confused at times with a bleeding ulcer. Various medications, especially salicylates, not infrequently may irritate the lining of the stomach, especially when taken in the absence of food. Bleeding may occur from the superficial ulcers produced on the surface of the stomach.

APPENDICITIS

The appendix is a blind-end tubular sac at the beginning of the large bowel (cecum), usually from two to five inches in length. Inflammation of the appendix (appendicitis) produces pain in the abdomen; at first the pain is diffuse, but within several hours, settles in the right lower portion of the abdomen. Usually low-grade fever accompanies the pain and the white blood cell count is elevated, indicating the presence of inflammation. Vomiting or diarrhea also may occur. On physical examination, the abdomen is tender in the right lower quadrant, with muscle spasm in this area.

An inflamed appendix must be removed before it ruptures and allows the content of the bowel to spill into the abdominal cavity, causing life-endangering peritonitis. Fortunately, not all appendicitis causes peritonitis, and the inflammation may subside. However, removal of the appendix, (appendectomy) is indicated promptly, once the diagnosis is made or strongly suspected. Often the appendix is removed routinely during an abdominal operation for another reason, a simple procedure that prevents further difficulties. However, removal of an appendix solely for vague digestive complaints usually is unwarranted and unrewarding.

REGIONAL ENTERITIS

Regional enteritis is a chronic inflammation of the small intestine, usually affecting its last portion, the ileum, but extending to all areas of the small bowel and colon in some cases. Ileocolitis is a descriptive term applied to inflammation of the last portion of small intestine and the first portion of the colon. Symptoms include abdominal pain, diarrhea, fever, and fatigue associated with anemia. The cause is not known. The disease is prevalent among young people and children, and a tendency is for the bowel to become narrowed, ultimately with partial obstruction of the intestine. Tenderness in the right lower quadrant of the abdomen often is present, and may be associated with a mass of inflamed bowel and adjacent tissue. Occasionally in children, fever, anemia, or weight loss may predominate, without diarrhea or abdominal pain. Regional enteritis tends to be chronic and recurrent. The treatment usually is diet, rest, and various medications to control inflammation. Surgery is needed for complications, such as obstruction and perforation of the bowel. The diseased loop of bowel is removed and the ends of the bowel are joined to provide normal continuity. While surgery is important and necessary for the complications, it does not cure the disease. The incidence of recurrence of the process after operation is high. All patients with this condition, therefore, require continued medical treatment after surgery, with a bland diet and medications to control infection and reduce inflammation.

HERNIA

A hernia or "rupture" is a weakness in the wall of the abdomen which allows a portion of the intestine to bulge through the defect. Hernias occur in a variety of locations; those due to a defect in a surgical scar, may occur anywhere in the wall of the abdomen. Occasionally, an internal hernia exists, with a loop of bowel extending through a defect in the inner structures of the abdomen. Hiatus or diaphragmatic hernias are discussed in the section on "Heartburn." In men, the most common place for a hernia is in the groin, with protrusion into the scrotum. The hernia usually is small, but without treatment, it may become large. In women, hernias can occur about the navel due to straining in childbirth. Children often are born with hernia defects, either in the groin or around the navel.

Usually a small hernia will not cause discomfort, but a large rupture will cause sharp pain or pressure, especially on straining, such as a cough, sneeze, or lifting. A large hernia, by its sheer bulk alone, may interfere with normal activities. When the opening to the hernia closes off the bowel within it, bowel obstruction results, and requires prompt surgery.

A truss is a mechanical device to prevent the bulging of a hernia by pressure against the defect in the wall of the abdomen. If the hernia does not enlarge, a truss can be worn for years, but it may cause scar tissue in the area of the pressure, making future surgery more troublesome. In addition, a large hernia is much more difficult to repair surgically than a small one; so that an enlarging, uncomfortable hernia should be controlled by operation. Surgical correction of the hernia is the preferred method of treatment.

DYSENTERY

Dysentery refers to an infection in the digestive tract, usually the small and/or large bowel. Diarrhea means loose stools from any cause. There are two common types of dysentery, one caused by tiny one-celled animals, ameba (E. histolytica) and the other by even smaller organisms, bacteria. Both types of dysentery can be spread from person to person and these infections, therefore, represent an important health hazard in areas where sanitation is poor.

Amebic dysentery may be associated with severe diarrhea, bloody stools, and high fever. Proctoscopic examination of the rectum demonstrates characteristic inflammation and ulcerations. The tiny, mobile amebae or their cystic forms can be visualized on examination of the stool under the microscope. Occasionally, the infection and diarrhea subside, but the amebae continue to live in the bowel, the patient thus becoming a carrier and making possible re-infection of himself and others. In the absence of treatment, the amebae may spread into the liver, causing liver abscesses. Medical treatment for amebic dysentery is constantly improving and currently is effective when properly supervised.

The dysenteries caused by bacteria usually appear as severe diarrhea, with fever but without the passage of blood. The most common class of bacteria associated with dysentery in the United States are salmonella, one type of which causes typhoid fever. Bacillary dysentery also is associated frequently with poor sanitation, and occurs in epidemics when the drinking water is contaminated with stool. These bacteria are detected by culturing the stool. Once the causative bacteria has been identified, different types of sulfonamide drugs and antibiotics may be given to determine the medication that will prevent growth most effectively in the patient. Treatment with the appropriate sulfonamides and antibiotics is effective in most cases. Prevention may be possible by "typhoid shots," which cause the body to ward off the infection if exposure has occurred. On certain occasions, a carrier state may exist wherein the patient feels well but salmonella remain in the stool. If such a carrier is involved in the preparation of food, there is danger of infecting the people who eat the food; such a person was "Typhoid Mary," a cook who infected many people. In other countries, as in the Far East, the bacteria identified as vibrio cholera cause catastrophic epidemics of severe dysentery, known as cholera. The loss of minerals and fluids from the body in this illness is enormous, with resultant shock and death. Treatment requires intensive replacement of the fluids and minerals and other supportive measures.

ULCERATIVE COLITIS

Ulcerative colitis is a digestive disorder of unknown cause which produces severe, bloody diarrhea, accompanied by fever and weight loss. Often the term "colitis" is applied rather loosely to conditions which do not involve actual inflammation and are not related to ulcerative colitis, such as "spastic colitis," or "mucous colitis." These latter disorders most commonly represent oversensitivity and overactivity of the bowel because of the effects of emotional tension or irritants in food or drink. Examination of the rectum with the proctoscope in patients with ulcerative colitis demonstrates a characteristic picture of inflammation, ulceration, bleeding, and purulent discharge. Ulcerative colitis also may be identified by X-ray examination, whereby barium is introduced into the large intestine and examined by the X-ray screen; this procedure reveals changes in the lining surface, alterations in the caliber of the bowel and its configuration, characteristic for the disease.

Treatment consists of a bland diet, sedatives, sulfa drugs to reduce the number of bacteria in the large bowel, and drugs to reduce diarrhea. If the ulcerative colitis is severe, adrenal steroids, related to cortisone, may be necessary to reduce the inflammation. When the disease is so severe that medical means are no longer effective or life-threatening complications develop, surgery must be performed. The operation usually involves removal of the entire colon and rectum (colectomy), with diversion of the waste products of the bowel through an opening made in the front of the abdomen, an ileostomy. People with an ileostomy are able to function well and live normal, useful lives.

DIVERTICULITIS

Diverticulosis, a condition especially common among the elderly, is characterized by the small, pea-sized outpouchings from the large bowel especially in the descending portion, on the left side of the abdomen. The mere presence of these pouches is not significant, except for the possibility of inflammation perhaps as a result of prolonged constipation in the presence of many bacteria in the bowel. Usually, a bland diet with avoidance of seeds and nuts is prescribed to prevent attacks of inflammation; together with regulation of bowel activity, utilizing mineral oil or gentle laxatives, if necessary. Inflammation of these pouches (diverticulitis) is manifested by pain in the left lower side of the abdomen, fever, constipation, or diarrhea. At these times, taking a laxative is dangerous since pressure within the bowel may cause one of the pouches to rupture and allow the intestinal content to spill into the abdominal cavity, producing peritonitis. Unfortunately, this complication may occur without laxatives or sometimes without warning; immediate surgery is necessary. The most common operation is to remove the inflamed portion of bowel and temporarily divert the digestive waste products from the area, by creating an opening for the colon in the front of the abdomen, a colostomy. After several weeks or months, the colon is replaced in normal continuity. In patients with recurrent severe diverticulitis and resultant narrowing, operative removal of the diseased area may be desirable.

HEMORRHOIDS

Hemorrhoids or "piles" are a common medical problem; they are dilated hemorrhoidal veins surrounding the anal opening of the rectum. They are subject to the same complications as other blood vessels, namely rupture and clotting. Bleeding hemorrhoids are the most common cause of visible blood in the stool; and the bleeding may be entirely painless. Clotting of the blood in the hemorrhoid causes severe pain because of the intense pressure upon nerve endings in the distended tissue around the vein; a situation that often requires incision of the distended vein releasing the clotted blood.

When hemorrhoids are too painful or persist in bleeding, they must be removed surgically. However, many hemorrhoid operations can be avoided with proper medical care. Initially, the pain of hemorrhoids may be relieved by sitz baths several times daily, i.e., sitting in a tub or basin of hot water for fifteen to twenty minutes so that only the painful area is immersed; this procedure relieves spasm and pain. In addition, medicated suppositories may be inserted into the anal opening to relieve pain. Long-term care consists in careful cleaning of the hemorrhoidal area with warm water and soap to remove tiny bits of stool which cling to hemorrhoids and adjacent tissue, causing irritation and inflammation. This procedure alone relieves the associated intense itching. The application of vaseline to the anal opening before and after each bowel movement insures that the area will be soft and pliable, so that hard stools will not tear the vulnerable hemorrhoids and cause bleeding. Finally, the avoidance of hard stools and straining at bowel movements is essential to prevent the hemorrhoids from further dilation and protrusion. Although hemorrhoids are the most common source of rectal bleeding, a thorough examination of the digestive tract always should be performed, to exclude other causes of bleeding, particularly cancer of the large bowel, in the older patients.

WORMS

Worms can live quite successfully in the digestive tract of man and they are common among primitive or less advanced people who lack good sanitation. Worms may live within the body and not cause difficulties; or symptoms may include pain in the abdomen, irregular bowel movements and anemia. Worms enter the body as eggs which are swallowed with contaminated food. The eggs hatch and the worms grow and attach themselves to the wall of the bowel. Common sources of worm eggs include poorly cooked or raw pork, beef, or fish.

The common types of worms are tapeworms, pinworms, roundworms, and hookworms. Tapeworms usually are several feet in length and are composed of multiple segments, like the cars of a train. Often, one or more segments will break off and be visible in the stool as movable, half-inch pieces of tissue. Pinworms are a common cause of itching around the anal opening of the rectum, particularly in children, and they may be spread easily from person to person.

The presence of worms in the bowel may be detected by examining the stool with a microscope for their characteristic eggs. Treatment consists of temporary avoidance of food, strong laxatives to purge the worms, and specific drugs to kill the worms. Appropriate treatment usually is effective in eradicating the worms from the bowel and eliminating the associated symptoms.

HEPATITIS

Hepatitis is inflammation of the liver. The most common cause is a virus infection, transmitted from person to person and often occurring in epidemics. In people exposed to hepatitis, the disease occasionally may be prevented by the injection of gamma globulin into the muscle, creating a temporary passive immunity. Another form of virus hepatitis may be transmitted by blood transfusions and by the injection of certain blood products. The first sign of hepatitis is severe fatigue, fever, and loss of appetite, followed by a darkening of the color of the urine and yellowing of the skin (jaundice). The treatment for hepatitis primarily is bed rest and a nutritious diet, with adequate calories and vitamins. Hospitalization may not be required, but, in any case, the patient should remain in bed at least until the jaundice is completely gone. The course of hepatitis may be mild or severe, depending upon the degree of injury to the liver. Every patient with hepatitis should be under the care of a physician, who can perform the necessary blood tests to determine the severity of the hepatitis and the response to treatment, and to differentiate hepatitis from other diseases causing jaundice. The vast majority of people with hepatitis recover without any permanent liver damage; however, a few retain a low-grade inflammation or later develop cirrhosis of the liver.

CIRRHOSIS

Cirrhosis means scarring of the liver, a situation that interferes with its normal function and with blood flow through the liver. The most common cause of the scarring is repeated injury to the liver from drinking large amounts of alcoholic beverages; but other known causes include poor nutrition, hepatitis, rare metabolic diseases in which large amounts of iron or copper are deposited in the liver, and, possibly, the long-continued effects of irritating or toxic drugs. People with cirrhosis may not have complaints, and the disease then is first detected by a physician on routine physical examination. The first sign of liver disease may be jaundice, fatigue, ankle swelling, enlargement of the abdomen, or a full feeling in the right upper part of the abdomen caused by the enlarged liver.

Cirrhosis may be suspected from the patient's history and the physical examination, but liver function tests are needed for confirmation. A biopsy of the liver, removing a small core of liver tissue with a special needle for examination under the microscope, may be desirable to characterize the liver problem more completely.

The treatment for cirrhosis involves, first, the complete abstinence from alcohol and other agents known to damage the liver. Additional important measures include eating a well-balanced, nutritious diet, and rest, especially bed rest. Since special medicines cannot dissolve the scars in the liver, the next best treatment is prevention of further damage. Those types of cirrhosis which are due to specific rare causes may respond to special drug treatment.

Repeated scarring of the liver interferes with normal blood flow through and beyond the liver, resulting in abnormally dilated, thin-walled veins in the esophagus (esophageal varices). These varices can bleed vigorously and produce a life-endangering hemorrhage, with vomiting of blood and the passage of black, tarry stools. The most permanent treatment for bleeding varices is an operation on the large veins leading to the liver to relieve the increased pressure within them (portacaval shunt). In addition, the portal hypertension contribute significantly to an accumulation of fluid in the abdomen (ascites) and in the legs (edema). Removal of this fluid can be accomplished with various drugs, called diuretics, which facilitate the elimination of excess fluid via the kidneys.

When the liver becomes so diseased that it cannot function at even minimal levels, liver failure results. The most serious consequences are coma, bleeding tendencies, and loss of kidney function, so that the urine output falls to small amounts. The coma or confusion of liver failure is treated by a diminished intake of protein, since the breakdown products of protein contribute to the coma, and the administration of antibiotics to decrease the number of ammonia-producing bacteria within the colon. The fundamental problem in the management of liver coma is the state of the liver cells and their capacity for regeneration to a sufficient degree as to permit adequate function.

GALLSTONES

Gallstones are accumulations of variably sized concretions in the gallbladder ranging in size from a tiny speck to a stone an inch or more in diameter. They are common; and by the time people reach the age of fifty or sixty years, perhaps half will be found to have gallstones. Many people apparently are never bothered by the gallstones, so that the removal of gallstones simply because of their presence is not always justified. In addition, the gallbladder should not be removed because of the fear that gallstones cause cancer; this is rare, in contrast to the frequency of gallstones. A low-fat diet often is suggested as treatment for gallstones but conclusive evidence that such a diet will prevent symptoms has not been found. Unfortunately, medical measures do not dissolve gallstones.

Gallstones are diagnosed by X rays of the gallbladder. After taking several capsules of special dye and eating a fat-free meal, a normal gallbladder is filled with dye. Stones can readily be detected within the gallbladder by this X ray. If the gallbladder is diseased because of chronic inflammation due to stones, it will not be visualized on the X-ray films.

The mere presence of gallstones does not cause digestive difficulty. However, once the stones move into the duct connecting the gallbladder to the common bile duct or into the bile duct itself, they may cause an intense cramping pain under the right rib margin that may travel to the right shoulder (biliary colic), often accompanied by nausea and vomiting. This pain can be extremely severe and require narcotic medication for relief. Biliary colic usually is treated best initially by allowing the irritation from the passage of a stone to subside. However, the occurrence of gallstone colic indicates a mechanical problem with the hazard of additional complications, and the gallbladder should be removed. Removal of the gallbladder containing gallstones also is often indicated in young people because of the longer period of time available for the development of complications and thus to avoid such problems.

If a stone blocks the common bile duct, the flow of bile will be obstructed so that bile will not flow normally into the intestine but back up in the circulation, producing jaundice. Sometimes, gallstone jaundice can occur without pain, increasing the initial difficulty in distinguishing this condition from hepatitis, cirrhosis, and cancer of the pancreas. Again, blood tests and perhaps liver biopsy will help to differentiate blockage of bile from other causes of jaundice. Surgery often is needed to relieve the jaundice but always should be performed once stones have moved into the bile duct. If surgery is not undertaken, repeated attacks of jaundice can lead to permanent liver damage.

Indigestion, with belching, gas, bowel irregularity, and vague abdominal discomfort, especially after fatty or greasy food, often is attributed to gallbladder disease; however, gallstones may or may not be present. When the gallbladder is removed for such vague complaints, the same complaints often return, indicating that the gallstones actually were not responsible for the symptoms. The cause of such digestive symptoms often is irritability and spasm of the digestive tract.

PANCREATITIS

Acute inflammation of the pancreas causes severe upper abdominal pain, often extending through to the back on the left side, accompanied by nausea, vomiting and, at times, shock. The two most common causes for pancreatitis are alcoholism and the passage of gallstones through the common bile duct. The immediate treatment includes narcotics for pain, suctioning the stomach contents with a rubber tube and administering fluids by vein. However, the long-term treatment must be directed toward the cause, by complete abstinence from alcohol or by removal of the diseased gallbladder.

Occasionally, repeated attacks of pancreatitis occur without obvious cause. These situations are treated by a bland diet and medication to reduce the flow of pancreatic juice. If this approach is not effective, surgery may provide some benefit.

CANCER

Cancer of the digestive tract initially may not evoke any symptoms or may produce many symptoms, such as loss of appetite, weight loss, anemia, blood in the stool, change in bowel habit, or pain in the abdomen. Repeated X-ray examinations to detect cancer before any symptoms or signs have proved impractical and expensive. Thus, an awareness of the early signs of cancer is most important if a curable condition is to be found. Experience already has demonstrated that while not perfect, regular examinations by the physician are the most effective approach to the early diagnosis of cancer.

Anemia causes fatigue and pallor and often is the first clue to a digestive cancer. It results from the repeated loss into the stool of small amounts of blood, invisible to the naked eye. Examination of the stool for hidden blood, therefore, is an essential examination in cancer detection. Iron-containing medicines or products should never be given for anemia without first identifying its cause, since iron may cure anemia but cannot cure cancer.

Cancer of the stomach and pancreas can go undetected for a long time, since it often does not cause recognizable difficulty until it has grown quite large. Stomach cancer may produce obstruction to the passage of food, with loss of appetite and vomiting. Occasionally, a stomach ulcer actually is due to an ulcerating cancer and careful testing, by examination of the cells in the stomach content and measurement of acid output by the stomach, is required to distinguish between a benign peptic ulcer and a cancer. The treatment for stomach cancer usually is removal of the stomach, which in itself can produce serious difficulties in handling food, because of the resultant decrease in the normal reservoir function of the stomach. Cancer of the head of the pancreas commonly produces jaundice as the initial symptom. Cancer of the body of the pancreas may produce abdominal pain without jaundice, and weight loss.

Cancer of the liver usually is due to spread from other organs and is a serious sign of advanced tumor. At this stage, surgery is not feasible, but newer chemical methods are being developed to stop the growth of cancer, relieve pain and to prolong life.

Cancer of the large bowel often causes anemia, the presence of visible blood in the stools or a change in bowel habit, such as the sudden appearance of constipation or diarrhea. Cancer of the colon or rectum is among the more curable tumors when detected early. Three-fourths of all large bowel cancers can be detected with the proctoscope, a simple metal tube with a light on the end, which is inserted into the rectum and colon for a distance of about 12 inches. For those cancers above this level, the large bowel may be studied with X ray by outlining the colon with barium.

Polyps of the colon should be removed if they exceed a half inch in diameter, because of the possibility that they may be cancerous, in addition to the possibility of bleeding. Smaller polyps need not be removed since they rarely become cancerous. However, they should be observed by periodic barium-enema examinations and proctoscopy; since the bowel wall in such cases may be more vulnerable to the development of cancer.

Cancer of the colon may be removed readily and completely at operation and the ends of the bowel sewn together to re-establish normal continuity. Cancer of the rectum requires removal of the rectum, so that the bowel content must be rerouted to the outside by placing the end of the colon into the abdominal wall as a permanent colostomy. A colostomy, after adjustment, requires little more care than the usual time taken for a bowel movement and should in no way be considered a handicap.

INDIGESTION

Indigestion usually refers to almost any symptom involving or related to the digestive system. The term in one sense is a misnomer, since usually digestion, the process of breaking food down into small particles for absorption, is normal. Some diseases directly interfere with certain digestive processes, but these are relatively uncommon.

Acute indigestion may occur after eating irritating or spoiled food. An example of the former might be illustrated by the eating of too many green apples with the occurrence of severe abdominal cramps and perhaps diarrhea. Spoiled food contains the products of germs which are extremely noxious to the digestive tract. Improperly cooked foods or those which are sweet and left without refrigeration may allow germs to grow in them and also to produce bacterial poisons. Food poisoning often occurs in epidemics wherein large numbers of people have eaten spoiled food, such as at a picnic or a banquet. Acute indigestion causes severe abdominal pain, vomiting, and diarrhea, and subsequently, dehydration. Fortunately, these difficulties subside within six to twenty-four hours. Some deaths from "acute indigestion" actually may be heart attacks, with pain experienced in the abdomen rather than in the chest.

Another type of food poisoning not producing digestive symptoms, called botulism, is caused by a toxic product from a certain bacteria which paralyzes the voluntary muscles. This serious infection can be rapidly fatal, if the muscles used in breathing are affected, unless an appropriate antitoxin is given promptly. Prevention may be practiced by avoiding food which is poorly packaged or home-canned with inadequate facilities.

Difficulties, such as belching, gas, abdominal rumbling and gurgling, passing gas by rectum, heartburn and vague feelings of discomfort, heaviness and unrest in the abdomen, often are termed indigestion or "gastritis." Gastritis actually is an inflammation of the stomach and usually causes none of the many difficulties often attributed to it. Except for eating too much food or eating too rapidly, the majority of these complaints are due to three causes: the excessive swallowing of air, the rapid movement of food through the intestine, or an exaggerated awareness of the normal intra-abdominal processes. The healthy person is unconscious of the existence of his stomach, whereas the person with indigestion rarely forgets it. These disorders often are designated as an irritable digestive tract or functional bowel disease.

The most common cause of an irritable bowel is emotional tension. The bowel is sensitive to fluctuations in emotion and mood; as, for example, the "sinking feeling" in the pit of the stomach during periods of fear or anxiety. Most people can describe an area of vulnerability in sensation which is activated by emotional tension; the digestive system commonly is "the sounding board of our emotions." Often, the digestive difficulties will not begin until the tension situation is concluded, since the intestinal tract usually is inactive during times of stress. The treatment for an irritable bowel includes the use of bland diet, adapted to individual requirements. Experience is the best guide as to those irritating foods to be avoided.

With clinical improvement, the diet is liberalized, and eventually it may be discontinued. Eating when upset or in a hurry may cause similar symptoms; meals should be as calm and relaxed as possible. A mild sedative and medication to decrease the activity of the bowel may be prescribed, such as phenobarbital combined with extract of belladonna. Often a vacation and change in routine will have a favorable effect upon digestive troubles caused by emotional tension.

Air swallowing produces a variety of distressing symptoms. Air ordinarily is swallowed with breathing, eating, drinking, speaking, and even unconsciously, as a habit. Once the swallowed air reaches the stomach, it accumulates as a gas bubble, then enters into the intestines and eventually is passed out of the rectum; ordinarily, such air causes no difficulty and most people are unaware of its presence. Belching simply is the release of trapped air in the stomach or lower end of the esophagus. The voluntary swallowing of air in order to produce a belch usually results in the swallowing of more air than the amount released; therefore, this maneuver rarely relieves the problem. Some methods of overcoming air swallowing are rather simple: chew food slowly and carefully; never eat or drink rapidly; never talk while chewing; avoid long periods of rapid talking, especially in tense or emotional situations; avoid smoking; and avoid chewing gum.

The production of gas by certain foods, such as onions, cabbage, and beans, and the passage through the rectum of gas which may have a foul odor probably is attributable to the action of bacteria in the bowel on the food, together with the accumulation of swallowed air.

TROUBLE IN SWALLOWING

When food "sticks" in the throat before passing onward or when solids cannot be swallowed properly, trouble in the esophagus, the muscular tube leading from the mouth to the stomach, may be assumed. Many diseases can produce swallowing difficulty, but the most common is spasm of the muscle layer of the esophagus, like a spasm in any muscle of the body. Spasm may occur when too large a piece of meat is swallowed, so that the food is held up in the esophagus. The esophageal spasm may produce a chest pain very much like that of a heart attack. Tense people who swallow frequently become aware of the upper swallowing muscles in the throat and the more they swallow, the increasingly sensitive they become, until a definite abnormality appears to exist, often described as though produced by a round ball.

Another important cause of swallowing difficulty is known as cardiospasm or achalasia. In this situation, the lower end of the esophagus fails to relax normally, preventing food from entering the stomach and allowing large amounts of undigested food to accumulate. The lower portion of the esophagus becomes narrowed and the upper portion dilates; as a result, the person may experience serious loss of weight and malnutrition because inadequate amounts of food enter the stomach and intestines for digestion. The condition is diagnosed readily by X-ray examination of the esophagus, supplemented by other procedures, such as inspection of the esophagus with a lighted tube (esophagoscopy), examination of the cells from the esophagus (exfoliative cytology) and probing of the channel through the esophagus (bougienage). Treatment of achalasia involves stretching of the narrowed area with an expandable balloon; and usually is successful. Infrequently, the condition requires an operation, which also may be effective.

The most serious cause of swallowing difficulty is cancer of the esophagus, a condition more prevalent in the older age groups and especially among men. Narrowing of the esophagus may occur after the intentional or accidental drinking of caustic chemicals, such as lye. The narrow esophagus causes difficulty in swallowing, but without the dilatation of the esophagus seen in cardiospasm. Stretching of the narrowed area provides relief, but often must be continued for long periods of time.

HEARTBURN

A burning sensation under the breastbone or in the pit of the stomach is a common complaint and usually is relieved by one of many antacid preparations. The most common cause is an irritable digestive tract, or the so-called "acid indigestion." The reason for this type of heartburn is not clear, but one possible explanation is that the tissues are overly sensitive to the action of normal amounts of acid produced by the stomach. In peptic ulcer disease, the pain may or may not resemble heartburn, but the acid content of the stomach is increased and, the acid producing a chemical inflammation, directly causes the pain of peptic ulcer.

When the junction between the esophagus and stomach is relaxed, the acid stomach juice can flow back into the esophagus and cause irritation of its surface (esophagitis). A common cause for this type of heartburn is a rupture or weakness of the diaphragm, separating the chest from the abdomen; this weakness is called a diaphragmatic or hiatus hernia, and it allows part of the upper portion of the stomach to move up into the chest. The hernia occurs on straining, increasing pressure upon the stomach from below and thereby forcing it toward the chest. The displacement of the stomach is not necessarily permanent; so that with decrease in intra-abdominal pressure, as may occur when an obese patient loses a significant amount of weight, the stomach may regain its normal position. Not infrequently, there is no actual rupture but rather a weakness in the tissues normally preventing backflow from the stomach to the esophagus. This "weakness" may be sufficient to permit acid reflux and thus cause spasm and heartburn. Many people with this condition do not have difficulties, the condition being recognized on cautious study, whereas others experience severe heartburn. Heartburn from hiatus hernia may occur after a large meal if the patient lies down or frequently at night when lying down. Simple measures to relieve the heartburn of diaphragmatic hernia are the use of antacids, avoiding or correcting obesity, eating smaller meals, avoiding highly sweetened foods such as orange juice and sweet rolls, and sleeping with the head of the bed raised.

ABDOMINAL PAIN

Establishing the correct source of pain in the abdomen is one of the most important and yet most difficult problems. In general, the type and the location of the pain are most helpful. Additional valuable clues are where the pain travels, its relationship to meals, accompanying nausea or vomiting, and relief with medications, and bowel movements. Usually a localizing pain is more serious than a pain extending diffusely over the abdomen. The pain of irritable bowel disease or indigestion may be severe, either generalized or in one specific location, and may mimic many other digestive diseases. Thus, true evaluation of abdominal pain quickly is often impossible without careful laboratory and X-ray examinations.

There are six common locations for abdominal pain, utilizing the navel as a point of reference. However, atypical location of pain is not uncommon and pain may be transmitted to any location within the abdomen and to areas outside the abdomen. Pain located between the breastbone and navel, in the "pit of the stomach," could signify peptic ulcer or pancreatic disease. Pain in the upper right part of the abdomen might reflect disorder of the liver, gallbladder, or bile ducts; whereas in the left upper quadrant, pain usually originates in the stomach and occasionally in the colon. Discomfort around the navel may originate in the small intestine. Pain in the lower right portion of the abdomen usually is due to the appendix or adjoining colon (cecum, ascending colon) or last portion of the small intestine. Left lower abdominal pain almost always is attributable to the large bowel. Keep in mind that disease of the kidneys, e.g., stones, may cause abdominal discomfort, and that inflammation of the chest or disease of the heart may manifest itself initially in the form of abdominal discomfort or pain.

Severe intermittent cramping pain usually is more serious and acute than steady or dull pain. Sudden pain or sudden increase in severity may be more serious than the gradual development of pain. A careful description of the pain pattern by the patient obviously is important for the identification of the cause of the abdominal pain.

DIARRHEA

Diarrhea signifies loose bowel movements; not necessarily frequent bowel movements. Thus, a person who has three formed stools daily does not have diarrhea, whereas one loose stool indicates diarrhea. Loose stools result from insufficient absorption of water by the colon from the bowel content. Colon disease itself, such as cancer or ulcerative colitis, will cause diminished water absorption. Irritability of the digestive tract propels food and bowel content so rapidly, as to impair the normal absorption of water. The inability to digest or absorb food, causes a large amount of undigested food, particularly fats, to be eliminated; this situation is characterized by a bulky, gray, foul-smelling stool which floats on the water of the toilet bowl and contains an excessive amount of fat.

The treatment of diarrhea depends on the cause. The most common cause of diarrhea is a viral infection of the bowel, the so-called "intestinal flu." This illness usually lasts for one to several days and responds to simple antidiarrhea medication, such as paregoric, temporary limitation of roughage in the diet, bed rest, and heat to the abdomen. Persistent diarrhea requires a careful medical evaluation, especially if accompanied by weight loss or fever, to exclude potentially serious organic disease.

CONSTIPATION

Constipation probably is the most common of all digestive complaints. In a strict sense, constipation signifies the elimination of small, hard stools; and may be related, in part at least, to the excessive absorption of water from the intestinal content, as a result of prolonged transit time and bowel spasm. Many people refer to constipation as any decrease in the number of expected bowel movements. Thus, if one bowel movement every day is not forthcoming, this situation erroneously may be considered constipation, even though the stool may be perfectly normal. The sudden onset of constipation should be evaluated by a physician, since it may be the first sign of serious bowel disease.

The absence of a daily bowel movement is not harmful. The body will not become poisoned by its own wastes if they are not eliminated. Many people attribute a variety of complaints to constipation, such as fatigue, headache, and fullness in the abdomen. These symptoms more often result from emotional tension than from any other cause. The real danger is establishing a chronic laxative habit in order to have one bowel movement per day.

The laxative habit is perhaps the most common addiction in the modern world. In the elderly, who are less active, the use of laxatives is almost universal. In younger people, the laxative habit often is initiated by an overanxious mother who expects a bowel movement daily. A laxative functions by irritating the digestive tract, increasing the propulsion of food and bowel content. If stool is not present in the rectum, there is no urge or need for elimination. A laxative forces elimination of intestinal content from higher up in the large bowel, if no stool is present in the rectum. It hardly seems rational to irritate the entire digestive tract in an attempt to influence only the last segment of bowel. After the repeated use of laxatives, the normal response of the rectum to defecation is blunted or lost temporarily; and the bowel becomes dependent upon the laxative for the irritation and subsequent propulsion of food. As the bowel becomes accustomed to a certain laxative, this preparation becomes ineffective and so a stronger laxative is chosen. Eventually, the bowel becomes lazy, with no tone or propulsive ability of its own.

The proper treatment for constipation depends upon diet, elimination of laxatives, occasional use of small enemas or anal suppositories and, re-education as to normal bowel function and reassurance as to the absence of serious disease. The strongest natural urge for bowel movements occurs after eating, particularly in the morning or if the meal is large. This is the time to attempt bowel movements, but so often, in modern life, rushing to work prevents the person from heeding this natural time of elimination. Suppression of the natural urge is common in children who do not wish to take the time away from play and they allow stool to accumulate. Since the large bowel continues to remove water from the stool, a hard bowel movement is produced. The person suffering from hard stools should drink at least eight glasses of water daily to provide extra water for the bowel to absorb and thus prevent the excess absorption of water from the intestinal content. Certain laxative foods, such as prunes or figs, are most helpful. Finally, if stool accumulates in the rectum and a bowel movement does not occur for several days, a small (pint) water enema or a glycerine suppository may be used; these agents stimulate the rectum rather than the entire bowel and they help to provide symptomatic comfort, at least until the program with diet and antispasmodics can become effective.

INTESTINAL OBSTRUCTION

When the flow of bowel content is blocked, intestinal obstruction results. This situation may be produced by many conditions. Adhesions, possibly from previous surgery, are the most common cause and usually block the small bowel; the loops of intestine become entangled in these strands and are kinked. Hernias (ruptures) contain bowel which can move freely back and forth from the hernia into the abdomen; obstruction occurs when the bowel cannot return into the abdomen. In children, one portion of the bowel may telescope into another and produce obstruction (intussusception). Tumors narrow the interior of the intestine by progressive growth, so that obstruction due to a tumor usually is gradual in onset.

Sudden obstruction produces severe cramping pain, followed by intense vomiting and dehydration. Since air cannot pass the blockage, all the swallowed air becomes trapped within the bowel and produces swelling of the abdomen. Often a long rubber tube is passed into the bowel through the nose or mouth to remove the air and intestinal juices, and, at the same time, relieve the pain.

Simple X rays of the abdomen may be helpful in determining the location of the blockage but surgery may be necessary to locate accurately and correct the obstruction. Often the cause of obstruction is apparent immediately and can be dealt with simply. In some cases, an artificial opening may be made above the obstruction to the outside, to permit drainage of the blocked intestine; another operation is performed later to correct the obstruction and re-unite the ends of the bowel. If the blockage is allowed to persist uncorrected, rupture of the intestine will occur, producing peritonitis.

JAUNDICE

The sudden appearance of yellow skin, with yellowing of the whites of the eyes and often darkening of the urine, is due to a pigment (bilirubin), entering the blood stream which normally is eliminated in the bile. There are many causes for jaundice, but the two main considerations are disease affecting the substance of the liver, such as hepatitis, cirrhosis, or toxic drugs and those conditions causing a blockage of the bile ducts, especially stones, tumors, and scar tissue. Hepatitis produces jaundice by injury of the liver cells so that bile is not formed properly and some products, usually in bile, are lost into the blood stream. Surgery during hepatitis is extremely hazardous, so every effort should be made to exclude hepatitis before performing surgery for jaundice. Cirrhosis causes jaundice due to scarring by preventing proper functioning of the liver. As in hepatitis, patients with cirrhosis may tolerate surgery poorly.

Many medications can produce liver injury and jaundice, among them antibiotics and sedatives; these possibilities must be identified in every case. Often it is very difficult to distinguish between drug jaundice and obstruction of the bile ducts initially; but continual careful study permits clarification of the cause.

Gallstones blocking the bile ducts will not allow bile to flow into the intestine. Bilirubin and bile salts present in bile accumulate in the blood stream; bilirubin will cause jaundice and bile salts, intense itching. Tumors of the pancreas, particularly those in the head of the pancreas, also can cause obstruction of the bile duct. Blockage of the bile duct should be treated surgically, if possible. The various means of distinguishing the types of jaundice are blood-chemical analyses, X rays and, occasionally, biopsy of the liver.

BLAND DIET*

VERY BLAND FOODS FOR ACUTE BOWEL DISTURBANCE

Weak tea
Plain Jello
Meat broth
Bouillon soup
Rice
Cream of wheat
Farina
Toast
Soft cooked eggs
Boiled milk
Custard

STANDARD BLAND DIET

Cereals (with milk)
Cream of wheat
Oatmeal
Farina
Corn flakes
Puffed rice
Puffed wheat
Rice Krispies

Pasta (with butter)
Noodles
Macaroni
Spaghetti
Vermicelli

Eggs
Soft boiled
Scrambled
Omelet
Poached
Hard cooked

Cheese
Cream
American
Swiss
Munster

Milk Products
Milk
Cream
Butter
Cottage cheese
Eggnog

* Generally, a bland diet omits all roughage and irritating foods such as spices and nuts but allows certain cooked fruits and vegetables plus some other "non-irritating" foods; individual experience is important in the selection of a diet.

Beverages
- Tea
- Sanka
- Postum
- Coffee (1 or 2 cups)

Breads
- White
- White toast
- Melba toast
- Bread sticks
- Plain sweet rolls
- Soda crackers
- Zweiback

Soups
- Consommé
- Bouillon
- Cream of rice
- Cream of potato
- Homemade vegetable

Fish
- Creamed salmon, tunafish, whitefish
- Baked whitefish, halibut, cod

Meats
- Steak
- Hamburger
- Beef
- Lamb chops
- Veal
- Chicken
- Turkey
- Crisp bacon
- Baked or boiled ham

Potatoes
- Baked
- Mashed
- Boiled
- Steamed
- Au gratin

Cooked or Canned Vegetables
- Asparagus
- String beans
- Carrots
- Spinach
- Sweet potatoes
- Peas
- Beets
- Squash
- Tomatoes

Cooked or Canned Fruit
- Peaches
- Pears
- Applesauce
- Plums
- Apricots
- White cherries
- Prunes
- Baked apples (no skin)

Raw Fruit
- Banana

Desserts
- Custards
- Puddings
- Plain Jello
- Creams
- Plain cake
- Sponge cake
- Plain ice cream

Miscellaneous
- Jelly
- Hard candy
- Oleo
- Mayonnaise

FOODS EXCLUDED ON BLAND DIET**

Cereals
- Grape Nuts
- Shredded Wheat
- Bran

** Additions to the diet from this list may be permitted as patient improves.

Eggs
Deviled

Cheese
Edam
Roquefort
Camembert
Limburger
Pimento
Gorgonzola
Cheddar

Raw Fruits and Vegetables

Milk Products
Buttermilk
Cocoa
Milk substitutes

Beverages
Soft drinks
Cocoa
Cider
Alcoholic drinks (beer, wine, whisky, etc.)

Breads
Hot biscuits or rolls
Whole wheat
Rye
Raisin

Soups
Split pea
Bean
Onion
Fish chowder

Fish
Canned (sardines, anchovies, herring)
Shellfish
Boiled, broiled or roasted seafoods

Meat
Canned meats
Sweetbreads
Brains
Tripe
Sausage
Smoked meat
Liver

Potatoes
French fried

Cooked or Canned Vegetables
Cabbage
Cauliflower
Onions
Mushrooms
Beans
Brussels sprouts
Broccoli
Artichokes
Corn
Green pepper
Eggplant
Hominy
Parsnips
Rutabaga
Turnips
Kale
Kohlrabi

Cooked or Canned Fruits
Berries
Fruit pies
Grapes
Pumpkin
Pineapple
Figs

CHAPTER 18

The Kidney—Diseases and Disturbances

ROBERT M. KARK, M.D.

The kidneys are two fist-sized glandular organs at the back of the abdominal cavity. They excrete urine and so remove waste products from the body. Even primitive man recognized this function of the organs from their ammoniacal odor and from their piquant taste when he ate them. He learned about their structure and function from the wild and domestic animals he killed for food and in greater detail from those animals offered for sacrifice to his gods. The kidney fat was the choicest morsel from sacrificial animals, hence the biblical term "kidney of wheat" to describe the finest grains (Deuteronomy XXXII:14). The interesting shape of the gland gave its name to the kidney bean, the kidney potato, to an ancient coin—the kidney piece—and to kidney cotton. To the boxing fraternity, a kidney punch is an underhand, unsportsmanlike blow delivered in the small of the back which produces a sickening pain.

The kidneys are really versatile, highly integrated and beautifully organized organs with many functions, not only urinary or excretory functions. They also act as nutritional guardians of the body. Their cells synthesize and break down circulating chemicals as needed. They produce hormones which control and stimulate the functions of other parts of the body.

Scarcely a hundred and thirty years have passed since Richard Bright of Guy's Hospital, London, recognized that dropsical patients with protein in their urine had something wrong with their kidneys. From this came the term Bright's disease. Bright tested for protein by boiling the patient's urine in a spoon held over a candle and watching for flocculent particles to appear. This was the first time that a chemical test was used to diagnose disease.

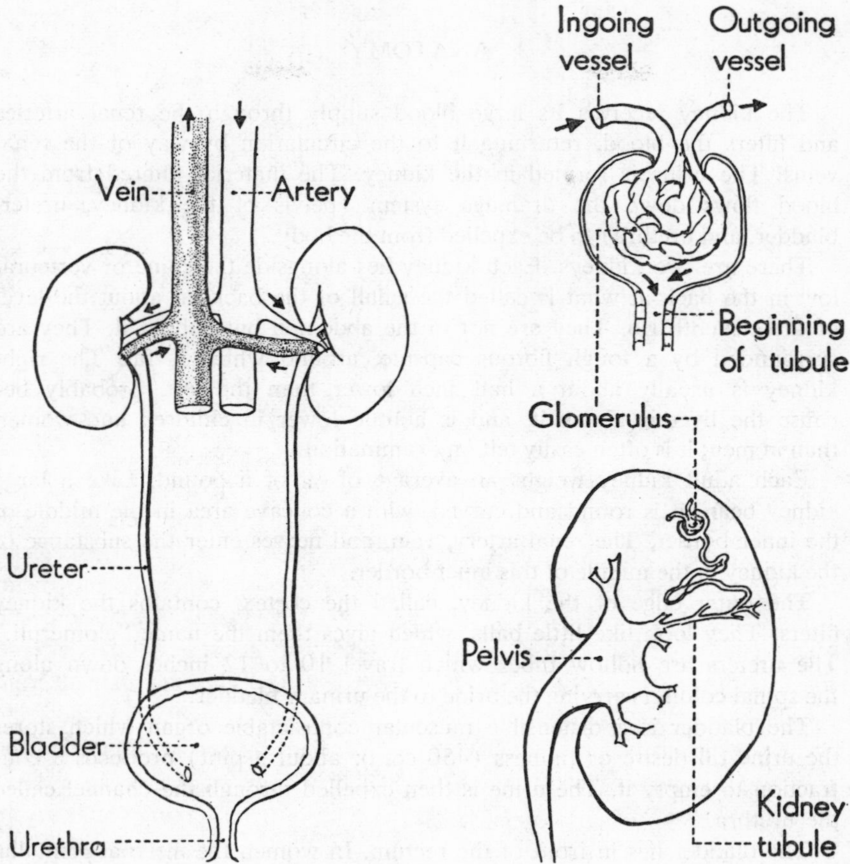

Fig. 49. (LEFT) "The master chemists of the body." The kidneys are located behind the abdominal organs. Descending from the kidneys are the ureters, which empty into the bladder. Illustration, courtesy of the National Kidney Foundation.

Fig. 50. (RIGHT) Each kidney contains about one million functioning units called nephrons. A nephron consists of a tuft of tiny blood vessels called a glomerulus and an attached tube called a tubule. Urine formation begins at the glomerulus, where blood traversing the glomerular vessels is treated by a process called filtration. There are roughly 140 miles of filters and tubes in both kidneys. Thus the kidneys perform their life-sustaining job of filtering and returning to the blood stream about three times the entire body weight in water and salts every 24 hours—about 200 quarts. Approximately two quarts are sent to the bladder to be flushed out of the body, and about 198 quarts are retained in the body. Illustration courtesy of the National Kidney Foundation.

ANATOMY

The kidney receives its large blood supply through the renal arteries and filters the blood, returning it to the circulation by way of the renal veins. The urine is formed in the kidney. The material filtered from the blood flows down the drainage system (pelvis of the kidney, ureter, bladder, and urethra) to be expelled from the body.

There are two kidneys. Each kidney lies alongside the spine or vertebra, low in the back at what is called the small of the back, at about the level of the eleventh rib. They are not in the abdomen but behind it. They are surrounded by a tough fibrous capsule, around which is fat. The right kidney is usually about a half inch lower than the left, probably because the liver is above it, and is a little lower in children and women than in men; it is often easily felt on examination.

Each adult kidney weighs an average of ⅓ of a pound. Like a large kidney bean, it is round and curved, with a concave area in the middle of the inner border. The renal artery, vein, and nerves enter the substance of the kidney in the middle of this inner border.

The outer edge of the kidney, called the cortex, contains the kidney filters. They look like little balls, which gives them the name "glomeruli." The ureters are hollow tubes which travel 10 to 12 inches down along the spinal column carrying the urine to the urinary bladder.

The bladder is a distensible muscular contractable organ which stores the urine till desire or fullness (450 cc. or about a pint) produces a contraction to empty it. The urine is then expelled through the channel called the urethra.

The bladder lies in front of the rectum. In women the internal genitalia, ovaries and tubes are between the rectum and the bladder. The female urethra is short. In the male, the long urethra runs through the penis to its tip. The male urethra is surrounded by the prostate near the base of the bladder. The ducts from the male genital apparatus which carry the sperm open into the urethra in the prostatic part.

STRUCTURE

The kidneys are not just two organs but really two million organs. Each kidney includes a million to a million and a half minute tubes called the nephrons. Each nephron is nourished by a separate tiny blood vessel.

The kidney is extraordinarily complex, but its structure is designed to serve its function.

The kidney has three functions: to develop the urine; to hold some chemicals and filter out others; and glandular or endocrine activity. In the urine the kidney expels excess water, sodium, potassium, calcium salts (solutes), waste products of metabolism (including urea, uric acid, creatinine, phosphorus, sulphur and hydrogen ions (protons), dead and dying renal cells, minute amounts of proteins—particularly renal mucoproteins—and ingested poisons. It maintains normal nutrition, the acid-alkali and electrolyte balance and the water economy of the body. The hormones secreted by the kidney are renin, which affects salt balance, and erythropoietin, which balances the hemoglobin or red-coloring material of the blood and production of red blood cells. A third hormone, found in the kidney of dogs and possibly in man, may act to preserve normal blood pressure.

METABOLIC AND SYNTHETIC ACTIVITIES

The metabolic and synthetic activities of the kidney are second only to those of the liver. The formation of ammonia in the renal tubules from glutamine and other amino acids is well-recognized; but the kidney is also the site of glucose formation. In addition, it synthesizes protein, mucoproteins, and fats. It uses energy for tubular transport and secretion of innumerable organic and inorganic substances. The kidney has the highest oxygen consumption (uses more oxygen to burn up food) of any organ. Particularly the oxygen consumption of the renal cortex is the highest of any tissue. The oxidation of fatty acids is the principal energy-yielding process in the work of the cortex of the kidney.

Formerly physiologists believed that three-fourths of the work of the kidney was involved in excreting urea; they advised restriction of dietary protein intake to "rest" the kidney injured by disease. Nowadays, dietary protein is restricted in the treatment of certain renal disorders but not to "rest" the kidney.

FORMATION OF URINE

The kidneys receive about one-quarter of the blood pumped out by the heart each time it beats. This is about 1000 cc. or one quart per minute. About one-tenth of glomerular filtrate is formed each minute to run down the 140 miles of tubules in the kidney to the renal pelvis. Some 99 per cent of it is returned to the body and only 1 cc. or fifteen drops get to the bladder per minute. Each day about 200 quarts of glomerular filtrate are formed. This fluid is mainly water but it contains vital nutrients such as sodium, calcium, potassium, glucose, amino acids, and water soluble vitamins.

This filtrate is essentially a protein-free extracellular fluid which passes into the tubules. If the tubules were absolutely inert, a person would theoretically void 172,800 cc. (nearly 173 quarts) in twenty-four hours. Since the total body water is approximately 45,000 cc., obviously a person would die quickly if the kidney tubules did not function.

Most of the organic nutrient materials like glucose in the material filtered are completely reabsorbed and returned to the body along the tiny loops of blood vessels which surround the tubules. Only about 80 per cent of water and inorganic salts are reabsorbed in this area, particularly sodium. The rest of it is handled in an adjacent part of the kidney. There the antidiuretic hormone of the posterior part of the pituitary gland works. Antidiuretic hormone allows excess water from the filtrate to be moved finally across the collecting duct cells into the blood; and this concentrates the urine. If, however, you drink a lot of fluid in excess of normal requirements, structures in the brain suppress the secretion of antidiuretic hormone. When this happens a large amount of dilute, pale urine is excreted.

Such bodily waste products as urea and uric acid are not completely returned to the blood stream. Some, like creatinine, go through the glomerular filter and pass down the tubules without much reabsorption. Others like uric acid pass into the tubules with the glomerular filtrate and are partially returned to the blood stream. Then part is returned to the filtrate and is actively secreted into the lower areas where it is excreted with the urine. Thus, during the formation of the urine the kidneys return necessary nutrients to the body.

Claude Bernard first pointed out that the body has two environments, an external environment which varies tremendously and to which man and other animals have adapted and in which they can live without ill effects; and an internal environment including much fluid and solid organs. The cells of the body are bathed in warm body fluids and grow and function well if the nourishing, fluid internal environment is unchanged or relatively unchanged. If, for example, the temperature of the fluid changes but slightly ill effects occur. If the blood sugar increases relatively slightly diabetes develops or if it is reduced somewhat convulsions may develop. The regulation of the internal environment of the body is a function of the kidneys and lungs. The kidneys conserve nutrients and excrete waste products from the breakdown of food from the wear and tear and repair of cells and tissues.

ENDOCRINE ACTIVITY OF THE KIDNEY AND EFFECTS OF ENDOCRINES ON THE KIDNEY

The kidney produces a substance called erythiopoietin which controls the production of red blood cells by the bone marrow. It also appears to control some aspects of blood pressure through another hormone. In the kidney also are large cells filled with renin. This hormone material is secreted in sodium deficiency and stimulates the adrenal gland to liberate aldosterone, an adrenal hormone which enhances salt (sodium) retention. Renin is also changed in the blood by enzymes into a polypeptide called angiotensin II which is a powerful blood pressure raising substance.

Reabsorption of sodium from the glomerular filtrate depends upon the presence of adrenal cortical hormones in the blood. For example, a decrease in the amount of adrenal cortical hormone, as in Addison's disease or insufficiency of the adrenal gland leads to an abnormal loss of sodium in the urine.

When a person is thirsty and dehydrated, the plasma is concentrated; this stimulates the release of a large amount of antidiuretic hormone from the pituitary gland. The antidiuretic hormone causes the tubular cells of the kidney to reabsorb relatively large amounts of water from the glomerular filtrate. This conserves body water and produces a concentrated urinary solution low in volume.

In diabetes insipidus, a condition of the pituitary gland with decreased production of antidiuretic hormone, an increase in daily urine output and an insatiable thirst occur; the daily urine volume may amount to twenty or more quarts per day. The secretion of the hormone is related to the fluid needs of the tissues. In the normal person urine output can be increased by giving large amounts of water and by drugs which stop the tubular cells from water reabsorption.

CLASSIFICATION OF KIDNEY DISEASES

There is no such thing as "kidney disease" just as there is no such thing as "heart disease." Many "diseases of the kidney" have been described. At least forty distinct types of diseases of the kidney may produce what physicians call the nephrotic syndrome. Any one of hundreds of different germs can infect the kidney. Some are transitory and trivial, many are serious and threaten life.

We can divide kidney disorders into two groups. First, there are those disorders produced by generalized disease of the body such as systemic lupus erythematosis which involves the kidney, and second, there are those diseases in which a local abnormality involves the kidney primarily, such as occurs in spongy kidneys (one form of congenital abnormality). Here entities or syndromes are discussed according to classification developed by the Kidney Disease Foundation.

TABLE 1
A CLASSIFICATION OF DISEASES OF THE KIDNEYS

This is one method of classifying the majority of diseases of the kidneys.

INFECTIOUS DISEASES OF THE KIDNEYS

- Pyelonephritis (including cases of "pyelitis")
- Focal embolic pyelonephritis (due to septicemia)
- Abscess within kidney; perinephric abscess
- Tuberculosis of kidney

NON-INFECTIOUS DISEASES OF THE KIDNEYS

PRIMARY, WITHIN THE KIDNEY

- *Glomerulonephritis, acute or chronic
- *Nephrotic syndrome, nephrosis
- *Interstitial nephritis
- Tumors
  - Benign
  - Malignant
- Congenital malformations
  - Polycystic disease
  - Congenital absence of one kidney
  - Specific disorders of tubules
    - Fanconi syndrome
    - Cystinosis
    - Renal tubular acidosis

SECONDARY TO OTHER DISEASE OF URINARY TRACT

- Renal Stones (nephrolithiasis)
- Obstructive disorders (uropathies) leading to Hydronephrosis
  - Enlargement of prostate
  - Congenital or acquired stricture
- Renal artery or vein constriction

SECONDARY TO OTHER DISEASE OUTSIDE URINARY TRACT

- Diseases of blood vessels (vascular diseases)
  - Malignant hypertension
  - Arteriosclerosis—(Nephrosclerosis)
  - Lupus erythematosus and collagen diseases
- Metabolic diseases
  - Diabetes mellitus
  - Parathyroid disease
  - Amyloidosis

* Bright's disease is the term formerly used to cover these and other apparently related intrinsic disorders of the kidney.

Acute Renal Failure due to severe injury or shock
Toxic effects on kidneys
  Mercury, carbon tetrachloride, and other poisons
Blood disorders
  Sickle cell anemia
  Purpura

SYMPTOMS AND SIGNS OF KIDNEY DISORDERS

Some kidney diseases progress silently and stealthily until death. The first sign of any kidney disease may be a single symptom like a broken rib, or blindness, or anemia, or headache, which at first glance does not seem even remotely connected with the kidney. Common symptoms which cause people to seek advice are swelling of the eyelids or ankles, drowsiness or fatigue, shortness of breath, a nasty taste in the mouth, thirst, headache and pain, particularly backache, unexplained abdominal pain, renal colic, pain in the penis or testicles, and fever, especially if chills and shivering are associated with it.

Passing urine more frequently than normal, either by day or night, noticing a change of color in the urine, such as passing a brown, red, or purple colored urine, inability to pass a normal stream, pain or discomfort on urination, such as burning at the tip of the urethra or spasm of the bladder; inability to pass urine or sudden marked decrease in the volume; passage of stone, gravel, or shreds of kidney tissue and discharge of pus from the urethra, are examples of conditions which should be referred to the doctor.

Anuria (no urine)–occurs in acute renal failure, but strongly suggests obstruction to urine flow below the kidneys.

Oliguria–exists when the urine flow is less than 300 ml. per day–a little over half a pint. In old people it may be diagnosed when less than $\frac{7}{10}$ of a quart is passed.

Nocturia or frequency of urination by night is dramatic; it wakes the patient. He has to get out of bed, grope around for a light and go to the lavatory. This bothers him much more than frequency by day. Patients can nearly always recall when they first started to get up at night; how many times they got up; changes in the new pattern of micturition and whether or not other symptoms, such as thirst, occurred.

Doctors ask about:

1. Whether the patient had scarlet fever, tonsillitis, hematuria, or previous renal disease (glomerulonephritis).
2. Pain in the loin or lower back associated with chills or fever (pyelonephritis).

3. Headache, drowsiness, paralysis, convulsions, dimness of vision, vomiting, dyspnea (uremia; hypertension).

4. Puffiness of the eyelids or face in the morning (acute nephritis; nephrotic syndrome; heart failure).

5. Swollen ankles (acute nephritis; nephrotic syndrome; heart failure).

6. Colic or pain in the back traveling down the front of the abdomen toward the genitalia (renal colic most often due to stones).

7. Weakness of the urine stream (an abnormality of the bladder or urethra, such as blockage by a large prostate gland).

Common abnormal observations in patients with kidney disease are high blood pressure, changes in the eyegrounds, enlargement of the heart, abnormalities in examination of the central nervous system, etc., but the doctor may find nothing wrong. Yet, when he comes to examine the urine or blood, he may find a clue like proteinuria—albumen in the urine—or an abnormal level of creatinine in the blood. Besides examining the urine, the blood, and its cells, doctors use X rays, cultures of the urine, urinary function tests, examination by the cystoscope, renal biopsy and many other tests to uncover the cause of disease involving the kidney. The most useful screening method is urinalysis.

LABORATORY TESTS

There are many methods of looking for disease in or investigating the urinary tract. Measurement of chemicals in the blood, particularly the distribution and levels of the plasma proteins (serum protein electrophoresis) and the levels of urea, creatinine, glucose, calcium, phosphorus, sodium, potassium, chloride, and carbon dioxide are made to diagnose disease. These laboratory studies are important. They represent a significant part of the increased cost of medical care.

The phenolsulfonphthalein excretion test measures both filtration and tubular secretory function. More physiologically rigorous clearance tests are done in attempting to diagnose renovascular hypertension (renal artery stenosis).

Many types of X rays are taken to study the kidney, ureters and bladders. Plain films without contrast medium will reveal dense materials like stones (calculi), calcium deposits in the kidneys (nephrocalcinosis) and other abnormalities, such as gas in the bladder.

Contrast dyes are injected into the blood stream for excretion by the kidney, and X rays are taken repeatedly to study how the kidneys handle the dyes (e.g., delay in filling the kidney with arterial obstruction). When the dyes are excreted into the pelvis, ureter, and bladder, they are radio opaque and all sorts of structural abnormalities in or outside the urinary tract can be seen and diagnosed when X-ray pictures are taken at the proper intervals after intravenous injection of the dye (intravenous pyelogram or IVP).

Experimental studies with trace amounts of radioactive substances combined with dyes (for example a combination of traces of radioactive iodine combined with the contrast dye "hippuran") are beginning to be used for studying renal function and promise to be more precise than the commonly used methods. Doctors are also beginning to measure blood flow and renal metabolism by collecting blood from the renal arteries and veins. This is still experimental.

Collection of twenty-four hours' urine is often made to measure total protein; glucose; sodium and potassium and other inorganic substances; and organic hormones or their breakdown products, such as catertrotamines, aldosterone, and glucocorticoids. Renal biopsy is a most useful method of getting a small piece of kidney tissue for examination.

The urologic surgeon is skilled in the use and interpretation of what he sees through the cystoscope, an instrument passed through the urethra to look at the bladder. He can also take a biopsy of tissue when necessary for special microscopic study by a pathologist.

THE URINE

Most adults usually pass between 1000 to 1500 ml. urine (a quart or three pints) per twenty-four hours in temperate climates, less in summer and more in winter. Except for the elderly who may urinate once during the night, healthy adults do not have nocturia unless fluids have been taken just before bedtime. During the day adults usually void between five and nine times and the urine volume for each voiding is between 100 and 300 ml. Freshly voided normal urine is usually transparent and its color varies from pale to dark yellow.

Each day the activity of the body produces an excess of acid. When acidosis occurs in people with healthy kidneys, acid phosphate excretion can increase relatively little but ammonium output may rise tenfold. When patients become acidotic in diabetes the kidney can increase and secrete ten times the amount of materials normally present to the urine. This also occurs during the high fat 'ketogenic diet' and during consumption of food and other chemicals which produce acidosis (e.g. methanol, ammonium chloride).

Healthy kidneys can produce urine with a wide range of pH (between 4.5 and 8) but the pooled daily specimen is usually acid (pH 6). Immediately following a meal, the urine becomes less acid (the "alkaline tide") and a few hours later it becomes acid again. During sleep, decreased pulmonary ventilation causes respiratory acidosis as less carbon dioxide is blown off and the urine becomes highly acid. The urinary pH varies widely in health.

Ingestion of different foods, various diets, and culinary chemicals (such as bicarbonate of soda) also affect the urinary pH. The usual diet of Western man, rich in animal protein, produces an acid urine. Predominantly vegetable diets, such as are commonly consumed in the East, in the tropics, and by economically depressed people, produce an alkaline urine.

The most important dissolved solids in the urine are urea, sodium, and chloride. These are derived mainly from ingested food and also from the metabolism of tissue protein and other substances. "Specific gravity," "refractive index," and "osmolality"—terms in the laboratory reports—of the urine are related to each other. They reflect the quantity of dissolved solids in the urine. All are used to assess the ability of the kidneys to maintain fluid balance.

The specific gravity of protein-free serum—and thus of the glomerular filtrate—is about 1.007. During the passage of the filtrate through the tubules and collecting ducts of the kidney this specific gravity is altered by tubular reabsorption or secretion of water and dissolved substances. By "concentration" and "dilution" we mean the ability to produce urine of specific gravity greater than or less than 1.010, respectively. In health this range is usually from 1.005 to 1.030, or higher.

Measurement of specific gravity in patients with healthy kidneys provides information about the state of hydration or water supply of the patient (e.g., postoperatively or during a febrile illness). Highly concentrated urine implies dehydration.

Normal urine also contains small amounts ($\frac{1}{200}$ mg. per 24 hours) of substances which chemically change alkaline copper solutions. These include glucose, sugars other than glucose (lactose, levulose, pentose, and galactose), and substances other than sugars (ascorbic acid). Some of these substances, which appear in the urine, are believed to be carbohydrates from the diet which are absorbed but poorly metabolized.

In health the urine contains small numbers of cells and other formed elements from the whole length of the genitourinary tract—casts and epithelial cells from the nephron; epithelial cells from the pelvis, ureters, bladder, and urethra; mucous threads and spermatozoa from the prostate. A few erythrocytes and leucocytes apparently reach the urine from any part of the urinary tract.

Two to three red blood cells, four to five leucocytes per high-power microscopic field and occasional hyaline casts are accepted as normal. Casts always originate in the renal tubules but red and white cells may originate anywhere in the urinary tract. Large numbers of erythrocytes, leucocytes, and casts may appear in the urine of healthy subjects who perform strenuous exercise or who are exposed to severe cold. Except under these conditions certain abnormal constituents always indicate renal disease, e.g., red cell casts and white cell casts.

Many substances may contaminate the urinary sediment. Fragments of cotton or other fibers, oil droplets from lubricants, bacteria or yeasts from unclean receptacles, and starch granules are common. Vaginal secretions, which may contain bacilli and trichomonads may also appear in the urine. Spermatozoa commonly appear in the urine of adult males.

METHODS OF COLLECTING URINE

For chemical and microscopic urinalysis, the patient will usually not need elaborate cleansing procedures. Precautions must be taken when the urine has been contaminated by vaginal discharge or hemorrhage. Properly collected, clean-voided specimens are preferable for virtually all examinations. Because it is concentrated, the first morning specimen is collected for examination in a clean receptacle.

Properly preserved twenty-four-hour urine collections give a more accurate quantitative measurement of the excretion of protein, glucose, or other constituents than can be obtained by analyzing random specimens.

COLOR AND SMELL OF URINE

Highly concentrated urines, such as are formed in hot, dry countries are usually deep yellow, strongly acid, and may be irritating.

Increasing amounts of bilirubin from the bile produces colors ranging from yellow-brown to deep olive green. Hemoglobin, red blood cells, porphyrins, some foods (e.g., beets and red candies), and drugs (e.g., amidopyrin and pyridium) produce various red hues. Urine containing old blood, hemosiderin, or myoglobin is brown to black; smaller amounts of red blood cells produce a characteristic smoky appearance.

Homogentisic acid (alcaptonuria) and malanin may make the urine dark brown or black, especially if the urine is alkaline. Blue-green colors come from drugs like methylene blue.

The sweet pearlike smell of acetone or acetoacetic acid can be recognized in uncontrolled diabetes. Heavily infected urine may have a particularly unpleasant odor.

CLINICAL SIGNIFICANCE OF MEASUREMENT OF URINE SPECIFIC GRAVITY

Unless adequate fluid is being ingested, the kidneys will not be able to concentrate to high levels, as occurs in patients on salt-poor or protein-deficient diets. In most cases of progressive renal disease, the range of specific gravity narrows with time, diluting ability persisting for longer, until ultimately the specific gravity of the urine is hardly altered by passage through the kidney.

In diabetes insipidus with deficiency of antidiuretic hormone, the urine specific gravity is consistently less than 1.005.

Compulsive water drinking occurs most commonly in neurotic women.

The kidney loses concentration ability with severe potassium deficiency; too much calcium in the blood (hypercalcemia) as a result of sarcoidosis, bone disease (e.g., multiple myeloma), vitamin D, intoxication or hypersensitivity, or hyperparathyroidism. This develops also with damage of the tubules, such as pyelonephritis, polycystic kidney disease, and hydronephrosis.

SUGAR IN THE URINE

Tests for glycosuria are part of the examination of any patient. Diabetes mellitus is a common disease. Tests for glycosuria should be done particularly in all health surveys, such as for insurance, or employment; as part of all periodic medical examinations in the doctor's office; in patients with recurrent infections (particularly staphylococcal or fungal); and in the following groups of patients in whom diabetes is common: relatives of diabetics, obese patients, patients over the age of forty, women who have given birth to heavy babies or who have unexplained stillbirths.

Alimentary glycosuria (sugar in the urine) is the excretion of traces of glucose after ingestion of large amounts of sugar. This occurs only in people who have had certain types of gastric operations, such as gastrectomy or removal of the stomach. Renal glycosuria is a primary familial renal disorder. Sugar appears in the urine with normal blood-sugar levels and with otherwise normal renal function.

During pregnancy reducing substances indicating sugar appear in the urine in 70 per cent of healthy women; this figure increases to 90 per cent during the post-partum period. Lactosuria or milk sugar in the urine is more common than glycosuria with glucose. Lactose alone occurs in 51 per cent, glucose alone in 24 per cent, and both in 16 per cent of pregnant women. After delivery glycosuria disappears, but the incidence and degree of lactosuria increases.

OTHER MATTER IN THE URINE

The term hemoglobinuria is used to describe the finding of free hemoglobin, the red coloring matter of the blood, or its immediate chemical derivatives in the urine, which are excreted by the kidney in states of hemoglobinemia. When erythrocytes are broken up in the urine, free hemoglobin appears and may be difficult to distinguish from that which arises in the serum.

Hemoglobinuria must be distinguished from hematuria, or blood in the urine, which is more common.

Hematuria varies from gross clots and obvious blood staining to amounts detectable only by microscopy or chemical tests. Bleeding without severe proteinuria, casts, or other evidence of kidney disease most often originates in the lower portion of the genitourinary tract, and massive hematuria is perhaps more common in surgical conditions such as tumor or lithiasis.

Hematuria is a prominent feature of acute hemorrhagic Bright's disease, and is often severe. The urine has a characteristic smoky appearance due to the red cells which are often crenated. Red cell casts are frequently present.

When pus is visible to the naked eye, or when leucocytes (the white blood cells) exceed about fifty per high-power field of the microscope, genitourinary tract infection almost certainly exists. Clumping of leucocytes in the urine also suggests infection.

Finding leucocytes in the urine is not diagnostic of urinary tract infection, because white cells may appear in any inflammatory condition in the renal tissues, notably acute hemorrhagic Bright's disease, systemic lupus erythematosus, etc.

Conversely, leucocytes are not always present in the urine when significant urinary-tract infection is shown by persistent bacteriuria or germs in the urine. In chronic pyelonephritis repeated examinations of the urine may be necessary before abnormal formed elements are seen, or pathogenic bacteriuria can be cultured.

Casts may be distinguished from other contaminants of the urine like mucous fibers, or crystals. Hyaline casts are formed in the tubules and their appearance in the urine depends on the rate of urine flow, urine pH, and the degree of proteinuria.

Except in certain special circumstances, the finding of crystals in the urine has relatively little medical value. Many crystals appear both in acid and in alkaline urine.

THE EFFECT OF NUTRITION, ENVIRONMENT, AND STRESS UPON URINALYSIS

Urine must be collected for analysis under standard conditions. In healthy young men, increasing amounts of proteinuria have been found with increasing severity and duration of exercise. Proteinuria also occurred in persons given low calorie diets with a relatively large proportion of fat. The proteinuria increased when the people lived in a cold environment.

Strenuous physical exercise such as football can cause the kidneys to excrete urine containing all of the formed elements found in acute glomerulonephritis, but the abnormal sediment clears over several days. Unbalanced diets, exposure to severe cold, and dehydration also cause increased urinary excretion of cells and casts.

THE URINE IN DISEASE

Proteinuria is generally evidence of the presence of renal disease, but evaluation of the significance of proteinuria may be difficult. Whenever it is first detected, the pattern of protein excretion may be determined by frequent urinalysis. Transient proteinuria is usually less likely to be significant than persistent proteinuria. The concentration of protein in a given sample depends on many factors including the concentration of the urine. The total protein excreted in a twenty-four-hour period may have to be estimated. Most insurance companies will offer standard policies to applicants with negative histories of renal disease if the proteinuria does not exceed 30 mg. per 100 ml. of urine.

Many proteins may be found in the normal urine which react similarly to proteins from the serum of the blood. However, the relative proportions of proteins in the urine are different from those in plasma, albumin being relatively less and globulin relatively more. The modern term "proteinuria" is preferred to "albuminuria" since, even in disease where albumin usually predominates, the urine also contains other proteins besides albumin.

Testing for proteinuria is part of the usual medical examination of a patient. In the hospital it is usually done on admission and at least once weekly thereafter. It is an essential part of examination of a person during health surveys such as are administered for recruits in the armed services, college students, and employment or insurance examinations.

When any test for protein in the urine is positive, the validity of the test should be confirmed by testing the urine again with another method. A common test is boiling of the urine in the presence of acetic acid.

CONDITIONS ASSOCIATED WITH PROTEINURIA

Proteinuria in the absence of organic disease affecting the kidneys or genitourinary tract is usually transitory and most commonly appears in young adults. It may occur

1. Following excessive exercise.
2. Following exposure to cold.

3. In Orthostatic proteinuria. In this condition, which occurs particularly in young adults, the patient passes protein while in the erect position but not when horizontal. Orthostatic proteinuria is thought to be due to increased pressure in the renal vein caused by an accentuated lumbar curvature of the spine.

Although the conditions mentioned are usually benign, they also may be indications of incipient renal damage, especially after adolescence. Patients with transient or orthostatic proteinuria should be examined periodically.

Transient proteinuria can occur with most acute diseases, especially those associated with fever, and in abdominal crises of various kinds. The urine may show some proteinuria in cardiac disease, central nervous system lesions, thyroid disorders, blood disorders, particularly severe anemia, or following the use of certain drugs such as gold or neomycin. Several systemic disorders may also produce renal lesions.

In pre-eclampsia and eclampsia, the pre-existing renal disease may be involved. Proteinuria may be the first sign and may vary greatly in amount.

Primary renal diseases include infections of the kidney and four syndromes: acute hemorrhagic Bright's disease, the nephrotic syndrome, chronic Bright's disease, and persistent proteinuria without symptoms.

Bacterial infections of the kidney, such as pyelonephritis, result in the presence of protein, pus, and bacteria in the urine. Usually the proteinuria is moderate. In pyelonephritis, especially of the chronic type, proteinuria as well as pus in the urine may be minimal or absent. A negative test for protein does not completely rule out pyelonephritis.

Acute Bright's disease may follow infection with streptococci such as the hemolytic streptococcus. Blood in the urine, high blood pressure, and a high blood urea nitrogen in the urine reported by the laboratory are usually found. After the diagnosis is made, testing and recording the urine each day is desirable. The outcome is indicated by disappearance or persistence of proteinuria.

Epidemic pharyngitis and hematuria, presumably viral in origin, may lead to epidemics of acute hemorrhagic Bright's disease in which evidence of streptococcal infection could not be found. In such cases patients had a mild nephritis and recovered rapidly.

The Nephrotic Syndrome. This group of symptoms appears with continued massive proteinuria (two or more grams of albumin a day). In addition to proteinuria, a high cholesterol level, and "nephrotic" edema or swelling develop.

Chronic Bright's Disease. Proteinuria is generally not massive in chronic Bright's disease, except in malignant or severe cases with chronic renal failure.

Asymptomatic Persistent Proteinuria. During routine examinations some people who feel completely well are found to have proteinuria. If proteinuria is persistent, most of these have been shown by renal biopsy to have some form of nephritis or kidney inflammation.

Proteinuria from the Lower Genitourinary Tract. (a) Vaginal discharge. Contamination of the urine by exudates from the female genital tract is a common cause of diagnostic confusion. By wiping the vagina and packing the entrance before collecting urine this confusion may be avoided.

(b) Prostatitis, cystitis, and other inflammatory conditions of the lower urinary tract may exude protein into the urine, usually in relatively small amounts.

Bence Jones Proteins. In serious diseases called multiple myeloma and primary macroglobulinemia, unusual proteins are present in the urine. They can often be detected in the urine by their unique quality of coagulating when heated to between 45°–55°C and partially or totally redissolving when the urine is boiled.

KIDNEY SYNDROMES

Most renal disorders have characteristic patterns (or natural histories). Each clinical pattern or syndrome can be the result of a variety of different causes or disease processes. For example, the "nephrotic syndrome" can be caused by any one of forty or more different causes. Listed below are some common clinical syndromes involving the kidneys.

Acute Nephritis (Acute Bright's disease; acute hemorrhagic glomerulonephritis)
Nephrotic Syndrome (Nephrosis; subacute Bright's disease)
Chronic Renal Failure (Chronic nephritis; chronic Bright's disease; chronic uremia)
Acute Renal Failure (Acute uremia)
Acute Pyelonephritis (Acute pyelitis; acute cystitis)
Chronic Pyelonephritis (Interstitial nephritis)
Obstructive Uropathy (Hydronephrosis)
Renal Tubular Failure (Fanconi syndrome)
Renal Colic Asymptomatic Proteinuria
Asymptomatic Proteinuria
Hypertension (High blood pressure)

ACUTE NEPHRITIS

Usually affects children but also adults and may be epidemic in military or other camps. The typical attack may follow a streptococcal infection, commonly of the throat. Some days to weeks after the infection began the patient passes brownish or tea-colored urine and may develop puffy eyelids, swollen ankles, backache, fever, high blood pressure, and convulsions. Complete recovery is usual in children. A few may become nephrotic (see below) or over the years show evidence of chronic renal failure. Occasionally, in severe cases, acute renal failure may develop. Recurrences of hematuria are not uncommon after the first attack and usually are associated with viral or bacterial infections of the respiratory tract. Of adults who are ill enough to come into hospitals about half make a complete recovery. The remainder develop persistent proteinuria or the nephrotic syndrome or chronic nephritis. Beside poststreptococcal nephritis, other causes of acute nephritis are Henoch-Schonlein purpura, lupus erythematosus, and other collagen diseases.

THE NEPHROTIC SYNDROME

The nephrotic syndrome (also known as "nephrosis" or "subacute Bright's disease" or "subacute glomerulonephritis") is the result of passage of large amounts of protein in the urine which depletes the body of protein stores, causes malnutrition and results in many biochemical abnormalities in the blood; the best known are low-serum albumin (hypoalbuminemia) and high-serum lipids, including a high cholesterol level. The nephrotic syndrome is manifested by the sudden or slow development of dropsy (edema). The patient rubs his eyes or notices puffiness on waking in the morning. The eyelids return to normal at the end of the day. Later, in the course of the illness, the ankles may swell and edema may spread to involve the whole of the legs. Ultimately the peritoneal cavity of the abdomen may be filled with fluid (ascites). Or all of a sudden puffy face, gross swelling of legs, and ascites may appear out of the blue. Such edematous patients are very prone to develop infections.

The causes of this syndrome, from infancy to old age, are legion. Among the causes are bee stings; clots in the renal veins; amyloid disease; diabetes; collagen disorders; etc. But, in most instances, no definite cause can be found and exact histologic diagnoses are made by renal biopsy. In children the course is often one of spontaneous remissions and relapses, usually ending in complete recovery if lipoid nephrosis is present. In adults the prognosis is best in those with histologic lesions of "lipoid nephrosis," particularly if there is rapid disappearance of proteinuria following treatment with steroids. Pure "membranous" glomerulonephritis also carries a good prognosis, despite resistance to all known treatments. On the whole the prognosis is much better with children than with adults.

Patients with nephrotic syndrome are treated by diet, diuretics, steroid hormones, and recently, with experimental immuno-suppressive drugs. When there is a known cause for the nephrotic syndrome which requires a special or specific treatment, this is also used. (E.g., an operation to relieve constrictive pericarditis; anticoagulant treatment for renal vein thrombosis [clots]; insulin for diabetes.)

CHRONIC RENAL FAILURE (UREMIA)

A healthy person, apparently vigorous, may fall asleep at inappropriate times. His eyes may be puffy or he may become easily fatigued, short of breath, and look pale, or he may complain of headaches and have a high blood pressure. He may have a stroke or complain of a nasty taste in the mouth, loss of appetite, twitching, or cramps in the muscles. He may be irritable, or perhaps be found one day in coma. The clinical disturbances described are often the result of slowly progressive symptomless failure of renal function. The kidney loses its reserve because of the relentless destruction of nephrons by life-long disease. In slowly progressive kidney disease, the body as a whole and the unaffected nephrons compensate for the piecemeal renal destruction as the kidney is destroyed. A time comes when the critical balance between compensation and decompensation can be disturbed by intercurrent noxious events, such as an operation or by injury or acute infection; by a new acute disease (e.g. a heart attack); and especially by conditions imposed on the person which disturb his critical internal water and chemical balance (homeostasis). In such persons if water and salts are lost by a bout of diarrhea or vomiting, the symptoms of uremia (poisoning by the products of metabolism) may appear. The loss of fluid from the gastrointestinal tract shunts water away from the kidney and little or no urine is formed. The patient's inability to drink aggravates dehydration and cuts down urine flow. Thus waste products are not excreted in the urine and pile up in the body. The loss of salts from diarrhea or vomiting further unbalances the already disturbed internal bodily environment and uremic poisoning appears.

Chronic renal failure with uremia is the end result of many disease processes and of course does not always arise out of the blue as described. It may be the end stage of obstructive changes of chronic pyelonephritis, of the nephrotic syndrome, or even of acute nephritis.

Unfortunately progressive renal disease can develop silently in some patients without abnormalities being obvious in the urine. This is why many doctors, in addition to examining the urine of patients during an annual examination and at other times, do chemical tests on the blood as well as a urinalysis. The most useful tests are the serum creatinine level or the blood urea nitrogen level. If these are both abnormally high, renal or urinary tract disease is usually the cause of the abnormality.

Treatment

Prevention of intercurrent infections, and prevention of water and electrolyte disturbances at and after necessary operations is one aim in the care of the patient with chronic renal failure. The doctor usually prescribes diets that minimize the production of bodily waste products and thus of uremic poisoning. Commonly these diets are low in protein, potassium, and phosphorus content, rich in carbohydrate and fat calories, in calcium, in sodium, and in other nutrients.

Intercurrent infections, if present, are treated with appropriate antibiotics, and water and electrolyte imbalances are corrected by appropriate infusions. Chronic anemia does not respond to iron or liver treatment and cannot be vigorously treated with transfusions. The reasons for this are that transfusions, which bring the blood level to normal in such patients, tend to increase the viscosity or thickness of the blood and thereby diminish filtration of blood through the few remaining glomeruli. Nonetheless, if the hemoglobin drops low some blood must be given to bring its level back toward normal.

In addition, tiding a patient over a critical intercurrent noxious event by using dialysis ("artificial kidney") is often necessary. A small number of patients with chronic renal failure are being kept alive by repeated dialyses two or three times each week or by transplantation of kidneys. These are still experimental procedures. All doctors hope for a scientific breakthrough that will allow transplantation of kidneys from donors or from the dead without rejection by the recipient's body. To date, the most successful transplants have been between identical twins. By 1965 about thirty-eight such transplants had been done in identical twins. Some such patients lived as long as eight years after the transplant. In seventeen of the thirty-eight twins operated on, generalized disease processes were responsible for the failure of their kidneys. In nine of these seventeen twins the healthy transplanted kidneys were destroyed by the same disease process that originally destroyed the patient's own kidneys. Unfortunately, at the time of writing (1964), most patients with transplanted kidneys had not lived for longer than a year after their operation. Treatment with repeated dialyses, whether done at home or in a hospital, appear to work best with young, highly motivated, self-disciplined patients of superior intellectual qualities. It requires great willpower to accept the vigorous dietary restrictions of the treatment program and the necessary regimentation of their work and social activities day after day, month after month, and year in and year out.

CONGENITAL OR HEREDITARY DISEASES OF THE KIDNEY INCLUDING POLYCYSTIC KIDNEYS

Structural defects of the blood vessels to and from the kidneys, of the kidneys themselves, or of the drainage system are common, occurring perhaps in one quarter of mankind. Usually they are not important and most people live with horseshoe kidneys or diverticula of the bladder or other congenital abnormalities without disturbance of health. Some rare defects are fatal, as, for example, complete absence of kidneys. A few, like stenosis of the renal artery or polycystic disease or tubular defects may or may not cause trouble.

Multiple cysts of the kidneys or polycystic kidneys result from structural defect in the formation of the nephron and are present at birth. If the defect is severe at birth, the infant with such a defect will die; if the defect is mild, it may not reveal its presence until adult life. In polycystic disease, the kidney tissue is filled with cysts, small holes or fluid-filled cavities. The cavities, or cysts, may range from pinhead to hen's-egg size. When the cysts become numerous enough and large enough, kidney function is impaired, the ability of the kidneys to excrete urine lessens and the symptoms of uremia develop. Sometimes there may be the symptom of pain over the kidneys, this being due to the pressure of obstruction, hemorrhage into one of the cysts, or from infection in one of the cysts. High blood pressure is frequently present in persons who have polycystic kidneys. If the disease progresses to an advanced state with uremia, then hospitalization may be necessary for more intensive care and relief. Most people with polycystic kidneys lead normal lives, die of some unrelated disease, and have the abnormal kidneys discovered only after death.

OBSTRUCTIVE UROPATHY

Local disease in the pelvis, ureter, bladder, or urethra may obstruct the flow of urine from the kidney to the outside of the body. Ureteropelvic junction abnormalities, stones in the ureter, scars of the ureter, retroperitoneal fibrosis, enlarged uterus, or tumors in the abdominal cavity, and especially enlarged prostate glands, may acutely or chronically block urine flow.

Obstruction can be acute as with renal stones and may or may not produce renal colic. It may cause anuria by blocking the flow of urine.

Chronic obstruction commonly causes a dilatation of the whole drainage tract above the site of obstruction. The pelvis gets big and the kidney is stretched around it. This is called hydronephrosis. The stagnant urine in the dilated pelvis often gets infected. Sometimes stones form in the hydronephrotic kidney. Enlargement of the prostate gland is the most common cause of obstruction to urine flow. This occurs in men at about fifty years of age or older. Why it occurs is still a mystery. Obstructive uropathy is treated by urologic surgeons who operate to remove the obstruction and repair the drainage tract.

ACUTE RENAL FAILURE

The causes of acute oliguria or anuria are legion. Acute obstruction of the urinary tract, dehydration, and various types of water and electrolyte disturbance, such as prolonged and severe water intoxication, may disturb formation and urine flow. Insults to the body remote from the kidney, such as an acute myocardial infarct–heart attack–may reduce glomerular filtration to such low levels that little or no urine is formed. And finally, transfusion reactions, nephrotoxins, renal disease, endotoxins, hemolytic crises, renal vascular damage, and acute allergic or immunologic reactions may disturb the function of the kidney, damage its cells, and produce acute renal failure.

The course of the illness may be short or long and can be divided into four phases: onset, oliguric or anuric phase, and early and late diuretic phase. The disorder may be mild or severe and, while the course can often be predicted initially from the type of disorder that has precipitated the failure, in at least thirty per cent of cases no diagnosis is made. The slope of the daily rise in the blood urea nitrogen is a good index of tissue breakdown and is one measure of mildness or severity. Potassium intoxication and pulmonary edema from sodium and water overload are the chief dangers in the early part of failure and depletion of water, potassium and salt in the diuretic phase.

The aims of treatment of acute renal failure are: to discover the cause and deal with it and its consequences; to keep tissue protein breakdown to a minimum; to maintain nutritional status; to control water and sodium balance; to treat symptoms of acidosis or alkalosis; to prevent or treat hyperkalemia, hypocalcemia, and uremia as they arise; and last but not least, to protect the patient from infection, which is the main cause of death.

Treatment may be conservative: mannitol may be used to prevent and treat the internal hydronephrosis of transfusion reactions or, the physician may elect to use peritoneal or extracorporeal dialysis. The trend is to earlier and more frequent dialyses, while at the same time providing limited meals to maintain nutrition and morale at optimum levels.

In conservative management when, for example, it is predicted that the course is to be short the aims of dietary treatment are to prevent accumulation of water and salt, to prevent and treat hyperkalemia, and limit the accumulation of nitrogenous end products to a minimum.

HYPERTENSION (HIGH BLOOD PRESSURE)

There are many causes for high blood pressure and many classifications or groupings of causes. Most commonly found as a result of the use of the blood pressure machine (sphygmomanometer) are persons classified as having "primary" or "essential" hypertension. Rarely is blood pressure raised because of an endocrine disease such as pheochromocytoma or Cushing's syndrome (both disorders of the adrenal gland). Renal disorders account for the remainder. When the kidneys are diseased by generalized abnormalities of their tissues, such as occurs in diabetic nephropathy, chronic glomerulonephritis, or interstitial nephritis, progressive hypertension commonly develops. In addition, when the blood supply to the kidney is compromised by local disease of one or both renal arteries renovascular hypertension may develop. This type of hypertension which, usually, is discovered in the young is often amenable to surgical treatment. The defect in the artery which causes obstruction to the blood flow can be excised at an operation. Arterial or plastic vascular grafts can also be inserted to by-pass the obstruction and restore blood flow to the affected kidney. Sometimes the affected kidney or part of it has to be removed.

Only a small proportion of patients with hypertension have reparable disorders. Renovascular hypertension is difficult to diagnose with certainty and the operation requires great skill on the part of the surgeon. Pre-eclampsia (toxemia of pregnancy) is also a potentially reversible hypertensive disorder. The hypertension which usually develops late in pregnancy nearly always returns to normal after delivery.

Hypertension may cause fatigue and nervousness. Irritability and headache are not uncommon. The heart enlarges and may later fail and the blood vessels of the brain may be damaged. These complications cause edema, shortness of breath, rupture of blood vessels (e.g., nose bleeds), and central nervous system complications such as strokes and blindness. Treatment with modern antihypertensive drugs have changed the outlook and health of the average hypertensive patient for the better but, as yet, there is no adequate treatment for those few patients who develop "malignant" hypertension, a fatal form of rapidly progressive high blood pressure.

Both genetic and environmental factors appear to play a role in hypertension, particularly in that form of hypertension formerly named "essential" and, nowadays, called "primary." For example, a tremendous incidence of hypertension occurs in northern Japan as compared to some other areas of the world and this has been related to the exceedingly high salt intake of the northern Japanese. Helmer and Page have developed the thesis that a renal hormone, renin, acting on a substrate released from the liver, produced a substance which was hypertensive. Braun-Menendez and Page named the polypeptide released "angiotensin." Interrelationships have been demonstrated between levels of dietary salt, the activity of the juxtaglomerular apparatus and the glomerulosa (aldosterone-producing) layer of the adrenal cortex. Much research is being done on various aspects of sodium metabolism as related to interaction between brain, kidney, adrenal gland, blood volume, and blood pressure.

The juxtaglomerular apparatus (JGA), its blood supply, and nerves, and the closely approximated macula densa of the distal convolutions of the tubule appear to be an interconnected renal-, chemo-, and baroreceptor which presumably act together to control the release of renin from the JGA. Renin in turn stimulates the adrenal gland to secrete aldosterone. This hormone acts directly on the renal tubules to conserve sodium and, thereby, affects the electrolyte economy of the body, the plasma volume and, presumably, blood pressure.

Besides stimulating the adrenal gland, renin also acts on the polypeptide renin substrate from alpha 2 globulin to form angiotensin I. This compound—a decapolypeptide—is split by converting enzyme into an active hypertensive octapeptide—angiotensin II. It is this latter compound which is thought to be responsible for the hypertension of patients and animals with significant renal artery disease.

A much higher sodium content prevails in the arteries of patients and animals with hypertension, and these levels return to normal when the hypertension is relieved. The sodium in the arteries, bound, presumably, to acid mucopolysaccharide in the wall, apparently provides the setting for the vascular response to vasoactive substances, presumably making the vessel more sensitive to hypertensive agents in the presence of excess sodium.

Patients with hypertension can be treated with diets alone which vary in their sodium content and ease of preparation. The lower the sodium content of the diet, the less palatable it is and the more difficult it is to prepare. However, at present rigid sodium restriction is not necessary. Patients are treated—when warranted—with a low-salt diet from which salty and pickled foods are excluded. Table salt is not used and only a little in cooking. With moderate restriction and use of modern diuretic drugs, large amounts of sodium are rapidly removed from the body. If this combination, with or without other antihypertensive drugs, does not reduce blood pressure, one can then embark on a trial of an 800 mg. sodium diet, along with hypertensive drugs. If this does not work, further reduction of sodium in the diet will not help. The hypertension can be considered resistant to sodium withdrawal, and other modes of treatment employed to treat the hypertension. A danger of sodium withdrawal is possible production of symptoms (the low salt syndrome).

ACUTE INFECTIONS OF THE KIDNEY AND UPPER URINARY TRACT

Acute infection of the urinary tract is particularly common in women during the childbearing age and in female infants and children. Apparently infection spreads from the urethral opening into the bladder where it may cause "cystitis." From there it may spread up the ureter to the pelvis of the kidney where it may produce "acute pyelitis." If the kidney becomes involved in the infective process this is then termed "acute pyelonephritis." Direct spread of the infection to the kidney may come from the blood stream or lymph and cause acute pyelonephritis and sometimes minute abscesses of the kidney. The infection then travels down the ureters to the bladder.

REFLUX

In some persons when it contracts, part of the urine held in the bladder may be squirted the wrong way. Instead of going out of the body it may be pushed backward up the ureters. This may or may not be harmful. If reflux causes hydronephrosis or recurrent infection it may have to be treated by operation. Usually it can be treated by training the patient to void repeatedly after the first emptying of the bladder.

In the early stages of the infection—usually by gram negative organisms, pus is not formed. Infection is detected by the doctor through culture of the urine.

The combination of pus and significant bacteria in the urine strongly suggests the diagnosis of urinary tract infection.

Infection may or may not cause symptoms. Common symptoms of infection are complaints of frequency and burning on urination. If inflammation develops, pus cells will be found in the urine. If the bladder is involved (cystitis), painful spasms of the organ may occur. With involvement of the pelvis (pyelitis) or the kidney (acute pyelonephritis) attacks of chills and fever, and backache as well as frequent, burning and painful urination follow. If the pelvis or the kidney is severely damaged by the infection, small pieces of tissue may break off. Renal colic and bloody urine may develop.

Antibiotics, bactericidal drugs, and supportive measures are prescribed for treatment.

Tuberculosis of the kidney may spread to the bladder and cause painful spasms of the organ. In Africa and Asia, a parasitic infestation called

Bilharzia is due to bathing in rivers and lakes infested with schistosomes which enter the body through the skin and cause bloody urine and backache.

UROLITHIASIS (STONES)

Renal stones occur with almost equal frequency in both sexes. Bladder stones, however, are far more common in men because of the additional factor of bladder orifice obstruction.

Crystallographic analysis of 2000 human urinary calculi demonstrated that approximately 30 per cent were composed of calcium oxalate, 40 per cent of calcium oxalate and apatite, 15 per cent of magnesium ammonium phosphate alone or mixed with apatite or with apatite and calcium oxalate, 4 per cent of apatite, 5 per cent of uric acid, and 2 per cent of cystine. Only one pure urate stone was found.

Some believe urinary calculi develop and grow when urinary crystalloids precipitate from supersaturated solutions in urine to either form a "stone nucleus" directly (on which the precipitating crystalloids can be further deposited), or when this urinary sediment deposits itself on a calcium (Randall's) plaque at the tip of the renal pyramid. They may act there as "stone nuclei."

Precipitations of urinary crystalloids occur when the limit of supersaturation is exceeded, either because of increased concentration of the crystalloids or because of a derangement of urinary solubility factors.

Two conditions can occur within the urinary tract which frequently accelerate the growth of a stone. (1) Urinary stasis, and (2) urinary infection. Urinary stasis gives more time for the urinary salts to precipitate. It also increases the incidence of urinary-tract infection and makes extremely difficult the eradication of such infections. Infection with urea-splitting organisms renders the urine alkaline. An alkaline urine favors the precipitation of ammonium magnesium phosphate hexahydrate and apatite calculi. Such stones are almost always considered to be secondary to infection.

In certain areas of the world, where the people usually take an improperly balanced diet, the incidence of urinary calculi is high. Such "stone areas" have been reported in China, India, and in Turkey and Thailand. In England and France during the last century, urinary calculous disease occurred chiefly in childhood (mainly in the lower urinary tract). At present, the disease is predominantly one of adult life and of the upper urinary tract. The elimination of deficiencies in the daily dietary in the Western countries apparently has brought about the changes of incidence and situation in calculous disease. Deficiency of vitamin A of animal origin and a deficiency of absorbable calcium in the diet are thought to have been demonstrated as the important faults.

If fluid intake is not proportionately increased, the excessive sweating which occurs in hot climates increases the concentration of the urinary crystalloids and thus favors formation of stone. In the United States the incidence of urinary calculi is greatest in Southern California and in Southern Florida. Stones are treated by increasing fluid intake night and day, by changing the pH of the urine with chemicals. This is difficult to do and often not satisfactory. The stones may have to be removed by an operation.

RENAL COLIC

Colic in the kidney is a severe pain, usually caused by a stone, blood clot, or piece of tissue from the kidney lodging in the ureter. This muscular tube contracts rhythmically trying to expel the object. This causes spasms of pain, starting in the back and going around the front and then down the abdomen to the tip of the urethra or penis. Renal colic is often a severe pain requiring injections of morphia and antispasmodic drugs and admission to hospital.

RENAL TUBULAR DEFECTS

A famous Swiss pediatrician, Fanconi, first proposed the concept that a defect in the function of the tubular cells could account for the set of signs and symptoms, a syndrome, which bears his name. Children afflicted with this disease have a genetically inherited abnormality of tubular reabsorption with wastage of glucose, amino acids and phosphates in the urine. The latter disturbance leads to rickets or osteomalacia (Milkman's syndrome) depending on the age of the patient. Fanconi's name has become generally used to describe the various types of "tubular failure," such as "the adult Fanconi syndrome" and "the secondary Fanconi syndrome" which occur in patients ill with renal disorders such as chronic pyelonephritis or multiple myeloma.

TREATMENT OF RENAL DISEASE

DRUGS

Treatment of renal disease is changing rapidly, and new drugs and devices are always being tested.

When people are edematous or dropsical—a common condition in patients with renal disease—the body must get rid of water and sometimes of salt. Digitalis acts as a diuretic when patients have heart failure. Most modern diuretics remove sodium and potassium with water and patients have to take potassium to prevent the development of potassium deficiency (which, incidentally, may cause interstitial nephritis).

Prednisone is the steroid drug commonly used to treat the nephrotic syndrome and is used to treat a wide variety of collagen diseases and other disorders involving the kidney. We do not know how it works, but it has greatly improved the chances of survival in children with nephrotic syndrome. Doctors are warned to use prednisone with caution and skill.

Antibiotics of different kinds are used to treat specific infections of the kidney. In some situations of infection in the urinary tract (e.g., large stag-horn stones in an infected renal pelvis) medications are prescribed which suppress bacterial growth by changing the acidity or alkalinity of the urine (potassium citrate) or which work by interfering with bacterial growth (mandelamine). Often these are used for long periods of time.

DIALYSIS AND "ARTIFICIAL KIDNEYS"

Membranes from animals (e.g., sausage casings from gut) and artificial plastic membranes like cellophane will allow water and small molecular weight chemicals (salts) to pass freely through them but will not allow large molecular weight substances like proteins or cells to pass across them. This is dialysis, the principle in artificial kidney machines. Blood from the artery or vein of a uremic patient is pumped through plastic tubes to a chamber lined with artificial membranes or through artificial membranes. As the blood flows from the body and runs over the membranes some of the water, salts and uremic poisons pass through the membrane and are removed from the body. Thereafter, the blood cells, the blood proteins and lipids are returned through a second series of tubes to the body. This is called hemodialysis. (See PLATE 101.)

Peritoneal dialysis is tried for a similar purpose. The natural lining of the abdominal cavity—the peritoneal membrane—will extract uremic poisons and toxic concentrations of salts (particularly potassium) or external poisons (aspirin) from the body. A small hole is made in the wall of the abdomen and a perforated plastic tube is inserted into the abdominal cavity. A specially designed mixture of water, glucose, salts, and other chemicals is run through the tube into the cavity and left there. "Poisons" pass from the body across the peritoneal membrane into the fluids in the cavity. After a time, the fluid, now containing the poisons, is allowed to run out of the abdominal cavity. This process of running fluid in and out of the peritoneal cavity may be repeated many times.

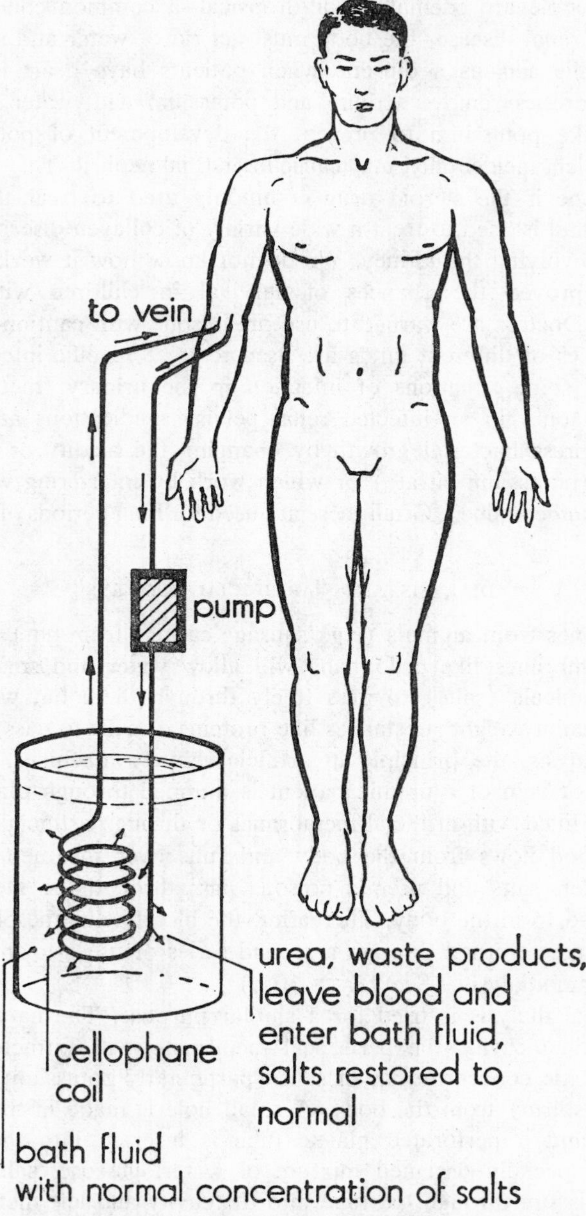

Fig. 51. The artificial kidney machine is a rather large, bulky piece of equipment which is attached to the individual periodically for only a few hours at a time. The machine is connected to an artery, usually in the arm, so that the patient's blood will flow through the machine. After completing the circuit, it is returned to the patient through a vein, usually in the same arm. In this sketch the

The use of different forms of dialysis in the long term management of chronic renal failure is still being intensively investigated. Doctors and engineers are working together to develop simple, foolproof, inexpensive machines which may be used safely in the patient's home to prolong life.

TRANSPLANTATION OF KIDNEYS

Still experimental for the treatment of patients whose kidneys have been irreparably damaged is transplantation. Kidneys from volunteer donors, from corpses (cadaver kidneys), and from animals have been grafted into patients. The natural immunologic defense mechanisms of the patient's body rejects and destroys the transplanted organ to a greater or lesser degree, except in the case of identical twins. The procedure is fraught with difficulties which are being debated from moral, ethical, legal, psychological, financial, technical, and immunologic points of view.

---

artificial kidney machine is simply a very long tube of cellophane, or similar material, wound upon itself so that it becomes a coil. The coil is placed in a large fluid bath, about 100 quarts, which has a composition very similar to that of blood plasma from a normal individual except that it contains no protein. The bath fluid is well stirred so that it continually moves over the outside of the cellophane coil. The two ends of the coil are then connected by tubes to the blood vessels of the patient so that the blood from the arm artery flows into the cellophane tubing, and returns to the patient by way of the arm vein. Illustration courtesy of National Kidney Foundation.

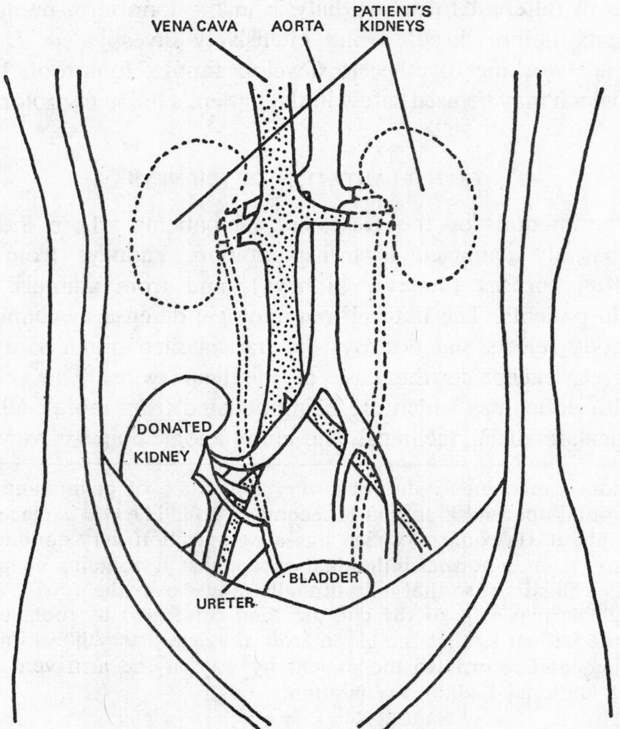

Fig. 52. The steps in transplantation of a kidney are illustrated in this simplified sketch. The patient's kidneys are removed about two weeks before the transplanting to allow for healing. Within minutes after removal from the donor, the new kidney is placed in the patient's pelvis and the artery, veins, and ureter joined. In some hospitals the ureter of the new kidney is joined directly to the bladder. Urine flow often begins immediately. Illustration courtesy of the National Kidney Foundation.

CHAPTER 19

The Blood and Its Diseases

ERNEST BEUTLER, M.D.

Blood is the red fluid which is driven by the pumping action of the heart through the blood vessels to all parts of the body. The various body organs (liver, muscles, glands, brain, lungs, etc.) depend upon each other for their proper functioning. They may be visualized as "factories" which require a constant supply of raw materials for turning out their special products, which, in turn, are in demand by other organs. Some waste material of the production processes also has to be eliminated. The blood vessels represent a well-developed network of highways and smaller roads connecting the different "factories." The vehicle which transports the raw material, the various end-products, and the waste on these highways to and from the various organs is the blood.

COMPOSITION OF THE BLOOD

Blood consists of the red cells, the white cells, and the platelets which are suspended in a pale yellow liquid called the plasma. The plasma also carries the blood proteins, blood sugar, blood fat, various salts, and many other substances which are needed in the well-planned economy of the body. Serum is the liquid part of the blood after it has been clotted; it is similar to plasma.

In health, the composition of the blood is kept remarkably constant. This stability is maintained because anything that is "used up" or "taken away" from the blood is immediately replaced. Because of this constant composition, the doctor knows the normal amounts of the various types of cells and substances present in the blood. When, however, an organ becomes involved in a disease, it may turn out either an increased or decreased amount of its regular products, or some abnormal factors may appear in the blood. The composition of the blood may thus become quite different from that of a healthy person, and the doctor may learn from such alterations which organ is diseased and to what extent.

THE MEANING OF A "BLOOD TEST"

Obviously, there is no such thing as a single "blood test." There are many different blood tests, each for a special factor. When you speak of a "blood test," you must really know what has been examined specifically. Thus, blood is tested for its increased content of sugar in patients with diabetes; for "uric acid" in instances of suspected gout; or blood is examined for the presence of specific "antibodies" which develop when an infection has occurred. One commonly performed blood test is a test for syphilis. If such a test is positive, a person may have had a syphilitic infection in the past. Sometime later in his or her life severe damage to the heart, the nervous system, or other parts of the body may develop if the hidden syphilis is not vigorously treated. Most states in the United States now require pre-marriage blood tests to discover slumbering syphilis in the prospective parents, since this disease may also seriously affect the health of future babies. By energetic treatment of the syphilitic bride or bridegroom with penicillin, the danger to the child can be prevented, and a cure or at least an improvement of the sick adult achieved.

RED BLOOD CELLS

The human red cell is filled with a red-colored matter named "hemoglobin." Its shape is something like an automobile wheel and tire, round and thicker at the rim than in the middle. The cell's diameter is about .0003 of an inch. Normally, women have about 4½ million, and men about 5 million of such red cells in one cubic millimeter of blood. One cubic millimeter is about a .0000034 part of one ounce. The red cells are manufactured in the bone marrow, which is located in the interior of the bones. In infants the marrow of all bones produces red cells, whereas in adults the bones of the arms and legs no longer perform this function. The red cells ripen in the marrow and are discharged into the circulating blood only when nearly mature. They remain in the blood for about 120 days before they are destroyed. The cells which are destroyed are replaced by new ones from the bone marrow. In this way the number of red cells in the blood always remains approximately the same.

When the physician wants to know whether the bone marrow functions properly, he can insert a needle into the cavity of the bone and draw out some particles from the marrow. This procedure is called "bone marrow puncture"; most commonly the breastbone or the hipbone are used for this purpose. Since the skin and the bone are made insensitive by an injection of a local anesthetic like Novocain prior to the puncture, this little operation is not painful, although some discomfort is experienced at the moment when the marrow is removed. The marrow particles obtained by such a puncture are spread out on thin glass plates, stained by special dyes, and examined under the microscope. A specialist can thus obtain considerable information about the composition of the marrow which may be helpful in diagnosing various diseases.

The main function of the red cells is to carry the hemoglobin. This red substance contains iron, which is built into a very complex chemical structure and has the ability to combine with oxygen from the air within the lungs. From the lungs, the hemoglobin within the red cells transports oxygen to the various organs which require it and take it up. Without oxygen no organ can function properly, and therefore an adequate oxygen supply is essential for life. When the number of red cells, or their hemoglobin content is appreciably diminished from any cause, the resulting state is called anemia. Anemia is not a disease any more than is fever or a pain. It is a symptom, and the physician must determine its cause before he can treat it effectively.

WHITE BLOOD CELLS

Normally each cubic millimeter of blood contains 5000 to 10,000 white cells. Some of the white cells, named granulocytes, are, like the red cells, manufactured in the bone marrow; others, called lymphocytes, are produced in the spleen and in the lymph nodes. Unlike red cells, the white cells can actively leave the blood stream and wander into the tissues. Indeed, at any one moment most of the white cells are in the tissues, and only a relatively small number are in the blood stream. These cells are able to digest bacteria which have been successful in invading the body. The white cells act, therefore, as the scavengers of the highway system as well as of the various factories of the body. When bacteria become lodged in an organ and begin to multiply there, the white cells move to this location and attempt to defend the body against their further spread. They first surround the bacteria, and then attack them and, by engulfing and digesting them, try to kill them. A collection of white cells and bacteria form the yellow fluid known as "pus." Many infectious diseases caused by bacteria show an increase of the white blood cell count because many more of these cells are mobilized under these circumstances and sent rapidly through the blood vessels and to the endangered area. The physician, by taking a white blood cell count, may thus get information that such an inflamed area exists somewhere in the body. This is of great diagnostic significance, since the symptoms of some harmless bellyache caused, for instance, by gas, may be quite similar to those caused by a bacterial inflammation, like appendicitis. The finding of an elevated white cell count in infection is also an important demonstration that this particular defense mechanism of the body is in good working order. In contrast to bacterial infection, infections caused by viruses are often associated with a normal or even diminished white blood count.

BLOOD PLATELETS

The platelet is a minute particle of protoplasm (the basic material of cells) which is much smaller than the red blood cell. The normal platelet count is 180,000 to 350,000 in one cubic millimeter of blood. One of the functions of the platelets is to maintain the texture of the smallest blood vessels (the so-called capillaries) in proper condition. In the absence of platelets, red cells often leak out from the capillaries, and tiny bleeding points may be seen. Furthermore, platelets help seal tears which may occur in the blood vessels due to injuries. People who do not have enough platelets, or poorly constructed ones, will bleed much longer than normal from a needle puncture. The time it takes for such bleeding to stop is called the "bleeding time" and is normally from one to three minutes.

When larger blood vessels are injured, the platelets alone are incapable of plugging a bigger hole. Under these circumstances the vessels contract and the rent in the wall is closed in part by means of a clot. To produce such a clot, the platelets and the injured tissues release a substance which acts on a group of proteins present in the plasma. From this interaction, a new factor, called thromboplastin, is formed, which through a series of complicated reactions causes a firm gel-like clot to form. One of the substances activated by thromboplastin is called prothrombin. When the amount of prothrombin in the blood is diminished, clot formation is decreased and delayed. The physician can measure the amount of prothrombin present by means of a test called the "prothrombin time." When blood is drawn from a vein into a plain glass test tube, it soon forms a firm clot, which then shrinks, or "retracts" squeezing out the straw-colored serum. The length of time it takes blood to clot is called the "clotting time." This may be greatly prolonged in some diseases, such as hemophilia.

Clot formation represents a defense mechanism of the body against blood loss from injured vessels. However, clot formation may also take place in a blood vessel which has been damaged by a disease. Then the clot may grow within the vessel to such an extent that it completely obstructs it and interferes with the blood supply to this particular region of the body. To make things worse, such a clot frequently becomes dislodged and travels in the veins toward the lungs, where it then may plug the vital lung vessels and cause sudden death. Drugs such as dicumarol or warfarin, which may be taken in pill form, depress the amount of prothrombin in the blood and thus counteract the tendency to undesirable clot formation in certain diseases. The history of the discovery of these drugs is quite interesting. Cattle, when fed spoiled sweet clover, began to bleed profusely. From this spoiled clover, dicumarol was extracted and chemically analyzed; it was found to have a composition similar to aspirin. Dicumarol is now often given to patients who have a small blood clot within one of the vitally important blood vessels which supply the heart (the coronary arteries); in this manner further growth of such a clot may be prevented. Excessive doses of such drugs can produce dangerous bleeding. Thus, the quantity prescribed must be carefully regulated by the use of the prothrombin time blood test. Another drug, heparin, also prevents clotting, but must be given by injection at frequent intervals.

THE ANEMIAS

"Anemia" is that group of disorders in which insufficient hemoglobin is present in the blood, either because the red cells contain too little hemoglobin, or because the number of red cells is diminished. When this occurs the heart will attempt to circulate the blood faster to make up for the lack of red coloring matter. Thus, the first sign of anemia may be a feeling that the heart is beating faster than usual. When a severely anemic person exerts himself, he may readily become short of breath, may pant on climbing stairs, and may think that he has a weakened heart, although his heart is normal. When the anemia is more severe and cannot be compensated by the increased activity of the heart, many organs send out danger signals indicating that they have not obtained enough oxygen. The brain will react with headaches, dizziness, a feeling of faintness, loss of memory, nervousness, irritability, and even drowsiness. Many people experience numbness and tingling in the fingers and toes. Ringing in the ears, black spots in front of the eyes, pallor of the face may occur, and the skin may take on a waxy color. However, some healthy people always look pale, and sometimes it is hard to tell the difference between the naturally sallow complexion of a person who lives mostly indoors and the pallor of anemia. Many of the symptoms which occur in anemia may, however, also be caused by different disturbances and only the blood count will permit a definite diagnosis of anemia to be made.

Anemia is never a disease in itself, but is always caused by other factors which the physician must recognize in order to start proper treatment. Sometimes the cause of the anemia is obvious; in other instances it may be difficult to find and require many special tests.

SUDDEN BLEEDING

When a patient loses a large amount of blood by being injured in an accident, by extensive bleeding from the nose, from a stomach ulcer, from hemorrhoids, by excessive bleeding from the womb or from any other organ, a sudden anemia may develop. If bleeding is gradual, occurring over a span of a few days, the lost blood is replaced with newly formed plasma. The remaining red cells are diluted by the new plasma so that severe anemia may result. The bone marrow then receives a signal, which tells it to manufacture more red cells. If no more bleeding occurs, the lost red cells will be replaced in a few weeks, and the blood will again be normal. If, on the other hand, bleeding is rapid, the total amount of blood in the body decreases suddenly. Shock, with pallor, sweats, and even unconsciousness may develop and blood transfusions may be life-saving.

Before a blood transfusion is given, a sample of the blood of the donor must be mixed with that of the patient to see that clumping of the red blood cells does not occur, since such clumps would block the small blood vessels. All human beings belong to one of four main blood groups, A, B, AB, and O, and only certain groups do not clump the red cells of other groups on mixing. Other blood groups are also important, however. When a person received several blood transfusions from a donor with the same blood group as the patient's, the first transfusion was sometimes well tolerated, but the second and third caused severe reactions. Another "blood group" besides the four already mentioned was found to be responsible. This new blood group system was demonstrated to be identical with a blood factor occurring in the Rhesus monkey, and therefore has been called the "Rh factor." About eighty-five per cent of all human beings have this Rh factor within their red cells, but fifteen per cent do not. When red cells containing the Rh factor are transfused into a recipient whose blood does not contain this factor, the body of the recipient develops an "anti-Rh" substance which clumps the foreign transfused cells. It is, therefore, not sufficient to type blood only for the four chief blood groups, but this also must be done for the Rh factor. Recipients whose red cells do not contain the Rh factor are called "Rh negative," and they should receive only transfusions of Rh-negative blood.

Before giving a transfusion one must also be sure that the donor is healthy, that he has not had an infectious liver disease (hepatitis) or syphilis. There is no way to be certain that any donation of blood is free from the hepatitis virus. Because of this and because of the rare accidents in which blood of the wrong type is given, doctors transfuse blood only when safer means will not correct the anemia of blood loss. Because blood should be given immediately in emergencies, hospitals now use "blood banks" in which blood of various types is stored in the refrigerator, ready for use. This blood is drawn into a preservative solution which contains citric acid to keep the blood from clotting. Blood may be stored in a suitable refrigerator for more than two weeks without harming the red cells. In some patients only the red cells are transfused, the plasma having been separated from the cells; other patients may require only a plasma transfusion.

ANEMIA DUE TO LACK OF IRON

By far the most common cause of anemia is iron deficiency. Hemoglobin, the red pigment of the red cell, contains iron. When there is a lack of iron, not enough hemoglobin can be formed. The number of red cells in the blood is then diminished, and the amount of hemoglobin in each red cell is greatly reduced. The normal diet contains only a limited amount of iron, and only a relatively small fraction of this can be absorbed. Thus, when the needs of the body for iron become increased, iron deficiency often develops. The most frequent cause for increased need for iron in adults is bleeding. Each red cell which is lost from the body carries away a small amount of vitally needed iron. The body's iron reserves are used up to replace this iron, and when no more reserves are left, iron, a necessary building block for hemoglobin, is lacking. Blood formation can then no longer proceed normally. Iron deficiency is much more common in women than in men. Menstrual bleeding robs many women of much more iron than they are able to obtain from their food. Furthermore, each pregnancy takes iron from a woman's body. Adult men develop iron deficiency from nose bleeds, bleeding hemorrhoids, ulcers, and any other cause of blood loss. Children may become iron deficient without bleeding because the rapid increase in their body size sometimes requires a larger supply of iron than may be obtained from their diet, especially if it consists largely of milk.

Iron deficiency is best treated with iron tablets or solutions. These must be kept out of the reach of children, since many children have tragically lost their lives through the eating of large numbers of candy-coated iron pills. Attempts to correct iron deficiency by changing the diet are usually unsuccessful because of the relatively low iron content of most foods when compared with iron medications.

THE ANEMIA OF CHRONIC INFECTION, CHRONIC INFLAMMATION, AND CANCER

People suffering from chronic infections such as tuberculosis or osteomyelitis, from inflammatory arthritis, or cancer will often have a moderately severe anemia. Their red cells are destroyed prematurely in the blood and the bone marrow is unable to increase its rate of red-cell production enough to make up for this loss. How this comes about is not known, but we know that iron, liver, and vitamins have no effect on this anemia. Only removal of the cause seems to be effective treatment.

MEDITERRANEAN ANEMIA

In some families who live in the southern parts of Italy or in Greece—countries which lie on the Mediterranean Sea—an anemia is found in which the red cells contain little hemoglobin and are thinner than normal ones. Iron treatment is not effective and may be harmful. This disease is caused by an inability of the body to build up normal hemoglobin. Mediterranean anemia is a hereditary disease (transmitted from the parents to the child). In the United States it may be found in native-born Americans of Italian or Greek ancestry. This disorder was first discovered, not in Italy, but in Detroit, Michigan, a city which has a large population of Italian stock. This variety of anemia is also often called—after its discoverer—"Cooley's" anemia. Blood transfusions may be necessary.

PERNICIOUS ANEMIA

In this type of anemia the red cells are larger than normal, oval-shaped, and well-filled with hemoglobin. However, these abnormal red cells live for only a short time in the circulation, and many are destroyed before they ever reach the blood stream. Pernicious anemia is a hereditary disorder which rarely occurs before age forty. Frequently pernicious anemia causes severe involvement of the nervous system. The patient may be unable to walk with his eyes closed, he may have a staggering gait and a feeling of "pins and needles" in his hands and feet. He may be unable to feed himself because of muscular weakness, and severe bladder disturbances may develop. In some patients the signs pointing to a disorder of the nervous system are much more pronounced than is the anemia, whereas in others the anemia may be severe, but the nervous manifestations are hardly noticeable. Patients with pernicious anemia are deficient in a complicated chemical substance, vitamin B_{12}. However, this vitamin lack is not caused by a deficiency of the diet; indeed, diets deficient in vitamin B_{12} are nearly impossible to devise. Rather, they are unable to absorb vitamin B_{12} from their diet because they lack a substance known as "intrinsic factor," which is normally secreted by the stomach. This substance is necessary for the absorption of vitamin B_{12}.

Formerly, such patients had to receive injections of liver extract. It is now known, however, that only vitamin B_{12} is required. Since this is cheaper and more convenient to give, most patients with pernicious anemia are now regularly given injections of the purified vitamin. Folic acid, once thought to be beneficial in pernicious anemia, is now known to aggravate the nerve damage in these patients, and is never given to such patients except as an adjunct to vitamin B_{12} treatment. When treated with liver extract or vitamin B_{12}, return of strength may occur in two or three days. The anemia responds dramatically and the patient may regain an almost normal blood count within a few weeks; however, the healing of the damage to the nervous system requires a much longer time. Sometimes permanent damage to the nervous system has occurred and cannot be repaired. Because of these nervous complications, an early diagnosis and rapid institution of treatment are most important in pernicious anemia.

APLASTIC ANEMIA

Occasionally the bone marrow stops almost entirely its production of all cells; this condition is called "aplasia" of the marrow. A severe anemia develops, and the number of white cells and of platelets in the blood is likewise seriously decreased. Such a damage to the marrow may follow exposure to some chemicals (benzine and others), or when certain otherwise useful drugs such as chloromycetin or atabrine are taken by susceptible individuals. Aplastic anemia may also be observed after extensive uncontrolled radiation with X rays or other powerful physical agents. The condition frequently developed in the Japanese who escaped immediate death after the atom bombing during the last war. Sometimes an obvious cause cannot be detected in patients with aplastic anemia. Specific treatment is not available for such a damaged bone marrow, but the life of such patients may be maintained for many years by numerous blood transfusions. Sometimes cortisone-like drugs and male sex hormones appear to speed recovery. Gradually recovery may occur even after several years of severe illness with this disorder.

HEREDITARY SPHEROCYTOSIS OR FAMILIAL HEMOLYTIC JAUNDICE

In this hereditary condition, the red cells are smaller and thicker than normal ones since their shapes changed from a disc to a sphere. These "spherocytes" do not stay for the usual 120 days within the circulation, but only for about 20 days or less. The red blood cell pigment, hemoglobin, is normally broken down to a yellowish substance "bilirubin" after red cells are destroyed. Because more red cells than normal are destroyed in hereditary spherocytosis, an increased amount of bilirubin is produced. As a result, the skin, and the whites of the eyes may assume a yellowish discoloration, jaundice. In hereditary spherocytosis the red cells are trapped in the spleen and destroyed there. The disease can, therefore, be cured by removal of the spleen. Contrary to popular superstition, the spleen is not necessary for life, and the people without a spleen may live as long as any normal person. The anemia that occurs in hereditary spherocytosis is called hemolytic because this term refers to a very rapid destruction of red cells, regardless of the mechanisms which are responsible for their destruction.

OTHER HEMOLYTIC ANEMIAS

In some people, for unknown reasons, the body develops a red cell destroying factor which circulates in the plasma. An anemia results which is quite similar to that found in hereditary spherocytosis. The red cells assume a round shape, and jaundice develops. Removal of the spleen may or may not have any curative effect. Treatment with cortisone or cortisone-like drugs or with 6-mercaptopurine has been successful in stopping the production of this red cell destroying factor.

Increased breakdown of red cells (hemolytic anemia) may also occur due to the taking of certain medications or vegetables. This is particularly true in people who lack a red cell enzyme, glucose-6-phosphate dehydrogenase. Enzymes are complex chemicals which are necessary for the proper utilization of fuels, such as sugar, by the red blood cell. Individuals with a lack of glucose-6-phosphate dehydrogenase are unable to burn sugar in a normal fashion. When they are given drugs such as primaquine (an antimalaria medicine), furadantin (a urinary tract antiseptic), some of the sulfanilamides, or sometimes when they eat broad beans, the red cells are rapidly destroyed.

A group of other red cell enzyme defects also lead to premature red cell destruction (hemolytic anemia). These are rare disorders. Patients with these disorders, in contrast to those with hereditary spherocytosis, are not benefited by removal of the spleen. Usually the red cells are not spherical in this group of diseases, and they are, therefore, known together as "non-spherocytic hemolytic anemia." Enzyme lacks which have been found to cause this disorder include a deficiency of pyruvate kinase, glucose-6-phosphate dehydrogenase, glutathione reductase, and ATPase.

Sickle cell anemia occurs almost exclusively in Negroes. The red cells assume a sickle shape, and in the severe form of this disease they break up much more rapidly than do normal cells. Approximately eight per cent of the Negroes in the United States have a hereditary tendency to develop these abnormally shaped cells. In most of the Negroes the disorder is mild (sickle cell trait) and anemia absent. However, if two people with this trait marry, some of their children may develop the severe form which is called "sickle cell anemia." The sickle shape of the red cells is caused by an abnormal type of hemoglobin. A cure for this disease is not known at present, and removal of the spleen is not effective. Other types of abnormal hemoglobins, usually designated by letters of the alphabet, e.g., C, D, etc. have also been found, and may cause anemia.

ERYTHROBLASTOSIS

The discovery of the Rh factor was not only important in increasing the safety of blood transfusion but has also led to an understanding of a severe anemia which may develop in newborn infants. When the mother is Rh negative, but the unborn infant produces Rh positive blood cells, blood from the infant may leak across during pregnancy into the body of the mother, and there stimulate the formation of the "anti-Rh factor." This anti-Rh factor may then flow back into the circulation of the unborn infant, and cause severe damage to his red cells. Such infants, when born, show all the signs of rapid blood destruction, and, therefore, this disease is called hemolytic anemia of the newborn. Serious brain damage, a condition known as "kernicterus" may result.

In the milder cases recovery may occur without treatment. In the severely sick infant, however, when a large amount of anti-Rh factor has entered the body of the baby from the mother, almost all its red cells may be damaged. In such cases the blood of the child may have to be completely exchanged with Rh negative blood. This time-consuming procedure, which often lasts for several hours, has been named exchange transfusion and has rescued the life of many infants.

POLYCYTHEMIA

"Polycythemia" means that the number of red cells in the blood is increased as many as 8 to 10 million in one cubic millimeter instead of the usual 5 million. Not only is the red cell count per cubic millimeter increased, but also the quantity of blood in the circulation, which is normally about 5 quarts, may increase to as much as 8 to 10 quarts. The blood is of a much thicker consistency than normal, and the heart has to work harder to keep the blood circulating. All tissues are overfilled with blood, and the movement of the blood within the organs is considerably slowed down. There is a kind of traffic jam in the highway system (blood vessels) of the body. Such patients have a ruddy complexion and look quite healthy, but they have many headaches, itching, and excessive fatigue.

Polycythemia occurs normally in people who live at high altitudes. Here, the body tries to make up for the low oxygen content entering the lungs by providing more red cells. Similarly, in certain types of lung disease, or heart disease, in which blood containing little oxygen gains entry into the general circulation, excessive numbers of red cells are made.

Another type of polycythemia is known as "true" polycythemia or "polycythemia rubra vera." In this disorder, the bone marrow overproduces not only red blood cells but also platelets and white blood cells. The spleen and liver participate in production and may become greatly enlarged. Ulcers of the stomach or duodenum, and gout are common complications of polycythemia rubra vera. Eventually, the blood-producing tissues begin to wear out, and after many years of polycythemia the patient may begin to develop anemia. In a few cases, leukemia develops in the final stages of the disease.

Polycythemia can usually be well-controlled for many, many years. This is accomplished by withdrawing excess blood from a vein in the same way that a blood donation is given to the blood bank. In addition, in polycythemia rubra vera, medication may be prescribed to slow the rate of blood production. Radioactive phosphorus is effective in this respect. Some physicians prefer to use chemical, rather than radioactive means of controlling blood production. Drugs such as Myleran®, Cytoxan®, or Leukeran® are sometimes quite effective.

LEUKOPENIA AND AGRANULOCYTOSIS

When the number of white cells in the blood is below 5000 per cubic millimeter, a state of "leukopenia" exists. Some infectious diseases, typhoid, undulant fever, influenza, and others show leukopenia. Leukopenia also frequently occurs when the spleen is enlarged. In such cases removal of the spleen may again provide the body with enough white cells, and thus strengthen its defense power against bacteria.

Complete disappearance of granulocytes, those white blood cells manufactured in the bone marrow may develop within a few hours in persons who are unusually sensitive to certain drugs. Because there are no granulocytes, this allergic reaction has been called agranulocytosis. Patients with agranulocytosis may develop sudden chills, high fever, pneumonia, and other signs of blood poisoning, since the bacteria unchecked by the usual defense activity of the white cells overwhelm the body. Before penicillin and the other powerful antibacterial drugs were available, this blood poisoning often led to death. Since agranulocytosis is most commonly caused by an abnormal reaction to drugs, any medicine taken prior to the onset of the disease has to be stopped immediately in such patients. A number of years ago it was discovered that pyramidon (aminopyrine), which was widely used in Europe as an excellent painkiller similar to aspirin, may cause agranulocytosis. In Denmark, with a population of 3½ million, about 350 deaths due to agranulocytosis were observed within one year. When the sale of pyramidon was prohibited, cases of agranulocytosis were not seen in the following year. Now this drug is only rarely used. Other drugs such as chlorpromazine (Thorazine®), a tranquilizer, and phenylbutazone (Butazolidine®), a pain-killer, may cause such reactions.

Although the number of people who may develop such a reaction is small, the potential danger of any drug must be realized. Many of the new, powerful remedies may occasionally cause agranulocytosis, and the physician must always be on the alert for such a possible complication.

LEUKEMIA

Leukemia literally means "white blood." The disease was given this name because the number of white cells in the blood may be so greatly increased as to give the blood a grayish-white color. Leukemia is not, as is commonly believed, a condition in which the white cells eat the red cells. In leukemia, the white cells are immature and develop abnormally. Not only can they not eat red cells, but they are unable to ingest bacteria, and thus perform their natural function in protecting the body against infection.

In leukemia the white blood cells multiply without restraint, overgrowing the marrow, spleen, liver, and lymph nodes and often preventing the normal production of red blood cells, platelets, and of normal, mature white cells. This disease occurs in two forms, acute leukemia and chronic leukemia. Each of these may be further subdivided, depending upon the type of cell which has escaped normal growth control. If it is the lymphocyte which has run amok, the patient has lymphocytic leukemia; if it is a granulocyte which is multiplying in an uncontrolled fashion, the patient has granulocytic (or myelogenous) leukemia. Leukemia is not, as is commonly believed, primarily a disease of children. Acute leukemia is the most common form of the disease in children, while chronic leukemia is more common in adults.

Acute leukemia is a catastrophic illness which was formerly uniformly fatal within approximately six months. The introduction of new drugs, methotrexate, 6-mercaptopurine, and cortisone in the treatment of this disease has slightly brightened the still dim outlook. Treatment results are especially favorable in children, where better than one-half may achieve a "remission." During a remission the patient's health, blood, and bone marrow return to normal, or nearly so, and he is able to lead a normal life. Unfortunately, remissions are almost always transient and only rarely last for more than a year. Occasional instances of long remissions, lasting for more than five years have been observed, and some of these patients have not yet shown a recurrence of their disease. These valuable drugs have not yet been in use long enough to be certain whether they can ever effect a complete cure of acute leukemia. Unfortunately, in the vast majority of cases, they do not. When the leukemia recurs, it eventually no longer responds to drugs, and the patient succumbs, usually to bleeding and infection.

Chronic leukemia has a more gradual course. Chronic granulocytic leukemia is generally treated with the drug, busulfan (Myleran®), which checks the growth of the leukemic white cells, sometimes for several years. Irradiation of the spleen and radioactive phosphorus have also been used with good success in controlling the disease. These treatments never effect a cure in chronic granulocytic leukemia, and the disease always recurs, eventually in a form which does not respond to treatment. The final stage of the disease closely resembles acute leukemia. Chronic lymphocytic leukemia may cause very little trouble for many years. Sometimes persons afflicted with this disorder are unnecessarily frightened because they mistakenly believe that any leukemia runs the devastating course which they associate with acute leukemia. Patients with chronic lymphocytic leukemia, in contrast with those with acute leukemia may live perfectly normal lives for as many as ten, fifteen, or even more years without any treatment. When treatment is required, irradiation, Leukeran®, Cytoxan®, radioactive phosphorus, and cortisone-like drugs are some of the treatments which may be useful. Persons with chronic lymphocytic leukemia have considerable difficulty manufacturing antibodies, proteins in the blood stream which help to fight infection. Thus, they are particularly susceptible to boils, pneumonia, and other infections.

The cause of leukemia is not known. In animals, leukemia is sometimes caused by viruses. Yet, leukemia is not contagious in the usual sense. In the case of chronic myelogenous leukemia there is a loss of part of a chromosome from the abnormal blood cells. Chromosomes are tiny strands of material which carry the hereditary blueprints of the cell. Apparently, when a critical portion of these blueprints are lost, the cell becomes leukemic and grows in an uncontrolled fashion.

ENLARGEMENT OF THE LYMPH NODES

The lymph glands or lymph nodes are small structures which are scattered throughout the body, especially in the neck, the armpits, the groins, and around the lungs and intestines. They produce a particular type of white cell, the lymphocytes, which they discharge into the blood stream. They also act as a sieve, filtering out bacteria which may try to enter the blood stream. Thus if one cuts his finger and bacteria enter the tissue below the skin through this wound, the lymph nodes of the arm and the armpit will swell and become inflamed as a result of their strenuous efforts to combat the invasion by trapping the bacteria. The tonsils are also lymph nodes, and frequently they become inflamed because bacteria are always present in the mouth and often try to invade the body.

In some diseases the lymph nodes are the site of the diseases themselves. A cancerlike growth may develop from them and spread all over the body. Such malignant diseases of the lymph nodes are called lymphomas (tumors of the lymph node). Hodgkin's disease, lymphosarcoma, giant follicular lymphoma, and reticulum cell sarcoma all represent special varieties of lymphomas. The diagnosis of lymphoma can only be made by having a surgeon remove an affected lymph node and then examine it under the microscope after suitable preparation. Some lymphomas respond well to treatment and cause very little trouble for many years. The patient can live a normal life, only occasionally visiting his physician for a check-up and requiring retreatment at intervals which may be measured in years. Other types of lymphomas are much more difficult to control. The tumors may fail to respond to irradiation or the drugs which are given, and may rapidly lead to changes such as fever, accumulation of fluid in the chest and abdomen, interference with breathing, loss of weight, anemia, leukopenia, bleeding, and finally death.

When lymphomas are limited to one or two areas of the body, they are usually treated with irradiation, either from an X-ray machine or from a radioactive cobalt source. When the disease fails to respond to this treatment, or becomes very widespread, a variety of other treatments are available. Nitrogen mustard is one of the older, and still one of the best of these. This medication must be injected directly into the vein and usually causes severe nausea and vomiting. The benefits of treatment may last for many months, or even years, and, thus, the temporary discomfort is fully justified. Newer mustardlike drugs which cause less nausea and vomiting have also been developed. Some of these, Leukeran®, triethylenemelamine (TEM)®, and Cytoxan®, can be given by mouth. Newer plant extracts, Velban®, Oncovin®, and cortisone-like drugs also may be beneficial.

Infectious mononucleosis is a relatively harmless disorder which may sometimes closely resemble leukemia or lymphoma, and thus give rise to temporary concern on the part of physician, patient, and family. This disorder is apparently caused by a virus and is most common among young people, particularly college students. It is thought that it may commonly be transmitted by kissing. The disease is characterized by fever, swelling of the lymph nodes and spleen, sore throat, and a marked sense of weakness and fatigue which may last for many weeks after the other symptoms have subsided. A characteristic large lymphocyte is found in the blood stream, and is often helpful in establishing a diagnosis. A special blood test, the heterophil agglutination test, is also generally positive in this disease, and helps the physician to distinguish it from leukemia. Antibiotics and other treatments have been found to be quite useless in patients with infectious mononucleosis. Bed rest and time appear to lead to recovery.

ENLARGEMENT OF THE SPLEEN

The spleen may be considered the lymph node of the blood. Its particular function, together with the white blood cells, is the cleansing of the blood of foreign matter, dead cells, and bacteria which may have entered the blood stream. When the spleen is removed, serious weakening of the body does not result, however, since other cleaners of the blood similar to the spleen (the liver and also parts of the bone marrow) take over. In the absence of the spleen, these cleansing stations work overtime.

Sometimes the spleen enlarges tremendously because it retains some disease-causing organisms which enter the spleen through the blood.

In some patients the spleen actively destroys the blood cells and thus becomes the slaughterhouse for these cells, causing severe anemia, or bleeding due to lack of platelets. In rare instances the spleen swells because it produces some fatty material. Such disorders have been called after their discoverers "Gaucher's disease," and "Niemann-Pick's disease," and occur quite often in Jewish people. Enlargement of the spleen is also encountered in many infectious diseases, particularly in malaria which is widespread in the tropics. Sometimes the spleen may become distended to such an extent that it tears and the patient may die from an internal hemorrhage if the spleen is not immediately removed. It is interesting that in the wars between the primitive tribes of the uncivilized tropical countries, in which almost everyone has a large spleen due to malaria, the warriors try to hit the enemy in the region of the spleen in order to produce such a rupture.

DISEASES WITH AN ABNORMAL BLEEDING TENDENCY

Patients are sometimes alarmed by bleeding into the skin or from one of the openings of the body (mouth, nose, rectum, womb). In most instances such bleeding is caused by a local disorder or a harmless minor injury which leads to the rupture of a blood vessel. There are, however, disorders in which the blood is changed in such a way as to bring about a bleeding tendency.

HEMOPHILIA

In hemophilia the blood will not form a clot for hours after removal from the body. This disease is hereditary and with rare exceptions manifests itself only in the male sex. Although sometimes homophilia may arise anew in a family which has never previously been known to carry this defect, boys with hemophilia generally acquire the disorder from their mothers. Mothers who transmit hemophilia to their sons are known as "carriers" or "heterozygotes." They themselves do not have bleeding disorder, but on the average, one-half of their sons will be affected. Some carriers may be fortunate, and have several sons without one being affected. Others, less fortunate, may transmit the disease to each of three or four sons. One-half of the daughters of a hemophilia carrier will also be carriers and it is sometimes, although not always, possible to tell which of the daughters are carriers and which are not. This determination can be carried out only in the most highly specialized laboratories. When a male with hemophilia survives long enough to have children of his own, his sons will always be normal (unless, of course, he has married a carrier of hemophilia), but his daughters will all be carriers. It is now known that there are really two types of hemophilia which have been called hemophilia-A (or classical hemophilia) and hemophilia-B (Christmas disease, named after the first patient who was found to have the disease). Patients with hemophilia-A lack an important blood-clotting factor, antihemophilic globulin; patients with hemophilia-B (Christmas disease) lack a clotting factor known as PTC (plasma thromboplastic component). Both of these factors are important in the first stage of blood-clot formation.

Patients with hemophilia have normal platelets and, therefore, do not bleed from a tiny cut; such injuries to the small blood vessels can be taken care of by the clumping of the platelets at the site of the trauma. However, if a larger vessel is injured, almost uncontrollable hemorrhage may follow, since clot formation is only achieved with the greatest difficulties. Frequently hemophiliacs bleed into the joints if somewhat larger vessels are injured by a sudden twist of the body, and then the joint may become severely damaged by the hemorrhage and stiff for the rest of the patient's life. Simple extraction of teeth is often a source of great trouble for hemophiliacs. Patients with hemophilia must refrain from athletic exercises and should lead a protected life. If they have a hemorrhage, blood transfusions will supply the clotting factor which the hemophiliac is unable to produce. Thanks to safe blood transfusions, surgery, if necessary, can be performed on hemophiliacs when they have obtained sufficient normal blood plasma prior to the operation to tide them over the danger period.

PURPURA DUE TO PLATELET DEFICIENCY (THROMBOCYTOPENIC PURPURA)

When insufficient platelets are present in the circulation small openings of blood vessels are not sealed properly and a bleeding disorder known as "purpura" occurs. In this condition many small reddish spots appear particularly on the legs and gradually turn brownish and disappear over a period of a few days. These spots are tiny areas of bleeding into the skin and are known as petechiae. In addition, large bruises may appear without any noticeable cause on any part of the body. A minor blow may cause the appearance of a large bluish bruise anywhere on the body. A low platelet count may be the result of the taking of some drug, for example, chloromycetin, an antibiotic, or quinidine, a heart medicine, or may be the result of a leukemia or lymphoma. In a large number of patients, particularly, a cause is not known for the disappearance of platelets; the disorder is then known as "idiopathic thrombocytopenic purpura."

Idiopathic thrombocytopenic purpura may arise suddenly, particularly in children following an infection, or may be present for long periods of time with relatively mild symptoms. The acute form is usually treated with cortisone-like drugs, and in the absence of serious complications from the bleeding, recovery is usually complete. The more chronic form of the disease may also be treated with cortisone-like drugs or by removal of the spleen.

CHAPTER 20

Deficiency Diseases

CLIFFORD F. GASTINEAU, M.D.

The lack of certain necessary substances usually found in food may result in conditions known as "deficiency diseases." The deficiency of a given necessary food substance results in a particular disease state. The food substances that are necessary for good health can be divided into the following categories: vitamins, minerals, proteins, fats, and carbohydrates.

A deficiency can occur in a number of ways. It can result from an unavailability of the substance. Much of the world's population suffers from chronic or recurring scarcity of many foods. Also, desirable foods may be available but may be avoided because of custom, prejudice, or taste preferences. Then, too, odd combinations and restrictions of food often are used in fat reducing diets in the hope that weight will be lost in some semimagical way. In some diseases of the stomach, pancreas, or intestinal tract, although foods can be eaten, they are digested or absorbed incompletely. Finally, there are inherited diseases in which certain substances cannot be utilized by the body tissues.

In our own culture an adequate selection of foods generally is available, and deficiency diseases are rare indeed. Our knowledge of the effects of diets that are deficient in protein, for instance, has been gained largely from studies in Africa and other areas in which the available foods contain very small amounts of protein.

The high degree of purification of some foods that is necessary to help prevent spoilage or to improve palatability has resulted in some loss of necessary food substances. However, the wide selection of cereals, fruits, vegetables, dairy products, and meats that is available in our stores at all seasons makes such losses from purification less important if you have a varied diet. Eating various foods probably is the single most important factor in good nutrition, since it is through variety that one can obtain all of the nutrients necessary for good nutrition. Furthermore, as a result of the bread and flour enrichment program begun in 1941 and the general practices of adding vitamin D to milk and of iodine to table salt, some previously common deficiency diseases have become rare.

A remarkable diversity of diets is compatible with good health and vigor. Many people try various food supplements in the hope of attaining greater vigor and resistance to infection, but generally these measures are disappointing. A sizable, and at times fraudulent, business in the selling of so-called health foods and vitamin supplements depends on such hopes.

The question, "What is optimal nutrition?" is becoming more difficult to answer as more is learned about nutrition. The raising of animals for market aims simply at producing the maximal amount of meat of a standard quality for the minimal cost. In human nutrition, the rate and extent of growth should not necessarily be a major criterion of good nutrition. Some evidence indicates that degrees of underfeeding which might retard growth may lead to longer life if the person survives the other hazards associated with undernutrition. The role of nutrition in the production of atherosclerosis (deposition of fat in the lining of arteries) and of osteoporosis (a thinning of bone structure) is not yet entirely settled.

VITAMINS

When nutritional deficiency is mentioned, one is likely to think first of vitamins. Although there is more to nutrition than vitamins, these substances have attracted much attention and at times have been regarded as possessing almost magical properties.

Vitamins are natural constituents of foods of which small quantities are necessary for normal nutrition. These substances are essential to normal functioning of the body and cannot be manufactured by the body from simpler substances. The lack of any vitamin interrupts some vital process in the body and leads to certain specific adverse effects.

If a definite vitamin is removed from the diet, a period of time ensues during which the reserve of that vitamin is gradually depleted. The time for this process varies for different vitamins and may be affected by infection, stress, and physical activity. Finally, when amounts of the vitamin have been depleted sufficiently for a certain period of time, symptoms of the deficiency appear. Biochemical studies for measuring amounts of some vitamins such as ascorbic acid in the serum and thiamine, riboflavin, and niacin in the urine are used for research purposes but are not generally available. Carotene (a substance that closely resembles vitamin A and which is converted to vitamin A in the body) in serum is commonly determined and is used as a measure of intestinal absorption of fats.

Vitamins important in human nutrition include: vitamin A, vitamin D, ascorbic acid (vitamin C), thiamine (vitamin B_1), riboflavin (vitamin B_2), nicotinic acid (antipellagric vitamin), pyridoxine (vitamin B_6), folic acid, vitamin B_{12}, and vitamin K.

Although pantothenic acid, vitamin E, inositol, and biotin are considered vitamins, deficiencies of these substances in man do not result in recognizable disease states.

Vitamin A or substances from which it can be formed (carotenes) are found in butter, egg yolks, milk, certain fish oils, and green leafy vegetables. This vitamin is added to most commercial margarines. Ordinary cooking does not destroy it, but oxidation does. Since vitamin A is a fat, its absorption is impaired in individuals with deficiency of pancreatic enzymes or with diseased small intestine such as occurs in sprue, celiac disease, chronic obstruction of the bile ducts, or cystic fibrosis of the pancreas. Vitamin A is stored in the liver in amounts that can suffice for as long as a year. Measurements of vitamin A levels in the blood are not an accurate measure of the size of the reserve.

Vitamin A is necessary for the normal functioning of the retina, the light-sensitive structure at the back of the eye. In the absence of vitamin A, the ability to see in dim light is lost (night blindness). Other results of deficiencies of vitamin A are dryness of the cornea and conjunctiva (xerophthalmia), which sometimes leads to blindness, and dry roughened change in the skin involving tiny nodules from which a central plug protrudes. The latter is sometimes spoken of as "toad skin."

Among the vitamins, only *vitamin D* can be formed in the body. It qualifies as a vitamin because the circumstances under which adequate amounts can be formed are lacking, at times, and deficiency states can occur. The use of ultraviolet light even on limited areas of the body enables the skin to manufacture vitamin D; but because of climatic conditions and protection of the body from the sun by clothing and shelter, deficiency states frequently occur when dietary sources of vitamin D are not available. As with vitamin A, deficiencies of vitamin D may occur in diseases of the pancreas and small intestine.

Eggs and fish oils are the primary sources of vitamin D. Vitamin D also can be made commercially for reinforcement of foods by irradiating certain oils. Commercially processed milk is almost always treated by the addition of vitamin D.

The need for vitamin D is greater in infancy and in pregnancy. The common practice of giving vitamin D to infants also has made deficiency states quite rare in this country.

A deficiency of vitamin D results in a condition known as rickets. Rickets is characterized by a softening of bones at the sites of growth (the epiphyses) near the end of the bones as well as in the shafts or central portions of the long bones of the extremities. Bowing of legs and knobbing of the ribs and ends of the long bones are common manifestations. Sometimes thinning of a portion of the skull results if there is continued pressure at that point. Permanent teeth are formed poorly. Rickets tends to appear after the first month of life, is most commonly seen from the first through the second year, and is encountered less frequently during the remaining years of growth.

The function of vitamin D and the minerals calcium and phosphorus are closely related. A major mechanism of action of vitamin D probably is the facilitation of absorption of calcium. Retardation of the excretion of phosphorus by the kidney is a second action. In active rickets, the concentrations of calcium and phosphorus in the blood tend to be low, and the concentration of alkaline phosphatase tends to be elevated. Vitamin D has a remarkably long action so that a single large dose may exert protection against rickets for 4 to 6 months.

Vitamin D-resistant rickets is a congenital, sometimes inherited, condition in which amounts of vitamin D 50 or more times that needed to prevent rickets in the normal individual care are required. This abnormality frequently is associated with other functional disorders of the body such as acidosis (Lightwood's syndrome), loss of glucose and amino acids in the urine (Fanconi's syndrome), and accumulation of cystine crystals in the body (Lignac-Fanconi disease).

Vitamin K includes a group of substances that prevent bleeding. This group is chemically classified as quinones. These substances are found in many foods and also are manufactured by bacteria growing in the intestinal tract. Vitamin K is necessary for the production of prothrombin by the liver. Prothrombin in turn is a substance necessary for the effective clotting of blood. Hence, in the absence of vitamin K, prothrombin is no longer available, the blood fails to clot, and minor injuries result in excessive bleeding and bruising. There is relatively little storage of vitamin K, and this sequence in clotting may take place within a short time. Synthetic forms of vitamin K are available commercially and are quickly effective in correcting this situation.

Deficiency of vitamin K occurs frequently during the first week of life before the intestinal tract has acquired its usual population of bacteria and after supplies of vitamin K obtained before birth from the mother have been depleted. However, bleeding of any consequence is uncommon, and the prophylactic use of vitamin K in newborn infants has made this problem relatively unimportant.

Conditions that interfere with absorption of vitamin K—such as obstruction of the flow of bile into the intestine or disease of the intestine itself—may result in vitamin K deficiency; but since only minute amounts of vitamin K are required to prevent bleeding, significant difficulty occurs uncommonly. Furthermore, evidence of vitamin K deficiency can be obtained readily by means of measurements of the amount of prothrombin in the blood, and the use of one of the synthetic forms of vitamin K (menadione) can correct this deficiency. Unfortunately in some instances, liver disease may prevent adequate formation of prothrombin even in the presence of vitamin K.

Thiamine (vitamin B_1 or antiberiberi factor) is necessary for the disposal of pyruvic acid, a substance that is a normal intermediate in the metabolism of carbohydrates. A lack of thiamine results in loss of appetite, muscular soreness and weakness, emotional changes, and impaired sensation over the extremities. Weakness, shortness of breath, light headedness on assuming the upright posture, and enlargement of the heart are other effects of thiamine deficiency. However, such symptoms also may arise from other causes and are not necessarily the result of thiamine deficiency. Proven instances of significant thiamine deficiency, known as beriberi, are rare. In the Orient, beriberi has been an occasional consequence of a diet of polished rice. The requirement for thiamine may be increased in diabetes, thyrotoxicosis, and chronic diarrhea and is increased with a greater caloric intake, growth, pregnancy, or lactation.

Pork, liver, yeast, whole cereals, and green vegetables are good sources of thiamine.

Riboflavin (vitamin B_2 or G) is found in milk and meats, and its lack results in inflamed cracks in the skin at the angles of the mouth (cheilosis), dryness of lips, crusting greasy eruption of the skin in the folds of skin at the lower part of the nose, inflammation of the tongue, and an inflammation of several structures of the eye. Riboflavin deficiency is most likely to occur when the diet consists mostly of cereals with little or no milk and meat.

Riboflavin is not usually destroyed by ordinary cooking, but it may be destroyed by exposure to light, for example when milk in bottles is left in the sunlight. This vitamin also may be dissolved in cooking water, and thus lost if this is discarded.

Nicotinic acid (niacin or antipellagric vitamin) is a component of two vital co-enzymes, triphosphopyridine nucleotide (TPN) and diphosphopyridine nucleotide (DPN). These co-enzymes serve as parts of the system of respiration for all cells. A deficiency of this vitamin results in a disease called pellagra—a term derived from an Italian expression meaning rough skin. Pellagra often is associated with deficiencies of thiamine and riboflavin, and in earlier periods the effects of deficiencies of these vitamins were confused.

Pellagra was relatively common in southern parts of the United States, but since World War II, the flour-enrichment program and improved economic condition have nearly eliminated this disease. Nicotinic acid can be derived in the body from the amino acid called tryptophane. Among foods supplying nicotinic acid are lean meat, fish, eggs, milk, fresh fruits, and vegetables. Pellagra was found in individuals who habitually had a diet consisting largely of corn, corn meal, and fat meat. Alcoholism, hook worm infestation, and malaria seem to favor the development of pellagra.

Symptoms of pellagra have been described as the "three D's," dermatitis, diarrhea, and dementia. Sometimes a "fourth D" in the form of death occurs. Before any of the three symptoms appear, the victim may experience soreness of the tongue and mouth, apprehension, nervousness, indigestion, and a general decline in strength, weight, and endurance. The dermatitis consists of roughened, scaling, reddened areas distributed symmetrically, frequently on the backs of hands, face, and neck. Characteristic swelling, redness, and ulcers of the tongue often enable the physician to suspect pellagra. Normal bowel habits or constipation may be present in the early phases of the disease, but diarrhea frequently occurs later. The nervous system is involved, producing symptoms of irritability, headaches, weakness, burning sensations in the limbs, tremulousness, and finally a form of insanity.

Prolonged dietary deprivation is necessary to produce pellagra, but factors such as excessive consumption of alcohol may facilitate the appearance of symptoms. Pellagra should be suspected among individuals who have food idiosyncrasies, erroneous dietary habits, or debilitating diseases that might interfere with a varied diet. Pellagra, like other deficiency diseases, is unlikely in the individual who consumes a reasonably varied diet.

Pyridoxine (vitamin B_6) is necessary for the metabolism of many amino acids and of some fats. Deficiency states are characterized by weakness, nervousness, irritability, and incoordination. A pellagra-like change in the skin has also been reported to occur. Infants who have been fed on formulas lacking pyridoxine have had convulsions.

Vitamin B_{12} (extrinsic factor of Castle, cobalamine) is necessary for normal maturation of red blood cells. A deficiency of this vitamin results in an anemia characterized by large red blood cells and at times a weakness and paralysis of the legs. Pernicious anemia is a classic example of this. In pernicious anemia, the lining of the stomach is unable to produce a substance (intrinsic factor) that normally permits the absorption of vitamin B_{12}. If intrinsic factor (derived from the lining of animal stomach) is given orally or if vitamin B_{12} is injected into the muscle, pernicious anemia is corrected. The injection allows the vitamin to enter the bloodstream without the need to be absorbed through the walls of the intestinal tract. In practice, pernicious anemia is treated by regular injections of vitamin B_{12}.

In diseases characterized by poor intestinal absorption such as sprue, vitamin B_{12} deficiencies may occur. Vitamin B_{12} is present in many foods, perhaps in greatest quantities in lean meat.

Folic acid (pteroylglutamic acid) is effective in correcting the anemia of pernicious anemia but is ineffective in preventing the neuritis seen in this condition, hence its use in pernicious anemia is not advisable. Folic acid will correct anemias characterized by large red blood cells seen in pregnancy, sprue, certain infantile anemias, and pellagra.

Folic acid is found in many foods and is present in large amounts in green leafy vegetables and in liver.

Ascorbic acid (vitamin C) is related chemically to the sugars. Its function in the body is to maintain the connective tissue and to facilitate formation of red blood cells. In the absence of ascorbic acid, the structure of the connective tissue becomes weakened. The linings of blood vessels as well as the sheath of connective tissue about them become weakened so that bleeding occurs. This bleeding frequently occurs in the gums, nose, and intestinal tract. Bones are softened, and sometimes there are spontaneous fractures. Growth of bone in children is disturbed, and tender swellings resulting from bleeding into the covering of the bones may occur in the extremities. The breastbone in infants may sink inward and give a beadlike appearance to the ends of the ribs, a phenomenon that has been called the "scorbutic rosary." Anemia develops; wounds fail to heal; teeth loosen and fall out; and finally death, sometimes after convulsions, fever, jaundice, and coma, may occur.

Such symptoms from deficiency of this vitamin have been known for many centuries and have been designated as scurvy. The course of history has been influenced by scurvy since this disease has limited the strength and endurance of armies and crews of sailing ships. After four months at sea, a ship's crew subsisting only on biscuits and salt meat would develop scurvy. During the eighteenth century, the properties of citrus fruits to protect against such deficiency were recognized, and the British navy began issuing one ounce of lemon juice daily to all members of its fleet.

Ascorbic acid is found in fruits and vegetables. Since this vitamin is susceptible to oxidation, the cooking of vegetables, if done to the point of palatability whether by steaming, boiling, or pressure cooking, preserve only about half of the vitamin. Freezing, canning, and dehydration also cause about the same degree of destruction. Continued heating in air tends to destroy the balance of the ascorbic acid rather rapidly, however. Citrus fruits and juices and tomato juice perhaps are the most convenient source of ascorbic acid, but some other fruits and vegetables are actually richer sources in the fresh uncooked state.

Pantothenic acid is found in many foods—meats, cereals, and milk. It is a component of co-enzyme A, a most important part of cellular metabolic mechanisms. Diets lacking this substance produce graying of fur or feathers in animals. Symptoms of burning feet in some prisoners-of-war have been attributed to deficiency of pantothenic acid. No definite deficiency disease associated with depletion of pantothenic acid has been convincingly demonstrated.

Vitamin E (alphatocopherol) is another vitamin that appears to be necessary for life in lower animals, but one in which there is no proven corresponding deficiency disease in humans. A deficiency of vitamin E in animals may produce a form of muscular dystrophy and sterility. There is some indication that diets high in polyunsaturated fats decrease the amount of vitamin E measurable in the blood, but harmful effects have not been shown to result from this.

Biotin is a curious vitamin that is neutralized by a substance in raw egg white called avidin. A deficiency of this vitamin is not encountered in nature but has been produced in human volunteers by the feeding of large amounts of raw egg white for five weeks. Symptoms consist of a skin eruption, lassitude, nausea, and anemia.

Inositol is a sugarlike substance that is found in large amounts in heart muscle. It appears to be necessary for the growth of yeasts and rodents, but any deficiency disease has not yet been demonstrated in man.

MINERALS

Calcium and phosphorus can be considered together since they are obtained from similar sources and are the principal chemical elements in the skeleton.

Deficiencies of calcium in the diet are exceedingly rare and occur most likely under circumstances of increased need. In infancy, pregnancy, and lactation, the need for calcium is increased and the amounts of calcium that ordinarily would be adequate are insufficient.

In certain intestinal diseases, for example as in sprue, the absorption of calcium is impaired. In rare kidney disorders, losses of phosphorus and calcium in the urine are excessive. Vitamin D deficiency also impairs absorption of calcium from the intestinal tract. In calcium deficiency in adults, a softening of the bones called osteomalacia occurs. In infants or young children, the lack of calcium results in rickets, in which there is bowing of the bones of the legs and deformity of bones of the spinal column. In growing children, distortion of the bones at the sites of bone growth is found.

In women who are more than fifty years old, a thinning and increased fragility of the bones of the spinal column known as osteoporosis is common. Some evidence exists that a generous consumption of calcium during the lifetime of the individual may prevent osteoporosis, but a low calcium content of the diet is not likely to be the sole cause of this condition.

Iodine is necessary for the normal functioning of the thyroid gland and is a major component of the "hormone" manufactured by and released from the thyroid into the blood. A lack of iodine results in enlargement of the thyroid gland, a condition described as a simple goiter. If the deficiency of iodine is severe enough, a deficiency of the thyroid hormone may result.

Such goiters were found most frequently where soils are naturally deficient in iodine. Examples of these "goiter areas" are Switzerland and the Great Lakes region in the United States. In recent times, although the importation of vegetables and other foods from lands that are not deficient in iodine make such goiters unlikely, the general use of iodized salt has given good protection against the development of such goiters.

Iron is an essential component of hemoglobin and certain enzymes. Deficiency of iron is manifested primarily as an anemia. Iron-deficiency anemia is characterized by a greater decrease in hemoglobin than in number of red blood cells. The need for iron is increased when growing takes place or when blood is lost. Heavy menstruation perhaps is the most common cause of iron depletion. Women during their menstruating life and growing children are in a precarious state with respect to iron supplies and the amount of iron absorbed from the usual diet barely balances the quantity needed. Thus, children and menstruating women should have adequate amounts of iron in the diet. Similarly, individuals who donate blood for purposes of transfusion are vulnerable to iron deficiency.

Sources of iron in food include eggs, meat, and bread made from fortified flour.

Copper deficiency has never been clearly demonstrated in man although it has been seen in animals. Copper is a part of the structure of some enzymes and is necessary for protection of red blood cells.

Cobalt is of interest biologically because of its part as a necessary component of vitamin B_{12}. No evidence exists that cobalt deficiency itself, however, causes any disorder in man.

Fluorine is necessary for the formation of dental enamel with maximal resistance to decay and also may contribute to resistance to osteoporosis. To be fully effective in the prevention of dental decay, fluorine must be available during the first several years of the child's life, although direct application of fluoride-containing pastes to the teeth may yield some protection against decay. Drinking water is now the usual source of fluorine, although in some areas the foods may contribute substantially. Fluoridation of water supplies carried out according to approved techniques appears to be safe and to exert a considerable protective effect against dental decay.

Manganese, selenium, zinc, and molybdenum, like cobalt and copper, have been found lacking in animals, resulting in deficiency states. However, this has not been true in man. Nevertheless, these trace elements probably have essential functions. The requirements for these elements are presumed to be so low that human diets, in all their varieties, meet these requirements by generous margins.

CALORIES

A food calorie is defined as the amount of energy or heat required to raise the temperature of 1 kg. (2.2 pounds) of water 1° C. (from 15° to 16°). Calories are derived from the metabolism of carbohydrates, protein, and fat, and an adequate supply is needed for growth, maintenance of weight, and for body heat, and activity. The need for calories is increased in periods of growth and muscular activity and is greater for men and for larger persons. The need for calories gradually decreases after the age of 30 so that a person may need about 15 per cent less food at age 60 than at age 30. Unfortunately, we frequently fail to recognize this decrease in need for food with aging, and the result is obesity.

A deficiency in calories in infancy or childhood leads to retardation of growth and to a lack of adipose tissue (fat). In adult life, caloric deficiency results in gradual loss of weight and of fatty tissue. There is intolerance to cold, lessened activity, irritability, loss of strength, and pre-occupation with thoughts of food. Some obese persons become stimulated and euphoric during periods of caloric restriction and are able to continue their accustomed activity. However, other obese persons become depressed, apathetic, or anxious under these circumstances. These differences seem to stem largely from the psychologic stresses involved in a weight-losing regimen.

While starvation from lack of available food is almost unheard of in our culture, remarkable degrees of emaciation sometimes are seen in a condition known as anorexia nervosa. In anorexia nervosa, psychologic factors cause a loss of appetite and distaste for many forms of food although physical activity often is maintained remarkably well.

CARBOHYDRATES

Carbohydrates, one of the most widely available and generally inexpensive of foods, are found in grains, fruits, and vegetables. Refined carbohydrate in the form of sugar may form at times a large proportion of some diets. Extreme restriction of carbohydrate may result in ketosis, the formation of organic acids known as ketone bodies. The degree of restriction necessary for ketosis is so great that it is extremely unlikely to be encountered as a result of dietary change alone. Furthermore, ketosis of simple dietary origin generally is not of sufficient severity to be of significance.

FATS

Fats are the most concentrated source of calories. They provide a sense of satiation and carry with them the fat soluble vitamins A and D as well as essential fatty acids. The essential fatty acids are linoleic, linolenic, and arachidonic acids. These cannot be formed in the body from other substances and must be obtained from food. In infants, a form of eczema has been seen when the diet was very low in fat. Adult humans, however, do not seem to suffer any definite ill effects from a lack of the essential fatty acids.

PROTEINS

Proteins are substances which constitute much of the structure of our bodies. Proteins are composed of strings of amino acids, which are simpler substances containing nitrogen and an organic acid group. Proteins derive their individual character from the selection, number, and sequence of amino acids that are linked together to comprise the protein molecule. Some of the amino acids can be produced by the body from more simple materials and are called nonessential. Another group cannot be synthesized by the body and must be obtained from the food. Protein obtained from meat, eggs, and milk products contain a good selection of these essential amino acids and are considered of high biologic value. Proteins derived from cereals or vegetables do not contain adequate amounts of all of the essential amino acids, being relatively deficient in one or another. If a mixture of various protein-containing foods is consumed, these deficiencies usually are compensated for by the other members of the protein mixture. An adequate amount of protein of reasonably high biologic value is needed for growth and for the repair of the day-to-day wastage of the protein structure of our bodies.

Protein deficiency usually does not occur alone but rather in combination with caloric, vitamin, and mineral deficiencies. In infancy and early childhood, lack of protein results in slow growth, anemia, susceptibility to infection, retarded development of the brain and nervous system, retarded healing of wounds, fatty change of the liver, and a reddish tint to the skin and hair. This condition, known as kwashiorkor, is common in tropical countries where diets are high in carbohydrate and low in protein. It usually occurs after the child is weaned or when he is subjected to the stress of injury or infection.

Although protein deficiency is more difficult to provoke in adults, it is similar in its manifestations to that seen in children. Protein deficiency is rare in the United States and it is most likely to occur in conditions of stress or infection. The substitution of alcohol for other nutrients, caloric deficiency, or interference with intestinal absorption of protein, as in sprue, also may contribute to protein deficiency.

TOXIC EFFECTS OF EXCESSES OF ESSENTIAL NUTRIENTS

Efforts to correct or anticipate deficiencies of essential nutrients occasionally may have serious effects.

Since iron poisoning is not an uncommon threat to the life of children, iron capsules should be kept safely out of the reach of children.

Vitamin D in excessive amounts may cause high levels of calcium in the blood and injury to kidneys. Usually, such toxic effects result only from the ingestion of more than 50,000 international units daily for a number of weeks or months. This is to be compared to the vitamin D content of most vitamin preparations of 400 to 1000 units per capsule. However, some vitamin D capsules intended for the treatment of parathyroid deficiency or vitamin D resistance contain 50,000 units and are usually the source of such poisoning.

Vitamin A in excess may result in jaundice, enlarged liver, and irregularities of the bones of the extremities.

Excessive amounts of fluorine over a period of years have been reported to cause increased density of the bones and impairment of the function of the kidneys. On the basis of animal studies, however, the amount of fluorine probably needs to be fifty times greater than that supplied by properly fluorinated water in order to produce such injury.

Exceedingly large amounts of nicotinic acid (a form of the antipellagra vitamin) may cause impairment of the metabolism of glucose in a manner resembling that in diabetes.

In certain industrial situations, exposure to large amounts of zinc or manganese may cause serious effects, but in amounts likely to be ingested in food there is no hazard.

Obesity is perhaps the most common and lethal result of all the excesses of nutrients. The ingestion of more calories than are expended leads to accumulation of adipose tissue and a series of hazards to health which, in the aggregate, shorten life appreciably.

CHAPTER 21

Allergy and Clinical Immunology

INCLUDING: HAY FEVER, ASTHMA, ALLERGIC RHINITIS, HIVES, SKIN ALLERGY, CONTACT DERMATITIS, MIGRAINE, GASTROINTESTINAL ALLERGY, ETC.

LEO H. CRIEP, M.D.

INTRODUCTION

Tremendous advances have been made in the field of allergy since 1940. Because allergic manifestations are common and because symptoms of allergy have a tendency to be persistent, people need to have an intelligent understanding of the whys and wherefores of this group of diseases.

INCIDENCE OF ALLERGY

About 10 per cent of the population suffer from major allergic disorders such as bronchial asthma, hay fever, nasal allergy, hives, and allergic eczema. Approximately 40 to 60 per cent of the population have minor allergies, such as intolerance and idiosyncrasy to certain foods, and other substances. It is thus seen that allergic diseases involve many patients. Furthermore, the symptoms of allergy are persistent.

WHAT IS ALLERGY?

A person is said to be allergic if he reacts to a substance in a manner different from the ordinary or normal person. Thus to most of us an egg is harmless and wholesome food—yet in certain persons even a small amount of egg may produce such symptoms as swelling of the lips, a skin rash, or even severe asthma. In a similar way most of us can inhale pollen or molds without showing untoward symptoms. Not so with the allergic patient. These patients may be normal in every other respect except for this peculiarity or idiosyncrasy. And so we say of such persons, who are hypersensitive to egg protein or to pollen or to molds, that they are allergic.

HEREDITY AND ALLERGY

The tendency to develop some types of allergy is in many instances hereditary, being handed down from parent to child. Such transmission, of course, cannot be prevented any more than could blue eyes or red hair. It follows, therefore, that the stronger the hereditary factor, the more likely it is that the offspring will show some form of allergic manifestation. All that can be done from a preventive point of view is to keep such children in the best of possible health and to treat any suspicious symptoms of allergy as soon as they appear. Although asthma and some allergic skin disorders are hereditary, none of these conditions is contagious or "catching," so there need be no fear of people coming into intimate contact with such cases.

EMOTIONAL STATES AND ALLERGY

There are those who instruct pregnant mothers not to eat highly allergenic foods such as milk or eggs, in order to prevent the occurrence of allergy. However, such procedures are neither practical nor effective.

Treatment will not be effective in instances in which an asthmatic child, for example, is exposed to much contention and tension in the midst of constant quibbling and screaming at home. In these cases something must be done to correct the environmental emotional situation. For this reason, some have advised what is euphemistically referred to as parentectomy, that is sending the child away to some hospital or home for asthmatic or allergic children. Such procedures, fortunately, are only necessary in extreme situations and then one must carefully weigh the advantages and disadvantages of such procedures. One must also remember that eventually the child will have to come back to his former environment, and unless something is done to correct it, his being away for a short period of time will not be of too great value.

HISTORY OF ALLERGY

The earliest mention of allergy is by Hippocrates, who comments on the appearance of a skin rash which no doubt was hives as a result of the ingestion of certain foods. In the second century, A.D., Galen mentioned the development of nasal symptoms from exposure to roses. A physician by the name of Bostock described in 1819 his own seasonal nasal symptoms, which he thought were due to heat and cold as well as to certain particles which he inhaled. He recognized these symptoms in himself and described them as hay fever, a term which came to be adopted in standard medical nomenclature. Sometime later Salter realized that he must be sensitive to cat hair because when playing with cats he developed wheals or welts at the point where he was scratched by the cat. In 1890, Koch, while working with tuberculosis, realized that patients and animals developed a sensitivity to tuberculin, the product of the tuberculosis germ. At present allergy is on a sound scientific basis, even though there are many things about the subject which remain to be learned.

HOW IS ALLERGY PRODUCED?

ROLE OF CONTACT

Previous contact with or to a substance is necessary in order for a person to develop allergy to that substance. Such contact is not always easily demonstrable. For example, one may question the occurrence of previous contact in the case of a baby who develops hives, eczema, or asthma upon ingesting cow milk for the first time. However, it may be demonstrated that the contact which produced sensitivity occurred before the baby was born and was caused by enough of the protein from cow milk ingested by the mother, reaching the baby through the placental circulation. That contact plays a role in the development of allergy is demonstrated by the fact that allergic individuals living in Europe where there is no ragweed pollen never develop sensitivity to this pollen. In the same way there is no sensitivity to poison ivy among Eskimos who are not exposed to poison ivy.

The next question is, how does such contact bring about allergy? This may be explained on the basis of an immunological reaction. Exposure to a given substance in a person who is predisposed to allergy causes certain tissues and organs—namely, the lymph glands, spleen, and bone marrow—to produce certain substances which are referred to as antibodies. These antibodies usually protect the person from the harmful effects of a second exposure to the same substance. For example, vaccination or infection with typhoid germs brings about the development of certain antibodies against typhoid. As long as these antibodies are present in the blood and tissues, additional exposure or infection with typhoid will bring about only mild if any symptoms at all, because the antibodies tend to neutralize or destroy the typhoid germs. So it is with many other infectious agents. However, in the case of non-living agents such as proteins, the story is quite different. An allergic person will develop antibodies against some of the proteins to which he is exposed. If, at any later date, he is exposed to the same proteins, a union occurs between this protein or antigen and the antibodies which have been previously produced by the same protein. This union or interaction between the protein, dusts, foods, animal danders, etc., and the specifically related antibody in the tissue is thought to liberate, at least in some instances, a chemical substance which is related to histamine. This chemical substance acts upon the tissues producing the symptoms of allergy. The action largely consists of spasm of muscle and dilatation of blood vessels. When this action occurs in the skin, dilatation of the blood vessels brings about oozing of the watery portion of the blood under the skin, so that there are localized welts, and hives result; if the interaction of antigen and antibody takes place in the mucous membrane of the nose, then the water comes out of the dilated blood vessels and swells up this lining membrane so that the nasal airway is reduced and there is nasal stuffiness and nasal watery discharge and sneezing. When this interaction occurs in the lung, the lining membrane of the tubes of the lungs, the bronchi, becomes swollen, and the openings of these tubes are reduced or may even be occluded. This narrowing is also contributed to by the spasm of the muscles of the walls of the bronchi and by the outpouring of mucus in the tubes; the patient, therefore, has breathing difficulty referred to commonly as asthma. The type of symptoms produced will depend entirely on the selective sensitiveness of the particular part of the body where the antigen antibody reaction occurs. It would appear, therefore, that although the symptoms are varied, the fundamental basis for the allergic condition is the same; that is, a swelling occurring in the sensitized tissue of the allergic patient. Some allergic reactions are somewhat differently characterized by inflammatory and connective tissue changes, but in general the basis is the same. These symptoms may occur, therefore, in various parts of the body, that is, in the nose, the bronchi, the gastrointestinal tract, or the skin. It is natural, then, for the allergic patient to seek relief by consulting various specialists, not realizing that while the manifestations are different, the cause is the same. Thus the person who has an asthmatic attack when he comes in contact with a cat, dog, or horse, and another who gets hives from eating strawberries really have the same trouble—both are allergic.

AGE OF ONSET

Allergy may develop at any age—in the young and in the old. The reason for this is not known. Of two allergic patients living in the same climate and area and exposed to the same vegetation and pollen, one may show signs of hay fever at the age of five, and the other may develop hay fever at the age of thirty-five.

DURATION

Once developed, an allergy, if untreated, usually lasts for many years. Occasionally complete disappearance may occur; this is called a spontaneous loss of sensitivity. Most frequently, though, complete loss of allergic symptoms is due to the fact that the patient no longer is exposed to the substances which produce his symptoms.

RELATION OF ALLERGY TO ADRENAL GLANDS

The adrenal glands are located one on each side at the upper pole of the kidney. These small glands produce certain substances referred to as hormones. The adrenal hormones, as discussed in the chapter on glands, have many important functions. Among these may be mentioned the regulation of water balance in the body, the metabolism of sugar and proteins, and finally the growth of certain white cells in the blood and some immunologic properties. The adrenal hormones have a profound effect on allergic conditions. The exact nature of this effect is not as yet altogether clear. At any rate, the administration of these hormones, namely cortisone, is beneficial in the treatment of allergy. In the same way ACTH, a hormone produced by the pituitary gland, which stimulates the production of the cortisone, has the same beneficial value. These cortisone products produce a dramatic relief from symptoms, but they are not without danger. They should never be taken without a physician's specific supervision. Allergic patients respond to much smaller doses of cortisone than other patients and cortisone will arrest development in children. Some obstetricians object to its being administered to allergic pregnant mothers.

CAUSES OF ALLERGY

In general, the causes of allergy may be grouped by the manner in which they become introduced into the body, that is, as inhalants, ingestants, contactants, injectants, and infectants.

INHALANTS

A large number of substances reach the body through breathing or inhalation. The fact that they are introduced through inhalation does not necessarily indicate that the symptoms will be only respiratory; for example, inhaled substances can produce hives, and conversely foods may cause asthma. Air-borne pollen and molds produce seasonal hay fever. House dust is a very important inhalant antigen. Animal hairs are frequent offenders, and for this reason allergic patients should avoid contact with or exposure to animals regardless as to whether they are skin sensitive to their hair. Contact with horses, especially riding behind a horse, or using horse blankets or being in the company of people who wear riding habits may produce severe allergic symptoms. A little boy, a physician's child, was sensitive, among other things, to horse dander and had severe asthma. With treatment his condition improved. On two separate occasions, however, the child had severe asthma. Once he attended a children's party at which one or two of the children were dressed as Indians, wrapped up in horse blankets. The second time he was feeling well. He and his mother were walking along the street when they met some friends who had just returned from horseback riding and were in an automobile. The car was stopped, the window was lowered while the conversation was carried on. A brief period of exposure to these people and their riding habits contaminated by horse dander brought about severe asthma. A social worker was also allergic to horses. Her asthma did not respond to treatment. Investigation into the possible causes of failure of therapy indicated that though this intelligent patient had been warned not to go horseback riding or come in contact with horses, she did not realize that the horse saddle which she kept under the bed in her small apartment bedroom was sufficient exposure to cause her to develop asthma, especially at night.

Infinitesimally small quantities of a substance can produce symptoms in an allergic patient. An egg-sensitive patient may develop symptoms if he uses a knife or fork that had previously been contaminated with egg and not washed properly. A child who was sensitive to potatoes could not enter the house without developing asthma if potatoes were being peeled. Another sensitive to sardines would get severe hives if present when a can of sardines was opened, and still another would get severe sneezing and asthma if present when fish was being cooked. House dust is a potent inhalant antigen. This accounts for the fact that so many allergic people sneeze and cough and develop other symptoms when they are exposed to house dust either through cleaning or sweeping. If a patient is sensitive to basement or attic dust, we suspect mold allergy. Feathers, especially old feathers, similarly are important in these conditions. Rabbit hair may be found in stuffed toys and cushions, and in various furs. Mohair contains goat hair, also a frequent offender. Until recently most cosmetics contained orris root, an ingredient which is seldom, if ever, used now in commercial cosmetics; it is no longer necessary to resort to specially high-priced so-called non-allergenic cosmetics in order to avoid orris root. Janitors are frequently sensitive to insecticides, the most common ingredient of which is pyrethrum. Among inhalants are insect emanations. This includes the caddis fly, moth, butterfly, mayfly, bee, and others. These insects give off certain hairs to which some people may be consistently sensitive. It is not uncommon, therefore, to find that there are people who develop manifestations in areas where sand flies predominate. Another important antigenic inhalant in respiratory allergy are molds or otherwise referred to as fungi. Inhalation of spores of these molds may produce severe allergic manifestations in sensitive individuals. These molds occur usually from spring until late fall in variable amounts in different localities.

It is important to have available information as to the growth of molds and of pollen in different parts of the country or of the world. A patient may leave his home for a vacation at a time when pollen is practically absent and go to another location where the same pollen to which he is sensitive is just beginning to be distributed.

Cattle hair is found in carpet or rug pads in the form of ozyte. Goat hair is found in clothes and rugs.

Pyrethrum is a frequent allergenic cause and may be found in such products as Gulf Spray, Flip, and Black Flag. Sensitivity to glue involves avoidance of various types of cabinets and furniture, toy airplanes and books.

Flaxseed is used in shampoos, in stock feed, wave sets, paints, tiles, etc. Allergy to burlap is frequently encountered. This is due to a sensitivity to jute, which is a fiber from a plant imported from India and used for the preparation or manufacture of burlap, rugs, carpets, carpet pads, etc.

INSECT STINGS

Sensitivity to insects particularly to bees, wasps, hornets, and mosquitoes can produce sudden, severe, and even fatal anaphylactic shock. For this reason it is imperative that the patient be tested and treated with a suitable set of such extracts. Such hyposensitization treatment is usually very effective. In addition, the patient should be given a prescription for a bee repellent which usually consists of propionic acid in aquaphor and an emergency kit. The emergency kit should be carried by the patient when he goes out in the country or to picnics or away from home. It should include several tablets of isuprel which can be taken under the tongue in case of an insect sting, of ephedrine which may be taken by mouth, and of cortisone and an antihistamine. The patient should be instructed that if stung by an insect he should seek medical advice as soon as possible because the injection of adrenalin and the placement of a tourniquet above the point of the sting usually may prove life saving.

INGESTANTS (FOODS)

People may be sensitive to single or to multiple foods. Here again are some foods which are botanically related, so that if a patient is sensitive to one food in this group, he is sensitive to the others. Examples of this may be cited in the case of cabbage, Brussels sprouts, and cauliflower. Many of the sea foods and fresh water fish are thus similarly related; so that if a patient is sensitive to one type of fresh water fish, he is likely sensitive to the others. The most frequent allergy-producing foods are common foods, namely, milk, eggs and wheat, fish and nuts. It is unfortunate that this is the case because these are also essential foods, and this avoidance becomes a serious problem in undernourished people and in children or infants. When a patient is definitely sensitive to one or two foods only, it is not difficult for him to realize it himself. The difficulty arises, however, when he is allergic to many foods. Under these circumstances he is likely to become confused and then he needs a physician's help. Allergy to a food may be of various degrees of severity. Symptoms of asthma or hives may not arise if only one food is eaten if the sensitivity is mild. However, if a number of such foods are ingested at one time, the symptoms may be pronounced. Another factor which is important in connection with the production of symptoms is the readiness with which a food is absorbed from the gastrointestinal tract. The quicker the absorption, the more rapid will the symptoms develop after eating.

In the case of sensitivity to eggs, the allergy, as a rule, is to the egg white and not to the egg yolk. Heating destroys, in many instances, the active part of the egg white by coagulating it. For this reason some people who are allergic to eggs may find it possible to eat hard-boiled eggs without developing symptoms. The same is true in the case of milk because heat destroys certain active principles in the milk and under given circumstances, some allergic people may find it possible to drink boiled milk. Patients who are sensitive to egg or milk or wheat find it impossible to take any foods which contain these various ingredients. The name of a proprietary food does not always indicate the presence of these substances; thus eggs are found in mayonnaise, waffles, ice cream, meringue icing, covering for bonbons, and bread. Certain vaccines, like the influenza vaccine, are prepared on egg media and should be avoided by such patients.

Similarly, milk-sensitive patients should avoid milk-containing foods: custards, candy, cake, cheese, and bread; nor can such people drink powdered or evaporated milk.

Cereals include many substances to which one may be sensitive. These are corn, rice, oats, rye, buckwheat, wheat, and others. Wheat is found in a large variety of foods: sauces, macaroni, spaghetti, noodles, bread, coffee substitutes such as postum, and many others. Corn may be used in the preparation of beer or whiskey. It is found in corn muffins, corn mush, or corn bread. Rice and rye go into the preparation of breakfast foods and many other foods.

Fish is a strong antigen because it usually produces severe symptoms. Some patients may develop asthma if they are exposed even to the odor of fish that is being cooked. The same is true of nuts. A variety of symptoms may result from the eating of nuts. These may include asthma, nose allergy, hives, or headaches. A physician, upon eating nuts, developed an eye condition which led to blindness in one eye as a result of a small hive occurring in the delicate structures of the eye. The same patient developed migraine headaches from the ingestion of peanut butter. This patient was extremely sensitive to peanuts (actually a legume, not a nut). Even the oils from nuts may contain sufficient nut protein to give symptoms, and this should be kept in mind because peanut oil is used in cooking and in the preparation of many products (candy, etc.).

Among the spices, perhaps mustard is the most frequent offender. Wieners and certain spiced meats contain mustard. Oil of wintergreen is another such agent. One patient developed severe asthma after eating a popular brand of candy bar. Then, it was discovered that this candy contained wintergreen oil. When a drop of diluted wintergreen oil was placed under the tip of the tongue of the patient, he developed severe asthma and hives. Allergy to seeds is not uncommon. This includes cottonseed and beans. A large group of asthmatic patients lived in the vicinity of a castor bean factory in Toledo; smoke from this factory contained sufficient castor bean dust to sensitize many of these people.

CONTACTANTS

These are substances with which the person comes in contact by touching or by external physical contact. A wide variety of such substances will be discussed later. These include various cosmetics, such as shampoos, face lotions, shaving lotions, mascara, and many others. Poison ivy is also a good example. Ointments which are prescribed for the relief of certain skin conditions may produce skin rashes.

INJECTANTS

Various drugs are injected into patients. These substances may elicit allergic reactions. A classical example is horse serum which has been used for a long time as a carrier for certain antitoxins and other immunity-producing agents. Not uncommonly people receiving such injections develop a reaction which is due to an allergy to the horse serum. Insect bites may also be classed under this heading. Patients may become sensitive to the proteins in the serum injected by bees, flies, or bedbugs. I saw an instance of severe hives in a nurse, thought at first to be due to foods; however, it was found later that this patient suffered with hives only when she slept in a rooming house where she boarded. She never had this difficulty when she went home. Further investigation revealed that she had severe allergy to bedbugs, with which her rooming house was infested.

PHYSICAL AGENTS

These include heat, cold, and sunlight. Severe skin reactions and other allergic manifestations may be produced by such agents.

BACTERIA AND FUNGI

Bacteria and fungi are known to be frequent sources of allergy. Infection in the nose may produce nose allergy or asthma. Intestinal parasites may similarly cause these conditions.

Patients allergic to molds may reduce their symptoms if they make sure there is no mildew or molds growing in their house. Molds growing in dark, damp, poorly ventilated basements are soon enough distributed throughout the entire house. Under these circumstances, see that your basement is properly heated and properly aerated and ventilated as well as dust free. Sponge all leather products with 1 per cent paranitrophenol and alcohol. Test this product out on a small piece of the leather first in order to make sure that it does not injure the material. Trioxymethylene, a form of formaldehyde, may also be used as a powder in order to prevent the growth of molds or mildew in basements. A small amount of powder, that is, say, about half an ounce or an ounce, is placed in an open jar in the clothes' cupboard where rabbit fur is found in felt hats, cheap furs, gloves, mattresses, and quilts.

HOW IS ALLERGY DIAGNOSED?

Many people who suffer with bizarre symptoms, or with conditions that have not responded to ordinary treatment, suspect that their condition may be allergic. The purpose of an allergic diagnosis is to indicate the specific causes of a patient's allergic symptoms. However, before doing this it becomes necessary to determine that the patient's condition is allergic in nature. In this way one may avoid disillusionment and unnecessary medical handling. We know in a general way that certain diseases are allergic; for example, we know that bronchial asthma, hay fever, hives, certain forms of eczema, skin rashes, and headaches are frequently allergic in origin. We also know that certain other diseases—for example, heart disease, cancer, or acne—are not allergic. Furthermore, allergic persons as a rule present a family history of some allergic disease; they present a past or present personal history of other allergic involvement. They frequently state that they have noticed that when they eat certain things, or when they are exposed to animals or to dust, they develop symptoms; and finally they respond in a characteristic manner to certain anti-allergic drugs. On examination of the blood, many of these patients will show characteristic cells (eosinophiles), which cells may suggest the possibility of allergic disease.

There is virtually no part of the body that cannot be involved in allergic manifestations. For this reason patients will frequently seek advice from nose and throat specialists or gastroenterologists or chest specialists for the relief of a condition which is allergic to begin with.

A well-qualified allergist will inform you as to whether the condition that you suffer with is or is not allergic in nature. Only within the last fifteen years have training courses for residents in allergy been given systematically by recognized institutions throughout the country. In most instances individuals who have received such training qualify and have passed the "Boards," as they are called—that is, Diplomate Boards of Internal Medicine or Pediatrics and Allergy. Such certification is, as a rule, presumptive evidence of the competence of the physician handling this type of work.

Of all the forms of investigation to which an allergic person is submitted, none is more useful than the story told by the person himself. This frequently reveals all-important clues to the diagnosis. For this reason it is important for the patient to become acquainted with the manifestations of allergy, so that he can become more observant about the relation between his environment, his occupation, food, and habits to his symptoms. For this reason patients are encouraged to read reliable information about allergy. Much time is consumed by history taking. The history includes a detailed analysis of the various symptoms. One inquires into the date of onset, course, and severity of the condition. The occupation of the patient may shed an important light; janitors are found to be sensitive to insect powder; florists to flowers; bakers to bakery sweepings; stablemen to horses; pharmacists, in some instances, to drugs, furriers to furs. Sometimes symptoms are related to the acquisition of new furniture such as upholstered chairs, or new carpets, or new bedding. Children may be found sensitive to stuffed toys; some people react to cosmetics, so that they develop bronchial asthma or nose allergy when they attend movies or go to church or are in crowds in confined places. Some patients are better at work, others at home, which suggests environmental factors. A husband may be sensitive to the cosmetics used by his wife. This has been called conjugal allergy. Allergic diagnosis sometimes requires actual detective work, and much patience on the part of both the physician and his patient. A business executive had an intractable rash on his forearms. Various tests revealed little, until one day the diagnosis was finally made. On walking into the examining room and turning the doorknob, the physician commented on the fact that the wax which was used in shining the door found its way to the doorknob. The patient, who was seated in the examining room, commented casually that in his office building they used the same wax for shining the desk tops; subsequently the dermatitis with which he was severely troubled for a long time was found to be due to this wax. The patient worked with his sleeves rolled up, and contact with the wax caused the rash.

PHYSICAL EXAMINATION

Every allergic person, especially those suffering with asthma, is entitled to a careful physical examination. This is important to make sure that the condition is not due to some disease with which allergy may be confused. Frequently nasal infection produces symptoms of nasal allergy. A careful examination of the nose will reveal the presence of such an infection and the necessity of combating it by adequate treatment. Similarly, not everything that wheezes is asthma. And so it becomes necessary to determine whether the patient has tuberculosis, tumor of the lung, or heart disease, or even a foreign body in the lung, of which conditions may well produce symptoms which are indistinguishable from those of bronchial asthma. Furthermore, a skin condition which may be thought to be allergic may actually be scabies or some other non-allergic condition.

SENSITIZATION TESTS

Sensitization tests include skin tests, eye and nose tests. Unfortunately, many people, including even many physicians, believe an allergic diagnosis is synonymous with skin tests. Actually, they form only a part of the allergic survey. Furthermore, certain types of skin tests are valuable and diagnostic only for given allergic conditions, and useless and misleading in others. The materials—or extracts, as they are called—which are employed for the performance of skin tests must be active and reliable. In addition, the interpretation of the results of skin testing is equally important. Hence these tests should be read by competent physicians. It is silly to test patients with substances they never eat or to which they will never be exposed. It serves little or no purpose, for example, to test a laborer to caviar, or a shop girl to sable. The number of skin tests to be carried out will depend on the conditions surrounding the situation with which the patient is confronted. When these tests are properly performed and critically and correctly interpreted, they are an important link in the chain of evidence which may unearth the cause of the allergy. The fact that a person has had skin tests without receiving much benefit casts no reflection on skin tests themselves as a procedure. This may indicate merely that the skin tests were probably not properly performed or interpreted. These important tests should not be relegated to a layman or to a lay laboratory where a technician performs them, reads them and sends the report to the physician. The allergist alone has a thorough acquaintance with the type of extracts which are useful, and he alone can decide whether positive tests are clinically significant or whether they are due to nonspecific irritation.

TYPE OF TESTS

In conditions in which the agent producing allergy is introduced into the body, such as through eating or inhalation, skin tests are performed by means of scratching the material into the skin or by injecting a small amount of the extract into the skin. After waiting for a period of five to ten minutes, one "reads" the reaction. The appearance of a localized swelling, wheal, or welt at the point of the scratch or injection surrounded by an area of redness indicates a positive skin test. Such a positive reaction merely indicates skin sensitivity and does not always mean that the patient cannot eat or inhale the substance.

When a person is sensitive through contact, the test of choice is a so-called patch test. For example, if we suspect a patient to be sensitive by contact to nail polish, it would serve no purpose to inject the nail polish with a needle; the proper procedure in such a case, or similarly in the case of poison ivy, is to apply a drop of the suspected material to the surface of the skin. After covering it with a small square of cellophane, it is held in place for forty-eight hours with adhesive. At the end of this period the material is removed; if an area of dermatitis or skin rash appears at the point of contact, we say that the patient is in all likelihood sensitive to the substance to which he was patch tested.

None of these tests are particularly painful. If properly performed they certainly are not dangerous. Infants as a rule do not have a very reactive skin; for this reason skin testing should be postponed until later in childhood.

Occasionally it may be useful to test for sensitivity of the lining membrane of the eyes or of the nose. In these cases a drop of a suitable liquid extract is introduced into the eye or nose. At the end of a waiting period of ten minutes, if the reaction is positive, the membranes become red and congested. Local symptoms appear—that is, watering and itching of eyes and nose—and we say that the patient is sensitive to that substance.

Another useful test in instances of suspected food allergy is the elimination diet or trial diet test. The patient is given a limited diet consisting of four or five foods for a period of five to seven days. The effect of such restriction on his symptoms is noted. Various items of food are then added to the diet every few days.

LABORATORY AND SPECIAL EXAMINATION

It frequently becomes necessary to expose the patient to additional medical studies; these may include an examination of the urine and of the blood; in cases of asthma the sputum is frequently examined for the presence of tuberculosis or of mold infection. X rays of the chest are necessary to eliminate co-existing or other diseases. In cases of heart disease an electrocardiogram is helpful. Various tests which determine the functional capacity of the lung may also be employed. Since infections of the nose are of great importance in connection with allergy of the respiratory tract, nasal secretions are examined carefully and X-ray studies are made of the sinuses.

CONSTITUTIONAL REACTIONS

Every allergic patient and his physician must appreciate that an occasional reaction of variable severity may occur following testing or treatment with allergenic extracts. As a rule, in competent hands such reactions are rare and relatively easily controlled. They occur because the patient has been exposed to too strong a dose of extract. Patients are kept waiting in the physician's office for about half an hour following testing or treatment in order to detect a reaction as soon as it occurs, because the effect of the treatment for a reaction depends entirely on the promptness with which it is instituted. The reaction may come on within a few minutes or a few hours. When it occurs more than a half hour or an hour after treatment, it is usually not severe and not a source of worry. The sooner it occurs, the more severe it is likely to be. At first the patient experiences the itchiness of the palms of the hands, the lips, the roof of the mouth and the nose. The patient's face is flushed; hives may appear; the nose may become stuffed and begin to run. There is a choking sensation accompanied by wheezing and choking. When treatment is instituted promptly, it is effective and all of these symptoms disappear in a matter of a half hour. It is well for the patient to carry with him capsules containing ephedrine and some antihistamine so that he may take one or two such capsules should he develop a reaction after he leaves the physician's office and before he has had a chance to contact him. Unfortunately, some patients have had unfavorable experiences with such reactions and have come to the conclusion that the treatment is worse than the disease. However, such experiences are usually avoidable and easily treated if necessary.

HAY FEVER

The term hay fever is a misnomer because the condition is not due to hay nor is it associated with fever. Constant usage, however, justifies its adoption. The symptoms are well known, including usually obstruction to nasal breathing, sneezing, lacrimation, itching of the eyes and nose, and a watery nasal discharge. Occasionally these patients may have asthma. Because the symptoms result from sensitivity to pollen, they will be seasonal and will coincide with the pollination dates in a given area, because pollen surveys indicate what pollens are prevalent in various areas. This information is of great value since patients have been known to leave the eastern seaboard, for example, and go to California, Florida, or Texas in order to avoid hay fever. They may, however, leave their home when the hay fever season is about over and reach their destination at the beginning of the pollinating season in that region of the country. Of course, in order for a pollen to be hay fever producing it is necessary for it to fulfil certain requirements; the pollen must grow in abundance in the given district; it must be light and wind-borne, and must be sufficiently widely distributed. Pollen that is heavy is carried by the wind with difficulty, and since it is not found in the air it will not produce hay fever. Goldenrod is an example. This pollen is conspicuous because of its color and because it is found in the neighborhood of ragweed, a common hay fever producing plant. Because of these reasons the patient frequently blames goldenrod as a cause of his trouble. Prevailing climatic conditions also control the abundance of pollen in the air and, therefore, the severity of the patient's symptoms. For example, heavy rain preceding the hay fever season naturally aids in the growth of vegetation and increases the supply of pollen. Sunshine in the early morning hours helps to dry the pollen and in this way renders it lighter for wind distribution. Heavy winds further help to distribute pollen and increase its concentration in the air. Some parts of the country are pollen free. These are usually areas in the northern parts of Canada. Pollen can be carried by the wind for a hundred miles or even more. Seasonal hay fever symptoms may be due not only to sensitivity to pollens, but also to sensitivity to the spores of certain molds and fungi which may be found in the air during certain seasons.

In spite of the fact that the symptoms of a hay fever patient are a source of great entertainment to non-hay-fever sufferers, hay fever patients are frequently quite miserable. Their symptoms may interfere with their happiness, with their ability to do their work, and to lead a normal life for several weeks or months out of the year. Just how seriously this condition may interfere with one's life may be gathered from reading a biography of Daniel Webster—a hay fever sufferer.

DIAGNOSIS OF HAY FEVER

The history as to the date of onset and the date of termination of symptoms is highly suggestive of the cause, because we know the date of pollination for the given areas. Skin tests are performed with dilutions of these various pollens to confirm the diagnosis. Occasionally eye or "sniff" tests are made. Patients frequently ask why it is that they have been "exposed for the last twenty-two years to ragweed and never developed hay fever." Contact is necessary in order to develop an allergy, and contact to ragweed pollen over a period of years produced the antibodies against ragweed in this susceptible person. People who live in Europe are not exposed to ragweed because ragweed does not grow there and therefore are never found to be allergic to ragweed.

TREATMENT OF HAY FEVER

Much can be done for the hay fever patient. The most rational and the most dependable form of treatment is still the "desensitization" treatment. This involves the injection of increasing doses of pollen extracts at variable intervals. The treatment is begun sufficiently before the beginning of the season so that the patient may receive a maximum dose at this time. The injections are spaced from three to seven days apart; each subsequent dose is increased in strength, provided the patient's arm does not swell and become sore as a result of the previous dose. After reaching the top dose, treatment is then continued at monthly intervals throughout the entire year. The responsibility of carrying out and adhering to this schedule is the patient's. Treatments may not be given at intervals longer than four weeks. Unless this is remembered, a constitutional reaction may follow, for there is a tendency for a patient to lose his tolerance for a given dose under these circumstances. This form of treatment is not only effective in ridding the patient of symptoms and making life more pleasant for him, but it is also helpful in avoiding the extension of the patient's hay fever symptoms into his chest and the development of asthma. As a result of lessening the hay fever symptoms, treated patients are less likely to develop sinusitis and other undesirable complications of hay fever.

The hay fever sufferer will do well to avoid drafts and winds. He should not travel through the country. Ventilation for his bedroom should be provided with a partly opened window in the next room. If it is necessary that the bedroom window be opened, a damp sheet should be stretched across it so as to catch the incoming dust and pollens. The use of a damp gauze mask or any of the other available masks may be helpful. Change of climate is effective provided it is definitely known that the offending pollen is not found at the patient's intended destination. Many resorts widely advertise that they are pollen-free, but on investigation are found to be no better than the patient's home town. The seashore offers relief only on days when the wind blows from the sea inland.

In addition, these patients are helped by certain drugs such as antihistamines, nose drops, and by ephedrine.

There are many hay fever resorts which are widely advertised; however, it is well to check up on these with the State Health Department and find out whether the pollen to which you are allergic is actually absent in that area.

More recently much interest has been shown in the so-called "one-shot" treatment of hay fever. This consists of the injection of an emulsion of the pollen or molds to which the patient is sensitive. It involves at least two to four treatments and not one. Many doctors doubt the safety of this form of therapy. At the present writing, this type of treatment must be considered in the experimental stage.

Patients frequently want to know for how long allergic treatment consisting of desensitization must be continued. Hay fever patients, as a rule, can get along well without any injection treatment after about five to six years of treatment. Asthmatic patients suffering with perennial bronchial asthma are gradually weaned away from such treatment after the first two years. If the patient gets along well, there is no need for continued treatment.

The treatment for hay fever as outlined is a long cry from that used during the life and time of Oliver Wendell Holmes, a hay fever sufferer himself, who said the only effective treatment for this condition was six feet of gravel.

PERENNIAL NASAL ALLERGY (ALLERGIC RHINITIS)

Nasal allergy is a condition associated with symptoms referable to the nose. These are obstruction to nasal breathing, stuffiness of the nose, sneezing, and a nasal discharge which is usually watery. Unlike hay fever which is seasonal, this condition is present throughout the year. It is frequently confused with the common cold.

THE DIAGNOSIS

If a person has frequent colds which last for a variable period of time, maybe a few hours to a few days, and recur again and again, one should suspect allergy involving the nasal membrane. This diagnosis may be corroborated by the examination of the nose and its secretions. It must be differentiated from sinusitis, which in reality is not an allergy but an infection. Nasal allergy may become complicated, if untreated, by sinusitis.

THE TREATMENT

This includes avoidance of causative agents, diet, and injection treatment or so-called desensitization. Correction of nasal deformity which blocks off the nasal passages may be necessary. If sinusitis is present, the condition is treated as though there were no allergy present, and then allergic treatment follows. Emotional factors should also be attended to. A man had typical nasal allergy. Because of his difficulty in proper breathing, he used nose drops constantly and this actually made him worse; he could not attend a dinner party or business conference without using his nose drops. He had just changed jobs and there was considerable insecurity in his new position. This instability made his nasal condition unbearable until it was remedied.

Nasal mucous membrane constrictors, while giving the patient relief for a few minutes, invariably cause the condition to become worse later because of the secondary swelling or congestion that follows. For this reason patients with nasal allergy should not use nose drops to excess. In instances in which emotional factors play an important contributory role, psychotherapy—that is, discussion of the patient's problems with him—in addition to allergic treatment is helpful. Antihistamine drugs are also valuable in the treatment of these conditions. People with allergic rhinitis should not sleep in a room the temperature of which falls below seventy, because chilling of various parts of the body produces nasal congestion.

PROGNOSIS (OUTLOOK)

In most instances of nasal allergy the outlook is fairly good; especially if the condition has not reached the irreversible stage in which there are various complications, and especially if nasal infection is absent. Because these complications occur so frequently, nasal allergy should be treated early.

BRONCHIAL ASTHMA

Bronchial asthma is a form of allergy which involves the lungs and its tubes—the bronchi. It is characterized by spells of coughing, wheezing, choking, and shortness of breath. In children the only manifestation may be an intractable, recurrent cough which is of unknown cause and which does not respond to ordinary treatment.

FACTORS AFFECTING ASTHMA

Climate seems to affect the asthmatic patient. This is particularly true of climate characterized by great variations of temperature and increased humidity. Under these circumstances an increased incidence of respiratory tract infections occurs, and these in turn precipitate asthma. Seasonal variations are present particularly in instances of pollen or mold sensitivity. The patient's occupation may play a very important role. Glandular disturbances such as accompany pregnancy, menstruation, and menopause may contribute to the severity of the asthmatic attack. Many patients are free or relatively free of asthma during pregnancy and are invariably worse during the menstrual cycle. Emotional factors are quite important in this connection; they affect all allergic patients to a great extent. Pungent and irritating odors, such as turpentine, gasoline, smoke, and fog, have a bad effect on the asthmatic symptoms.

DIAGNOSIS

An allergic patient should be studied carefully from a medical as well as an allergic point of view. This is necessary because wheezing, choking, and shortness of breath may be caused by conditions which are not allergic. Heart disease, tuberculosis, tumor of the lung, foreign bodies, and many other conditions may cause symptoms which are indistinguishable from those of bronchial asthma. A young man had severe asthmatic manifestations for three years. He had various studies, including allergic studies followed by treatment which proved ineffective. It developed that he had a small foreign body at the base of the right lung. This was later removed by bronchoscopic treatment. Shortly before the onset of his asthma, the patient was in a brawl in one of the local night clubs. He was bounced out of the night club unceremoniously, and during this procedure he had several teeth knocked out. He aspirated one of these which was attached by a small metal clip. Following bronchoscopic removal of the tooth, the patient's condition improved.

The allergist should be not only a physician well-versed in immunologic problems, but also a competent internist or a competent pediatrician. Otherwise, he will not recognize some of the conditions which may masquerade as allergic but which in reality are not allergic. Furthermore, he can decide whether the patient's asthma for example is accompanied by such complications as infections in the lung or emphysema and under these conditions will provide the patient with additional needed treatment.

TREATMENT OF ASTHMA

Treatment of bronchial asthma includes removal of the offending substance from the patient's environment, desensitization, and the administration of certain drugs.

Patients suffering with chronic asthma, especially if this condition is complicated by distention of the lungs commonly referred to as emphysema, should abstain from smoking.

"DESENSITIZATION"

Increasing doses of extracts of the substance to which the patient is sensitive are administered. Most of these patients are allergic to house dust. Some of them are sensitive to molds. Suitable mixtures of these may be prepared, including also other inhalants which the patient finds impossible to avoid; the patient is then treated with such extracts in a manner similar to that adopted in the treatment of the hay fever.

Asthmatics are susceptible to frequent colds, and because they usually have an associated bronchitis, they also receive suitable help toward controlling these conditions.

So-called desensitization treatment, more correctly called hyposensitization treatment, consists in the administration of increasing doses of a product to which the patient is allergic, at weekly intervals. Such a product may be pollen or it may be dust or molds. Under these circumstances the patient must follow faithfully the directions given to him by his physician and stick to the schedule religiously. The patient must himself be impressed with the importance of following a line of treatment which invariably will give him relief. This treatment of necessity is painstaking, time consuming, and of long duration. A condition which has been present for years cannot suddenly disappear following the performance of a series of skin tests or some other procedures.

Nor is it fair to blame allergy for failure of treatment in instances in which the patient received so-called "shots" without any benefit. Even more important is to know what material was given by injection, what the dosage was, and whether the patient was actually allergic to this material. The same holds good for skin tests. We frequently find patients who have lost faith in skin testing because skin testing they say is not successful. Again, it depends on the materials that are used and who performs and interprets these tests.

DRUGS

Medicinal treatment includes the use of many drugs; perhaps the most important of these is epinephrin, or, as it is sometimes called, adrenalin. There are now available adrenalin preparations which may be used by inhalation with a nebulizer as well as by injection, in accordance with the following directions: Remove stopper from throat tube and drop solution in as directed in the instructions with nebulizer. Place throat tube inside teeth and inhale deeply while compressing the bulb. Do not press bulb while exhaling. Only press on bulb three to five times at each treatment, and only use nebulizer about every three hours. Replace stopper after each use so that solution does not spoil, and return nebulizer to box. Add solutions only when necessary. Clean instrument according to instructions which are inclosed. A clean nebulizer and knowledge of how to use it are essential for maximum benefit. Ephedrine capsules and iodides are also helpful in loosening up the secretions which clog the bronchi.

In instances in which the asthmatic attack does not respond to such treatment, it may be necessary for the patient to be hospitalized. It is amazing to see how quickly improvement takes place under those circumstances. Oxygen as well as ACTH and cortisone may also be given if necessary.

Antibiotics are employed if infection is present.

In many instances the asthmatic patient's symptoms are due to difficulty in bringing up sputum. The act of coughing is nature's attempt to expectorate and to get rid of mucus which has accumulated in the bronchial tubes. In some instances this mucus becomes thick, dry, and viscid and sticks to the walls of the bronchial tubes. Under these circumstances it becomes necessary to give the patient an expectorant. Iodides are time-honored expectorants. They are prescribed in the form of drops. If, however, while taking this drug the patient develops a runny nose or swollen parotid glands or an acne-type of eruption the drug must be discontinued or at least the dose must be reduced.

Another drug which has a bronchodilator effect in asthma, thus relieving the spasm in the bronchial tubes is aminophylline. Your physician will prescribe this drug for you in the form of rectal suppositories, one of which may be taken at bedtime. The dose and the frequency of administration should be carefully gauged when this drug is given to children. One must at all times avoid self-medication. Many of these drugs are two-edged swords. They produce what is referred to as side effects and they may actually be contraindicated in certain conditions. The physician alone can decide whether the use of any of the drugs recommended may be helpful or actually may be harmful.

NASAL INFECTION AND ASTHMA

Nasal infection should be treated conservatively at first and by surgery if necessary.

BRONCHIAL ASTHMA AS A SURGICAL RISK

As a rule, it is safe to proceed with any surgery during the period between asthmatic attacks. Precaution should be observed with regard to the anesthetic and drugs employed.

PROGNOSIS (OUTLOOK)

The results from treatment are usually dramatic in patients who have asthma due to one or two substances. It is comparatively easy for these patients to avoid these offending agents. If there are no complicating factors, the results are even better. This is especially true in children. However, when there are complications such as infection and changes in the structure of the lung, the outlook is not quite as good. Even in these cases proper and prolonged treatment accompanied by co-operation on the patient's part is helpful. The asthmatic person must realize that the condition from which he has been suffering for a period of many years cannot disappear overnight; and that a great deal of effort, co-operation, and painstaking treatment is necessary to bring about desirable results. Fortunately, death occurs but rarely from asthma. The younger the patient, the better is the outlook. As the patient's condition lasts longer, certain complications result; these include infection in the lungs (bronchitis and bronchiectasis) and pulmonary fibrosis.

SKIN ALLERGY

The incidence of skin allergy is high. There are many different kinds of skin allergy. These may be divided into allergic skin conditions due to sensitivity to substances which reach the body through contact from without and those which produce allergy as a result of distribution following eating or inhaling of certain other foods or material. The skin is an important organ of the body; it takes a great deal of punishment. It is exposed constantly to all sorts of changes in temperature and humidity, to pressure, pull, tear, rubbing, infection and many mechanical and chemical factors.

CONTACT DERMATITIS

The outstanding example of contact dermatitis is poison ivy dermatitis, which affects a large segment of the population. This type of skin rash is due to an allergy or sensitivity to the oily fraction in the poison ivy plant; since symptoms are produced by contact, the dermatitis or rash occurs on the exposed surfaces of the body. However, it is not unusual to find these manifestations also on covered parts of the body. The explanation for this is that the material to which the person is sensitive is carried by the fingers to these areas. To indicate the frequency with which this type of mechanism can play a role in contact dermatitis, Dr. Sulzberger, some time ago, carried out the following experiment: He painted fluorescein on the fingers of a number of his patients and instructed them not to wash their hands or to take a bath for twenty-four hours. At the end of this time he exposed these patients, in the nude in a dark room, to ultraviolet rays. Now ultraviolet rays cause this material to fluoresce. This took place not only on the previously painted fingers, but also on various parts of the body that were covered.

CAUSES OF CONTACT DERMATITIS

There are many substances that produce contact dermatitis. I have already mentioned plant oils. Occasionally there are people who develop a contact dermatitis during certain seasons of the year. Closer investigation reveals that these people are sensitive to oily fraction of seasonal pollens and plants. Contact dermatitis may also be due to occupational substances such as chemicals, furs, dyes, leather, cosmetics, and many drugs.

When confronted with a condition that is suspected as being contact dermatitis, we try to find out as much information as possible to shed light upon the possible causes.

In the case of factory workers sensitive to given substances, certain preventive measures must be employed. These include forced circulation which gets rid of the dust to which the person may be sensitive, compulsory showers, protective clothing, gloves, etc. In some instances it may be necessary for the person to change his occupation. In these instances the amount of local application which is intended to relieve the itching is reduced to a minimum. At first these local applications do give the patient some relief, but eventually in many instances they may make him worse, because he may actually become allergic to the ointment which is prescribed for his relief.

In some instances treatment with the offending agent is employed, such as in the case of poison ivy dermatitis where the patient is given increasing doses of a poison ivy extract in the hope of increasing tolerance to this material. One must exercise care in such treatment for fear of distributing and aggravating the condition. It has not been found necessary to treat patients with poison ivy dermatitis with the so-called desensitization treatment. Some serious doubts prevail as to whether or not this treatment is actually effective. In acute cases the administration of cortisone for a few days and local treatment usually help to control the condition.

COSMETICS

Among cosmetics, nail polish and mascara are a frequent cause of contact dermatitis. Nail polish contains tin oxide and some abrasive powder. It may be colorless when used for men, or it may be slightly tinted. Nail enamel or liquid nail polish contains a large variety of ingredients. Dermatitis in these instances does not necessarily occur on the hands, but usually occurs on the face, especially on the eyelids because of the habit of some people to rub their eyelids with the back of their fingers. Various preparations which are applied to the face or to the hair may produce contact dermatitis, among which two of the most important are hair dyes and permanent wave preparations. Hair lacquer shellac is a frequent offender. It would, therefore, seem desirable to test people for sensitivity to the substances when they have dermatitis of unknown origin. Certainly no one who has a tendency to contact dermatitis should use hair dyes without first making sure that he is not sensitive to these dyes. A woman who was emotionally unstable dyed her hair. She had dyed her hair some years previously and following this second experience she developed a severe dermatitis of the entire scalp, face, and neck; the itching and subsequent nervous manifestations became so serious that in her despondency she committed suicide.

Other causes of such psychodermatitis are perspiration detergents and deodorants. In men, after-shaving lotions, shaving creams, and shaving soaps may produce dermatitis of the face. Plastics have been known to be a frequent offender in this connection, and of course numberless articles contain plastics. Artificial teeth, telephone receivers, cigar holders, varnishes, cheap jewelry, stockings, steering wheels, dishes, water containers, and other devices are made of plastic.

INFANTILE ECZEMA (ATOPIC DERMATITIS)

Skin eruptions which may occur at any time in life but which usually are found in infants and children may be eczema. The condition at first appears on the face and on the back of the wrists. Later in childhood it may be found in the bends of the elbows and the region back of the knees. At first the skin becomes red. Later small blobs or vesicles appear. As a result of scratching, these break open and oozing takes place. There is severe itchiness, and this constitutes the most disturbing feature of the disease. Allergic factors play a rather important role in this dermatitis. Most of these people have a family history of allergy. They may present other allergic manifestations, such as hay fever or asthma. Indeed, in some instances it is realized that the infant or child cannot tolerate certain foods or is sensitive to certain substances in his environment. One two-year-old boy had eczema on the inner surface of the elbows and back of the knees. The child would lose his voice following the ingestion of potatoes, peas, chicken, and eggs. Playing with stuffed toys produced paroxysms of asthma. He was quite sensitive to spices. Once while in the kitchen, he got hold of several boxes of spices which he emptied into a pot and pretended he was going to bake a cake for his father. He immediately developed a severe attack of asthma and a severe flare-up in his eczema. There is also evidence which emphasizes that nervous influences play an equally important role in the causation of this disease. If the cause of infantile eczema is not recognized and treated properly and early, there may occur, as a result of continuous scratching and skin injury, certain secondary changes in the skin. The skin becomes thick and leathery, and fissured or infected.

Because the skin of infants is not suitable for skin testing, it is important to arrive at a diagnosis by trial and elimination. As a rule, it is best to study such cases in the hospital. By so doing, the patient is most likely to be removed from the environmental sources of his difficulty; these factors may be dust, household inhalants, and many other substances which are present in his home, and to which he may be allergic. Elimination diets are tried. After the age of twelve months however it is feasible to perform skin tests on the infant with atopic dermatitis.

LOCAL TREATMENT OF ALLERGIC DERMATITIS

Most persons who suffer with allergic dermatitis have accumulated numberless lotions, salves, ointments, and other local preparations. These have either been prescribed for them or suggested to them by their family or friends. For the most part, the effects of these long-continued local applications is to further irritate and traumatize the skin, so that in the end more harm than good is done. First take away all these various drugs and prescribe only such bland preparations as are least likely to injure the skin. These must be cautiously and carefully applied, observing their changing effect. Indeed, at times it is necessary to use the preparation on one area of the skin only, such as one arm or one leg, and observe the difference between the dermatitis on that area and on the area of the body where no preparation has been used. Furthermore, an allergy may develop to the very preparation or substance that has been prescribed for the alleviation of the patient's disturbing itch. All local irritants must be avoided. The most important of these is soap. The patient is urged to employ a non-irritating cleansing substance, of which there are many on the market, such as Lowella Cake or Phisoderm Basis Soap. The patient must, of course, avoid washing dishes. If that is absolutely essential, she should use thin white cotton gloves over which may be worn thin rubber gloves. One avoids the use of rubber gloves directly on the skin because the heat and the sweat which is thus generated may macerate and further hurt the skin.

In the case of infants it must be remembered that the severe itchiness disturbs the child and renders him sleepless and fussy, causing him to lose weight. As a result of scratching, secondary infection appears, and this requires special treatment. In view of the fact that the mother's emotional attitude so frequently reflects itself on the child's reaction to his condition, it is often necessary to direct one's effort toward the proper handling of the mother. She must be reassured that the child's skin condition is not infectious and contagious and that it will in no way affect the infant's general health. The mother must learn to be more patient and less anxious about the child's condition. With older children it is important to take time out to discuss the nature of the condition and give some hope and encouragement as to the final outcome.

One should, of course, avoid the irritating effects of rough clothing and blankets, particularly wool. Feather pillows should be covered, or, better still, rubber foam pillows should be procured. If the child comes in direct contact with the mother, she should avoid the use of irritating and allergenic cosmetics and perfumes. The room should be kept at a steady temperature because constant changes in temperature will affect the skin also. Excitement should be avoided insofar as possible. Digestive disturbances and the effects of irritating fumes and odors should be eliminated. Diapers should be boiled in boric acid in order to remove traces of soap. This also helps to counteract the irritating effects of ammoniacal urine. In infants it is frequently necessary to immobilize the arms, especially at night, in order to avoid scratching. This is done by placing cardboard cylinders around the elbows. The nails are filed and the fingers are taped. If the baby has an intolerance to milk, boiled skimmed milk or, better still, goat milk should be given. One should watch for such symptoms as diarrhea and loss of weight and evidence of infection, which conditions should be treated as soon as they appear. At times it is necessary to give the child some form of sedation which the doctor will prescribe.

The development of contact dermatitis to a dye in a dress or clothing material is no reflection on the product. It does not indicate that the product is poisonous. All it indicates is that the patient has developed a sensitivity to this product, which sensitivity manifests itself in local symptoms.

Occasionally the use of cortisone lotions locally is helpful if the lesions are spread over a limited area of skin. The product helps to allay the itching and in this manner prevents further injury to the skin.

URTICARIA AND ANGIOEDEMA (HIVES)

Hives consist of wheals and welts of various sizes occurring throughout the entire body. These are accompanied by severe itching. At times these may be massive so that the swelling may involve the lips or the eyes. Indeed, the eyes may become shut, or the tongue may become swollen. A glue-sensitive patient developed tremendous swelling of the tongue after licking stamps so that he had difficulty getting his tongue back in his mouth. These swellings may occur in the throat so that the patient may have difficulty in swallowing or difficulty in breathing. When this occurs one may have to deal with a serious emergency. A young college student was found sensitive to sulfa drugs. In spite of being warned about this, he chose to chew some sulfa gum when he thought he was developing a sore throat. Soon after that he developed edema or swelling of the throat and uvula so that he began to choke. He was brought to the emergency room where the condition was found to be so critical that the intern did not take the time to take him to the operating room, but immediately performed a tracheotomy—that is, made a hole in the patient's windpipe in order to permit him to breathe and thus dramatically saved his life.

In about one third or one half of all cases of hives, some form of allergy may be demonstrated. Once the cause is found, treatment becomes rather simple. It consists largely in avoidance. Careful dietetic treatment is often necessary. In addition, the patient is frequently relieved by the administration of the antihistamine drugs. These should be taken only as prescribed by the physician.

SERUM DISEASE

There are occasions when it is necessary to treat patients with serum obtained from some animal, usually horses. These horses are immunized against certain diseases, and their serum contains the specific antibody which will help fight the disease in the patient. However, serum injection may lead to a train of symptoms referred to as serum reaction. This is a form of allergy. Two to twelve days following the administration of serum, the patient develops hives, a slight elevation of temperature, joint symptoms, and nausea and vomiting. As a rule, however, these symptoms are easily treated with antihistamines and adrenalin, and in a few days the patient is well. There is nothing dangerous about this type of reaction.

Rarely, however, a patient who has had serum before may, upon receiving serum for the second time, develop much more serious reactions. For this reason asthmatic patients, especially those who give a history of sensitivity or allergy to horses, must avoid such serums.

ALLERGY TO DRUGS

A similar type of reaction to that which occurs following the administration of horse serum may also occur following certain drugs. Almost any kind of skin rash may develop as a result of drug allergy; or the patient may develop asthma or hay fever. Whenever a patient develops a skin rash or unexplainable symptoms during the course of some illness, keep in mind the possibility that these symptoms are produced by a drug which the patient is receiving. Not infrequently the elimination of these drugs will cause a sudden disappearance of the symptoms. Sulfa drugs, aspirin, coal-tar products, iodine, bromine, belladonna, antibiotics such as penicillin, insulin, liver extract, and many others are frequent offenders in this connection. These reactions are so common that the question arising now during the course of treatment is not what drug to prescribe, but which drug to omit. The serum disease type of reaction described occurs not only after the administration of a foreign serum but may occur also after the administration of almost any drug. Penicillin is a good example. Because of its wide usage this drug has become an important cause of drug allergy.

It is possible in some instances to carry on tests which determine the presence of such sensitivity to certain drugs. Most drugs, however, do not lend themselves readily for the performance of these tests.

Certainly, a history of a reaction to a previous administration of a given drug with or without positive skin tests should be sufficient warning not to use the same drug again unless the drug is really a life-saving procedure. Under these circumstances caution must be employed.

PHYSICAL ALLERGY

Some persons, when exposed to changes in temperature such as cold or heat or when exposed to sudden effort or sunlight, may develop allergic manifestations, such as asthma, hay fever, or hives. In these instances the cold or heat acts as an antigen, much the same as milk or pollen may produce allergy. The demonstration of the presence of such sensitivity requires special tests. In the case of a patient sensitive to cold one tests the patient by attaching a small tube containing ice water to the skin of the arm. The tube is held in place with adhesive. Sensitivity to cold is determined by the appearance of a large welt or hive at the point of contact. A similar test may be carried out with hot water. Undoubtedly, under this classification of allergy are also included those patients who when exposed to a draft or a cold breeze develop nasal symptoms followed by severe so-called sinus headaches.

Physical allergy is relatively not serious. Under unusual circumstances it may prove to be serious. Some instances are reported in which a child, after diving into a swimming pool, died suddenly. Examination after death did not reveal water in the lungs. Obviously the child did not drown. He was a good swimmer. There was no history of pre-existing heart disease or other conditions which might explain such a sudden death. Death in these cases is usually due to asphyxia, brought about by the sudden swelling or hivelike formation in the throat, shutting off the air passages so that the patient cannot breathe. These hives or swellings are produced by sensitivity to cold. The change in temperature brought about by the sudden diving into the cold water is responsible for symptoms in cold-sensitive patients.

Similarly other patients develop hives or certain forms of skin rashes upon exposure to a small amount of sunlight. This type of skin reaction is unusually severe. It occurs upon minimal exposure as compared with the sunburn which most people develop upon prolonged sunlight exposure. A directress of nurses was sensitive to sunlight. She sought a position in one of the Pittsburgh hospitals because she had heard that Pittsburgh has little sunlight. A few days after her arrival in Pittsburgh she found out otherwise. She continued to develop severe dermatitis on exposed surfaces, in spite of the fact that she protected herself by wearing a large picture hat, and using newspapers or a parasol when walking during the daytime from the nurses' home to the main hospital building.

There is no specific and effective treatment against physical allergy. Antihistamines are of some help. However, such patients must be taught to protect themselves against exposure. Sometimes a tolerance may be developed by continued exposure to small doses of cold, heat, or sunlight, whichever the offending agent may be.

ALLERGIC HEADACHE

Certain types of headache are allergic in origin. In these cases patients develop headaches of variable severity when exposed to substances to which they are allergic. These may be food or inhalants. The symptoms vary with the person. As a rule, the pain is deep and sometimes throbbing, or it may acquire the characteristics of so-called sick headache or migraine. Not all instances of migraine are allergic in nature. When one realizes that chronic headaches interfere with the patient's happiness and productivity, a serious effort must be made in each case to discover its cause. It must by no means be assumed that every case of headache is allergic, because most frequently the cause of headache is something other than allergy. In the case of chronic recurrent headache one must always rule out some serious systemic condition like kidney disease, anemia, infection, or brain tumor.

As a rule, sick headaches are accompanied by pain which is located on one side of the face and head. The patient may be sick at the stomach, and the very thought or odor of food nauseates him. He usually cannot tolerate light and prefers to be lying down. He does not want to be disturbed. He does not invite sympathy. A young physician would invariably get these sick headaches on holidays. Not until he had an allergic survey was it discovered that he was very sensitive to chicken. These two facts were then correlated. There was usually a family dinner on holidays, and chicken was invariably served at these functions. As a matter of fact, this patient could not eat any soup which had chicken stock in it, nor could he eat any food which had been cooked in pots that had previously contained chicken unless they were thoroughly scrubbed. By scrupulously avoiding chicken, he managed to reduce the frequency and severity of his headaches. The patient's "nerves" may also have a bearing on the occurrence of his headaches. Most of these persons have a characteristic personality. They are usually perfectionists. They burn the candle at both ends and usually also in the middle. They demand a lot from themselves, as well as from those by whom they are surrounded. They have tremendous drive. Treatment involves, in addition to allergic management and improvement in general health, an attempt at change in the patient's philosophy of living and attitude toward his environment. He must learn to take things a bit easier. He must learn to enjoy leisure time. Conflicts and the cause of emotional upsets must be resolved. Some form of psychotherapy is often helpful. Those who suffer with chronic recurrent intractable headaches are miserable. There is no class of more grateful people than these—if they experience relief from their distressing symptoms; hence they are entitled to every bit of help they can get.

BACTERIAL ALLERGY

A person may be allergic not only to foods and inhalants, but also to the bacteria or germs which may infect him. Particularly is this true of bacteria which produce infection in the nasal sinuses, so that one may well develop asthma or nose symptoms as a result of such bacterial allergy. Indeed, it is thought that rheumatic fever symptoms are produced by an allergy to the germ that is found associated with this condition. Another example of bacterial allergy is tuberculosis. Symptoms of tuberculosis have been shown to develop from allergy to the products of the tuberculosis germ, namely tuberculin. For this reason present or past tuberculous infection may be demonstrated by skin testing with tuberculin.

ALLERGY OF THE EYES

Many eye conditions are possibly due to an allergy. This includes not only involvement of the eyelids—that is, both the inner and outer surface of the eyelids—but also of the eyeball and of some of the delicate structures within the eye. An elderly physician experienced a "blind spot" in one eye and swelling of the fingers after eating fish. Contact dermatitis of the eyelids is not uncommon. Eye symptoms are frequent in hay fever.

ALLERGIC DIZZINESS

Many are the causes of dizziness. However, if a person is otherwise allergic and after a careful examination no other causes are found for his dizziness, then it is well to think of the possibility that this condition is produced by allergy. There may or may not be associated ringing in the ears and various degrees of loss of hearing. In certain conditions a person may break out in a cold sweat; the duration of the condition may vary from a few minutes to a few hours. There may be vomiting. When due to allergy, dizziness is caused by hives or swelling of the delicate structures of the internal ears. A clerk developed these symptoms for the first time after he was engaged in licking stamps and envelope flaps on a large number of items that were to be mailed. Subsequently it was found that this patient was sensitive to sweet potatoes, and we discovered that stamp glue is made from sweet potatoes. Absorption of this material into the blood produced ear involvement and the resulting dizziness. A civil engineer was found sensitive among other things to garlic. After he received his report and on thinking it over, it occurred to him that he had been having many of his attacks of dizziness after his evening meal. Further inquiry revealed the interesting information that they were using garlic in a shaker for seasoning foods at the table. Doing away with the garlic shaker, his evening attacks of dizziness almost completely disappeared.

GASTROINTESTINAL ALLERGY

Gastric symptoms often follow the ingestion of certain foods. Children are particularly prone to develop vomiting and abdominal pain from foods to which they are allergic. If the food is an essential one like milk or eggs, and one does not realize that the child is allergic, the parents are likely to insist that the child continue to drink milk or eat eggs in spite of these symptoms. As a result, the child continues to become worse. The manifestation of such allergy may be only gastrointestinal—namely, nausea, vomiting, cramps, and diarrhea. There may be skin lesions about the mouth, namely, eczema; or there may be ulcerations in the mouth, in the throat, or of the stomach or the intestines. Any or all parts of the gastrointestinal tract may be involved. Mucous colitis is frequently due to an allergic condition. The elimination of the offending foods frequently brings about an almost miraculous change in the patient's condition. Skin tests, careful history, and trial and elimination diets are frequently helpful.

URINARY BLADDER SYMPTOMS

Urinary bladder symptoms may on occasion be produced as a result of allergy. Careful examination fails to reveal any evidence of disease, and yet the patient has serious local symptoms; eliminating the offending factors may bring about almost immediate relief.

JOINT INVOLVEMENT

Swelling and pain in the joints may occur because of an allergy to foods or other substances. Joint involvement is a frequent accompaniment of allergy to serums and to drugs. Similar symptoms may also be found after ingestion of foods. The wife of a physician had severe hives at various times in her life. The last attack of hives was associated with excruciating pain in the region of the back of the neck. The patient had severe pain in the neck and limitation of motion. X ray and other examinations of this region failed to reveal any evidence of disease. The patient was anxious, restless, and sleepless. Because of this it was thought at first that these were nervous manifestations, and the patient was diagnosed as a psychoneurotic. An allergy survey revealed that she was sensitive to several foods and particularly to grapes. On several occasions she noticed that drinking champagne, or grape wine, brought about an attack of hives as well as an attack of pain in the neck. Proper allergic treatment gave her complete relief from all of these disturbing symptoms.

EPILEPSY

Several instances are on record of convulsions which have been relieved by removal of offending foods from the patient's diet. These instances are rare. The epileptic patient who is otherwise allergic, and has a family history of allergy, is entitled to an allergic survey and allergic management in the hope that such investigation may bring about some improvement in the condition.

ALLERGY IN CHILDREN

The importance of an early diagnosis of allergy cannot be overemphasized. This diagnosis should be made in infancy or early childhood. This involves not only recognition that the condition affecting the child is allergic, but also a serious attempt at discovering the cause of the allergy. In doing this, however, one meets frequently with a great deal of resistance by the mother because she does not want to see the child hurt, or because she somehow has a vague suspicion that skin testing endangers the child's health. The mother must understand the importance of such an early diagnosis. She must realize that delay is equivalent to neglect, and that neglect needlessly exposes the child to the dangers of complications which may result from an untreated allergy. When handled early, it is comparatively easy to diagnose and treat effectively a case of hay fever or a case of asthma in a child. After a few years, however, this condition becomes complicated by nasal infection or by bronchitis, or by changes in the tissues of the lungs. These changes become refractory to treatment, so that even if the allergy is discovered, treatment of complications becomes difficult if not impossible. The mother must also understand that skin testing, if properly done, is not dangerous and does not affect the child's physical condition.

Bronchial asthma is frequently preceded in infants and in children by an unexplainable persistent cough which occurs in spasms and does not respond to ordinary treatment; furthermore, because asthma in infants and children is frequently associated with fever, the condition is misdiagnosed as due to pneumonia. If a child has frequent unexplained cough accompanied by wheezing and high fever, he probably does not have pneumonia, but has bronchial asthma. If the child's nasal or chest symptoms are seasonal, always suspect that he is sensitive to pollen or to seasonal molds. These patients are not uncommonly said to suffer with frequent so-called summer colds, when in reality they are allergic. A little girl had attacks of asthma especially severe in the early summer when she was taken to the lake where her parents had a cottage. Investigation revealed her to be sensitive not only to certain foods, but also to dust and to fungi. The cottage was closed during the winter and became dusty and mildewed due to increased humidity and to lack of ventilation. Her allergy to these molds found in the cottage was responsible for her summer asthma.

Furthermore, infants are frequently sensitive to many foods. Many different ingredients are included in the numerous proprietary baby foods. In the case of breast-fed babies the infant may be sensitive to some food ingested by the mother and passed into mother's milk in quantities sufficient to produce symptoms in the baby. Nasal allergy is common in children. The child experiences considerable itchiness of the nose. His delicate nasal membranes are swollen, and he finds it difficult to breathe through the nose; the child makes an attempt at scratching the tip of the nose with the palm of his hand, pushing the tip of the nose upward and backward, in that way spreading the nasal walls apart so that he can also breathe more easily. Nose rubbing and nose wrinkling are some of the common mannerisms developed by these children, and have been dubbed "the allergic salute."

Because little was known about allergy some twenty years ago, it was not an uncommon practice for physicians to dismiss an allergic infant or child with the remark, "The child will outgrow his condition." On rare occasions spontaneous recovery does result. Most frequently, however, when recovery results, it is because of a fortuitous coincidental removal of the patient from environmental substances to which he is allergic. As a rule, in spite of wishful thinking and endless temporizing, if untreated, the allergic child continues to suffer, and as a result of this neglect he frequently develops complications and secondary changes which make difficult the solution of a problem which was comparatively simple in the beginning. For this reason the parents of allergic children have a direct and immediate responsibility, to seek competent and adequate attention for their allergic children.

In the case of children suffering from allergic skin conditions do not attempt to vaccinate the child during the active phase of the skin condition because such a procedure may lead to a widespread involvement and aggravation of the skin condition.

IMMUNIZATION PROCEDURES IN CHILDREN

Children must be vaccinated against smallpox, diphtheria, and tetanus. In certain regions of the country typhoid vaccination is indicated. A tuberculin test should always be done. Rabies vaccine should be used when necessary. Tetanus toxoid should be given to children who have been previously immunized against tetanus when exposure demands it. Immunization procedures are essential, necessary, and effective. They carry with them no danger whatever. In many instances they are, indeed, lifesaving.

Vaccination against smallpox should be carried out between the ages of three and twelve months. This vaccination should be repeated between the ages of seven and eleven years, especially if there is an epidemic or if the patient is to leave for another country. Tuberculin tests should be performed at the age of three years, and later if needed. Possible combined vaccines are being used successfully now against diphtheria, tetanus, and pertussis, starting at the age of three months.

A Schick test is done between the ages of eighteen and twenty-four months in order to determine whether the child has developed immunity against diphtheria. Re-immunization should be performed if needed. Tetanus toxoid may be given at any period, although booster doses are repeated every one to three years. Typhoid fever vaccine is administered if the child is to travel to areas where there is typhoid fever or there is a possible danger of such exposure.

TREATMENT OF ALLERGY

The general principles of allergic treatment are somewhat similar for all allergic diseases. Every allergic patient should have an understanding of what this treatment implies. Following the completion of the diagnostic procedures, the patient is given to understand that his complete co-operation is essential. Unless he is willing to help, any effort at allergic management is bound to lead to disappointment. The nature and duration of the patient's condition itself indicates the necessity of prolonged and careful treatment.

GENERAL PROCEDURES

The patient's health is cared for. There must be a sufficient amount of rest. Foci of infection, such as diseased teeth and tonsils, are removed. If the patient is anemic, an attempt is made to correct this condition.

PSYCHOTHERAPY AND PSYCHOSOMATIC APPROACH

There is little doubt that emotional factors have a profound effect upon an allergic condition. The reverse is also true, allergic diseases affect the patient emotionally. A patient who suffers with a long-standing chronic condition like asthma, or a patient whose normal life is seriously interfered with during a good portion of the year because of hay fever, is bound to become nervous and upset. These patients develop emotional disturbances which in turn contribute to or aggravate their condition. The person who has been the subject of repeated asthmatic paroxysms, or one who experiences continuous itching from an allergic skin condition, naturally becomes disturbed, irritable, and nervous. The more severe the condition, the more profound are the emotional changes which are brought about in that particular patient. If the disorder starts early in life, the child's personality may become definitely affected. He may become submissive or introverted and lead the life of an invalid, demanding a great deal of attention and sympathy from his family and refusing to partake of his normal responsibility; or, the child may overcompensate and become extroverted and aggressive.

There are many instances which indicate that emotional upheavals have had either an indirect or even a direct effect upon the patient's allergic condition. The power of suggestion may bring about allergic symptoms. This is exemplified by the instance of the hay fever patient, sensitive to ragweed, who began to sneeze violently in the winter when shown a ragweed plant framed under a glass cover. Every physician has seen patients develop severe attacks of asthma under severe emotional strain, or patients with allergic eczema whose dermatitis flares up under similar circumstances. Under the impact of fear, anxiety, or some other emotional explosion, the patient's wheezing, cough, and shortness of breath, or his itching may become unbearable. The patient becomes dissatisfied with life and discouraged. He loses sleep, his appetite is poor, and he loses weight. All these symptoms may contribute to and make worse his already existing allergic symptoms. Real improvement may result following psychotherapy, that is an attempt to discuss the patient's condition with him and give him an opportunity to express himself. Everyone knows that emotions may affect certain normal bodily functions. Examples of this are palpitation, vomiting, blushing, sweating, diarrhea, and insomnia, all of which normal functions may be exaggerated and brought about by nervous influences. However, in some patients various conflicts, frustrations, anxieties, and other nervous states may lead to maladjustment and contribute to and emphasize the allergic symptoms. These patients do not respond to medical treatment unless the nervous condition is also properly cared for. Physicians find it increasingly necessary to devote more and more time to careful discussion with the patient so that an understanding may be obtained of the patient's personality and of his domestic, social, and business problems. A realization of such problems and such conflicts will influence profoundly the clinical course and the outcome of treatment. The person who is maladjusted cannot be well and happy, and an unhappy person will not respond to even the most effective form of medical treatment. At the same time it is unwise to assume that just because an asthmatic patient is nervous, his asthma is due to his emotional difficulties.

ASTHMA DUE TO FOREIGN BODIES

A patient had severe asthma which did not respond to usual medical treatment. It was of three years duration and occurred in a relatively young man. The physician who knew him well brought up the possibility of psychosomatic factors playing an important part in producing the asthma. The patient showed emotional instability and was poorly adjusted. His family was wealthy. He had never followed a definite line of work. He took up drinking. Attempts at rehabilitation were unsuccessful. Obviously strong psychogenic influences were at work. Since all examinations inducted at one of the clinics failed to show a cause for the asthmatic condition, psychoanalysis was suggested and adopted. The results were poor. He was re-examined. Bronchoscopy was advised. This examination revealed nothing of note, although it was not satisfactory because the patient jumped off the table before the bronchoscope was introduced. The chest X ray was repeated and at this time closer examination of the film showed a small metal clip at the base of the right lung. The mere presence of emotional conflicts and psychosomatic problems in an asthmatic patient is no proof that these factors are always the important causative factor in producing his condition.

AVOIDANCE OF CAUSATIVE FACTORS

The prime and basic principle of allergic treatment is to avoid the cause of the allergy. Allergic treatment cannot be carried out without an accurate allergic diagnosis. This may frequently involve a visit to the patient's home in order to discover whether there are many factors in the home which produce the allergy. People who are sensitive to goat hair may have their symptoms as a result of exposure to mohair furniture. The person's occupation should be carefully investigated. Allergic people are frequently sensitive to house dust and this makes it desirable to render the living room and bedroom dust-free, if possible.

INSTRUCTIONS FOR PREPARATION AND MAINTENANCE OF A DUST-FREE ROOM

In order to avoid house dust, an allergen of particular importance in respiratory allergy, the patient is given a list of directions which will help him as much as possible in ridding his house of dust. A suggested set of directions follows:

The bedroom should be entered seldom by others. Cleaning should be done only when the patient is out of the room. Remove all hangings, carpets, and extra furnishings from the sleeping room, as they are dust catchers. There should be no overstuffed (upholstered) furniture in the room. Clean the walls and ceilings. Scrub the woodwork (floors, baseboards, closets, etc.); scrubbing should be repeated each week. Scrub the bedsteads and all open coil springs at least once each month. A scrubbed wooden or metal chair may be used. Use cotton rag rugs and plain light curtains, and wash them weekly. Window shades (blinds) of the pull type are desirable. Mattresses, pillows, and upholstered box springs are inclosed in dustproof covers. Use only washable blankets and washable cotton bedspreads (use no chenille or tufted candlewick type); blankets should be washed at least once each month. (For woolen blankets this washing may be done in the bathtub in a simple manner. The use of "Dreft" suds is recommended, as they remove fiber dusts rapidly.) If there is sensitivity to wool, ordinary cotton blankets may be put into sheets (old, soft, well laundered) before being brought into the room. These sheets should be changed only outside the room.

Do not store household objects or outer clothing such as shoes and overcoats in the clothes closets. When possible, the ventilation is to be obtained from outdoors. A suitable ventilator with a filter should be installed in the window. All doors leading to other rooms should be kept closed. If furnace heat outlets exist, a dust filter must be installed and changed frequently.

GENERAL AVOIDANCE INSTRUCTIONS

General directions are given to each patient emphasizing certain avoidance advice as follows: Use no insect powder in any part of the house without specific permission. This includes fly sprays, roach and ant powders, dog flea powders, and certain other types of mothproofing preparations. As far as it is possible, none of the substances to which the patient is sensitive should be found in his home.

The patient should avoid exposure to inhalants, particularly animal hairs and insecticides. This necessitates an understanding of the various toys, hats, furs, carpets, that may contain such hairs. Foods to which the patient is sensitive should also be eliminated. In this connection, and especially in the case of children, keep in mind the possibility of the development of deficiency diseases because certain minerals and certain vital vitamins may have been eliminated from the diet. Therefore, allergic treatment sometimes must be supplemented by the administration of vitamins and a proper combination of the various constituents of a healthy diet. The weight should be carefully watched. An asthmatic woman spoke English with difficulty. She was definitely food sensitive. Treatment therefore included some dietary restrictions. She was instructed to report to the clinic at intervals of two weeks, so that her diet might be properly adjusted. However, her asthma disappeared. She properly attributed this to her dietary treatment and of her own will proceeded to restrict her food intake further. Though asthma-free, she continued to lose weight and finally was hospitalized with pellagra.

No fresh or artificial (dust catcher) flowers should be kept in the house. Use only washable toys (remove all stuffed or hair fabric toys). Avoid contact with irritating odors from leaking stoves and electric refrigerators, kerosene lamps, fresh paint, tobacco smoke, camphor, tar, etc. Do not keep any animal pets in your home unless specifically permitted. Do not indulge in any physical exertion which makes you short of breath or causes you to become overheated. Do not hurry; walk slowly and stop occasionally. Protect yourself against exposure to changes in weather so that you do not catch colds. Do not use mustard plasters or flaxseed poultices. Take drugs only when prescribed, for harmless medicine may be injurious to you. Avoid perfumes, face powders, sachet, and scented talcum powders, shaving and shampoo soaps, toothpaste, toilet water, and scented soaps. Many of these contain orris root and rice powder. Use only those specifically recommended. Avoid all dusty and musty places (basements, storerooms, attics, etc.). Avoid all contacts and foods listed for you. Avoid swimming unless specifically permitted. Do not overload your stomach with heavy meals. Avoid carbonated waters, such as seltzer, cola, pop, ginger ale, etc. Consult your physician if troubled by constipation. Use no condiments, spices, peppers, sauces, mustards, pickles, or any other highly seasoned foods.

Foods to which you are found to be allergic must be avoided. The Ralston Purina Company will supply upon request wheat-free, milk-free and egg-free diets including recipes which are most palatable and which may be used in these cases. In the case of dietetic restrictions in children it is important that the child receives suitable vitamins. The crux of all allergic therapy is still avoidance. Having found out what the patient is allergic to, it is imperative that he should avoid exposure to or contact with the antigens to which he is allergic. There is no drug or desensitization substitute for avoidance.

DESENSITIZATION

Desensitization is an accepted form of treatment, in which doses of the substance to which the patient is sensitive are injected. In this manner, an increased tolerance to this substance is frequently produced. Such treatment is usually effective, and carries little danger if properly carried out. The method is employed in hay fever, asthma, etc. Patients are "desensitized" to dust, pollen, molds, etc.

DRUG TREATMENT

Many drugs are used in the treatment of allergy. Since histamine seems to be at the bottom of all allergic reactions, medical scientists searched for a long time for a chemical which could destroy histamine, hoping that in such a drug would be found the final answer to the treatment of the allergic patient.

For the past ten years intensive research has centered on work with many such drugs, commonly referred to as histamine antagonists. In 1937 certain substances such as histadine, cystine, and arginine were found which seemed to inhibit to some extent the action of histamine on animals. However, these could not be used in man because of their poisonous action. In 1942 a new series of related chemical compounds were discovered which proved effective against histamine and yet not too toxic in man. This investigation was carried on first by several Frenchmen working in their laboratories in France, then by a twenty-six-year-old chemist in Cincinnati and finally by several pharmacologists in other parts of the United States. Many chemicals were studied by rearranging their molecular structure, and each of these seemed to have certain advantages over the other until a final compound was discovered which seemed to meet all objections. The drug appeared to be the answer to the long struggle and search for a suitable antihistamine chemical. This substance is called beta dimethylamino-ethyl-benzhydryl-ether-hydrochloride, and is named "Benadryl." Another drug which serves practically the same purpose but has a slightly different chemical composition is "Pyribenzamine." Both drugs have been used extensively in the laboratory and in medical practice. Experimentally, they will protect sensitive guinea pigs against the shock produced by injecting them with the proteins to which they are sensitive. In other words, if one administers to an animal a small amount of Benadryl or Pyribenzamine and then injects the animal with either the protein to which it is sensitive or with histamine itself, the animal will be found protected by the administration of the drug. These new chemicals in some way interfere with the action of histamine on certain cells and tissues of the body, both in animals and in man, and in that way prevent the usual histamine effect. They bring about satisfactory results in the palliative treatment of certain allergic conditions particularly hives and nasal allergic disorders, such as hay fever. The patient obtains relief from his sneezing, nasal obstruction, or from his itching. The effect of the drug, however, is only transitory so that it must be taken continually. It has no effect on the basic allergic condition or in reducing the patient's sensitivity to pollen, dust, foods, or other substances to which he is allergic. As soon as the medication is stopped the symptoms recur.

Antihistamine agents are effective in connection with the treatment of nose allergy and hives and are ineffective in asthma. These drugs unfortunately have some side effects, namely, nausea, vomiting, dizziness, and drowsiness. The drowsiness may lead to serious accidents in industry or in persons driving a car while under the influence of the drug. A young lady took a capsule of "Benadryl" after dinner for the first time for the control of her hay fever symptoms. By the time her "date" showed up an hour later to take her to the theater, she was so sleepy that she insisted they abandon their plans to go out and remained at home for the evening. Some of these drugs are more effective than others. They should be taken only on a physician's prescription. They must not be used as a substitute for proper allergic diagnosis and effective rational treatment. Some of the present available antihistamine drugs are "Neohetramine," "Benadryl," "Pyribenzamine," "Histadyl," and "Chlortrimeton." These may be had in capsules, pills, or liquid form. Their effect is transitory. Patients also become used to them so that after a while the drugs are ineffective and a change is made to another antihistamine.

A milestone has been reached in the fight against allergy with chemicals. These discoveries may well forecast the development of a new era in the approach to the management of the allergic patient. However, these drugs are effective only as palliative, transient, and temporary measures, and then only for some and not all allergic disorders. Epinephrin or adrenalin is a useful drug in the treatment of many allergic disorders. It is used in asthma extensively, by injection under the skin or by inhalation through a nebulizer. It may be used as nose drops in nose allergy. Occasionally it is administered mixed with gelatin or oil by injection because it is more slowly absorbed and has a longer lasting effect. Its prolonged use has not been shown to produce heart damage. The drug has an immediate beneficial effect. However, it has a tendency to produce side reactions such as palpitation, nervousness, insomnia, blanching of the skin, and other disturbing symptoms. Since it may exaggerate or precipitate heart pain in already existing heart disease, it must be employed with caution in such instances.

Ephedrine has much the same effect as adrenalin. It has the added advantage of being more stable and can be taken by mouth in the form of capsules. Because it has powerful side effects, especially because it produces nervousness and sleeplessness, it is given in conjunction with one of the sedative drugs. There are, in addition, a host of other drugs related or derived from adrenalin and ephedrine. These may also be used as drops or by injection. A few are "Neosynephrin," "Propadrine," "Privine," "Paredrine," "Benzedrine" and others. These are marketed in various strengths and are supplied occasionally mixed with antibiotics such as penicillin and others to be used intranasally when there is local associated infection. These should be used sparingly and always only on the prescription of a physician.

ACTH and cortisone are valuable additions to the drug armamentarium. They are employed in acute emergencies, such as severe asthma and allergic dermatitis that has not responded to usual treatment. These hormones should not be taken routinely. Careful examination is necessary before their administration. The presence of stomach ulcer, tuberculosis, acne, furunculosis, and certain mental and emotional disorders contraindicates the prescribing of these products. Since certain side reactions may occur and since some of these may be serious, the person is kept under observation while ACTH or cortisone are given. The patient's weight, blood pressure, blood, and other studies are followed. After such a period of observation, these hormones may be taken at home as maintenance treatment. In many instances these drugs are lifesaving and will tide the patient over an acute fulminating stage of the disease. They are, however, not a substitute for careful and adequate investigation of the allergic patient.

Sedatives are frequently necessary. The choice of the proper drug is important in this connection. "Aminophyllin" is occasionally prescribed in the form of rectal suppositories and is useful in the treatment of asthma. Iodides form the basis for an old and useful remedy in the treatment of asthma. The drug helps in loosening of the cough and aids in liquefying the sputum so the patient has less difficulty in bringing it up. Oxygen may be necessary in severe asthma. If infection is present in the nose or chest, the physician may wish to give the patient antibiotics. Some of these may produce allergic and other undesirable symptoms. Many other drugs are used with various success in the treatment of allergic symptoms. They are employed, however, only as adjuncts and only to help tide the patient over the acute manifestations of his allergy. The basic and most useful form of treatment consists in discovering the source of the patient's allergy and removing it as thoroughly as possible from the patient's environment.

Many so-called cures, many quackeries and nostrums have been advocated and promoted to the public, from time to time. These, for the most part, are advanced by unscrupulous money-seeking agents. The medical profession can only warn the patient that most of these products are not only useless and ineffective, but are actually harmful because they give patients a false sense of security. Furthermore, they invariably and inevitably lead to disillusionment and the neglect of early proper treatment, neglect which breeds needless complications and structural irreversible changes in the affected organs. If you suffer with an allergic condition, you should consult your family physician and ask him to refer you to a board certified, well-trained internist or pediatrician who is qualified in allergy. Do not listen to what your friends and neighbors advise. They are ill-equipped to give you responsible, helpful information. Only your physician should be the source of such help.

OTHER SKIN TESTS

One form of bacterial allergy is sensitivity to tuberculin. Patients who have had tuberculosis become allergic to the products of growth of the tubercle bacillus. For this reason when these patients are skin tested with tuberculin they will give a positive reaction or a positive test. This is being used as one of the diagnostic aids for tuberculosis.

Skin tests are used also in the practice of medicine for the diagnosis of many conditions. Among these may be mentioned infestations with echinococcus, trichinosis, and other worms. These tests are used in many mycotic diseases, that is where molds are involved in producing actually a diseased condition; also for the diagnosis of tularemia and of undulant fever. Skin tests are also used to determine the presence of immunity to diphtheria toxin, namely the Schick tests; or, to determine by the so-called Dick test the presence of immunity to scarlet fever.

HOMOGRAFT REJECTION

Another type of allergic response deals with the phenomenon of rejection of a skin or organ transplant. Normally, if one transfers a small piece of skin from one part of the body of a patient to another part of the body of the same individual the skin graft will "take" and will become part of the local tissues. However, transplantation of tissues such as skin from one individual to another (homograft) is characterized by a transient "take" of the transplant. This "take" lasts for several days and then it sloughs off and is discarded. The reason for this rejection is the production of antibodies against the transplanted skin in the recipient. The only exception to homograft rejection is in the case of identical twins or of uniovular twins and twins in cattle. A great many attempts have been made to transfer not only skin but actually organs such as lung or kidney from one person to another. Except in instances of kidney transplants in identical twins most of these procedures have not been successful. Surgery has made tremendous progress in the development of technical skills. Difficulty with this type of surgery is not lack of progress and development of surgical technique, but lack of means or procedures which one can employ to prevent the production of antibodies and the reaction of the antibodies thus produced in the patient receiving the graft against the organ grafted. In this connection X-radiation and various drugs intended to suppress immunologic mechanisms have also been used.

AUTOIMMUNITY

Still another field of interest in clinical immunology is the group of diseases referred to as autoimmune diseases. Normally, the body does not react with the production of antibodies against its own tissues. This is referred to as a "recognition of self." However, as soon as tissue or a protein is introduced into the body which is foreign, then antibodies are formed, the purpose of these being to fight off the invader. Apparently under a given set of conditions certain body tissues or components of organs become affected by infection or other influences so that they also become antigenic and produce antibodies. Under these circumstances disease processes will occur in those organs. Examples of autoimmune diseases are thyroiditis, certain reactions to Pasteur rabies vaccine, conditions involving the eye and a group of diseases which involve destruction of red blood cells, platelets, and white blood cells. Evidence indicates that diseases such as rheumatic fever, rheumatoid arthritis, systemic lupus erythematosus, and polyarteritis nodosa may be autoimmune or allergic diseases. This field is rapidly expanding because of the tremendous amount of research work which is being done in this connection.

CHAPTER 22

Endocrinology
The Gland Conditions

SHELDON S. WALDSTEIN, M.D.

The activities of the living body are carried on through a multitude of chemical reactions. Growth, development, reproduction, locomotion, thinking, communication, repair of injury—all the attributes of life and of living appear to be reducible ultimately to chemical terms. By a series of interrelated chemical events the foodstuffs we ingest are transformed within the body into basic chemical compounds which are then used as the building blocks for structural material and the sources of energy. Such chemical events, described in general by the term *metabolism,* are facilitated by a number of diverse enzymes. Among the mechanisms which provide for the coordination of these intricate processes are the *hormones.* Hormones can be thought of as chemical substances which regulate the chemistry of the body for the orderly achievement of biological purposes.

Understanding of the role of the hormones is a relatively modern development. Centuries ago removal of the testes was recognized to profoundly affect the sexual characteristics of males, both of lower animals and man. Investigation of this phenomenon was sporadic and incomplete until the middle of the nineteenth century. By this time, experiments in animals had shown that although removal of the testes severs their nerve connections to the body, regrafting them immediately into another part of the body prevents the usual changes of castration. Such studies led to the realization that the effects of castration are due to chemical changes rather than nervous mechanisms. By the turn of the century, the great English physiologists Starling and Bayliss developed the general theory that the glands of the endocrine system regulate other parts of the body by producing chemical compounds which are circulated by the blood to the tissues, where their effects occur. They coined the term "hormone" for such chemical messengers. (The word is derived from a Greek word meaning to stimulate or to excite.)

An organ which releases (secretes) a chemical substance is called a gland. The word "endocrine" means internal secretion, that is, secretion directly into the blood stream. Thus, the organs which secrete hormones are known as endocrine glands since they release their products directly into the blood. This is by contrast to the exocrine glands or glands of external secretion which secrete their products through ducts (tubes) rather than into the blood stream. Structures which serve to remove the poisonous materials of infections from the lymphatic vessels have been called the lymphatic glands. These often become enlarged during infections. Such structures should be termed lymph nodes, not glands.

For coordination of the metabolic processes, the nervous system is also vitally important. However, the accomplishment of this end by action of the nervous system differs from that by the endocrine system in several ways. First, nerve action begins and ends abruptly, whereas hormone action is best adapted to long-sustained effects. Second, nerve impulses are directed to a few places at one time, limiting the results to certain parts of the body. Hormones are distributed to all tissues alike, and the responses depend on the capacities of various tissues to act under such stimulation. Third, nerve impulses may set in motion processes which were previously dormant, or stop completely action which had been going on. Hormones act to accelerate or to slow down processes which are already going on, but they do not start new processes. In some respects this action may be compared to lubrication of machinery so that it will run more swiftly and easily. Thus, both nerves and endocrine glands are involved in the orderly correlation of the processes of life, but each system has its special functions.

A natural question concerns the links between the two systems, by which their separate functions are made to fit appropriately together. The details of such interactions are not well understood. Certain portions of the brain appear to influence the function of the pituitary gland, and through it, the function of other glands. Emotion and mental stress can alter the degree of hormone secretion of several endocrine organs. Excess or deficiency of one of several of the hormones may cause nerve or mental disorders. The hormones are concerned with the more primitive biological processes, such as keeping warm, mustering reserves to meet emergencies for defense, and making sure of the reproduction of the species, in addition to the controls on the use of sugar, protein, and fat foods, and the balance of salts and water in the body. Since our mental state depends to such a large extent on our comfort, sense of security, and the satisfactions of our several appetites, the activity of the endocrine glands has important consequences on our mental and emotional life.

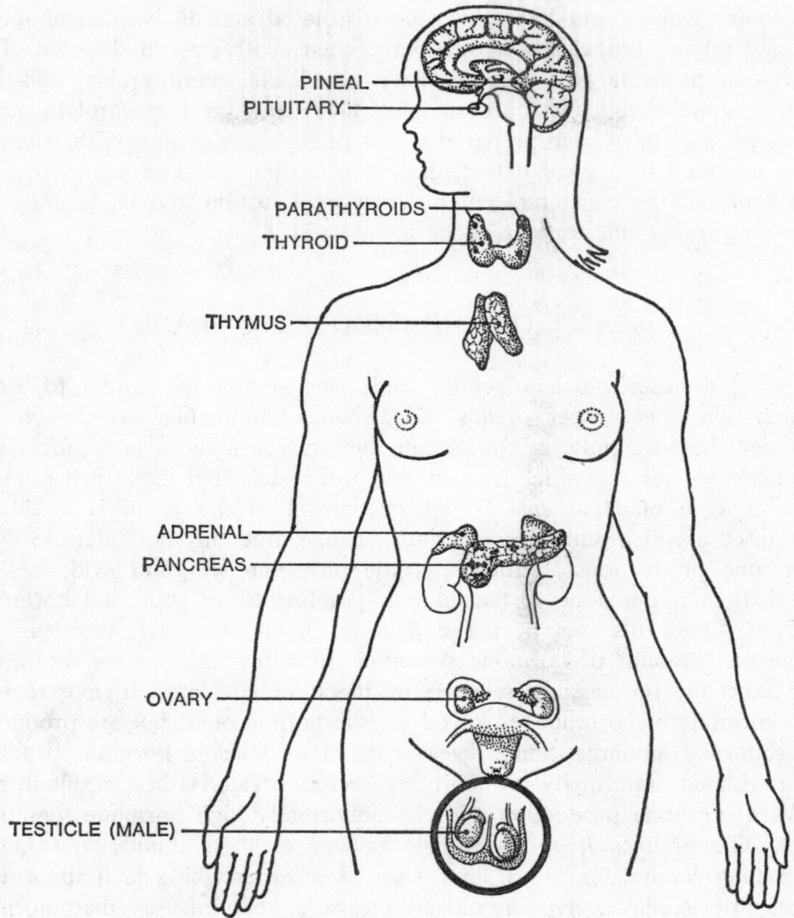

Fig. 53. A most significant change in glandular functions occurs at the age of puberty. The hypothalamus, a structure in the brain, and the hypothysis or pituitary gland, which it controls, appear to be less concerned with growth of the body than they are with the secretion of the sex hormones. Illustration by Lou Barlow.

The endocrine glands are the pituitary, the thyroid, the adrenals, the testes, the ovaries, the pancreas, and the parathyroids. During the present century remarkable progress has been made in endocrinology, as in other areas of modern medical knowledge, because of the close cooperation in research between physicians, biologists, and chemists. Up to World War II, chemists had discovered how to make synthetically six of the hormone products of the body. In the postwar years progress has been even more rapid and a number of natural hormones, particularly those of the thyroid, adrenals, ovaries, and testes have been isolated and analyzed, and many closely related artificial hormones have been synthesized and tested. The hormone products from the pituitary gland, the parathyroids, and the pancreas are chemically more complex, since they are large protein products, yet they have been prepared with a high degree of purity, their structure analyzed to a great extent, and even partial synthesis achieved. The discovery of the exact molecular structure of insulin and its recent synthesis represent milestones in endocrine chemistry.

DISEASES OF THE ENDOCRINE GLANDS

Some diseases which affect the endocrine glands are similar to those which can affect other organs of the body. Inflammations, infections, deficient blood supply, non-malignant tumors (swellings), and cancer are examples of disease which may involve this specialized tissue just as they may involve other organs. If only a portion of the gland is involved, the disease will produce an anatomic change, but may not interfere with hormone production. In this case, the physician will find evidences of local disease, but none of the findings pointing to an abnormal hormone output. Other diseases of the endocrine glands, however, result in an abnormal amount of hormone secretion. In a few instances, a hormone not normally produced is released by the diseased gland. In most cases, the hormone or hormones involved are the normal ones, but are produced in abnormal amounts. Some diseases result in deficient hormone production with an abnormally low hormone-secretion rate. Others result in excessive hormone production with an abnormally high hormone secretion rate. The prefixes *hypo* (meaning "under" or "less than") and *hyper* (meaning "above" or "more than") are used in describing such abnormalities. For example, hypothyroidism means a state of less than normal thyroid function, and hyperthyroidism means a state of more than normal thyroid function.

HORMONE DEFICIENCIES

A deficiency or excess of a given hormone will usually produce characteristic symptoms and physical changes which the physician skilled in endocrinology can recognize. Of course, these changes vary in degree depending particularly upon the severity of the disturbance and the length of time it has existed. Many physiological and biochemical changes also occur which can be detected by appropriate tests. Several types of tests are used to confirm diagnoses or assess results of treatment. It is possible, for example, to measure with great accuracy some of the hor-

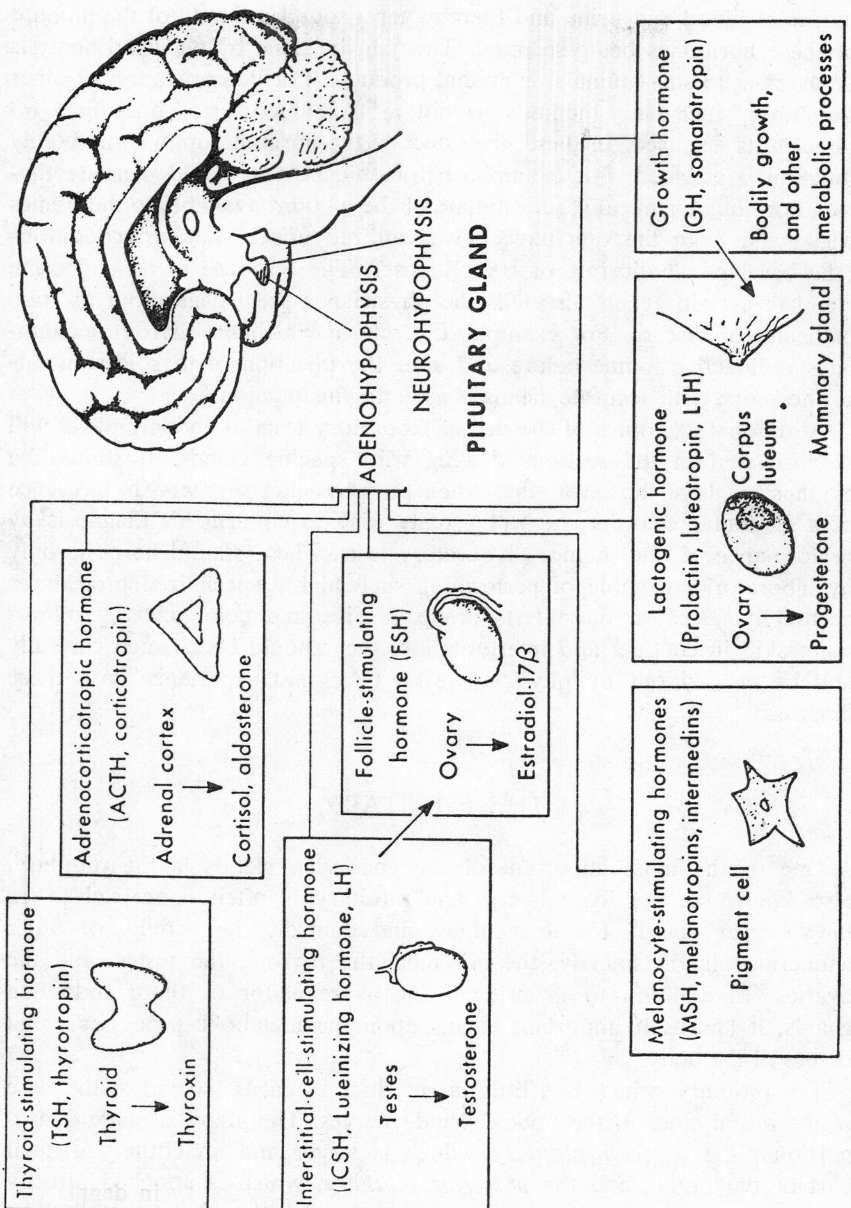

Fig. 54. Diagrammatic Summary of the Biologic Properties of Adenohypophyseal Hormones. This illustration shows how the pituitary gland is responsible for stimulating the activities of other cells and glands in the body. *Bulletin of The New York Academy of Medicine*, March 1963, paper by Dr. Choh Hao Li.

mones in blood and urine and thereby get a sound estimate of the amount of these hormones being secreted. This can be done by chemical analysis or by assays using animals or animal products. For determination of other hormones, since assay methods are not yet developed for all hormones, indirect tests are used. In these, the effect of the hormone upon some bodily function is assessed. For example, before biochemists could measure thyroid hormone chemically, an estimate of the amount available to the tissues was made from the rate oxygen was utilized under standard conditions (the basal metabolic rate or B.M.R. test). The response of an endocrine gland to certain agents also tells the physician a great deal about its state of health or disease. For example, the rate at which the thyroid accumulates radioactive iodine before and after the injection of thyroid-stimulating hormone is an accurate means of assessing its function.

Additional examples of the use of laboratory tests in endocrinology will be discussed in the sections dealing with specific glands. It should be emphasized here, however, that when the physician suspects the presence of a glandular disorder, he will usually wish to confirm his diagnosis by performance of one or more laboratory tests. These should be done only by laboratories capable of performing such highly specialized procedures accurately. Because these tests are expensive and complicated, and require skill in conduct and interpretation, they should be selected carefully and be carried out by physicians who have had experience with these diseases.

THE PITUITARY

One of the most important of the endocrine glands is the pituitary, also known as the hypophysis. The pituitary is often conceived to be the "master gland" for it regulates and controls the activity of other endocrine glands, namely, the adrenals, the thyroid, the testes, and the ovaries. In addition to its critical role as regulator of these endocrine glands, it has itself important effects upon the metabolic processes of all tissues of the body.

The pituitary, which is a little larger than a pea, is located at the base of the brain, close to the optic (visual) nerves. The gland is made of two portions: the *anterior pituitary,* which is larger and an entirely distinct part of the organ, and the *posterior pituitary,* which is attached directly to the brain by nerve connections passing through the pituitary stalk. The intimate association of the pituitary and the brain apparently is important to the coordination of the nervous system and the endocrine system. Recent evidence indicates that the adjacent portion of the brain (known as the hypothalamus) directs anterior pituitary hormone release by chemical means (releasing factors), as well as by nerve impulses. The pituitary responds by varying the amount of the regulator hormones it secretes.

These regulator hormones are called *tropic hormones* or *tropins* and are named for the endocrine gland which is affected. Thyrotropic hormone (thyrotropin, TSH) regulates the thyroid gland; *a*drenocorticotropic *h*ormone (corticotropin, ACTH) regulates the adrenal cortex, and gonadotropic hormones (gonadotropins) regulate the testes in man or the ovaries in woman. Tropins cause increased hormone secretion. For example, when ACTH is secreted by the pituitary, the adrenal cortex is stimulated to secrete its hormones. When secretion of ACTH is decreased, the adrenal decreases its hormone output. By a delicately controlled series of checks and balances, the pituitary directs the other endocrine glands to maintain the appropriate blood levels of their hormones.

In addition to secretion of tropic hormones, the anterior pituitary also secretes hormones which affect the tissues directly without the mediation of other endocrine glands. These include growth hormone, which regulates body growth in general, a hormone which controls the amount of pigmentation of the skin, and a hormone which stimulates secretion of milk after delivery of a baby. Through the interaction of the various hormones of the pituitary, there are also effects on the metabolism of sugar and of fat.

The hormones of the pituitary, like those of the pancreas and parathyroid, are proteins. Proteins are chemically made of many subunits, called amino acids, strung together to form large and complex molecules. Most mammals have been found to have essentially the same hormones as man. However, there appears to be some difference among animal species in the *exact* chemical composition of the protein hormones, including those of the pituitary. For some hormones, such as ACTH and thyrotropin, the differences between species are so minor, that hormone derived from one is effective in another. Thus, ACTH extracted from the pituitaries of slaughterhouse animals is suitable for human use. This is fortunate because ACTH has important medicinal uses (*See* section on Adrenals). Its availability from animal sources assures an ample supply. Growth hormone is more nearly species specific. By this is meant that its action is limited to one or a few closely related species of animals, and that it is ineffective in more distant species. This is probably due to more definite differences in chemical structure. Thus, growth hormone extracted from pituitaries of slaughterhouse animals has little or no effect in man, although the hormone extracted from apes has considerable effectiveness. Growth hormone extracted from human pituitaries is fully effective in humans. The supply of growth hormone for human use is sharply limited, the source being deceased donors, but it is possible that chemists in the future will learn how to synthesize it or at least how to alter the species specific portion, so that hormone derived from animals can be used in humans.

DISEASES OF THE ANTERIOR PITUITARY

The stimulation of growth by the anterior pituitary is one of its best known functions, though the exact manner in which this action is effected is still not fully understood. Normal growth and development is a complex process in which most of the endocrine glands participate. This will be discussed in greater detail later. The prime importance of growth hormone, however, is apparent from the fact that, if growth hormone is deficient, the child grows much too slowly and he remains dwarfed throughout life. If there is no other abnormality, the body of a *pituitary dwarf* is well-proportioned and his intelligence is normal. Often, however, persons with pituitary dwarfism have deficiencies of other pituitary hormones as well and, therefore, have disturbed function of several endocrine glands, for which treatment is required. Within recent years purified human growth hormone has been tried in children who are suffering from pituitary dwarfism. The hormone must be given by injections. Its effects appear slowly, and treatment must be continued for many years if accomplishments are to be significant. Obviously treatment needs to be directed by a physician who knows what to expect of the procedure, and when it should be stopped. The supplies of human growth hormone are limited, but when available, this hormone has proven to be effective treatment for this condition.

If, however, the growth hormone is secreted by the pituitary in excessive amounts, the stature increases faster than normal, and the person will be unusually tall, or even a "giant." If the excess secretion of growth hormone does not begin until after maturity, the height will not be increased because the bones no longer have a capacity for growing longer. But the bones will grow thicker, and the head, hand, and foot sizes grow larger. The features become coarse, the tongue large, and all the internal organs increase in size. This rare condition is called *acromegaly*. It is usually due to a tumor (or enlargement) in the anterior pituitary which is producing excessive amounts of growth hormone. Sometimes this has to be removed surgically, but in other patients it is possible to stop the overproduction of hormone with powerful X-ray treatments.

Pituitary tumors also occur which do not secrete hormones. They share one important feature with those tumors which cause acromegaly: being immediately in contact with the optic nerves passing from the eyes to the brain, they may press on these nerves and damage vision. Especially for this reason any pituitary tumor deserves prompt and expert treatment. Even if damage to the optic nerves does not occur, untreated pituitary tumors may enlarge to the point where they crowd out the normal pituitary cells. This results in loss of pituitary hormone secretion. Another cause for loss of pituitary function is destruction of pituitary tissue by infection or by loss of its blood supply. Destruction of sufficient pituitary tissue leads to a condition known as *hypopituitarism* (underfunction of the pituitary), wherein the symptoms and physical changes are caused by lack of normal amounts of pituitary hormones. Deficiency of the gonadotropins or hormones which stimulate the sex glands results in declining sex function in men and cessation of menstrual periods in women. ACTH deficiency results in shrinkage of the adrenals with symptoms of adrenal deficiency (*See* section on Adrenals). In like manner, deficiency of the tropic hormone to the thyroid results in the shrinkage of this gland and symptoms of thyroid deficiency (*See* section on the Thyroid). Children with hypopituitarism also suffer from the loss of growth hormone and consequently are dwarfed. In adults, the loss of growth hormone which occurs with hypopituitarism is not reflected in change in stature, for once grown the body does not shrink. But growth hormone deficiency may account for the tendency for the skin to wrinkle, the muscles to become flabby and weak, and for weight to be lost in this disease.

To establish the diagnosis of anterior pituitary disease, the physician takes X rays of the skull bones which surround the pituitary in order to detect the presence of tumors. Examination of the visual fields helps to detect encroachment of tumors on the optic nerves. Tests of the function of the sex glands, the adrenals, and the thyroid gland are made to detect deficiency of the tropic hormones. These studies require specialized laboratory facilities. Although hypopituitarism may be treated by daily injections of preparations of pituitary tropic hormones, this method is uncomfortable for the patient, expensive, and not really practical. Instead, the sex hormones, adrenal hormones, and thyroid hormone can be supplied in the form of pills taken by mouth daily. This therapy is inexpensive, convenient, can be maintained throughout life, and the results are quite satisfactory.

THE POSTERIOR PITUITARY

The posterior pituitary is supplied with a large number of nerve fibers, originating in a part of the brain which is concerned with the unconscious regulation of temperature, weight, water retention, sleep, and muscular coordination, as well as of emotional activity. If these nerve fibers are severed, the posterior pituitary will atrophy and be inactive. In this case, or if the posterior pituitary is destroyed by a tumor or injury, a condition follows called *diabetes insipidus*. The term is used because of the passage of large amounts of urine (*diabetes* means to "run through" and the word *insipidus* means the urine lacks the sweet taste of sugar, in contrast to the urine voided by a diabetic of the mellitus type). The posterior pituitary secretes a hormone which stimulates the kidneys to conserve water by the formation of concentrated urine. The supply of this hormone is increased whenever the blood begins to become concentrated by the loss of water. In the person with diabetes insipidus this regulatory mechanism is inadequate. The kidneys continue to excrete water until the blood is seriously concentrated. Before genuine danger occurs, a second line of defense is set into motion: conscious thirst appears and compels the person to drink more water. Of course this avoids damage to the body, but at the expense of unusually frequent drinking and unduly frequent voiding of urine. Diabetes insipidus can be kept under control by the use of extracts of the posterior pituitary, which may be injected hypodermically from one to four times daily as required to avoid frequent passage of urine. Fortunately this hormone may also be absorbed through the lining of the nose, although it is destroyed if swallowed. Pituitary glands that have been dried and ground to a fine powder have been used as a snuff a few times a day to control the loss of water. Recently, the hormone from the posterior pituitary has been prepared synthetically. A few sprays into the nose of a solution of the synthetic preparation several times a day has been shown also to afford effective control. This method of treatment undoubtedly will be popular in the future. Treatment must be continued indefinitely.

THE THYROID

The thyroid is a U-shaped gland which lies in the lower front portion of the neck on either side of the windpipe, crossing it just below the Adam's apple (the cartilage which encloses the larynx or voice box). Ordinarily, the normal thyroid is so small as to fit beneath the neck muscles without being seen. Normally, the gland can be barely felt where it crosses the windpipe, or it may not be felt at all. If the thyroid becomes enlarged so that it is visible and can be felt easily, it is called a *goiter*. The term goiter is applied to any enlarged thyroid gland. Several types of goiter are known which have different causes and different significance for health. Therefore, occurrence of a goiter should lead one to seek medical examination to determine its cause and to decide whether treatment is necessary.

The thyroid gland is regulated by the thyroid stimulating hormone (TSH, or thyrotropin) of the anterior pituitary. This tropic hormone stimulates the thyroid to secrete *thyroid hormone* (*thyroxin*). When there are normal amounts of thyroid hormone circulating to the tissues, the pituitary secretes normal amounts of TSH. When there are insufficient amounts of circulating thyroxin, the pituitary releases large amounts of TSH in an attempt to stimulate the thyroid. This causes the thyroid to enlarge, as well as to increase its manufacture of hormone. When an excess of thyroid hormone circulates, the pituitary slows down its output of TSH, and the thyroid decreases its manufacture of thyroxin and tends to get smaller.

GOITER

Simple goiter, which is an enlargement of the thyroid gland without a disturbance of its net hormone output, is often caused by a deficient supply of iodine in the food and drink. Iodine is an indispensable element used by the thyroid to manufacture its hormone. Not more than 0.05 mg. of iodine per day is required for this purpose. (A drop of water weighs 1300 times this much.) In most parts of the world, ordinary water and food provide more than this small amount of iodine and goiter is infrequent. In certain regions remote from the sea, particularly high mountainous areas, surface and well water and locally grown plant and animal food are markedly deficient in iodine content. In the United States, the glaciated region of the Great Lakes is iodine deficient and goiter formerly occurred with great frequency. The explanation for the occurrence of this type of goiter seems to be that deficiency of iodine decreases the amount of thyroxin manufactured. The low output of thyroxin results in secretion of large amounts of TSH by the pituitary. The gland enlarges, under this influence, and traps avidly whatever small amounts of iodine become available. Thus, the thyroid is able to make sufficient thyroid hormone only by becoming larger. Because this type of goiter is usually uniformly enlarged, it is also known as a diffuse goiter.

Since the relationship of goiter to iodine deficiency was recognized, it has been possible to prevent the occurrence of this disturbance simply by furnishing iodine. This can be done by providing the element as a medicine at regular intervals, such as daily or for a few days each week. The thyroid gland is able to store iodine for periods of weeks to months and to draw on this reservoir as needed. Introduction of iodine into the municipal water supply has not been utilized because it is uneconomical. The most practical means has been the introduction of iodine into table salt. Iodized table salt as a source of supply has a number of features to recommend it. It is used principally for human food; it is used by almost everyone; the iodine content of the salt can be determined with ease; and the cost is very small. When iodized salt is used in the home, all members of the family including infants and children will receive enough iodine in their food to prevent iodine-deficient goiter. Therefore, iodized salt should be used in those geographic areas where iodine deficiency and goiter are known to be common. With the advent of nationwide transportation of foods, many foods consumed in goiter areas have actually originated in regions with ample iodine. Thus, iodine deficiency and iodine deficient goiter are declining.

During periods of rapid growth, the body requires more than the usual amount of thyroid hormone. Such an increased need may exist also at other times, as during severe infections or during pregnancy. Under such circumstances the need for iodine is also increased and the physician may wish to prescribe some form of iodine to meet the temporarily increased demand.

Not all goiter is due to simple iodine lack. In many people beyond the age of thirty, the gland gradually enlarges and develops many irregularities and nodules (lumps). The reasons for the occurrence of *multinodular goiter* with advancing age are not yet fully understood. Episodes of iodine deficiency followed by ample supplies, so that the thyroid is stimulated to enlarge, then shrink, then enlarge repeatedly, may explain some. In others, factors which impair thyroxin manufacture at irregular intervals may play a role. In some patients, by a succession of changes not well understood, a single local area of the thyroid enlarges, forming a benign tumor mass, known as a *solitary nodule* or *adenoma.* Uncommonly *cancer of the thyroid* may occur. There is no definite relation between nodular goiter and cancer of the thyroid. However, since cancer begins in a localized area, the physician may be unable to distinguish between a benign, solitary adenoma and early cancer. In this situation, it is often advisable to remove the nodule surgically so that microscopic examination can determine with certainty whether it is benign or cancerous.

Besides being unsightly, both diffuse and multinodular goiters may become large enough to cause discomfort when collars are worn, or to cause pressure on the windpipe or to disturb swallowing. Therefore, goiters should not be neglected when small. Treatment with iodine or with thyroxin may prevent some small goiters from becoming larger, and occasionally may cause the goiter to shrink. The effect of these medications on any particular goiter is not easy to predict and medical guidance is important for adequate dosage, discrimination as to which patient should be treated, and the decision as to other treatment. If the goiter has become large enough to cause pressure symptoms, surgical removal may be necessary.

Goiter also may be produced by inflammation. This condition is called *thyroiditis.* In one form of thyroiditis, the goiter occurs abruptly and is painful and tender. This type of inflammation which may be caused by bacteria, by viruses, or by other agents tends to subside spontaneously, but also has a tendency to recur for several episodes. Eventually the disease disappears and the thyroid becomes normal. When pain and tenderness are severe, the physician may prescribe cortisone or other medication to hasten the subsidence of the inflammation. A second type of thyroiditis is a chronic condition which leads over a period of months to years to a firm, often large goiter. Eventually, the function of the thyroid gland may be destroyed. Treatment of chronic thyroiditis often includes thyroxin in order to replace the amounts of hormone the diseased gland fails to manufacture.

Because not all goiters are the simple type, the patient should seek medical attention whenever a localized lump or diffuse enlargement of the thyroid gland appears. Only the physician, on the basis of his examination and on the basis of the results of laboratory tests of thyroid function, can determine with certainty whether the goiter is due to iodine lack or whether it is one of the other types of goiters. He can then decide whether the proper treatment is with medicine or whether surgical intervention is necessary to remove the goiter.

EXOPHTHALMIC GOITER—THYROTOXICOSIS

A common disorder of the thyroid gland is that in which a goiter is associated with overproduction of thyroxin with the development of symptoms and physical changes due to the excessive amounts of the hormone. This disorder is called by a variety of names. One is *exophthalmic goiter* because of the frequent though not universal association of protrusion of the eyeballs (exophthalmos). Another is *hyperthyroidism* meaning the thyroid gland is overactive and producing more than the normal amount of its hormone. It is called *thyrotoxicosis* or *toxic goiter* because the symptoms are the same as if the patient were poisoned with an excessively large dose of thyroid. The disease has also been called by the names of the men in various countries who first recognized its nature.

Hyperthyroidism is most common in young and middle-aged adults, particularly women, but it has occurred in early infancy and childhood and as late as the ninth decade of life. The symptoms of thyrotoxicosis are produced by the excess thyroid hormone. Thyroid hormone stimulates the rate at which the metabolic processes of the body occur. When there is excess thyroid hormone, the over-all rate of metabolism is accelerated. As a result, the patient loses weight despite an increased appetite, which is often voracious. There is a feeling of nervousness and increased muscular activity. The hands shake. The heart accelerates and the patient is often aware of palpitations. The person cannot tolerate heat, complains of warm weather, and sweats a great deal. Frequent bowel movements may occur. Women may have menstrual irregularities. Often there is an anxious look and the eyes appear to be bulging or actually protrude. If the disease is not far advanced, the physician may have difficulty distinguishing between an early case of thyrotoxicosis and simply an unstable nervous system. Under these circumstances, great care must be exercised in making the diagnosis. The physician will confirm the hyperactivity of the thyroid gland by measurements of the accumulation of radioactive iodine by the thyroid gland, the blood protein-bound iodine (PBI), and the basal metabolism rate. When these tests of thyroid function show increased activity, the physician can diagnose hyperthyroidism with certainty.

Treatment of patients with toxic goiter is most important because this condition may cause serious damage to the heart, the central nervous system and other systems of the body. In recent years, treatment has been simplified considerably. Formerly, the only treatment was the surgical removal of about nine-tenths of the thyroid gland. Although this was effective, it necessitated a major surgical procedure with the risk of certain complications of the surgery in a small per cent of cases. Then physicians found it possible to block the formation of thyroid hormone by the use of any one of several drugs, thereby inducing a remission of the thyrotoxicosis. The most common drug employed is propylthiouracil. In some patients, particularly young children, a remission may be maintained by such medical means for months to years, and eventually a permanent cure of the disease achieved. In other instances, propylthiouracil or a similar drug is used to bring about improvement in the hyperthyroidism so that surgical removal of the gland is safer, with fewer complications. This is a form of treatment which is particularly used for adolescents and young adults. Such drugs occasionally cause reactions, so it is important that they be used only under the supervision of a physician.

Today, most toxic goiter patients above the age of twenty-five are treated with radioactive iodine. Radioactive iodine is handled by the body in the same manner as ordinary iodine. It is quickly collected in the thyroid gland after it has been administered, where the radioactivity delivers a destructive dose of radiation to the thyroid cells. By careful measurement of the dose of radioactive iodine, an overactive, enlarged gland may be reduced to one that is normal in size and function. The destruction is entirely painless and occurs in six to twelve weeks. After successful treatment with radioiodine, the goiter shrinks gradually. Occasionally, second or third courses of treatment are necessary. During this treatment, however, the patient is able to be up and about and hospitalization is not necessary. This method was first employed about 1945 and is now known to be effective and safe. It has largely replaced surgery for the treatment of thyrotoxicosis in the adult. Such treatment should be undertaken only by a physician who has special training in the use of radioactive materials, and particularly radioactive iodine.

HYPOTHYROIDISM

In a small proportion of cases, after operation or after radioactive iodine treatment, the remaining thyroid tissue is found inadequate to meet the body's needs for thyroid hormone. This occurs in about eight per cent of patients. In these, a condition will develop gradually which is known as *hypothyroidism,* that is, the state of deficiency of thyroid hormone secretion.

Hypothyroidism may also occur spontaneously. Children may be born without adequate thyroid tissue to maintain normal growth and development. Unless these children are recognized and are treated promptly, their growth and development will be severely retarded and a feebleminded dwarf of the type known as a *cretin* will develop. Some children have sufficient amount of thyroid tissue to grow normally for the first few years, but thyroid tissue may not be sufficient to keep up with the growing body later in development. A condition known as *juvenile myxedema* develops. In the adult, hypothyroidism with *adult myxedema* may appear as a result of chronic thyroiditis or as a result of gradual shrinkage and disappearance of the thyroid due to unknown cause. The term myxedema refers to a curious accumulation of a material beneath the skin and in other tissues, which gives a swollen appearance to the face and the extremities, resembling in some respects edema or dropsy.

The patient with hypothyroidism manifests symptoms and physical changes explainable by a slowing of the metabolic processes because of the lack of normal amounts of thyroxin. Sluggishness is the outstanding symptom. Movements, mental processes, and speech are slow. The voice is coarse and froglike because of myxedema of the vocal cords. The patient is intolerant of cold and may wear sweaters or sleep under covers even in warm weather. The heart rate is slow and bowel action may be so sluggish as to lead to severe constipation and even bowel obstruction. The physician can confirm the clinical findings by finding a low metabolic rate, a low protein bound iodine, and the virtual absence of accumulation of radioactive iodine by the thyroid gland when a tracer dose is given.

The specific treatment for any of these forms of hypothyroidism is the daily administration of tablets of dried thyroid, made from the thyroids of slaughterhouse animals. These tablets contain not only the active hormone, thyroxin itself, but a variety of other substances which are inactive. Recently, chemists have been able to produce pure thyroxin. These products are not destroyed by the digestive tract and, therefore, may be taken by mouth. The effects occur slowly. Results of a daily dose become increasingly evident during succeeding months of continued treatment. The patient being treated for hypothyroidism should take such replacement doses of thyroid hormone for the remainder of his life. If he does, he can be returned to an entirely normal state. He should, therefore, be under the continuous care of a physician so that evaluation of his status can be made and adjustment of dosage made whenever necessary.

TESTS OF THYROID FUNCTION

The basal metabolism test is a method for measuring how much oxygen the person uses per hour. The person breathes through a closed system in which the decrease in the amount of air is due to the consumption of oxygen by the tissues of the subject. From the rate oxygen is consumed in the short period of the test, the oxygen consumption per hour is calculated. When there is an inadequate supply of thyroid hormone, the rate of oxygen use is reduced and the basal metabolism rate may be as much as 40 per cent below the normal for the age, height, and weight of the person. When there is an excessive amount of thyroid hormone, the rate of oxygen use is much exaggerated and the basal metabolism rate may be as much as 80 to 90 per cent above normal for the age, height, and weight of the person tested. As a diagnostic test, the basal metabolism test is not infallible. Not only do other diseases affect it, but it is subject to distortion by excitement of the subject and by errors in the preparation for or the conduct of the test. Such tests should be conducted only by trained personnel and only after careful explanation to the patient of the way in which his cooperation is required. The test is most useful for following the course of treatment. After taking the test for one or two or more times, the patient becomes quite used to it and the values obtained become more accurate. In hyperthyroidism under treatment, a decrease in the metabolic rate is a good measure of the progress being made in the treatment. In hypothyroidism, the test helps the physician to judge the amount of thyroid hormone treatment to be given and the adjustment of dose necessary from time to time.

Determination of the blood protein-bound iodine (PBI) requires a special laboratory, but from the patient's standpoint, the test is simple, since the physician merely has to draw a sample of blood. Although a number of substances may interfere with the accuracy of the test, under usual circumstances the level of protein-bound iodine estimates accurately the amount of thyroid hormone circulating, and helps the physician evaluate thyroid function and judge the efficacy of treatment. As hyperthyroidism comes under control, the protein-bound iodine which was previously high will decrease toward normal, and as hypothyroidism is treated adequately with thyroid, the previously low values of protein-bound iodine will increase towards normal.

Determination of the uptake of radioactive iodine by the thyroid gland is a direct measure of how well the thyroid gland is able to function. A number of substances may interfere with the accumulation of iodine by the thyroid gland. Most common is excess iodine itself. Large amounts of iodine are found in cough mixtures and various patent medicines. When interfering substances are not present, however, the radioactive iodine test is one of the most accurate and most useful measurements of thyroid function. The test is quite simple. The patient is given a small amount of radioactive iodine to take orally. This may be contained in a small capsule or a colorless and tasteless water solution. The amount taken for a tracer test is so small as to be undetectable chemically and does not represent any radiation hazard whatsoever to the patient. Tiny infants may safely be given tracer doses of radioactive iodine. At an interval after the ingestion of radioactive iodine, most commonly in twenty-four hours, the patient returns to the laboratory where a radiation detector counts the amount of radioactivity contained within the thyroid. This is a measure of the iodine which has been trapped by the gland. When the gland is overactive as in toxic goiter, the amount of iodine trapped is far in excess of normal. When the gland is underactive as in myxedema, far less than normal amounts are found in the thyroid. The test is simple to conduct and can be used repeatedly to follow the state of thyroid function.

THE ADRENAL GLANDS

The adrenal glands are a pair of small structures placed just on top of the kidneys, and made of two different types of tissue. The outer layers of these glands are so important that death may occur in a few days if they are destroyed or removed. However, the inner portion of these glands are not essential. This portion, called the *medulla,* is really a part of the sympathetic nervous system. When impulses pass down the sympathetic nerves, as during any emotional experience, the medulla of the adrenal gland is stimulated and secretes the hormones, epinephrine (adrenalin) and norepinephrine (noradrenalin). These hormones cause a series of events which are essentially preparations to meet various emergencies. Included are increases in heart rate, in breathing, in blood pressure, in the amount of sugar in the blood, in the speed with which blood will clot, and in the strength which can be exerted by the muscles. These rather striking phenomena are to be viewed as adaptations by which primitive man, when frightened, enraged, or endangered, could summon greater strength for combat and better avoid death from blood loss if wounded. In the relatively quiet existence of modern civilized life this mechanism is seldom important since the sympathetic nervous system can achieve much the same results even in the absence of the adrenal medulla. The tendency of emotional reactions to increase blood-sugar concentration, however, is frequently helpful. When blood sugar decreases for any reason a slight stimulation of the sympathetic nerves results. The epinephrine secreted by the adrenal glands causes the liver to release some of the sugar stored there as glycogen. This probably happens daily in such a smoothly adjusted fashion that most people never know of the reaction. It is an example of the nicely balanced forces with which the body is equipped to maintain stable conditions from hour to hour.

One medical use of epinephrine is based on the ability of this hormone to cause puckering of the tiny blood vessels in any region where it is applied, thereby limiting the oozing of blood from wounds. Another important value of the hormone is its capacity to relax the muscles in the bronchial tubes. It is used for this purpose by patients who suffer from asthmatic attacks. Norepinephrine is sometimes used to raise the blood pressure in certain types of low blood pressure. But there is no established use for these hormones as substitutes for deficient secretion by the adrenal glands. In fact, physicians do not recognize any condition which can be considered as lack of secretion by the adrenal medulla.

The situation is far different in the case of the outer portion of each adrenal gland, called the *cortex*. This vitally important tissue constantly secretes hormone substances. Although chemists have identified well over twenty-five related compounds in extracts prepared from adrenal glands of animals, there are probably not more than four or five which are circulated and act in the body, the remainder being precursors used in the formation of the major hormones.

One of these hormones, *hydrocortisone* (cortisol), makes it possible for the liver to change protein food into sugar, thus sustaining the normal blood sugar concentration even during fasting. This hormone permits the body to withstand environmental and physical stresses such as cold and injury. Without it, trivial injury could result in collapse and death. The hormone participates in the normal responses to infection and immunity and also helps regulate skin pigmentation. In fact, this hormone is so fundamental to health that when the adrenal glands are destroyed by disease or removed, death occurs unless hydrocortisone or a similar hormone is supplied. A closely related hormone secreted by the adrenal cortex is *corticosterone*. *Cortisone,* one of the first adrenal hormones to be isolated and used widely in medicine, is practically identical to, and can substitute entirely for, hydrocortisone. Both are readily available for prescription.

Another important adrenal hormone is *aldosterone,* which enables the body to retain a sufficient amount of salt, and therefore of water also, to maintain the normal fluid conditions within the cells as well as the blood, and to maintain a proper blood pressure. Certain synthetic compounds, notably desoxycorticosterone (DOC), have effects in the body similar to aldosterone and can be used therapeutically to substitute for the natural hormone when it is deficient.

The adrenal cortex also secretes the *adrenal androgens*. These hormones resemble the male hormone, testosterone, chemically and in their biologic effects. (The term "androgen" means "male producer.") In men, of course, the adrenal androgens supplement the supply of testosterone from the testes. The small amounts of androgen found normally in women are produced primarily by the adrenals and are thought to be necessary for the growth of the sexual (pubic and axillary) hair found in normal women. Some of the androgen produced by the adrenal cortex is converted to estrogen (female sex hormone). This supplements the ovarian hormones in women, and accounts for the small amount of estrogen found in normal men.

With the epochal discovery that cortisone can improve rheumatoid arthritis, a new era of therapeutics was begun. Adrenal hormones, particularly those related to hydrocortisone, or ACTH from the pituitary (which stimulates the adrenal glands to secrete hydrocortisone), are useful for the treatment of acute and chronic inflammation, allergic disorders, skin diseases, and certain diseases of obscure cause such as lupus erythematosus and nephritis. For these purposes, adrenal hormones are employed as *drugs*. To obtain the desired effect an amount far in excess of that normally present is needed. The excess hormone may produce undesired effects not unlike those seen in spontaneous overactivity of the adrenal glands. For this reason, a vast array of synthetic compounds related to the adrenal cortical hormones have been invented by pharmaceutical chemists in the search for drugs which retain the desired properties and do not have the undesired effects. Although the perfect drug has not yet been found, much progress has been made and the physician now has available to him a number of compounds, cousins to the naturally occurring adrenal cortical hormones, which have truly advanced medical treatment in a major way and have saved thousands of lives. Obviously, such potent drugs must only be used under strict medical supervision.

ADRENAL DISEASES

Naturally occurring adrenal disease which results in underactivity or overactivity of hormone secretion is not common. Adrenal deficiency is the more frequent. Adrenal deficiency produces a disease complex known as *Addison's disease* (after the physician who recognized it over a century ago) in which the symptoms can be explained by the lack of sufficient amounts of the adrenal hormones. Various degrees of severity are seen. In typical cases, the lack of aldosterone results in the inability to retain salt so that the body fluids are deficient, and the blood pressure is low. The lack of adrenal androgens results in loss of pubic and axillary hair. The lack of hydrocortisone is most significant, resulting in weakness, poor appetite, a tendency to low blood sugar after the overnight fast, an increase in skin pigmentation, and most important, the propensity to sudden and exaggerated attacks of collapse and vomiting from minor infections, injury, or overwork ("adrenal crisis"). When the latter occurs, prompt treatment is necessary lest a disastrous and irreversible shock ensue with a fatal outcome.

The diagnosis of Addison's disease can be established with certainty by the determination of adrenal hormone levels in blood and urine under baseline conditions and in response to ACTH. These complex tests must be done by special laboratories. Although expensive, the importance of knowing whether Addison's disease exists warrants the performance of these tests when the physician suspects it. Addison's disease may be caused by tuberculosis of the adrenals, which destroys them, by spontaneous shrinkage, or by unusual destructive processes. Whereas treatment of this condition formerly was difficult and unsatisfactory, and often could not prevent adrenal crisis, the availability of hydrocortisone has dramatically changed the prognosis. Daily doses of moderate amounts of this hormone taken by mouth in pill form, with or without salt-retaining hormone as needed, have enabled patients with Addison's disease to regain their health and lead lives which are virtually normal in all respects. The hormones must be taken regularly; in times of injury, infection, or stress, additional amounts are necessary. Here, the natural hormone hydrocortisone (or cortisone) is needed, not the altered hormones used for the non-adrenal diseases discussed. Medical supervision is of paramount importance. The saving and rehabilitation of patients who have Addison's disease is an important achievement of modern medicine.

Overactivity of the adrenal glands is known as *Cushing's disease,* after the late Dr. Harvey Cushing who first recognized it. This disease is rare, although a number of patients suffering from it are seen yearly in large clinics. The overactivity may be caused by a tumor of one of the glands, or by enlargement of both of the glands. What causes these changes is not certain, but the result is an excessive secretion of one or more of the adrenal cortical hormones, with loss of the check-and-balance system the pituitary normally maintains. When hydrocortisone is the hormone secreted in excess, the signs and symptoms are similar to those seen in patients taking large doses of hormones, as for arthritis. The face becomes round, the trunk obese, the skin bruises easily, purplish stretch marks appear, and the patient develops diabetes and hypertension. When adrenal androgen is secreted excessively, masculinization occurs. Virilism in women should always arouse the suspicion of an adrenal tumor which is oversecreting androgen. The menstrual periods cease, the voice deepens, acne appears, hair growth becomes excessive, the musculature becomes heavier, and the genitalia show alterations. Excessive hair alone, known as hirsutism, is common and does not mean an adrenal tumor is present. The other signs of virilism have more significance. (*See* section on Hirsutism.) When aldosterone is secreted in excess, an unusual type of hypertension (high blood pressure) is produced. The diagnosis of adrenal overactivity is complicated and the physician must employ many varied tests, including hormone determinations under a variety of conditions. Treatment depends on the type of overactivity found. Some types require surgical removal of the adrenal glands. The patient will have adrenal deficiency after operation, but the availability of adequate treatment in the form of hydrocortisone to replace the vital normal amounts of this hormone has permitted adrenal surgery to be carried out when necessary.

THE TESTES OR MALE SEX GLANDS

Among the first structures to be suspected of secreting hormones were the testes or male sex glands. The striking change induced in young men who were deprived of these organs was the basis of this belief. The testes produce at least one hormone, which is known as *testosterone*. Its chemical structure is known and it can be made synthetically by the chemist without the use of animal glands. Some investigators believe that at least one other hormone is made by testicular tissue, but the evidence is still uncertain. The testes also produce sperm cells which are the essential testicular product for the fertilization of the ovum of the female and necessary for reproduction. Production of sperm cells and secretion of testosterone are regulated by the pituitary gonadotropins. This is another example of the check-and-balance system between the pituitary and an endocrine gland, for the amount of testosterone secreted determines, in turn, how much gonadotropin is released.

The activity of testosterone is seen in many different parts of the body. This hormone is first produced in significant amounts as a boy approaches puberty. It is the stimulus which makes the external reproductive organs grow to their adult proportions. It is also the factor which leads to the growth of the prostate gland, situated at the bottom of the bladder. Effects of testosterone are found also in every kind of tissue of the body. The bones of adult men are heavier and stronger than those of women because of this stimulus. The muscular development of men is brought about in large part by this hormone. Growth of the cartilages in the larynx is accelerated so that the vocal cords become longer and the voice achieves a lower pitch. Testosterone stimulates the growth of hair on the face and on other body areas. There are definite effects on mental and emotional life also. The obvious increase in sex interest, leading ultimately to marriage and reproduction, is the most direct effect of the hormone on behavior. Less obvious although just as real effects are seen in the complicated group of ambitions, interests, and personality traits which teachers and parents recognize as the evidence of developing adult character in boys. Testosterone is the hormone which is required to stimulate development from boyhood to manhood, and to maintain typically manly qualities thereafter.

Deficient production of testosterone may be caused by diseases of the testes or of the pituitary which occur during fetal development, during infancy and childhood, or during adult life. Certain inherited malformations of the testes limit testosterone secretion and impair sperm-cell production. Sometimes, the testes fail because of injury or infection or for unknown causes. When there is pituitary disease the normal stimulation of the testes to secrete is lacking.

Lack of testosterone in boys for any reason is followed by failure to achieve full masculine development, and in men, by a regression from a normal to a less virile physique and mental status. Males with subnormally active testes, or those who have lost these glands, suffer not only physical handicaps, but also may have psychological difficulties associated with their consciousness of being different from others. Testosterone can be injected into such men, and thereby much of the lacking testicular hormone replaced. Most of the features of adolescent development and adult interest can be induced in this way, as long as the treatment is maintained. This type of treatment cannot substitute for the exocrine function of healthy testes in producing the sperm cells. Nevertheless, the general well-being induced by testosterone injections in men whose testes are deficient warrants such replacement.

Rarely do testes produce so much testosterone that a person can be termed oversexed. This term, as applied to conduct, indicates a psychological rather than physical disturbance. Hormone-secreting tumors do occur in the testes, but their dangers are due to factors other than overproduction of the hormone. By analogy with the overactivity of other glands of internal secretion, overactivity of the testes without tumor might be expected, but is rarely encountered.

THE OVARIES OR FEMALE SEX GLANDS

The ovaries have a dual task just as do the testes: they produce ova, or egg cells, for reproduction, and they secrete hormones. Like the testes, the ovaries are regulated by the pituitary gonadotropins, and, in turn, determine gonadotropin release. The ovaries are now known to produce two types of hormone, both available in chemically pure form as a consequence of the intensive work of many investigators during the last forty years. The first type of hormone belongs to the class of compounds known as estrogens or "female sex hormones." The naturally secreted estrogen is *estradiol.* Several estrogens related to estradiol occur in the body, and are excreted in the urine. A few of these are so nearly like estradiol that they can substitute for it in experimental work or in treatment of women who have a deficiency. Estradiol is the most powerful of all the naturally occurring estrogens. A second ovarian hormone, chemically distinct, and having different functions, is called *progesterone.* It is excreted in the urine as the related chemical compound, pregnanediol.

With the onset of puberty and thereafter, the ovaries produce both these hormones until the occurrence of the *menopause* ("change of life").

The physiological effects of estrogens are varied. They cause growth of the uterus and development of the lining of the vagina to their adult types, stimulate the growth of the external genital parts to adult proportions, and stimulate the growth of the duct system in the breasts. Besides these effects on the reproductive apparatus, estrogen causes the development of the typically feminine contours, with narrow shoulders, broad hips and pelvic bones, and the deposition of fat in those areas which contribute to the graceful lines of the young adult woman. Furthermore, this hormone is apparently the one which is responsible for that psychological development of ambitions and interests characterizing the adolescent young woman as contrasted to the girl.

The ovaries, like the testes in males, may fail to develop normally during growth of the fetus, or may be subject to disease during infancy and childhood. They may also fail to function because of pituitary disease. In these instances, normal puberty does not occur and menstruation does not begin. If the onset of menstruation is delayed, the child should be examined thoroughly to determine whether there is disease or malformation of the female organs or a lack of female hormones due to failure of the ovaries. If the latter, administration of female sex hormones can bring about normal development of feminine characteristics and will often establish a menstrual cycle. As with other problems of the endocrine system, careful and competent advice and supervision of therapy can correct or compensate for many hormonal deficiencies.

MENSTRUATION AND PREGNANCY

One of the important tasks apparently associated with estradiol is the development of the lining of the uterus in partial preparation for the reception of a fertilized egg. Before such an egg can become implanted in the uterus, the second hormone, progesterone, must have been available for several days. Progesterone induces a further change in the uterine lining, enabling it to form certain protein and carbohydrate materials which are needed for the egg cell when it arrives. Without this latter step, pregnancy cannot occur. Progesterone has been named for this action, i.e., it is in behalf of (*pro*) pregnancy (*gestation*). Progesterone has another important effect, namely, reducing the muscular contractions of the uterus, thereby preventing expulsion of the fertilized egg and a miscarriage. It also makes milk glands develop in the breasts. Evidently, therefore, these two hormones of the ovaries are concerned with the direct and indirect provisions for reproduction of the species.

The production of ovarian hormones is almost continuous from near the beginning of the second decade of life to near the end of the fifth decade. Variations occur in the amounts secreted from week to week. The usual

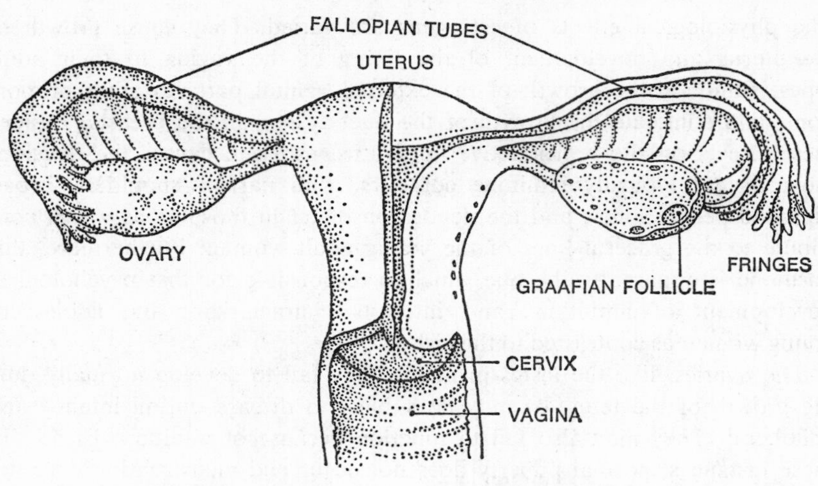

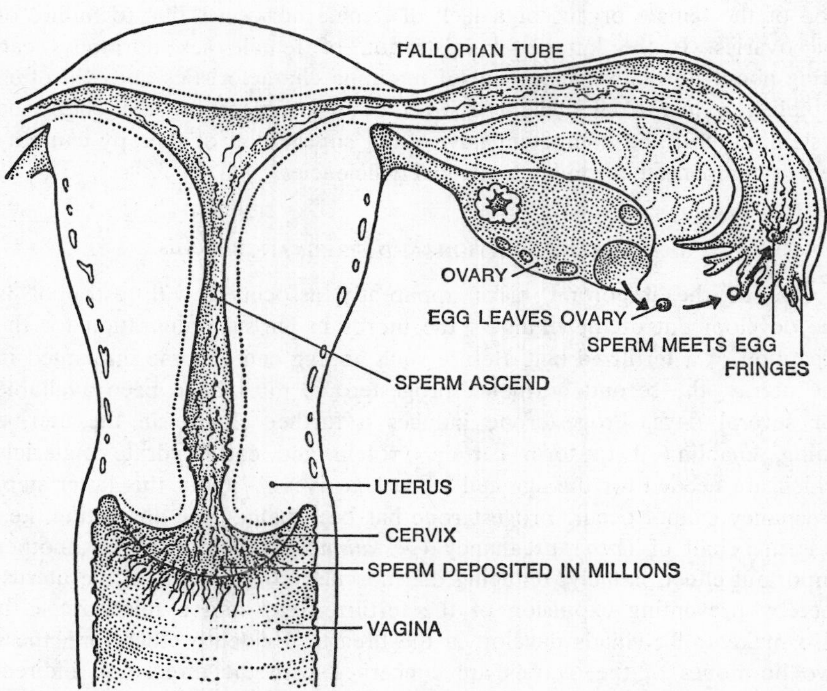

Figs. 55 & 56. Ovulation and Fertilization. During ovulation the ovary releases an egg which is picked up by the end of the Fallopian tube and carried downward to the uterus. Fertilization occurs if the egg is impregnated by male sperm cells. Illustration by Lou Barlow.

cycle of events lasts about four weeks. The ovaries secrete estradiol in increasing amounts for about two weeks. Then, an ovum is liberated from an ovary. After this has occurred the ovaries begin to produce progesterone in addition to estrogen. Progesterone is secreted for ten to twelve days. If the egg is not fertilized and implanted within this time, the secretion of progesterone subsides and a few days later the highly developed lining of the uterus is washed away, together with some bloody discharge. This flow of bloodstained material is termed menstruation (because it occurs about once per month). Following this flow, which lasts a few days only, the cycle of events is repeated again.

If a fertilized egg cell is implanted in the lining of the properly prepared uterus, a different chain of events occurs. The ovary is caused to continue the secretion of progesterone, so that the egg may continue to have its nutrient material and so that the uterus will not expel it. Soon the egg develops into an embryo or fetus and forms a specialized structure called the *placenta.* This resembles a root system, which brings the circulation of the fetus into intimate contact with that of the mother, in the wall of the uterus. The placenta also produces a special hormone (*chorionic gonadotropin*) to maintain progesterone secretion by the ovaries, and also to prevent the ovaries from liberating more ova. Later the placenta develops its own supply of progesterone and estrogen, and then the ovaries are quiescent during the remainder of the pregnancy. A production of these hormones by the placenta continues throughout the nine months of pregnancy. At the end of this period changes in the proportions of these hormones occur. These hormonal changes seem to be responsible for the onset of the muscular activity in the uterus which brings about the birth of the baby.

During pregnancy the increased supply of estradiol and progesterone brings about an increase in the number of glands in the breasts. The beginning of actual secretion of milk is dependent on a special hormone from the pituitary, but this is counteracted during pregnancy by the placental hormones. Within a day or two after the birth of the child and the removal of the placenta, the sudden withdrawal of the supply of this placental hormone allows the pituitary hormone to stimulate the secretion of milk. This continues under the stimulation of suckling, but fails rapidly if the mechanical stimulus is absent.

THE MENOPAUSE

Except during pregnancies, the ovaries continue the cycles of producing ova and the accompanying hormone secretions until the fifth decade. Then a gradual decrease in the intensity of ovarian secretion occurs, ova fail to be produced, and progesterone is not manufactured. Still later estradiol is formed in decreasing amounts, until finally no hormone is produced. As these changes occur, the menstrual rhythm is subject to a variety of alterations. Periods may become irregular in rhythm, frequency, and amount of flow. A change in menstruation from the usual pattern makes the menopause the first consideration for any woman who has reached the fifth decade of life. Unfortunately, any of these changes may occur as evidence of other disturbance in the endocrine activity of the ovaries, or of growth of fibroids or other types of tumors in the uterus. Therefore, whenever women note any shift from their usual routine of menstruation they should report promptly for medical examination to determine the cause.

If the flows are becoming irregular due to the menopause, there is no need to attempt to change this course of events. For a great many women there is little other evidence of the decline in the activity of the ovaries. But often women find that parallel to these objective changes there are a number of disturbing sensations, such as surges of heat ("hot flashes") followed by sudden sweating and coolness, feelings of tenseness, headaches, consciousness of heart action and difficulty with breathing, dizziness, numbness, and odd sensations on the skin. Many women undergoing menopause are easily disturbed by minor vexations and have weeping, worrying, and periods of depression. Difficulty in sleeping is common. Women who undergo these symptoms, when they have had good health previously and have not had obvious illness to explain their discomforts, may begin to think their mental stability is disappearing. Yet nothing other than the subsiding activity of the ovaries may be occurring. It is not safe to make this assumption without medical advice, however, for any or all of these complaints may be associated with other types of illness. Therefore, whenever any of these bothersome symptoms become noticeable to a woman she owes it to herself and her family to give her physician the opportunity to do a careful medical examination. Incidentally, this is usually at a time of life when several diseases occur with increased frequency, and such a health examination will serve to detect, or, still better, disprove the existence of such other disease.

One of the most widely applied benefits of research in hormones has been the relief of many of the symptoms associated with the menopause. After it became possible, beginning in 1927, to prepare ovarian extracts of purity and definite strength, these were administered to women undergoing the menopause. An important advance in hormonal therapy had been made. When the dose of ovarian hormone is adequate in size and in frequency, most of the unpleasant symptoms of the menopause can be relieved. If the doses are large enough, the uterus can be made to produce menstrual flows again. There is no advantage in this latter feature, however. Fortunately it is almost always possible to secure relief from the subjective difficulties without using a dose large enough to restore flowing. At first the treatment was given by hypodermic injections, but now natural or related synthetic estrogens can be administered by mouth. There is a rather prompt destruction of estrogens by the liver, immediately after absorption, but if the doses are large and frequent enough, oral treatment is entirely satisfactory. The choice of drug, frequency with which it should be taken, dosage, duration of treatment, and other variations are matters upon which every woman will need professional advice. For these reasons it is unwise for any woman to attempt to purchase ovarian materials for treating herself for such complaints, except with a physician's prescription. When the ovaries have been removed surgically, or when radium or X-ray treatment has been applied to the pelvic organs, similar symptoms are as apt to occur as during the menopause which develops spontaneously. Treatment is just as helpful under these circumstances.

An old belief prevails that removal or inactivation of the ovaries will make a woman gain weight. The same has been said of the menopause. Since this does not occur in all cases, women may be assured that weight gain is not a necessary result of change in ovarian secretion. Treatment with the ovarian hormones will not prevent or cure obesity. The frequent tendency to obesity in middle life has several factors which may contribute to the one result. Those who tend to gain need to revise their habits of eating and of exercise, again with medical advice. For those women who follow sound rules of hygiene, using medical treatment when really necessary, the passing of the menopause usually means reaching a period of greater stability of health and comfort than before.

THE PANCREAS

Just one year before thyroid deficiency was first treated by the feeding of dried animal thyroid gland, two German investigators proved that removal of the pancreas from dogs caused the animals to become diabetic. Not until thirty-three years later was it possible for the Canadians, Banting and Best, to prepare an extract from the pancreas of animals which would lower blood sugar and counteract diabetes in human patients. This extract contains one of the hormones made by the pancreas, to which the name *insulin* was given. This name is derived from a Latin term for islands, since the part of the pancreas which makes insulin is a group of specialized cells collected into small "islands" distributed throughout the pancreas. Under the chapter on diabetes further consideration of this hormone is available.

Subsequently, a second hormone secreted by the islands was discovered. This is *glucagon,* a hormone which raises blood sugar by causing the liver to release sugar from its stores. The larger part of the pancreas is an exocrine gland, or gland of external secretion, which produces an important digestive juice for use in the upper part of the intestine. The pancreas is, therefore, two glands in one. In certain fish these two glands occur in separate parts of the body, which makes these fish a convenient source of insulin. Insulin must be injected, for if it is given by mouth the digestive juices destroy most of it.

Insulin is a substance whose structure, after more than forty years of intensive study is now known exactly. The discovery of its structure and its synthesis from simpler chemicals is a testimony to the great strides that have been made by modern chemistry. Synthetic insulin is scarce, expensive, and is presently reserved for experimental purposes. Naturally occurring animal insulin, prepared from the pancreas of cows, pigs, sheep or fish, can be prepared in a high degree of purity, and is available for use by diabetic patients in all countries of the world. The cost for enough to maintain excellent health in a human with even the most severe type of diabetes seldom exceeds twenty-five cents per day. Since there are many diabetics in the United States, and since more than half of these patients must use insulin daily, the importance of this contribution to medicine cannot be overestimated. Probably no other single step in endocrine research has been of equal significance.

The action of insulin cannot yet be described with entire exactness in chemical terms. This hormone is necessary if the body is to make prompt and thorough use of sugar in the several ways which are involved in normal metabolism. Deficiency of insulin, leading to impaired ability to use sugar, handicaps the brain, heart, liver, kidneys, the muscles, and other tissues. Every tissue in the body requires sugar in some fashion. If the utilization of sugar is interfered with, other fuels are consumed in greater amounts than usual. This leads to the burning of stores of fat and to the consumption of tissue proteins. When the disease is severe, the attempt of the body to use fats as fuel is so extensive that there is an accumulation of a dangerously large amount of acid residues of fat, leading to acidosis. This process may become so overwhelming that death results. Yet these disturbances can be corrected by the injection of appropriate doses of insulin.

The proper term for diabetes is *diabetes mellitus*. Diabetes which means to "run through" was applied because the body appeared to melt down into urine and flow away. Mellitus means "honey" and was applied because the urine was found to be sweet. This is due to the presence of sugar. Finding sugar in the urine is frequently the means for detecting diabetes, and the absence of sugar in the urine of one who is known to have diabetes is one of the best evidences that he is keeping his difficulty under control. The presence of sugar in the urine of the diabetic is the consequence of his inability to use sugar. The unused sugar accumulates in the blood, and the kidneys remove it when it rises above approximately twice the normal level. However, diabetes is not diagnosed simply by the appearance of sugar in the urine. Sugars other than the normal blood sugar, glucose, may appear under unusual circumstances. This is not ordinarily serious, but obviously may be confused with diabetes.

Fortunately, there are now simple chemical tests available to determine whether the urine sugar is glucose or some other compound. Some persons have a tendency to excrete glucose in the urine even though the blood level is normal. This kidney condition is harmless, but also may be confused with true diabetes mellitus. For these reasons, the physician will check the significance of glucose in the urine by determining the blood level of glucose. Since the essential defect in diabetes is the inability to maintain a level of blood sugar that is within normal bounds during fasting and after eating, he will determine not only the blood-sugar level after an overnight fast, but also after a meal or glucose load, the so-called glucose tolerance test. This helps him diagnose diabetes with certainty. In milder forms of the disease, very little sugar may appear in the urine so that an abnormal tolerance test may be the only means of diagnosing the condition. Much more detail is given in the chapter on diabetes.

The disturbances produced by diabetes mellitus may be of all degrees of severity, from mild to severe and life-threatening. In mild cases, the deficiency of insulin is slight and occurs only when unusual demands for insulin are made as by the ingestion of large amounts of sugar. Such a disturbance might be met by merely restricting the intake of sugar and other carbohydrates (sugar-forming foods). An increased amount of fat might be used to make up the deficit in calories. This method is satisfactory for many mild diabetics. Diabetes frequently occurs in middle-age or later and is commonly associated with obesity. Current evidence indicates that the pancreas of a patient with onset of diabetes in middle age does secrete insulin in response to blood sugar elevation but does so in a disordered fashion. If left untreated for a protracted period of time, the insulin reserves may be temporarily exhausted and acidosis may occur. In this event, insulin must be supplied by hypodermic injection at least until the acidosis is corrected. If the condition is recognized sooner, however, the pancreas may be stimulated to secrete its insulin more normally by the administration of one of the *sulfonylurea drugs*. Thus, many middle-aged or older diabetics may be treated satisfactorily by weight reduction, careful diet, and the ingestion of one or more pills per day. These patients require as close medical supervision as more severe diabetics. Only the physician can determine whether the diabetes is suited to treatment with pills, and for this reason, these drugs cannot be obtained without a physician's prescription.

Diabetes in children or young adults ("juvenile diabetes"), is usually the result of a nearly total lack of insulin production by the pancreas. Diabetes of this type cannot be satisfactorily managed by diet or by diet and oral drugs alone. Without sufficient insulin, the liver will make sugar from sources such as protein even though there is already an excess of sugar in the blood. Therefore, the blood sugar remains abnormally high, even without excessive carbohydrate food. The only remedy for this situation is the daily hypodermic injection of insulin. Lacking this treatment, this type of diabetic will gradually lose weight and strength, and eventually die. With insulin therapy, restoration of metabolism toward or to normal is possible, with consequent good health. Dietary management is adequate for some diabetics, others require drugs to stimulate insulin secretion, and still others require daily injections of insulin.

At first hope prevailed that the use of insulin would make diet limitation entirely unnecessary for diabetics. This hope has not been realized. On the contrary, the use of careful diets is more important with the injection of insulin than without. This is not due to any inability of insulin to accomplish desired results. The difficulty is that the insulin once injected continues to have an effect, stimulating the body to use sugar rapidly. If there is not a sufficient supply of sugar coming from food, blood sugar concentration will fall and the brain will be deprived of an essential nutrient. As a consequence, hunger and nervous irritability occur, which should serve the diabetic as a warning to procure food. If this warning is not understood or heeded, still further brain disturbances may occur, with sweating, trembling, slurring of speech, and lack of coordination of muscles. The person may act as if ill or intoxicated with alcohol. If relief is not obtained, brain activity may be suppressed to the point of unconsciousness. The remedy for all these disorders is a quick supply of sugar. If the results have been allowed to proceed to a point where the patient can no longer take food by mouth, a physician may have to inject glucagon to mobilize sugar from the liver, or administer a solution of pure glucose intravenously. Under these circumstances recovery is dramatically prompt.

As a result, diabetic patients are trained to estimate their food intake carefully so that they eat uniform amounts of carbohydrate food daily. The number of pills or the amount of insulin is then adjusted to the point where the blood sugar concentration is nearly normal, but care is taken to avoid unduly low blood-sugar levels. The diabetic orders his life between two limits: too little blood sugar, which can produce the reaction described, or too much blood sugar, which will be followed by loss of sugar in the urine, and a tendency to acidosis. If the amount of food is adjusted to maintain proper weight of the body, this routine of carefully limited diet and the ingestion of pills or the hypodermic injection of insulin is only a slight inconvenience. By following these directions the diabetic can remain otherwise in excellent health, pursue his usual occupation, and expect to live a normal life.

Originally, insulin had to be given two to four times daily. This followed from the rapid but brief activity of the material injected. If a whole day's supply was given at one time, the results would be too intense within the first few hours, and would have disappeared before the day had passed. A few years later it was found possible to combine insulin with a protein called protamine and with zinc in small amounts. This preparation of *protamine zinc insulin* is not soluble in water, but is used in a milky suspension which can be injected hypodermically. Under the skin, such insulin is slowly absorbed, so that it becomes available throughout the day. Later, protamine zinc insulin was prepared according to a method which allows it to act like a mixture of the slow- and quick-acting types, called *isophane* or *NPH insulin.*

Recently, by the controlled crystallization of insulin, insulins have been prepared with intermediate or long duration of action without the need to add other proteins like protamine. These are known as *lente insulins.* Because of the different durations of action of various insulins, most diabetics who require insulin may be treated with only one injection per day. This is a great convenience for the diabetic and enables him to inject his insulin himself every morning, and thus manage his disease under the supervision of his physician.

The discovery of insulin and the understanding of the consequences of the injection of an excessive amount of insulin led to the recognition of a condition which had not been previously known. This is the spontaneous occurrence of unduly low blood-sugar concentrations with distressing symptoms resembling epilepsy or other brain disturbances. It was suspected that some individuals with this problem might be found to have pancreatic tumors secreting large amounts of insulin. This has been proven in many patients, and with removal of such tumors these patients have been cured.

Of even greater importance has been the realization that a large number of otherwise healthy persons have excessive reductions in the amount of circulating blood sugar temporarily two to four hours after a meal which was rich in sugar and starch. When these foods are being absorbed from the digestive tract, the amount of sugar in the blood is sharply increased. The immediate reaction of the pancreas is to secrete more insulin into the blood, to facilitate the use and storage of this sugar. The production of insulin under these conditions is generous, and may be slightly in excess of the needs. Under these circumstances sugar is withdrawn from the blood more rapidly than it can enter from the intestine. This produces a slight deficit of sugar in the blood, hunger follows, and if the process goes a bit farther, the individual may become irritable, nervous, and feel weak. This process will be accentuated if vigorous exercise is being undertaken. Such a chain of events is especially common in children, and is responsible for the need of frequent feedings. Adults who respond in this way to sweet food will find they are more comfortable with several small meals per day. Another alternative is the use of meals with exceedingly small portions of carbohydrate food, and larger amounts of the protein and fat foods which are more slowly digested. Also, the presence of these latter materials in the intestine prevents too rapid absorption of sugar and helps avoid rapid changes in blood sugar. Not infrequently the occurrence of this type of hunger is the cause for lunching between meals, and for use of sweet and rich foods at every opportunity. The result is a steady gain in weight. When obesity results from exaggeration of the normal response to intake of sugar, it is easy to plan a diet which limits the amount of carbohydrate in each meal. The person who follows this diet is not only able to lose weight, but actually will be less hungry on less food.

THE PARATHYROIDS

At the edges of the thyroid gland are found four small glands which are entirely different, called because of their location, parathyroid ("around the thyroid") glands. Their task is to control the amount of calcium and phosphorus which circulates in the blood. A decrease in activity of these glands (*hypoparathyroidism*) is followed by a decrease in blood calcium but an increase in phosphorus. Under such circumstances muscles become more easily stimulated; when the change is sufficient certain muscles begin to contract or exhibit spasms spontaneously. This is called tetany (not to be confused with tetanus, which is the result of a specific infection). In tetany, the commonest spasms are of the hands, arms, legs and feet, but the most dangerous contractions can occur in the muscles of the larynx, closing the passage through which the breath passes. This emergency can be relieved quickly by the injection into a vein of a solution of calcium salts. The decreased amount of circulating calcium is the cause of the increased irritability of the muscles. Hypoparathyroidism may occur from naturally acquired disease of the parathyroids, but this is uncommon. Most cases are the result of destruction or removal of the glands during the operative treatment for goiter. Surgeons are careful to avoid these small glands during thyroid operations, but the parathyroids are small, difficult to identify during an operation, and are occasionally removed unavoidably by even the most experienced surgeons.

The treatment of tetany by means of extracts of animal parathyroids became possible in 1925, when this potent material was discovered simultaneously by two investigators. Unfortunately, the continuous use of even the best of the extracts is not satisfactory, since the treatment gradually loses its efficacy after a number of weeks to months. Several other measures help make the relief of tetany possible. If the diet is selected so that there is a minimum of phosphorus, if calcium salts are added in frequent doses, and if vitamin D is used liberally, most patients with tetany due to hypoparathyroidism can get along well enough. Vitamin D increases the body's ability to absorb calcium from the digestive tract. Recently a chemist prepared a vitamin D derivative which is especially potent in keeping up the calcium and assisting the kidneys to eliminate phosphorus. This is named dihydrotachysterol. Vitamin D appears to be equally useful. Either drug can be taken by mouth every day, whereas the parathyroid hormone had to be injected hypodermically. Because the use of dihydrotachysterol or vitamin D does not become less beneficial as time goes on, this is the preferred method of treating tetany.

In some persons the parathyroid glands become overactive, secreting an excessive amount of the hormone, usually as the result of the development of a functioning tumor (parathyroid adenoma) of one or more of the glands. This condition is known as *hyperparathyroidism.* The consequence is an increase in the amount of blood calcium and a decrease in phosphorus. These changes result from the action of the excess parathyroid hormone upon the bones, releasing excessive amounts of calcium and phosphorus, and upon the kidneys, causing them to remove too much phosphorus from the blood. The bones of the entire body are gradually weakened. Sometimes the dissolving of calcium occurs in spotty fashion, and the X rays of these bones look as though local excavations had been made. Sometimes, one or more of these local areas develop into large cysts which may produce swelling of the bone. In other instances, the bones become less dense throughout. However, only in rare instances do the bones become so soft as to be deformed or broken.

More commonly, the patient with hyperparathyroidism develops kidney stones, with painful kidney colic and the passage of gravel or stones. In others, kidney calcification occurs and leads to progressive impairment of the kidneys' ability to excrete waste materials. Kidney failure and death from uremia may result. The formation of calcium stones in the urinary tract and the calcification of the kidney tissue is the result of the excessive load of calcium the kidney is called on to excrete as a consequence of the high blood level of calcium. *Not all cases of kidney stones are due to overactivity of the parathyroids;* indeed, in only a small per cent will a parathyroid disturbance be found. Yet, because hyperparathyroidism is a curable condition if treated before kidney damage is far advanced, but fatal if untreated, the investigation of all patients with kidney stones for parathyroid disease is necessary. The physician makes repeated determinations of blood and urine calcium and phosphorus, and from these and other specialized tests is able to decide whether a parathyroid disturbance is likely. A certain diagnosis can often not be made without surgery.

Cure of hyperparathyroidism is dependent on the surgical removal of the tumors. If there are no distinct tumors, the surgeon must remove one, two, or even three of the four parathyroid glands. Since they are so difficult to identify, this is a task for a surgeon who has made a special study of the field. After successful removal of a parathyroid adenoma, kidney function usually improves rapidly and the bones recalcify. When parathyroid trouble is suspected, studies should be carried out by specially trained physicians and surgeons in hospitals equipped for the special investigations required.

COMMON PROBLEMS RELATED TO ENDOCRINOLOGY

Several conditions often considered to be due to glandular disturbance are known in which specific and recognizable disease of the endocrine system is usually not found. These are obesity, excessive body hair in women (hirsutism), slow or rapid growth in children, and delay in the appearance of adolescence. The inability to discover underlying endocrine gland disease may be due, in part, to present imperfect knowledge of the fine workings of these glands and their interrelations. More often, the problem is simply one extreme or another of the normal condition and should not cause concern. Sometimes, non-endocrine factors are responsible for the apparent endocrine abnormality. In any event, a thorough examination and investigation should be made so that specific causes can be recognized if they exist. If specific causes are not discovered, advice and reassurance can be given.

OBESITY

Many people, including many physicians, have come to believe that an abnormally low basal metabolism is the cause of obesity. This is rarely true. Associated with this belief has been the use of thyroid as a means to reduce excessive weight. Such treatment seldom produces significant weight loss unless the doses of thyroid are so high that the person is made definitely ill. Nevertheless, a number of "reducing remedies" which are mixtures containing thyroid have been sold without prescription. Use of such preparations is to be avoided for at least three reasons. First, these remedies are usually not helpful, hence they are wasteful expenditures. Second, if the doses of such drugs are large enough to cause definite effects, genuine illness is apt to be produced. Finally, excessive weight may come from any one of several causes. Appropriate dietary schemes and exercise for the needs of the individual patient require the advice of a physician who has been adequately trained in the problems involved. Obesity is a sufficient reason for requesting medical advice. There is no simple and safe way to reduce excessive weight except by the time-honored use of less food and more work. The details of such a program need to be prescribed just as definitely as do medicines for other diseases.

HIRSUTISM

Excessive body and facial hair in women is known as hirsutism. The amount of hair a normal woman has varies considerably and depends, among other factors, upon racial and familial inheritance. What is excessive hair for some women may be normal for others. When a woman notices hair growth, which is excessive for her, she should consult her physician and have a thorough examination. Physicians distinguish simple hirsutism from *virilism* which is due to overactivity of the adrenal glands or to rare tumors of the ovaries. Virilism is associated with cessation of the menstrual periods, acne, development of a receding hairline and baldness, deepening of the voice, changes in the genitals, and an increase in the size of the muscles. In the majority of patients noticing hirsutism, such signs do not occur, and the menstrual periods continue in a regular fashion. Whereas virilism interferes with fertility, the majority of women with simple hirsutism do not have difficulty conceiving or carrying a pregnancy. Determination of urine hormone levels will confirm the absence of virilism and the presence of normal femaleness in simple hirsutism.

What causes hirsutism without virilism is not known for certain. Some evidence indicates that slight alterations in adrenal androgen production may be an important factor. This possibility is currently under intensive investigation. For the present, there is no medical treatment that is applicable to the majority of women with hirsutism. Medical examination should be sought. When the physician has completed his examination and studies and does not find any overt hormonal imbalance, the patient can be assured virilism will not develop and can then safely undertake appropriate cosmetic measures.

PROBLEMS OF GROWTH

Growth is a complex process regulated by the endocrine glands. When there is no malnutrition or chronic, serious disease to interfere, such as heart or kidney disease, growth proceeds normally during childhood at the rate of one to two inches per year. All hormones play a role, but pituitary growth hormone, thyroid hormone, the sex hormones, and the adrenal androgens are particularly important. When growth hormone is deficient, dwarfism results. When thyroid hormone is deficient, not only is growth impeded, but body proportions remain of the infantile type.

With the onset of adolescence, the pituitary begins to stimulate the action of the testes or ovaries. The sex hormones, acting in conjunction with growth hormone and thyroid hormone, produce an acceleration of growth of three to four inches per year, the so-called "growth spurt" characteristic of adolescence. When the individual reaches maturity, he normally stops growing at the height expected from his heredity even though these hormones continue to be secreted throughout adult life. As a rule, linear growth stops before age twenty or age twenty-five at the latest. This is another of the automatically balanced control systems which keep the human body in what is called the normal condition.

The explanation of this endocrine balance is important to those who are concerned with the growth and development of children. The growth of the long bones in the arms and legs determines the body's eventual stature more than other factors. These bones grow at both ends, by means of two centers of bone formation. These centers are attached to the shaft of the bone by actively growing cartilages, in which the bone is being made. The pituitary growth hormone and the thyroid hormone stimulate this bone-building process. The sex hormones, which enter at adolescence, potentiate these effects and stimulate the growth spurt. At the same time, the sex hormones increase the rate at which the growth centers tend to unite with the shaft. Eventually, the growth centers and the shaft fuse, after which further elongation of the bone does not occur. Thus, the secretion of testosterone or estradiol during adolescence ultimately determines the adult stature for the individual. It is of prime importance that the pituitary stimulate growth to nearly adult proportions before it begins to stimulate the hormone production of the reproductive organs. The way in which this sequence of affairs is regulated is still a mystery.

From these facts it is evident that if any treatment is to be directed toward altering the growth process, it must be undertaken in the years before adolescence is completed. X-ray pictures of the long bones are valuable in determining when growth can still be expected because they show whether the growth centers are active or whether union with the shafts has occurred.

A frequent cause of concern to parents are children or adolescents who appear to be slow-growers. The physician, on examining these children, usually finds they do not have evidence of pituitary or other disease. In the majority of instances, such slow-growing children eventually reach normal height. Often, the childhood history will show that for a period of six months to two years virtually no growth occurred, then it resumed. Children with such a background drop behind their contemporaries, but their growth usually proceeds at a normal rate once it begins again and they eventually catch up. Another common cause of slow growth is delayed adolescence. This is because the growth "spurt" induced by the sex hormones is lacking because of the delay in sexual maturation. When adolescence finally does occur, growth will accelerate and normal height will be reached.

In slow-growing children or those with delayed adolescence, a variety of treatments to induce growth have been tried, usually with disappointing results. As explained previously, growth hormone derived from slaughterhouse animals is not effective in humans. Whether human growth hormone will prove useful is presently unknown. The supply of human growth hormone is necessarily limited since it must be extracted from the pituitaries of persons who have recently died. For this reason human growth hormone has been reserved for true pituitary dwarfs and has not yet been tried extensively in slow growth. The sex hormones have been used, testosterone in the male and estrogens in the female, in an attempt to mimic the spurt in growth which normally occurs during adolescence. Although growth acceleration may be induced, the long bone growth centers are usually matured so rapidly that premature union with the shaft occurs. The end result is an individual whose adult height is less than might have been attained had not sex hormone therapy been used. Recently, chemical compounds related to testosterone have been synthesized. These chemicals differ from testosterone in that its protein-building properties are preserved, but the masculinizing properties are absent. In some instances of slow growth, these compounds may induce a growth spurt without the undesired effect on the bone growth centers.

The child with unusually rapid growth also concerns parents. If there is no evidence of a pituitary overactivity, growth can be expected to stop when the height common to the family is attained. Examination of the growth centers of the bones by X ray will help the physician determine when growth is nearing completion. Parents who are tall often seek advice to see if a daughter's growth can be brought to a halt if it appears that she may also be unusually tall. Unusual height is a social problem for women, though not for men. Female sex hormones have been tried in these tall girls in an attempt deliberately to close the bone centers prematurely, but results have not been successful with regularity.

The child with unusually slow or rapid growth should be investigated thoroughly by a physician experienced in handling these problems. Treatment must be selected with care and be carried out only under the most careful medical supervision.

DELAYED ADOLESCENCE

The normal supply of anterior pituitary hormones to stimulate the reproductive system begins gradually and comes to full intensity by the early years of the second decade of life. The development of testes and ovaries to fully adult activity requires a few years to be completed. The transformation in physical type as well as emotional attitudes and intellectual interests continues at a pace which seems rapid to the parent, often slow to the youth. It is probably well for the health of both body and mind that the process does not go on more rapidly. In fact, some individuals develop so rapidly that the coordination of processes is temporarily imperfect. It is common in this adolescent period to find awkwardness of muscles, instability of emotions, and minor disorders of the skin such as acne, or of the nervous system, such as sweating or irregular and fast heart action. Usually these are only evidences of a temporary imbalance, but medical supervision of such children is wise to make certain there is no disease concerned. Unusual leanness or excessive weight is frequently encountered at such periods, and these may necessitate instruction in appropriate habits of eating and of exercise.

The age at which puberty occurs varies considerably in normal children. Although it usually begins by the early teens, it may begin normally as late as seventeen to eighteen years of age. If evidences of adolescence are not seen by the age of fifteen, the child should be examined thoroughly. Inquiry about the time of maturity of the parents and other relatives will be made, for there may be a family tendency to early or late adolescence, which must be taken into account. If there is an inherited tendency to late adolescence, without physical abnormalities or disease, treatment may be unnecessary and observation for a period of time may be advised. During this observation period, the physician may detect the onset of puberty from urine hormone levels before visible changes are seen. If there are evidences of psychologic disturbance because of the delay, however, the patient should be treated. Injections of gonadotropin for a short period of time will often get puberty started, and it will progress normally thereafter. In selected instances, sex hormones will have to be used, testosterone in the male and estrogens in the female. Careful selection must be made of the time appropriate for treatment and of the type of treatment. Much can be accomplished by careful management for young people who are developing too slowly or incompletely.

OTHER GLANDS

The pineal, a small structure attached to the upper surface of the brain, and the thymus, occurring in the upper portion of the chest, just in front of the trachea, have long been suspected of being glands of internal secretion. The evidence is meager and lacking in consistency so that these structures are not presently recognized as definite endocrine organs. However, most recent evidence indicates the thymus is concerned in developing immunity to infection.

In the digestive tract are several hormones produced during the processes of digesting food. One of these stimulates the flow of pancreatic juice when food leaves the stomach. Another hormone derived from the lining of the intestine stimulates contraction of the gall bladder, forcing out some of the stored bile. A third hormone from the intestine serves to reduce the activity of the stomach, slowing down its emptying and thereby extending the time available for digestion in both the stomach and the intestine. These digestive hormones seem different from the hormones of the endocrine glands already described in that they have only local actions in the digestive system and do not affect other tissues of the body.

CHAPTER 23

Diabetes Mellitus

HOWARD F. ROOT, M.D. (Deceased)

INTRODUCTION

Deaths from diabetes in the United States have risen to nearly three times that of the rate in 1900. In the United States, for example, the rate per 100,000 population in 1900 was 9.7. In 1949, it was 29.1. More women have been dying of diabetes than men. The death rates for men and women were about the same until about 1905. Then the rate among women began to rise more rapidly, so that by 1932 about twice as many women as men died of diabetes. Sound conclusions regarding diabetes, however, cannot be drawn, because insulin was introduced in 1923, and diagnosis has become more frequent. Diagnosis has improved and women are being examined more frequently and regularly than they were before.

Not all the people who have diabetes get an early diagnosis. Moreover, a laboratory examination is required to make a positive diagnosis. This, and the fact that women are appearing more frequently in positions requiring physical examinations, explain some of the increase in diabetes as found in women. Another reason is the aging of the population. Thus in 1901 the expectancy of life for white men was 48.2 years and for women 51.1 years, but in 1965 for men it was 70 years and for women 75 years. This growing older of the population increases the number of liabilities, because two thirds of all the cases begin after forty years of age.

A remarkable change has been brought about by the use of insulin in the causes of death of diabetics. Formerly, people who died of diabetes died from coma—a form of unconsciousness which resulted from chemical changes in the body. The number of deaths from this cause has decreased greatly. Persons who have diabetes live much longer nowadays than those in former years. This explains why diabetics die of other conditions.

The person who develops diabetes has a lifelong problem. He must watch his condition carefully if he is to gain the maximum benefit from methods of treatment. In some cases the changes that have taken place in the body resulting from diabetes are hereditary. By use of insulin, children with diabetes—which used to be especially fatal to youngsters—now live and are likely to have children. Hence the question of heredity in diabetes will, in the future, be increasingly important.

In the attack on diabetes in the United States, one of the most important contributors was Dr. E. P. Joslin. He wrote a popular handbook on the subject, as well as a scientific text widely used by physicians throughout the world. While recognizing that the average person may be competent to regulate his own diet under the advice of the doctor and also to administer remedies to himself, Dr. Joslin did not suggest either self-diagnosis or self-treatment as safe for anyone suffering from this disorder.

M. F.

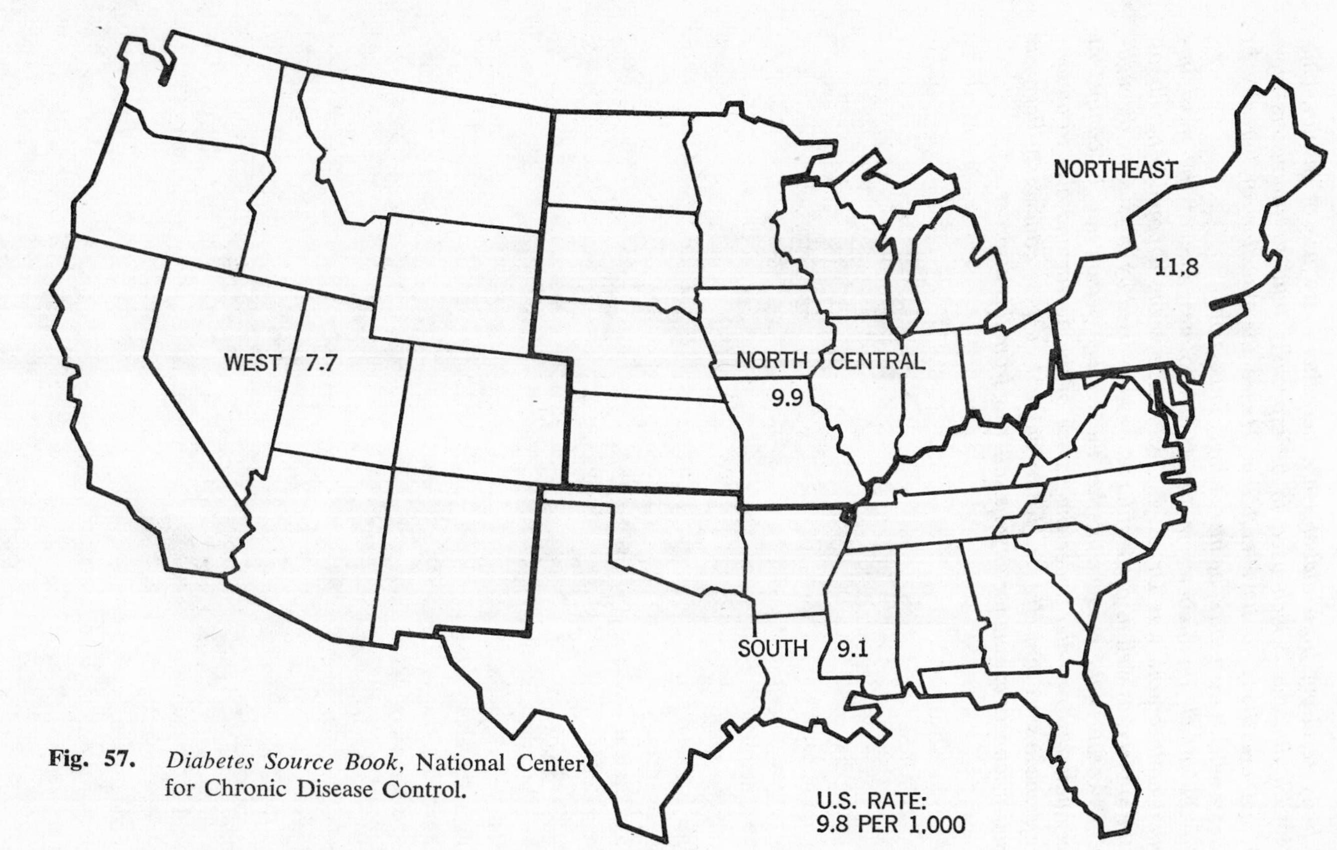

Fig. 57. *Diabetes Source Book*, National Center for Chronic Disease Control.

CURRENT CONCEPTS

All those interested in diabetes, especially diabetic patients and their relatives, should have a new understanding of diabetes as a result of the many studies in research laboratories and medical clinics in recent years. Old ideas with relation to the causes of diabetes and its prevalence in the community are being modified. Diabetes mellitus is an hereditary disease of metabolism progressing insidiously or in some cases with relatively great rapidity, and eventually including the stage characterized by the presence of sugar in the urine, high blood-sugar values, and a loss of the normal ability to utilize food and especially foods containing sugar and starch. Stages in the development of diabetes have been classified in various ways.

1. Prediabetes, the stage beginning with conception and lasting until the demonstration of lowered tolerance for glucose by means of tests showing sugar in the urine and increased sugar in the blood.
2. Chemical diabetes is that stage at any age when the patient who does not have symptoms nevertheless shows abnormal tests of the blood and urine for sugar under conditions of stress, such as pregnancy, of infection, or through a special glucose tolerance test.
3. Clinical diabetes (overt, acute) is the well-known stage when symptoms such as increased thirst, increased passing of urine, blurred vision, skin infections, loss of weight and strength, or even acidosis occur.
4. Chronic diabetes is the stage when minimal changes in the small blood vessels seen in earlier stages have advanced so that serious alterations in the arterial system in the kidneys and the eyes may occur.

Formerly the onset of diabetes was thought to be due to the failure of the pancreas, which produces insulin. Indeed, many investigations clearly showed that within a few years after the onset of diabetes the blood of young diabetic patients and even of adults contained a greatly reduced amount of insulin. However, in recent years, new methods of measuring insulin or the insulin-like activity in the blood (ILA) have shown clearly that in early diabetes, even in childhood, it may actually be increased two or three times the normal level. This increased blood insulin may be bound to mysterious protein substances which at present are the object of intensive investigation.

Prediabetes, as it has been studied in the children of diabetic parents, is a phase lasting sometimes for years, during which the body is coping successfully with forces tending to produce diabetes. In this stage, recent research has shown some changes in the small blood vessels but otherwise the patient feels and seems entirely well without any sugar in the urine or increased sugar in the blood. One of the main objects of research laboratories is to discover a means by which a patient in this stage can be treated and prevented from really advancing into a stage of active diabetes. Treatment during this stage should emphasize, first, a proper diet adequate for growth, normal muscular activity, and the avoidance of obesity.

During the chemical stage of diabetes, diagnosis can be made from special tolerance tests which will be described later. Again, research is aimed at finding methods of treatment including some of the newer drugs which will prevent progression into more advanced stages.

In the two later stages, overt and chronic diabetes, the most important basic need is the provision of a proper diet suited to the needs of the patient, the avoidance of obesity, and the use of remedies such as the new oral drugs or insulin under careful and continuing medical care. The need for institutes providing for further research into the causes, cure, and prevention of diabetes with provision for instruction of patients and the care of special problems such as the diabetes of childhood, surgical complications in diabetes, and pregnancy must be met in various parts of the world.

Diabetes has become a world health problem. Due to the underlying factor of heredity, at least one person in four now carries one (or two) genes by which the disease can be transmitted from parents to their descendants. Fortunately, not all the carriers of the diabetic gene will develop the disease; but, nevertheless, a large number of carriers exist (perhaps one fourth of these) who are susceptible to diabetes and who will need diagnosis and treatment.

Diabetes is one of the most common ailments in the United States and

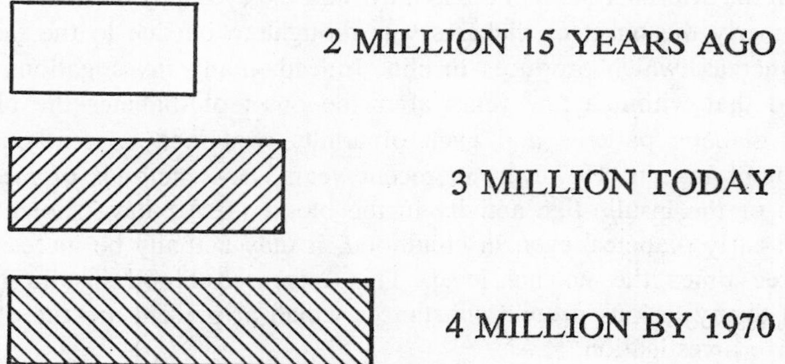

Fig. 58. Prevalence. Today, more Americans are living longer, and more are estimated to have diabetes—over three million, compared with two million some fifteen years ago. Furthermore, present indications are that unless some unforeseen cure or preventive is found, the number may exceed four million by 1970. *Diabetes Source Book,* National Center for Chronic Disease Control.

ranks seventh among the causes of death. Approximately nine million Americans of all ages have now or will develop the disease in later life. Tragically, half of those already diabetic are unaware of their condition since their cases have not been carefully studied by newer diagnostic methods. Approximately one-fourth of the American population is touched by the disease, either directly by acquiring it or indirectly by being a carrier of the diabetic gene.

THE INCREASING PREVALENCE OF DIABETES

Although diabetes is found in all parts of the world, only in industrialized countries are reliable data obtainable. The number of cases increases rapidly, first because the total population in such countries as the United States is increasing; second, the increasing number of older people brings more patients to the age when diabetes develops most frequently; third, diabetic patients live so much longer; fourth, great improvement in diagnostic measures and the examination of larger numbers of persons. In 1900, diabetic patients lived on the average a scant five years, according to the experience of Dr. Elliott P. Joslin, pioneer in the study of diabetes whose name has been given to the Joslin Research Laboratory and Clinic of the Diabetes Foundation in Boston.

Now diabetic patients expect to live indefinitely and indeed, many do live longer with the disease than one would expect them to live without it. Community studies in various countries, in which both blood and urine tests are made, indicate a much greater prevalence than was expected on the basis of past experience.

Mortality statistics on diabetes are more readily available than statistics on the number having the disease. However, the evidence based on mortality statistics is notably unreliable since it is well known that in various communities from 20 to 30 per cent of diabetic patients may die from some other cause without having the word "diabetes" appear on the death certificate. In the closing twenty years of the last century, the death rate from diabetes in the registration area of the United States trebled and trebled again in the next forty-nine years.

There are wide international variations in the prevalence and mortality of diabetes, no doubt the result of many factors such as differences in the quantity and quality of medical care and the public health programs and facilities available to the population. Genetic factors are probably of great significance. The frequency of overweight and the food consumption in various countries is an important element.

Among the first of the community surveys was that conducted in 1946 by the U. S. Public Health Service. Examinations of the urine and blood of most of the people in the community gave evidence of the number of tion by age and sex was approximately the same as that in the United existing cases of diabetes instead of depending on hearsay evidence by a house-to-house canvass. They chose the country town of Oxford, in Worcester County, Massachusetts, with 5000 inhabitants in which the distribu-States. As a result, Dr. H. C. L. Wilkerson and Dr. L. P. Krall found that among the 3500 inhabitants out of the 5000 inhabitants, there was one unknown diabetic for each one known. This survey has been followed by many others in various nations with usually somewhat similar results. According to the survey, "Diabetes in 1964—A World Survey" by P. S. Entmacher and H. H. Marks, read at the Fifth Congress of the International Diabetes Federation, the incidence in countries formerly thought to have little diabetes has been at least equal to that in the United States.

DIABETES EIGHTH LEADING CAUSE OF DEATH

RANK	LEADING CAUSE OF DEATH	RATE PER 100,000 POPULATION	
		1962	1950
	All	954.4	963.8
1	Diseases of heart	370.3	356.8
2	Malignant neoplasms, including neoplasms of lymphatic and hematopoietic tissues	149.9	139.8
3	Vascular lesions affecting central nervous system	106.3	104.0
4	Accidents	52.3	60.6
5	Certain diseases of early infancy	34.6	40.5
6	Influenza and pneumonia, except pneumonia of newborn	32.3	31.3
7	General arteriosclerosis	19.8	20.4
8	DIABETES MELLITUS	16.8	16.2
9	Other diseases of circulatory system	12.2	4.9
10	Cirrhosis of liver	11.7	9.2

The effect of the increasing length of life of diabetic patients is shown in Table 1. Since the period 1937–43, the duration of life even in patients dying from other causes such as auto accidents has more than doubled for children with onset under 20 years of age and actually increased materially in patients whose diabetes began at 60 years and over.

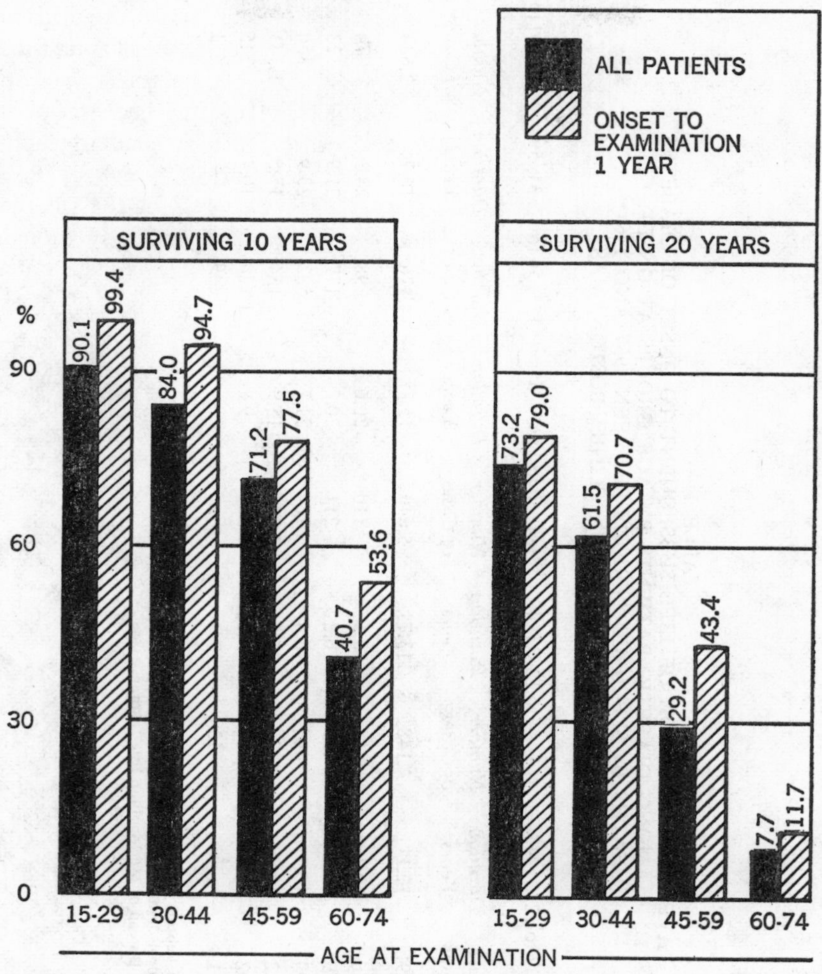

Fig. 59. Survivorship and Life Expectancy. After decades of experience in treating diabetics, the Joslin Clinic reports that those who receive treatment shortly after the onset of their disease live longer than diabetic patients in general. This is true at every age level. From *Diabetes Source Book,* National Center for Chronic Disease Control.

The survivorship of diabetic patients in which the percentage of diabetic patients surviving 10 and 20 years since the first visit has been traced. The extraordinary increase in the length of life of young patients with

TABLE 1

AVERAGE DURATION OF LIFE SUBSEQUENT TO ONSET OF DIABETES AMONG DIABETIC PATIENTS BY AGE GROUPS AT ONSET. DEATHS IN SPECIFIED PERIODS BETWEEN 1937 AND 1964* EXPERIENCE OF THE JOSLIN CLINIC, BOSTON, MASS.

	1/1/37 to 12/31/43		1/1/44 to 12/31/49		1/1/50 to 12/31/55		1/1/56 to 12/31/59		1/1/60 to 2/19/64*	
Age Groups at Onset	*Number of Cases*	*Duration Years*	*Number of Cases*	*Duration Years*	*Number of Cases*	*Duration Years*	*Number of Cases*	*Duration Years*	*Number of Cases*	*Duration Years*
All Ages	3,639	12.1†	4,148	13.7†	5,640	15.3†	4,176	16.7†	2,634	16.9†
0–9	36	10.3	58	18.5	110	20.6	98	24.3	74	25.6
10–19	79	11.4	125	16.2	211	20.2	177	21.9	123	23.1
20–39	399	16.9	465	18.8	764	21.7	582	23.9	350	24.0
40–59	1,922	13.4	2,230	14.9	2,986	15.9	2,134	17.5	1,341	17.6
60 and over	1,202	8.6	1,257	9.2	1,564	9.8	1,176	10.4	745	10.3
Unknown	1	–	13	–	5	–	9	–	1	–

* Deaths reported through February 19, 1964.
† Based on cases with known duration.
Prepared by the Statistical Bureau of Metropolitan Life Insurance Co.

diabetes today gives an unbelievably better outlook for the future. The causes of death for diabetic patients have shown a tremendous change in the last 50 years. Coma, which formerly caused the death of 64 per cent of all diabetic patients, is now only 1.1 per cent of all causes. The cardiorenal vascular causes have increased from 65.7 per cent in the earlier period to 77.9 per cent in the four years from 1960 to 1964. Infections as a cause of death have declined owing to the use of the new antibiotics. Tuberculosis has almost disappeared whereas cancer as a cause of death remains in the neighborhood of 10 per cent. See Table 2.

In the United States, diabetes still ranks as the seventh cause of death, being preceded by heart disease, cancer, cerebral hemorrhage, accidents and violence, diseases of early infancy, influenza and pneumonia, tuberculosis and kidney disease.

At present diagnosed diabetes, that is, recognized and treated by a physician is ten times more prevalent at the age of 45 and thereafter in the United States. Diabetes rates also rise as the weight increases as shown in Figure 61.

The known frequency of diabetes differs in different states in the United States and in different countries. The reason for this was demonstrated by Dr. Elliott P. Joslin when he found that differences in age, sex, and occupation reduced the differences between the frequency of diabetes in Arizona and Rhode Island greatly. However, it is difficult to explain the variations in the prevalence of diabetes in such countries as The Netherlands and England. Probably the explanations for the differences are connected with the reporting of the disease by physicians in these various countries on the death certificates. Thus, in the United States by the methods of the Fifth Revision of the United States Census the death rate was estimated at 29.1 per 100,000 for 1949, but by the Sixth Revision in which doctors reported the actual cause of the diabetic death and not diabetes alone, it was only 16.9 per 100,000. The Sixth Revision Census described methods nearly like those in Florida, England and Wales where the death rate was 8.4 in 1950.

WHAT IS DIABETES?

Diabetes is a chronic disorder but with various acute manifestations. It is hereditary, controllable, but not curable. The exact cause continues to escape research scientists. In certain patients the insulin which is released by the beta cells of the pancreas is prevented from doing its normal job of transferring the sugar from the blood into the tissues. This defect may be followed by failure to produce adequate amounts of insulin and then any of the complications of diabetes may follow, including acid poisoning which may be fatal unless properly treated.

TABLE 2
CAUSES OF DEATH AMONG DIABETIC PATIENTS.
DEATHS IN SPECIFIED PERIODS BETWEEN 1937 AND 1964
EXPERIENCE OF THE JOSLIN CLINIC, BOSTON, MASS.

	1/1/37 to 12/31/43		1/1/44 to 12/31/49		1/1/50 to 12/31/55		1/1/56 to 12/31/59		1/1/60 to 2/19/64*	
Cause of Death	*Number of Deaths*	*Per Cent of all Causes*	*Number of Deaths*	*Per Cent of all Causes*	*Number of Deaths*	*Per Cent of all Causes*	*Number of Deaths*	*Per Cent of all Causes*	*Number of Deaths*	*Per Cent of all Causes*
All Causes	3,639	100.0	4,148	100.0	5,640	100.0	4,176	100.0	2,634	100.0
Diabetic Coma (Primary)	102	2.8	72	1.7	60	1.1	35	0.8	29	1.1
Cardio-renal-vascular	2,392	65.7	2,958	71.3	4,336	76.9	3,182	76.2	2,053	77.9
Arteriosclerotic	2,375	65.3	2,931	70.7	4,298	76.2	3,150	75.4	2,030	77.1
Cardiac	1,496	41.1	1,958	47.2	2,835	50.3	2,123	50.8	1,404	53.3
Coronary and Angina	825	22.7	1,115	26.9	1,904	33.8	1,461	35.0	1,061	40.3
Renal	167	4.6	239	5.8	507	9.0	372	8.9	243	9.2
Diabetic Nephropathy	–	–	–	–	281	5.0	229	5.5	160	6.1
Cerebral	430	11.8	529	12.8	746	13.2	520	12.5	327	12.4
Gangrene	192	5.3	121	2.9	111	2.0	84	2.0	33	1.3
Site unassigned	90	2.5	84	2.0	99	1.8	51	1.2	23	0.9

Other circulatory and rheumatic heart disease	17	0.5	27	0.7	38	0.7	32	0.8	23	0.9
Infections, total	377	10.4	246	5.9	294	5.2	212	5.1	154	5.8
Pneumonia and respiratory	202	5.6	151	3.6	163	2.9	99	2.4	79	3.0
Gall Bladder	21	0.6	13	0.3	19	0.3	10	0.2	12	0.5
Appendicitis	19	0.5	6	0.1	8	0.1	4	0.1	–	–
Carbuncle	18	0.5	1	0.0	2	0.0	2	0.0	–	–
Kidney, acute	32	0.9	27	0.7	34	0.6	34	0.8	32	1.2
Abscesses	29	0.8	9	0.2	8	0.1	7	0.2	2	0.1
Other infections	56	1.5	39	0.9	60	1.1	56	1.3	29	1.1
Cancer	327	9.0	402	9.7	569	10.1	459	11.0	249	9.5
Tuberculosis	79	2.2	69	1.7	40	0.7	16	0.4	3	0.1
Diabetes–(i.e., unknown)	127	3.5	109	2.6	36	0.6	18	0.4	7	0.3
Accidents	69	1.9	86	2.1	108	1.9	81	1.9	45	1.7
Cirrhosis of the liver	33	0.9	51	1.2	52	0.9	51	1.2	26	1.0
Suicides	23	0.6	24	0.6	23	0.4	10	0.2	7	0.3
Insulin reactions	10	0.3	10	0.2	12	0.2	10	0.2	7	0.3
Other diseases	100	2.7	121	2.9	110	2.0	102	2.4	54	2.1

* Deaths reported through February 19, 1964.
Note: Figures for 1950 and later are not strictly comparable with those for earlier periods because of changes in the basis of classification.

In diabetes the patient fails to get the benefit of the food which he eats, particularly the sugar and starch (carbohydrate foods), and to a lesser degree of the meat, fish, eggs, and cheese (protein foods), and even of the fatty foods such as the fat in meat, cream, butter, oil, and nuts. As a result of interference with the action of insulin or of insufficient insulin from the pancreas, much of the food including most of the carbohydrate, a notable portion of the protein, and only a small portion of the fat, changes to sugar "glucose," and this sugar accumulates to excess in the blood and tissues. In diabetes the normal routine is broken and the sugar spills over and passes out of the body through the kidneys and escapes into the urine.

Years ago it was noticed that the urine of a diabetic was sweet, as sweet as honey, and so the disease was called *diabetes mellitus,* in contrast to a much rarer disease, *diabetes insipidus,* in which the urine is simply watery. The sugar is thus lost to the body, and from this fact anyone can imagine what most of the symptoms of diabetes must be. The untreated patient loses weight, because he loses the sugar in his urine. This sugar may amount to as much as one pound or even more in a day. He is thirsty because he must excrete the sugar in soluble form, and to do this he drinks large quantities of water. As a result he voids large quantities of urine. Of course he is thirsty, of course he loses weight, of course he becomes weak and debilitated, and years ago, when treatment was unsatisfactory, he became a prey to almost any disease. Thanks to a better knowledge of diet and the discovery and use of insulin, the diabetic patient can live the average life expectancy. There are many times as many diabetics as fifty years ago, but this is largely because the treatment has correspondingly improved and kept alive those who have it for years—children fifteen times as long, and all patients on the average at least three times as long. A goodly percentage live longer with the disease than they were expected to live without it, because of their following the rules and living a more hygienic life.

Growth-onset diabetes, seen in childhood or adolescence, is usually rapid in its development. Thirst, loss of weight and strength are definite and the family can recognize the onset easily. This is the so-called "brittle" type (the labile type) in which the sugar in the blood rises easily after food or during infections and sometimes falls easily and rapidly following the administration of insulin, especially if extra exercise is taken. This instability with also the tendency to develop acidosis and coma is probably related to a greatly reduced power of the pancreas to make insulin.

Maturity-onset diabetes is the milder diabetes occurring in persons above the age of forty years. The symptoms may develop so gradually or be so mild that the condition may actually exist for years before it is recognized. Such patients are most frequently obese. They do not so easily get low blood-sugar reactions and are less likely to develop acidosis and coma.

Diabetes is not a bad disease, because it is clean and not contagious, and the patient who learns the rules of treatment and follows them can keep it largely under control. Many of the most celebrated people in the world have had diabetes. There is some ground for the belief that the diabetic is born more capable than the usual person. Be that as it may, certainly, through the training of his mind to control his condition, he acquires character. Therefore the diabetic should be encouraged. There may be compensations. With courage and persistence he can prove himself to be the master of his fate.

PREVENTION OF DIABETES

BLAMABLE DIABETICS (INFLUENCE OF OVERWEIGHT)

Richard Wagner, formerly of Vienna, who has had many diabetic children to treat and has written an excellent book with Richard Priesel on the disease,[1] divides diabetics into two classes according to the origin of the disease: the blameless diabetics and the blamable diabetics. Let us consider the blamable diabetics first.

If a man gets smallpox today, we say he is to be blamed for it; he is blamable. If he gets drunk and has an accident, we blame him; if he is an adult and gets typhoid fever, we say he could have avoided it, he is blamable. No man needs to get smallpox, needs to get drunk, needs to get typhoid fever, because he can be vaccinated against smallpox, leave alcohol alone, and be immunized against typhoid. So it is with a large group of diabetics. Needless overweight precedes their diabetes. Most of those who have diabetes in middle life have overeaten and were fat before they got it. Take any group of diabetics of the age of fifty years or more, and the highest weights of most any ten of them before they developed the disease would have added up to a ton.

Years ago we frequently assembled at our diabetes classes ten diabetics whose maximum weights totaled a ton, but now fat people are less common. This fat type of diabetes contrasts sharply with *blameless* diabetes, in which overweight is insignificant and the chief factor is heredity. Overweight should be avoided particularly by relatives of diabetics, among whom diabetes is much more apt to occur. Overweight at all ages above the second decade predisposes to diabetes, but it is of little account among

[1] *Die Zuckerkrankheit und ihre Behandlung im Kindesalter*, George Thieme, Leipzig.

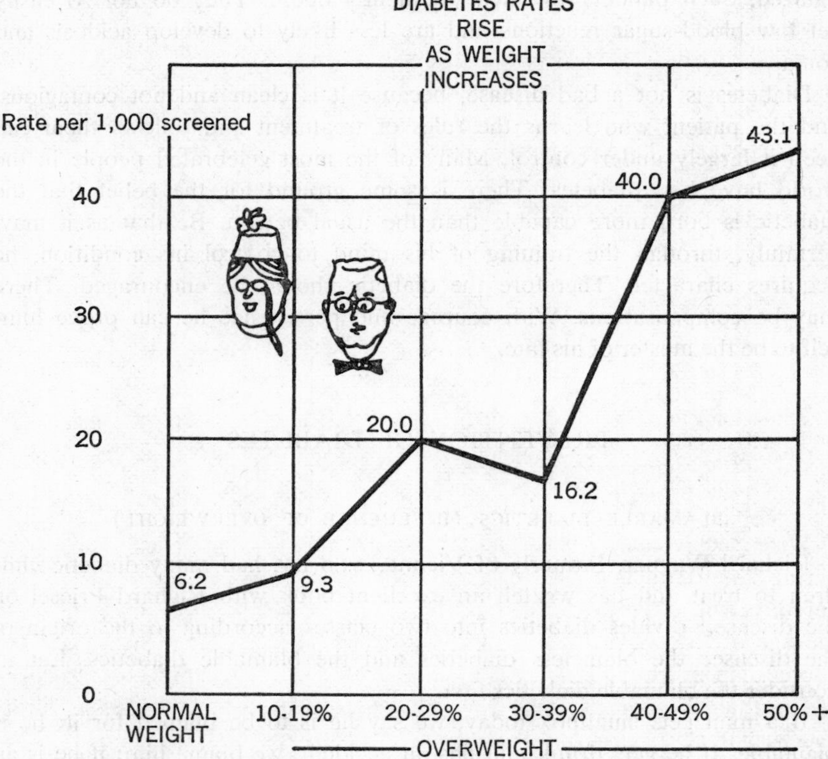

Fig. 60. Diabetes Rates Rise as Weight Increases. Obesity is reported to precede diabetes in 85 per cent of the cases and is considered by some to be second only to heredity as the most activating factor in its development. Mass screening surveys demonstrate the pronounced prevalence of diabetes among persons who are overweight. Joslin, Elliott, P., et al., *The Treatment of Diabetes Mellitus,* Philadelphia: Lea and Febiger, 1959. From *Diabetes Source Book,* National Center for Chronic Disease Control.

those who develop it until middle life. Eighty per cent of diabetics with onset above twenty years of age are overweight. In Jewish adults the figures are still higher, and among Jewish women reach no less than 94 per cent. Of diabetics in the Joslin Clinic with onset between fifty-one and sixty years of age, only one in 1,000 gave a history of always having been underweight. Diabetic children are overheight rather than overweight, and the contrast shows from the earliest years of onset. When I see a diabetic who, I suspect, is overweight, I look up the age, weight, and height table and, if overweight is present, I make a large red cross on the history sheet along with the pounds in excess to attract his and my attention. I always weigh the relative of a diabetic coming to the office, if overweight seems probable, as a warning.

TABLE 3
VARIATION FROM NORMAL OF MAXIMUM WEIGHTS AT OR PRIOR TO ONSET OF 1000 CASES OF TRUE DIABETES, CALCULATED FOR HEIGHT, AGE AND SEX

Age, Years	*Number of Cases*	*Percentage in Normal Average Zone (+5 to −5 Per Cent)*	*Percentage of Each Decade*	
			Below Standard Weight	*Above Standard Weight*
0 to 10	43	37	44	19
11 to 20	84	39	29	32
21 to 30	112	19	10	71
31 to 40	172	6	5	89
41 to 50	244	12	3	85
51 to 60	252	12	1	87
61 to 70	79	10	6	84
71 to 80	14	14	7	79

Wise people, and particularly the wise relatives of a diabetic, remembering the frequency of diabetes among the fat and the possibility of heredity, will strive to keep their weight under control. If they are under the age of thirty-five, they should not try to be underweight, because the young man or young woman who is underweight has a shorter expectancy of life than the one of normal weight or slightly above, and, furthermore, overweight as a cause of diabetes is not so important in the young. But being wise people, when they reach thirty years of age, they will keep their weight under control. To do this, exercise helps. Avoidance of overeating of any kind of food helps. And particularly and most easily can one control body weight by limiting sugar and starch, and most safely by lowering the fat in the diet, such as the butter, cream, oil, and the fat on meat.

When do people get fat and then get diabetes? They get fat when exercise ceases and a sedentary life begins. The policeman is promoted from his beat to an office chair and develops diabetes; a laborer is promoted, lessens physical activity, adds pounds as well as diabetes. An officer in the field is given an assignment at headquarters, and diabetes begins. A boy breaks his leg, his activity ceases, and friends place a box of candy at his elbow, and diabetes appears. A woman has gallstones, is successfully operated on, and her friends send food instead of flowers; she rapidly becomes fat, and diabetes breaks forth. It develops particularly with patients after operations in which underactivity is accompanied by overeating, after operations which lead to overweight because of the removal of an organ like the thyroid which lowers the metabolism; and, above all, in women when the tendency to diabetes is greatest, namely, at the menopause and especially after hysterectomy.

The surgeon should always warn his patients against putting on excessive weight after an operation.

One is on sure ground when preaching and exhorting against overweight. The insurance companies realize this and are spending millions of dollars to prevent it, so that those they insure will live longer. There is no doubt about the handicap of overweight to one with heart disease. If you are fifty pounds overweight, apply for insurance and see how much more you must pay to get insurance than you would if your weight were standard. Overweight shortens life for everyone, but it is especially dangerous in diabetes, because it helps to bring on the disease. If you are the relative of a diabetic, never be overweight, because in this way you may escape developing diabetes.

BLAMELESS DIABETICS (INFLUENCE OF HEREDITY)

Blameless diabetes is the diabetes pre-eminently of children and those under thirty years of age. This rule of obesity, as provocative of diabetes, does not hold in the first two decades of life, and there is evidently another reason for the breaking out of diabetes in the young. Blameless diabetes is the diabetes, then, of the child, and why is his diabetes blameless and that of the poor old man or woman blamable? The diabetic child could not follow Oliver Wendell Holmes's rule and pick out his parents. Although Naunyn suspected and recognized heredity as the cause of diabetes, it is only recently that the proof of its influence has arrived. At first heredity did not seem to be of great importance, because in only 20 per cent of our cases in children could we trace a relative who had the disease. We did not realize years ago that this was simply because the children only lived a year or two and so we lost track of them. Their families were so sad at the death of their children that one did not feel justified in seeking information in after years about the later appearance of the disease in the parents or other members of the family. But today we have a sufficiently large group of diabetic children for statistical purposes who have already lived twenty years. And now we find that, instead of one child in five, or 20 per cent, having a relative with the disease, today, according to Dr. Priscilla White, every other child (actually 55 per cent) has a diabetic relative. As the parents of many of our diabetic children are still young, they have hardly entered the diabetic zone of fifty years, the year in which diabetes is most common, and therefore it is probable that still more may show it before they die. Dr. Priscilla White has studied this most carefully in association with Dr. Gregory Pincus, formerly of the Biological Department of Harvard University, now of the Worcester Foundation for Experimental Biology.

TABLE 4
INCIDENCE OF DIABETES IN THE FAMILIES OF DIABETICS.
PERCENTAGE OF CASES REPORTING HEREDITARY
AND/OR FAMILIAL TYPES OF FAMILY HISTORY.

	No. of Cases	*Per Cent with Family History of Diabetes*
Joslin, 1920–1928	4831	25.6
Joslin, 1941. Hospital Cases	1619	41.0
Joslin, total children, 1946	2191	35.0
Joslin, 1946. Children of 20 or more years' duration	249	55.0

The diabetic child is born with a tendency to diabetes. The facts correspond with the theory. Consequently, if you do not want diabetes, first of all pick out non-diabetic parents. The tendency to diabetes appears to be transmitted as a so-called recessive characteristic. If the tendency is strong, the disease comes on soon after birth; if the tendency is slight, it takes some secondary cause to make it develop, and of these secondary causes obesity stands first. Perhaps, after all, our fat friend is not so blamable as we may have thought: he may have been born with a tendency to diabetes. However, if he had kept thin, perhaps he could have avoided it.

The rules, therefore, for the prevention of diabetes as far as heredity is concerned are quite definite and can be summarized as follows:

To prevent the transmission of the disease to the offspring:

1. Two diabetics should not marry and have children, because theoretically all their children would have their disease.
2. If a diabetic marries a non-diabetic, but in whose family there is a close diabetic relative, half of the children are liable to have diabetes.
3. If two individuals marry who do not have diabetes, but in whose families the disease exists, the chances are that one in four of the children will develop the disease.
4. If a diabetic marries a non-diabetic who is of a non-diabetic family, no diabetic children should be expected, although their children could transmit the tendency.

For *practical* purposes, the liability of the offspring of diabetics to diabetes is not quite so strong as indicated above. It is only about *half the theoretical,* because those born of diabetics, like those of non-diabetic parents, die from other causes before the time arrives at which they would develop diabetes. Thus we know that only one diabetic in three develops the disease under forty years of age, one in three between forty and fifty-five, and the remaining one in three between fifty-five and one hundred years.

A diabetic child, therefore, is always a blameless diabetic. It is rather the parents who may be blamable. But the parents of a diabetic child are not always blamable, because they may not have been aware of the extent of diabetes in their families and may not ever have heard that diabetes is hereditary.

If you want to dodge diabetes, therefore, pick out your ancestors, don't get fat, and keep active; and if you have diabetes, or if it is in your family and you do not want to hand it down, fall in love with someone who does not have the disease or whose family is free from it. Of course, this may be a hardship, because you may not find anyone to marry who is as nice and bright as a diabetic, but still there are compensations, because your grandchildren may rise up and call you blessed. Remember there are about 200,000,000 people in the United States, and only one fourth of them have a diabetic tendency. So there are left some 150,000,000 for you to choose from.

Every once in a while a diabetic discovers diabetes in a relative, and, contrary to his expectations, he is rewarded by finding that his relative does better with treatment than he himself. The reason may be that he has discovered the relative's disease at an earlier stage than that at which his own was recognized, and so treatment was started early, which is always a help. Furthermore, any diabetic who picks up the disease in a relative can be encouraged, because the treatment of diabetes is improving so rapidly that his relative, who develops it a few years after his own disease began, will be able to begin the treatment under improved conditions and so will do particularly well. I have seen this occur in various families where a second child has come down with the disease, and recently it was a great comfort to me to note the attitude of the parents when they found out that their second child had diabetes. They were sorry but not overwhelmed, because from their experience with their older boy they were confident they could keep the disease under control.

The diabetic, if he is fond of his family, will not only point out to his relatives the dangers of being fat, but will go a step farther and along with the tests which he makes of his own urine he will make similar tests for the rest of the family whenever their birthdays occur.

Today the diabetic children are the pathfinders for the diabetic adults. Every honest diabetic day which a child lives teaches a lesson which helps a feeble old diabetic man or woman to live more comfortably. Children are exploring unknown diabetic regions. Today, the younger the child the longer can be the length of his life, and instead of saying, as we used to do, the older you are the milder the diabetes, now all agree the younger you are the greater the diabetic life expectancy.

ORGANS IN THE BODY INVOLVED IN DIABETES

In recent years it has been shown that diabetes is not at first a lack of insulin *per se* but rather an interference with its action. It appears that the presence of one or more factors in the blood alter the insulin and render it unable to play its usual effective role. The hereditary nature of diabetes suggests that this factor may be carried by a single gene but requires a double dose for the development of the symptoms of diabetes. Therefore, intense interest exists in a search for the mysterious protein causative factor. Nevertheless, later on the amount of insulin produced by the pancreas does fall to a low level. Therefore, for many years it has been felt that diabetes centers around the pancreas.

The pancreas is commonly known as the sweetbread and lies behind the stomach and just in front of the backbone. It was not until 1889 that the discovery was made by Minkowsi and von Mering that by removing this gland from a dog diabetes developed. In the pancreas are groups of cells called islands of Langerhans. Their work was described by a young German doctor in 1869 and given his name, but no one appreciated what they were for until in 1901 Opie and Sobolew discovered that when they were destroyed diabetes was present. It is not the whole pancreas but these collections of cells in it, which weigh not more than two and a half to five grams, or the weight of a dime or a nickel, that are responsible for diabetes. In them, insulin is made; and when we do not have insulin, diabetes exists. But there are other glands which influence the secretion of the Langerhans islands which make insulin. The most important is perhaps the pituitary gland situated in the center of the head and protected by a bony case. This is a tiny gland, the master gland of the body, which makes many hormones. It controls growth and sexual development and has many other functions. Inject an extract of it into a sound animal and diabetes will eventually appear, because it destroys the insulin-producing cells of the islands of Langerhans. Remove it and the diabetes gets milder.

Another gland situated on the upper pole of each kidney also influences the secretion of insulin. One of its powers is to interfere with the secretion of insulin, another is to accelerate the rapid breakdown of glycogen (animal starch) and protein in the liver and thus increase their change to sugar, thus making the diabetes more severe, providing insulin is not available to control the rate of change.

The thyroid gland in the neck, if overactive as in that type of goiter which is manifest by rapid pulse, protruding eyes, sweating and tremor, and rapid consumption of body tissue–increased metabolism–is another gland which affects the diabetes and makes it much more severe. Fortunately, by its partial removal this unfavorable action can be eliminated.

The liver is the storehouse of animal starch–glycogen–and is the factory where this can be broken down into sugar for the body to use or be converted into fat and then either stored in the liver or transported for storage to other parts of the body. The liver is very important in diabetes because in it one kind of food is interchanged with another. We need to know much more about its many activities.

EXPERIMENTAL DIABETES

Dunn, in Scotland, while experimenting to learn the cause of shock, was so observant as to note that when alloxan, one of the many chemicals he was testing, was injected into an animal the islands of Langerhans were singled out and destroyed almost immediately, leaving the remainder of the body uninjured. He deserves great credit for having observed this, because grossly there was no change in the pancreas and it was disclosed only by microscopical examination. Alloxan is a derivative of uric acid, which is a common component of the body. If it were true that alloxan and uric acid were found in excess in diabetes, then we would be a step nearer to an explanation of its cause. However, this is not the case; for as yet alloxan has not been found in human beings, although studies revolving around it have taught us much.

In certain animals, diabetes-like states may be induced experimentally by means of growth hormone, glucagon, corticosteroids, or ACTH.

An extraordinary discovery occurred in 1964. Sand rats, imported for kidney studies, became acutely diabetic on the standard American laboratory chow diet. In Egypt, these creatures live in the desert and survive by nibbling green leaves and burrowing for plant roots. This diet is low in carbohydrate. When brought to laboratories in this country, it was found that when, given a more nutritious diet, rich in starch which American animals are fed, they developed spontaneous diabetes in less than ten days. Blood sugar levels rose from 100 to 700 milligrams and without immediate treatment, the animals would die. Insulin production by the pancreas rapidly declined.

A colony of such animals in our research laboratory are being studied with the hope that this discovery will give new insight into the relation of diet to the onset and treatment of diabetes.

There are two kinds of cells in the islands of Langerhans—the beta cells, which are the more numerous and the ones which produce insulin, and the alpha cells, which are less abundant and apparently secrete something which raises the blood sugar and makes the diabetes worse. Quite recently it has been found that just as alloxan will destroy the beta insulin-producing cells, a mineral—cobalt—will destroy the alpha cells and thus abolish the action of the alpha cells which makes the diabetes worse. The properties of alloxan and cobalt are wonderful and almost past belief. Alloxan is so specific that it is as though a bomb dropped from an airplane high up over a city with 800,000 blocks would invariably always select and destroy the same block!

What hours, days, months, and years must be spent to unravel the mystery of the marvelous action of these chemicals! Each diabetic should have a hand in furthering research. Think of what might be learned if each of the 1,500,000 diabetics in the country gave a dollar yearly for this purpose!

DOGS AND DIABETICS

The diabetic child does well because he leads a routine life, having regular hours for meals, exercise, and sleep. Note this, you older diabetics. You will do well to follow the example of a child, just as he in turn follows that of his dog and cleaves to him. In fact, every diabetic should own a dog, because a dog is a diabetic's thoughtful friend. A dog never says to a diabetic, "You are thin," never speaks about his diet, never tempts him to break it and to eat a little more, never refers to the delicacies he himself has eaten or the good bones he expects to eat; in fact, never implies by any sign or action that he knows his master has diabetes. A diabetic is never embarrassed by his dog. How often he wishes his friends were as considerate!

A dog is a diabetic's teacher. His dog shows the diabetic how to rest and sleep at odd moments, shows him how to exercise and play, indicates the value of sunshine, and sets him a good example by cleaning his paws every night. A dog is cheerful. The friends of a diabetic sometimes wish that he would take lessons from his dog.

From experiments on a dog Minkowski found out that diabetes originated in the pancreas. From experiments on a dog Allen learned that undereating helped and overeating harmed diabetes. From experiments on a dog Banting and Best discovered insulin, and from experiments upon a dog Young found that diabetes could be produced by injections of the pituitary gland, and Best showed that it could be prevented by the prompt administration of insulin.

So deeply did Dr. Elliott Joslin feel our indebtedness to animals for advances in medicine that in the foyer of the Joslin Clinic in the Diabetes Foundation building has been placed a plaque, suggested by the War Memorial Chapel in Edinburgh, with its memorials to men and women as well as to birds and beasts who also served and died.

DETECTION AND DIAGNOSIS OF DIABETES

The earlier the discovery of diabetes, the better will be the results of treatment with modern remedies, diet, exercise and insulin or the oral remedies. This conviction led to the establishment of the countrywide efforts of the Diabetes Detection Program—Annual Diabetes Week in November—of the American Diabetes Association. Approximately one child under 15 years of age in 2500 was found to have diabetes but among adults, over 65 years of age the frequency of diabetes is very great. Two-thirds of the cases begin after 40 years of age and the mean age of onset for men is 45 years and for women, approximately 50 years. Diabetes is much more common in females than in males after the age of 50 years but this increased frequency is predominantly among married women. Married women weigh on the average more than single women. All studies in various parts of the world have agreed that the prevalence of diabetes in middle and late life is associated with obesity. If you don't want diabetes —never get fat. Especially is this true if you are related to a diabetic.

We are now interested in recognizing persons who are susceptible to diabetes and who are most likely to develop diabetes later, even though there are no abnormal blood-sugar tests or no sugar can be found in the urine. This is the state of prediabetes and as yet we can only be certain that the prediabetic state exists in a few situations: *A*. The identical twin of a diabetic patient; *B*. Persons with diabetes in close relatives. Thus if both parents are diabetic, 100 per cent of the children will be susceptible to diabetes but not necessarily develop it; 50 to 80 per cent of individuals with one diabetic parent and a diabetic brother or sister. *C*. Women with a tendency to have large babies, usually considered as in excess of 10 pounds. Not all future diabetic mothers do have large or stillborn babies but the majority of mothers in the prediabetic years have produced at least one baby over 10 pounds at birth. Repeated miscarriages and the toxemias of pregnancy should be suspected and should be included in the group of patients described above who should have regular medical examinations at least once a year.

In 1964 the International Diabetes Federation voted to encourage detection programs throughout the world. In the same year, the World Health Organization in Geneva has appointed a Committee of Diabetes Experts to consider the world problems of diabetes, diagnosis, and detection.

URINE TESTS IN DIAGNOSIS OF DIABETES

Every diabetic should learn how to test the urine for sugar. Then he knows whether his disease is controlled and, to a great extent, becomes the master of his diabetes. The urine on rising—the fasting urine—is the one most apt to be sugar free; the urine voided after a meal is the one most apt to contain sugar. If the fasting urine contains sugar, test another specimen half an hour later, because that urine may be sugar free. The reason for this is that the urine is constantly being secreted by the two kidneys day and night, and then passes through two tubes, called ureters, into the bladder. This has no compartments. Therefore, if a urine containing sugar was secreted at 2:00 A.M. by the kidneys, it would collect in the bladder, and even if no sugar was secreted by the kidneys at 7:00 A.M., when the bladder was emptied, the voided urine would contain sugar, because it would have been mixed with the 2:00 A.M. specimen.

The Benedict Test. The Benedict test is the test most generally employed for the detection of sugar in the urine. It requires a single solution and this keeps indefinitely. The test is sufficiently delicate to detect quantities as small as 0.08 or 1.10 per cent sugar, in which case a faint pea-green change in color takes place. This green color changes to a yellowish-green when the urine contains about 0.5 per cent sugar. When the solution loses the greenish tint entirely and becomes yellow or brown, the urine contains over 1 per cent sugar. Above this percentage the color of the solution gives very little aid in estimating the amount of sugar in the urine, although large amounts of sugar will produce an orange, brown, or red test.

The test is carried out as follows: Four (exactly 4) drops of urine are placed in a test tube and to this are added 2.5 cc. (an ordinary teaspoon holds about 5 cc.) of Benedict's solution. Eight drops of urine and 5 cc. of Benedict's solution are often employed, but the use of half quantities is just as satisfactory and more economical. The tube is shaken to mix the urine and solution, and then placed in water that is already bubbling boiling. In the presence of glucose (sugar), the entire body of the solution will be filled with a precipitate, which may be greenish, yellow, or red in color, according to whether the amount of sugar is slight or considerable. Particularly if 4 drops are used with 2.5 cc. of Benedict's solution, the test should be carried out in boiling water for five minutes rather than over a free flame, because of evaporation of the solution. If 5 cc. of Benedict's solution and 8 drops of urine are employed, as in the original test, the solution may be boiled over a free flame for two minutes, in which case a Pyrex test tube should be used. This latter method is liable to error because, unless one has a test-tube holder, the test tube gets too hot to hold with the fingers, and therefore the specimen may not be boiled for the whole length of time.

Other methods of testing the urine sugar exist. The Clinitest is carried out by dropping a tablet into a measured amount of urine and water and watching the change in color which denotes if sugar is present. It depends upon the same type of copper reduction as occurs in the Benedict's test. Tes-tape is a simple test carried out by dipping a strip of test paper in the urine and the change in color from yellow to blue or green indicates sugar in the urine. It depends on what is called the "glucose oxidase" method. Patients frequently use the Tes-tape while traveling. Both Tes-tape and

Clinitest or Clinistix materials must be kept dry and preferably in a dark place.

Occasionally, rare sugars such as levulose or pentose are found in the urine. They do not indicate true diabetes. Only glucose in the urine suggests diabetes and requires a blood-sugar test for final diagnosis. Many persons, particularly in the older age groups, have increased sugar in the blood without sugar in the urine. Occasional patients have normal sugar in the blood with sugar in the urine and they do not require treatment if it can be proved that the condition is renal glycosuria.

THE BLOOD SUGAR (GLUCOSE)

All of us have sugar (glucose) in our blood. Glucose is grape sugar, and because a ray of light passing through a solution of it is turned to the right, it is said to be dextrorotatory and is called dextrose. The normal percentage varies between about 0.080 to 0.120 per cent fasting (usually reported 80 and 120 milligrams) and does not exceed 160 milligrams after a meal. In diabetes the blood sugar is above normal after an ordinary meal and usually rises to 200 milligrams or more. If the sugar in the blood is above normal, it is termed *hyperglycemia;* if the blood sugar is below normal, it is termed *hypoglycemia.* The fasting blood sugar is usually elevated in diabetes, but may not be in the very early stages of the disease, particularly in children. The sugar in the blood corresponds to that in the urine only when compared with a specimen of urine which has been secreted by the kidneys and voided in the preceding few minutes—half an hour—the bladder having been previously evacuated.

DIAGNOSIS OF DIABETES

The fasting blood sugar is usually elevated in active diabetes, but it may be of no value in the diagnosis of early diabetes, especially in children. A test by giving an extra load of carbohydrate may be necessary to show the early defect of diabetes. This load can be supplied by a meal containing 100 grams of carbohydrate in the form of bread, potato, and dessert, or two candy bars or a measured amount of glucose as prescribed by the doctor. The blood sugar taken one, two, or three hours after eating such a meal may be above normal, exceeding 160 mg. together with sugar in the urine and this identifies diabetes. Blood-sugar tests therefore taken after a meal are most valuable, particularly when the patient is under stress. However, a single abnormal blood-sugar test should be regarded merely as an indication for a more complete study to determine whether true diabetes exists or not.

A diagnosis of diabetes is made when in addition to glucose in the urine, a fasting blood sugar is 130 mg. or when after food the blood sugar is 160 mg. or more. These are borderline values and caution must be observed in making a diagnosis until the tests are confirmed by special tolerance tests. The 100-gram oral glucose tolerance test carried out for three hours is one of the commonest diagnostic procedures in recognizing true diabetes. The patient should be tested after being on a liberal diet for three days before the test. Sometimes special diets are prescribed during this period. Then the patient should have taken no hypoglycemic agents such as insulin or the oral drugs for a few days before the test. Complications such as infections, fever, disorders of the thyroid or pituitary gland, and certain gastrointestinal conditions must be absent if the test is to be reliable.

TREATMENT OF DIABETES

DIET

1. Reduce the Total Amount of Food. In diabetes there is an excess of sugar in the blood and a loss of sugar in the urine. To bring the blood sugar down to the normal level of 0.1 per cent (100 milligrams per cent) fasting, or below 0.17 per cent (170 milligrams per cent) after meals, and to prevent this loss of sugar in the urine, the earliest method known, and still the best, is the diet. Fasting, living entirely without food, will make most any diabetic sugar free, but naturally that can be employed only temporarily. In the very severest cases it would be dangerous, because even out of the body tissues sugar would be formed and lost in the urine, and the individual would burn up so much of his own body fat that he would develop acid poisoning—acidosis—which might result in diabetic coma and death. Nevertheless, the avoidance of overeating of any kind of food is helpful, and that alone in the mildest cases will prevent the diabetes growing worse. The diabetic therefore should never overeat, should never be fat, but today we do not need to fast a diabetic to control his disease.

2. Lower the Carbohydrate. If reducing the total quantity of food does not stop the loss of sugar in the urine, the next step is to limit the sugar and starch—carbohydrate—in the diet, because from sugar and starch, sugar is most readily formed. This will result in lowering the sugar in the blood and the escape of sugar in the urine. Today we need not omit all the carbohydrate, because one can take insulin to help utilize part of it. It is seldom necessary to reduce the carbohydrate below that contained in a slice of bread and a medium-sized orange at each meal, four portions of vegetables in the low 3 per cent and 6 per cent carbohydrate groups (Table 5), a portion of cereal, and oatmeal is the best because it contains

Dietary Essentials for Diabetics

TABLE 5. CARBOHYDRATE, PROTEIN, FAT, AND CALORIES IN COMMON FOODS

30 Grams 1 oz. Contain Approximately	*Carb. C. Gram*	*Protein P. Gram*	*Fat F. Gram*	*Calories*
Bread, 1 large slice	15	2.5	0	70
Oatmeal, large portion	20	5	2	118
Crackers, 2	10	1	0	44
Vegetables, 3% + 5% 4 large portions	20	6	0	104
Potato	6	1	0	28
Milk	1.5	1	1	19
Egg, 1	0	6	6	78
Meat, lean	0	7	5	73
Chicken, lean	0	8	3	59
Fish, fat-free	0	6	0	24
Cheese	0	8	10	122
Bacon	0	5	15	155
Cream, 20% light	1	1	6	62
Cream, 40% heavy	1	1	12	116
Butter	0	0	25	225

Vegetables and Fruits Arranged According to Content of Carbohydrate

Water, clear broths, coffee and tea, can be taken without allowance for food content

VEGETABLES, fresh or canned	
Reckon average carbohydrate, utilized, 3%; 6%; 20%	
3 per cent	
Lettuce	Tomatoes
Cucumbers, raw	Radishes
Spinach	Water cress
Asparagus	Snap beans
Celery	Cauliflower
Mushrooms	Cabbage
Rhubarb	Egg plant
Sauerkraut	Broccoli
Endive, raw	Green peppers
Swiss chard	Kohlrabi
Beet greens	Kale
Dandelions	Summer squash
6 per cent	**20 per cent**
Turnip	Potatoes
Carrots	Shell beans
Okra	Baked beans
Pumpkin	Lima beans
Onions	Corn
Squash	Boiled rice
Brussels sprouts	Boiled macaroni
Beets	
Green peas	

FRUITS, fresh or canned (water packed) *Food*	*Carb. 10*	*Grams 15*
Grapefruit pulp	150	225
Strawberries	150	225
Watermelon	150	225
Cantaloupe	150	225
Blackberries	120	180
Orange pulp	100	150
Pears	90	135
Peaches	90	135
Apricots	80	120
Raspberries	80	120
Plums	80	120
Pineapple	70	105
Apple	70	105
Honeydew melon	70	105
Blueberries	70	105
Cherries	60	90
Banana	50	75
Prunes (cooked)	50	75
Ice cream	50	75

1 gm. carbohydrate, 4 calories
1 gm. protein, 4 calories
1 gm. fat, 9 calories

1 kilogram (kg.) = 2.2 lbs.
30 grams (g.) or cubic centimeters (cc) = 1 oz. A patient "at rest" requires 25 calories per kg.

TABLE 6. DIABETIC DIETS IN GRAMS

Diets	Total Diet				Carbohydrate (C)						Protein and Fat (PF)				
	Carbo-hy-drate	*Pro-tein*	*Fat*	*Calo-ries*	*Vege-tables 3%-6%*	*Or-ange*	*Oat-meal*	*Po-tato*	*Bread*	*Milk*	*Egg*	*Meat*	*Bacon*	*20% Cream*	*But-ter*
C1 PF1	137	60	61	1337	600	450	0	0	90	300	1	120	0	0	30
C2 PF2	149	65	74	1522	600	450	15	0	90	300	1	120	0	60	30
C3 PF3	167	78	86	1754	600	450	15	90	90	300	1	150	15	60	30
C4 PF4	184	89	103	2019	600	450	15	90	120	300	1	180	15	120	30
C5 PF5	199	101	116	2244	600	450	15	90	150	300	1	210	30	120	30
Acute Illness	160	52	52	1316	0	450	15	0	90	960	1	0	0	0	15

To add carbohydrate 15 grams, add bread 1 slice, potato 75 grams or 1 medium orange; to add 75 calories, add bread 1 slice, milk ½ glass, meat 1 oz. or 1 egg. One oz. bacon contains C.0 P.5 F.15 155 calories; one oz. butter 225 calories.

the least carbohydrate, a glass of milk, and a few biscuits–4 saltines, 3 Uneedas, or 4 graham crackers. The balance of the diet would be made up of the usual quantity of protein–meat, fish, eggs, cheese–for the age, weight, and height of the individual, and finally of fat sufficient to maintain a normal weight or bring it to normal. Liquids are unrestricted, and as for minerals and vitamins, there are usually enough in the foods above mentioned.

The above diet can be increased or decreased according to age and size and activity, but there are few who would eat twice as much, and only rapidly growing boys and girls and very hard-working men three times as much carbohydrate.

COMPOSITION OF THE ABOVE DIET

What is the composition of the above diet? How much carbohydrate, protein, and fat does it contain?

Carbohydrate

The carbohydrate content in this diet is easily reckoned if one will remember that a slice of bread, if it weighed one ounce, or 30 grams by the metric system, would contain approximately one-half carbohydrate, one-half ounce, or 15 grams. A half ounce is equivalent to a tablespoonful of sugar, or 3 large lumps. A nickel weighs 5 grams.

The diet is easily learned by examination of Tables 6 and 7.

Table 5 shows the vegetables which contain the least carbohydrate utilized by humans. Even four liberal portions of 3 per cent and 6 per cent vegetables contain only about 20 grams of carbohydrate, which is so little that few diabetics show sugar in the urine if they eat them alone without insulin. They are good for diabetics because they furnish bulk, contain many vitamins, and satisfy hunger. The vegetables in the 20 per cent carbohydrate group, like potatoes, contain much more carbohydrate, and about one third as much as bread. Many diabetics eat no potato when they take bread. Remember that sugar and starch are 100 per cent carbohydrate, bread 50 per cent, potatoes 20 per cent, fruit about 10 per cent, except bananas which are 20 per cent, and vegetables 3 to 6 per cent.

Vegetables in the 3 and 6 per cent carbohydrate groups were formerly listed as 5 and 10 per cent vegetables. They do contain these amounts, and animals eating them get 5 or 10 per cent value of carbohydrate from them, but human beings are not able to secure their full value. A cow gets nourishment from hay and grass, and even Nebuchadnezzar, when "he was driven from men, and did eat grass as oxen," acknowledged its good effect by saying "mine understanding returned unto me" (Daniel 4: 33–34).

Diabetics like to eat. Therefore, give them bulky foods in which the percentage of sugar and starch, the so-called carbohydrate foods, is low. Such foods are the vegetables (the green vegetables, those which generally grow above the ground), termed 3 and 6 per cent vegetables. These bulky vegetables require a long time to be eaten, their use permits many minutes of happiness.

Diabetic vegetables, however, have other advantages in addition to the pleasure one derives while eating them. The sugar and starch in these low-carbohydrate vegetables take so long to get from the stomach into the blood that when the patient takes them, his blood is not suddenly swamped with sugar, which would be the case if he took pure carbohydrate such as sugar or cornstarch. I often tell my patients that the carbohydrate in vegetables *creeps* into the blood, the carbohydrate in potatoes and in cooked rice or macaroni *walks* right into the blood, whereas actual sugar in the diet *runs* into the blood, and if the blood is overloaded with sugar, it spills over and leaks out through the kidneys. Still another great advantage which comes to the diabetic who eats freely of green vegetables and fruits is due to the vitamins which they contain. Perhaps it is because of all these vitamins in vegetables and fruits that diabetic children have such good teeth.

Fruit is desirable, and most kinds contain between 10 and 20 per cent carbohydrate. The equivalent in grams of various fruits which contain 10 or 15 grams is shown in the table at the top of the fruit columns. A few fruits, like grapefruit and strawberries, can be taken in greater amounts than oranges to make up 10 or 15 grams carbohydrate. A medium-sized orange, peeled, contains 15 grams carbohydrate. An apple of similar size contains nearly half as much more. Diabetics must always be careful to compare an apple with its thin skin to an orange without its thick skin.

Fruit is the diabetic's best dessert.

Grapefruit is the safest fruit for a diabetic in that it contains only about 7 per cent carbohydrate. The sugar in half a medium-sized grapefruit is equivalent in weight to two nickels, or 10 grams. Oranges contain 10 per cent carbohydrate, and a small orange, peeled, weighs 100 grams and its sugar content is therefore equal to 10 grams, which is the same as in the half medium-sized grapefruit. A banana contains 20 per cent carbohydrate, and as the ordinary banana weighs about 100 grams, the carbohydrate in half a banana would be equivalent to that in a small orange or half a medium-sized grapefruit. Bananas vary so much in size that, as with potatoes, it is safer to weigh out the allowed portion. Potatoes and bananas, weight for weight, are alike in the percentage of carbohydrate, and it makes no difference whether they are cooked or not so far as the carbohydrate is concerned.

Protein

Tiny cells make up our bodies, and the essential component of these is protein. A horse likes his oats because there is more protein in the oats than in the straw. Protein we must have to replace old cells and to add new ones. Diabetics need protein just like the rest of us. Protein is found in concentrated form in meat, in fish, in eggs, and in its purest state in the white of an egg. The baby gets his protein in the curd or cheese of milk. The younger you are, the more protein you require, because not only have children worn-out cells to repair, but they need new cells to grow. Instinct teaches the baby to take three or four times as much protein for his weight as the old man. (Milk is an ideal food partly because it contains so much protein, and again because of its high content of calcium [lime] for the formation of bones.) Fortunately, diabetics can have as much protein as the ordinary individual and only seldom should have more.

Fat

Fat is the third component of the diet. This is to be found in a pure state in oil. Butter is 85 per cent fat, and cream is a transition from this percentage to the 3 per cent in milk as established by law. There is fat in meat and fish, and one should never forget that in nuts and cheese the percentages of fat are usually high. Oleomargarine can be reckoned as butter. A generation ago we doctors reduced the carbohydrate (sugar and starch) in the diet of our diabetic patients so low that we were compelled to raise the fat to furnish them enough nourishment to keep alive, and we overdid it. What happened? We satisfied their hunger, but we poisoned them with fat, because in the fat lurked danger. Soon we found out through the painstaking work done in many laboratories that if the proportion of fat to carbohydrate in any diet was unduly high, the patient's individual tolerance for fat was exceeded, acetone bodies accumulated in amounts greater than he could oxidize, which in turn caused acid poisoning and death from coma. For this reason today the fat in the diet of diabetics is watched quite as closely as the carbohydrate, and for this same reason we are testing the fat in the blood as well as the sugar to be sure it is not in excess.

As a rule, the diabetic is given as much sugar and starch (carbohydrate) as he can take without sugar appearing in the urine. If he cannot tolerate a considerable quantity—the 150 grams mentioned above in the form of bread 3 slices, oranges 3, 3 per cent and 6 per cent vegetables very freely, oatmeal one portion, milk 1 glass, biscuits 3—he is given insulin to help him get the benefit of it. He takes as much protein as the ordinary individual. As for the quantity of fat, he regulates that by what he needs to hold his weight, which seldom if ever should long remain above normal standards.

In the table are recorded foods with varying percentages of carbohydrate, and, for certain commonly used foods, the quantities of carbohydrate, protein, and fat per 30 grams or one ounce. The values are approximate and not absolute.

A DIABETIC'S MENU

The average diet prescribed for a diabetic in the United States today, I suspect, is about as follows, and if it is not tolerated, the patient's doctor will probably give him insulin.

Breakfast:

Half a grapefruit, a medium portion of oatmeal or a little less of any other cereal, one egg, a pat of butter, one slice of bread, coffee and cream.

Dinner (noon):

A moderate portion of meat or fish, two liberal portions of 3 per cent vegetables or somewhat less of 6 per cent vegetables, a slice of bread or a medium-sized potato, a pat of butter, an orange or its equivalent.

Night:

A similar meal to that at noon.

During the day:

Half a pint of milk and ¼ pint medium rich cream.

With such a diet as a working basis, it is easy to add to it or detract from it according to the needs of the individual patient and to make definite the quantity of carbohydrate, protein, and fat. Such a diet probably contains carbohydrate 150 grams, protein 65 to 75 grams, and fat 80 grams. The food and caloric values are shown in Table 7.

If one wishes, such a diet can be reckoned in calories.

Food	*Calories per Gram*	*Carbohydrate in Diet*	*Total Calories*
Carbohydrate	4	150	600
Protein	4	70	280
Fat	9	80	720
			1600

Calories

Just as coal and gasoline furnish heat which can be reckoned in heat units, so the food we consume contains heat, and this can be estimated

TABLE 7. THE BASIC DIABETIC DIET IS SIMPLE

Food	*Unit Portion*	*Grams in Each Portion*				*Total Portions*	*Total Grams*		
		Weight	C	P	F		C	P	F
Bread	1 slice	30	18	3		3	54	9	
Oatmeal	1 large	30, dry	20	5	2	1	20	5	2
Orange	1	150	15			3	45		
Vegetables, 3–6%	1 cup	150	5	2½		4	20	10	
Milk	¼ pt.	120	6	4	4	1	6	4	4
Cream, 20%	¼ pt.	120	4	4	24	1	4	4	24
Egg	1	60		6	6	1		6	6
Meat	1 small	60		16	10	2		32	20
Butter	1 square	10			8	3			25

Grand total grams (approximate) C150 P70 F80
Calories per gram x 4 x 4 x 9
Total Calories – 1600 = 600 + 280 + 720

also in heat units, or calories. A calorie is a standard unit of heat and is equivalent to the quantity of heat necessary to raise one kilogram of water one degree centigrade, or approximately one pound of water one degree Fahrenheit.

All of us need calories—heat—to live. Babies and children need more heat than adults, because they are more active and must grow. A baby grows so fast that it requires about 100 calories for each kilogram—2.2 pounds; an adult requires about 30 calories with moderate activity, and an old man or woman less. Exercise greatly increases the need for calories and similarly rest in bed decreases it.

The caloric—heat—value of food varies with its composition, just as does the heat value of coal, whether it is of high or low grade. Pure carbohydrate and protein give off 4.1 calories for each gram burned; fat yields 9 calories. Therefore, if we reckon up the grams of carbohydrate, protein, and fat in the diet, we can easily determine the calories. (See Tables 5 and 6.)

A person always eats, never truly fasts. He always requires heat—calories—and if he does not get calories from food, he eats up his own body: first, that part of it which is in the form of carbohydrate—glucose and glycogen, or animal starch; next, the fat; and, last of all, the protein which composes the various tissues.

A person needs from 100 to 25 calories per kilogram (2.2 pounds) body weight, according to whether he is a baby or an old man. The above diet would be about right for an adult who weighs 110 pounds, or 50 kilograms, because it would furnish a little over 30 calories per kilogram body weight.

Bouchardat, a hundred years ago, did not weigh diets, but he did almost better by teaching his patients to examine the urine. If, after eating a certain food, sugar showed, his patients knew that food contained too much carbohydrate—sugar or starch—for them. This is worth while doing today, and the oftener the urine is examined the better. Especially is this necessary if the diabetes is hard to control and it is difficult to keep the urine sugar free. One should never give up testing the urine.

EXERCISE IN THE TREATMENT OF A DIABETIC

The second steed in the diabetic's three-horse chariot of treatment is exercise. Regular physical activity, whether at work or play, not only promotes health and strength but, in the presence of insulin, helps lower the blood sugar. Many patients have found that on days of outdoor activity their urine tests will improve and especially during a vacation spent camping or canoeing in the woods. Not only will the urine and blood tests improve but the insulin dose could be reduced. However, particularly in children and in adults with unstable diabetes, exercise may not be an unmixed blessing. To drive this horse, Exercise, along with Diet and Insulin, requires judgment, and one must often lower the load for Exercise and increase it for Insulin. Exercise is good for the diabetic of mild or moderate severity, but for the severest diabetics before we had insulin, exercise did harm, and only recently a few patients told me they got along better if they stayed abed. Exercise to be advantageous requires insulin. The mild diabetic has enough insulin of his own available; the moderately severe diabetic produces some insulin; but the severe diabetic who manufactures practically none of his own must buy it and inject it, and then he can undertake as strenuous exercise as any healthy man or woman. In general, however, any patient who cannot exercise is handicapped. One reliable patient tells me a game of golf is worth five units of insulin. Today doctors are careful to provide exercise in one form or another for their diabetics who must stay abed as a result of operations or for other reasons. Exercise should be utilized in the treatment of nearly every case of diabetes, but this steed must not be overdriven.

Exercise lowers the sugar in the blood just as does lack of food (fasting) and insulin. If one's diabetes is well controlled and exercise is greatly increased, while diet and insulin remain the same, the blood sugar may fall so low as to lead to an insulin reaction. The diabetic always should remember he is driving a three-horse team and he must think how to make Diet, Exercise, and Insulin pull together.

INSULIN IN TREATMENT OF DIABETES

The announcement of the discovery of insulin in Toronto in 1921 brought hope to the diabetic, and its general introduction in 1922 gave him life. The addition of protamine to it by Hagedorn of Denmark in 1936, and subsequently of zinc by Scott and Fisher in Canada, and more recently the new protamine insulin (NPH), devised also by Hagedorn, have led to his comfort and joy, because these improvements have reduced treatment from two, three, or four injections a day to once in twenty-four hours. It is one of the four major medical discoveries thus far of the twentieth century. Even today none of us wholly realizes the good which insulin has done. *First of all, insulin enables a diabetic child to live, but, best of all, to grow and be happy.* Insulin protects the diabetic mother. Insulin allows the diabetic doctor, lawyer, teacher, laborer to resume his occupation and again to play an active part in the community. Years ago, before we had insulin or knew as much as we do now about diet, nearly one fifth of all diabetics died the very first year of their disease, and most of them were invalids. Today less than one in fifty die the first year, and this number is made up almost exclusively of old men and old women, with whom the date of onset of diabetes is uncertain, and of diabetics who have sustained medical or other accidents. Even if we do not grant to insulin the whole responsibility for the prolongation and protection of the lives of diabetics, it surely is responsible for 99 per cent of their health, because it affords them the opportunity to satisfy their longing for food and their desire to act as live men and live women and, if children, to rejoice in their play.

Insulin comes from a gland, the pancreas or the sweetbread, which lies behind the stomach in the upper abdomen. No one can live without insulin. Insulin regulates the percentage of sugar in the blood. If this percentage is too high, insulin removes the excess sugar and stores it as starch —glycogen—in the liver and muscles and skin, or helps in its change to fat for deposit throughout the body. Starch is an insoluble form of carbohydrate and thus is suitable for storage just as sugar is soluble and, if not used, is lost in the urine. For most of us our own pancreas suffice. The cells of the pancreas are so closely in touch with the demand and supply of insulin in the body that if there is ever a surplus or deficit of insulin in a normal person we consider it an anomaly. If we eat carbohydrate, the pancreas makes insulin to care for it, and the insulin factory is so delicately adjusted to the amount of sugar which should be in the blood that it does not allow this to vary as much as a teaspoonful, which, by the way, is the normal amount of sugar in the blood of the entire body in the fasting state. If 0.1 per cent, or 100 milligrams per cent—another scant spoonful —collects in it, sugar begins to appear in the urine. (The body contains about 5 quarts of blood or [5x32] 160 ounces [1 ounce = 30 cubic centimeters] or 160x30 = 4800 cubic centimeters or grams, and if multiplied by 0.1 per cent, we have 4.8 grams–and a spoonful is equal to 5.0 grams.) Sometimes normal individuals, who during violent exercise burn up most of their reserve starch (glycogen) and sugar in the body as a result of a Marathon run, a football game, or a four-mile boat race, suffer because exercise has done the work of insulin. Today trainers give to such athletes carbohydrate, tea with sugar, orange juice, etc., to offset the deficiency. Even a healthy child may go without a meal, and his pancreas may not stop manufacturing insulin soon enough, and as a result the blood sugar is reduced so low that he becomes unconscious. Recently four such cases were reported. The diabetic differs chiefly from the normal person in that his pancreas produces too little insulin, and to make up for the lack of insulin he must buy it. Few persons' intelligence is equal to their instinct, and so it is not strange that the diabetic occasionally gives himself an overdose of insulin. He is the one above all others who must learn what he needs, and no doctor can decide as well as the patient himself, provided he understands his diabetes and the workings of diet, exercise, and insulin. Few patients at first recognize the symptoms which demand an increase or decrease in the dose of insulin, but the diabetic of several years' duration does know these, and with the help of his physician he finally arrives at the proper amount which his system requires from day to day. The diabetic can test his urine one or more times daily and thus determine whether it contains sugar or is sugar free, and so whether he needs more or less insulin or no insulin. Unfortunately, as yet he cannot test the sugar in his blood with perfect accuracy, but a helpful approximation is now possible with a paper test (Dextristix).

At one time it was the belief that a diabetic got worse the longer he lived, but today we know that this is not necessarily true. Diabetics can improve, and now it is a fact that the doctor must be as alert to detect his patient's getting better as he was formerly to note a downward course. Fortunately, every diabetic manufactures some insulin, even though the quantity is small, but we cannot tell yet how much a diabetic pancreas can be repaired, renewed, or how much it can grow when conditions are favorable. The possibility is still open that someone will discover a means by which the beginning destruction of the cells of the islands of Langerhans will be reversed and that the beta cells in the islands which make the insulin will again fill with granules and go to work.

Insulin can now be bought all over the world and has a fixed standard of strength in accordance with an International Standard adopted in 1935. The dose varies with each patient, but the total amount employed for the day ranges, as a rule, between ten and forty units, rising above this in the severer cases, and especially when the diabetic has a complication due to an infection or to diabetic coma. Under such circumstances a patient may

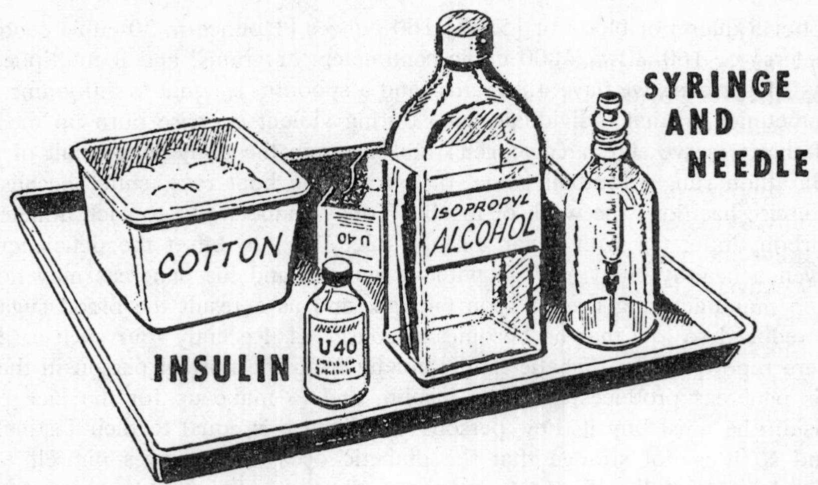

Fig. 61. Insulin and Its Use. If the body does not have enough insulin, a doctor may prescribe it. The body can use bottled insulin only when it is injected through the skin with a syringe and needle. The diabetic must be careful to use only the kind and amount his doctor prescribes. *Taking Care of Diabetes,* National Center for Chronic Disease Control.

require several hundred units of insulin in the twenty-four hours. An infection, whether general like influenza or local like a boil, always makes the diabetes worse, and in diabetic coma the insulin also acts less efficiently.

The cost of insulin should be kept as low as possible. One uses it to save life and not for fun. I hope the price can be kept low by wholesale methods and by allowing hospitals and clinics to sell it at a minimum profit. Everything should be done to encourage the purchase of insulin, so as to avoid giving it away, because that promotes wastage to an enormous degree.

The size of the dose, the number of units of insulin, not only varies with the severity of the disease, but with the amount of carbohydrate in the diet and also its relation to the fat as well. There is no absolute rule. Theoretically, one can reckon the total carbohydrate or glucose, sugar-forming material in the food, as follows:

Food	*Per Cent Sugar-forming*
Carbohydrate	100 grams × 100% = 100 grams
Protein	100 grams × 58% = 58 grams
Fat	100 grams × 10% = 10 grams

However, this will not indicate how much insulin is required, because sometimes the carbohydrate from carbohydrate alone appears to be better utilized if the fat in the diet is relatively low.

Today with new knowledge about the chemical structure of insulin and new methods for modifying insulin, there is greater hope than ever for the discovery of a form of insulin which can be taken by mouth instead of injected under the skin.

Varieties of Insulin. The duration of the action of insulin varies with the type employed. Regular insulin acts for six or seven hours and most powerfully at the end of one hour. Globin and NPH insulins are intermediate insulins and have a duration of action of about twenty and twenty-two hours respectively. Protamine zinc insulin, the long-acting insulin, acts up to twenty-eight and even forty-eight hours.

Since the introduction of the NPH and Lente insulins, protamine zinc variety has been used to much less extent. This is due largely to the fact that in usual dosages, regular insulin and protamine zinc insulin cannot be given in a single injection. The "Lente" family of insulins consist of semi-Lente, Lente insulin and ultra-Lente; the most widely used is Lente insulin. It has the advantage that crystalline insulin can be mixed in the same syringe and the effect will be that of the combined units.

The immediate effect of regular or crystalline insulin is to lower the blood sugar rapidly for the first four or five hours after it is injected, while protamine zinc insulin acts slowly, and the blood sugar may not reach the lowest point for twelve hours. The intermediate globin and NPH insulins act most successfully in about eight hours, and so if injected before breakfast have the greatest effect in the late afternoon. Insulins fortunately do not accumulate in the body.

TABLE 8

ACTIONS OF VARIOUS INSULINS

Name	*Duration of Action in Hours*	*Peak of Action after Injection in Hours*
Regular	6–7	1
Globin	20–22	8
NPH	20–22	8
Protamine	28–48	12–16
Lente	20–22	8–10

Sterilization

Equipment: 1. Saucepan 2. Strainer

1. Place syringe, plunger, and needle all disconnected in strainer. If no strainer used, place a cloth in bottom of pan.
2. Cover completely with cold water; heat to boiling and boil 5 minutes.
3. Lift strainer out of pan and pour out water. Place strainer back in pan.
4. Fill a clean dish or bottle with iso-propyl alcohol.
5. Pick up plunger by knob only and fit into cylinder. Handle needle by hub (thick end) and fasten to syringe by a twist to left or right to secure. Be sure nothing touches needle or plunger where they will touch insulin.

6. Place syringe with needle attached into covered dish or bottle containing alcohol to cool. (Steri-tubes to hold syringe and needle may be purchased.)

Entire equipment should be sterilized by boiling every week, or daily if iso-propyl alcohol unavailable.

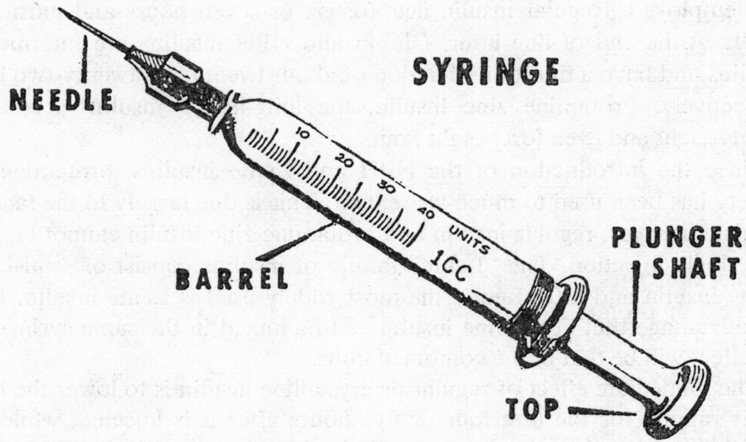

Fig. 62. The diabetic becomes familiar with the parts of the syringe. He learns how to read the markings on the barrel so he will always use the right amount of insulin. *Taking Care of Diabetes,* National Center for Chronic Disease Control.

Loading

1. Mix insulin by rotating bottle between hands. Clean rubber top of insulin bottle with alcohol.
2. Remove syringe from alcohol. Work plunger back and forth several times to expel any alcohol.
3. Draw air into syringe to equal insulin dose.
4. Cautiously but firmly push needle through center of rubber top. Push plunger down to expel air into bottle.
5. Invert the bottle. Pull down plunger to withdraw insulin. If air bubbles are present, holding syringe and needle point upward, expel insulin into bottle and slowly again withdraw dose. Remove needle from bottle.

Injection

Areas used: top and outsides of legs or arms. Abdomen. Never inject into same spot more often than once a month.

1. Clean skin with alcohol sponge where you plan injection.
2. Pinch up skin at site between thumb and forefinger. With syringe held at 45-degree angle to the skin, quickly insert needle its entire length. (The more quickly the needle is inserted, the less will be the pain.)

3. Force insulin from syringe. Cover area with alcohol sponge and remove needle.
4. Rinse out syringe with boiled water.
5. Replace syringe with needle in alcohol container.

Insulin, as already mentioned, acts by removing the sugar from the blood and storing it in the liver, the muscles, and the skin in the form of an insoluble carbohydrate, animal starch (glycogen), so that it can be utilized when required by the body. The sugar in the blood rises to its highest level from half an hour to an hour after meals, and to offset this insulin is usually administered one quarter to three quarters of an hour before a meal. This is necessary if regular or crystalline insulin is used. In fact, if insulin is given when the stomach is empty, it may lower the sugar in the blood so quickly that the symptoms of an overdose, the so-called insulin reaction, appear. Many patients can keep the urine free from sugar if they take one injection of protamine zinc insulin a day, but if they use the quick-acting but shorter-duration regular insulin they will require it twice, a few three times. Rarely is it necessary to give it four times.

When only the original regular insulin was available, how frequently with children mothers would be obliged to waken with an alarm clock at 2:00 A.M. in order to inject the fourth dose into the child. During infections the patient may require insulin every three or four hours, in pregnancy three times daily, and in the treatment of a patient unconscious with diabetic coma it is often administered every thirty minutes until improvement begins to take place. Truly insulin is wonderful, and I know of nothing more dramatic in medicine than to watch an unconscious diabetic-coma patient come back to life with the use of insulin.

Protamine zinc insulin when given before breakfast day after day will act strongly enough to control the diabetes in about half of all cases for the entire twenty-four hours. In other words, it enables the patient to get the full benefit of (1) the food stored in the body as it changes from glycogen (animal starch) to sugar, or from protein, which yields 58 per cent sugar, and from fat, out of which 10 per cent can be formed, and (2) also takes care of the sugar which comes from the different foods at mealtimes. In the severer types of diabetes protamine zinc insulin is unequal to the task of utilizing the food which the patient eats rapidly enough. In such instances one supplements it with the quick-acting regular or, better, crystalline insulin plus protamine zinc insulin also before breakfast, and the effect of this quick insulin plus the slow protamine zinc insulin will protect the patient for the periods of meals.

When regular insulin is given in the same syringe with protamine zinc insulin, a part of the regular or crystalline insulin changes to protamine zinc insulin because there is an excess of protamine in protamine zinc insulin. Fortunately, no such change takes place when the quick-acting insulins are added to NPH insulin, Lente, or globin insulin, so that a single injection of insulin (both the rapid-acting and slow-acting being mixed in the same syringe) can be employed before breakfast.

During the course of infections or after operations, when patients eat irregularly, one usually depends upon an anchor dose of protamine zinc insulin once a day or a mixture of NPH insulin and regular insulin, and also gives insulin every four to six hours as needed according to the following formula:

Red	Orange	Yellow	Green	Blue
16	12	8	4	0

The results of the Benedict tests are recorded in the numerator of the fractions, and the corresponding units of insulin to be given in the denominator.

Insulin is given by injection just under the skin. The patient should be

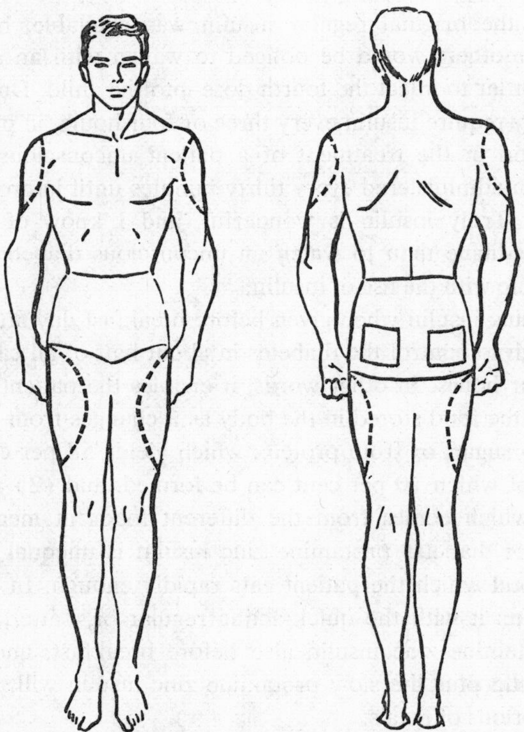

Fig. 63. Sites of the body where insulin can be injected. *Diabetes Mellitus, a Guide for Nurses,* National Center for Chronic Disease Control.

systematic about this and not use the same spot of the skin for an injection oftener than once a month. A little planning will provide for this. If insulin is always injected in one place, lumps may appear, because the tissues are injured. As a result the insulin is incompletely absorbed, and the patient does not get his money's worth. And this is not the whole story, because in the injured tissue an infection may start. Abscesses from the injection of insulin, however, are extraordinarily rare and usually are due only to gross neglect.

The proper dose of insulin is not always easily determined because of the uncertainty as to when or how much the patient will eat or the amount of exercise that he has had or is to take. Obviously the trained patient who injects his own insulin can decide all this better than the doctor. Furthermore, sometimes people eat a meal but fail to digest it—and this especially occurs with children—or, if seasick, lose it, and so the insulin which may have been given with the expectation that the patient would eat has no food to work upon. If food remains in the stomach and so does not reach the blood, it is the same as if no food had been taken at all. For all these reasons it is not uncommon to see a patient who has had an overdose of insulin with a resulting "insulin reaction." Insulin is a drug, and symptoms will result from an overdose of any drug.

INSULIN ATROPHIES

In children and in women, rarely in men, insulin injections are sometimes followed by the disappearance of small portions of the fat layer of the skin. These make depressions in the surface of the body, and this hollowing out of the skin causes deformities. These are disagreeable but not dangerous. Eventually, if no insulin is injected in the neighborhood of such a fat-atrophied area, it will fill up. Treatment consists in using scrupulous care in the administration of insulin. Never inject near the same site twice in a month, use concentrated U-80 insulin, and employ sharp, perfect needles. One never needs to give up insulin on account of insulin atrophies. One can take advantage of the abdomen and lower back for injections.

When insulin was first discovered, its strength was weak and to get an effect it was necessary to inject several teaspoonfuls at a time. Gradually it has been made stronger and stronger, and so smaller quantities are necessary for an effect. At one time a syringeful—usually holding 1 cubic centimeter or one fourth of a teaspoonful—contained 10 units, but now insulin is usually dispensed in four times that strength, or 40 units in a cubic centimeter, known as U-40 insulin, although sometimes only twice as strong, as U-20 insulin, or eight times as strong, as U-80 insulin. At any rate, one unit is always the same no matter what the strength, even if as many as 500 units are contained in one cubic centimeter. Sometimes syringes holding two cubic centimeters instead of one cubic centimeter are used. Obviously, one must always be very careful to note the strength of insulin to be injected as well as the type of syringe employed, so as to be sure of the number of units.

The one-cubic-centimeter syringes may be divided into ten parts, and then one tenth of one cubic centimeter would contain 1, 2, 4, or 8 units according to whether the strength of insulin was U-10, U-20, U-40, or U-80. Some syringes are marked for U-40 or U-80 insulin, and then one can read the desired number of units on the side indicated for the strength of insulin. U-10 insulin, now seldom available, comes in a bottle with a blue label, U-20 insulin in a bottle with a yellow label. U-40 insulin is sold in red-labeled bottles, and U-80 in green-labeled vials. NPH insulin comes in a bottle with four sides instead of in a round vial.

Be sure you know the kind of insulin you are supposed to use and the number of units. Show your insulin bottle and your syringe to your doctor to be sure you are making no mistake.

HYPOGLYCEMIC REACTIONS DUE TO INSULIN

The symptoms which result from low blood sugar (hypoglycemic) attacks due to an overdose of insulin resemble symptoms which occur under such conditions as a long-delayed meal when hunger and faintness may even be accompanied by emotional changes. If one has been without food for hours or even fasting, the amount of sugar in the blood may be lowered with the result that faintness, nervousness, and other symptoms may occur. Insulin reactions arise whenever there is an overdose of insulin, too long an interval between insulin and food, too little or poor absorption of food and physical or muscular activity unusual for the individual. The common symptoms of an insulin reaction appear on the average in patients receiving insulin, when the blood glucose falls from the higher level to 50 mg. or below. Occasionally, reactions occur with blood sugar values within a normal range but usually only when there has been a rapid fall in the blood sugar level. The most frequent symptoms of a reaction are weakness, faintness, hunger and trembling. Sweating, numbness, tingling of the lips and even unconsciousness can come on rapidly. If the dose of insulin has been extreme, the patient may have a convulsion. Reactions due to regular insulin appear three or four hours after the insulin has been given, whereas reactions produced by the slowly acting insulins such as protamine zinc insulin, are more apt to occur within eight to twenty-four hours after the administration, depending upon the type of depot insulin used. Consequently, in patients receiving insulin before breakfast, reactions from regular or semi-Lente insulin are apt to occur during the forenoon or early afternoon; those due to globin, NPH or Lente insulin are more likely to occur in the afternoon or evening; those due to protamine zinc or ultra-Lente insulin commonly cause difficulty during the night or before breakfast. However, a great variation occurs with regard to the time of reactions, depending upon diet and muscular activity. Unusual manifestations include inability to move muscles as desired, inappropriate crying, smiling, or laughing, difficulty in forming words, unsteady gait.

A diagnosis of the condition is quickly made by examination of the blood for sugar. This will show the true nature of the condition. It is extremely important to differentiate this condition in a patient who is drowsy or semiconscious and not make the mistake of giving insulin on the supposition that the unconsciousness is due to diabetic acidosis. Such an error may have serious results.

Reactions without the usual warning symptoms are occasionally seen in patients who after taking insulin for ten years or more, begin to find that the reactions occur without the characteristic symptoms which they formerly experienced. Mental confusion may be unrecognized by the patient. Such patients need special and careful planning of the diet so that the food is taken 6 or 7 times a day. Occasionally patients need to take saltines or a cracker every 60 minutes but such patients are really rare.

In Table 9 are summarized the symptoms which serve to differentiate diabetic coma and insulin reactions. Emphasis should be laid not only upon the symptoms and the course but particularly upon the prevention of reactions; when driving a car, a diabetic who takes insulin should take carbohydrate 10 grams every 2 hours.

The treatment of insulin reactions is usually simple if begun promptly. Frequently, a child lying unconscious on the floor with an insulin reaction, will within 2 or 3 minutes after given a teaspoonful of syrup, rise and resume playing with his toy trains. Five or 10 grams of carbohydrate by mouth in the form of sugar, orange juice, ginger ale, candy, or syrup are usually sufficient unless the reaction has not been recognized. Then if the patient has been unconscious for some time, intravenous administration of glucose may be necessary. The families of diabetic children, or in whom the patient though an adult is of the youth onset type, should have on hand ampules of glucagon. Mixing the glucagon in the solution provided results in a preparation which when injected like insulin, 1 mg. at a time, will usually raise the blood sugar to a level where the patient can be roused and can then begin taking food containing carbohydrate.

TABLE 9
DIFFERENTIAL DIAGNOSIS BETWEEN DIABETIC COMA AND INSULIN REACTION

	Diabetic Coma	*Insulin Reaction*
Cause	**Acid poisoning due to** 1. Insufficient insulin 2. Overeating 3. Fever	**Low blood sugar due to** 1. Too much insulin. 2. Too little food or delay in eating after taking insulin. 3. Unusual exercise.
Onset	Gradual over a period of hours or days.	**After regular or crystalline insulin.** Sudden, usually in a few hours after taking. **After protamine zinc globin or NPH insulin.** Slow, usually some hrs. after taking.
Signs and Symptoms	A feeling of serious illness, thirst, nausea, vomiting, deep and difficult breathing, pains in the abdomen, drowsiness, often fever.	**After regular or crystalline insulin.** Hunger, tremor, sweating, nervousness. **After protamine zinc globin or NPH insulin.** As above, though at times headache, nausea, drowsiness, malaise.
Prevention	Test urine regularly. **NEVER** omit insulin except under doctor's orders when urine is repeatedly sugar free. **If you feel ill** 1. Send for a doctor. 2. Go to bed. 3. Drink a cupful of hot liquid hourly. 4. Keep warm. 5. Get nurse or friend to give care. 6. Take an enema.	Meals at regular hours. Those taking protamine zinc globin or NPH insulin should eat something between meals and on retiring. When driving a car, a diabetic should take carbohydrate 10 grams every two hours to prevent low blood sugar. Repeated reactions call for readjustment of the patient's daily routine with respect to insulin, diet and exercise.
Treatment	Must be carried out by the physician, preferably in a hospital.	Give sugar immediately. Patients using protamine zinc globin or NPH insulin may need sugar more than once. Diabetics should always carry two lumps of sugar for use if an insulin reaction occurs. Adrenalin ½ cc. may be injected under the skin.

The diabetic's best insurance against both coma and insulin reaction is to see the doctor as often as the latter thinks necessary and always every three or four months.

A patient using insulin should always carry his name, address, and directions for treatment of a reaction so that he can be protected if such a reaction comes on in strange surroundings.

I AM A DIABETIC

If I am found unconscious or behaving abnormally, my condition probably is the result of an overdose of insulin. ***I am not intoxicated.*** **Place sugar or candy in my mouth. If this fails to revive me in 15 minutes, call my physician or send me immediately to a hospital.**

Physician's name ....

Address .... Telephone ....

Name ....

Address ....

Fig. 64. Diabetic identification card. National Center for Chronic Disease Control.

RESISTANCE TO INSULIN

Occasionally, patients with diabetes require extraordinarily large amounts of insulin in order to control the diabetic state. As an example, a physician treated at the Joslin Clinic some years ago was not sugar free even with 100 units of insulin daily. And a few months later the insulin had to be increased until finally he was taking 1600 units of insulin a day. In his case, as in other remarkable patients, sometimes specific complications or causes explain the resistance. Thus the development of infection or of acidosis sometimes will be followed by an increase in the resistance to insulin so that patients may require 200 or 500 units of insulin daily. In many instances, however, no complicating cause requiring special treatment is found. In such patients, usually this insulin resistance develops rather rapidly. A high dose must be continued for weeks or months and then in the great majority of our patients the high dose gradually can be reduced until after a year or two the patient is often back on the former dose of insulin. The important thing is that the patient should know by reason of his urine tests when this condition of insulin resistance is developing. Unless he does so, if the requirements for insulin increase rapidly and no change in his ordinary dose is made, then the patient runs the risk of developing serious acidosis or even actual coma.

The cause of insulin resistance has been studied in many research laboratories. In many patients there have been found antibodies to insulin in the blood serum. These antibodies can be studied by special research methods. In many patients who take insulin for a period of some years, moderate amounts of antibodies do explain the increasing requirement for insulin each day. In occasional patients, the amounts of such antibodies are very large and the result is that the requirement of insulin may be great. In such patients, the use of the usual U-40 and U-80 strength insulin is not sufficient. Fortunately, U-100 and even U-500 strengths of crystalline insulin are available on prescription and help greatly in the treatment of this problem of insulin resistance. It must be remembered that when using insulin of such strength as U-500 that the action of insulin is often much prolonged and that special care and medical instruction under these conditions is important.

SENSITIVITY TO INSULIN

It is well known that diabetic patients are sometimes quite sensitive to insulin. In certain patients, particularly those with the juvenile or "growth onset" type of diabetes, the blood sugar tends to respond quickly and markedly to an injection of insulin and in these patients insulin reactions are common. On the other hand, in older patients with mild diabetes, such sensitiveness to insulin is the exception, although it is true that among such older patients marked sensitiveness to insulin does occasionally occur. In patients with insulin-sensitive diabetes, often special dietary programs are necessary. Thus such patients frequently need a diet divided into three meals with three snacks about two or three hours after each meal. The insulin dose needs frequently to be divided into a morning dose and a second dose at bedtime or before the evening meal.

ORAL HYPOGLYCEMIC AGENTS

One of the great recent advances has been the discovery of substances which can be taken by mouth for the reduction of the sugar in the blood, instead of insulin. Over the last 80 years, many substances beginning with salicylates, vegetable extracts, have been known to exert some hypoglycemic action in mild cases of diabetes but in fact, investigations indicated that one could not conclude that reduction of the blood sugar with these substances was necessarily associated with the correction of the real trouble in diabetes. However, beginning in 1913, certain sulfonamide derivatives were shown to be capable of blood-sugar-lowering effects. The same proved true of certain guanidine derivatives. The result has been intense activity and the discovery of a series of substances which can be used with diabetic patients of mild degree effectively. At present, Orinase®, also known as tolbutamide, has been widely used in adults usually with diabetes of rather short duration and of such severity that only 15 to 25 units of insulin would have been required. A similar product, chemically a biguanide, known as DBI® has had similar effects but has the additional advantage that, in some patients, even in children, with unstable diabetes subject to frequent insulin reactions, this substance can be taken at the same time with insulin. The result is in some instances that the amount of insulin can be reduced so long as the DBI® is taken. Low blood sugar reactions will be less frequent.

A third preparation, Diabinese®, is also, like Orinase®, a sulfonylurea compound with similar action. Acetohexamide (Dymelor®) has approximately the same therapeutic value as Orinase®, although the dosage is somewhat less.

Important in the use of these oral remedies is the proper selection of patients with diabetes beginning chiefly after the age of forty, of rather short duration, without any acidosis and most important of all, the cooperation of patients in carrying out a carefully planned diet. Without careful dietary treatment, the use of the oral remedies is fraught with danger.

THE USEFULNESS OF DIABETES IN PUBLIC HEALTH

That a disease should be useful seems like a contradiction of terms. Actually, diabetes is a disease which really serves the public health. We need our diabetics. The diabetic sets an example of cleanliness to his family, his friends, and in fact to all his neighbors. He is taught to be the cleanest citizen in the community, because if he keeps his skin in good condition, the chances for complications are slight, and in this way he avoids the carbuncles and boils and inflammations of the skin which years ago were a most annoying accompaniment of the disease. The diabetic is useful because he sets an example for temperance in eating, for control of body weight. He is an instructor in dietetics, and he diffuses through his family a practical knowledge of the properties and values of foods. He understands the meaning of a balanced diet. He knows that his 3 per cent vegetables, his fruit, his cream, his egg, his meat, and his cod-liver oil contain priceless vitamins. Diabetes is particularly useful because it is so evidently associated with overweight that it directs attention to the dangers of overweight in general, for these are by no means limited to diabetes. For years the insurance companies have pointed out that the expectation of life of the fat person is far less than that of the one of standard weight, because the fat person is more liable to diseases of the heart and the arteries. Lately they have shown that if a fat person loses weight and regains a normal value, his expectancy of life, which was shortened, will again rise.

Diabetes is useful because it brings before the public the advantage of cooperation between the physician and patient in the treatment of a chronic disease. The diabetic patient who does the best is the one who knows the most about the disease, and this soon becomes apparent to all onlookers. He thus demonstrates that it is desirable for the ordinary individual to know something about diseases, and particularly his own disease, so that he and his doctor can work in partnership. The diabetic is useful because today we know that diabetes is to a certain extent hereditary, and, having the disease, the patient must stop and think before he gets married. Not only must he consider whether he can take care of himself or herself, but he also must consider the health of his future partner before he gets engaged, because one diabetic should not marry another diabetic. In other words, the diabetic will spread the knowledge of eugenics, and when we remember the known and unknown three million diabetics in this country and the millions now living who will acquire diabetes before they die, the necessity of thoughtfulness on the part of diabetics before they have children will be taught them and through them pass to the community as a whole. One can see the necessity of great care in contracting marriages. Almost any thoughtful father today demands a report of the physical examination and Wassermann reaction of the suitor of his daughter before he consents to her marriage.

For the doctor, the diabetic is a challenge because no group of patients is under closer supervision; therefore cancer should be detected earlier, more cures obtained, and tuberculosis always caught in its incipiency.

Dr. Elliott P. Joslin said:

"I feel that the diabetic who lives long lives usefully and that he deserves recognition. Unless he had used judgment in diet and treatment and care of his body, his duration of life would have been short. Therefore, I believe a diabetic who has lived longer with his disease than he was expected to live without it at the time it began should be given a medal in recognition of it. Such a practice has been followed, and for the encouragement of patients I can say that I know of more than two thousand diabetics who have earned such medals. Amelia Peabody, the designer, placed on the reverse side of the medal a child in a boat sailing toward the rising sun with this inscription, *"Explorers of Diabetes,"* because it is the child who is leading the way for improvement in the treatment of diabetics."

Quarter Century Victory Medal. A medal of greater distinction was created in 1947 by the Advisory Committee of the Diabetic Fund at the Boston Safe Deposit and Trust Company. It is awarded to that diabetic who after twenty-five years of known diabetes is perfect on physical examination; has eyes and blood vessels free from complications, as certified by a recognized ophthalmologist and a roentgenologist. Application for the Quarter Century Victory Medal should be sent to the Advisory Committee, Diabetic Fund, Boston Safe Deposit and Trust Company, Trustee, 100 Franklin Street, Boston, Massachusetts, or to Dr. Howard F. Root, Chairman, Advisory Committee, 81 Bay State Road, Boston 15, Massachusetts.

If your physician or you think that you deserve a Quarter Century Victory Medal after your proved twenty-five years of diabetes, just get a complete examination by your family physician; if he thinks you will pass, second, secure an examination of the eyes by an eye specialist; if they are reported all right, then, third, secure X rays of the blood vessels.

The letter of application should briefly summarize your history, with age and date of onset and course of diabetes, together with a statement of your physician about your physical condition. If he considers this perfect and that you are eligible, the report of the examination of the eyes by an eye specialist should accompany the doctor's report. In case you pass these tests by your family physician and the eye specialist, then X rays should be taken to demonstrate whether there is calcification of the arteries. By experience we have found it necessary to have an X-ray examination of (1) the heart and aorta in the chest; (2) the abdominal aorta (film taken laterally to avoid the spine); (3) pelvic arteries; and (4) a lateral view of the lower legs, including the vessels about the ankles.

These medals are so rare and the discovery of such cases so important that eye and X-ray specialists, as well as the family physician, often will do the tests at minimum fees.

Already one hundred ten such diabetics have been granted medals. It is significant that the histories of these patients showed that they carefully followed treatment in their early years and that none was neglectful of treatment, although they may have controlled their disease in different ways. So far, no patient living on a free diet and careless of his diabetes has been able to pass the above tests.

A diabetic in the home after all may be an asset. To sum up, he knows about cleanliness, diet, the dangers of overweight, the use of a drug, the importance of heredity, and hence it is no wonder that often he lives long. He and his confreres constitute a great experimental laboratory for the benefit of the human race. I tell my diabetic children that each honest diabetic day they live is a great help to some diabetic old man or old woman, because from their young lives we learn how to treat those whose vitality and recuperative powers are less.

EMPLOYMENT OF DIABETICS

If a diabetic can secure employment which involves exercise, it is most advantageous, because exercise helps to utilize the diet and thus benefits the patient. If the diabetic must accept employment which does not involve exercise, then he must make up for it by taking exercise out of hours. I remember well those diabetics who progressed most satisfactorily while active in athletics in college, but who, after they graduated and took jobs which did not involve exercise, such as postgraduate work in the law school or in medicine, or in an office, found they did not do well unless they resumed exercise out of hours. These diabetics will not do as well as they might unless they arrange to secure exercise, even if it is only walking daily and a short period for calisthenics. Bouchardat was very insistent that his patients should exercise until they sweat. He said they should earn their bread by the sweat of their brows. He wanted them to use all the muscles of the body.

If a diabetic can work independently and be his own boss, that is often advantageous. Theoretically a diabetic who is a farmer should do especially well, because he can regulate his exercise according to his work and ask no questions of anyone.

Opportunities for employment of diabetics are many. Particularly was this true during the war when they were given positions which did not involve combat activities. More than one thousand types of positions in the United States Civil Service are open to diabetics. Whereas more than one diabetic doctor, nurse, technician, secretary, or camp counselor was seldom employed by the Joslin Clinic. Fourteen held such paid positions recently. (I hope a million diabetics will not apply for a job, because already we have quite a diabetic labor pool of our own.)

Employers in general are kind to diabetics. It is very important that any diabetic seeking or holding an appointment should do his or her work not only as well as but better than a non-diabetic so as to increase the opportunities for other diabetics to get a job. Diabetics may need to give up certain pleasurable activities, but if they can demonstrate their good health and their skill, then they will not need to fear for a position.

Certain occupations are unsuitable for diabetics. Recently the American Diabetes Association has suggested standards for the employment of diabetics, and below I record abstracts from these standards.

1. A diabetic seeking employment should be required to present a note from his physician or the personnel manager, stating that he is a controlled diabetic and is examined at regular intervals.

2. Diabetics are capable of performing any type of work for which they are physically, mentally, and educationally equipped. Those diabetics who are taking large doses of insulin should not, however, be assigned work in which hypoglycemic attacks might result in injury to themselves and others.

3. An effort should be made to see that diabetics work the same hours on a steady shift; or, if they must work on a rotating schedule, that they avoid the "graveyard" shift from midnight to 8 A.M. This is the only concession in terms of hours that a well-controlled diabetic should ask.

4. Diabetics should carry cards or tags identifying their condition at all times, particularly when on the job.

5. The plant physician can save time for the company and also help the employee by performing blood sugar and urine examinations, whenever the patient's usual laboratory facilities are available only during working hours. Ordinarily, of course, this should be done only after consultation with the family physician.

6. A complete physical examination of each diabetic should be made regularly, at least once a year.

7. A plant physician is within his rights if he reassigns a diabetic employee to other work whenever the arising of new complications creates new risks for himself or for other employees.

8. The diabetic requiring insulin should be considered controlled if the fasting blood sugar is not below normal limits and not above 150 mg. per 100 cc. by Folin Wu method and the blood sugar three hours after a meal is not higher than 250 mg. per 100 cc. by the Folin Wu method and if the patient is under regular medical supervision. Although these or more nearly normal blood sugar levels are desirable, greater hyperglycemia alone, if not extreme or habitual, need not be considered a disqualification for employment in those cases where the patient's personal physician and the industrial physician both feel that other limits should be observed.

Naturally if diabetics have frequent reactions or develop diabetic coma, their chances for continuance in their occupations or for promotions are lessened. In a way this is fortunate, because it forces diabetics to study their diabetes thoroughly and to control it.

INSURANCE AND DIABETES

The first offer to insure the life of a diabetic patient was extended twenty-five years ago. Not until the last ten or fifteen years, however, has life insurance become widely available to selected diabetic patients through most of the life insurance companies in the United States and Canada. As more experience accumulates with regard to the life expectancy of diabetic patients, probably more patients will be accepted. The insurability of an individual person is determined by insurance companies by select characteristics which will affect their length of life. The age at the onset of diabetes, the duration of diabetes, and the quality of medical treatment are all factors to be considered. Dr. Frank A. Warner, Medical Director of the John Hancock Mutual Life Insurance Company, emphasizes control of the diabetes with the following basic goals:

Maintaining normal weight and good nutrition; promoting health and well-being;
Maintaining blood-sugar levels as near normal as possible, avoiding hypoglycemic reactions;
Prevention of complications.

The physician has a large role in assessing the insurability of patients when it is clear from the physician's report that the patient is on a well-planned treatment schedule which he understands and adheres to, it becomes possible to classify the risk properly.

In 1964, a new program to provide life insurance for youngsters with diabetes was established, proposed by the Connecticut Diabetes Association. Any diabetic child between 5 and 17 can be covered by a policy which runs to the age of 21 and then the value of the policy will automatically be increased.

Health and accident insurance has long been available for those diabetic patients fortunate enough to be included in policies for large groups.

DIABETES AND ADVANCING AGE

The frequency of diabetes increases with age. Two-thirds of the Joslin Clinic cases begin above the age of 40 years; the median age for its onset in males is 45.1 years and for females, 50.1 years. About one-half of our cases begin between 40 and 60 years and one-fourth between 45 and 54 years. In the Joslin Clinic series, the onset of diabetes is rare after 70 years and extremely rare after 80 years.

General experience shows the highest mortality rates being in the age groups 80 to 84 years. In the community, the prevalence rate of diabetes shows that 80 per cent of diabetic patients are 40 or more years of age and 40 per cent are over 65 years.

The patients live long, and the average age at death, which between 1898 and 1914 was forty-four years, is now about sixty-five years. The expectancy of life of a ten-year-old diabetic child is to pass his fiftieth birthday, even if no discoveries in treatment occur. Finally, medals have been given in our clinic alone to more than 2000 patients who have lived longer with the disease than they were expected to live without it when it was first acquired. But despite all this it is regrettably true that up to the present time it has been the rule for diabetics to grow old too fast. This had long been suspected for the middle-aged diabetic, but it is in the children that the proof appeared. When the children lived only two or three years, of course this was rarely evident, but as improvements in diet came and children lived longer, the very same changes were noted in them which one sees in aging adults. Their arteries began to harden, and one could not only feel the hardening, but see the deposits of lime by X-ray examinations of the blood vessels of the legs. More important than the changes in the blood vessels of the legs were those in the arteries of the heart, and in comparatively young people it was found that clots in these vessels (coronary thrombosis) caused death just as in mature individuals. Sadder by far was another change of old age, which came on in the eyes, and diabetic children showed cataracts, hemorrhages, and exudates impairing the vision. I should hesitate even to record all this if it were not possible to add that in the last few years we know that in children this early aging has been deferred, and in some patients who have carefully followed treatment for even twenty-five years it has not appeared.

Old age has been deferred, because insulin permits the diabetic today to eat more nearly the diet of the normal individual. How can we help advancing the argument that if modern treatment has halted arteriosclerosis in diabetic children and is deferring it in the middle-aged diabetics, there must have been something in the disease itself or perhaps in its treatment by us years ago which was responsible for this arteriosclerosis?

First of all, the evidence points to overeating. It appears to be not so much the particular character of the food, because all the foods break up into quite similar components which enter a common pool and are more or less interchangeable. For a long while the insurance companies have insisted that a man or woman above fifty years was not a good risk if he or she were fat, and although this has appeared to be due to the overweight alone, it is possible the additional fat tissue itself in the body has been the reason. At any rate, since our diabetic children have eaten less fat and have assimilated it better, and had it replaced with more carbohydrate food, which insulin has permitted, we have noticed less hardening of the arteries. At the moment excess in total calories rather than in those derived from fat appears to be the crucial factor.

In recent years the fat in the diet, particularly that known as cholesterol, has been thought to be of major importance in the development of hardening of the arteries. This fat is found in the walls of the blood vessels and is especially common in the blood of diabetics with arteriosclerosis. Nothing would appear easier than to exclude it from the diet and thus keep young. But it is not quite so simple. It happens that only 10 per cent of the cholesterol in the body comes from the diet, and the remaining 90 per cent is manufactured by the body itself. It would seem queer for the human body to produce so much cholesterol normally unless it was useful and surely harmless. One is on safer ground today to urge restriction of total calories rather than to urge extreme restriction of cholesterol alone.

Other fatty components of the diet have been studied extensively with relation to diabetes and vascular disease in recent years. In many diabetic patients, though not all, a diet containing large amounts of fat derived from meat, dairy fats, and eggs is associated with an increase in fatty substances in the blood. On the other hand, a diet that is rich in the essential fatty acids which are polyunsaturated has been employed with some success by many doctors in the attempt to reduce the increased amount of cholesterol and other fatty substances in the blood. Such diets replace about one-half of the fat ordinarily obtained from meat and dairy products by corn oil or soy bean oil. Thus an increased amount of the essential fatty acids, Linoleic, linolenic, and arachidonic may be obtained. Control of the diabetes by diet, exercise, and insulin is our best deterrent of degenerative disease of the blood vessels.

HEREDITY AND MARRIAGE OF DIABETICS

HEREDITY

Diabetes is an hereditary disease. Probably about one in four of all the people in the United States has a diabetic relative and therefore harbors a tendency to diabetes. Among Jewish people it may be one in three. Proof that diabetes is hereditary is shown in various ways. When our diabetic children first come to us for treatment, the known heredity of these children is 20 per cent, but after the children have lived fifteen or twenty years, enough other of their relatives have developed the disease to show their diabetic heredity is over 50 per cent. Years ago Dr. White found that diabetes was seven times as frequent among the relatives of those of our diabetics whom she examined as among the non-relatives; and a few years ago in the United States Public Health Service studies in Florida, diabetes among the relatives of diabetics there investigated was five times as common. The most convincing argument that diabetes is hereditary is based upon twins. If the twins are similar, exactly alike (identical), one finds that if one of the twins comes down with the disease, it is not long before the other twin develops it. The non-diabetic twin of non-identical twins is no more liable to diabetes than the brother or sister of any diabetic.

Diabetes is considered to be *recessive* rather than *dominant;* it may skip a generation. As yet there are very few instances on record in which it has been shown to be present in four successive generations.

In studying heredity among diabetics, one must remember that about one-third of all diabetic patients begin to show diabetes under forty years of age, another third between forty and fifty-five years of age, and the remainder between fifty-five and one hundred years. These figures are only approximate.

It always takes two to make a diabetic, but if there is no heredity in one parent and none of the relatives of this non-diabetic parent has ever had the disease, then theoretically the children of such a marriage will never show it. Of course, with diabetes being so common that one in four in the United States has a relative with it and so carries a diabetic gene, there is always the possibility that it may have been in an ancestor without its being recognized. Consequently, if a diabetic marries a non-diabetic in whose family there is no known history of diabetes, theoretically it would be impossible for their children to have the disease. If they did develop it, it would be because, so far as we can tell now, some member of the non-diabetic parent's family had had it.

Realizing that heredity is so common in diabetes, how can one prevent the disease, and particularly how can the relatives of diabetics, who are more prone to it, avoid it? The best rules I know are that the relatives of a diabetic should never be overweight, always should work (exercise), and should avoid excesses of any kind of food, but particularly sweet foods. When one realizes that it is extraordinarily rare for diabetes to appear in middle life unless an individual has been overweight, one can see the reason for such advice.

MARRIAGE OF DIABETICS

As late as 1885, Bouchardat, the leading diabetes clinician in the world up to that time, said he had never seen a pregnant diabetic woman. Insulin has changed all this, and diabetic women now become pregnant as readily as non-diabetic women; and it is most exceptional for any pregnant diabetic woman today to lose her life on account of diabetes. On the other hand, even up to twelve years ago nearly half of the pregnancies of the diabetic mothers resulted unfavorably even with the use of insulin. Today results are far better, and it is reasonable to state that approximately 70 per cent will give birth to live children.

Pregnancies in very mild diabetics should result as favorably as in non-diabetics. In general, the outlook is good for live babies if the disease has gone on for less than ten years, whether the pregnancy is the first or a subsequent one. Danger begins when there are changes in the blood vessels, the kidneys, or the eyes. Consequently, no diabetic woman should become pregnant unless assured that her physical condition in these respects is good.

It is true that patients who have had diabetes fifteen, twenty, or twenty-five years can bear a healthy child, but until recent years it certainly has been rare for a diabetic mother who had had the disease twenty years to have a successful outcome of her pregnancy. Dr. Priscilla White has had an unusual opportunity to follow such cases, and she has given me permission to state that between 1936 and November, 1964, she has had 1399 treated pregnancies; 87 per cent of the viable pregnancies resulted in live births. Among these there have been 210 cases of diabetes of twenty years or more duration and 25 of twenty-five years or more.

Two diabetics should not marry one another, because theoretically if they had a hundred children, all of their children would develop the disease. However, the outcome would not be quite so black as this. Actually only about forty-four of one hundred such children would ever develop diabetes, because only that number of children in either diabetic or non-diabetic families live to the period in life at which diabetes breaks out. The remainder would succumb to the ills to which all of us are exposed. Fifteen of the theoretical forty-four would be destined to develop diabetes before forty years of age, another fifteen to develop it between forty and fifty-five, and the remainder not until the age period of fifty-five to one hundred years. I have often thought that if a foreign ruler should issue a decree that diabetics in his country should not have children, my diabetics easily could conquer him, because two-thirds of them would not develop the disease until after forty years of age, and therefore would make good soldiers, and the chances also are that a good many of those under forty also could serve in the army.

PREVENTION AND TREATMENT OF DIABETIC GANGRENE

With pride we describe the changes with respect to the prevention and treatment of diabetic gangrene which have occurred over the last forty years. Once infections and gangrene of the extremities were a common cause of death. In spite of the greatly lengthened life of diabetic patients and the large number of patients in the age period when hardening of the arteries and the duration of diabetes itself might be expected to produce and actually does result in many infections and gangrene, the results of treatment both preventive and surgical have now vastly improved. When with Dr. L. S. McKittrick we described 322 operations upon diabetic patients between 1923 and 1926, the mortality in amputations was 18 per cent. Today, diabetic patients understand far better the importance of early treatment and early admission to the hospital for infections of the feet. In the following table it is shown that 442 patients out of 1981 patients admitted to the surgical wards (excluding patients in Hospital Teaching Unit) at the New England Deaconess Hospital on the Joslin Clinic Service had serious lesions in the feet. Nevertheless, many had come sufficiently early so that modern treatment of infections of the feet with the antibiotics such as penicillin and other newer drugs could prevent extension and in the majority of cases, major surgery was not necessary.

DIABETES MELLITUS WITH DISEASES OF LOWER LIMBS
New England Deaconess Hospital
1962–1963

Osteomyelitis	63
Gangrene	161
Infection	68
Ulceration	149
Charcot's Joint	1
Total	442

The preventive treatment for lesions of the feet including gangrene is better understood now than ever before but not yet sufficiently emphasized. Gangrene occurs in the elderly patient with mild diabetes of long duration, often with low insulin requirements, usually with inadequate diabetic treatment. Modern patients understand that earlier use of insulin and diet is the first step in the prevention of gangrene. Second comes the prevention of obesity; it is in the obese patient that serious foot lesions are most frequent. Instruction in the care of the feet, particularly treatment of corns and calluses with the aid of the chiropodist, will be of the greatest value. Hardening of the arteries is the underlying factor of greatest importance. Patients who find that they have cramps in one leg or both legs on walking one or two blocks must be instructed in the care of the feet. These hardened arteries make the circulation and nutrition of the foot or leg poor. An injury to the skin and particularly a burn may result in a lesion which heals very slowly. The skin must be kept clean. Hot water bottles must be avoided. The chiropodists on the Staff of the New England Deaconess Hospital have been of great help to our patients. They know the dangers involved and they have made fitted shoes of the newer types to avoid the pressure points where calluses and areas of infection will easily develop.

CARE OF THE FEET

Injuries to the feet in both old and young patients must be avoided. New shoes should first be put on at night and worn for an hour or two only. Shoe linings should not be broken. One should carefully avoid protruding nails in the shoes. Every diabetic should keep his feet as clean as his face. Every older diabetic should show his feet to his doctor at each visit.

Today, amputation of an extremity above the knee has become rare because of the skill of the surgeons who can overcome infections and gangrene with local treatment and minor operations. The following sheet of instructions has been given to patients at the New England Deaconess Hospital for a number of years.

CARE OF THE FEET FOR DIABETIC ADULTS

1. Wash feet daily using a mild soap and warm water. Dry carefully, especially between the toes.

2. If skin is dry, apply Lanolin. Do not put Lanolin between the toes or around the toe nails. Avoid excess of Lanolin.

3. Cut nails straight across and file carefully to avoid rough ends. Do this only under good light and after the nails have been washed. If nails are too thick or tend to split or crack when you cut them, have them cared for by a chiropodist.

4. Treatment of corns and calluses. After washing feet, rub gently with a turkish towel. If these areas cannot be removed by this method, have a chiropodist care for them. Do not use patented corn remedies. Do not use a knife or razor blade.

5. If feet tend to sweat, apply a mild foot powder daily after careful washing and drying.

6. Buy new shoes carefully. Make sure they fit and are comfortable. Shoes should support, protect and cover the feet. Break them in gradually. Wear for one-half hour the first day and increase this by one-half hour every day. Wrap a small amount of lamb's wool around the toes when breaking in new shoes to prevent blisters. Avoid tight and ill-fitting shoes.

7. Do not go barefooted. Always protect your feet, especially when on the beach or in swimming.

8. Do not soak sore feet in hot water. If your feet ache, remove shoes and sit with legs elevated to hip level.

9. When visiting a chiropodist, be sure he knows you are diabetic.

10. Inspect feet daily. Examine around nails, between toes and the bottom of the feet. If your eyesight is poor, have someone in your family do this for you. Look for corns, calluses, redness, swelling, bruises or openings in the skin.

11. First-aid treatment. Wash area immediately with ST-37. Cover with a dry sterile dressing, but do not put adhesive tape on the skin. Get off your feet. Go to bed, if possible. Call doctor if area does not improve in 24–36 hours. Do not use strong antiseptic solutions.

12. Do not use hot water bottles or heating pads on your feet.

13. Pain, redness, swelling, pus and tenderness are danger signals. See your doctor immediately.

14. Avoid any antiseptic solution with dye in it. Use no Tincture of Iodine or solutions of Boric Acid or Epsom Salts.

Do not forget that in many diabetic patients, both old and young, numbness of the feet or reduced sensation so that the patient does not feel heat or even slight injury, may be present. Many such patients are not aware that their sensation is reduced and therefore forget that a burn may occur from hot water bottles, an electric pad, or even hot water when the temperature is much lower than would be required for such an injury in a person without diabetes. Never should the feet be soaked in hot water for long periods. Patients, especially elderly individuals with diabetes of long duration, should never obstruct the circulation with round garters or by crossing the knees. Patients should move about and then after walking, place the feet on a chair or a stool. In patients who suffer pain in the calves of the legs upon walking, special exercises have been recommended.

The patient who has deficient blood supply in the legs should avoid the use of tobacco in any form. Smoking is harmful.

Gangrene most frequently occurs in the elderly patient with mild diabetes of long duration, with low insulin dosage and delay in treatment. Earlier use of insulin and diet is important as the first step. Of chief importance in the diet is the prevention of obesity. The care of calluses and corns is often best carried out under the direction of a chiropodist, and hospitals which treat diabetic patients should have a chiropodist on their staff.

Complications in the feet are so serious that every preventive measure should be employed. In the Deaconess Hospital, a special beauty parlor for diabetic feet was made possible by a gift of many friends. On one morning each week at 7:30 A.M., a combined medical and surgical conference is held to discuss lesions of the feet for patients who are then under treatment in the hospital.

INFECTIONS

Diabetes is made temporarily more severe by an infection. The patient with uncontrolled diabetes has less than normal ability to withstand infections and therefore infections have been over the years a very frequent cause of death, especially prior to the discovery and use of insulin. The use of the newer antibiotics has enabled many patients to combat infections successfully. Thus in the Deaconess Hospital experience, prior to 1938, nearly 40 per cent of deaths were attributed to infections. Since that time however, with the discovery of new antibiotics, deaths from infection have become rare. During infections it may be necessary to double or quadruple the dose of insulin. Yet with recovery from infection, frequently the insulin requirement will return to its previous level. Nevertheless, whenever possible, infections should be avoided and the source of infection removed. Abscessed teeth should be extracted; seriously infected tonsils should be removed; infected gall bladders or appendix should be eliminated; boils or "run-abouts" about a nail or a callus on the foot or hand should receive prompt attention. The diabetic patient is susceptible to tuberculosis and to infections in the urinary tract and skin. In general, this decreased resistance seems to be related to the bodily insult of diabetic acidosis. Therefore, in relation to the prevention of infections, the early diagnosis and the continued control of diabetes is of primary importance.

Infections do not cause diabetes except in rare instances where infections seriously involve the pancreas itself.

The need for vaccination against smallpox, diphtheria, pertussis, typhoid, poliomyelitis, influenza and tetanus are the same for diabetic patients as for nondiabetic individuals.

Common skin infections due to staphylococcus, streptococcus, and fungi may result in boils or in the case of fungi, epidermophytosis. This last condition, commonly known as "athlete's foot" is common in diabetic patients and requires effective treatment.

Tuberculosis has fortunately greatly declined in frequency among our diabetic patients. Today in addition to sanitarium treatment, drug treatment consisting of the anti-tuberculosis remedies is often suggested.

When an infection is in progress in a diabetic it may be necessary to give the insulin every three or four hours; it is administered according to the results of the tests of the urine for sugar. Thus some doctors prescribe fifteen units for a red test with Benedict's solution, ten for a yellow test, five for a green test, and no insulin if the test is blue, showing no sugar. Mothers soon learn to vary the dosage of insulin which even so mild an infection as a common cold in a child may demand. Fortunately, when the infection subsides, the dose of insulin can be reduced to its former level. This makes us conclude that infections do not permanently injure the pancreas or indeed cause diabetes, but in some other way interfere with the diabetic state. By having all his lurking infections promptly treated, the diabetic may score a few points of health over the non-diabetic who is neglectful or careless about the same.

Get rid of all infections.

DIABETIC ACIDOSIS AND COMA

Lack of diabetic regulation is the cause of the condition known as diabetic acidosis terminating in coma. This condition may be present in newly discovered diabetes, in patients who omit the usual insulin dosage, and in those who fail to increase the insulin dosage when requirements for insulin rise or finally, in those who rely on the oral drugs when insulin is needed. Increases in the need for insulin frequently occur during prolonged inactivity, infection, insulin resistance, pregnancy, surgical operations, and other strains. Errors in diet, with or without emotional disturbances will lead to an increased need for insulin, which, if not recognized, will result in coma.

Half a century ago, at least 64 diabetics in each 100 died of diabetic coma but today a death from diabetic coma is as needless as a death from diphtheria. Today only 1 in 100 of all Joslin Clinic diabetic patients, wherever in the world their lives end, now succumbs to coma.

All patients must learn how to avoid coma and acidosis. If you are the patient or if you are a relative or friend of a diabetic and wish to prevent it, the following rules have been effective.

RULES TO AVOID AND PREVENT DIABETIC COMA

If you feel sick, take no chances, but call it diabetic coma and

1. Go to bed.
2. Call the doctor.
3. Test the urine for sugar every 2 to 4 hours.

4. Never omit insulin if the urine contains sugar, even though you cannot eat.
5. Take one cupful of a hot drink—water, coffee, tea, broth, gruel—every hour.
6. Get someone to care for you.
7. Move the bowels with an enema.
8. Keep warm.

The symptoms of the onset of diabetic coma are notoriously obscure. It comes on like a thief in the night. The patient usually feels "sick" and has discomfort or pain in the abdomen, nausea or vomiting; often he has given up insulin or broken his diet; he may have developed an infection and not realized that he required more insulin; he may have drawn too heavily on his own body fat because of extreme exercise or lack of food. Too much fat is bad for a diabetic, no matter whether it is his own body fat or some other kind of fat. Perhaps he has been seasick, or had diarrhea; perhaps he has goiter and thus, not getting enough food, he is living on his own body fat for nourishment to the exclusion of carbohydrate, which either he has not taken or has been unable to utilize because of want of insulin, either his own or that which he buys. He is weak, irritable, tired, nervous, and begins to have difficulty in breathing. All this comes on slowly and slyly: that is the reason for telling him if he feels sick to go to bed, get the doctor, and to call it the onset of diabetic coma until the doctor proves it otherwise. The cupful of hot liquid every hour will help to wash out of the body the fatty acids which cause the coma.

The onset of coma is slow, but its course is fast, and its outcome in death or recovery may take place in twenty-four hours, so that treatment must be prompt and active. Hence the patient needs a nurse or someone to care for him at once. As one patient put it, even get your mother-in-law, because it is touch and go. What is done in treatment the first two hours is worth more than what can be done the next twelve hours. The children know this. So do the well-trained hospital patients. When they get sick they telephone their doctors and start treatment immediately, and thus the coma is stopped before it gets a headway. If the patient becomes advanced so far in coma that he is nearly unconscious, then it means a day-and-night job for the doctor and the nurse to bring him out of it and maybe a week or two to convalesce. An hour of prevention or early treatment saves weeks of hospitalization.

Diabetic coma is due to lack of insulin. If this is given promptly in the course of the first three hours, we have found that ten times as many patients recover as do if the same amount is given in the course of the next twelve hours.

The treatment of diabetic coma is complicated, and whenever the diagnosis is made it is safer to send the patient into a hospital. Here tests of the blood, as well as of the urine, for sugar can be performed, and the extent of the acid poisoning determined. Usually several hundred units of insulin are required. For the extreme dryness of the body, normal salt solution is given and several quarts may be administered in the first few hours. There are many details of treatment which contribute to recovery from this complication which before the discovery of insulin was almost uniformly fatal.

To make an accurate diagnosis is the first and essential step. The patient may be unconscious and yet not have diabetic coma, but be unconscious from other causes, and the danger is then imminent that he may be treated for the wrong condition. Accidentally he may have taken too much of a drug to produce sleep or relieve pain. He may have taken too much insulin. He may have had a stroke of apoplexy or some temporary nervous trouble which has made him unconscious. Children not uncommonly are unconscious at the beginning of various diseases, or even in health if long without food. Diabetic coma may be confused with a beginning appendicitis, and that is why it is so desirable to remove the appendix in a diabetic when there is a history of its being diseased, so that the question of appendicitis will not arise to confuse the picture if signs of acid poisoning, diabetic coma, appear.

The consequences of a wrong diagnosis between the unconsciousness of diabetic coma and an overdose of insulin (insulin shock) are tragic, and, I regret to say, in a few instances fatal. Therefore every diabetic should carry an identification card in his pocket, so that if by accident he should become unconscious from any cause, the strange doctor who first sees him will be given a hint of his condition. If a diabetic has symptoms of coma or does not recover from an insulin reaction within fifteen to thirty minutes, it is safer to send him to a hospital. An example of such a confusing situation is shown by the following incident. An old Negro preacher whose kidneys were bad and blood pressure high in pipestem arteries became unconscious, and his wife thought he was having a stroke. At first, on reaching the hospital, this appeared to be the diagnosis, but a bright young house officer examined his blood and found the blood sugar to be below normal. He injected a little sugar into the vein and—a miracle—the unconscious preacher was brought back to life. If that doctor had made a mistake and treated him for diabetic coma and injected insulin instead of sugar, in the place of a miracle there might have been a funeral. What happened was this: The pious old preacher took his insulin as usual before breakfast and then went into his garden. He worked hard, so hard, in fact, that his steed Exercise did all the work of his steed Insulin. Insulin ran away with his blood sugar and sent it away below normal. The patient should have realized that the diabetic who takes unwonted exercise is entitled to an orange or a little additional carbohydrate in some other form. The extra carbohydrate would have protected him.

In diabetic coma the blood sugar is high and the urine contains sugar.

In an insulin reaction the blood sugar is low and the urine is either sugar free or a second test in thirty minutes will be sugar free.

Diabetic patients will never go into diabetic coma if they live on their diets, keep the urine sugar free, and are careful about their insulin. They must remember, however, that infections make a diabetic worse and so make changes necessary in the doses of insulin. Patients must not omit a regular dose of insulin without testing the urine within six hours to note its effect. A little experience will protect them.

If a diabetic patient can get into a hospital with a laboratory in which tests can be performed by night as well as by day, his chances for recovery from coma are good, and the younger he is the better the outlook for recovery. Of twenty-three children with diabetic coma recently treated in the New England Deaconess Hospital, none died, but we have had only one person as old as seventy-seven recover.

There are easy tests of the urine for the detection of acid poisoning by examining it for acetone and diacetic acid. Many doctors teach their patients how to make these tests. In general, I emphasize keeping the urine sugar free, and then coma does not appear; but one must remember that a patient voiding a urine which gives a green test with Benedict solution for sugar may in a few hours void a specimen which gives a red test. The tests for acetone and diacetic acid are recorded below.

The test for acetone is readily performed with Nitroprusside, which conveniently is put up in tablet form ("Acetest" manufactured by the Ames Company, Inc., Elkhart, Indiana).

The test for diacetic acid is also easily performed:

To 5 or 10 cc. of freshly voided urine carefully add a few drops of a 10 per cent aqueous solution of ferric chloride. A precipitate of ferric phosphate first forms, but upon the addition of a few more drops is dissolved. The depth of the Burgundy-red color obtained is an index to the quantity of diacetic acid present. The intensity of the reaction may be roughly recorded as 1, 2, 3, or 4+. If the color does not disappear on boiling, it is not a true test for diacetic acid, and is due to aspirin or some similar drug.

THE NERVOUS SYSTEM

Many diabetic patients or their families ask advice with regard to "nervous" symptoms. Some patients especially in the first two or three decades of life have emotional difficulties or problems in personal development for which helpful treatment can be given. On the other hand, the great majority of diabetic patients have no trouble with "nerves" but accept their lot courageously and strive to overcome any handicaps connected with the disease. Careful studies have been made of the intelligence and personality of diabetic patients when compared with other persons of the same age. The diabetic patient showed no greater deviations than their nondiabetic friends. Some diabetic patients have shown superiority in mental achievement. On the whole, diabetic patients do not have any greater personality problems than nondiabetic patients of similar ages.

DIABETIC NEUROPATHY (NEURITIS)

Neuropathy means the diabetic effect upon nerves which supply the various tissues of the body. In some instances the result is a painful neuritis of the legs. However, the condition may involve the stomach, the intestines, the urinary bladder, or the eyes. The nerves contain many fibers, both motor and sensory. Thus occasionally there may be a paralysis of one of the motor nerves which controls the movement of the eyes, especially the sixth nerve which supplies the external rectus muscle—then one sees "double." Rarely a nerve may be involved which supplies the muscle of the forehead and the resulting condition suggests a shock but it is entirely different. In the lower extremities, weakness of the muscles, such as the iliopsoas, may make it difficult to rise from a chair, or the peroneal nerve is involved, a toe drop and shuffling gait will result. These conditions may be painless because only the motor fibers of the nerve are affected and in time recovery occurs.

The sensory fibers may be involved with or without the motor fibers. Then pain may result in the legs which is severe. It may be worse at night and relieved only by walking. Instead of pain there may be numbness, prickling, pins-and-needles feelings which are most annoying. They may be quite general or localized to a small area of the body.

When the nerves to the digestive and urinary tract are involved, there may be a severe and troublesome diarrhea or on the contrary, a severe constipation. Involvement of the urinary bladder is not rare. In these cases, the patient may have difficulty in emptying the bladder. Then it is frequently difficult to interpret the urine tests because some of the urine remains for hours in the bladder. This is the reason why it is so often necessary to test a second specimen of urine rather than the first voiding. Even then, interpretation of the test may be difficult.

THE EYES

Blurring of vision in diabetics may occur when treatment is about to begin and frequently this disturbance in vision is the first sign which is recognized by the patient. The high blood-sugar content is reflected in chemical changes in the eye which gradually return to normal with prompt treatment. Usually this condition lasts for a few weeks. It is advisable therefore in the first few weeks of treatment of diabetes not to have new glasses fitted because they would serve only temporarily. Usually within a month the eyes will become adjusted and then correct new glasses can be fitted. Cataracts develop more often in diabetics than in patients without diabetes. Occasionally cataracts develop in diabetic children. However, it is not yet definitely certain that in later life diabetes produces cataracts or whether cataracts are actually more frequent in diabetics. Operations can be performed successfully even on persons of advanced years.

Hemorrhages and exudates occur far too commonly in the eyes of diabetics. If these involve the macula in the retina, vision is seriously impaired. The best known way to avoid such conditions is to control the diabetes from the very beginning. Tobacco is harmful. Medicines may be of some value in preventing the hemorrhages.

CAMPS FOR DIABETIC CHILDREN

The treatment of diabetic children in summer camps is an invaluable supplement to home, hospital and office management. Although the lot of diabetic children is steadily improving and they now enter into all the activities of a normal child, they carry heavy responsibilities. Teaching is carried on at their own age level; and the benefits of group teaching and important contacts with resident doctors, nurses, dietitians, and laboratory technicians increase the child's knowledge and understanding of his condition. Self-management when the child is ready is encouraged as well as the emphasis upon other activities. Searching for and developing the child's special aptitudes is important. Those children and those families in whom overanxiety, dependence, or resentment are factors, can be helped with regular emotional support. At each meal the diabetic child is reminded of his disease and must have insulin once or twice a day. Apprehension is relieved by understanding.

The first camp for diabetic children was planned by the late Dr. Wendt in Detroit. In the following year, 1926, Mrs. Devine of Ogunquit, Maine, opened a camp for diabetic children and little by little these camps have sprung up in various parts of the country. Under the supervision of Dr. Priscilla White and Dr. Alexander Marble, some 200 diabetic girls go to the Clara Barton Birthplace Camp for girls in Oxford, Massachusetts and 150 diabetic boys to the Elliott P. Joslin Camp in nearby Charlton, Massachusetts. These camps have proven most advantageous.

I am informed by the American Diabetes Association that in 1967, 39 such camps for diabetic children were maintained in 27 states in the USA,

7 camps in Canada, and 9 abroad. The countries known to have such camps are Denmark, England, France, Germany, Israel, Japan, The Netherlands, Switzerland, and Turkey.

Further information can be obtained by writing to the American Diabetes Association, 18 East 48th Street, New York, New York 10017.

The change of food and surroundings, which a trip away from home involves, and the contact with many others who have the same disease, along with the pleasures of camp life, are splendid for the children. The revision of diets and dosage of insulin while under supervision which is as close as that in a hospital and yet not so obvious gives an excellent opportunity to improve treatment. But these camps soon disclosed another useful feature of almost equal value, and that was the vacation they provided for the children's parents and households. It is no joke to have the responsibility of a diabetic child day and night for years, and we soon learned that the mothers were quite as thankful for the freedom from care and the vacation they received as were the children themselves.

CHAPTER 24

Blood Pressure

ARTHUR M. MASTER, M.D.
AND RICHARD P. LASSER, M.D.

Within the last decade, many profound discoveries have been made regarding the causes of high blood pressure (or hypertension), making available new methods of diagnosis to uncover these underlying diseases. Medical and surgical treatment of hypertension has been greatly improved resulting in an increasingly favorable life span for those suffering from this prevalent condition. Consequently the care to the patient has changed from a more or less passive attitude, where treatment was regarded with considerable nihilism by many physicians, to an active one where exact diagnosis is carefully sought, and treatment prescribed and carefully followed. There is still much unnecessary fear and anxiety generated concerning what are really only minor elevations of blood pressure. Dr. Arthur M. Master pointed this out as early as 1950 and tried to break the rigid interpretation of "normality" which had labeled a large number of healthy adults as hypertensive.

MECHANISM OF BLOOD PRESSURE

Blood pressure refers to the pressure within the arteries throughout the body, i.e., the blood vessels carrying the blood from the heart to the organs and tissues. The pressure in the arteries is produced by the beating of the heart. Each time the heart contracts (this part of the heart beat is called systole), the left side of the heart or left ventricle propels the blood within it into a large artery called the aorta. From this vessel the blood flows into many arterial branches which become smaller and smaller until they are exceedingly fine and connect with the veins through the capillaries. Because of the force with which the left ventricle ejects the blood into the aorta, it flows with considerable speed, and a pulse wave is sent ahead through all the arteries. This pulsation is easily felt at the wrist, but may also be felt in the neck and feet and in other parts of the body. The arteries are elastic and flexible; in their walls are muscle fibers which contract and help send the blood along. The combined effects of the force of the pumping action of the left ventricle and the elastic contraction of the arteries serve to maintain a pressure within the entire arterial system. This is the blood pressure.

Furthermore, the blood pressure is regulated automatically to maintain it at normal levels despite varying circumstances encountered during daily life. Tiny pressure "gauges" are situated in the arteries leading to the head and these act, for example, to raise the pressure when it falls, by stimulating the heart to pump harder and faster and by constricting the blood vessels throughout the body. This occurs every time one changes from a lying to a standing position. A sudden rise in blood pressure due to an emotional outburst, however, is quickly corrected back to normal levels by this same automatic regulation.

The pressure in the arteries is not the same throughout each heartbeat; it is highest during the period of contraction, or systole, and lowest during the relaxation phase, or diastole. As a result, each person has an upper systolic pressure and a lower diastolic blood pressure, e.g., 124 over 82. Usually the diastolic pressure is about two thirds the systolic, but, as you grow older and the arteries tend to lose their elasticity and become rigid, the systolic pressure is apt to rise considerably whereas the diastolic increases only slightly.

Both the systolic and diastolic pressures can be recorded. The instrument used to measure them is technically termed a sphygmomanometer. This name, derived from the Greek, literally means a measure of the pulses but is rarely used even by doctors. Most of them merely say blood-pressure machine. The device consists of two parts connected by a rubber tube. One part is a long cloth sleeve containing a rectangular rubber bag at one end. Two rubber tubes lead out from this bag through the cloth sleeve. One leads to a rubber bulb which inflates the rubber bag and has a valve which regulates the inflow and outflow of air. The second tube is long and is attached to the second part of the apparatus, which consists of a glass tube containing a column of mercury. The glass tube is graduated in millimeters from 0 to 300. These days many doctors use a spring-type pressure gauge (aneroid) in place of the mercury column. The gauge is as accurate and more convenient.

When your doctor takes your blood pressure, he winds the cloth sleeve around your right or left arm. He places his stethoscope in the crease of the elbow on the artery and squeezes the bulb. As he continues to do this, the pressure in the rubber bag on the arm increases, causing the mercury to rise in the glass column and the needle to move on the gauge-type machine. When this pressure exceeds the systolic (upper) pressure in the artery, the pulse at the wrist disappears and the doctor can no longer hear the sounds of the pulse through his stethoscope. The doctor then opens a small valve in the bulb allowing the pressure to fall gradually. The precise point at which the sounds of the pulse are again heard and the pulse can be felt at the wrist is the systolic pressure. At a certain point the sounds again disappear or diminish markedly. This is the diastolic pressure.

NORMAL BLOOD PRESSURE

In the past, normal people were supposed to have systolic pressure less than 150 mm. mercury and the diastolic under 90. These figures applied to all people over 40 regardless of their exact age, sex, or build. Therefore, if a man or woman of 55 or 65 had either a systolic pressure of 160 or a diastolic pressure of 95, they were considered to have high blood pressure or hypertension. As a result, these people were treated as if they were ill or potentially sick. As might be expected, this caused considerable emotional disturbances and even physical invalidism.

However, doctors observed that many of these people who were supposed to have high blood pressure remained in good health for many years. Therefore, in collaboration with Dublin and Marks, and later with Lasser and Jaffe, Dr. Master began a new investigation into what was a normal blood pressure at various ages.

It was found that blood pressure actually increases gradually with age and differs by sex. Table 1 shows the range of normal pressure established by these studies. Note that the blood pressure of women is lower than that of men at younger ages; but after about age 49 (female menopause), it exceeds that of the men, and at age 65, the systolic pressure in women is 10–12 mm. mercury higher. The diastolic pressure, on the other hand, is essentially the same in both sexes. Some representative average values are: at 20 years of age, for men 123/76 and for women 116/72; at 40 years of age, for men 129/81 and for women 127/80; at 60 years of age, for men 142/85 and for women 144/85; at 80 years of age, for men 145/78 and for women 154/83. This is not the entire story, however, since it is known that people whose pressures are consistently lower than the normal, actually have a better-than-average life expectancy and suffer less frequently from diseases of the heart and circulatory system. This is not true, of course, when the low pressure is due to severe malnutrition, chronic or acute anemia, advanced tuberculosis, inadequate glandular function, heart attacks, or rheumatic heart disease (*See* section on hypotension).

However, in general, as the blood pressure rises above 150 mm. systolic and 95 mm. diastolic, a certain number of people go on to real high blood pressure and suffer from an increased number of heart attacks and diseases of the blood vessels and kidneys. Therefore, on the average, the life expectancy of this group as a whole is somewhat reduced. The higher the pressure, that is, the further away from normal it is, the greater is the risk of reduced life expectancy. However, to repeat, the variation among people is so great that one must not become apprehensive even if the pressure is somewhat above normal, but leave the decision to the doctor as to what measures, if any, must be taken to combat it.

Most people think of the blood pressure as being fixed and assume that the exact height of the pressure determines how they feel. Neither of these ideas is true. Many people, particularly those who are inclined to be nervous and apprehensive, have a variable or labile blood pressure. It may suddenly rise considerably in any situation of excitement, such as visiting a doctor, preparing for an examination, or experiencing pain. Because of this, the physician takes the blood pressure again if the first reading or two is high. If he wishes, the physician can obtain the "basal" blood pressure by placing the person being examined at rest or in bed for several hours or days and taking frequent blood-pressure readings. In extreme cases the pressure may rise 40 or 50 mm. temporarily. As a rule, the systolic pressure rises more than the diastolic. One of our patients has a normal blood pressure of 124/74 mm. but when she comes to the office, the first reading at times is up to 170 or 180 systolic and 110 to 120 diastolic. There is some difference of opinion among doctors concerning the importance of these transitory increases in blood pressure. Some doctors believe that such patients have a tendency to high blood pressure and probably will develop it later on. In our experience, however, many of them retain a normal blood pressure over the years.

WHAT CAUSES HIGH BLOOD PRESSURE?

High blood pressure in itself is not, strictly speaking, a disease. It is an abnormal finding caused by some disease process. At present, however, though many different specific causes have been identified, in over 80 per cent of cases the ultimate cause is unknown. In these patients the high blood pressure is called Essential Hypertension. The next decade will probably see the elimination of this term with the discovery of the, as yet, unknown underlying disease which results in the high blood pressure. The past decade has seen the identification of certain curable cases of hypertension which have now been estimated at up to 15 per cent of all cases.

TABLE 1
NORMAL RANGE OF BLOOD PRESSURE

	Systolic mm.		*Diastolic mm.*	
Age	*Male*	*Female*	*Male*	*Female*
16	105–135	100–130	60–86	60–85
17	105–135	100–130	60–86	60–85
18	105–135	100–130	60–86	60–85
19	105–140	100–130	60–88	60–85
20–24	105–140	100–130	62–88	60–85
25–29	108–140	102–130	65–90	60–86
30–34	110–145	102–135	68–92	60–88
35–39	110–145	105–140	68–92	65–90
40–44	110–150	105–150	70–94	65–92
45–49	110–155	105–155	70–96	65–96
50–54	115–160	110–165	70–98	70–100
55–59	115–165	110–170	70–98	70–100
60–64	115–170	115–175	70–100	70–100
65–94	115–175	120–192	70–95	65–102

First among the "curable" cases of hypertension is that which results from disease of the main artery to one of the two kidneys. If the principal artery to one kidney is narrowed, and does not bring a sufficient blood supply, the deprived kidney secretes a hormone into the blood stream which has the effect of raising the blood pressure. This is a compensation since the higher blood pressure will then force more blood into the deprived kidney. The diseased artery may be narrowed from several causes —malformation with which the person was born (congenital), hardening of the arteries (arteriosclerosis), and certain other rarer conditions. This type of high blood pressure responds promptly to surgical repair of the artery and restoration of its natural diameter. Where this is impossible the kidney is removed. Other "curable" forms of high blood pressure resulting from kidney disease are tumors of a single kidney and also infection or stones confined to a single kidney. Removal of the diseased kidney often results in restoration of blood pressure to normal. The gratifying cures obtained in such cases now makes necessary restudy of many patients with so-called essential hypertension to discover the curable ones due to single-kidney involvement. When both kidneys are involved by these same processes, the hypertension is no longer curable; obviously both kidneys cannot be removed, and in such instances where repair of arteries to both kidneys was attempted, results were not entirely satisfactory. Great strides in the identification of such cases has been made. Tests consist of special kidney X rays ("timed intravenous pyelogram"), and visualization of the arteries to the kidneys by direct injection of an opaque substance and simultaneous taking of multiple X-ray films (angiography). It is generally advocated that all patients with high blood pressure who are under the age of 40 years be studied routinely in this fashion, as well as those in whom blood pressure rises suddenly to great heights, or those with rapid progression of the disease. Patients in older age groups with high blood pressure for less than 5 years may also be studied. Usually patients with hypertension due to involvement of one kidney have very high blood pressure, 240/140 mm. for example. Therefore, what we have said does not apply to patients whose pressures are only slightly or moderately elevated above the average or normal value. Remarkably, we have now found the human and natural counterpart to the great experiment of thirty years ago, where high blood pressure was produced in dogs by Dr. Goldblatt in the same manner, i.e., by partial narrowing of the artery supplying one kidney. As the search for curable cases is widened and if early diagnosis is made, more and more cases will be cured. Possibly most cases of hypertension will ultimately prove to be due to some subtle narrowing of small arteries within the kidney itself.

In children and young adults and even occasionally in older adults, high blood pressure proves to be due to an inborn defect, namely, a narrowing or stricture of the aorta. This is called *"coarctation of the aorta"* and is a curable form of hypertension since surgical removal of the narrowed portion of the aorta and re-establishment of its normal width results in restoration of the pressure to normal. This condition is readily diagnosed, if looked for, since blood pressure is high in the upper half of the body, i.e., the arms, but is low in the legs. There is usually a heart murmur and characteristic findings in the X-ray film.

New advances have been made in the diagnosis of hypertension due to tumors of the adrenal gland (a small but vital gland lying just above the kidney). This gland normally secretes "adrenaline" and "noradrenaline," substances designed to aid the body in times of stress by raising blood pressure, heart rate, and general strength of the heart. However, tumors of these adrenaline-secreting cells occur and release large quantities into the blood stream resulting in attacks of severe high blood pressure, palpitations, sweating, dizziness, and headache. These attacks sometimes are precipitated by bending down and squeezing the tumor. Reliable tests of blood and urine have now been developed to identify these tumors and should be performed on all patients in young and middle adult life with severe hypertension, i.e., 220/120 mm. or more, whether they have typical attacks or not, and also in those with marked fluctuations of blood pressure, i.e., varying from normal to very high values suddenly. The cure is surgical removal of the tumor. Such cases are rare. Even rarer are tumors of another part of the same gland which normally secretes a substance concerned with salt metabolism—aldosterone. These tumors also cause marked hypertension, and can be identified through certain alterations in the amount of sodium and potassium in the blood, urine, and saliva. Direct tests are available but are very expensive and not suitable now to routine use for screening purposes. These cases are still medical curiosities. Surgical removal is the treatment, and cures the hypertension entirely.

Hypertension also is seen in other diseases of the kidneys such as nephritis—a diffuse inflammation which may follow sore throats or scarlet fever. It is diagnosed by the finding of albumin and abnormal elements in the urine. Fewer cases are seen now than formerly because of the more effective treatment of sore throats with antibiotics.

During pregnancy, blood pressure may rise suddenly during the last three months. This is called toxemia of pregnancy and is associated with a high incidence of spontaneous abortion and stillborn infants. While the cause is unknown, these consequences can be prevented by careful observation of pregnant women for early signs of toxemia, and effective treatment against high pressure with a salt-free diet, rest, and medication.

Blood pressure is usually high (but rarely exceedingly high) in patients with an overactive thyroid. Here, treatment of the thyroid disorder automatically returns the pressure to normal.

Elevation of the systolic pressure alone (normal diastolic pressure) is a form of hypertension which is seen usually in the older age group when the arteries have become hardened with age and arteriosclerosis. These patients are usually without symptoms from the blood-pressure elevation and only rarely require medication to lower pressure. In fact, medication to lower pressure often has deleterious effects in this older age group.

ESSENTIAL HYPERTENSION

After the doctor has completed a search for known causes of high blood pressure and they have proved negative, he says that the patient has Essential Hypertension. This is just another way of stating that the only abnormality to be found is the high pressure itself. Such patients still make up over 80 per cent of all the cases with hypertension. Although the reason is unknown in these people, the smallest branches of their arteries throughout the body are narrowed or constricted. This increases the resistance in these tiny vessels, and the blood pressure must rise to keep the blood flowing through them.

A number of theories have been proposed concerning the cause of Essential Hypertension. The most popular view is that people who develop this disease are emotional and react more tensely and sensitively to the conditions of life. They meet most daily happenings, big and small, with anxiety and restraint. They tend to repress their conflicts. These inner tensions set up impulses in the brain which travel through a special part of the nervous system to all parts of the body, causing the arterioles to tighten. When this happens repeatedly, day in and day out, these small vessels may become scarred and thickened. The resistance within them rises, and the blood pressure increases permanently.

Many situations in everyday life may cause emotional strain and anxiety in tense people. Among the commonest are financial difficulties, dissatisfaction with the job, failure to advance in work, jealousy, disagreement among members of a family, and physical disability or illness of a beloved one. Many people are full of fears about various things, many of which do not have any basis in fact.

Since anxiety and tension are almost universal, you may wonder why all people do not have hypertension. Likely there is another factor in people with hypertension, in addition to the specific type of nervous reaction already mentioned. This localizes the effect of nervous sensitivity in the arterioles, resulting in hypertension, whereas other nervous people develop ulcer of the stomach, colitis (disease of the large bowel), or other diseases. This tendency to hypertension is more common in some families than in others. For example, we have observed a family in which the grandmother, her four daughters, and a grandson developed a high degree of diastolic hypertension at a relatively early age. As is not uncommon even in advanced hypertension, one of the sisters is alive at 77 and the others did not die until they were 69, 63 and 61—life spans not much different from the average. This is perhaps an unusual instance, but in a considerable number of families one not infrequently finds high blood pressure in one parent and one or two children. Hypertension is not hereditary, and the specific factor which predisposes certain families to develop it is not clear.

Observations have led some doctors to believe that there is a relation between high blood pressure and race and climate. Hypertension, according to some reports, rarely occurs in some parts of China and the Orient, and among people, particularly the natives, living in the heat of the tropics. These statements remain to be proven, and the results may not be comparable with those in the Western World because the life span of the people in the tropics may be much shorter. If hypertension is less common among tropical people, it is probably because of their type of diet, which is low in proteins, fats, and salt and because of the mode of life, which is slow and less tense than ours. When these people have lived among us, they develop hypertension pretty much as we do.

Overweight or obesity tends to increase the blood pressure and therefore favors the development of hypertension. Although it is an aggravating factor, it probably is not a direct cause, because many people with high blood pressure are of average weight or even thin. The popular conception of a person with hypertension is someone who is obese and emotional and has a florid complexion. Although this is often true, many such people have a normal blood pressure. However, obesity is significant and often serious when high blood pressure exists, and merely reducing weight is often sufficient to lower the blood pressure. Overweight increases the amount of work which the heart must perform, and loss of weight lessens the burden on the heart, allowing the blood pressure to fall. This was observed during wartime when malnutrition and starvation were common in many countries and the frequency of hypertension fell sharply.

Recently it has become evident that the endocrine glands play an important role in regulating the blood pressure and form a link in the development of hypertension in many cases. We have already mentioned how a tumor of the inner portion or medulla of one of these glands, the adrenal, causes bouts of high blood pressure or even constant hypertension. Similarly, high blood pressure may be caused by a tumor of the outer portion of the pituitary gland, another endocrine gland, which is situated in the under surface of the brain above the nasal passages. The endocrine glands, which also include the thyroid, pancreas, and ovaries, secrete substances directly into the blood stream which are called hormones. The latter control many functions of the body such as growth, sexual development, menstruation, metabolism, and the distribution of salt and water in the body. Each gland secretes a specific hormone, but the functions of all the glands are interrelated, with the pituitary gland acting as the regulator of many functions.

One factor connecting the endocrine glands with hypertension is that many women develop high blood pressure during or after the menopause. At this period the activity of the endocrine glands undergoes a great change. In many of these women the blood pressure later falls. The factor of anxiety about their changed state, however, is often the most significant element in menopausal hypertension.

In the past a variety of other factors have been suggested as causes of hypertension. They include focal infections, such as diseased tonsils, abscessed teeth, or infected hemorrhoids, also syphilis, gallbladder disease, constipation, alcohol, tobacco, and coffee. These conditions do not cause high blood pressure. Excessive smoking or drinking of coffee or soft drinks containing caffeine may help to maintain high blood pressure. During the recent war it was not uncommon for officers to drink ten to twenty cups of coffee a day, and sometimes their blood pressure rose above normal. When they drank only two or three cups, the hypertension disappeared. People with hypertension should follow their physician's advice concerning tobacco, alcohol, and coffee.

SYMPTOMS

There is a popular misconception that high blood pressure itself always causes symptoms and that the severity of these depends upon the actual height of the pressure. Patients often come to a doctor's office because of a headache, dizziness, or noises in the head which they are certain indicates a jump in the blood pressure. Usually the doctor finds the blood pressure the same as in previous examinations. High blood pressure in itself often does not cause symptoms. There is, however, a peculiar type of persistent morning headache which may signal the presence of severe hypertension. Other patients complain of inability to concentrate, or of insomnia, or generalized weakness. Nose bleeds may occur but are not really frequent. In some patients, sudden and transient weakness of an arm or leg or numbness of the face or extremities ("dead fingers") may bring them to the physician. In the majority of instances the elevated pressure is discovered on routine examination. Many people with a blood pressure, for example, of 200/110 mm. feel well. This is particularly true if they are unaware of their high blood pressure. Moreover the knowledge of having hypertension often produces a state of anxiety and tension which causes symptoms. For example, a man of 55 conducted a large business and had not visited a physician for some years. When the Red Cross called for donations of blood, he volunteered but was rejected because his blood pressure was found to be 180/100 mm. Almost immediately he began to feel tired and dizzy, and these symptoms persisted even though at times his blood pressure fell to 160/96. Examination of his heart and blood vessels was negative; his symptoms were nervous in origin.

Dr. Paul D. White has said that hypertension is the most important of all human illnesses. The reason for this statement is that it often leads to, or accelerates, hardening or sclerosis of the small arteries in various parts of the body. This does not always happen; many people with high blood pressure remain well for years without developing significant arteriosclerosis. Also, men and women differ in their tendency to develop arteriosclerosis. It occurs in men whether their blood pressure is normal or high, whereas in women it is usually found in those with hypertension. It is also apt to occur in both sexes when diabetes is present.

The commonest and most important organs affected by arteriosclerosis are the heart, brain, and kidneys. Recording the blood pressure is, therefore, only the beginning of the examination. The major part is the search for symptoms and signs of inadequate circulation to, or diseases of, these organs.

When the arteries which supply blood to the heart, the coronary arteries, become hardened and narrowed, the person affected may experience two types of symptoms. The first consists of temporary heart pain (angina pectoris) when he walks or is excited, or a serious heart attack (coronary thrombosis). The second type may include shortness of breath, cough, and swelling of the ankles. These are due to congestive heart failure.

Hypertension often causes another change in the heart, i.e., enlargement. This happens because the heart must work against an increased pressure in the arteries and resistance in the arterioles. As a result, each muscle fiber in the heart increases in size, and the heart as a whole is enlarged. At first, the enlargement of the heart is not harmful, but beyond a certain size the heart becomes inefficient. At this stage sclerosis of the coronary arteries has usually developed, and both factors may produce shortness of breath, swelling of the ankles, and poor effort tolerance.

When the arteries in the brain are hardened, a change in personality and judgment may follow. The person may gradually become irritable and stubborn and his memory may be impaired. He may complain of weakness, headache, dizziness, noises in the head, and unsteadiness in walking, or he may suddenly have a stroke as a result of a hemorrhage or clot in one of the arteries. If it is severe, coma or stupor sets in; in less serious cases there is a paralysis of one or more parts of the body, usually the face and an arm and leg on one side (hemiplegia). Occasionally only the speech is affected. In most cases the paralysis recedes slowly.

When the kidney is damaged by arteriosclerosis, the person is apt to be weak and anemic and to vomit occasionally. His ankles and face may be swollen. The diagnosis is confirmed by making tests of the urine and blood.

Other evidence of hardening may be found in the arteries in the legs. There is a special type of hypertension, called malignant, which occurs in younger people and progresses rapidly into severe diseases of the arterioles. In these cases treatment must be started at once.

To repeat, when hypertension is discovered, it is imperative that the patient have a complete examination to determine whether the heart, brain, or kidneys have been affected.

TREATMENT

In caring for people with high blood pressure, the doctor always looks for some condition which may be causing the hypertension (*See* section on Causes of High Blood Pressure).

The vast majority of patients have primary or Essential Hypertension. Although its cause is not definitely known, we have already emphasized the importance of the nervous and psychological elements. It is essential to find out the patient's anxieties and fears. If his tensions can be released, his blood pressure may fall.

Since most people are filled with a dread of hypertension, the first step is to give them a true picture and clear understanding of the condition. The newly determined limits of normal blood pressure are of great importance; many people who are supposed to have hypertension may now be assured that their blood pressure is normal for their age. For example, a man, sixty-five years old, has had a blood pressure of 170/100 mm. for four or five years; he may now forget about his blood pressure instead of worrying about it and having it checked frequently. This habit of frequent taking of the blood pressure should be discouraged since the blood pressure normally varies a great deal from day to day, and even from hour to hour. Anyway, the exact level of the pressure is not significant. The remainder of the examination is far more important than the blood pressure reading.

Even if you have hypertension, you should realize that many, if not most, such people remain well and lead normal lives; they run a benign course similar to people with normal blood pressure.

It is often possible and valuable to modify the personality of hypertensive people. Many of them are full of drive and suppressed resentment; they have a tendency to flare up suddenly over unimportant matters. Pointing these facts out to them may alter their behavior and approach to life. They can learn to do things at a slower tempo and under less strain; in this way they can reduce the pressure of life. This approach is important also in younger persons who show occasional elevations in blood pressure and come of families predisposed to hypertension. If they can be taught to live with less intensity and more equanimity, it is likely that many of them can be prevented from developing hypertension later on, just as this approach can cause a drop in blood pressure in people with hypertension.

The person with an ordinary degree of hypertension should not consider himself an invalid and should go on working. People with hypertension perform their work as well or even better than those with normal blood pressure. Naturally, people with hypertension should abide by their doctor's advice concerning hours and type of work, rest periods, and vacations. In many cases significant restrictions are unnecessary. Ordinary work is not harmful and often prevents anxiety.

The importance of avoiding or correcting overweight in people with hypertension cannot be overemphasized. The frequency of illness and death is directly proportional to the amount of overweight. When a reducing or low-calorie diet is indicated, the doctor will prescribe one suitable for each patient. All reducing diets are low in fats and starches or carbohydrates and high in proteins; they include fruits, vegetables except potatoes, lean meats, fish, and pot cheese; they avoid butter, sweet or sour cream, bread, cake and other desserts, dressing with oil, nuts, spaghetti, puddings, and custards. Such diets are listed elsewhere in this book.

DRUGS FOR HYPERTENSION

The past decade has seen a change in approach to treatment with the advent of new drugs which really are effective, and with the increasing evidence that lowering the blood pressure does prolong life and help to avoid complications such as strokes and heart failure. The new emphasis on drug treatment does not eliminate the necessity for avoidance of excess nervous tension, for slowing down the pace of life, for reducing weight in obese patients, for reduction of coffee drinking, for elimination of smoking and for living at a more moderate pace with occasional vacations.

The dietary treatment of hypertension is still important, but drastic regimes, such as a rice diet, are only rarely employed. The rice diet was one of the really important innovations in the treatment of hypertension and rigid adherence to a diet composed of rice products and fruit did produce lowering of the blood pressure in many patients. However, the effect is largely due to the low salt content of this diet and to weight reduction. Low-salt diet or elimination of salt by medication is still a cornerstone of treatment. Salt or particularly sodium is thought to cause swelling of the walls of small blood vessels to produce increased resistance and consequent elevation of blood pressure. Removal of salt from the body does lower an elevated pressure, but it does not seem important whether this is accomplished by drastically restricting the amount of salt which is eaten, or by use of medications which cause the kidney to eliminate salt in the urine. The latter treatment is the one most widely used and the drugs are termed diuretics. A diet low in salt must also be prescribed with the diuretics otherwise their effectiveness is lost. The list below indicates some foods with high content of salt which should be avoided.

Salt-Rich Foods

Bacon	Chili sauce	Pastries
Beer	Corned beef	Pickles
Beets	Cornflakes	Popcorn
Bouillon cubes	Crackers	Potato chips
Bran	Dried fruits	Prepared desserts
Cakes and cookies	Duck	Prepared flours
Candies	Frankfurters	Pretzels
Canned fish	Ham	Relishes
Canned meats	Kale	Salad dressings
Canned soups	Kidney	Salt butter
Canned tomato juice	Malted Milk	Salt pork
Canned vegetables	Mayonnaise	Sardines
Catsup	Meat soups	Sausage
Caviar	Muffins	Smoked foods
Celery	Mustard	Spinach
Celery salt	Nuts, salted	White bread
Chard	Oleomargarine	Worcestershire sauce
Cheese	Olives	

More and more foods are appearing on the market prepared without salt. These include bread, milk, and canned vegetables, soups, tomato juice, etc.

Some of the names of diuretic drugs are Diuril® (chlorothiazide), Hydrodiuril® (hydrochlorothiazide), Esidrex® (hydrochlorothiazide), Hygroton® (chlorthalidone), Naqua® (trichlormethiazide), and many others. When given over protracted periods of time, a supplement of potassium is also given since these drugs tend to deplete the body of potassium. The specific dosage of these drugs and of potassium naturally is regulated by the family physician who is aware of precautions to be taken and also of side effects of medication. A general precaution is that such treatment should not be used when kidney disease is present.

In a few instances, removal of salt or sodium from the body is enough to produce a satisfactory lowering of blood pressure. In the majority, however, the fall is most modest, somewhere between 20 to 40 mm. lower systolic pressure and 15 to 30 mm. lower diastolic pressure. The diuretic drugs are then combined with the derivatives of Rauwolfia serpentina, an Egyptian plant root, known for thousands of years, recently purified and shown to be a highly effective drug, capable of producing moderate decrease in blood pressure when given by itself and greater decreases when combined with diuretics or other drugs to be discussed. These rauwolfia drugs act on the brain to modify certain effects of the sympathetic nervous system. The names of some of these Rauwolfia serpentina (Raudixin®) derivatives are Serpasil® (Reserpine), Rauwiloid®, Singoserp® (Syrodingopine), etc. The choice of drug and dosage is left to the family physician. The most important side effect of these drugs is the occasional occurrence of nervous depression, particularly seen in older people. This should be quickly recognized and the medication should be discontinued at once.

For the patients with high pressure not responding satisfactorily to diuretic therapy combined with Reserpine, one may add a drug called Apresoline® (hydralazine) or Aldomet® (alpha methyl dopamine).

The best drugs for the patient with serious hypertension are those which act to block the spasm of blood vessels produced by actions of the sympathetic nervous system. The experience of the past few years has seen the proof of the benefit of these potent blood pressure lowering drugs. At present only three are in wide use: Guanethidine® (Ismelin), Ansolysin® (Pentolinium tartrate), Inversine® (Mecamylamine hydrochloride). These are usually used with diuretic drugs and/or Reserpine. Side effects of the potent drugs consist of a too rapid lowering of blood pressure with consequent dizziness or even fainting. This usually is seen on standing because these drugs block the normal constriction or narrowing of the small arteries in the body which accompanies the standing position. Constipation and difficulty with urination may occur. These side effects can be controlled. Difficulties with sexual performance in males sometimes necessitates cessation of therapy. When these drugs are necessary, very careful control of blood pressure is necessary to arrive at the correct dose.

Some patients, under special conditions, are permitted to take their own blood pressures at home in order to regulate the dosage.

Drug treatment in older patients with hypertension is to be approached with great caution. It is rarely necessary to treat any but those with considerable hypertension (i.e. 240/140 mm.) or those with severe angina pectoris or heart failure. In these, the serious complications can be improved by lowering blood pressure.

Treatment of hypertension depends upon the age of the patient, the elevation of blood pressure, whether the hypertension is present constantly (fixed hypertension), or whether it varies up and down (labile hypertension).

Labile hypertension (where blood pressure jumps up suddenly and then falls back to normal quickly) is the least serious of all forms and there is some question as to whether it should be considered real hypertension at all. Rarely is it necessary to treat elevated pressure in these patients, since relief of nervous tension with tranquilizers is usually all that is necessary. Rarely a Reserpine product is given.

OPERATIONS FOR HIGH BLOOD PRESSURE

Another method of treating high blood pressure is to perform an operation in which many of the "sympathetic" nerves are cut. These nerves run in a chain on each side of the spine and carry the impulses from the brain which cause the arterioles throughout the body to tighten. When these nerves are severed, this constriction is prevented and the blood pressure falls.

At first, this operation, which is called sympathectomy, was popular because many patients felt better afterward. However, as time went on, the blood pressure was found often returning to its previous high level. Also the operation is a major procedure requiring an experienced surgeon and a lengthy stay in the hospital. However, the operation is often successful and should be considered seriously when a patient has many symptoms which have not been relieved by adequate medical therapy.

LOW BLOOD PRESSURE OR HYPOTENSION

Many people believe that low blood pressure or hypotension is a common, even serious, condition capable of causing many symptoms. This notion is untrue! Low blood pressure in the true sense is uncommon and usually is the result of some condition, e.g., anemia; acute and chronic infections, such as grippe, disabling diseases like tuberculosis, or following heart attacks or certain forms of rheumatic fever.

What is ordinarily considered hypotension, e.g., a systolic pressure of 100, 110, or 120 mm., is, in fact, normal at any age. A significant number of normal women have a systolic pressure of 96 to 100 mm. While normal people with hypotension tend to be thin and narrow-chested, to feel weak, to tire easily, and to lack stamina, some are well developed and even athletic. Indeed, people with a low normal blood pressure have a greater life expectancy than the average. Their symptoms are not the result of their lowered blood pressure, but are part of their nervous, constitutional make-up.

We do not wish to give the impression that true hypotension, i.e., a systolic pressure under 96 mm. does not exist or that a low normal blood pressure may not be associated with some type of heart disease. As in the case of hypertension, a complete examination of the patient with a low blood pressure is essential to determine whether or not it is significant.

The lowest blood pressures, 40 to 80 mm. are found in a rare disease causing destruction of the outer layers or cortex of an adrenal gland. It is known as Addison's disease after the man who discovered it. It can be corrected by giving the patient salt and a drug (DOCA).

Following a heart attack or coronary thrombosis, a small number of patients maintain a blood pressure between 90 and 100 mm. for months or years. They usually feel well, and their heart function is satisfactory.

Narrowing of the aortic valve (aortic stenosis) is often associated with a blood pressure of 100 to 120 mm.

There are also several conditions in which the blood pressure or the heart rate suddenly falls, causing dizziness or fainting. This happens because the flow of blood to the brain is suddenly reduced, and that tissue is sensitive to a lack of blood and oxygen. This type of fainting in young people is usually nervous, but in others it occurs only when they stand up. Usually when people get up after sitting or lying down, the blood pressure rises. In certain people, however, it falls and they feel faint. This can usually be avoided by getting up gradually, by wearing an abdominal belt, or by drug therapy.

These sudden drops in blood pressure are not serious, but fainting may also be caused by heart disease and other illnesses. The correct diagnosis requires a thorough examination.

Hypotension may occasionally be induced by medication to lower high blood pressure. This manifests itself when the patient stands up and he experiences a sensation of weakness, spots in front of his eyes, and may faint. Such symptoms must be called to the attention of the treating physician. Other drugs such as tranquilizers may also have this undesirable effect.

SUMMARY

Hypertension is one of the most prevalent diseases of mankind. In most instances, however, only mild to moderate elevation of the blood pressure is found and much unnecessary anxiety could be avoided if such patients were treated with reassurance, weight reduction, and mild sedation or tranquilizers. Actually the studies of the authors reveal that such patients have a normal life span in the vast majority of instances. Patients with fixed, markedly elevated blood pressure, should first be carefully studied to see if the disease is in the "curable" category, such as a narrowed main artery to a single kidney, stones, infection, or tumor of a single kidney, stricture of the aorta, adrenalin-secreting or aldosterone-secreting tumor of the adrenal gland. For these, the treatment is surgical repair of arteries or removal of diseased kidney or tumors. Curable cases constitute 10 to 15 per cent of all patients with high blood pressure. For the remaining patients, effective drugs are now available. The use of such drugs, naturally, must be initiated and controlled by the physician. With successful therapy, blood pressure actually can be lowered to normal.

CHAPTER 25

Cancer

HAROLD S. DIEHL, M.D.*

Cancer is a dread disease responsible for almost 800 deaths a day, 300,000 a year in this country. The chance that a person under the age of 20 will develop cancer at some time during his or her lifetime is about one in four for males and slightly higher for females. Thus, at present rates, more than 45 million Americans now living will eventually get cancer and almost 30 million will die from it, many after prolonged illness, disability and suffering.

While there is much about cancer that is still unknown and therefore mysterious, each year we learn more about what can be done to prevent and cure it.

In 1940, one person in seven who developed cancer was saved; in 1965 the ratio is one in three and, if presently available medical knowledge were widely and effectively utilized, at least one out of two persons who develop cancer could be cured. This would mean the saving of about 100,000 lives a year, in addition to the 1,300,000 Americans now living who have been cured of cancer. And this is not all, for many are convinced that at least 50,000 lives a year might be saved by prevention of the cancers due to cigarette smoking.

Much can be done to protect one's self and one's family from cancer but to do so requires an understanding of the disease and of personal responsibility and initiative in cooperating with physicians and health organizations for prevention, early diagnosis, and proper treatment.

* Senior Vice President for Research and Medical Affairs, American Cancer Society, Inc., New York, N.Y. Prepared for *Modern Home Medical Adviser,* Doubleday & Co., Inc., Garden City, N.Y. Adapted in part from publications of the American Cancer Society, Inc., and in part from the sections on Cancer, on Tobacco, and on Medical Quackery, in *Healthful Living,* 7th edition by Harold S. Diehl, M.D., McGraw Hill Book Company, 1964.

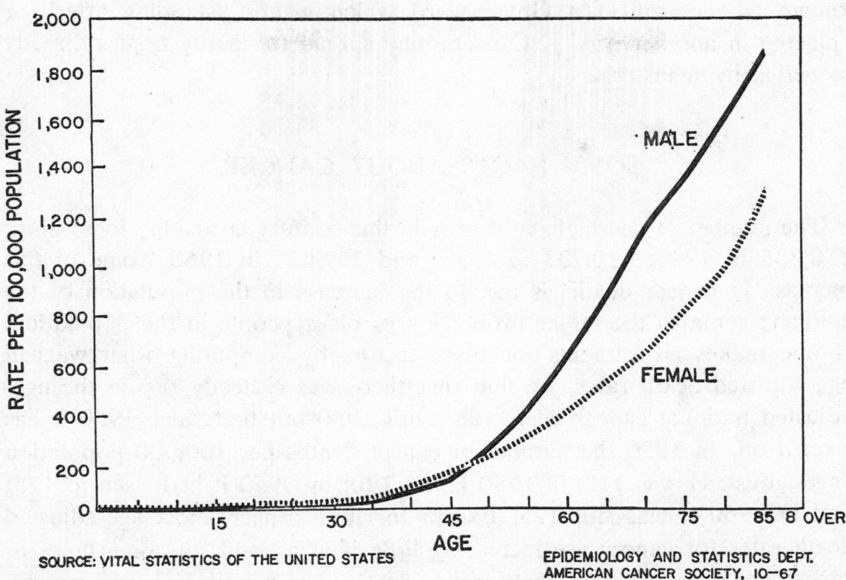

Fig. 65. Cancer death rates by age and sex, United States, 1965. From Epidemiology and Statistics Department, reprinted by permission of the American Cancer Society.

WHAT IS CANCER?

Cancer is a condition in which cells in certain tissues of the body reproduce wildly and without limit. This disease, or rather group of diseases, has been found in all ages and all races of man. Early Egyptians knew of it many centuries ago and the Romans were well acquainted with the appearance of cancer, noting how it extended into surrounding tissues. The word "cancer" in Latin means "crab," and from its crablike appearance the disease derived its name: the columns of cancer cells invading tissues resembling the appendages of a crab, and the center of growth the body of the crab.

The words "cancer" and "tumor," though frequently confused, are not synonymous. A tumor (or neoplasm) is a new growth or an overgrowth of tissue which does not serve a useful purpose. Tumors may be benign or malignant. Benign tumors never spread to distant parts of the body and, unless they cause pressure on vital organs, they are not generally dangerous to life. Malignant tumors, which we call cancer, infiltrate the tissues, destroy them and often spread to distant organs when cancer cells enter blood vessels and lymph channels. This process of colonization is known as metastasis (a Greek word which means "standing after" or "placing in another way"). Cancers may spread to nearby tissues directly as well as by metastasis.

SOME FACTS ABOUT CANCER

The number of deaths from cancer in this country is steadily increasing: 158,335 in 1940; 210,733 in 1950; and 267,627 in 1960. Some of this increase in cancer deaths is due to the increase in the population of the country; some to the larger proportion of older people in the population. If one makes adjustments for these factors by computing what we call age-adjusted death rates, we find that there was a steady rise in the age-adjusted national cancer death rate until 1950 but that since 1950 it has leveled off. In 1930 the number of cancer deaths per 100,000 population (age-adjusted) was 112; in 1940 it was 120; by 1950 it had risen to 125; and in 1960 it was still 125. Except for lung cancer, most age-adjusted death rates for cancer are increasing little if at all and for some types of cancer are decreasing. In fact, cancer death rates among women have decreased in almost every age group but this improvement has been offset by the increase in cancer deaths among men—primarily due to cancer of the lung.

Although cancer is primarily a disease of older people, it causes more deaths than any other disease among persons between 1 and 35 years of age and is the leading cause of death of women aged 30 to 54. Approximately half the cancer deaths in children are due to leukemia, a type of cancer involving the white blood cells.

During 1965 more than 830,000 Americans were under medical care for cancer and more than 500,000 new cancer cases were diagnosed for the first time.

THE EPIDEMIOLOGY OF CANCER

Studies of factors related to the occurrence of cancer are exceedingly interesting, are contributing to a better understanding of cancer and help to provide basis for the development of preventive measures. Among these are the high rates of stomach cancer in Scandinavia, Iceland, and Japan; the high rates of liver cancer in South and West Africa; the high rates of cancer of the nasopharynx in China; the high rates of cancer of the oral cavity in India; the high rates of urinary bladder cancer in certain parts of Africa and of cancer of the esophagus in other parts of this same continent; the low rates of breast cancer in Japan, and in this country the higher rates among unmarried women and among married women who have not nursed their children; the low rates of cancers of the cervix and of the uterus in Israel and in Jewish women of other countries; the high

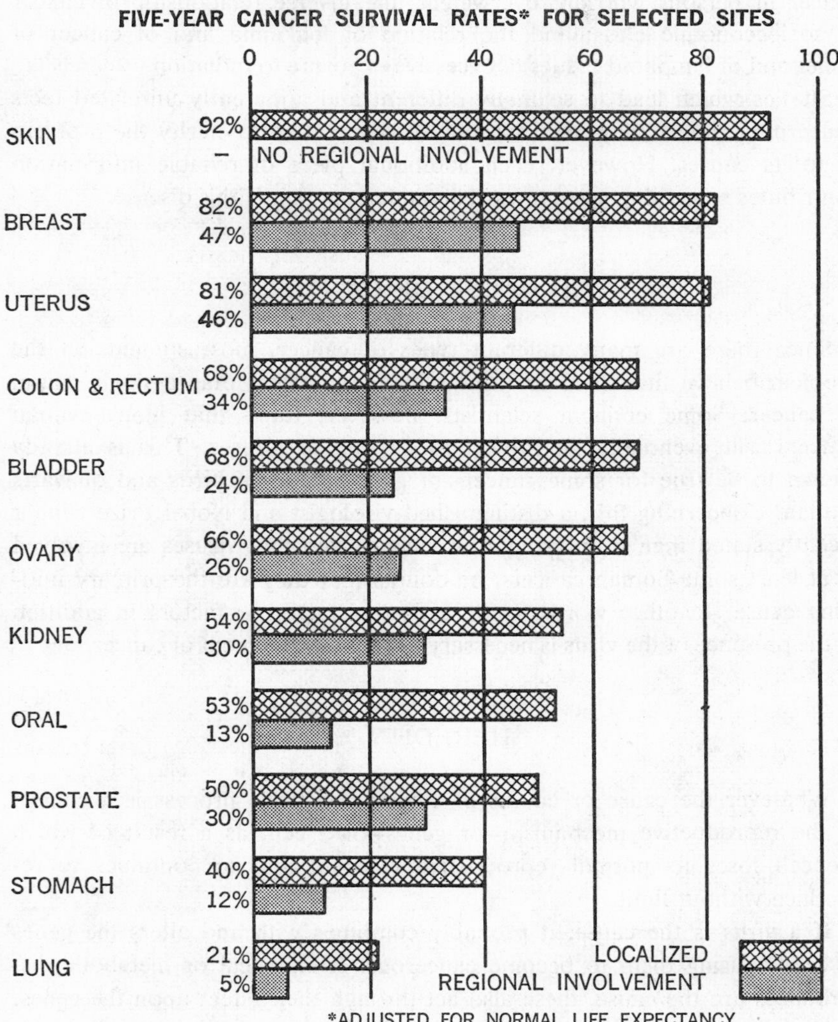

Fig. 66. Five-year cancer survival rates for selected sites. Reprinted by permission of the American Cancer Society.

degree of association between cigarette smoking and cancer of the larynx and of the lungs; the almost complete absence of cancer of the penis in males who have been circumcised; the higher incidence of cancer of the skin among Caucasians who have excessive exposure to sunlight and the very rare occurrence of skin cancer among Negroes; the higher rates of cancer in persons who are overweight; the inverse relationship of cancer to socioeconomic class; and the relation of leukemia and of cancer of bones and of lymphoid tissues to excessive exposure to radiation.

Studies which lead to so many different and apparently unrelated facts concerning cancer may seem to confuse rather than to clarify the problem as to its causes. However, each additional piece of reliable information contributes something more toward an understanding of this disease.

THE CAUSE OF CANCER

Since there are many different types of cancer, most students of the problem believe that there are multiple causes, rather than a single cause, of cancer. Some eminent scientists, however, think that many human cancers will eventually be proved to be due to viruses. This is already known to be true for some cancers of animals and of birds and of warts in man. Concerning this, a distinguished virologist and Nobel Prize winner recently stated that, even though he feels certain that viruses are involved in at least some human cancers, he doubts that they are the primary initiating cause. In other words, some causative factor or factors in addition to the presence of the virus is necessary for the development of cancer.

HEREDITY

Whatever the cause or causes of cancer, the basic process is a change in the reproductive mechanism—or genes—of a cell, as a result of which the cell loses its normal reproductive restraint and so continues to reproduce without limit.

If a virus is the cause, it probably combines with and alters the genes of cells causing them to become cancerous. If chemical or metabolic disturbances are the cause, these also act through their effect upon the genes.

If viruses may cause cancer, one naturally wonders whether cancers are communicable. Careful studies do not show evidence of communicability. The probable reason is that if a cancer virus is involved, like certain other viruses, it may be present in our bodies from birth, living in equilibrium with our body cells; and only when this balance is disturbed does it cause disease. This possibility is not without precedent, because it happens with herpes labialis, or cold sores. This condition is caused by a virus which is continuously present in the body but which causes disease only when there is irritation from a "cold" or from exposure to sunlight.

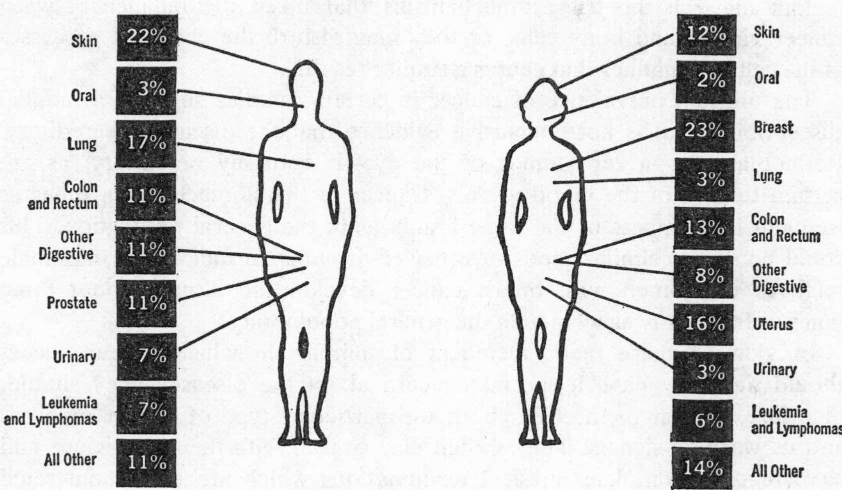

SITE	ESTIMATED NEW CASES 1968	ESTIMATED DEATHS 1968	WARNING SIGNAL WHEN LASTING LONGER THAN TWO WEEKS SEE YOUR DOCTOR	SAFEGUARDS	COMMENT
BREAST	65,000	28,000	LUMP OR THICKENING IN THE BREAST.	ANNUAL CHECKUP. MONTHLY BREAST SELF-EXAMINATION.	THE LEADING CAUSE OF CANCER DEATH IN WOMEN.
COLON AND RECTUM	73,000	45,000	CHANGE IN BOWEL HABITS; BLEEDING.	ANNUAL CHECKUP, INCLUDING PROCTOSCOPY.	CONSIDERED A HIGHLY CURABLE DISEASE WHEN DIGITAL AND PROCTOSCOPIC EXAMINATIONS ARE INCLUDED IN ROUTINE CHECKUPS.
LUNG	61,000	55,000	PERSISTENT COUGH, OR LINGERING RESPIRATORY AILMENT.	PREVENTION: HEED FACTS ABOUT SMOKING, ANNUAL CHECKUP. CHEST X-RAY.	THE LEADING CAUSE OF CANCER DEATH AMONG MEN, THIS FORM OF CANCER IS LARGELY PREVENTABLE.
ORAL (INCLUDING PHARYNX)	15,000	7,000	SORE THAT DOES NOT HEAL. DIFFICULTY IN SWALLOWING.	ANNUAL CHECKUP.	MANY MORE LIVES SHOULD BE SAVED BECAUSE THE MOUTH IS EASILY ACCESSIBLE TO VISUAL EXAMINATION BY PHYSICIANS AND DENTISTS.
SKIN	105,000	5,000	SORE THAT DOES NOT HEAL, OR CHANGE IN WART OR MOLE.	ANNUAL CHECKUP, AVOIDANCE OF OVEREXPOSURE TO SUN.	SKIN CANCER IS READILY DETECTED BY OBSERVATION, AND DIAGNOSED BY SIMPLE BIOPSY.
UTERUS	44,000	14,000	UNUSUAL BLEEDING OR DISCHARGE.	ANNUAL CHECKUP INCLUDING PELVIC EXAMINATION AND PAPANICOLAOU SMEAR.	UTERINE CANCER MORTALITY HAS DECLINED 50% DURING THE LAST 25 YEARS. WITH WIDER APPLICATION OF THE "PAP" SMEAR, MANY THOUSAND MORE LIVES CAN BE SAVED.
KIDNEY AND BLADDER	32,000	15,000	URINARY DIFFICULTY. BLEEDING—IN WHICH CASE CONSULT YOUR DOCTOR AT ONCE.	ANNUAL CHECKUP WITH URINALYSIS.	PROTECTIVE MEASURES FOR WORKERS IN HIGH-RISK INDUSTRIES ARE HELPING TO ELIMINATE ONE OF THE IMPORTANT CAUSES OF THESE CANCERS.
LARYNX	6,000	3,000	HOARSENESS—DIFFICULTY IN SWALLOWING.	ANNUAL CHECKUP, INCLUDING MIRROR LARYNGOSCOPY.	READILY CURABLE IF CAUGHT EARLY.
PROSTATE	35,000	17,000	URINARY DIFFICULTY.	ANNUAL CHECKUP, INCLUDING PALPATION.	OCCURS MAINLY IN MEN OVER 60, THE DISEASE CAN BE DETECTED BY PALPATION AND URINALYSIS AT ANNUAL CHECKUP.
STOMACH	20,000	17,000	INDIGESTION.	ANNUAL CHECKUP.	A 40% DECLINE IN MORTALITY IN 20 YEARS, FOR REASONS YET UNKNOWN.
LEUKEMIA	19,000	15,000	LEUKEMIA IS A CANCER OF BLOOD-FORMING TISSUES AND IS CHARACTERIZED BY THE ABNORMAL PRODUCTION OF IMMATURE WHITE BLOOD CELLS. ACUTE LEUKEMIA STRIKES MAINLY CHILDREN AND IS TREATED BY DRUGS WHICH HAVE EXTENDED LIFE FROM A FEW MONTHS TO AS MUCH AS THREE YEARS. CHRONIC LEUKEMIA STRIKES USUALLY AFTER AGE 25 AND PROGRESSES LESS RAPIDLY.		
			CANCER EXPERTS BELIEVE THAT IF DRUGS OR VACCINES ARE FOUND WHICH CAN CURE OR PREVENT ANY CANCERS THEY WILL BE SUCCESSFUL FIRST FOR LEUKEMIA AND THE LYMPHOMAS.		
LYMPHOMAS	22,000	17,000	THESE DISEASES ARISE IN THE LYMPH SYSTEM AND INCLUDE HODGKIN'S AND LYMPHOSARCOMA. SOME PATIENTS WITH LYMPHATIC CANCERS CAN LEAD NORMAL LIVES FOR MANY YEARS.		

Fig. 67. Cancer incidence: (*a*) Leading cancer sites, 1968, by site and sex, (*b*) Estimated new cases, estimated deaths, warning signal, safeguards. From *1968 Cancer Facts and Figures*. Reprinted by permission of the American Cancer Society.

In spite of the fact that the fundamental cause of cancer is a disturbance in the genes of cells, contributory factors are also considered causes of cancer. Prominent among these are cigarette smoke in the production of lung cancer; sunlight, soot, or other irritating substances in skin cancer; and radiation in leukemia and in cancer of the bones. Such contributory factors may be the trigger mechanisms that upset the balance between cancer viruses and body cells, or they may disturb the chemical processes of the cell in a manner that causes a similar result.

The unusual prevalence of cancer in certain families suggests a familial susceptibility but is not conclusive evidence that the disease is hereditary. Retinoblastoma—a rare tumor of the eye—is certainly hereditary, as are certain tumors of the blood vessels. Cancer of the stomach is ten times as frequent in members of the same family as in the general population. This could be due to similar foods or other environmental factors. Close female relatives of women with breast cancer develop the disease about three times as frequently as women in the general population.

In view of these facts, members of families in which cancer occurs should naturally have a special concern about the disease. They should, therefore, inform themselves about the particular type of cancer involved and its warning signals. They should also consult with their physicians and have regular, complete physical examinations which are of demonstrated value in detecting most cancers in an early and usually curable stage.

THE CONTROL OF CANCER

The prevention of cancer depends primarily upon the avoidance of exposure to substances or conditions that cause cancer. This was first demonstrated in 1775 by Sir Percival Pott, a British physician, who noted that cancers of the scrotum occurred with great frequency among chimney sweeps and then proved that these cancers could be prevented by regular washing after exposure to soot.

A most important environmental cause of cancer, however, is cigarette smoking and to a less extent the use of tobacco in other forms, such as cigars, pipes, snuff, and chewing tobacco. The avoidance of excessive exposure to sunlight, particularly by blonde persons, will prevent many cases of cancer of the skin. Avoidance of excessive exposure to radiation will prevent certain cancers. And the reduction of exposure to cancer-producing substances has virtually eliminated the cancers associated with certain occupations, such as bladder tumors in the aniline dye and the rubber industries; skin cancers from pitch, coal tar, paraffin, and certain plastics and lacquers; and lung cancer among arsenic, beryllium chromate, and asbestos workers.

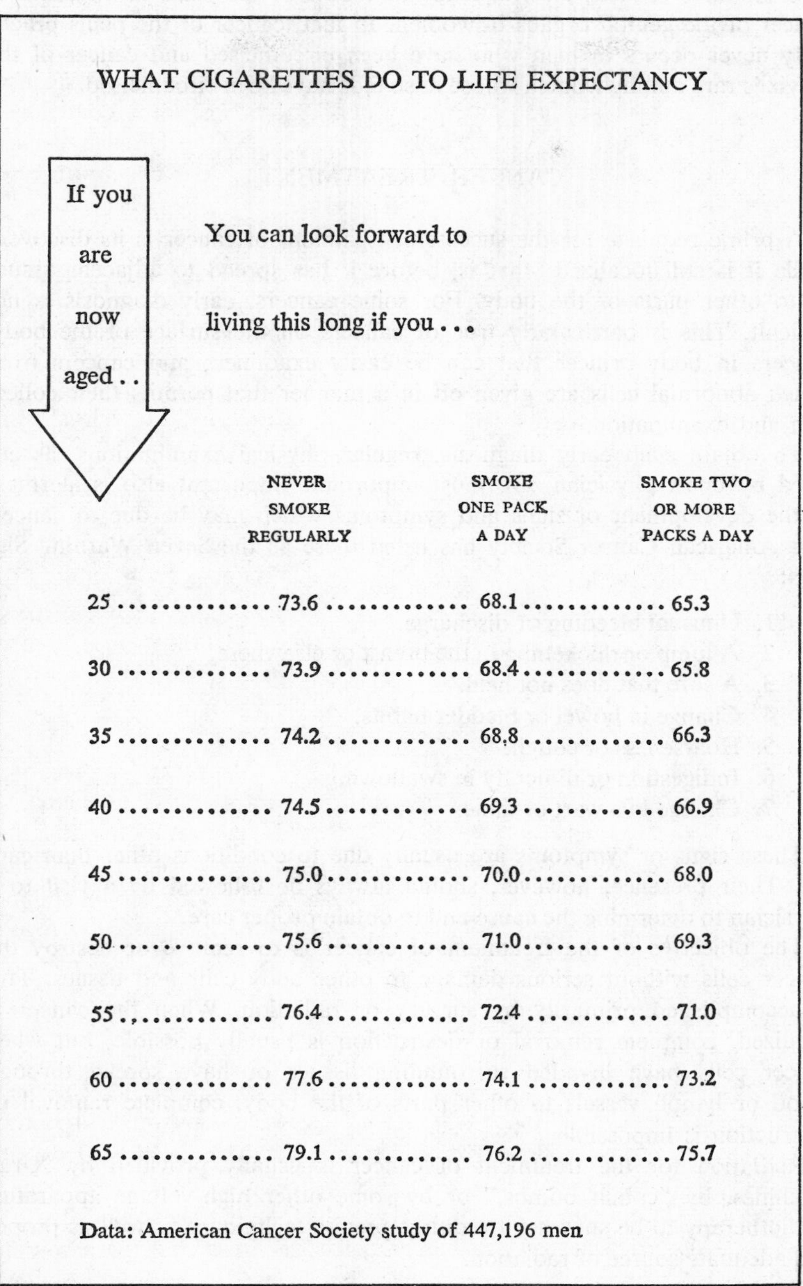

WHAT CIGARETTES DO TO LIFE EXPECTANCY

If you are now aged . . You can look forward to living this long if you . . .

If you are now aged . .	NEVER SMOKE REGULARLY	SMOKE ONE PACK A DAY	SMOKE TWO OR MORE PACKS A DAY
25	73.6	68.1	65.3
30	73.9	68.4	65.8
35	74.2	68.8	66.3
40	74.5	69.3	66.9
45	75.0	70.0	68.0
50	75.6	71.0	69.3
55	76.4	72.4	71.0
60	77.6	74.1	73.2
65	79.1	76.2	75.7

Data: American Cancer Society study of 447,196 men

Fig. 68. What cigarettes do to life expectancy chart. Site pictures.

Cleanliness reduces the frequency of cancer of the penis in men and of cancer of the genital organs in women. In fact, cancer of the penis practically never occurs in men who have been circumcised and cancer of the cervix is rare among women whose husbands have been circumcised.

CANCER TREATMENT

A prime requisite for the successful treatment of cancer is its discovery while it is still localized: that is, before it has spread to adjacent tissues or to other parts of the body. For some cancers, early diagnosis is not difficult. This is particularly true of cancers on the surface of the body, cancers in body orifices that can be easily examined, and cancers from which abnormal cells are given off in a manner that permits their collection and examination.

To obtain such early diagnosis, regular physical examinations, as advised by one's physician, are most important. Important also is alertness to the development of signs and symptoms which may be due to cancer. The American Cancer Society has listed these as the Seven Warning Signals:

1. Unusual bleeding or discharge.
2. A lump or thickening in the breast or elsewhere.
3. A sore that does not heal.
4. Change in bowel or bladder habits.
5. Hoarseness or cough.
6. Indigestion or difficulty in swallowing.
7. Change in a wart or mole.

These signs or symptoms are usually due to conditions other than cancer. Their presence, however, should always be followed by a visit to a physician to determine the cause and to obtain proper care.

The objective of the treatment of cancer is to remove or destroy the cancer cells without serious damage to other body cells and tissues. This is accomplished primarily by surgery or radiation. When the cancer is localized, complete removal or destruction is usually possible; but when cancer cells have invaded surrounding tissues or have spread through blood or lymph vessels to other parts of the body, complete removal or destruction is impossible.

Radiation for the treatment of cancer is usually provided by X-ray machines, by "cobalt bombs," or by some other high-voltage apparatus. Radiotherapy to be successful requires precise techniques as well as proper and adequate source of radiation.

Radiation is sometimes used in conjunction with surgery to destroy cancer cells that may not have been removed by the operation. It is useful also to retard the growth and decrease the size of cancers that cannot be removed, thereby relieving pain and giving to the patient added months or years of life. In some instances, extremely high voltage radiation causes some advanced cancers, even of the lung, to regress and in a few instances to disappear.

Certain drugs, antibiotics, chemicals, and hormones are also utilized for the treatment of cancer, particularly for cancers like leukemia which affect the body as a whole or have spread from the original source throughout the body. One of these drugs, called methotrexate, has cured a considerable number of patients with choriocarcinoma, a rare but usually fatal cancer that occasionally follows childbirth. In the treatment of certain other cancers, drugs or hormones give dramatic results. Patients who are incapacitated, and even near death, regain their health. Unfortunately, after varying intervals of weeks, months or years, the disease usually recurs and progresses. In some instances, cancers which have become resistant to one drug will respond favorably to another drug—but again only temporarily.

The chemotherapy of cancer is under extensive and intensive investigation. Each year brings some progress and it is hoped that increasingly effective drugs will be developed. This hope, however, must be tempered by caution against unjustified claims for drugs or preparations that are promoted for the treatment of cancer without adequate testing and evaluation.

SOME COMMON CANCERS

Although cancer may develop anywhere in the body, it rarely originates in certain tissues and organs, such as muscle, fat, the spleen, or liver. In this country, the largest number of newly diagnosed cases of cancer in men and in women arise in the digestive system. In men, cancers of the respiratory system, genital organs, and skin are next in frequency. In women, the most frequent origins of cancer after the digestive system are genital organs, breast, and skin.

Cancer death rates are similar in frequency to diagnosed cases except for skin cancer which is a relatively minor cause of death. Among men, the leading causes of cancer deaths, as estimated for 1965, by specific sites of origin are lung, 40,400; colon and rectum, 20,800; prostate, 15,800; stomach, 11,400; urinary organs, 9500; pancreas, 9500; lymphomas, 8800; and leukemia, 8300. Among women, the corresponding order of cancer deaths is breast, 26,100; colon and rectum, 22,100; uterus, 13,900; ovary, 8900; stomach, 7000; pancreas, 6800; lung, 6600; lymphomas, 6500; and leukemia, 5900.

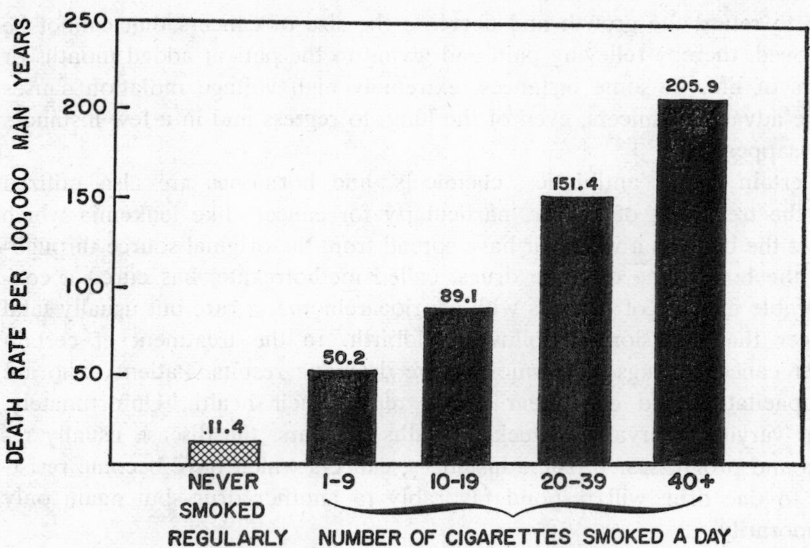

Source: Hammond, E. C.: Smoking in relation to mortality and morbidity. Findings in first thirty-four months of follow-up in a prospective study started in 1959. J. Nat. Cancer Inst. 32: 1161-1188, 1964

Fig. 69. Lung cancer age standardized death rates, age range 40–89. Reprinted by permission of the American Cancer Society.

CANCER OF THE LUNG

Cancer of the lung, a leading cause of cancer deaths in this country, has increased with such rapidity in recent years that some refer to it as an epidemic. In 1940, cancer of the lung caused 7121 deaths in the United States; in 1950, 18,313 deaths; in 1960, 36,420 deaths, and in 1965 it caused approximately 47,000 deaths; 40,400 of men and 6600 of women. Although lung cancer is much more common in men than in women, the rate of increase has recently become greater among women than among men.

The technical name for this type of lung cancer is bronchogenic carcinoma, meaning that it arises in the lining of the bronchial tubes through which air passes to various parts of the lungs. The principal types of bronchogenic carcinoma are called epidermoid carcinoma, undifferentiated carcinoma, and adenocarcinoma. The great majority of cases are of the first two types, both of which are highly related to cigarette smoking. The third type, adenocarcinoma, is far less common and less related to smoking.

By far the greatest contributing cause of lung cancer seems to be cigarette smoking, with the degree of risk related to the amount of smoking, the degree of inhalation, and the age at which smoking was begun.

This is the conclusion of significant studies of this subject. Of these studies, the most extensive was the report of the U. S. Surgeon General's Advisory Committee on Smoking and Health. This report, prepared by a panel of distinguished scientists, and released in January 1964, affirmed the earlier conclusions of the American Cancer Society by stating that:

> Cigarette smoking is causally related to lung cancer in men; the magnitude of the effect of cigarette smoking far outweighs all other factors. The data for women, though less extensive, points in the same direction. The risk of developing lung cancer increases with duration of smoking and the number of cigarettes smoked per day, and is diminished by discontinuing.

The report stated that not only lung cancer is involved; the mortality ratio of cigarette smokers over nonsmokers is particularly high for a number of other diseases including bronchitis and emphysema, cancer of the larynx, oral cancer, cancer of the esophagus, and peptic ulcer. Smoking cigarettes was also cited as a factor in heart and circulatory diseases.

The high degree of relationship between the development of lung cancer and cigarette smoking is indicated by the fact that cigarette smokers of less than ½ pack a day have 15 times the risk of dying of lung cancer as nonsmokers; smokers of ½ to 1 pack, 17 times the risk; smokers of 1 to 2 packs, 42 times the risk; and smokers of 2 or more packs, 64 times the risk of nonsmokers. These ratios are based upon cases of lung cancer in which the diagnosis of lung cancer has been well confirmed, usually by microscopic examination or by X ray or by both.

The death rates from lung cancer among cigar and pipe smokers are much less than among cigarette smokers, probably because cigar and pipe smokers rarely inhale.

Cigarette smokers who say that they inhale deeply have almost twice the risk of dying from lung cancer as smokers who say that they do not inhale and one and a half times the risk of those who say that they inhale slightly. Also those who begin to smoke cigarettes before the age of 15 have a 50 per cent greater risk than those who do not begin to smoke until 25 or older.

The greater frequency of lung cancer among men than among women could be due to a sex difference in susceptibility or resistance, as is true for coronary artery disease, for diabetes, and for certain other diseases, as well as for leukemia, for cancer of the tongue, the stomach, and the urinary organs. The probability is, however, that the difference is due to the fact that women have not smoked so long and usually do not smoke so much or inhale so deeply as men. Supporting this are the facts that the rate of increase of lung cancer deaths among women parallels that among men and that the differences between death rates for women who smoke and those who do not smoke are similar to the corresponding differences for men.

Another suspected cause of lung cancer is general air pollution. Polluted air may contain various cancer producing chemicals from motor car exhausts and from the burning of coal, oil, and other materials, and death rates from lung cancer increase with the size of the community in which the individual resides. Studies in California, however, did not show any difference in frequence of lung cancer among nonsmoking men in the Los Angeles area where the air is heavily polluted and in areas of the state where there is little or no air pollution.

In normal breathing at least 75 per cent of suspended matter in inhaled air is removed by filtration in the nose: a protective mechanism which is bypassed in cigarette, cigar and pipe smoking. Furthermore, the risk of lung cancer, even in large cities, is only about one-sixth as great for nonsmokers as for cigarette smokers.

Lung cancer may be caused also by prolonged inhalation of several different substances; such as dust containing radioactive material, chromates, nickel and asbestos. Exposure of the general population to these substances, however, is negligible and precautionary measures have eliminated dangerous exposure of workers in industries in which such dusts occur.

The mechanism by which tobacco smoke causes lung cancer is not entirely understood. However, tobacco smoke contains, in addition to nicotine and carbon monoxide, a mixture of chemicals, commonly called tars, which are able to produce cancer. These tars produce the brown stain when cigarette smoke is blown through a handkerchief or similar material.

The bronchial tubes of the lungs have a remarkable protective mechanism. The cells lining these tubes and tubules secrete mucus, a sticky fluid which collects particles of soot, dust, and other substances in inhaled air. This mucus is carried up through the bronchial tubes and the trachea by the action of the cilia and is either swallowed or expectorated. These cili are little hairlike structures which protrude from the inner surface of the respiratory passages and are continually in motion. Their movement causes mucus to flow up and out of the lungs. Particles of inhaled dust and other substances trapped in the mucus are thus removed. This keeps the lungs clean and protects the bronchial tubes from damage. If the pollution of the inhaled air is more than this system can remove, or if the cilia are destroyed or fail to work, this protection is lost. Cigarette smoke first slows then stops the action of the cilia and eventually destroys them.

Symptoms of cancer of the lung are usually vague and frequently considered as "only a cigarette cough." Occasionally, blood-streaked sputum is the first recognized symptom. Unfortunately, when any of these symptoms occur, the cancer is frequently well advanced.

Diagnosis is most commonly made or at least confirmed by an X ray. If such X-ray examinations are made routinely—at least every six months for regular cigarette smokers—the possibility of discovering the cancer at an early stage is vastly greater than if one waits for such an examination until suggestive symptoms occur.

Treatment is surgical removal of the lung or lobe of the lung in which the cancer is located. X-ray treatment is frequently used following surgery or if surgical removal is impossible. The over-all five-year survival or so-called cure rate for cancer of the lung is discouragingly small—only 3 to 5 per cent of those in whom this disease is diagnosed. If the cancer is discovered early, usually by routine X-ray examination before symptoms have appeared, and promptly treated, the recovery rate is increased to between 25 and 35 per cent.

Fortunately, prevention of most of this prevalent and highly serious cancer is possible: first, by avoiding the cigarette habit, and, second, by discontinuing the habit if it has already been acquired. Various long-time studies show that the lung cancer death rate of cigarette smokers who discontinue smoking, even though they have smoked heavily for many years, at the end of five years is only half as great as of those who continue to smoke and at the end of ten years is essentially the same as those who have never smoked.

Furthermore, if parents hope that their children will not be exposed to this risk of lung cancer, they should not smoke. Various studies have shown that the most important influence upon smoking by children is the smoking habits of their parents.

CANCER OF THE COLON AND RECTUM

Cancer of the colon and rectum is responsible for about 70,000 new cases and 40,000 deaths annually in this country, with the number of deaths approximately equally divided between men and women. This represents approximately the same death rates as existed twenty years ago.

This type of cancer is frequently diagnosed as a result of bleeding from the rectum or the discovery of blood in the stool. Unfortunately, when bleeding occurs the disease is usually advanced and the cure rate only about 35 per cent. However, more than half of these cancers could be discovered sufficiently early for complete cure, if adult men and women, particularly those over forty years of age, would have regular annual examinations of the lower bowel with the proctosigmoidoscope—a lighted tube which enables the physician to examine visually the lining of this portion of the bowel and to recognize abnormalities which are early cancers or may develop into cancer. Sometimes an X-ray examination is ordered by the physician to investigate the possibility of tumors too high up in the colon to be seen with the proctosigmoidoscope or to get more information concerning abnormalities lower down.

The cause of cancer of the colon and rectum is unknown. Some differences in its frequency may yield a clue or clues. For example, cancer of the rectum is more frequent in men than in women, while cancer of the colon is more frequent in women than in men; also, these cancers are more common in the United States than in the countries of northwest Europe, Japan, certain areas of Africa, and probably in Latin America; and in the United States they are more frequent in the North than in the South and more frequent in urban than in rural residents.

Furthermore, some of these cancers develop in polyps—that is, small grapelike growths—in the intestine. Physicians, therefore, recommend removal of these polyps when they occur. Intestinal polyps tend to run in families, so if one has a parent or grandparent who has had polyps, regular examinations, including an X ray, are especially important.

Early cancers of the large intestine give rise to few, if any, symptoms. More advanced cancers are usually associated with unusual quantities of gas and with varying degrees of abdominal discomfort or pain. These cancers frequently cause bleeding, but the bleeding may be slight or so mixed with feces that it is not noticeable. Blood from high up in the colon usually is black rather than red when it appears in the stool. Continuous or frequent bleeding may result in sufficient loss of blood to cause paleness, weakness, fatigue, and even shortness of breath. So commonly does bleeding occur with cancer of the colon that every person with unexplained anemia should have a sigmoidoscopic and X-ray examination of the large intestine. Other suggestive symptoms are changes in bowel habits, such as alternating constipation and diarrhea. Usually these symptoms are due to other causes, but if they persist, a thorough examination of the lower bowel is essential.

CANCER OF THE STOMACH

In 1940 cancer of the stomach was the leading cause of cancer deaths in the United States. In some parts of the world it is still the leading type of cancer. In the United States, however, cancer of the stomach has been decreasing steadily until the current death rate is less than half what it was thirty years ago. In spite of this, 21,000 new cases and 18,400 deaths—11,400 of men and 7000 of women—are estimated for 1965.

We do not know the cause of cancer of the stomach nor the reason for its decline in this country. Neither do we know why cancer of the stomach occurs more frequently in men than in women; why it is more frequent in certain countries, such as Japan, Chile, Iceland, Russia and the Scandinavian countries than in the United States; why it is more frequent in certain states than in other states of our own country; nor why countries which have high death rates for cancer of the stomach usually have low rates for cancer of the colon and rectum and vice versa. Diet may be a factor for at least some of these differences but this is as yet only speculation. We do know, however, that cancer develops much more frequently in persons with pernicious anemia and in other people who have little or no hydrochloric acid in the gastric juices. There is no truth to the rumor that food cooked in aluminum utensils may give rise to cancer.

Unfortunately, cancer of the stomach rarely produces definite symptoms early in the disease, at the time that the possibilities of cure would be the greatest. In fact, early symptoms are commonly only mild "indigestion." Eventually a physician is consulted and a diagnosis made, but all too frequently–and tragically–precious time is wasted trying the suggestions of friends or preparations advertised for the cure of indigestion.

If cancer of the stomach is treated surgically when the disease is still limited to the stomach, the possibility of complete removal and therefore cure is vastly greater than after the disease has spread to adjacent tissues or lymph nodes: In the former circumstance, the cure rate is 40 per cent as compared to 5 per cent in the latter.

Although many people have mild stomach complaints from time to time due to functional disturbances, these should not be neglected. Persistent indigestion should be carefully investigated by a physician: whether this be loss of appetite, a feeling of fullness or bloating, heartburn, eructations of gas, gaseous distention, nausea, vomiting, pain, or weakness. It is only by careful examinations, frequently including determination of the amount of hydrochloric acid in the gastric juice and X rays of the stomach, that one can diagnose cancer of the stomach at the stage that successful treatment is possible. In fact, for people past middle life, a regular annual or semiannual investigation of the digestive system is worthwhile insurance against serious disease.

CANCER OF THE BREAST

With 62,000 new cases and 26,300 deaths–26,100 of women and 200 of men–estimated for 1965, cancer of the breast continues as the leading cause of cancer deaths among women in this country.

Breast cancer is most likely to develop after the age of 45 but is not infrequent in women in their thirties and may occur in still younger women. Early it begins usually as a painless lump but as it progresses it may cause changes in the shape of the breast, retraction or bleeding from the nipple. If untreated it may result in large, ulcerating masses. Such cancers also spread–metastasize–through the lymphatic system or the blood stream to other parts of the body, there to grow and spread still further, eventually destroying life. Some breast cancers grow slowly, while others grow rapidly and metastasize early.

Almost 90 per cent of breast cancers are first noted as lumps in the breast by women themselves. However, not all lumps in the breast are cancers. Some are cysts, some are masses of fat, some are fibrous changes that occur with age; and some are benign tumors: that is, new growths which develop for a time but then cease growing and do not spread to other parts of the body. All lumps, or suspected lumps, however, should be examined by a physician. In some instances, a small bit of tissue must be taken for microscopic examination to determine whether or not a lump is a cancer or a benign tumor (biopsy).

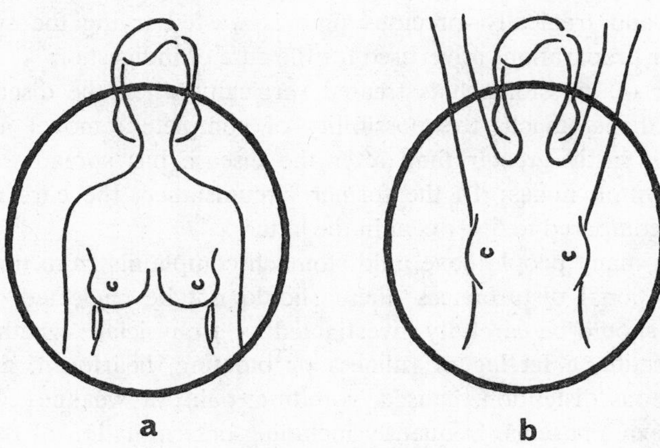

Fig. 70. Breast Self-examination.

a. Sit or stand in front of your mirror, with your arms relaxed at your sides, and examine your breasts carefully for any changes in size and shape. Look for any puckering or dimpling of the skin, and for any discharge or change in the nipples.
b. Raise both your arms over your head, and look for exactly the same things. See if there's been any change since you last examined your breasts.
c. Lie down on your bed, put a pillow or a bath towel under your left shoulder and your left hand under your head. (From this step through Step h you should feel for a lump or thickening.) With the fingers of your right hand held together flat, press gently but firmly with small, circular motions to feel the inner, upper quarter of your breast, starting at your breastbone and going outward toward the nipple line. Also feel the area around the nipple.
d. With the same gentle pressure, feel the lower inner part of your breast.
e. Now bring your left arm down to your side, and still using the flat part of your fingers, feel under your armpit.
f. Use the same gentle pressure to feel the upper, outer quarter of your breast from the nipple line to where your arm is resting.
g. And finally, feel the lower outer section of your breast, going from the outer part to the nipple.
h. Repeat the entire procedure, as described, on the right breast.
Your own doctor may want you to use a slightly different method of examination. Ask him to teach you that method.

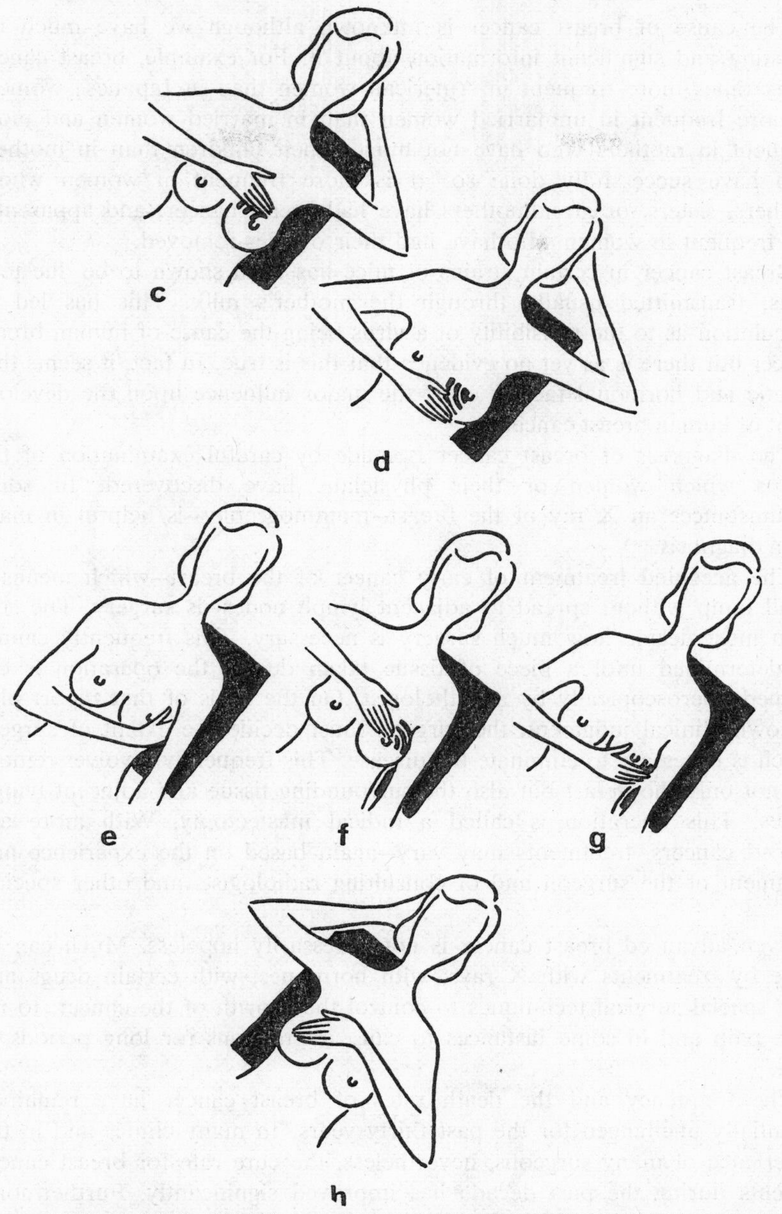

Examine your breasts every month, just after your period. Be sure to continue these checkups after your change of life.

If you find a lump or a thickening, *leave it alone* until you see your doctor. Don't be frightened. Most breast lumps or changes are not cancer, but only your doctor can tell. Reprinted by permission of the American Cancer Society.

The cause of breast cancer is unknown although we have much interesting and significant information about it. For example, breast cancer is six times more frequent in American women than in Japanese women; is more frequent in unmarried women than in married women and more frequent in mothers who have not nursed their children than in mothers who have successfully done so. It is more frequent in women whose mothers, sisters, or grandmothers have had breast cancer; and apparently less frequent in women who have had their ovaries removed.

Breast cancer in certain strains of mice has been shown to be due to a virus, transmitted usually through the mother's milk. This has led to speculation as to the possibility of a virus being the cause of human breast cancer but there is as yet no evidence that this is true. In fact, it seems that genetic and hormonal factors exert the major influence upon the development of human breast cancer.

The diagnosis of breast cancer is made by careful examination of the lumps which women or their physicians have discovered. In some circumstances an X ray of the breast–mammography–is helpful in making a diagnosis.

The accepted treatment of early cancer of the breast–which means a small lump without spread to adjacent lymph nodes–is surgery. The surgeon must decide how much surgery is necessary. This frequently cannot be determined until a piece of tissue taken during the operation is examined microscopically by a pathologist. On the basis of that report plus his own clinical judgment, the surgeon must decide the extent of surgery which is necessary to eliminate the disease. This frequently involves removing not only the breast but also the surrounding tissue and adjacent lymph nodes. This operation is called a radical mastectomy. With more advanced cancers, treatments may vary–again based on the experience and judgment of the surgeon and of consulting radiologists and other specialists.

Even advanced breast cancer is not necessarily hopeless. Much can be done by treatments with X rays, with hormones, with certain drugs and with special surgical techniques to control the growth of the cancer, to relieve pain and in some instances to cause regressions for long periods of time.

The frequency and the death rates of breast cancer have remained essentially unchanged for the past thirty years. In many clinics and in the experience of many surgeons, nevertheless, the cure rate for breast cancer patients during the past decade has improved significantly. Furthermore, the cure rate for breast-cancer patients whose disease is discovered early and treated promptly and properly is almost double that for those whose cancer is not discovered until it becomes advanced. The University of Minnesota reports that 18 out of 19 women (94.7 per cent) were alive and well five years after operations for breast cancers, which had been discovered on routine cancer-detection examinations and which had not spread to local lymph nodes. The 5-year cure rate after surgery reported by the National Cancer Institute for 15,444 patients is 85 per cent. This series, however, included women who did not consult physicians until after the appearance of signs or symptoms and in whom the disease was more advanced than in the University of Minnesota group. If the cancer has spread to adjacent lymph nodes, the 5-year cure rate is substantially reduced but still far from hopeless: 80 per cent (4 out of 5) for the Minnesota series and 37 per cent for the general average.

The major reason that the general death rate for breast cancer has not declined is that not enough breast cancers are discovered early. The responsibility for this rests primarily with the patients themselves. Although most breast cancers are found by patients, many are discovered too late, or the women wait too long to bring the symptoms, usually a painless lump, to the attention of their doctors.

Women can learn to look for and find these lumps when they are small, less than ½ inch across. The American Cancer Society has published a pamphlet called "Breast Self-Examination"—available from local units—and has produced a motion picture on the subject. Many millions of women have learned how to examine their breasts through these media. A California college that makes a practice of showing this film to its undergraduate women students reports that even in this young age group several breast cancers have been found.

In addition, women should have a careful examination of their breasts as part of their regular annual physical examinations. Research on the cause, the prevention, the early diagnosis, and the treatment of breast cancer needs to be accelerated and supported. But, many lives can be saved and much suffering and disability prevented if women will learn to examine their breasts, will do so regularly and conscientiously, and will report promptly to their physicians and cooperate with them in the investigation of any suspected abnormalities.

CANCER OF THE UTERUS

Cancer of the uterus attacks about 44,000 women and causes the deaths of 14,000 women each year in this country—most of them unnecessarily. Of these fatal uterine cancers, about 4000 arise in the body of the uterus and 10,000 in the cervix: that is in the lower necklike portion of the uterus which extends into the upper end of the vagina.

This type of cancer is twice as frequent in nonwhite as in white women, and is less frequent in single women, notably nuns, than in married women. Its occurrence seems to be related to early marriage, early pregnancy, low social-economic status, and to sexual promiscuity.

Cancer of the uterus is infrequent among Jewish women and among women of certain other religious groups in which all males are circumcised. This probably is because circumcision prevents the accumulation and thus introduction into the vagina of secretions which may contain irritating and carcinogenic substances. Cleanliness of the sex organs of males and females reduces the likelihood of cervical cancer. This is the probable reason that though Indian women usually have a high rate of cervical cancer, it is rare among the Navajos who have exceptionally high standards of personal hygiene.

The most common symptom of cancer of the uterus is abnormal bleeding or discharge, either between menstrual periods or after the menopause. Any evidence of this should be investigated by a physician without delay.

Far better, however, than to await the appearance of symptoms is for every adult woman to have a "Pap test" or a "Pap smear" each year, preferably as part of a regular pelvic and general physical examination. This test or rather examination is named for Dr. George Papanicolaou who developed it after years of painstaking research. The test consists of a microscopic examination of cells which have been shed from the cervix of the uterus. Several simple, painless procedures are used for obtaining these cells, which are smeared on a glass slide, stained and examined under a microscope. If abnormal cells suggestive of cancer are present, a further examination is essential, usually including a biopsy; that is, a microscopic examination of a piece of tissue from the area from which the cells have come. By this examination, beginning cancers can be discovered and completely removed, frequently by means of a relatively minor operation.

The development of this "Pap test" is most important in the control of cancer of the uterus. If women would utilize it regularly and follow through with any suspicious findings, the suffering and the deaths caused by cancer of the cervix could be completely eliminated and many other cancers of the uterus could be diagnosed when still curable. Progress in this direction is substantial and heartening; the age-adjusted death from uterine cancer declined from 22.7 per 100,000 women in 1947 to 12.9 in 1962. Yet only about half of the women in the United States have ever had a "Pap test" and many of those who have had one or two do not have them regularly. The American Cancer Society has available informational pamphlets for individual distribution and films for showing to groups about the prevention of uterine cancer.

CANCER OF THE PROSTATE

The prostate is a gland about the size of a small walnut which surrounds the beginning of the male urethra—the tube that carries the urine from the bladder to the outside of the body. Cancer of this gland, with an estimated 33,000 cases and 16,000 deaths in 1965, is one of the most common cancers of men. It occurs most frequently in men past 60 years of age and is more common in married men than in single men. Its cause is not known.

The most frequent early symptoms of cancer of the prostate is difficulty in urination. This is due to the pressure of the growing cancer upon the urethra. It often begins with a narrowing of the stream, a lessening of its force, and dribbling after urination. Later, urination may become exceedingly difficult and blood may appear in the urine. Difficulty in urination, however, does not necessarily mean cancer, for it may be due to a benign enlargement of the prostate. In either case, early diagnosis and immediate medical attention is essential.

In a considerable proportion of patients with this disease, the first symptoms are pain in the back or other parts of the body to which the cancer has metastasized without producing symptoms referable to the prostate itself. Early diagnosis is usually possible in these cancers, as well as in those that obstruct urinary flow, by a rectal examination in which the physician, with his index finger, can feel the size and the shape of the prostate.

Treatment of localized cancer or other enlargement of the prostate is surgical removal. If the cancer has metastasized, X-ray treatments, the administration of hormones or castration are usually effective in controlling the development of the disease, frequently for long periods of time.

Cancer of the prostate is the third cause of cancer deaths among men. Yet, many of these could be prevented and much suffering alleviated if men over fifty would have an annual or semiannual rectal examination by a physician.

CANCER OF THE PANCREAS

One of the leading causes of cancer deaths in this country is cancer of the pancreas with an estimated 16,300 deaths—9500 men and 6800 women—for 1965. This represents an almost threefold increase over the past thirty years. Neither the reason for the increase nor the cause of cancer of the pancreas are known.

Unfortunately, cancers of the pancreas do not produce distinctive early symptoms. The disease therefore is frequently advanced before it is discovered. This fact and the difficulty of surgical removal of these cancers result in a low cure rate.

The symptoms most commonly produced by cancer of the pancreas are pain in the upper part of the abdomen, loss of appetite, loss of weight, weakness, indigestion, and sometimes nausea or vomiting. These symptoms are rarely due to cancer, but when they occur they should be carefully investigated.

CANCER OF THE OVARY

Another important cancer in women, one that causes about 9000 deaths a year, is cancer of the ovary. These cancers, like a number of other internal cancers, rarely produce recognizable early symptoms. Regular annual pelvic examinations of women and prompt attention to pain in the lower abdomen and to vague gastrointestinal disturbances may lead to the discovery of ovarian cancers when they are early enough to be successfully treated.

LEUKEMIA

Leukemia, which literally means white blood, is a malignant disease in which white blood corpuscles are produced in overwhelming numbers. In 1965 leukemia will cause the death of about 8000 males and 6000 females in the United States. Of these about 1 in 6 will be children under the age of 15. The leukemia death rate has increased by 50 per cent over the past 20 years, with the greatest increase among adults. Childhood leukemia is most frequent at 3 or 4 years of age with a gradual decrease at 9 or 10. In adults, leukemia begins to appear at about thirty-five and becomes increasingly frequent throughout life. It is more common in men than in women and more common in whites than in Negroes.

The cause of human leukemia is unknown; although, in mice, excessive exposure to X rays will produce leukemia, as will the injection of a mouse leukemia virus. Some investigators believe that viruses may also cause leukemia in man. Although this is still unproven, research on this possibility is being greatly intensified. In human beings, it is estimated that 5 to 10 per cent of leukemia cases are due to radiation, about half of which is from the environment and about half from exposure to radiation for medical purposes. According to an extensive three-year study reported in 1964, an increased risk of leukemia is associated with irradiation of mothers even before the children are conceived, with irradiation of expectant mothers during pregnancy, and with irradiation of the children themselves. This risk, however, is small and does not warrant the avoidance of necessary radiation for either treatment or diagnostic purposes.

Early symptoms of leukemia in children may simulate a respiratory infection or rheumatic fever. In the early stage it is most often detected during a routine laboratory examination of the blood before the patient has symptoms. Leukemia should be suspected when a patient is anemic, pale, easily fatigued or has a tendency to hemorrhages.

In 1950 only about 5 per cent of children with acute leukemia survived a year. By 1965 approximately 50 per cent survive for more than a year, and some continue in good health for a number of years. Patients with chronic leukemia, which usually occurs after the age of thirty-five, survive much longer.

The treatment of leukemia is one of the most active and important areas of cancer research. Several drugs or combination of drugs result in the complete disappearance of symptoms in nearly 90 per cent of patients who have been critically ill with this disease and a few are reported to have survived for more than five years. Unfortunately, this improvement, although frequently dramatic, is only temporary; for after a time, the disease becomes resistant to the drug. Research workers hope that modifications of these drugs or new drugs may result in lasting cure instead of only temporary improvement.

LYMPHOMAS

This group of malignant tumorlike growths causes approximately 15,300 deaths a year; 8800 of men and 6500 of women. Although there are several distinct diseases in the group, they are all composed of lymphoid tissue: that is, tissue similar to that which occurs in lymph nodes. They may arise in various parts of the body but are most commonly first noted in enlarged lymph nodes of the neck or armpit.

Some of them, notably Hodgkin's disease, if recognized early, can be treated successfully with high-voltage radiation. In others, various anticancer drugs may be helpful.

CANCER OF THE SKIN

Currently, about 80,000 cases of skin cancer with 4000 deaths occur annually in the United States. Skin cancer develops more frequently in persons with light or ruddy skins than in persons with dark skins. It is rare in Negroes.

Some cancers seem to develop from normal, healthy skin tissue, but many of them develop in areas where abnormal conditions have been apparent for a long time. These conditions are called "precancerous" because, while not cancerous themselves, they sometimes develop into cancer.

Excessive exposure to sunlight, ultraviolet light, coal tar, pitch, paraffin, certain lubricating oils, arsenicals, and other irritants may cause cancers of the skin. Fortunately, these cancers are on the surface of the body where they can be observed. Consequently, early diagnosis and prompt treatment usually result in cure.

Keratosis. This is the most common of the precancerous skin conditions. It is a dry, scaly patch, or clump of patches, usually darker than the surrounding skin, which appears on exposed surfaces such as the face, neck, ears, and hands of older people particularly those who have been excessively exposed to the sun. When the top, scaly layer is removed, the base is seen to be made up of red, thickened "new skin." Especially if bleeding occurs, there is a possibility of early cancer. Keratoses vary greatly in different people and frequently cannot be distinguished from cancer without removal of a small bit of tissue for microscopic study by a pathologist—a procedure known as biopsy.

Moles. Moles are an overgrowth of the deeper pigment layers of the skin. Most moles are harmless, but occasionally one develops into a rare but extremely serious form of skin cancer known as malignant melanoma. The usual freckles, skin-colored moles, or reddish birthmarks are not precancerous. The ones to keep under observation are the dark brown or blue-black moles, slightly raised from the skin. These are particularly dangerous when they are on the feet or so located that they are irritated by friction such as by a collar or belt. If moles are irritated or show a tendency to change in color or size, they should be examined without delay.

Leukoplakia. This is a white, scaly thickening on the lip or membranes of the mouth, which may predispose to cancer. If this condition is present, it should be examined by a physician.

Basal-Cell Cancer. This is the most common type of skin cancer. It rarely, if ever spreads to distant parts of the body. In its simplest and most common form it appears as a small, firm, translucent gray nodule or bump on the skin, usually on the forehead, cheeks, nose, or other exposed areas, such as the backs of the hands. Since it is painless and rarely bleeds, this form is often unnoticed until it begins to grow more rapidly and its size calls attention to it. Another form of basal-cell skin cancer appears as a raised scaly patch of keratosis which is noticed because it bleeds easily when rubbed or scratched. A fully developed basal-cell cancer is easily recognized. It has a central area of ulceration circled by a raised, gray, pearly edge. It is a painless, slow-growing ulcer which does not heal.

Epidermoid Cancer. Epidermoid (or squamous-cell) cancer is another common form of skin cancer. This type may appear much like basal-cell cancer, but it spreads more rapidly. The epidermoid type of skin cancer usually starts in the form of a warty, crusty keratic area or several such areas on the cheek, ear, neck, or back of the hand. These may be tender and often become infected. The ulcerating form of epidermoid skin cancer is usually a shallow, nonhealing ulcer which spreads on the surface of the skin—sometimes over a wide area—but rarely grows into the deeper tissues. On unexposed areas of the body, epidermoid skin cancer may arise in old scars of burns or infections, appearing as a nontender, raised, firm, pinkish, flesh-colored, small area on the normal skin. Attention may be drawn to epidermoid cancers of the skin because of their rapid growth or because they become infected, tender, nonhealing sores.

Malignant Melanoma. The most dangerous but fortunately a rare type of skin cancer is malignant melanoma. This type spreads early to other parts of the body. Malignant melanoma may arise from a mole, particularly one subjected to constant irritation or injury. The common tan moles almost never become cancerous. The dark brown or bluish-black moles rarely become cancerous, but when malignant melanoma does occur, it usually develops from this type of mole. One of the most definite signs of danger in a mole is the appearance of a dull, diffuse brownish zone spreading from it. If a mole is irritated and becomes larger, blacker, or bleeds, it should be seen at once by a physician. Moles between the toes or on the soles of the feet are constantly being irritated but are easily overlooked.

Early Diagnosis, Prevention and Treatment. In looking for the signs and symptoms of skin cancer, one should remember: Any increase in size, change in shape, deepening of color, bleeding, or ulceration of a painless sore or mole which does not heal may be cancer unless proved otherwise.

From what is known about skin cancer, certain rules of skin hygiene help guard against the development of the disease. These rules include:

1. Ample use of soap and water by workers in industries utilizing materials suspected to be cancer-producing, to cleanse the skin of these irritating substances.
2. Avoidance of overexposure to the sun. This rule applies particularly to light-complexioned people. All outdoor workers should wear protective clothing and use skin ointments to prevent the skin from becoming cracked or thickened.
3. Protection of the skin from suspected cancer-producing substances. Workers should wear clean gloves and avoid long use of sooty, tarry, or greasy clothing.
4. Careful shaving by men with scaly patches or moles on their faces to prevent injuring such areas of the skin.
5. Frequent examination, by a physician, of skin blemishes which may be subject to constant irritation or friction from clothing.

If skin cancer develops, it can be treated effectively by surgery, cautery, or radium. The particular form of treatment depends on the type of cancer and the stage of the disease. Selection of the proper treatment can be made only by a qualified physician.

CANCER OF THE MOUTH

Cancers of the mouth are responsible for approximately 4000 deaths each year in this country: 3000 of men and 1000 of women. Yet, most of these cancers could be prevented or cured.

A century ago, Bouisson reported a clinical study of 68 cases of cancer of the oral cavity in a hospital in France. Two-thirds of the cases were cancer of the lip, the others were cancer of the mouth, tongue, internal surface of the cheek, tonsil and gum. He was able to ascertain the habits of 67 of these patients and found that 66 smoked tobacco and the other chewed tobacco. Bouisson noted that cancer of the lip ordinarily occurred at the spot where the pipe or cigar was held. Similar findings were reported by many other physicians during the next eighty years.

Cancer of the lip attacks men more often than women and affects the lower lip more often than the upper one. Too much heat and overexposure to the sun's rays creates conditions that favor the development of lip cancer. Smokers, who have a history of holding on to the hot short end of a cigar or who favor the old-fashioned clay pipe, seem prone to develop this kind of malignant tumor. So do men who make their living out-of-doors —farmers, for example, and sailors.

A cancer of the lip is easy to see. The first sign may be a crack in the skin that does not heal properly, or a wartlike, scabby lump that does not become progressively smaller and disappear. From either of these, a bleeding sore may develop, with or without pain. Finally, the flesh at the base of the sore may feel firm and swollen.

Cancers of the gums, cheeks, and tongue also show a "sex preference" for men. Persons who smoke or chew tobacco or who do not keep the mouth and teeth clean may develop malignant tumors in this location. Other kinds of irritation also suspected of favoring cancer in this site are jagged teeth, poorly fitting false teeth, or teeth that do not meet properly when the mouth is closed. Good dental care and regular examination by a dentist are important safeguards against mouth cancer.

Cancer of the gum or inner cheeks starts in much the same way as cancer of the lip, and with similar symptoms. Running or wartlike sores, and white spots, anywhere in the mouth, are danger signals. Soft, puffy gums that bled easily, often for no apparent reason, may be an early sign of a malignant growth.

On the tongue, also, cancer may develop from a sore that fails to heal either by itself or after a short period of simple medication. A malignant tumor in this location may appear as a lump on the tongue. Such a lump may be topped by a whitish, painless scab, or a painful, open sore.

Sudden paralysis of the tongue, particularly if it is accompanied by pain, is another danger sign. So is bleeding or the discharge of pus from the tongue, since these may be the product of a cancerous sore that has become infected.

Lip cancer, provided it is treated soon enough, can be cured in all except most unusual cases. Whether treatment is by surgery or radiation will depend on the individual case. Many lip operations are comparatively minor and leave little or no blemish. Wartime developments in plastic surgery enable surgeons to restore normal contours even after the most radical operations.

Cancer of the mouth is more difficult to treat than lip cancer, but it, too, can be cured provided it is discovered early and receives prompt, adequate treatment.

OTHER CANCERS

Many other cancers, which though less common also are important, can be prevented or diagnosed early enough to be treated successfully. Cancer of the larynx is frequently the result of smoking and early causes hoarseness. Cancer of the esophagus which may be associated with smoking or with heavy drinking of hard liquor early causes difficulty in swallowing. Cancer of the bladder may be associated with stones in the bladder, with certain chemicals, particularly aniline dyes, and with cigarette smoking. Blood in the urine is often the first suggestive sign. These are illustrations of how important it is that people keep informed about cancer and alert to the possibilities of prevention and of early diagnosis.

UNPROVED CANCER TREATMENTS

Cancer patients and their families are almost certain to be urged to try some "new cancer treatments." This may be suggested by well-meaning friends or it may be promoted by cancer quacks or by organizations with something to sell.

The medical quack may be a physician, he may be a practitioner of one of the cults, or he may lay no claim to any sort of medical education whatsoever. His only purpose is to exploit human misery for personal gain.

The usual earmarks of a purveyor of unproved or worthless treatments are:

1. His method of treatment is known only to himself, or the drugs or preparations which he uses are manufactured according to a secret formula or method or are available only from one private source.
2. He does not report his results in reputable scientific journals but promotes his methods by advertising, testimonials, planted stories in the general press, and/or organized campaigns.
3. The substances or treatments he uses are usually controlled by a high-sounding research organization or foundation.
4. He often claims that the "medical trust" is against him.
5. His records are scanty or secret.
6. He is quick to threaten legal proceedings when anyone questions his methods.

7. His chief supporters are rarely reputable medical men or researchers. He relies for support on politicians, actors, writers, lawyers—as well as the general public—all of whom are untrained and inexperienced in the natural history of diseases and have no way of judging whether diagnoses are accurate and whether reported improvements are real or are merely a stage in the usual course of the disease.

No medicine, diet, or serum is known that will cure cancer. Ointments and plasters are worthless, and massage and manipulation tend to disseminate cancer cells throughout the body. The cancer quack is the most despicable of all the vultures who prey upon human misery. He alleges to cure cancer without surgery, using electrical treatments, salves, light, diet, injections, or pills. His treatment is worthless; but worse still, while the patient relies on his treatment, the cancer progresses until even the best of medical care is unavailing.

The reasons that some people follow irregular forms of treatment for cancer are (1) cancer is a capricious disease; it has many forms; it does not always run a predictable course; (2) cancer can be accurately diagnosed only by a biopsy, but this procedure is not always followed and people may be told that they have cancer when they do not have it at all; (3) the recognized treatments—radiation and surgery—do not always yield immediate results on which their ultimate success can be evaluated; and (4) patients with cancer occasionally, though very rarely, recover from the disease spontaneously. In these cases, the immune mechanism of the body apparently destroys the cancer.

People who attribute their apparent recoveries from cancer to unorthodox treatments are offered as "living proof" of the value of the treatments. Most, though not all, of these are entirely honest in their belief that the injection, the pill, or the tonic actually cured them. These "living cures" give the quack strong support.

PROTECTING YOUR FAMILY AND YOURSELF AGAINST CANCER

Cancer is a serious disease that over the years will develop in approximately two out of three American families. Yet, the following simple precautions may save your life or the life of ones dear to you:

ONE: Every year pick a regular date on which you and everyone in your family will have a thorough medical checkup. In adults it should include a proctoscopic examination of the rectum and lower bowel, where cancer strikes more frequently than in any other part of the body. This examination with the proctosigmoidoscope—a lighted hollow tube—can save more lives from cancer than any other step in the physical checkup.

Remember, your annual physical could prove your most valuable form of insurance because it can detect cancer at a very early stage before it causes symptoms.

TWO: Learn the seven warning signals that may mean cancer . . . These have been mentioned earlier but they are of such importance that they merit repetition:

1. Unusual bleeding or discharge.
2. A lump or thickening in the breast or elsewhere.
3. A sore that does not heal.
4. Change in bowel or bladder habits.
5. Hoarseness or cough.
6. Indigestion or difficulty in swallowing.
7. Change in a wart or mole.

None of these means you have cancer. More than likely you do not. (Hoarseness or cough could be due to an infection and occasional rectal bleeding does not necessarily mean cancer.) However, if a signal lasts longer than two weeks, it is serious enough to call for a visit to your doctor. It could be cancer. Any blood in the urine or bleeding after the menopause should be immediately investigated.

Pain is seldom an early cancer signal. Don't wait for pain if signs or symptoms persist.

THREE: The health risk of cigarette smoking is established. Scientific studies have demonstrated that cigarette smoking is a major cause of lung cancer and a factor in other diseases. In general, those who smoke fewer cigarettes live longer. Quitting cigarettes even after years of smoking improves health, decreases the risk of cancer, and saves lives. Studies show that the children of smokers are most likely to smoke themselves. Your example is of vital importance. Studies show that those who begin smoking cigarettes before fifteen, smoke more, inhale more, have a higher death rate than those who do not begin smoking until after twenty-one. Therefore, if you don't smoke cigarettes, don't start; if you do smoke cigarettes, stop; if you can't stop, cut down. Pipe or cigar smoking is far less hazardous than cigarette smoking because the smoke is usually not inhaled.

FOUR: Avoid home remedies, secret or quack cures. Depend only on a reputable doctor. Wasting your time with others may keep you away from proper treatment until it is too late. If you are offered a secret cure, check with the American Cancer Society or your county medical society. Your county medical society will also be able to help you select a family doctor if you do not have one.

A SPECIAL WORD TO WOMEN: Be sure your annual examination includes a "Pap" test. Because of this test, more progress has been made against cancer of the uterus than against any other cancer. Since 1937 the death rate has dropped 50 per cent.

Learn how to examine your breasts—it takes only a few minutes—and make this examination yourself once a month. Your doctor will show you how. You can learn also from the American Cancer Society film and pamphlet on "Breast Self-Examination." Millions of women have seen these and from them obtained information which is helping to save many lives.

ABOUT CHILDREN: Fortunately, cancer in children is rare—in any given year, only one child in 7000 is likely to develop cancer. Yet, more school children die of cancer than any other disease.

Regular physical examinations and prompt investigation of any suspicious conditions by a doctor are cornerstones of cancer control in children.

Any out-of-the-ordinary symptoms which do not subside in two weeks should be reported to the doctor. Thus, should any of the danger signals listed last for more than two weeks in either child or adult, the condition should be investigated.

ACT NOW FOR YOUR FAMILY: More people are being cured of cancer than ever before: at least half of all cases can be cured if they receive treatment in time. Some 1,300,000 living Americans once had cancer and have been cured. Many hundreds of thousands more should and could be saved by early diagnosis and proper treatment. In addition, more than 100 deaths a day from cancer could be prevented by avoiding cigarette smoking.

You alone can take the steps that will make the best medical skills and knowledge available to you and your family.

CHAPTER 26

Occupational Health

HENRY F. HOWE, M.D.

INTRODUCTION

The greatest natural resource supporting America's stupendous economic prosperity is not its wealth of raw materials, the ingenuity of its inventors and scientists, or the efficiency of its managers. All these are expendable and replaceable. Its single greatest resource is its industrious and enthusiastic body of healthy working people, who get the millions of jobs done that comprise the complex economy of the nation. This zest for work which is characteristic of Americans is continuously dependent on an abundance of good health. Without health the zest and industriousness would disappear. Maintenance of good health among wage-earners is therefore a keystone in the arch of our country's productivity. Without health, none of our booming economic development could have happened.

Some employers, in the middle of the nineteenth century, established medical services for their employees in areas where satisfactory medical services were not readily available. Since 1911, workmen's compensation laws requiring employers to compensate employees or their heirs for occupational disability or death and to provide medical care for occupationally injured employees have been enacted in all states. In addition, most of these laws require employers to provide medical care for employees with occupational disease. These and other laws have given employers a greater incentive, as well as an obligation, to maintain safe and healthful working places. The problems associated with the increasingly complex technology of industry, with ever-new, hazardous physical and chemical substances, have served as an important stimulus to the development of occupational health programs. From these developments the earlier idea of curative occupational medicine has been broadened to include and emphasize prevention, safety, and health maintenance, and there has gradually emerged the occupational health program, now utilized in all large industries.

Health maintenance is primarily the responsibility of the person himself. However, the employer is required to provide a safe workplace for his employees, and he has a real interest in the prevention of loss of work time and of work efficiency resulting from his employees' ill health. Diagnosis and treatment of nonoccupational injury and illness are not responsibilities of the employer, but he may provide certain preventive health measures on the job where the employee, the employer, and the community all stand to benefit, by avoidance of lost time, lost wage-earning, lost production, and ill health.

Two types of health programs are available for those who work. The one that most concerns us is the *occupational health program* that deals with the health of employees in relation to their work and is largely preventive. The other type is a *medical care program* for nonoccupational illnesses and injuries, provided by various forms of hospital- and medical-care insurance. These two types of programs differ in methods of financing and amounts and kinds of services. Failure on the part of employers, employees, and physicians to distinguish properly between these two types of programs sometimes gives rise to misunderstandings.

The objectives of an *occupational health program* are:

1. To protect employees against health and accident hazards in their work environment
2. To help job placement and make sure that people are put to work in jobs that are suitable to their physical capacities, mental abilities, and emotional make-up which they can perform with efficiency and without endangering their own health and safety or that of their fellow employees
3. To assure good medical care and rehabilitation of the occupationally ill and injured
4. To encourage personal health maintenance.

The achievement of these objectives benefits both employees and employers by improving employee health, morale, and productivity.

In order to attain these objectives the following activities are essential:

1. Maintenance of a healthful work environment.

   Personnel skilled in industrial hygiene and safety perform periodic inspections of the work premises, including all facilities used by employees, to detect health and safety hazards. Such inspections, together with the knowledge of processes and materials used, provide current information on health conditions of the workplace. This information is used for appropriate recommendations for preventive and corrective measures to develop an effective safety program.

2. Health examinations.
   a. Preplacement examinations.
   These examinations determine the condition of health of the worker to aid in suitable job placement. They are not intended as a mechanism for rejection of applicants for work. They often result in improved job performance, less absenteeism, and decreased likelihood of injury. They are an excellent example of good preventive medicine.
   b. Periodic examinations.
   These health examinations are similar to preplacement examinations and are carried out at appropriate intervals to determine whether the employee's health is still suitable for his job assignment and to detect any evidence of ill health which might be connected with his employment. They are particularly useful for employees exposed to dangerous hazards, for people over forty, and for workers contemplating changes in job assignments.

All health examinations are conducted by a physician. The examination may be made at the place of work or elsewhere. The physician discusses the results of the examination with the worker, explaining to him the importance of further medical attention for any significant health defects found.

Unrealistic and needlessly strict standards of physical fitness for employment defeat the purpose of health examinations.

3. Diagnosis and treatment.
   a. Occupational injury and disease.
   Diagnosis and treatment in occupational injury and disease cases is prompt and is aimed at rehabilitating the patient so that he gets back to work in good health again quickly. Workmen's compensation laws usually govern the payment for medical services for such cases.
   b. Nonoccupational injury and illness.
   Diagnosis and treatment in nonoccupational injury and illness cases are not responsibilities of an occupational health program with these limited exceptions:

   (1) In emergency the employee is given the attention required to prevent loss of life or limb or to relieve suffering until placed under the care of his personal physician, and

   (2) For minor disorders, first-aid or palliative treatment may be given if the condition is one for which the employee would not reasonably be expected to see his personal physician, or to enable the employee to complete his current work shift before consulting his personal physician.

Every employee is encouraged to have a personal physician for diagnosis and care of nonoccupational illness or injury.

4. Immunization programs.

   An employer may properly make immunization inoculations available to his employees, particularly where the job may expose workers to infection which is preventable by immunization.

5. Medical records.

   The maintenance of accurate and complete medical records of each employee from the time of his first examination or treatment is a basic requirement. These records, including the results of health examinations, are kept confidential. Such records remain in the exclusive custody and control of the medical department. Disclosure of information from an employee's health record is not made without his consent, except as required by law.

6. Health education and counseling.

   The industrial physician and nurse educate employees in personal hygiene and health maintenance.

The occupational health program is tailored to each employee group according to its needs. These needs are determined by the number of employees, the nature of the industry and extent of the hazards to which they are exposed, and the availability of community medical services. The staff required in an occupational health program may include, in addition to physicians and nurses, engineers skilled in various technical procedures of the safety and health program, laboratory technicians, other specialized personnel, and clerical help.

Nurses in occupational health programs are graduates of accredited schools of nursing, registered and legally qualified to practice nursing where employed. Training and experience in occupational health are desirable.

In establishments which do not have a nurse, one or more employees should be qualified in first aid and available throughout the working hours.

Occupational health personnel cooperate also with voluntary and official community agencies providing health, safety, employment, and welfare services.

THE SAFETY PROGRAM FOR EMPLOYEES

Many advantages are gained from a survey of the workplace. The information obtained permits the industrial physician to prevent or to diagnose and treat occupational disease in the employee. As an example, a persistent hepatitis may be caused by exposure to carbon tetrachloride.

Only after this exposure is confirmed and brought under satisfactory control can the patient's disease be treated and, of equal importance, development of hepatitis in his fellow workers avoided.

Similarly, the survey permits the physician to become familiar with the physical and mental demands of each job. He becomes acquainted with materials and operations, the nature of exposure to substances, and conditions that may injure health, and the actual circumstances that may be the cause of accidents.

The purpose of the survey is not only to determine what conditions are wrong but to learn also what constitutes safe procedure. A safety-inspection checklist is often used to assist in the survey of working areas and production processes to locate actual or potential hazardous conditions. The following checklist is an example of the procedure:

1. Housekeeping, control of waste, oil spills, etc.
2. Floors, stairs, platforms, railings, work surfaces
3. Aisles, walkways, exits, clearances, etc.
4. Ladders, stability, etc.
5. Material handling equipment, types, traffic control, etc.
6. Storage and material piling
7. Machinery–guards and maintenance
8. Tools–use and care of, etc.
9. Electrical and welding equipment, shielding
10. Pressure equipment, steam lines, tanks
11. Overhead pipes, valves, and superstructure
12. Hot materials and heat
13. Chemical hazards, estimate of employee exposure, availability of emergency showers and eyewash facilities
14. Flammable or explosive substances–storage and handling
15. Solvents used for maintenance and cleaning
16. Dusts, fumes, vapors, and gases
17. Fire-fighting equipment, drills and training (including rescue drills)
18. Smoking areas, regulations
19. Personal protective equipment–hard hats, safety glasses, goggles, safety shoes, respirators–and whether workers really are using them
20. Washrooms and locker rooms–sanitation, towels, soaps, etc.
21. First-aid equipment–availability, contents, training in use
22. Ventilation
23. Noise
24. Illumination
25. Ionizing radiation–X ray, alpha, beta, gamma, or neutron, personal monitoring devices
26. Electromagnetic radiation–microwave, infrared, ultraviolet, etc.

27. Job-permit procedures
28. Unauthorized job transfers
29. Food handling
30. Miscellaneous unsafe practices

The physician and the nurse thus cooperate with management and safety personnel to investigate the true causes and preventive aspects of industrial injuries. An effort is made to investigate routinely each disabling and near serious accident. At the time of treatment the physician discusses the circumstances of the accident with the patient to determine clues to the cause of the accident.

The effectiveness of a safety program depends upon the continued interest of both management and employees. Management assumes the responsibility in carrying out the program. Management demonstrates to the employees its interest in accident prevention by investigating the causes of accidents and eliminating them, and by persuading workers to take an active part in safety. The employees become cooperative in such programs when they see that it is in the interest of their own safety. A safety program is no better than the persistent cooperation of the workers themselves in carrying it out.

SAFE WORK CLOTHES FOR EMPLOYEES

Workers should wear clothes designed not to create a hazard. Long, loose sleeves, neckties, or loose garments around the waist may be tangled in moving machinery. Cuffs on pants can catch sparks from such operations as cutting or welding.

Machine operators should wear short-sleeve shirts. Long sleeves buttoned at the wrist may be worn for other jobs. Pant legs should be at ankle length, either cuffless or with cuffs sewed up.

Women employees should wear slack suits or well-fitting work uniforms and low-heeled shoes. A cap should be worn to prevent entanglement of hair in moving machinery. Hair nets or scarves may be worn for other work.

Synthetic fabrics resist acids, many solvents, mildew, and abrasion. However, because of their ability to release static sparks, they should not be worn in explosive or high-oxygen atmospheres. Chemical treatments are available to prevent sparking in some synthetic fabrics, but some of these have to be applied at each laundering.

Protruding rings, bracelets, wrist watches, and neck jewelry should not be worn on any job involving moving machinery, electrical equipment, or moving vehicles.

PERSONAL PROTECTIVE EQUIPMENT

Companies with good occupational health and safety programs provide protective equipment when and where it is needed to prevent injury to workers. Physicians, industrial hygienists, and safety personnel are knowledgeable in the need, selection, limitations, and use of protective clothing and devices. They recommend the protective equipment and devices which meet the requirements of the job. Workers are taught why and how the equipment and devices must be used.

The following is a brief description of some of the protective clothing and devices used in industry in hazardous situations which may be the source of injury.

Head—A protective hard hat, resistant to impact, fire, moisture, and insulated against electricity, will provide protection against impact of falling objects, sparks, splashing or spattering material, splashing liquids and chemicals, heat, and cuts or abrasions. Many industries have zoned areas in which hard hats must be worn by all personnel, workers and visitors.

Eye and Face—Safety glasses should be worn on any job in which there is possibility of injury to the eyes. The nature of the job and eye hazard determines the selection of eye protection. Face shields are used where face and eye protection is required.

Welding helmets and hand shields also provide protection for eye and face. Hoods and nonrigid helmets with window arrangements can be equipped with air line when exposure is to toxic dusts, fumes, or gases.

Eye protection devices can be supplied with special filter lenses for protection against glare of visible or ultraviolet light.

Many tragic eye losses have occurred to workers who have the habit of removing their eye protection for just a few minutes. There is a long list of members of the Wise Owl Club whose eyes have been saved by safety glasses.

Ear—Hearing protective devices are of three types: inserts or plugs, muffs, and helmets. Cotton will not provide any appreciable reduction of noise. Helmets with muff-type protectors frequently are worn in exposure to jet noise at airports or engine test areas.

Respiratory Protective Devices—The selection of a respiratory protective device depends upon the desired protection, which may range from nuisance conditions to those which are immediately dangerous to life. The general types of respiratory equipment are canister gas masks, chemical cartridge respirators, mechanical filter respirators, supplied air equipment —hose mask and air line respirators, and self-contained apparatus supplying oxygen and air.

Respirators must be properly maintained, cleaned, and inspected on a periodic basis to give satisfactory protection when it is needed. Training of workers who will wear respirators, and of their supervisors, is essential for intelligent, confident, and safe use.

Finger, Hand, Arm, Body, and Leg—Protection of the upper extremities may be provided by finger cots, hand pads, gloves or mittens, and sleeves. The body may be protected by aprons, cape sleeves, jackets, coats, coveralls, and overalls, or complete suits designed for fire fighting, radiation protection or chemicals. Protection for the knees, legs, and ankles is by knee guards, shin guards, leggings, pants, or spats. The type of exposure determines the choice of garment and material of construction.

Feet and Toes—Safety shoes provide protection for the feet and toes. The hidden steel cap is often the difference between a crushed foot or injured toe and no injury at all.

Other Equipment—Safety belts or harnesses with life lines may be required for normal or emergency use for structural steel and bridge workers, window cleaners, public utility linemen, forestry workers, crane men, miners, mechanics, builders, drivers of vehicles, or workers entering tanks, bins, and underground passages. Belts and harnesses must be selected for the particular job.

ENGINEERING CONTROL IN THE SAFETY PROGRAM

Accidental injuries result from human or mechanical failures or exposure to dangerous hazards. Personal protective equipment may reduce injuries but will not completely eliminate hazards. Engineering design and controls to eliminate hazards are an important objective of a preventive program. This is accomplished by the installation of mechanical devices or control methods such as: guards to prevent flying or falling objects; exhaust fans to remove hazardous dusts, mists, vapors, fumes, or gases; material handling equipment to eliminate hand handling; enclosing a hazardous area to lessen exposure to the hazard; and substitution of a less hazardous process, such as welding for riveting when noise is the hazard. Good preventive programs also consider the human factor. Equipment is designed to allow for limitations in human capabilities. Such machine controls as switches and handles can be designed to fit the stature and reach of the operator.

Some hazards cannot be completely controlled and still produce the product; in these situations, engineering design is supplemented by personal protective equipment. Hazards such as chemical splashes, radiant heat, ultraviolet radiation, and low-oxygen atmospheres require specialized protective devices and clothing.

Training of workers in the use of mechanical safeguards and personal protective equipment is part of the on-the-job training program. Workers should know how to clean and maintain individual protective clothing or devices assigned to them, and develop self-discipline in seeing to it that they are used.

The following are examples of occupational hazards requiring engineering control, personal protective equipment, and training of the worker.

Material Handling—The major cause of injuries in industry is improper material handling. Almost one-fourth of all accidents are back injuries due to improper lifting. Stooping with the back arched with the load out at the end of the arms causes the injury. When lifting in this manner, the whole strain is put at the bend of the back, the muscles of which are not made to take it.

There are simple rules to lifting. The object to be lifted should be inspected for weight and size. Help should be secured if the load is too heavy or awkward. The worker should plant his feet firmly, well apart. He then should squat with knees bent and get a good grip on the object. He should keep his back as straight as he can and lift slowly, without jerking, by pushing up with his legs. The strong leg muscles should do more work than the back muscles. The body should never be twisted with the load. Lowering an object to the floor or ground requires the same careful procedure.

Falls—Falls are responsible for one-fifth of on-the-job injuries. They may be the result of stumbling, slipping, or losing balance. They can be caused by slipping on oil, grease, water spills, waxed floors, icy walkways, or objects left in the aisles or stairs. Serious injuries are often caused by jumping from work stages, trucks, or loading docks, or falling from ladders. Stairs should be walked up or down slowly with feet firmly planted on each step and handrail used. Ladders and stagings should be solidly built and firmly placed.

Impact of Falling Objects—Overhead hazards exist in excavations, demolition, construction, steel or foundry operations wherever objects may fall from building structures, cranes, roofs, elevators, hoists, ropes, chains, or slings. Constant vigilance is needed by all those working in such areas, together with compulsory use of hard hats.

Flying Particles and Objects—Flying particles may result during the scaling and grinding of metals, woodworking, or from blown dust in operating tractors or power shovels. Large flying particles may originate from power presses, forging or machine operations, lathe work, chipping or finishing of iron and steel castings, or from use of chisels, jack hammers, rock drills, and sledges. Flying particles or objects act as missiles and can produce severe injuries, especially to the eyes. Protective devices can prevent injury, if supplemented by thoughtful care.

Sparks, Metal Spatter, and Splashing Metals—Metal sparks fly from arc welding, metal work, or during the use of hand tools. Operations involving metal pouring, casting, and tinning may result in injuries from spatter or splashing. Careful procedure and protective devices or clothing are the preventives.

Splashing Liquids: Chemicals—Almost every industry has laboratories or processes in which there may be exposure of workers to burns from handling corrosive chemicals. Limited protection can be provided by eye, face, and body protective devices and clothing. Whenever possible, the hazard should be eliminated by engineering design. The severity of burns from accidental spills or splashes can be reduced by immediate washing of the skin with large quantities of water. Only a deluge shower will provide sufficient water for rapid flushing of the chemical from the skin. To prevent extensive eye damage, the eye should be irrigated immediately with large amounts of low pressure water from an eye-wash fountain, drinking fountain, shower bath, hose, or any type of water container. Thorough training of employees in the location and prompt use of these facilities is essential.

Dusts, Fumes, Vapors, and Gases—Industrial materials may enter the body by inhalation, skin contact, or by mouth. Inhalation is the most hazardous because the surface area of the lung tissue exposed by breathing is much greater than the total area of the skin. Most chemicals are not easily absorbed through the skin but those that reach the air sacs of the lungs easily enter the blood stream and thus reach the entire body. Poisoning by mouth is rare in industry, except for a few strong poisons introduced by the unwashed hands during eating of food.

Most of the industrial dusts have little effect on health and are only a nuisance type. The principal dangerous one is silicosis, which may result in a disabling lung condition. It can only be caused by dust containing free silica such as found in quartz, granite, sandstone, and sand. Only the fine particles reach the air sacs of the lungs. These particles are too small to see. The visible ones do no damage because they are trapped in the nose and throat from which they are blown out, expectorated, or harmlessly swallowed.

The important factors producing silicosis are high concentration or quantity of the fine dust, the duration of exposure and the susceptibility of the individual. Silicosis is often not produced until ten years and sometimes only after twenty-five years of exposure.

Other types of dust to which prolonged exposure in high concentrations may cause disabling lung conditions are asbestos and sugar-cane stalks.

Metals and Their Compounds—As an occupational health hazard, the most prominent industrial metal is lead, which may be present alone or in a wide variety of compounds. The chief means of entry of lead into the body is inhalation of dust or fume. Absorption through the skin of metallic lead and inorganic lead salts is insignificant, but tetraethyl lead and a few other organic forms of lead may be thus absorbed in dangerous amounts. Molten lead ordinarily does not present a hazard unless its temperature is well above its melting point.

Lead compounds may be known by a number of names, not including the word lead. Litharge, the common name for one of the oxides of lead, is found in the paste of lead storage battery plates, in certain cements, in "doctor" solution in petroleum refining, and in pigments. Measurement of exposure to dusty lead compounds is made with the aid of laboratory analysis of the air and of samples of the blood or urine of exposed employees.

Other toxic metals used in industry include antimony, arsenic, beryllium, cadmium, cobalt, manganese, mercury, and phosphorus. Exposure may occur in mining, metal refining, fabrication, and metal-cleaning operations. Welding or high-temperature cutting on cadmium-plated surfaces can be particularly hazardous. The toxicity of beryllium is extreme. Mercury is of special importance because hazardous concentrations of vapor can be released from the liquid metal even at room temperature. The dust of various mercury compounds is also toxic. Chromium exposure as mist or dust is commonly found in chromium electroplating and may cause ulceration of the skin or the nasal septum. Zinc oxide fume exposure, arising from molten zinc at a galvanizing operation, may cause the temporarily disabling illness known as metal fume fever.

Solvents—Many solvents used in industry present hazards dependent on the volatility, the concentration, the toxicity, and the duration of exposure.

One of the frequent uses of solvents in a great variety of plants is in a vapor degreaser. Such equipment can be used without excessive exposure to the operator, but poor practices can result in dangerous exposure. Benzol (benzene), carbon tetrachloride, carbon disulfide, and methanol (wood alcohol) are other industrial solvents that may cause serious illness if not used under properly controlled conditions.

Gases—Potentially hazardous exposure to gases is often not detectable by the worker in the shop. Carbon monoxide may occur by moderate leakage from a pipe line, or by impingement of a gas flame upon a cold surface, or by its use in a heat-treating department. The only warning of its presence may be when a number of workers complain of headaches. Accidental liberation of high concentrations of carbon monoxide can result in asphyxiation.

This same undetectable characteristic applies to exposure to a number of other hazardous gases. The early symptom of excessive exposure to hydrogen sulfide is irritation of the eye rather than headache, but the danger of rapid asphyxiation is even greater. The odor of hydrogen sulfide is no safeguard because even brief exposure often results in the loss of the ability to smell it.

A number of gases are brought into plants in cylinders in the form of liquids under pressure. These include hydrogen fluoride, used in certain oil-refining processes and in the chemical industry; hydrogen cyanide and methyl bromide, both used for fumigation; and chlorine, widely used for bleaching, in water treatment, and as a disinfectant. Other toxic gases include ozone, nitrogen dioxide, and sulphur dioxide. Careful engineering control and prompt investigation of early symptoms are the basis of safe use of the toxic gases.

Heat and Hot Materials—In many industrial plants, the problems of heat in summertime are no different from those in the nonindustrial environment. For purposes of evaporation of perspiration, usually the better the air movement, the greater the comfort. Although high humidity in itself creates no harmful effects, it does limit evaporative cooling and intensifies the discomforts of high temperatures. Heat sources are found wherever there are flames, ovens, furnaces, heat-treating baths, or molten metal.

Many plants have local "hot spots." In steel, glass, foundry, and other similar industries, control of radiant heat is a major problem. Radiant heat passes through the air without heating it until it strikes some object such as the human body. Air movement will not reduce this heat load. Shielding with some reflective material, such as aluminum, may be required.

In hot occupations the plant physician advises how much water supply, with salt, is needed for the prevention of heat cramps and exhaustion. Thirst is not an accurate indicator of how much water a man needs when working in extreme heat.

Cold—Exposure to extreme cold may occur in meat-packing plants, in deep-freeze food-producing and -storage operations, and sometimes in flying at high altitudes. Proper clothing must be provided to prevent muscle and joint pains and respiratory diseases.

Cuts and Abrasions—Protection by gloves and training procedures against cuts and abrasions should be provided when handling sharp and rough materials or from sharp-edged tools. The safety program includes prompt first aid to prevent infections of even minor injuries.

Dermatitis—Industrial skin diseases may be caused mechanically by friction; by physical agents such as heat, cold, or radiation; by such chemical agents as acids, alkalis, irritant gases or vapors, and cutting oils. Dermatitis can also result from plant poisons, bacterial fungus, or parasites, or as a result of removing the natural oils of the skin by solvents, soaps, detergents, or other chemicals.

The best methods of control are elimination of skin irritants, personal hygiene (frequent washing or showers and change of clothing) and protective gloves, clothing, and devices. Personal cleanliness of workers exposed to skin irritants is the most essential measure for the prevention of dermatitis. The plant physician recommends the specific washing procedures and advises on the use of barrier creams and protective equipment.

Electricity and Electric Shock—Specialized rubber clothing protects workers such as linemen and electricians on energized and high-voltage electrical equipment. Such clothing should supplement, and not substitute for, safety devices and procedures.

Machinery—Injuries from mechanical equipment may result from direct contact with moving parts, the work processes themselves, mechanical or electrical failure, and human failure. Safeguarding of machinery can be achieved primarily by engineering design. Protective equipment should only supplement engineering design.

Welding and Cutting—Welding and cutting operations may require both engineering control and personal equipment for eye, respiratory, and body protection. Exposures to workers and helpers may include hazards of material handling, falling objects, eye injuries, burns, electric shock, and inhalation of toxic metallic fumes and gases. Opaque shielding should be used around welding or cutting operations to protect nearby workers especially from "welders flashes" of the eyes.

Radiation—Microwaves found in radar, communication, and diathermy operations may be of sufficient field strength to cause heating of body tissue or cataract of the eye.

Infrared radiation does not inflict deep injuries. However, there is evidence that continual exposure to infrared may result in cataract. Eye protection is therefore required.

Germicidal lamps and electrical welding arcs are producers of ultraviolet radiation. Ultraviolet light produces effects similar to sunburn; the severity depends upon the wave length, the intensity and duration of exposure. Protective eye glasses and skin protection are required.

X rays and radioisotopes are used for radiography testing, tracers, friction and lubrication studies, static eliminators, thickness gauging, and nuclear energy. Protection varies with type and intensity of radiation. Engineering design and control procedures, specialized clothing and devices, decontamination facilities, and fire-fighting equipment are part of the protective program. Personal monitoring devices, such as film badges, pocket dosimeters, and ionizing chambers, provide techniques for measurement of exposure to ionizing radiation and recording of the degree of hazard.

Lasers may be used in space communication, high-temperature welding, electron accelerators, and biomedical and surgical tools. The possible hazard in the handling of lasers is the inadvertent exposure of the eye to the reflected beam.

Excessive Noise—Prolonged exposure to excessive noise levels may cause loss of hearing. Noisy areas where one must shout within an inch or two of the ear to make one's self heard are potentially injurious conditions. When such areas exist, the physician recommends a study of the noisy environment and perhaps advises practical noise-reduction measures and an audiometric examination program. Hearing protective devices are recommended when adequate reduction of noise at the source is not possible or practical.

Extremes of Atmospheric Pressure—Extremes of atmospheric pressure include those encountered in foundation and tunnel construction and in diving operations, and the low pressures of flying at high altitudes. "The Bends" may occur whenever the body is subjected to rapid changes in pressure. Prevention is through graduated return to normal pressure.

WORKMEN'S COMPENSATION LAWS

The workmen's compensation program in the United States was adopted primarily to meet certain needs of employees or their survivors resulting from disability or death of an employee arising out of and in the course of employment. In general, the program sought to remedy inadequacies in earlier common law by providing new laws based upon the principle of insured liability regardless of negligence by either employee or employer. The first of the new laws provided cash payments to replace a part of the wages lost by disabled employees. Little or no attention was paid at first to providing medical care and rehabilitation for the disabled worker.

Substantial progress has been made recently in the extension of medical care and other aspects of rehabilitation, including vocational training and selective placement of the disabled in kinds of work suited to their limited physical and emotional capacity. It is a matter of growing concern that a considerable gap still exists between needed services to the occupationally disabled and what is actually available to them under the laws.

The basic goals of workmen's compensation today are:

1. Rehabilitation of the occupationally disabled
2. Sure, prompt and adequate payment to the disabled workers or their survivors
3. Minimal cost to employers and society to provide the above provisions.

The essential elements in the implementation of these goals are described in the following paragraphs.

REHABILITATION OF THE OCCUPATIONALLY DISABLED

Rehabilitation implies the effective use of all skills for the conquest of disability. Current experience shows that the provision of rehabilitation services results in substantial savings in both medical and compensation costs, just as the development of medical care provisions has resulted in lower compensation costs.

The establishment of workable rehabilitation programs calls for new provisions in some of the workmen's compensation laws; planned and improved cooperation from the medical profession; and intelligent, forceful administrative supervision.

The disabled employee is entitled to all services, appliances, and supplies required by the nature of his disability or the process of his recovery and that will promote his restoration to employment. Services include medical, surgical, dental, hospital, and nursing attendance and treatment, as well as the training necessary to rehabilitation. Appliances and supplies include medicines; medical, surgical, and dental supplies; crutches; artificial members; and apparatus. Services, appliances, and supplies are to be paid for by the employer under the supervision of competent professionals responsible to the administrative agency. Vocational counseling, training, transitional employment and placement services, require prompt reporting of occupational disabilities to the administrative agency. When necessary procedures for such a system of rehabilitation do not exist, steps should be taken to provide them.

The amount and method of compensation payments have a direct and important bearing on an effective rehabilitation program. While overgenerous compensation can dull the injured worker's desire for rehabilitation, inadequate compensation can destroy an employer's incentive to support rehabilitation by providing him with a cheaper alternative. More important, inadequate indemnity can lower patient morale or force return to gainful employment before medically indicated. Inadequate cash indemnity encourages "lump-summing" of payments, which tends to interfere with rehabilitation.

Workmen's compensation is not a relief program. The real purpose of the program is that a disabled employee and his family should not suffer a serious reduction in normal living standards during the rehabilitation period. This requires that the benefit level be maintained at an adequate percentage of usual wage and include reasonable personal expenses to support the rehabilitation process. Effective rehabilitation can drastically reduce the number of permanently disabled employees, which now constitutes the heaviest burden on workmen's compensation systems.

Various methods of compensating employees with pre-existing permanent impairments have been devised. In these cases liability is apportioned generally between the employer at the time of subsequent injury and a state fund ("second injury fund") established for this purpose. In recent years increasing consideration has been given to cases where the pre-existing condition is an organic disease that, combined with a subsequent injury, results in increased or total permanent disability. While the medical complexities surrounding this problem are difficult, intensive study is currently being given to the fair resolution of the whole problem.

EMPLOYMENT OF THE HANDICAPPED

Employers have not, as yet, fully recognized the presence of a large reservoir of unused manpower, which has a valuable contribution to make. Comprehensive and documented studies of the performance of handicapped people have repeatedly shown excellent job performance, as well as less absenteeism and better safety records than in comparable groups of able-bodied workers. In most circumstances, such employment does not lead to increased workmen's compensation costs.

The principle of evaluating ability, rather than disability, of a potential employee deserves continued emphasis. The phrase "an equal opportunity employer" should not relate solely to race or creed, but also should apply to those who have some physical or mental impairment. Strict placement requirements are unavoidable for certain jobs, but if the type of work permits, the handicapped individual should receive equal consideration with any other worker. The handicapped have a strong motivation to succeed.

Present trends in manufacturing indicate progressively less need for physical labor, particularly in the unskilled or semiskilled groups. Physical impairments, therefore, will have decreasing importance, and concurrently the importance of brain power will increase. Many so-called handicapped persons already have needed skills, or have the potential to develop them as readily as the nonhandicapped.

Successful employment of the handicapped involves:

1. Proper medical evaluation of the physical and mental condition of the applicant
2. Evaluation of the applicant's physical and intellectual capacity for work
3. Proper job placement in which the employee can utilize his maximum functions and skills without affecting adversely his own health or exposing his fellow workers to increased hazards
4. Periodic re-evaluation of the employee's health status to protect his capabilities for continuing satisfactory employment.

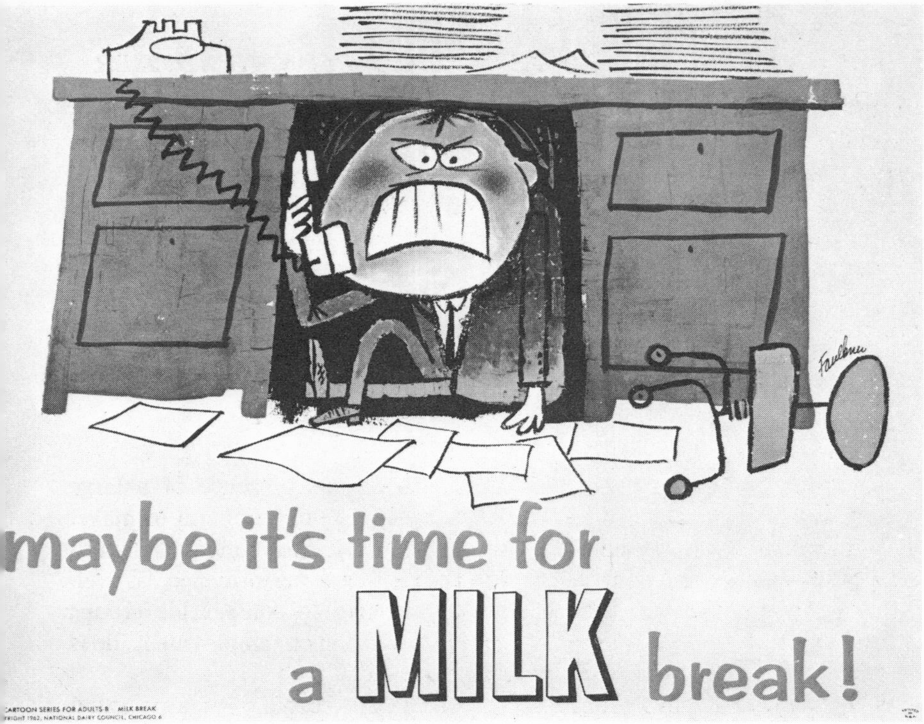

maybe it's time for
a MILK break!

CARTOON SERIES FOR ADULTS B   MILK BREAK
RIGHT 1962, NATIONAL DAIRY COUNCIL, CHICAGO 6

PLATE 65. Maybe it's time for a milk break! *(National Dairy Council.)*

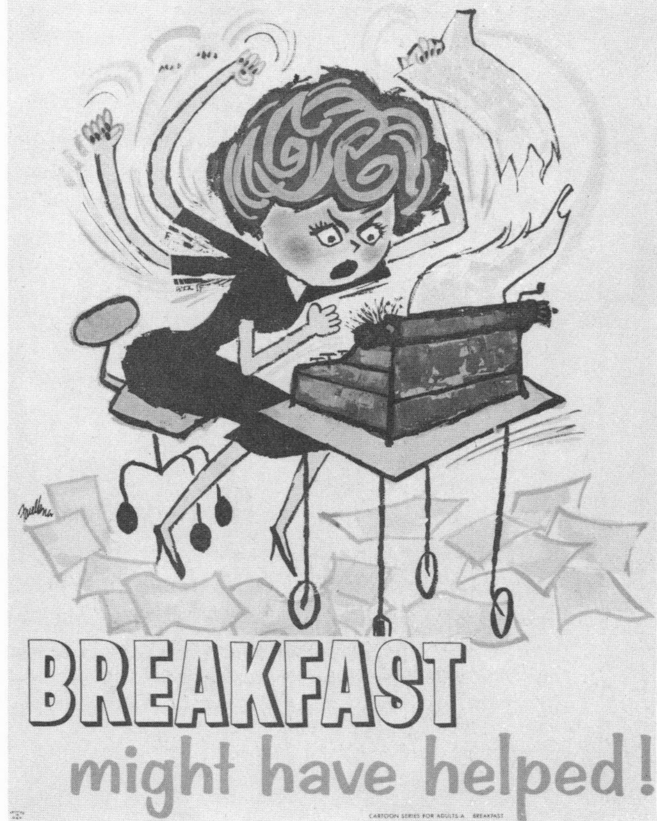

PLATE 66. Breakfast might have helped! *(National Dairy Council.)*

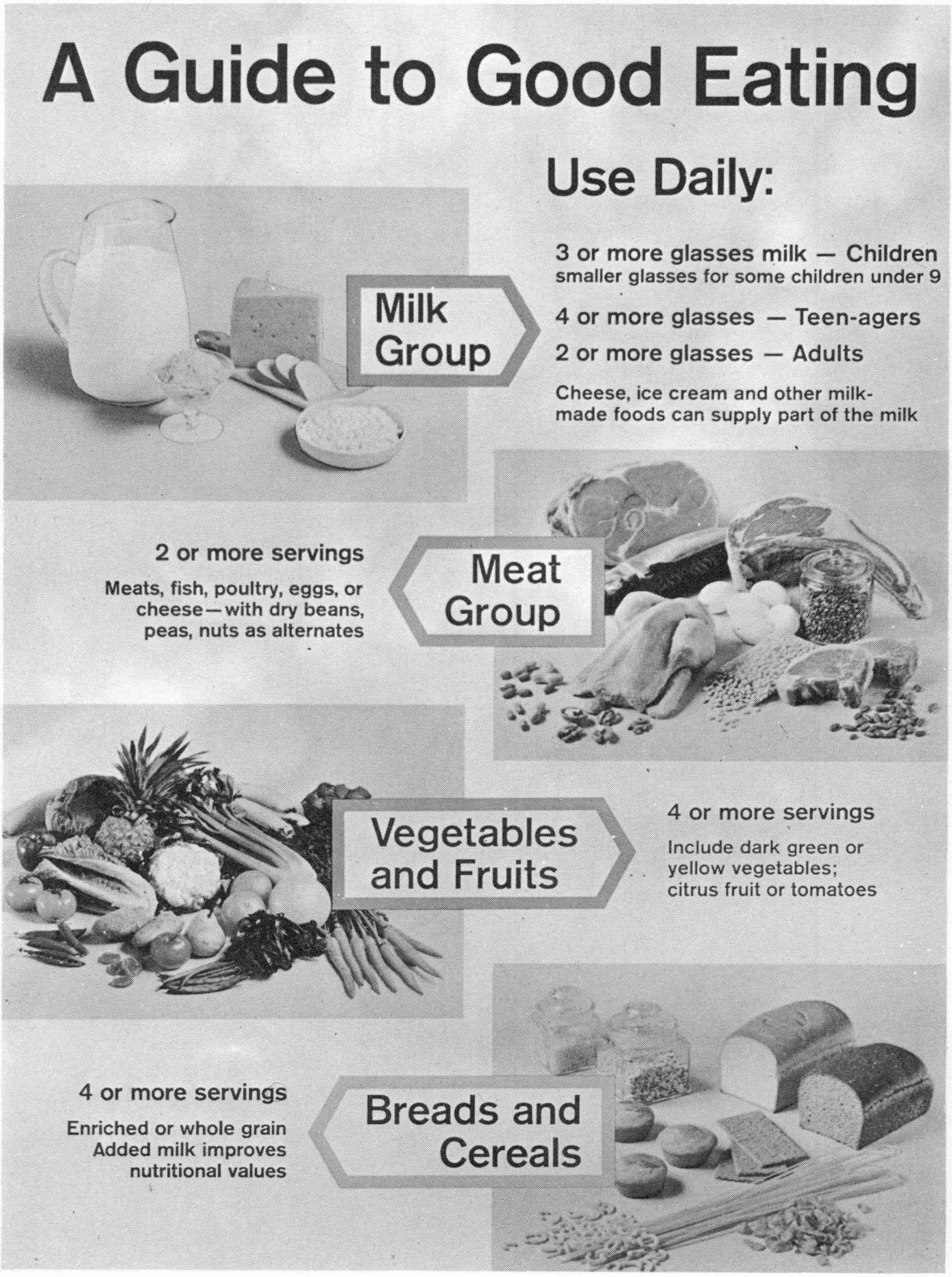

A Guide to Good Eating

Use Daily:

Milk Group

3 or more glasses milk — Children
smaller glasses for some children under 9

4 or more glasses — Teen-agers

2 or more glasses — Adults

Cheese, ice cream and other milk-made foods can supply part of the milk

Meat Group

2 or more servings

Meats, fish, poultry, eggs, or cheese—with dry beans, peas, nuts as alternates

Vegetables and Fruits

4 or more servings

Include dark green or yellow vegetables; citrus fruit or tomatoes

Breads and Cereals

4 or more servings

Enriched or whole grain
Added milk improves nutritional values

PLATE **67.** A guide to good eating. This is the foundation for a good diet. Use more of these and other foods as needed for growth, for activity, and for desirable weight. (The nutrition statements made in this chart have been reviewed by the Council on Foods and Nutrition of the American Medical Association and found consistent with current authoritative medical opinion.) *(National Dairy Council.)*

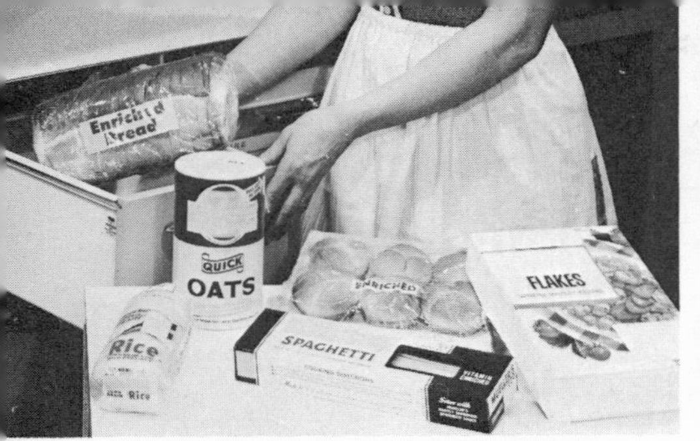

PLATE **68.** The bread and cereal group furnishes worthwhile amounts of protein, iron, several of the B vitamins, and food energy. Four servings a day from this group are recommended.

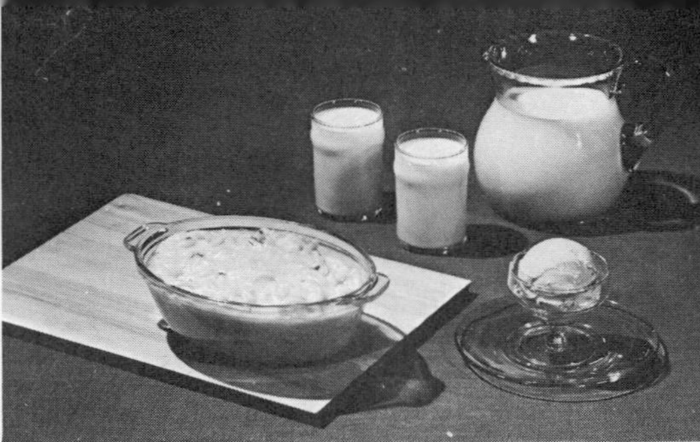

PLATE **69.** The United States Department of Agriculture Daily Food Guide suggests that part of milk concerned may be whole or skim milk, buttermilk, evaporated or dry milk.

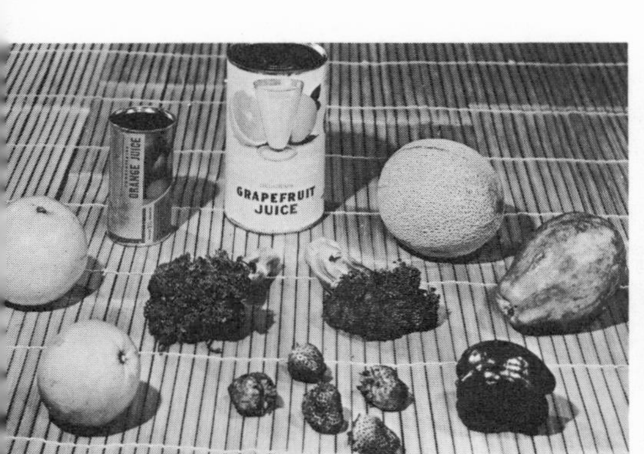

PLATE **70.** Good sources of vitamin C. Grapefruit, orange, cantaloupe, papaya, raw strawberries, broccoli, green pepper. Good sources not shown are guava, mango, sweet red peppers. The new food guide suggests one serving a day from this group.

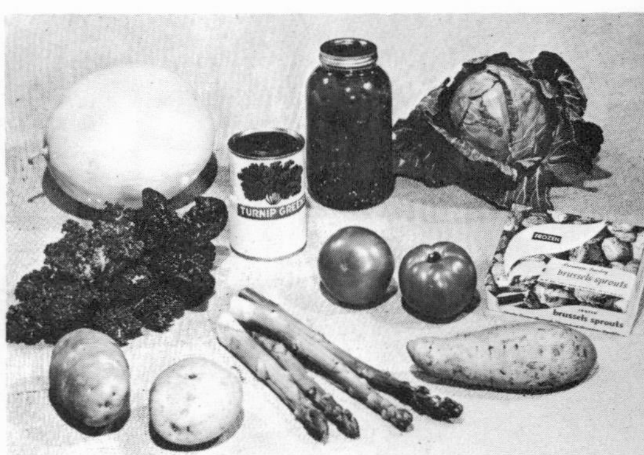

PLATE **71.** Fair sources of vitamin C shown are honeydew melon, asparagus, Brussels sprouts, cabbage, kale, spinach, turnip greens, potatoes, sweet potatoes, tomatoes. Others are watermelon, tangerine, kohlrabi, garden cress, and mustard greens.

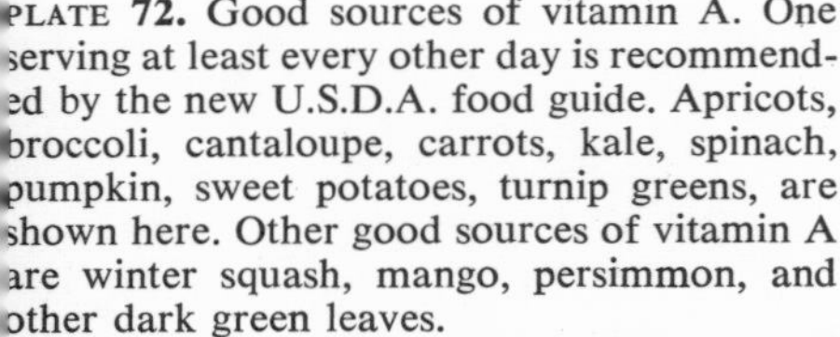

PLATE **72.** Good sources of vitamin A. One serving at least every other day is recommended by the new U.S.D.A. food guide. Apricots, broccoli, cantaloupe, carrots, kale, spinach, pumpkin, sweet potatoes, turnip greens, are shown here. Other good sources of vitamin A are winter squash, mango, persimmon, and other dark green leaves.

PLATE **73.** These count as servings in the meat group: 2 to 3 ounces (figuring without bone) of lean cooked meat, poultry, or fish; 2 eggs; 4 tablespoons of peanut butter; one cup cooked dry beans or lentils (not shown).
(U.S. Department of Agriculture, Agricultural Research Service.)

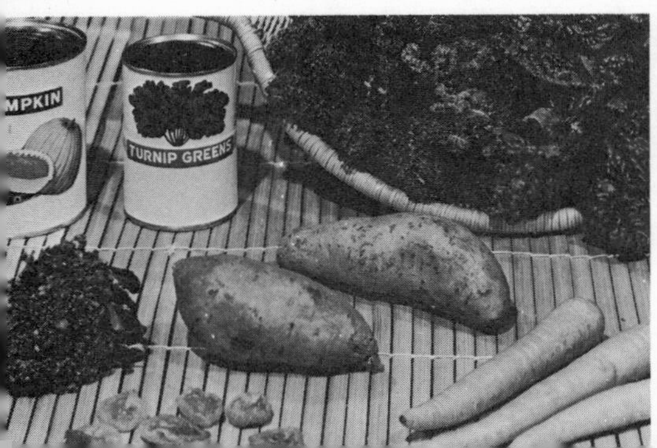

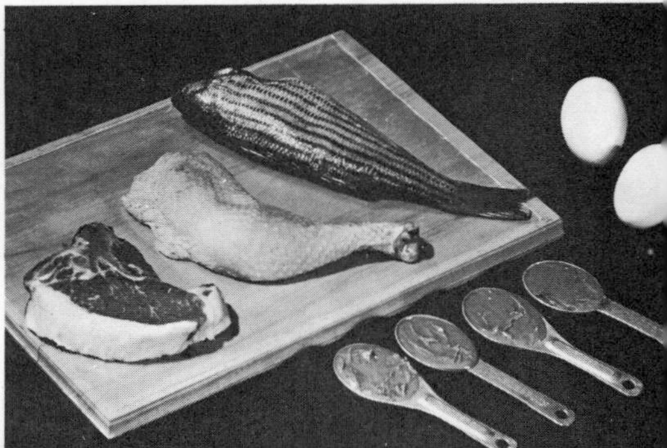

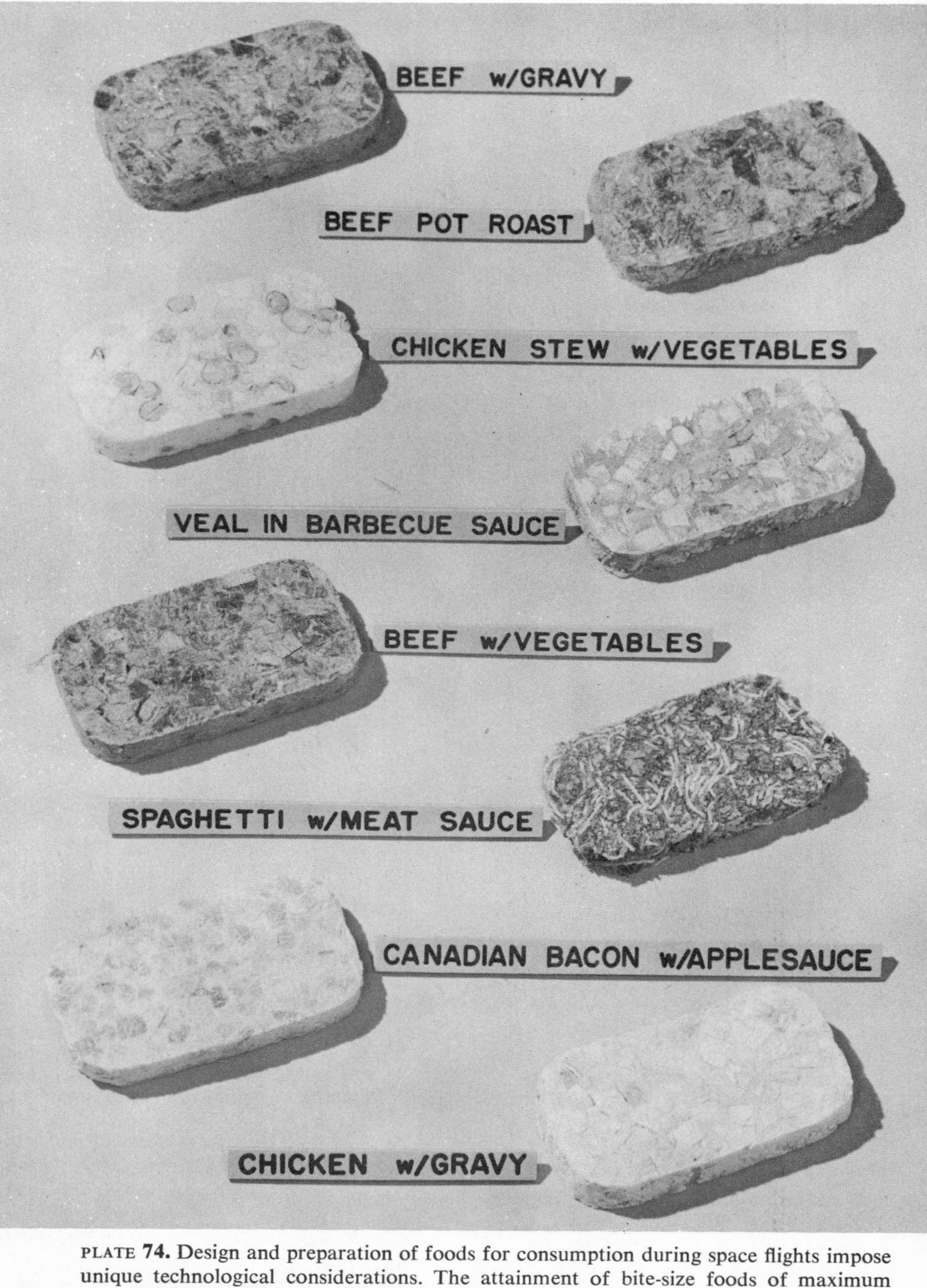

PLATE **74.** Design and preparation of foods for consumption during space flights impose unique technological considerations. The attainment of bite-size foods of maximum caloric density and the control of fragmentation, impact, and pressure resistance, cohesiveness, stickiness, microbiological safety, retention of moisture or flavor, and migration of fat under high vacuum have posed a great challenge to our space food technologists. *(U. S. Army Photo, U. S. Army Natick Laboratories.)*

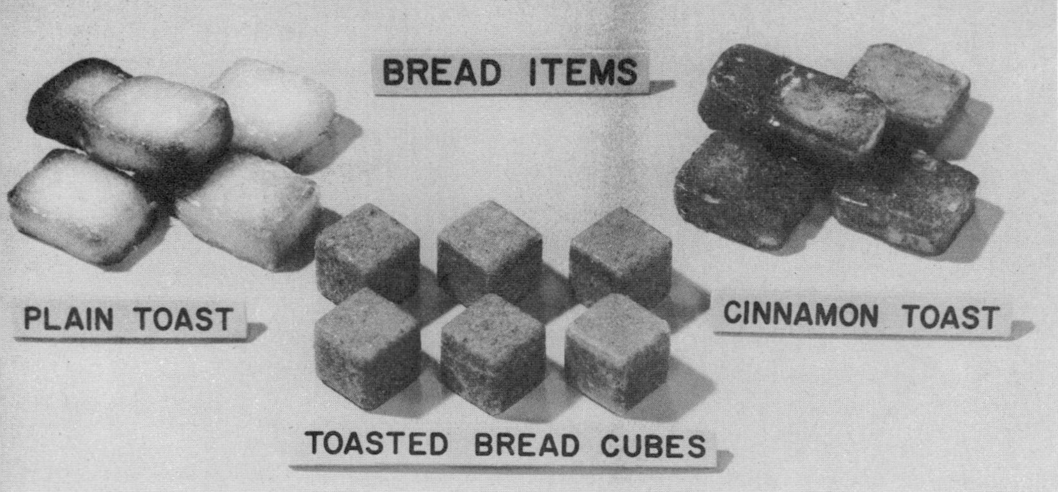

PLATE **75.** Space food in cubes. Meat items are cooked and then diced into cubes not over ¼″ (1 cm) in size; the gravy or sauce is prepared separately and then combined with the other ingredients; the combination is placed in molds, frozen, sliced into bars, and freeze-dehydrated. Each bar, approximately 3½″ x 27/32″ (90 x 50 x 21 mm) thick, constitutes one portion. *(U. S. Army Photo, U. S. Army Natick Laboratories.)*

PLATE **76.** Astronaut eating specially prepared food from plastic tubes. *(U. S. Army Photo.)*

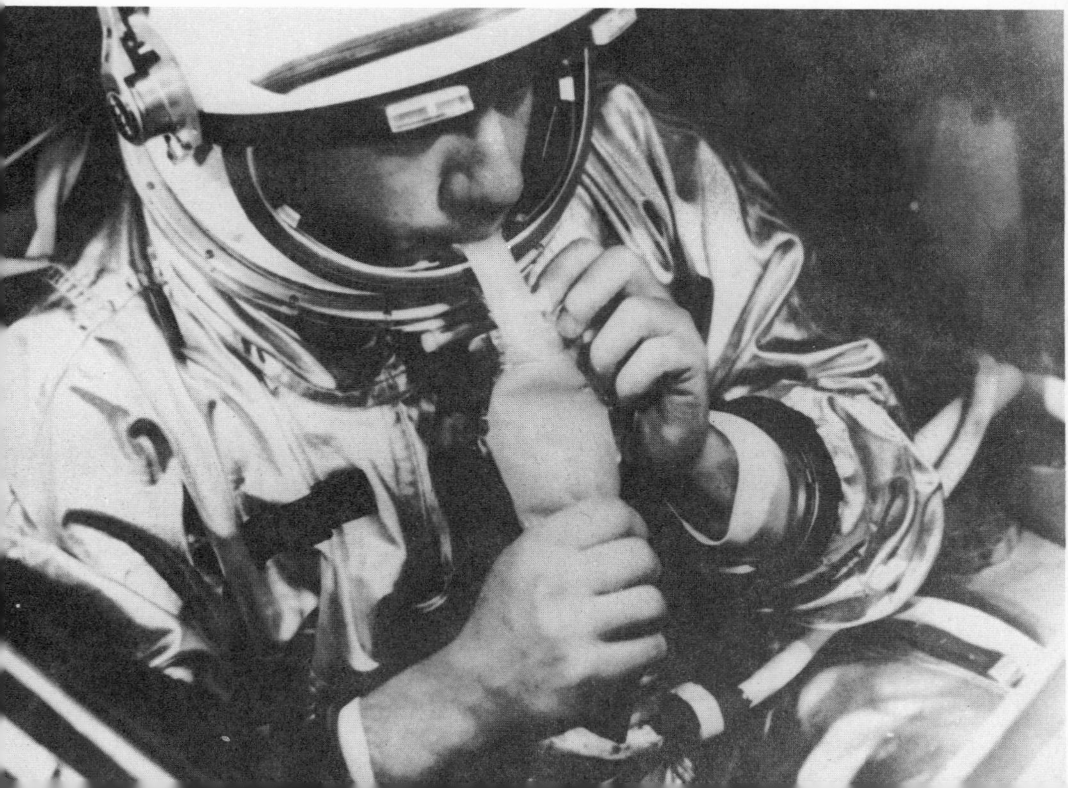

PLATE **77.** Do you keep your teeth clean? Whenever possible, do you brush them after you eat, or rinse your mouth with water? *(National Dairy Council.)*

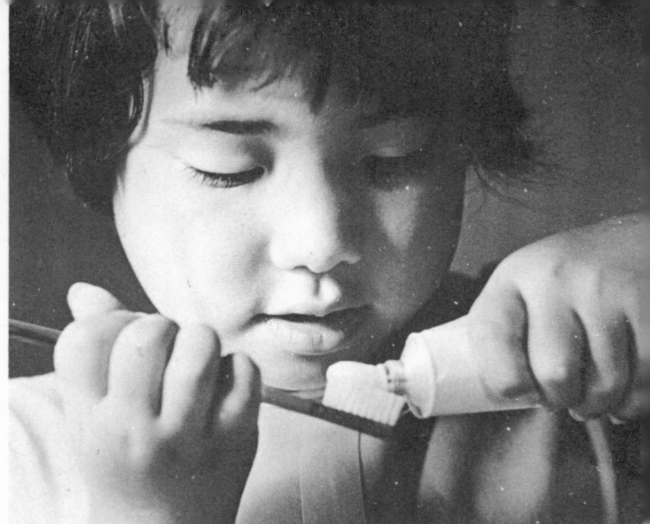

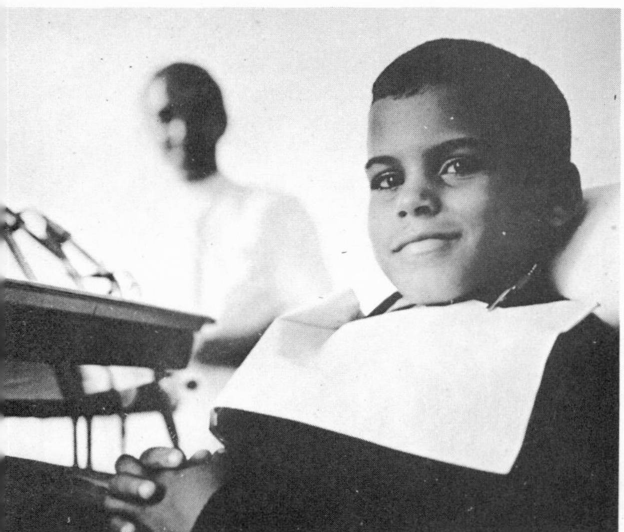

PLATE **78.** Do you visit your dentist as often as he suggests? He will check your teeth. Follow the rules he gives you to help keep your teeth healthy and clean. *(National Dairy Council.)*

PLATE **79.** Do you eat good food? You know that you need your teeth to chew your food. Your teeth also help you to look your best, and talk clearly. So, start now to take care of your teeth. *(National Dairy Council.)*

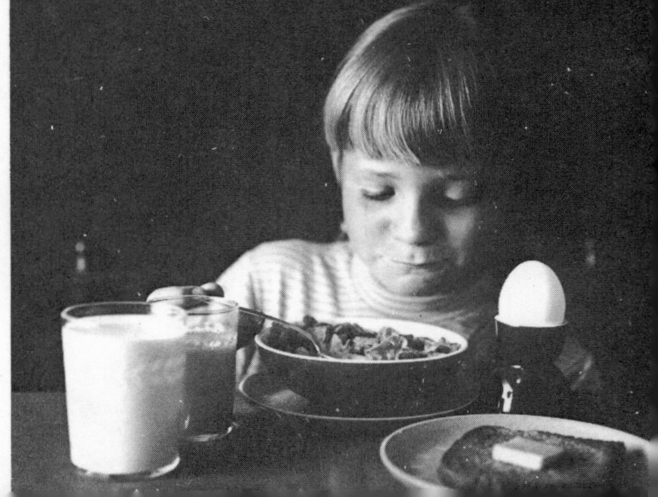

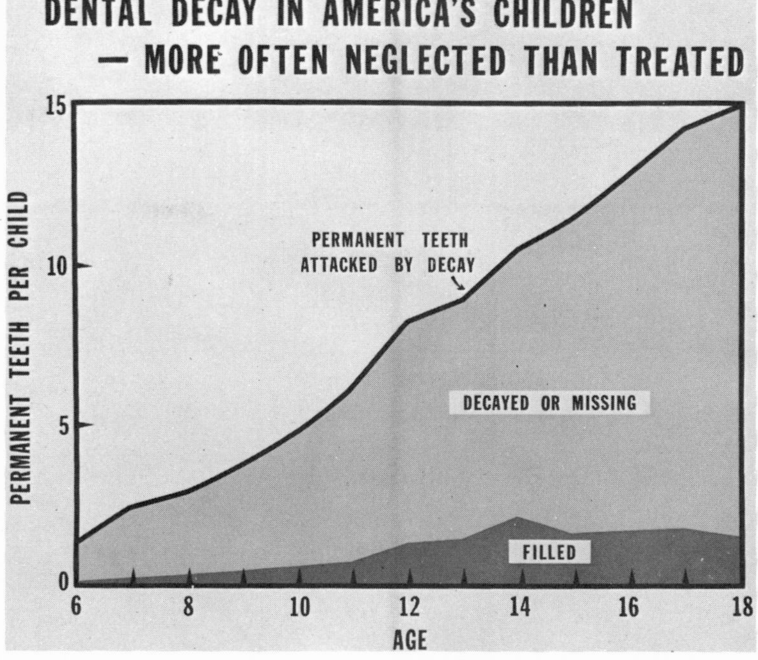

PLATE 80. The most prevalent disease in the United States, afflicting 98 per cent of our population is tooth decay. **PLATE 81.** *(below)* When the upper and lower teeth do not meet evenly, the result is an incorrect bite or malocclusion. An even bite is important for good speech, good nutrition, and good looks. Early attention to a child's first teeth through regular visits to a dentist from the age of 2½ or 3 years and after that regularly at least every 6 months can help detect and treat such conditions. *("Healthy Teeth," Division of Dental Health, U.S. Public Health Service.)*

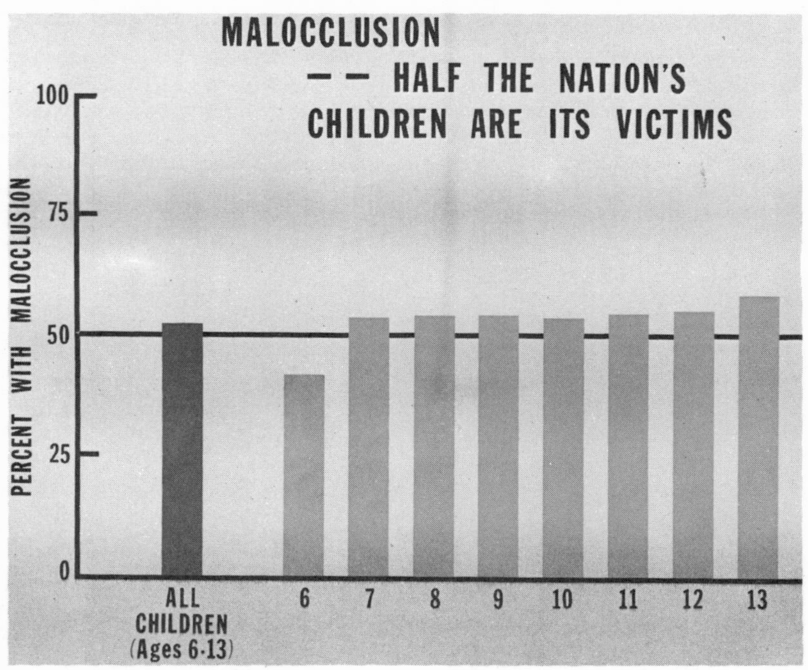

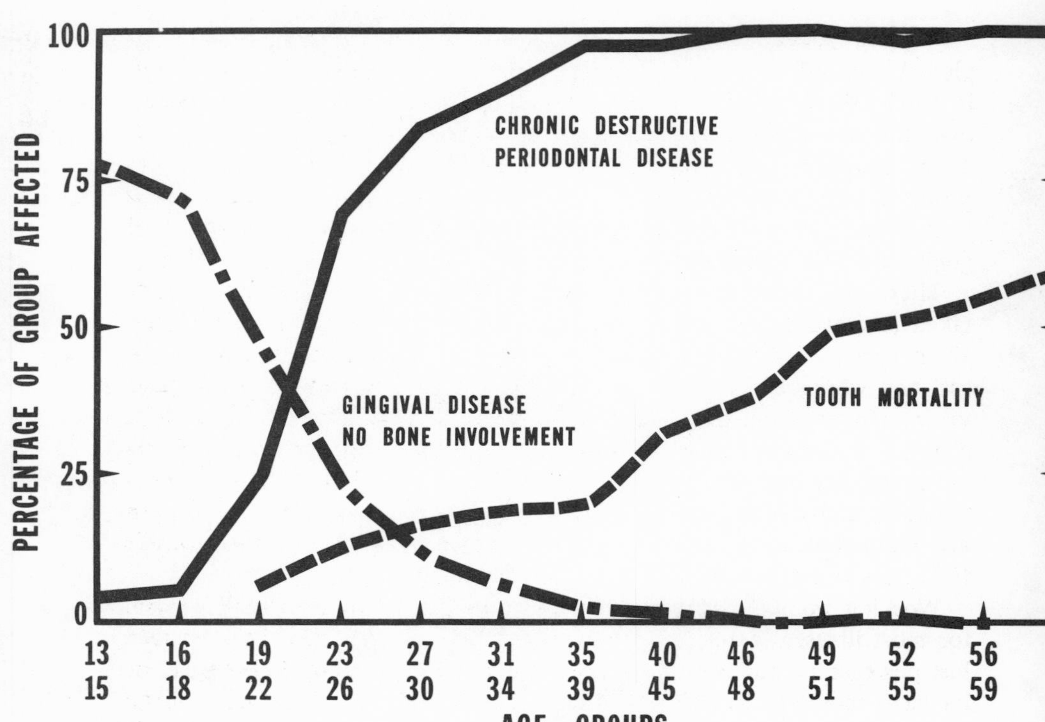

PLATE **82.** Periodontal disease (the severe form of which is sometimes referred to as pyorrhea) is the chief cause of tooth loss in adults. Beginning with gingivitis or inflammation of the gums, it then causes inflammation or destruction of the soft tissue and bone that surround the roots of the teeth. Thorough brushing to remove the accumulation of debris at the gum line and between gum and tooth surfaces will help prevent the disease and the eventual loss of teeth. *("Healthy Teeth," Division of Dental Health, U.S. Public Health Service.)*

WOMEN EMPLOYEES

Women, young, middle aged, and older, single and married, are employed in an infinite variety of jobs in almost all industries. They numbered in 1965 over 24 million workers, constituted about a third of all females over the age of fourteen and about a third of the nation's labor force. These numbers will undoubtedly continue to increase. Certain health problems exist in connection with the employment of women. These problems, while not so difficult as generally believed, do require sound medical guidance for their satisfactory solution.

There are few differences between men and women that have to be taken into account in the placement and utilization of women employees. Women generally are not as strong physically as men and should not be assigned work beyond their strength. Certain physiological states peculiar to women are sometimes disturbed by complications that may require changes or interruption of their work. The most important of such states are pregnancy and the weeks after childbirth; of less importance are menstruation and the menopause. There is a belief widely held that women are temperamentally and emotionally better suited for certain specific tasks, less well suited for other tasks, than are men.

Working women lose more days per year due to sickness than do men for most illnesses common to both sexes. The severity rate, i.e., the time lost per case is, however, lower for women than for men. Moreover, studies have shown more sickness absence among married than among single women. Probably home and family responsibilities are in part responsible for this excess.

PROBLEMS RELATED TO SEX FUNCTION

Women present problems peculiar to their sex which have to be reckoned with in their placement and utilization, which account for considerable absence from work and require changes and interruption in their work. These problems are associated with the physiological states of menstruation, pregnancy, the time after childbirth, and the menopause.

Menstruation—Normal menstruation does not present a problem; abnormal menstruation may do so. The commonest menstrual abnormality encountered seems to be painful menstruation. Some women lose considerable time from work on account of it. Of these, many appear to "give in" unnecessarily and take more time off from work than is warranted. Extensive studies have been made of painful menstruation in large women-employee groups. These have shown the value of simple exercises and other individual and group measures for its correction. These measures, supplemented with sound group and individual instruction in feminine hygiene, will generally control satisfactorily the problem of time lost from this cause.

Pregnancy—The healthy woman during a normal pregnancy can, with proper medical supervision, be employed in a wide variety of positions, with minimal limitations imposed for health, safety, and other considerations. It is imperative that the worker make her pregnancy known promptly to the appropriate person at her place of work. The company policy should be such as to encourage and in no way discourage a worker's reporting her pregnancy. Concealment of pregnancy invites harmful consequences, particularly during the first three months when concealment is easy. The pregnant employee, having reported her pregnancy, should be encouraged to seek care and guidance by her personal physician. Special report forms have been found useful for encouraging the pregnant employee to utilize the care of her personal physician and for the latter to report to the company.

A woman should be considered physically able to work during at least the first twenty-eight weeks of pregnancy. Should complications or other health impairments occur, the personal physician and the company physician have a joint responsibility in determining whether the pregnant employee's work assignment should be changed or she should stop work. Indeed, women in exceptionally good health and with only light housework to do may continue until the thirty-second or even the thirty-sixth week of pregnancy in certain types of work, such as stenography, and in keeping with individual company policies. Conversely, a pregnant employee with an unstable blood pressure, for example, may have to be relieved before the twenty-eighth week of pregnancy from work involving excessive physical activity or emotional tension. There may be nonmedical reasons that make leave of absence or a change of work advisable although the pregnancy per se remains uncomplicated. Nonmedical reasons accounting for a pregnant employee's absence from work should be recognized, and work absence due to them should not be permitted to masquerade as sickness absence.

As a safeguard, however, certain restrictions should be placed on the hours and the nature of the work permitted a woman during even a normal pregnancy. These are dictated as much by common sense as by obstetrical considerations.

Awkwardness in movement and the shifting of the body's center of gravity with advancing pregnancy must be taken into account. Such changes will inevitably require that the pregnant worker not be assigned tasks requiring her to climb a ladder, to stand or work on a scaffold, or in other ways incur the risk of falling. She should not be assigned tasks involving undue stretching or reaching, with the danger of losing her balance. She should be afforded maximum protection against moving machinery. Particular care should be taken to minimize the amount of lifting that the pregnant employee is required or permitted to do.

It is necessary that the pregnant woman observe good personal health habits for the sake of her own and her unborn baby's health. Insofar as practical, a pregnant woman should work on the normal daytime shift, in order to have sufficient evening and night hours at home to care adequately for her family and to get the required amount of sleep with as little interruption as possible. However, a pregnant woman with other children may be permitted to work on other shifts if her husband or other adult is in the home to care for her children. The pregnant employee should be allowed a rest period of at least fifteen minutes during the first and second halves of her work shift and a mid-shift break long enough to permit her to visit the rest room and the lunch room and eat unhurriedly the sort of meal she requires. She should not work more than five days or forty hours a week.

Where practical, a place should be provided, preferably in the medical department, where the pregnant worker can lie down if she is uncomfortable or experiences symptoms possibly indicative of complications in her pregnancy, and where she can be observed medically and referred to her personal physician if this appears to be indicated. If the pregnant employee is under the continuing care of her personal physician, the likelihood of serious complications in her pregnancy is reduced.

A healthful work environment should be provided for women. There are certain harmful substances, forms of energy, and conditions from which, according to available scientific evidence, the pregnant woman should be spared to an even greater extent than the male or the healthy nonpregnant female worker. Among such substances are those which may damage the liver or kidneys, like carbon tetrachloride; those which may cause anemia, such as benzol and lead; and those which may reduce blood oxygen, such as carbon monoxide. Another occupational exposure which may exert a harmful effect on pregnancy is ionizing radiation which can produce injury to the baby.

After Childbirth—The length of time that a woman should be kept off work after delivery should be determined by agreement between her personal physician and the company physician. This will depend upon her previous general health, the nature and severity of any complications of her pregnancy or delivery, her convalescence, the nature of her work, and the conditions in her workplace. Ordinarily a woman should not return to work for at least six weeks after delivery. She may have to postpone her return to work beyond the six weeks for a period depending upon the degree and severity of any unfavorable factors. If she nurses her baby, this may still further delay her return to work. This or other nonmedical considerations, such as having to care for her children, may influence her decision as to whether or when to return to work.

Menopause—The normal menopause is a physiological state, not a disease. Its symptoms are more emotional than physical. Generally incapacitation is only slight and of short duration, if it occurs at all. The reassurance and care of her personal physician generally enable her to pass promptly and with minimal distress and disability through the menopause and regain stability and comfort.

Women can be employed successfully in an infinite variety of jobs, provided that in their placement and utilization reasonable care is taken to avoid overtaxing their physical strength and to change or interrupt their work during pregnancy and after childbirth as required by medical and valid nonmedical considerations. In all other respects, in the lines of work for which they are suited by their physical strength, women can work with only those measures being taken for their health protection and safety that should be taken for male employees.

AGRICULTURAL WORKERS

Until recently, "industry" excluded farming. The farmer is an independent operator, often working alone, or sometimes cooperatively with his neighbors, employment of hired help being the exception rather than the rule. The farmer has his home and workshop together.

However, a change is taking place, in that little farms (80 acres and less) are being abandoned or combined to produce farms of 160 acres to a section in size. The change has been hastened by technological advances in machinery which make it unprofitable to engage in farming under 160 acres. There is availability of better fertilizers, of farm chemicals such as pest destroyers, and of growth stimulators such as hormones and antibiotics, which make large farm operation more possible and economical.

FARM ACCIDENTS

Accidents play a leading role as the principal causes of death for people in all occupations. From ages 1 through 34, the leading cause of death is accidents, and in farm accident compilations, farming as an industry ranks third in the number of deaths by accidental means—only mining and construction work rank above it. Motor vehicle accidents are responsible for the greatest share of the deaths from farm accidents.

During the growing season, the farmer is not on a 35- or 40-hour week, and, although he has the opportunity to take breaks while working with farm machinery, he frequently does not take them, particularly when the weather makes it appear desirable to complete the job. When farm machinery was horse-drawn, periodic rest periods were necessary for the horses, and the farmer, of necessity, also rested. Now he can demand of his machinery work which takes him into the night, sometimes as long as sixteen hours with only a lunch break.

In how many instances in industry would one expect a worker to hold a young child in his arms while running a lathe or any other piece of machinery; to allow a child of eight or ten to ride in a cab of a crane or on the seat beside the driver of an earth mover; or to permit a child to stand on the scaffold with his bricklayer father? Yet the farmer evidently has no qualms about carrying a two-year-old on his lap while driving a tractor in the field or on the highway, allowing a ten-year-old to drive a tractor or car on the farm premises, using the highway for travel between field and the farm home, or allowing the boy to cross a busy highway to reach home. The farm worker's idea is to get the job done as quickly as possible, and this invites shortcuts and unnecessary risk-taking involving health and accident hazards.

There are other penalties which might be considered in relation to the hazard of working with farm machinery. The farmer takes shortcuts while hurrying to get the job done which may lead to tipping of the tractor sideways or backward. A person becomes careless when tired. Farmers often stand on tractors while driving and may hit an unseen boulder or chuckhole. The only place to stand is on the axle, and this gets hot. On encountering an obstruction, they are in more danger of losing balance than when sitting.

Farm machinery is being improved, but there is a long way to go. A local physician reported the fact that three cornpicker accident victims who had been injured on the same type and make of machine were in the same hospital at the same time. The manufacturer of the cornpicker involved was supplied with the findings and photographs of his tractor-mounted cornpicker with unshielded gears. Six months later, plans had been made to equip all new cornpickers of this manufacturer with shields to protect the operator.

ZOONOSES

Zoonoses are infections of animals which may be transmitted to man, and some eighty have been described as occurring in the United States. Few animal diseases are reportable, and the impact of the zoonoses is not yet fully appreciated. The health of the farmer and of the consumer of farm products is affected by control of infection in animals on the farm. The key people in the prevention of the zoonoses are veterinarians and general physicians. Each should immediately report disease when and where it is found.

PESTICIDES

The large number of pesticides and other agricultural chemicals introduced into the farming industry have produced new problems. Carelessness and misuse of many of the chemicals have produced poisoning either through skin contact, inhalation, or accidental swallowing. Not all are as toxic as the organic phosphate pesticides such as parathion, TEPP, Thimet, but all call for sound safety practices when stored, mixed, or applied. If precautionary measures and correct procedures are followed, the user is not in danger of being poisoned.

The user should read the labels and follow directions. Pesticides should never be transferred to unlabeled containers. These chemicals should be kept under lock and key away from food items and out of reach of children. The user should avoid skin contact and inhalation of dust or vapors when handling, mixing, or applying the chemicals. The hands should be thoroughly washed after use and before eating and smoking. Protective clothing such as goggles, gloves, coveralls, respirators, and masks should be worn as directed. Spraying equipment should be maintained and regularly cleaned. Spraying should not be done into the wind. If clothing or skin becomes contaminated, the skin should be washed immediately and a change should be made to clean clothing. In case of an accident, a physician should be contacted or the patient taken immediately to a hospital.

Physicians in agricultural communities are equipped to provide educational materials to their patients on the safe use of pesticides and agricultural chemicals. Such information can also be obtained from local agricultural, safety, and health agencies who consult with physicians in establishing adequate health and safety measures to be taken in the use or control of pesticides and other agricultural chemicals.

FOR FUTURE HEALTH AND SAFETY

This chapter has described the ways in which medical and safety programs have been developed to make people's employment safer and healthier. A program of industrial health examinations, elimination of unsafe procedures and chemical hazards, and health education has made the worker and his shop much safer than they used to be. Safer clothing, protective equipment, and engineering safeguards have been provided. The various special hazards that still cause some accidents have been described. The workmen's compensation laws now usually include payments for medical care, and often for rehabilitation of the injured worker.

The desirability of employment of handicapped people, and the special problems of women employees and farm workers have been presented.

The success of all these efforts to preserve the health of working people depends on the careful cooperation of the workers themselves. Nowadays more accidents are caused by human carelessness than by machine defects or unsafe conditions in the shop. Every accident or occupational disease is a disaster to the wage-earner's family. The occupational safety program depends on careful workers. We have the knowledge to prevent accidents; all that is needed is employees who make that special extra effort to work safely, and carry into their homes, the farms, and on to the highways, the same safety practices that are taught in industry. If this kind of cooperative effort can be attained, there will be much less suffering, sickness, and human tragedy in our American communities.

CHAPTER 27

The Skin

HOWARD T. BEHRMAN, M.D.

Many people think of the skin as a sort of envelope into which the rest of the body has been stuffed. This is far from true, as the skin is essentially one of the most important parts of the body and performs many functions which are necessary for both life and health. This complex and sensitive organ shows many different variations, depending upon age, sex, climate, and race; and, in addition, it shows considerable changes in different parts of the same person. For example, in some parts of the body such as the lips and the eyelids, the skin is soft, smooth, and exquisitely sensitive. On the hands and feet, as well as over the surfaces of the joints, the skin is tough and dry and sometimes even on the rough side. The skin is a useful part of the body. In its far-flung stretches, there are millions of minute factories at work producing oil, sweat, hair, and nails. So too, there are numerous waste-disposal stations where busy little cells and groups of cells are at work getting rid of waste products, bringing blood to the surface of the skin so that the temperature will be regulated, helping absorb or neutralize various substances from the surface, and trying to protect the skin from the ravages of various bacteria, chemicals, and all sorts of external irritants. In many ways the skin is a mirror of what is going on inside the body and will often show changes along its surface which indicate the presence of some internal illness. These illnesses vary from the minor ones, such as a sore throat beginning with a fever blister, all the way to the covering of the entire body by the ugly spots of smallpox. The skin plays a part of great importance as far as the human being is concerned, and the following paragraphs will show how these activities are specifically regulated.

STRUCTURE OF THE SKIN

The skin consists of two main divisions, an outer layer called the epidermis, or outer skin, and an inner layer called the corium or true skin.

The corium is a sort of meshwork support for all the important little organs, blood vessels, and nerves which supply and nourish the skin. Underneath the skin itself is a third layer called the subcutaneous tissue, which also contains additional fat and fibrous supporting structures.

THE OUTER LAYER OF THE SKIN (EPIDERMIS)

The epidermis, or cuticle, is made up also of several layers. The main layers are the corneous or horny outer layer, and the mucous or deepest layer of the epidermis. The corneous or horny layer is the very top covering of the skin, and it is composed of practically lifeless cells which are being constantly shed from the surface as new cells from below move up and take their place. Its chief function is the protection of the skin. The deep or mucous layer is the most important layer of the epidermis because it is the living one and the one which produces new cells. It is composed of several layers of cells which are many-sided and joined to each other by tiny bridges of cell substance under which flow minute canals. As the cells in the deep mucous layer grow, and push those above them toward the surface, the top cells become flatter, dryer, and more shriveled in appearance. When they finally reach the surface, they are dried, horny, and wrinkled and are constantly shed from the surface as new cells from below take their place. The other two layers of the epidermis are called the clear layer and the granular layer. Their functions are relatively minor in importance.

The pigment cells, which are responsible for the color of the skin, are also produced in the mucous layer of the epidermis. These cells may vary from merely a few in number, or none at all, as in the albino, to the concentration of many cells heavily laden with pigment as in the darkly colored races. Pigment cells may also be found in the inner layer or corium of the skin. This is especially true in the colored races, in whom the pigment cells are more highly developed and the corium itself is deeply pigmented.

THE INNER LAYER OF THE SKIN (CORIUM)

The inner or connective tissue layer of the skin is its most important part. It is composed of parallel fibers forming a meshwork support for the blood vessels, nerves, oil and sweat glands, and hair which travel through it. As seen under the microscope, the line between the outer and inner layers of the skin is not a straight one because of the presence of little nipple-like prominences in the corium called papillae. These little structures dovetail into depressions on the under surface of the epidermis, thus serving to fasten the two layers together securely and increasing their flexibility. The papillae in general have two main functions, depending upon their origin. One type of papilla carries blood vessels and is responsible for the nutrition of the skin and all its minute parts. The other type of papilla carries various specialized types of nerves and is responsible for the feelings of touch, pressure, pain, and any of the many other sensations that originate in the skin. Even the sensation of tickling has a special type of nerve ending which notifies its owner that he should laugh. Estimates indicate that there are approximately five thousand of these specialized papillae to the square inch of skin surface. In addition to the papillae, the true skin is composed primarily of bundles of stringy fibers arranged in the form of an intricate mesh and forming sort of a crisscross network. This network runs directly into the third layer or subcutaneous tissue, and in many places is composed of a great deal of fat as it gets farther down in the skin. These layers form a comfortable cushion on which the skin rests and protects the delicate glands, vessels, and nerves from injury. In addition, it also gives the rounded appearance to the body which adds so much to beauty, provided it is not too rounded. Scattered through these layers are also found many little elastic fibers, which act like a layer of rubber bands in the skin. These fibers are primarily responsible for the elasticity of the skin, and if these fibers are numerous and healthy, the skin is likely to be smooth and have a good tone. If they are few in number, or shriveled because of age, the skin becomes saggy and wrinkled. Because of these fibers, the skin can accommodate itself to a moderate degree of stretching, such as occurs during exercise, and still return to its original smooth condition. However, there are limits to which the skin can be stretched, and this is demonstrated during certain states such as pregnancy, when the elastic fibers often stretch to the breaking point, and subsequently return almost to normal, leaving the white lines often seen on the abdomen of women who have had children. It is also common these days to see these white lines in the skin of women who have undergone periods of rapid reducing. The skin which had been stretched to the extreme, as in the very obese, cannot accommodate itself rapidly enough to the contraction of the fatty layer and hangs in apronlike folds. A similar process is in operation as we get older and the skin loses its elasticity, so that normal lines deepen and wrinkles become more apparent and noticeable.

Advancing age is inevitably associated with a certain degree of wrinkling of the skin. The only way really to escape wrinkles would be never to move a muscle in the face. Even such pleasant functions as eating and drinking require the use of facial muscles, and the inevitable appearance of lines and wrinkles in the face. This brief survey of the anatomical reasons for wrinkling and aging of the skin will not suffice to deter women from spending millions of dollars a year in attempts to lessen or minimize the ravages of time. Within the past few years, numerous "hormone" creams have been marketed with claims of skin rejuvenation, wrinkle removal, and the like. Unfortunately, the skin shows little, if any, change after their usage. Other creams are also available which may temporarily smooth out small wrinkles; this effect may last for minutes or hours and may be likened to the stiffening action which occurs when the white of an egg dries on the skin. Wrinkles are also being treated with injection of a fluid silicone into the skin, but only time will prove the safety and efficacy of this method.

SWEAT GLANDS

The sweat glands are corkscrew-shaped tubes beginning in the true skin and spiraling up to the cutaneous surface. Their openings in the skin surface are called pores, and literally millions of them are scattered over the surface of the skin, especially on the palms and soles. The larger sweat glands are found in the armpits and are primarily responsible for various types of body odor. The secretion of sweat is one of the most important functions performed by the skin.

SEBACEOUS OR OIL GLANDS

The sebaceous or oil glands are composed of a number of baggy pouches grouped together, along the sides of the hair shafts. They produce an oily, semifluid material of a whitish or yellow color, which is excreted directly along the upper part of the hair follicle onto the skin surface. This semisolid, greasy secretion lubricates the hairs and the skin surface, protecting it in part from all external agents and keeping it in a constant well-oiled state. As we grow older the oil glands function less and less adequately; for this reason the skin becomes dried with advancing age. Several million glandular oil factories are scattered over the body surface; the largest of these are found in the free margins of the eyelids, where they are called Meibomian glands. Beneath the sebaceous gland is a small involuntary muscle which is also associated with the hair follicle. During periods of stress or fear this muscle squeezes the gland and at the same time is responsible for the erection of the hair. Thus your hair can actually stand on end, as all of us who have had "goose flesh" at some time or other are well aware.

SKIN TEXTURE

The normal texture of the skin is smooth and fine, because the scales covering it are minute, oiled, and covered with delicate hair. The skin may be coarse, like that on many noses, because of large sebaceous ducts. Often faces that are scarred are referred to as having large pores. This is incorrect, as the scars are actually little pits unrelated to the pore openings. On the skin, as best seen on the palms and soles, there are many fine ridges arranged in patterns which are characteristic for each person and are often used for identification (fingerprints). On these ridges the sweat pores open. Coarser, less regular lines are caused by motion and stretching of the skin with eventual folding of the skin along these lines. Still larger lines are caused partly by motion and partly by the attachment of the skin to the underlying tissue about the joints and under the breasts. Dimples are caused by the attachment of the skin to the muscles of expression, thus drawing in the skin at this point when they contract. It almost seems a shame to break down the bare anatomical reasons for a dimple, but there you have it!

COLOR OF THE SKIN

The color of the skin depends upon the amount of pigment in the lower layer of the epidermis and by the color of the neighboring blood and the size of the surface blood vessels. Through the skin of the average blonde (if there is such a woman as an *average* blonde), the red color shows diffusely as through ground glass, with just enough effect of the pigment to make the color creamy. Brunettes have even more pigment, and other races than the white race have still more, until in the black race the red color of the blood is largely concealed. In many instances the skin may be quite light at the time of birth and become progressively darker with age. As is well known, the babies of the colored race are born with a comparatively light skin, and the pigmentation becomes progressively darker during the first few months of life, until the final skin color has been attained. In a few instances, when experiments have been performed with skin grafts, it has been found that a white man's skin grafted to the skin of a Negro will rapidly become dark and vice-versa. Such grafts are usually nonpermanent in nature as compared to homografts where the skin is grafted from one part of the same body to another part.

The color of the skin may be temporarily affected by flushing or blushing of the skin surface. This momentary change in color is due to the opening of the small blood vessels near the surface and a flooding of the skin itself with blood. This may occur as a result of exposure to excessive heat or as a result of some local inflammatory change. However, the skin is so readily influenced by the emotions that even a mild degree of embarrassment will result in temporary redness of the face. Now you know what the humorists meant when they said that "your skin is showing." The skin reacts so vigorously to an emotion that we can see an immediate redness of the skin as a result of embarrassment, "goose flesh" as a result of fear, excessive sweating of the palms and under the arms prior to an interview with the boss or that quarrel with your in-laws, and so on down the line. The unusual person can develop a poker face. These examples illustrate how the skin readily mirrors not only the health and functions of the body but also of the mind.

NUTRITION OF THE SKIN

The skin feeds on the blood which seeps into its layers from the small blood vessels in the corium or true skin. These blood vessels also bring all nutritional necessities to the glands, the hair follicles, and the papillae. In the papillae the smallest blood vessels, which are called capillaries, exude a serum which passes into the little canals of the epidermis and circulates between the cells. As it circulates it gives up its nutritive substances and picks up the waste products, and flows down again to the papillae where it finds its way back to the blood vessels or lymph vessels, and is carried away. From this description of the structure of the skin it is obvious that food for the skin does not come from its outer surface. The skin receives its nourishment from the blood stream and from the essential ingredients of the blood stream. There is actually no such thing as a skin food because, like every other part of the body, the skin feeds on what is brought to it by the blood stream. Yet millions of dollars are spent yearly for nourishing creams, skin foods, and the like, under the mistaken impression that these preparations feed the skin and are responsible for its health and beauty. It would be almost as unintelligent to attempt to increase knowledge by rubbing the head with some learned treatise as it is to attempt to feed the skin from the outside.

THE FUNCTIONS OF THE SKIN

The skin has many uses and important functions. In general, these include the protection of the rest of the body from injury, to minimize the absorption of dangerous substances, to act as an organ of sensation and touch, to excrete waste products, and to regulate heat. Besides this, some of its nerve organs are connected with sexual gratification and other physiological stimuli.

The chief function of the skin is protection. A dry skin is a good insulator against all but high-voltage electrical currents. Insulation against body cold is aided by the contraction of the tiny muscles of the hair follicles, which lift the skin to form "goose flesh" and at the same time close off the surface pores and blood vessels, thus preventing the loss of the body's heat.

The prevention of evaporation of the body fluids is also of great importance. This provision against drying out made it possible, millions of years ago, for living beings to emerge from the sea and risk the drying effect of air, a bitter enemy of life.

Not less important than the loss of fluids from within is the prevention of the entrance of water and other harmful substances from without. The normal skin is almost entirely waterproof, but when its surface has been injured, water is readily absorbed. Usually, however, only small quantities of water filter through, and when this happens the cells of the outer layer "drink" it up and swell in the process. Have you ever weighed yourself before and after a long tub bath? The change in weight is due to the extra fluid absorbed by the cells in the top layer of the skin.

The skin can protect itself during long-continued slight exposure to mild acids but not to prolonged contact with a strong acid. Against alkalies the protection is only fair, for the alkalies soften the horn cells and, together with other chemicals of a fat-removing nature, they can reduce the resistance of the skin and favor penetration.

Radiation of heat is one of the chief functions of the skin, protecting it against the harmful effects of fever. In hot weather or during a fever the surface blood vessels become opened or dilated, thereby increasing the amount of blood exposed to the cooling air, and at the same time increasing the production of sweat which helps in the evaporation of heat. The production of sweat is also one of the important functions of the skin. Its value as an eliminant of waste products from within the body is slight, for only volatile bodies are eliminated in the perspiration. The odor of the sweat is the chief source of body odor, now popularized as "B.O.," about which so much is said by the advertising profession. The odor is due partly to these volatile substances from within and partly to the fatty acids in the skin. While sometimes unpleasant, giving the unfortunate possessor much mental distress, cases are also on record of a pleasant, violet-like odor of the sweat, but don't count on it! Several published statements and advertisements refer to the value of chlorophyll and other substances in lessening mouth and body odor. While such agents cut down some mild odors, they will not really lessen the obnoxious odor of large amounts of garlic and similar dietary indiscretions.

Under ordinary circumstances, absorption through the outer skin is slight even for greasy substances. By friction, fats may be forced into the hair follicles and absorbed, carrying other substances with them. The quantity of such absorbed substances is so small that while it may be valuable when strong medicines are applied to the skin, for the purpose of "skin food," it is too slight to be of consequence and must be redigested by the internal organs before the skin can use it. The popular idea that oils applied to the surface can feed the skin is a fallacy. Oils or creams thus applied only serve a useful purpose by keeping the skin supple, preventing scaling and cracking, and maintaining the resistance of abnormally dry skins, even though small portions of these creams or their ingredients may be absorbed. Recently, a chemical derived from wood pulp has been found capable of absorption through the skin, and it has even been possible to add other chemicals and drugs to this substance so that they can be absorbed with it. However, several years of study will be required to evaluate the safety and long-effectiveness of this interesting chemical.

The nerves of the skin protect the body against harm by warning us of the dangers of excessive heat or cold or sharpness. They also help us to become acquainted with the world about us, and provide one of our sources of pleasure in the feel of marble, fine woods, smooth skin, velvet, and the like.

By pigment formation the skin can protect the body successfully against exposure to ordinary sunlight and ultraviolet rays. The skin cannot protect itself from overexposure to X rays and the rays of radium, and its efforts, though often manifested by pigmentation, are of no avail because these rays penetrate the pigmented skin as easily as they do the non-pigmented. And when it comes to the atomic bomb, the skin has no protective defenses whatsoever. If compensatory changes of evolution continue, we can conceive of centuries of exposure to atomic radiations resulting in a thick, bombproof skin if the human race has not been wiped out by some type of chain reaction.

Besides these more or less obvious functions of the skin, it has also the ability to clear its surface of germs within a short time. The mechanism of this action is not completely understood. Against some bacteria the skin is powerless; it cannot rid itself of them. Even against these germs the normal skin is an important first line of defense. Further, if germs do gain entrance to the skin, whether from without or through the blood stream, the normal skin can produce chemical substances which may inhibit their growth or wholly destroy them. Of course, some agents of infection are too strong to be controlled in this way, and the resistance of the skin is futile. These efforts of the skin to protect itself and the whole organism against infection often take the form of an inflammatory reaction in the skin. This skin reaction is the basis for many of the tests used to develop or determine resistance or immunity to tetanus, tuberculosis, diphtheria, scarlet fever, or other infectious diseases. Various skin tests have also been devised to detect allergic causes in asthma, hay fever, hives, and eczema. They are all of more or less value in diagnosis. Thus the skin has become a useful bureau of information, ready to report on the state of affairs in relation to protection against these diseases or on the presence of unusual sensitivities to organisms, chemicals, drugs, and the like, whenever requested to do so by the physician. Here again, we can understand why it is often referred to as the mirror of the body. In addition to its ability to protect against infection, the skin produces the vitamin (vitamin D) that protects against and cures rickets. This explains in part the beneficial effects of sun baths and ultraviolet light baths, particularly for infants. Nevertheless, the sun is a two-edged sword and although it may have beneficial effects on some skins, it may have deleterious effects on others—especially those with fair skin, red, or blond hair and light-colored eyes.

Of course, there are still many functions connected with the skin about whose purpose we can only speculate. For example, we know that the secretion of the oil glands or sebum is of primary value in keeping the skin normally lubricated and also to supply a small amount of lubrication for the hairs. Another function of the oily secretion is to prevent the absorption of any toxic or poisonous material through the surface of the skin. Accordingly, if we wish to treat a certain area of skin with some drug or medication in a grease, it is important to wash the area thoroughly to remove its normal oily secretion and thus to get penetration of the specific drug contained in the externally applied grease.

Finally, one of the most unusual and important functions of the skin is to renew itself after it has been injured. The human being cannot quite compare with the lobster which can regrow a claw after it has lost one, but the skin certainly does show remarkable powers of regeneration. Very frequently extremely extensive areas of the skin will have been lost or injured, as in an accident or a severe burn. In many instances, these areas will completely regrow without leaving a trace of the original injury. However, if the injury has been extensive and deep, the normal skin will not regrow but the area will be replaced with a different type of tissue called scar tissue. Sometimes it is necessary to help the regrowth of this tissue by performing grafts with skin taken from other parts of the body. Modern science has made great strides in this direction and even now there are many ways in which ugly and disfiguring scars can be made almost insignificant in appearance.

NUTRITION

From a general point of view, proper diet is fundamental as far as the health of the skin is concerned. Faddist regimes and so-called health diets are not essential as far as the skin is concerned. A well-balanced diet, with proper attention to balanced meals and adequate vitamin and mineral intake is of fundamental importance. As shown in the chapter on diet, certain foods are required for health.

Special diets should be avoided unless you are allergic to some particular component of a diet. There are also certain diseases in which special diets are indicated, and the skin has its share of such disorders. In the last few years there has been much research concerning the fact that the skin is often the first indicator of a serious deficiency in the diet, and much has been written concerning the role of vitamins in the skin health.

In the following brief survey the vitamins are considered primarily from the point of view of their internal administration related to the skin and not from external application.

VITAMIN A

When vitamin A is missing from the diet, the effect on the entire system is pronounced. Some of these effects of vitamin A deficiency are lowered resistance to infection, poor appetite, disturbed digestion, eye disease called xerophthalmia, and loss of hair. The condition of the skin is also changed in deficient states. Generally, it becomes dry, rough, and darker than normal. Small spots, resembling goose flesh, appear on the arms and thighs, and gradually spread to involve the leg, abdomen, buttocks, and neck. Sometimes these tiny lumps resemble acne. Confirmation of the diagnosis of A deficiency may be obtained by various technical means, such as the biomicroscopic examination of the eyes under slit lamp illumination. Estimation of the vitamin A level in the blood is also helpful in diagnosis. The minimum daily requirements of vitamin A are approximately 4000 U.S.P. units. The treatment dose ranges from 10,000 to 300,000 units daily. Large amounts of vitamin A should not be taken over long periods of time without medical supervision because an excess of this vitamin may give rise to toxic manifestations. Surprisingly enough, one of these symptoms may be loss of hair.

VITAMIN B COMPLEX

Slight deficiencies of this vitamin lead to a decreased appetite, fatigue, and burning sensations of the hands and feet.

Vitamin B_2 or riboflavin is well distributed in our diet, and so deficiency states are not too common. A deficiency of it leads to itching and burning of the eyes, dimness of the vision, and a sensitivity to light. The skin shows characteristic changes as a result of a deficiency of riboflavin. These changes include scaling and redness of the lips, cracks at the angles of the mouth, and an oily scale on the nose and ears. These changes about the eye and mouth have been called "sharklike" in appearance. The tongue is usually bright and red and shiny. The minimum daily requirement is 2 milligrams.

Vitamin P-P, or niacin or nicotinic acid, is still another member of the B complex. A deficiency of it leads to the disease known as pellagra. In medical parlance, this disease is known to produce the three D's—dermatitis (skin rash), diarrhea (intestinal upsets), and dementia (mental changes). The victim is usually nervous, restless, and easily fatigued, and complains of vague aches and pains. The skin changes are present on the exposed parts of the body (hands and face) and vaguely suggest sunburn. The minimum daily requirement is approximately 25 milligrams.

Vitamin B_6 or pyridoxine is considered necessary to the body because of its role in aiding in the use of certain essential fats in the food. This may be the reason for the lessened secretion of fat from the skin when pyridoxine is given to persons with oily and greasy faces. It may even help clear up the excessive oiliness and blackhead formation of a sufferer from acne or "pimples." Nothing is known of the minimal daily requirements of this vitamin. Therapeutically, as high as 1000 milligrams daily have been used.

Pantothenic acid, another part of the B complex, is of interest in view of its alleged effects on hair. Also, a deficiency of it may be a factor in the development of gray hair. This effect may occur indirectly through its effects on the glands, as its exclusion from animal diet leads to the destruction of several of the glands of internal secretion. Workers in the field have not been able to demonstrate an exact relationship between the results in animals and in human beings. Accordingly, its value in the treatment of color changes of the hair is very questionable, as is discussed subsequently under the heading of gray hair. The daily requirements are not known, although 1000 milligrams are tolerated therapeutically.

Inositol, a little known factor of the B complex, is a substance of extreme interest to scientists engaged in the study of hair growth. Experimental investigation has shown that inositol will cure baldness in mice. This dramatic change can sometimes be produced within as short a period as three days. This definite growth response has been checked by workers in different laboratories. The relationship of inositol to human baldness has been investigated and proved of no value. Effects produced in laboratory animals cannot be applied directly to human beings. Perhaps the future will unveil some agent which will prove to be a specific stimulant to hair growth but the mystery remains to be solved.

Biotin, or vitamin H, is a term employed in the past to designate a number of different substances, but it is now considered a member of the B complex. Biotin concentrates prevent a scaly rash in chicks, but its importance to the human still remains to be clarified.

Para-aminobenzoic acid, still another B-complex factor, has also received widespread publicity as a cure for gray hair. This publicity followed the announcement that this vitamin restored the black color to the hair of rats which had become gray on a diet deficient in the substance. This is another of those unfortunate examples of the ease with which a gullible public may be misled by results obtained in animals. Well-controlled studies on human beings have failed to substantiate the claims advanced for this substance. No drugs have been discovered, as yet, which will restore gray hairs to their natural color.

Choline is the last member of the vitamin B complex of any importance at the date of the present writing. It is related to growth, the metabolism of food, and the prevention of fatty livers in animals. It is still in the investigative stage.

VITAMIN C

Lack of this vitamin is the cause of scurvy. The value of foods containing it, as being anti-scorbutic, was recognized long before the vitamin principle was known. Whalers and other ships bound on long voyages kept supplies of lime juice and lemons and potatoes aboard as preventives of scurvy. The British sailor was called a "limey" for this reason. This disease manifests itself by bleeding gums, hemorrhage into various joints, swelling, and bloody diarrhea. The skin changes are of particular interest because they are easily seen and enable the doctor to make an early diagnosis. The changes consist of red spots around the hair follicles and openings of the sweat pores. This is most common on the legs and thighs or wherever pressure exposes the extreme weakness and fragility of the small blood vessels. Irritability, lack of stamina, and retardation of growth may be due to insufficient amounts of this substance, and there also results a susceptibility to infectious diseases. The minimal daily requirement is 600 U.S.P. units.

VITAMIN D

Vitamin D is abundant in the liver of fishes, chiefly the codfish. The discovery of this vitamin disclosed the secret of rickets. This disease is characterized by enlargement of the wrists, knees, and ankles, bowed legs, and other bony changes. It is closely tied with the absorption and use of the minerals, calcium and phosphorus. Accordingly, it is of importance in the growth and development of normal teeth. A very interesting fact here is that ultraviolet rays can produce the same effect on the bodily health and growth as vitamin D; and, as a matter of fact, children suffering from rickets improve miraculously under the ultraviolet-ray therapy, provided other necessary minerals and substances are present in the body. The minimal daily requirement is 400 to 1200 U.S.P. units.

VITAMIN E

The wide distribution of vitamin E in natural foods has led to the belief that human deficiency of this vitamin is not likely. This vitamin was reported of value with respect to the healing of wounds and ulcers of the skin, but such reports have not been substantiated. The normal requirements of this vitamin are unknown. It is usually prescribed in the form of mixed tocopherols.

This brief discussion of the vitamins is merely intended to show that they are of importance as far as the health of the skin is concerned. It must always be remembered that vitamins are essential to health as accessory food factors and that they are not the *only* important factors from a dietary standpoint, despite the tremendous advertising campaigns which might lead us to believe otherwise. To maintain proper health of the body and the skin, proteins, carbohydrates, and fats and a number of mineral salts are also necessary. Some of the minerals of particular importance as far as the skin is concerned are calcium, phosphorus, iron, sulfur, and other substances.

INTESTINAL FUNCTION

The health of the skin is definitely influenced by the functions of the intestinal tract. Failure to eliminate waste through the bowels and absorption of toxic substance from the bowels injures the proper sanitation and nutrition of the skin. For many years great stress has been laid upon the importance of inner cleanliness to skin health. Although this is true in great measure, it must be realized that the term "constipation" is a much overworked and little understood word. A slight degree of constipation is preferable to looseness, although healthy evacuation is more important. The irritative effect of cathartics on the bowels may favor the absorption of the so-called toxic agents they are intended to eliminate. Obviously, the routine administration of laxatives is to be deplored as it leads to looseness of the stools with consequent lack of muscular effect and tone, with resultant aggravation of the very condition which it is desired to cure. Today it is known that there is little absorption of poisonous toxins if the bowel contents are solid, but that unhealthy absorption of such contents may occur when they are rendered on the soft or even loose side, and that in this state bacterial decomposition is even greater. As far as the skin is concerned, the proper functioning of the intestines is important, and this should be regulated by diet and medical guidance, rather than by the constant use of cathartics. People who take mineral oil for constipation must recognize that mineral oil depletes the body's source of vitamin A, a vitamin, as we have already learned, of considerable importance as far as the skin is concerned. Where it is essential that the mineral oil be continued (and its medical usage has greatly decreased) the intake of vitamin A should be considerably increased.

THE ENDOCRINE GLANDS

The last decade has witnessed great strides in the direction of knowledge of the glandular secretions and their functions as far as the skin is concerned. These glands supply substances known as hormones which have profound effects on the skin and the structures within the skin.

THYROID

If hypothyroidism develops early in life, the individual remains small; the hair becomes dry, thin, and brittle. If an adult develops hypothyroidism, the condition is usually known as myxedema. The skin develops a peculiar swollen appearance, especially over the forehead, cheeks, nose, and lips. The skin is sallow or yellowish in color and dry, coarse, and cold to the touch. The nails are thin and brittle, and sweating is much diminished. The hair tends to fall out or is short, thin, and dry. It is often entirely absent on the chin, under the arms, and around the sex organs. The outer third of the eyebrows is frequently missing.

Overactivity of the gland leads to hyperthyroidism or excessive secretion of thyroxine. This produces an increased metabolism, loss of weight (body fuel is burned up too rapidly), and a rapid pulse. In addition, excessive sweating, shortness of breath, and nervous symptoms are usually present. The latter include trembling of the hands and fingers, restlessness, fidgety motions, mental irritability, and troubled sleep. The eyes occasionally protrude and the heart may become enlarged. The skin becomes hot and flushed. The hair is usually thin and silky. The nails are frequently lined and ridged. Treatment consists of the proper use of iodine (especially the newer radioactive salts), and surgical removal. Milder cases respond to sedation and drug therapy, especially to drugs of the thiouracil group.

PARATHYROID

These glands are small bean-shaped masses located in pairs above and below the thyroid. A deficiency of the secretion from these glands gives rise to a condition known as tetany. In this disease the nerves become irritable. The nails are ridged and brittle and the teeth show defects of the enamel. In animals the hair frequently falls out, and this occasionally occurs in humans.

ADRENAL

The cortex, or outer part of the adrenal glands, has a direct relationship to the skin and to hair growth. A deficiency of the secretion of the cortex produces a condition known as Addison's disease. In this disease the victim shows extreme fatigue following a slight exertion. A peculiar pigmentation often develops which first attracts the patient's friends. The degree of color ranges from a bright yellow to a bronze-brown or tan, so white persons are often mistaken for mulattoes. The pigmentation may be difficult to distinguish from "sun tan," for, in both, the color is deeper on exposed parts. The patient gradually loses weight, the blood pressure drops, and diarrhea occurs. If treatment is not instituted, death may result. Primarily, it is in conditions due to hyperfunction (overactivity) of the adrenal cortex that we see effects on the hair structures. Overactivity of this gland gives rise to a peculiar chain of symptoms. In affected people there is an increase in hair over the entire body. This hair growth may be very heavy. The eyebrows are usually bushy and thick. The skin becomes thick and the sweat glands large. It is the overfunction of this gland in children which produces the so-called "infant Hercules." These children are much taller than their age, of broad stature, great muscular development, and especially well-developed sex organs. A boy of five may require daily shaving and have the hairy chest and mature sexual organs of an adult. A girl of five may have well-developed breasts, hair around the genital region, and may even menstruate. An adult woman may show the secondary sex characteristics of a man (growth of a beard, deep voice, and flat chest). The new wonder drug, cortisone, is produced by the adrenal cortex. It has been found helpful in the treatment of certain skin diseases. It must be taken with great caution because of certain side effects. As far as the skin is concerned, these side effects include the development of acne and the growth of facial hair.

PITUITARY

In those people who suffer from an oversecretion of the anterior pituitary growth factor, in addition to their tremendous increase in size, the skin becomes dry and yellowish in color. The entire body usually shows an increased growth of hair. In individuals who show an oversecretion of the pituitary sex hormone, a peculiar group of symptoms may develop. These symptoms also appear when ACTH (one of the pituitary hormones) or cortisone is administered in the treatment of disease. These symptoms include a rapidly progressing weight increase of the face (moon face), neck, and abdomen (buffalo type). In addition, these individuals develop high blood pressure and peculiar purplish lines on the abdomen. An extreme degree of hairiness is present. In conditions due to an undersecretion of this pituitary sex hormone, the individuals are known as Fröhlich types. Pickwick's "fat boy" is an example of this disorder. The victims are fat around the face, breasts, abdomen, and hips. The skin is delicate, soft, and cool. Dryness, falling hair, and nail changes are rare. The genitals remain undeveloped and infantile. Even when maturity is reached, the men have a distinctly feminine appearance and manner. The face remains hairless, fat deposits occur about the hips, and the voice remains high-pitched.

The posterior lobe of the pituitary has various effects on the blood pressure, lungs, intestines, and kidneys, but it bears no known relationship to skin changes or hair growth.

The pituitary gland has been the target of intensive research over the past few decades. It has been found to contain new and fascinating hormones such as the melanocyte stimulating hormone (MSH) which has specific effects on skin color, a sebotropic hormone which affects oil secretion and several other amazing substances. Perhaps in the future we shall be able to control skin color, oil secretion, and even hair growth with one or several pituitary hormones. What a way to solve racial problems!

MALE SEX GLANDS

The testes are the primary sex glands of man. They produce secretions which are responsible for the male appearance and development. They also produce the sperm cells, which are responsible for the propagation of the race following fertilization of the eggs produced by the female organs of reproduction. The secretion produced by the testes include the androgens or male sex hormones. These hormones are extremely potent, and a study of their behavior effects in animals is amusing; female canaries given male hormones sing like males, and hens crow; the social order of chickens can be manipulated, because birds receiving the hormone become very domineering and quarrelsome. A deficiency of this hormone in humans leads to retention of a high-pitched voice, reduction of hair growth, particularly around the sex organs and the chin, a slim figure, and poorly developed sex organs. The extreme form of this deficiency is evident in castrated individuals or eunuchs. It is extremely interesting to note that these people rarely if ever lose the hair from their head. Whether this fact is due to a deficiency of androgen or to other secretions contained in the testes, or through remote effects on other organs, is discussed in detail under the heading of hair growth. An excessive amount of male hormones is also considered to play a causative role in the development of acne or "pimples," and this fact must be considered when treating resistant or severe cases of this disease.

FEMALE SEX ORGANS

The ovaries are two in number and are located on each side of the lower abdomen. The ovaries usually produce one egg each month. Fertilization of the egg leads to pregnancy. The ovarian hormones are responsible for the characteristics of the female and influence the development of the breasts, uterus, and accessory female organs of reproduction. At the time of puberty these secretions lead to slight alterations in the voice, the enlargement of the breasts, and the acquisition of feminine characteristics. They also influence the development of hair under the arms and around the genitals. The average woman goes through several periods of glandular change. The first of these occurs at puberty, then at sexual maturity, and finally following the menopause or change of life. During the first cycle, an irregularity of the secretions may lead to acne of the face, chest, and back, and an increased hair growth on the face. The hair may also be affected at the time of the menopause when there is frequently an increased fall of hair from the scalp and a thinning of the individual hairs. Due to lessened activity of the oil glands, dryness of the skin may also accompany the menopause. Pregnancy may also be followed by a diffuse loss of hair, which is usually due to a temporary lack of hormones almost in the nature of a "miniature menopause." The hair lost during this period usually grows back. Pregnancy may also be accompanied by an increased growth of facial hair. Certain tumors of the ovary and the adrenal cortex are frequently accompanied by masculine changes in the affected women, as shown by an increased growth of hair over the entire body but especially on the face, under the arms, and around the genitals. This is due to an excessive production of male hormones similar chemically to cortisone and ACTH, and the same changes may also be produced by these drugs.

ALLERGY (HYPERSENSITIVITY)

Many skin conditions are produced or aggravated by a peculiar idiosyncrasy to a food, a drug, or some external application. Many people show an unusual susceptibility in their reactions to various foods and develop annoying rashes on their skins if they eat these foods. The most common offenders are eggs, strawberries, fish, chocolate, and related substances. In the majority of cases these foods produce a skin reaction known as "hives" or urticaria, which shows itself as itchy, raised "bumps" frequently shifting to involve different parts of the body. This is not always the case, as there are various other forms of skin reactions to foods and drugs. Sometimes it is possible to determine the offending agent by performing so-called skin or allergy tests. The suspected agent is either injected into the skin or scratched into the surface of the skin, and the sensitivity of the individual is determined by the development of an irritative patch of skin around the tested site. These tests are not infallible, and in many instances the allergic manifestation can only be brought out by swallowing the food or actually taking the drug, rather than by the performance of skin tests. The doctor must always be on the lookout for these drug eruptions as there are many old and new drugs which are capable of producing such reactions. In the early days of penicillin therapy this wonder drug was considered completely harmless, but as time went on numerous people were found to be sensitive to penicillin in various forms. Many of the newer drugs which are constantly being discovered are heralded in the beginning as completely harmless and incapable of doing damage. As their usage continues for long periods of time, many side effects and complications are observed to develop, and the skin is often the first to show these complications.

NERVOUS TENSION AND EMOTIONAL DISORDERS

Many eruptions on the skin are related to nervous tension, emotional upsets, and the like. We have all become familiar with the term "psychosomatic" and recognize the fact that it means the interplay of body functions with emotional or psychic factors. At present many diseases are called psychosomatic or "nervous" which are not entitled to the use of this term. Before dismissing a skin complaint as being due to nerves or emotions, it is advisable to obtain the opinion of your doctor first. The great strides that are being made in medicine are still due to the early recognition of disease rather than dismissing it on the basis of some emotional upset. Nevertheless, relaxation and rest are helpful in the treatment of many disorders of the skin, and understanding and insight into your own emotional background is also of great benefit. We have advanced too far in the treatment of ulcers, heart disease, and similar illnesses from the standpoint of their origin along the lines of emotional difficulties ever to dismiss the subject lightly in the matter of long-standing and resistant skin conditions. Our modern daily life provides many factors of tension and strain. The nerves especially suffer from the tension under which we live, and the skin is indirectly affected by it. Where skin disturbances are associated with an accompanying emotional disturbance, the physician can be of great help in assisting the patient to express his fears and worries, and to bring them out in the open for a frank discussion and understanding of their nature. It is amazing how much benefit can be observed in some chronic skin conditions following a reassuring discussion and a helpful adjustment in a life situation.

THE CARE OF THE NORMAL SKIN

It is of importance to understand how to take care of the skin and how to apply external preparations to keep it healthy and free from disease. The measures discussed in the following paragraphs are those accepted as adequate for maintaining a healthy skin.

BATHING

Local care is, of course, of great importance to the skin. Besides the removal of grease and dirt, bathing, particularly if the bath is ended with a cold shower, has a beneficial effect on the circulation. This is accentuated by the rubbing necessary to drying, especially because of the feeling of vigor consequent on the cold shower. Frequency of bathing is an individual problem. Some find frequent bathing enervating, while on others it has the opposite effect. Some people do not react well to cold baths and therefore should not take them. Often such persons react better to a mild application of cool water and can train themselves to the cold shower by gradual increase in the duration and decrease in the temperature of the bath. People with dry skins should not bathe frequently because constant washing removes their own meager supply of oil and merely degreases and defats a skin which desperately requires all of its own available oil supply.

The use of soap in the bath is to be regulated according to the kind of bath and the kind of skin that is being bathed, and according to the season of the year. In the summertime we perspire so profusely that soap can be used more freely by most of us. In fact, we usually start to produce more sweat and oil immediately following the bath, and there is no danger of depriving the skin of the oil necessary to its welfare. In winter, however, the skin secretes less sweat and oil, the cold air is dry, and so is the warm, overdried air of our steam-heated dwellings. Frequent bathing only serves to aggravate the dryness of the skin. The skin resents it by becoming flaky and itchy, especially after a bath. This can be corrected by limiting the use of soap during the winter months to the armpits and groin and to the parts that get the dirtiest, the hands and feet.

Some women and a few men find that their abnormally dry skins will not tolerate soap on the face at any season. The skin becomes scaly and itches and, if the irritation is carried farther, becomes red in patches, the condition known as chapping. For such people cold cream is a justifiable substitute for soap. More refreshing, however, is oatmeal water, made by boiling oatmeal for five minutes in a bag made of several layers of gauze. A handful of oatmeal should suffice in a gallon of water. It removes dirt better than plain water, taking the place of soap to a considerable degree, and can be used on some irritable skins with impunity. The introduction of sulfonated oils as soap substitutes for cleansing the skin has given us another method, valuable for those whose skins are sensitive to soap. The best of these oils are acid in reaction, as is the surface of the normal skin, and they cleanse without forming suds and without drying the skin. Those with greasy skins, however, must recognize that these methods are not for them; but that their skins are best cared for by vigorous washing with hot water and soap, followed by a cold shower.

For long periods of immersion in water, as in the use of a tub bath containing some medication intended to soothe the skin, the water temperature is best kept lukewarm. Ordinarily, both hot and cold baths are stimulating, and the greatest effect of this kind is obtained from a hot bath followed by a cold shower, which stimulates the circulation, preventing chilling and increasing resistance against infection. Rubbing the skin with the hands or the washcloth while in the water and vigorous rubbing while drying assist in obtaining this effect. The duration of the bath should be short, unless a soothing effect is desired. We are all aware of the relaxing and soothing effects of a warm bath at night. On the other hand, a short cold shower in the morning is stimulating and helps wake one up in preparation for a day of activity. Sweat baths, among which the Turkish bath is the most popular, are not essential and are, in fact, enervating. If benefit can be derived from them, they should be taken with the approval of the physician. The same rule applies to medicated baths, mud baths, and sulphur baths, for under some circumstances they may prove to be too much of a strain and should, therefore, not be taken indiscriminately. Certain types of skin conditions are made worse by excessive sweating, and this type of bathing is absolutely contraindicated in the presence of these disorders.

Open-air bathing is one of the most popular of the sports of today and of past ages, and deservedly so. At the beginning of the season care should be used to avoid too long exposure to the sun, and the same warning applies to those who go to the southern beaches during the winter. The skin, long protected from light, cannot stand much of it at first. Severe sunburn damages rather than benefits and should be avoided. This applies particularly to people with blue eyes and light complexions, inasmuch as constant exposure of such skins to strong sunlight may eventually lead to extreme dryness, warty growths, and even cancer of the skin.

SOAP

The surroundings of our present-day life, with constant exposure to the smoke and dirt of the cities, make frequent washing and the use of a good soap a necessity rather than a luxury.

As the result of the application of modern scientific research, there have been tremendous advances and changes in the formulation of soaps. A good soap must cleanse the skin thoroughly without irritation and without removing all of the skin oils. It should not be harsh nor excessively alkaline. It should preferably produce a thick creamy lather in both soft and hard water, without leaving an insoluble scum in the water. The manufacturing chemist has set his sights on the production of such a preparation, and there are several excellent soaps on the market. When fats are boiled with a solution of an alkali, they are split into glycerin and fatty acids and the latter unite with the alkali to form soap. The glycerin is a valuable by-product. Potassium hydrate forms soft soap, of which the green soap used in the hospital is the familiar example. Sodium hydrate forms hard soaps such as ordinary laundry or toilet soap. The solution of these in water is viscid, that is, it has the power of holding together, illustrated by the formation of bubbles, which are globules of air separated from the rest of the air by a film of soap. This viscid character of soapsuds enables it to emulsify the grease on the skin, carrying with it the dirt, and they both then dissolve in the water and are carried away.

In the making of soap there is always a part of the alkali not combined with the fatty acids, and this is the "free alkali" so often mentioned in connection with toilet soap. It makes the soap strong, loosening the dirt and grease so that it can better be removed. For rough work considerable free alkali is needed; but for the average skins it is desirable that the free alkali should be reduced to the minimum. Strong soap removes more fat from the skin than is good for its health and leaves it red and irritated, an easy victim to skin eruptions and infection. In good toilet soap the free alkali should not exceed ¼ of 1 per cent. For dry and delicate skins superfatted soap is made by removing as much as possible of the free alkali and adding wool fat. This does not become rancid and leaves a film upon the skin to replace that removed in washing. These superfatted soaps are only a little less efficient as cleansers than the regular soaps and are particularly recommended for infants and for older persons with dry skins. There are also available a number of new soap substitutes and milder cleansing agents for the dry and sensitive skin.

Green soap is strong; that is, it contains a considerable amount of free alkali. The surgeon prefers it because of this fact, in order to get his hands and arms as free from germs as possible. Not uncommonly, however, he suffers from its irritating quality. Pure green soap is not green but yellow. At present most hospitals have discontinued green soap because of its harsh reactions on the skin after long periods of use. Some of the newer antiseptics, such as hexachlorophene, are even more germicidal in action, and may be incorporated in a mild soap mixture, thereby minimizing the dangers of skin irritation.

Hard water soaps are often only ordinary soaps with an excess of coconut oil. This oil enables them to form suds more readily with water containing too much calcium. Coconut oil is an ingredient of most soaps and is not harmful as long as the amount is small; but in excess it may be irritating to delicate skins.

There are now available various types of water softener. When these substances are added to hard water, they prevent the combination of calcium and soap, thus softening the water and enabling it to form soapsuds more readily. The solution of such a salt in hard water prevents the deposit on the skin of a scum which holds and protects bacteria. Thus the water softener aids in ridding the surface of the skin of infectious agents. Sodium hexametaphosphate is one of the best softening agents.

Soap is not only cleansing in its action, but actually kills most of the ordinary germs. Unfortunately, two, the typhoid bacillus and that cause of most of the boils and other skin infections, the ubiquitous staphylococcus, are able to resist it. At present we maintain the normal germ-killing efficiency of the skin by proper care but we also attempt direct action upon the bacteria with antiseptics combined in soap.

The best soaps usually contain approximately 20 to 30 per cent of water. The best type of soap is a comparatively neutral form containing no more than ¼ to 1 per cent of free alkali. Transparent soaps contain more water, 25 to 35 per cent. Floating soaps also contain large amounts of water, although their brilliancy is due to the air stirred into them during their manufacture. Superfatted soaps are milder and less irritating due to the fact that the alkali has been neutralized by the addition of lanolin. A good soap need not be expensive, as the well-known brands put out by the leading manufacturers are usually priced within a reasonable range. For the average skin they are adequate. The highly perfumed soaps made up in expensive packages and given misleading names are not superior to the average inexpensive toilet soap. As a matter of fact, they are frequently less effective from the standpoint of cleansing and minimal irritation. Choose a soap adapted to your need and made by a leading manufacturer, and it should be adequate for the average skin.

POWDERS

Dusting powders and face powders are soothing, cooling, and drying, as well as protective and decorative. Each tiny particle of powder acts to increase the available surface for the evaporation of insensible perspiration, thus cooling and drying the skin. It also protects against the irritation of cold air or sunshine and the rubbing of clothing. The requirements for a good powder are that it be fine and non-irritating. Talcum is the best known and most widely used powder. It is of light weight, very fine texture, and adheres well to the skin. Zinc stearate is heavier and also a good adherent. The starches, potato, wheat, or corn, are useful but absorb moisture and swell, making them less desirable where moisture is present in any quantity. Boric acid in small amounts is often added to dusting powders for its action in deterring the growth of germs. Stout people and babies are the chief beneficiaries of dusting powders. Without them, they are apt to suffer from irritation in the folds of the skin (armpits, groin, buttocks), known as intertrigo. In applying powder to the infant, great care should be taken to have it in one of the patent containers made to prevent the possibility of the baby getting the open end of the container into its mouth, for severe consequences have been caused by the baby's shaking an antiseptic powder (boric acid) into its mouth and inhaling it. For this reason I prefer a bland type of baby powder with a minimum of added antiseptic ingredients. Where the skin folds are irritated (as in the diaper region), a powder of a more adherent nature with water-repellent powers is advisable.

Since powders are widely used on account of the smooth and cooling feeling which they give to the skin, they must be correctly formulated in order to exert this cooling effect. Although a good powder could be made from talc alone, it would not have good absorbing properties, and for that reason various metallic salts are usually added. In addition, when powders are used as aids to the complexion, they must have additional chemicals added in order to cover defects of the skin and to lessen the shine of the oil secretion. Unfortunately, the trend in recent years has been to mask completely the shine due to the secretions of the sweat and sebaceous glands, and the resultant powder gives a smooth, masklike appearance to the face. Aside from the appearance, the use of these heavy powders (cake make-up, theatrical bases) results in the undesirable side effect of blocking the skin secretions for a period of time. The constant use of heavy foundations and cake make-up, without adequate cleansing of the skin, often results in the appearance of blackheads and other minor complexion difficulties, much to the distress of the wearer. If a woman must use a heavy type of make-up base, she should apply it infrequently and cleanse her skin thoroughly following its use.

LOTIONS

Most lotions are actually water solutions containing powder. The usual preparation often requires thorough shaking prior to its use. The lotion is then spread on the skin and allowed to dry. The evaporation of the fluid leads to a cooling off of the skin, and the residual coat of powder which it leaves on the skin continues its action and so soothes both normal and inflamed skin. The well-known calamine lotion is just such a mixture. Part of its effectiveness is due to the fact that it is extremely bland and cannot irritate or aggravate an already inflamed skin. If most home remedies applied to the skin were of a similar bland and harmless nature, the doctor would see fewer cases of aggravated and irritated skin disorders.

COLD CREAM

The oil in the skin is an important ingredient. It keeps the horny layer of the skin soft, flexible, and watertight and forms a thin protective film on its surface. When oil is deficient the skin becomes rough, dry, and scaly, often inflamed, and much more liable to infection. The owner of such a skin is notified of this condition by a feeling of stiffness or even itching or pain. In common words, the skin is chapped. This happens most often in the winter, when cold dry winds are prevalent. To counteract it, oil may be supplied to the skin in the form of cold cream, supplementing nature. Creams are oils that contain water. When applied to the skin, the water evaporates and the cream absorbs water from the skin. If there is inflammation present, this results in a cooling of the skin, whence the name, cold cream. To avoid the overly frequent removal of oil by ordinary washing with soap and water, cold cream is rubbed on the skin and wiped off, removing much of the dirt with it. This does not compare, of course, with the cleansing attained by the use of soap, but is fairly efficient. Cleanliness may be next to godliness, but is not an unmixed blessing for those with dry skins. It can be overdone, or, rather, it can be done in the wrong way. In those with greasy skins, however, cream is harmful if it takes the place of hot water and soap cleansing. Cream adds to the grease already too plentiful in the skin, and in cases of blackheads and acne increases the tendency to form pus pimples.

Many different fats are available for anointing the skin; but cold cream, ointment of rose water, a perfumed emulsion of fat and water, is deservedly the most popular. There are many formulas for it; but all have about the same effect upon the skin. Light, soft creams are called cleansing creams and are sometimes advertised as "skin foods," which of course is a misnomer and a false claim, for the skin is fed only through the stomach, as the rest of the body is fed. Other preparations advertised as greaseless cold creams and recommended as cleansing creams are not creams at all but soaps made with sodium carbonate. Of course, they cleanse better than real cold cream, but they also defeat the purpose of creams, for they take oil out of the skin instead of adding to it. Some cold creams become rancid in time. This can be delayed by adding a small amount of boric acid, 5 or 10 per cent, to the cream. Many of the commercial cold creams are now made with petrolatum (mineral oil) in place of animal fats. Petrolatum is not a fat, but a derivative of petroleum which has many of the properties of fats but does not become rancid.

Creams are best used at bedtime following thorough washing of the skin with soap and water. From the point of view of their true value, the chief use of creams is to cleanse and protect the skin as well as to supply a small amount of oil and fat when the skin is on the dry side. In recent years there has been a great deal of discussion concerning the value of hormones in creams as an aid in minimizing the aging process. Up to the present time there has been no specific proof that hormones in creams will halt or lessen the process of wrinkle formation and maintain or produce a constant state of rejuvenation. If you are actually deficient in sex hormones, they should be administered in adequate dosage by your physician. It is very difficult for the average person to read between the lines of a skillful advertisement proclaiming an easy method for obtaining glamour and facial beauty. Experts in the field can do no more than advise caution and intelligence in reading highly publicized reports concerning a new easy road to perpetual youth and a beautiful complexion.

ANTISEPTICS

For application to small wounds, tincture of iodine is probably the most widely known antiseptic. It should be painted on, one coat only. More than this does not add to the good effect and increases the danger of irritation. The bottle must be kept tightly stoppered, preferably with a rubber stopper, for if the tincture is exposed to the air it evaporates and becomes so strong that even one application may cause a severe reaction. After iodine has been applied, no preparation of mercury should be used on the same area for several days for fear of an unpleasant skin irritation. The stain of iodine can be removed by alcohol, and it is usually advisable to follow an iodine application with an alcohol application.

Boric acid in saturated solution is a popular household remedy. Though it does not kill germs, it limits their growth and is soothing rather than irritating to inflamed skin. It should be made by filling a clean (boiled or scalded) fruit jar or large bottle one fourth full of the boric acid crystals, then adding boiled water to fill the jar. When this has cooled, it is a saturated solution, and what is needed can be poured off. By keeping crystals at the bottom, water above, a saturated solution is always ready for use. These bottles must be carefully labeled and kept in a safe place out of the reach of a child, as the solution is poisonous if swallowed. For infections, the boric acid solution should be heated and applied on a large dressing covered to retain heat as long as possible. For most acute skin irritations, however, it is best applied cool on a thin compress, allowing for evaporation. The compress should be kept thoroughly saturated if it is to be effective.

The solution of hydrogen peroxide is a useful household remedy. It does not kill germs, except those that cannot grow in the presence of oxygen. These occur in the mouth and other cavities of the body. More often, peroxide is used for cleansing wounds. It attacks and destroys pus and blood, and at the same time gets into small crevices where it forms oxygen gas and loosens dirt so that it can be wiped or washed away. It should not be applied too frequently as it may delay the healing of a wound. Care must be taken not to put peroxide into a cavity from which it cannot easily escape, for under these circumstances the gas may form under pressure and cause great pain and actual damage to the tissues.

Carbolic acid, often used in the household, is a dangerous chemical. It does not dissolve well in water, and when the attempt is made to make such a solution, concentrated carbolic acid often comes into contact with the skin and burns it. It should be used only under the direction of the doctor.

Within the past few years many new drugs and chemicals have been discovered. These agents have the common effect of killing or at least inhibiting many of the organisms which are present on the surface of the skin. A partial list of their names would have to include the sulfa drugs, penicillin, bacitracin, streptomycin, terramycin, aureomycin, chloromycetin, and many others. Although these drugs are effective from the standpoint of sterilizing the surface of the skin, they should be taken only under the supervision of a physician because of their capability of producing undesirable toxic or allergic reactions. Also their use in a skin cream for a minor infection may result in the development of an allergy to the drug, thereby preventing its use at some later date, for a more serious internal infection.

WET DRESSINGS

Wet dressings are helpful in the treatment of minor skin disorders, and some of them have already been described under the heading of antiseptics. Sometimes the application of a wet solution to an inflamed area of skin will accomplish a remarkable degree of healing and soothing action within a short period of time. In most instances it is important to apply the wet dressing every few hours for at least twenty to thirty minutes. Wet dressings are one of the most effective ways of removing crusts and dried secretions from the surface of the skin and in maintaining some drainage from infected areas. They serve as very effective local applications of heat, and may also be used to prevent rapid changes in the temperature of the skin surface. They are very useful in the treatment of skin eruptions with extensive blister formation, in that they tend to open these blistered sites and bring the effective medication in the wet dressing to the irritated area. The most widely used and effective wet dressings are a weak salt solution, Burow's solution (usually used in solutions containing ten to twenty times as much water), potassium permanganate solution in a weak form (approximately 1 part of potassium permanganate to 5000 parts of water), a 2 to 5 per cent boric acid solution, and a magnesium sulfate or Epsom salt solution containing approximately ½ to 1 tablespoon of the salt to a quart of water. There are two main types of wet dressing, and it must be realized that their effects are considerably different. The open type of wet dressing, in which the solution is merely soaked in several layers of cotton or gauze and applied to the skin, is used when cooling is desired and maceration of the underlying skin is not advisable (poison ivy, burns). The so-called closed type of wet dressing, in which the layers of gauze or cotton are covered with oiled silk or cellophane, is used where local heat and maceration of the top layer of the skin are desired (boils, carbuncles).

It is important that the dressing be kept sopping wet by constantly changing the entire thickness of gauze or cotton, or applying a completely new and fresh application. The hands and feet can also be treated by merely soaking the affected part in a basin containing the solution.

MASSAGE

Massage, including rubbing and kneading, is a well-established means of maintaining circulation in those prevented by disease from exercising, and of restoring circulation to parts of the body in which it is deficient. The face, however, seldom lacks exercise. Our days are full of facial exercise. At mealtimes we chew our food thoroughly (let us hope), and between meals we talk and allow the play of our emotions to find expression on the face. The rubbing in of cold cream is not necessary, for it exerts all its benefit on being applied gently. Massage is refreshing, however, and if followed by a good washing, as it always should be, does no harm in most cases. In any active inflammatory condition of the skin massage is harmful. In acne it is of doubtful benefit, and the grease that always accompanies its application is harmful. In any real infection, such as boils, it is dangerous, particularly on the face.

STEAMING

Steaming the face or other involved parts of the skin (back, chest) is a valuable measure in greasy skins containing blackheads. It causes increased perspiration and acts more vigorously than washing with hot water. It should not be carried to the point of causing the face to get very red and should always be followed by a cold application to restore tone to the vessels. Like the hot bath, if used too frequently, it may cause drying or even chapping of the skin.

SUN BATHS AND ARTIFICIAL SUBSTITUTES

The use of arc lights and quartz mercury vapor lamps in the home is being popularized. There is no doubt of the beneficial action of these rays and of the sun's rays under proper conditions and control. Light baths of any type should be given cautiously, allowing the skin to become accustomed to the light and to respond with pigmentation, instead of being burned. People with blue eyes and fair skins should exercise particular care to protect the skin from the harmful effects of light. The overly frequent exposure of the normal skin to ultraviolet rays for the purpose of a temporary cosmetic effect is not without the possibility of ultimate harm to the skin. There are some abnormalities and diseases of the skin, as well as some internal conditions, in which light is actually harmful.

On the water or snow the reflected rays may greatly increase the degree of the skin's exposure to ultraviolet irradiation. Hats are no protection against these rays, which contain the ultraviolet rays that are most active in producing irritation. Particularly at high altitudes, their penetration is great, and the effect of sunlight much greater than its visual intensity indicates. At low altitudes these rays are largely absorbed by the atmosphere, and comparatively few of them reach us. People who are strongly sensitive to the sun may now protect themselves by the use of creams and lotions containing physical or chemical sun screens. The most effective sun screens include red veterinary petrolatum, para-aminobenzoic acid and its derivatives incorporated in greasy or greaseless bases (which may be used under make-up) and several new chemical, light protectants.

CARE OF THE SKIN AT VARIOUS PERIODS OF LIFE

INFANCY

The skin of an infant requires gentle treatment. Soap should be of the mildest superfatted kind, and even this should be employed only when absolutely necessary. It is preferable to clean an infant's skin with a bland oil containing small amounts of one of the newer and less irritating surface antiseptics such as hexachlorophene. After the bath a bland powder should be used, care being taken that the baby cannot get the opportunity to shake the powder into its mouth and lungs. The folds of the body should receive more powder than the rest of the skin. The clothing should be soft, carefully rinsed after washing, and not too heavy. Many infants are kept too warm and suffer from heat rash, which may, as a result of scratching, become infected and eventuate in more serious skin disease. Infants frequently develop chafing of the skin in the diaper region due to prolonged contact with urine and feces. This area may be protected by the application of soothing creams of a slightly water-repellent nature.

CHILDHOOD

The same rules apply as in infancy, except that the young child and the older small boy or tomboy girl require for their hands (and too often for other parts of the body) more soap and water. The mother should not, however, let her love of cleanliness carry her too far with the scrubbing process, for it is better that the child be a little less than perfectly clean rather than hampered in its exercise. Precautions against overcleanliness can be safely left to the defensive power of the child in most cases. Both boys and girls, if they have blond skin that freckles, should be urged to wear hats in the sun and to protect the skin before going outdoors. Modern sunburn protection includes the use of red veterinary petrolatum or preparations containing para-aminobenzoic acid and derivatives, as well as salol, menthyl and benzyl salicylates, and other agents. The average sunburn is effectively soothed by applications of cold, weak boric acid solutions and a mild lotion such as calamine containing 1 per cent of phenol. The fair-skinned youngster should be taught in childhood that severe sunburn is dangerous and should be taught how to protect the skin from the sun's rays.

ADOLESCENCE

The chief change seen in the skin at puberty is the greasiness which appears in so many skins at this time, often accompanied by blackheads and pimples. The measures to be described later under the heading of acne must be instituted at once, and include frequent washing with hot water and soap and the insistence on good habits of hygiene.

MIDDLE LIFE

This is the active, strenuous time, when health is most often neglected for the sake of work or even sometimes for the sake of play. Loss of sleep, irregular meals, worry, all have their effect upon the health of the skin, as well as on the rest of the body. Worry, hurry, and impatience hasten the onset of age, which is often announced too early by the condition of the skin. The use of cold cream upon the female skin becomes more generally justifiable because of lessening oil production and decreasing glandular activity.

AGE

Age brings lessened nutrition to all parts, including the skin, and the latter loses both elasticity and oil to become wrinkled and rough. The skin loses its resistance and tolerance to the sun and various chemicals such as soap. Oil should be applied artificially, soap used sparingly, and the skin protected as much as possible. If hormones are necessary, they should be used only under the guidance of a physician.

INFLAMMATIONS OF THE SKIN

ECZEMA

Years ago almost any skin disease involving a patch of red, scaling, itching, and weeping skin was attributed to eczema; no one really knew what produced the symptoms. Accordingly, at some stage in development more than half of all skin diseases were called "eczema."

Eczema is a common inflammation of the skin. Its symptoms are: redness, itching, small blisters, and the discharge from the skin of a fluid that stiffens linen and tends to dry into scales and crusts. Incidentally, eczema is *not* catching.

This sounds specific enough—but, unfortunately, many other skin diseases have exactly the same symptoms. Actually, a skin disease is called eczema when it has all the features just mentioned, and is apparently caused by some unknown agent, either inside or outside the body.

For example, a man visited his physician and complained of an eruption of this type on the outside of his thigh. Without modern scientific investigation, it was classified as eczema of an unknown origin. Later, when the eruption had spread to the hands, face, and neck, the patient became seriously worried. Again he consulted a physician, this time a specialist in diseases of the skin. The second doctor made a detailed investigation. It revealed that the patient always carried a box of matches of foreign manufacture in his trouser pocket. The box rested against his thigh at the spot where the trouble began. The doctor found that the sulphur and phosphorus mixture on the striking side of the box and also on the match heads had an irritating effect on this particular patient's skin.

This man's reaction to these chemicals was so violent that he would have become a hospital case, with an entire body rash, had the cause not been discovered and the matches removed from his pocket.

Another instance, also an actual case, concerned a woman who asked her physician about an itching, red rash on her hands and forearms, a type of irritation that many chemicals and substances produce. This woman did not normally come in contact with strong chemicals, soaps, or other irritants. She was the sort of woman who used her hands for holding cocktails, waving people out of her way, and playing Mah-Jongg (before the days of Canasta). After questioning, the doctor discovered that a friend had given her a beautiful set of Mah-Jongg tiles, made in Japan. It was finally discovered that these Japanese tiles were covered with a lacquer made from a distant relation of poison ivy! The Japanese Mah-Jongg sets sold well, and, as a result, many women developed skin rashes from playing with the "poison ivy" tiles.

Neither the woman nor the man mentioned here had eczema. If the cause of their skin eruptions had not been discovered or determined, it would have been diagnosed as eczema, for want of a better explanation.

There is a lesson to be learned from these illustrations. It is of the greatest importance for patients to provide their doctors with all details of their daily lives when consulting them about skin condition.

There are other examples of specific skin diseases.

Among these are those fellow Americans who would develop a rash on Sunday nights, after a relaxing, restful day spent on the golf course. This rash improved during the week and flared up again on Sunday night.

"Aha, my friend," exclaims Sherlock Holmes the dermatologist, "you recently purchased a new set of golf clubs."

"Yes—so what?" replies our fellow American.

Well, you've guessed it! The upper part of the club shafts were beautifully covered with a new synthetic rubber which improved his grip. Unfortunately, he had become allergic to this substance and developed a rash on his palms whenever he played golf. In fact, he subsequently became sensitive to the steering wheel of his car (synthetic rubber) and even to the non-slip rubber mat he sat on in his bath tub. This last discovery was an uncomfortable one.

From the foregoing examples, there are irritants that affect certain people and not others. Likewise, there are certain substances that affect only certain parts of the body. For example, the scalp, face, and neck may react to a hair dye, a cold wave lotion, or to a perfume; the forehead to hat bands, especially those recently cleaned; the ears and nose to plastic or metal eyeglass frames; and the eyelids and neck to nail polish. The latter may sound strange—but the damage is done by contact with the fingernails.

Underwear shorts may affect the thighs or abdomen. Plastic watch straps may inflame the wrists. Even, forgive me, nylon stockings might affect the legs!

I can hear the American housewife say: "Just give me the nylons; I'll take my chances."

And, she is right. Ill effects from wearing nylons are infrequent. Yet the few women who are susceptible can develop an annoying and itching eruption from wearing these stockings.

There are innumerable other instances where diagnoses could not be made until after long and detailed investigations. A baffling case was that of an attractive young woman on whose lips a severe itching and burning broke out. Many tests were made, with lipsticks, cosmetics, foods, and other substances. Yet these and other procedures produced no effect. At long last the cause of the irritation was tracked down—her fiancé's mustache wax!

We seem to be concerned not with what eczema is, but with what it is not. This is necessary. The importance of the cases described is that there are some diseases classified as eczema that are due to specific agents. These agents can only be discovered by means of painstaking examinations.

The number of cases classified as eczema has been shrinking steadily. It will continue to do so as our methods and means for ferreting out hitherto unknown causes improve.

For our purposes, eczema can now be defined more exactly. It is a skin eruption in which there are certain complex internal factors more important than the local existing cause. In other words, though there may be a local existing cause, such as a matchbox, Mah-Jongg tile, or mustache wax–the removal of this cause, while essential, may not effect the cure. What is more, a skin irritation due to some such simple cause may develop into an eczema. Even though you track down and remove the primary cause, the irritation process goes on as eczema.

Again heredity comes into the picture. Some people are apt to develop eczema because of family tendencies. Blondes and redheads usually have sensitive skins that are irritated by sun, wind, and other agents. People with dry or oily skins may be predisposed to skin eruptions. People with dry skins are easily irritated by soap and, in general, lack sufficient resistance to skin infections. There are people whose sweat glands do not function well. Consequently, they don't perspire enough to remove irritants from the skin or cool the body.

Poor nutrition may also cause eczema. Lack of vitamins may lower skin resistance to the disease. Lack of vitamin A can cause a type of eczema complicated by pus formation. Lack of vitamin B can cause scaling of the nose and lips. Deficiency of various elements of the vitamin B family can cause a peculiar eruption on the arms and legs.

Various internal parts of the body influence the skin in the development of eczema. Among these are poorly functioning glands, such as the thyroid and others; and upset stomachs, livers, and kidneys. Often a good doctor tracks down some unsuspected disease elsewhere in the body following an eczema clue.

These conditions, and others, can predispose a man or woman to eczema. In other words, they are indirect causes. There are also causes directly responsible for it. Some people are hypersensitive, or allergic, to drugs or proprietary remedies which may do others good. If the hypersensitive individual takes these drugs, it may easily produce a skin disorder, or predispose him to it.

If you have a skin eruption, it may be possible that a supposedly harmless laxative, tonic, or blood purifier in your medicine chest is either the cause or part of the cause of your trouble. Perhaps you get a rash in the spring or fall of the year. You probably attribute it either to the weather or astrology. It's more likely to be caused by the insect spray or moth destroyer you use during these seasons.

Of course, there are many more factors which bear on this disease than can be briefly mentioned. Nerves also enter the picture. A period of emotional tension can produce inflammation of the skin. Does this sound far-fetched? If so, reflect on what happens when you are embarrassed–

your face gets red. What happens when you're nervous or excited?—you break out in little pimples, known as "goose flesh." So—you see—mere thoughts and emotions do produce definite skin changes. When these thoughts and emotions take firm hold, they can also play an important role in the production of skin eruptions.

The patient, on being convinced that he has eczema, next wants to know the answer to the question that doctors hear many times a day, "All right, what can you do for me?"

The answer is—a great deal. One of the first jobs is to determine the cause and to eliminate it.

Another decision the doctor must make is whether the condition is acute or chronic. If it is acute, the itching must be relieved and the inflammation reduced as soon as possible. Normally, the patient will be given wet dressings and soothing lotions at this stage. The doctor will urge him to avoid such irritants as soap and water. If there are any predisposing factors—such as the matchbox, Mah-Jongg tiles, hair dyes, or hat bands—and also specific worries or digestive troubles—these must be eliminated or modified.

In chronic or long-standing eczema, the skin becomes thick and leathery. The irreverent medical student calls it "pigskin" or "elephant's hide." When this stage is reached, the cure becomes a long and difficult task. It is important for the doctor to study the patient minutely, to eliminate all potential irritants. Each person presents an individual problem. The doctor must decide what investigation and laboratory tests to make and he must analyze and interpret the results.

In recent years, cortisone and its derivatives have been found to be of great value in certain chronic skin disorders. This drug may be given by mouth, by injection directly into the diseased area, or applied locally in the form of an ointment or lotion. When applied locally, the doctor may advise covering the total area with an occlusive plastic film in order to insure the effectiveness of the drug. This method is usually reserved for chronic, resistant patches of skin disease.

A word of warning—if a local remedy is prescribed—the greatest care must be exercised in applying it. To apply it skillfully is often as important as to choose the right remedy. It is also essential to carefully follow instructions. Strong remedies require careful judgment, and you may be sure your physician has assessed your requirements.

Eczema, then, occupies a unique position in the field of dermatology. It is not only the wastebasket for all unexplained eruptions with characteristic symptoms, but it is also the keystone of skin diseases. The specialist in this subject deals with the commonest and most distressing skin disorder. If he knows how to treat this disease, you may be certain that he is able to treat most skin disorders.

DRUG RASHES

Within the past few years rashes on the skin due to drugs taken for some reason or other have become one of the most important causes of skin disease. Every doctor who prescribes a drug is well aware of the many problems which arise both on the skin and elsewhere on the body, as a result of the same drugs which may do so much good internally. Although the physician may be well aware of the pitfalls and disadvantages of these drugs, the patient usually is not. This is especially unfortunate in view of the fact that many drugs may be bought in the neighborhood drugstore without the necessity of a prescription. Accordingly, the occasional person may be taking some proprietary remedy which is doing him more harm than good. As far as the skin is concerned, while many of the drugs embodied in these various remedies are harmless, many others produce skin eruptions varying from an occasional attack of hives to an extremely serious rash involving almost the entire body. At the present time, it is probable that the single most important cause of drug eruptions is penicillin. Even a drug as simple as the salicylates (most popular member of which is aspirin) may be the cause of a troublesome itch or recurrent eruption, often baffling to both the patient and to his doctor.

This brief paragraph cannot be regarded as adequate in view of the vast importance of the role played in chronic eruptions of the skin by one or several drugs. It may, however, serve to impress upon the reader that he must seek the services of a physician for advice concerning any chronic skin disorder and, of even greater importance, as to the necessity of continuing some highly vaunted home remedy or drug mixture. Many people, on being asked whether they take a drug, state that they do not. On further questioning, it develops that the remedy they have been taking over a period of years for constipation or for their liver, or whenever they have a headache, is just the drug that is producing the trouble with their skin. Even that so-called "harmless" hang-over remedy may be the cause of their troublesome rash, and that special cure of Grandma's may not only irritate the skin, but affect various other parts of the body even including the blood cells and certain vital structures. Don't take any of those home remedies unless you know exactly what is in them and the mixture has been approved by your physician.

DERMATITIS FROM EXTERNAL IRRITANTS

The common example of this type of rash is the inflammation caused by poison ivy, poison oak, or sumac. The plants, chemicals, fabrics, and other substances that may cause this form of dermatitis are as numerous as those causing eczema, and in fact the two are closely related, so that it is at times impossible to say definitely where one leaves off and the other begins. Children should be taught to recognize the appearance of poison ivy so that they may avoid it in their excursions to study nature. It has glossy foliage, arranged three leaflets on a stem. In the fall among the first to change color, the leaves turn a beautiful red, and are often collected for this reason by uninformed enthusiasts. A good working adage is: "Leaves of three, let it be!"

If contact with the plant has been unavoidable, the next procedure should be to wash thoroughly with soapsuds and hot water, followed by rinsing with strong grain alcohol. If the dermatitis has hardly begun, this may lessen the severity of the attack; but when it has become well established, this treatment comes too late and will irritate the skin and result in a more severe skin reaction. It should be employed preferably within a two-hour period following exposure to the plants.

Among house plants the primrose is a common cause of dermatitis. Tincture of iodine that has been allowed to become strong by evaporation, or the too enthusiastic application of the fresh preparation, often is responsible for it. One coat of a fresh preparation is all that is necessary, and more will not have any better effect but may have a bad one. In bygone days the mustard plaster also was a common cause, but today it is scarcely used. However, there are many new household cleansers, chemicals, and cosmetics which may result in skin irritation.

Severe cases of dermatitis may be caused by contact with certain chemicals. The conditions are just about the same as those caused by poison ivy. Paraphenylenediamine and mercury are among the most important of these chemicals, as they are contained in many hair dyes and toilet preparations. New York City has an amendment to the Sanitary Code prohibiting the sale and distribution of preparations containing these chemicals, except with certain precautions.

Paraphenylenediamine is a coal-tar derivative and a strong poison. It is commonly used in hair dyes and has recently become a source of exposure due to the popularity of home hair dyes. The scalp may react shortly after the hair is dyed, with severe itching, followed by swelling and blistering of the scalp and surrounding skin. On the other hand, the reaction to a hair dye may not appear for several days, depending on whether the reaction is due to irritation alone or to an allergy to the dye. Fortunately, the newer hair dye preparations have been carefully formulated and the incidence of hair dye dermatitis has decreased considerably.

Mercury is another chemical often used in antiseptics, ointments, and lotions. Most freckle removers contain mercury. While it is a valuable agent for many purposes, it is sometimes an acute irritant, and it should not be used except when specifically prescribed by a physician.

Another frequent source of inflammation of the face and neck is traced to dye used on furs, a dye similar to that in hair dyes. The inflammation is usually severe, prolonged, and recurrent. Another form of dermatitis on the forehead is caused by the action of sweat on the dye and other chemicals contained in cheap sweatbands in hats. Mouth washes, lipsticks, and toothpaste may cause a dermatitis around the mouth, face, and neck. Many cosmetics and cosmetic applicators (rubber sponges) may also be the cause of unpleasant and uncomfortable facial rashes.

For these forms of dermatitis the treatment consists in the detection and removal of the source of irritation, whatever that may be. The doctor must really do some detective work in order to ferret out the cause of some of the more obscure skin eruptions. After the cause has been eliminated, soothing remedies are all the treatment that may be required.

CHAPPING

Chapping is one of the simplest forms of inflammation of the skin. It is seen commonly in the wintertime, on the tender skin of children and on the hands of housewives who do not protect their skin from constant contact with soap, detergents, and other household chemicals. The combination of a cold, dry, wintry climate and a dried-out, steam-heated room conspire with hot water and soap to remove the oil from the skin, causing red, dry, scaly areas. Ordinarily such areas, when spared the irritation of soap and lubricated with some oil, will promptly return to normal. This same combination of overdried and steam-heated rooms together with the winter season not only dries out the skin but the mucous membranes of the nose and throat. Do you have a very dry and rough skin during the winter together with frequent colds and sore throats? If so, get hold of a monkey wrench and fix the radiators so that no one can heat your rooms to that blood-drying level where your skin, nose, and throat literally pant for a little atmospheric moisture. Or at least keep a pan filled with water on the floor so that the hot air can pick up some of the fluid. The Eskimos hardly ever catch cold, and their skins are in excellent condition—and all this without steam-heated igloos.

Some people have a distinct tendency toward chapping. Usually their oil and sweat glands do not function adequately. Accordingly, it is important for them to wash as infrequently as possible, and to minimize their contact with harsh, strong soaps. They are far better off using bland oils, either mineral or vegetable in nature, for cleansing purposes, and lubricating their skins whenever possible with a soothing cold cream. Some of the new lotions and emulsions containing ingredients whose purpose it is to increase the oil content of the surfaces of the skin are also very helpful.

CHAFING

This occurs commonly in babies and obese adults. It is caused by the rubbing together of parts moistened by sweat, offering an excellent opportunity for infection to take place. The parts should be kept scrupulously clean and well powdered. If this does not suffice, a flat bag made of gauze may be filled with talcum powder and suspended between the opposing surfaces to prevent rubbing. Of value also are various lotions and pastes which absorb some of the excessive secretions and excretions from these sites. In women with heavy thighs, chafing between the legs may be minimized by wearing a light, porous pantie specially designed to lessen friction in this region. If these simple measures are not successful, it is advisable to consult a physician because some form of infection may have been superimposed on the simple chafe.

SUNBURN

Sunburn is an inflammatory reaction of the skin to the rays of light, not to heat rays. It occurs on snow fields as well as in the hottest climates. The redness does not appear at once, but several hours after exposure to light. If given an opportunity, most skins can produce enough pigment to protect themselves against any ordinary exposure to the sun; but when they receive a large dose of light without any preparatory hardening, they react with an acute inflammation. Some skins do not produce pigment in all parts but only in small scattered patches—the well-known freckle. And the albino has a skin that apparently cannot produce pigment at all; sunburn in the albino can be a very serious malady.

People vary in their reaction to the sun's rays. Blondes, as is well known, are apt to grow very red, to burn instead of tan. Brunettes frequently do not redden at all but merely take on a tan color, due to increased pigmentation in the skin. If the exposure to the sun is prolonged or if the redness (erythema) has lasted for some time, the skin becomes dry, harsh, and what is called "dead." The top layers scale or peel off. Very sensitive skins, or those exposed to intense sunlight, may become severely inflamed. There is much swelling, blistering, oozing, and disfiguring. The eyelids, mouth, and nose swell greatly. Some persons react so severely to sunburn that after a short exposure which is only sufficient to cause a slight burn in the average person, they are generally upset and nauseated. Stronger exposures lead to more violent reactions with fever, chills, and severe surface burns.

Brunettes as a rule do not suffer from these reactions nearly so acutely as do blondes. The normally high percentage of pigmentation in brunette skins is what protects them. Pigmentation is the skin's chief protection from the sun's rays. The pigment-containing cells are called chromatophores, literally meaning "color-loving cells." Blondes have fewer chromatophores than brunettes. The colored races, naturally, have the greatest number of chromatophores, and therefore have greater resistance to the sun's rays.

Prevention against sunburn is worth many pounds of cure to those who react. Large, wide-brimmed hats should be worn. Parasols and the large type of beach umbrella are of great help, especially at the seashore, where the strongest rays are felt. Applications of oils, lotions, and creams keep the rays from penetrating the skin to some extent. Para-aminobenzoic acid in various liquid or solid forms is a very efficient protection against sunburn, as is red veterinary petrolatum (a very effective preparation). Salol (5 to 10 per cent) in a vanishing cream base is also pleasant and efficient. Other new drugs are effective and not unpleasant for application, but when trying a new sunburn cream, use it carefully for the first few times. It may not protect sufficiently, or the very chemical designed to protect your skin may do just the reverse if you are allergic to it.

When the first signs of sunburn appear, a cold cream should be applied. If there is swelling, a wet dressing of a slightly astringent and cooling solution, such as 5 per cent of Burow's solution, boric acid, or witch hazel, should be applied, followed by a powdery liquid such as calamine lotion. These reduce the heat, cool the skin, and help absorb the water in the skin.

The action of cold creams is excellent. They cool, soothe, and protect the skin, and counteract the drying effect of the sun. They do not make hair grow on the face, as some people would have us believe. (If cold cream did that, it would do as much for the scalp, and every bald-headed man in the country would be frantically massaging his scalp with his wife's newest and most expensive cold cream.)

Exposure to strong sunlight occasionally results in a very severe burn, usually of a first- or second-degree character, but never third degree. The so-called first-degree burns are really comparatively mild and produce only a redness of the skin. Second-degree burns occur simultaneously with the first-degree type, and in addition to redness, there are many blisters scattered over the burned area. The second-degree burns do not destroy the complete thickness of the skin, so that the remaining tissue can spontaneously regenerate the burned areas. It is only in third-degree burns, which practically never occur from sunburn, which cause complete destruction of the entire skin, and are far and away the most serious in that the burned victim is seriously ill and requires various types of plastic operation in order to correct the permanent damage to the tissues. First- and second-degree burns occur not only from some sun exposure, but primarily as a direct effect of exposure to heat. This heat may be due to exposure to fire, hot liquids, steam, and flash burns. Although we worry to a certain extent about the dangers of atomic bombs, the real medical problem of exposure to the atomic bomb is not the atomic radiation but the direct effect of heat.

Although the principal measures involved in the treatment of burns are primarily medical problems, their main features are the relief of pain, the prevention of shock and infection, and the actual treatment of the burned areas. With sunburn, the ordinary first-aid measures are adequate, such as the use of a simple mineral oil ointment containing a mild cooling agent such as menthol in a very weak concentration, in order to help relieve the pain. If not available, the application of a heavy paste made of water and sodium bicarbonate is also a useful first-aid measure. The more severe burns resulting from the direct effect of heat rather than sunburn should only be treated by a physician. While waiting, however, the victim may be made more comfortable by the application of a cool wet dressing, minimizing contact with the hands so that infection is not apt to occur. These extensive second- and third-degree burns are best covered with a clean, freshly ironed towel or sterile dressing moistened with a weak bicarbonate of soda solution until the doctor arrives. The newest method of treatment includes the surgical removal of all blisters and dead tissue, preferably in a sterile operating room. Subsequently, the burned area is washed with an antiseptic soap and sterile water, but in a very mild fashion, in order not to remove any of the still living tissue. The soap is then removed by rinsing with a sterile salt solution. There are many variations in the treatment of severe burns, depending upon the training of the physician. At the present time the most popular methods include the use of pressure dressings over a simple mineral oil application to the wound itself. Although many authorities feel that the ointment should contain some antiseptic or antibiotic, it would seem as though the best results have been secured by using the antibiotic internally, rather than locally. Another strange thing that has been found out is that it is preferable to leave the dressings in place for several days rather than to change them frequently. The reason for this is that there is less chance of infection developing, and the tissues seem to heal better when they are not disturbed.

Certain people are extremely sensitive to sunlight and should never expose themselves unnecessarily. Still others, particularly those suffering from a skin disease known as lupus erythematosus, should avoid sunlight as they would a plague. One strong exposure might initiate a fatal flare-up of the disease. People with a tendency toward skin cancer must also avoid the sun.

FROSTBITE

The skin may become irritated as a result of exposure to extreme cold. Usually it is most evident on prominent parts, such as the cheekbones, tip of the nose, ears, and chin. This is frostbite or chilblain, and it usually begins with a painful whiteness of the frozen part. Subsequently, the skin becomes cold, dark red, and painful. It may then lose all sensation. If the exposure is prolonged, the extremities may turn a black color, and in extreme cases the skin becomes gangrenous or dead.

The last war resulted in a considerable knowledge concerning the treatment of frostbite. These measures were learned, unfortunately, by the observation of aviators whose hands were frozen at high altitudes, and also from poor "G.I. Joe," who developed trench foot due to exposure of the feet to cold and wet for days at a time. Formerly we were all aware of the age-old custom of massaging the skin with snow, but this has long since been thrown out. In fact, massage of these almost brittle areas of the skin may actually lead to gangrene. The present methods of treatment of frostbite include gradual increase in the skin temperature by putting the patient first in a cool room and allowing the frozen part to thaw out slowly. It is of the utmost importance that the frozen tissue be thawed out slowly, because any rapid increase in the skin temperature will result in death of the skin cells and gangrene of the tissue. Gradually the frostbitten victim is warmed up with hot stimulating drinks, and if the freezing is extensive, transfusions of blood or plasma are usually necessary. Very little is done with the skin itself, other than keeping it extremely clean. The trend has been to give all the necessary antiseptics and antibiotics internally rather than locally, and this procedure has resulted in fewer cases of lost fingers and toes.

EXCESSIVE AND ABNORMAL FUNCTIONING OF THE SKIN OR OF ITS OIL AND SWEAT GLANDS

EXCESSIVE SWEATING

Excessive sweating may prove annoying, and the pads worn in the armpits and the various chemical applications to this area are not fully satisfactory remedies. Many chemicals act as deodorants when externally applied, and some are also anti-perspirants. The most effective antiperspirant preparations are the aluminum salts, although some people may be allergic to these chemicals and they must be tried out with caution. As a deodorant, plain bicarbonate of soda as a dusting powder is effective. It has also been discovered that the addition of an antibiotic (such as neomycin) to an antiperspirant mixture will give it deodorant properties. Some internally acting drugs such as banthine have been successfully used for the control of excessive sweating, but only under medical supervision because of their effects on other parts of the body.

BODY ODOR

Body odor is usually synonymous with the odor of the sweat. Certain perfumers advise the use of perfume suited to the body odor of the client, but that sounds rather unpleasant. Foul-odored sweat is a great affliction, fortunately not common. Some of the newer soaps and deodorants are effective in the control of unpleasant body odors. Many of these preparations contain antibiotics, hexachlorophene and other effective antiseptics.

PRICKLY HEAT

Heat rash (prickly heat) is an acute inflammatory disorder due, obviously, to an inability of the skin to adapt itself to an increase in temperature. It occurs more often in infants than in older persons, and is most prevalent during periods of heat and humidity.

The eruption consists of tiny elevations ranging in size from a pinpoint to a pinhead and usually containing a clear fluid. Actually, these tiny elevations are present over the pore openings and are due to the fact that the sweat secretions have been blocked by a surface inflammation of the skin. The surrounding skin is usually of a pinkish shade. The prickles may remain separate, but not infrequently they join with one another and form large patches of irritation, as in eczema. If these areas are not properly treated, secondary infection may result with pus formation and rapid spread.

Prickly heat is best prevented by the avoidance of too heavy clothing and frequent use of bath and dusting powder. Air conditioning, especially during the summer months and in hot climates, is a major deterrent to the development of prickly heat. Do not dress babies and children too warmly during the summer months. Bathe them frequently, and make certain that they drink enough water and other fluids. After the eruption is present, it will frequently yield promptly to cooling measures such as weak, cold applications followed by the use of a bland dusting powder or calamine lotion. The skin should not be cleansed with soap, which is very apt to irritate the condition. For the purposes of cleansing, mineral or vegetable oils may be employed in alternation with the local applications of powder and soothing lotions. If possible, the sufferer from heat rash should spend as much time as possible in an air-conditioned room. If these simple procedures fail to improve the condition, a physician should be consulted, as such eruptions afford an excellent invasion center for infections of the skin.

EXCESSIVE OILINESS

Excessive oiliness of the skin is one of the commonest causes of large pores and a generally poor complexion. It is most common around the age of puberty or adolescence, and this may be considered due to the increased activity of the sex glands during this period of life. The oiliness of the skin occurs about equally in both sexes, although it is presumed to be due to the secretion of male, rather than female, sex hormones. It is usually referred to medically as seborrhea, and is characterized by the presence of an excessive amount of oily secretion on the face and the scalp, and occasionally elsewhere on the body. This greasy secretion appears as oily droplets oozing through the pores of the skin and often on the scalp. The result is a greasy layer of oil droplets which can be wiped off the surfaces of the skin with a handkerchief at frequent intervals. In time the pore openings become blocked with oily secretion which can be squeezed out in the form of little wormlike bodies. In addition, these oily droplets serve as sort of a catch-basket for all the dirt floating in the air, and so the surface of these oil droplets or the secretion in the pores themselves is often of a blackish color and is referred to as "blackhead." The black color is not actually dependent on dirt, as certain chemical changes are responsible for the blackish color. The scalp is always affected, and the free oily material results in a glistening and shining appearance of the scalp. In women with long hair the secretion may be so extreme as to mat the locks together in a sort of glue-like paste. Although in former years this was believed to be responsible in great measure for early baldness, the relative importance of oil secretions in producing baldness is very slight.

Although the glands of internal secretion are primarily responsible for the excessive greasiness and oiliness of the skin, other predisposing causes include any internal change which lowers the vitality and general nutrition. Seborrhea may appear following any one of a number of infections and may be associated with constipation, lack of fresh air and exercise, and poor diet. When seborrhea has persisted for a long time, it may be responsible for the formation of crusts and scales on the scalp and around the ears and nose. This may even go on to a more severe form of the disorder, often referred to as seborrheic dermatitis.

In the average case of seborrhea frequent washing with soap and water and the use of a mild astringent may be all that is required. However, in the usual instance it is important to take care of both the external and internal factors if an effective cure is desired. Ordinary common-sense hygienic measures are indicated. Sunlight, nutritious food, and plenty of fresh air and exercise are important. An adequate intake of vitamins, especially of members of the B-complex family, is especially indicated. The latter vitamins contain substances which have been shown to lessen the greasiness and scaling of the skin both in animals and human beings. For the direct treatment of the skin, frequent use of soap and water on the face and frequent shampooing of the scalp are highly recommended. Bland soaps or soap substitutes such as sulfonated oils are of value in many instances, especially if the skin is sensitive and easily irritated. In some instances, however, more efficient and drying types of soaps and shampoos are required. One thing that is definitely contraindicated is the use of massage by the beautician and barber, both of the face and scalp. Massage of the face is not only valueless in this condition, but will often increase the local irritation and accentuate the blocking and oil secretion of the skin. In addition to frequent washing of the skin, the use of a mild astringent at frequent intervals is effective.

Where the condition is more of a rash, rather than merely excessive oil secretion, various drugs have been employed and recommended, and these include sulfur, resorcin, salicylic acid, and similar agents. They are usually made up in the form of flesh-colored mixtures of various types, although greaseless creams or lotions are better adapted to some skins. Repeated application and patient care of the face and scalp are necessary to secure complete relief in the case of a disease as essentially chronic as seborrhea. These conditions require the services of a physician, as the local and internal measures require close watch and frequent change.

EXCESSIVE DRYNESS

This condition is the exact opposite of seborrhea, in that there is an inadequacy of the secretions of the oil glands. As a result, the skin is not satisfactorily lubricated, and this may occur as a natural phenomenon or as a result of constant bathing of the skin, or as a result of immersing the body in strongly alkaline solutions in the course of various occupations. Dryness of the skin frequently occurs in the wintertime in cold climates, and is often aggravated by the lack of humidity in heated rooms. It is often associated with other disturbances of the skin, and is not infrequently a forerunner of eczema. In extreme instances the skin is not only dry but becomes cracked, chapped, and split. Dryness of the skin is more typical of the older age groups, but it must be realized that various internal factors may also produce this state. For example, when the thyroid gland does not function adequately, the skin often becomes extremely dry and scaly.

If the dryness is merely due to various external causes, the condition can usually be simply remedied by the use of oils such as lanolin, almond oil, mineral oil, and other agents. The skin should be bathed as infrequently as possible, and soaps confined primarily to the skin under the arms and in the groin. Even the face should be cleaned with oils rather than soaps, and a protective layer of cold cream should be left on the skin overnight. Other effective solutions for the face include glycerin in rose water and the occasional local application of the white of an egg rubbed gently into the skin. If the condition does not respond to simple applications of creams and oily lotions, a search for some internally causative factor, such as a hormone deficiency, may be rewarding.

ITCHING

The skin is the source of many peculiar sensations, including smarting, burning, prickling, tingling, creeping, and crawling. However, one of the most common sensations in the skin is itching. As a result of this sensation, we are provoked into rubbing and scratching the affected area in an attempt to relieve the undesirable sensation or to change it almost preferably to one of pain. When the itching is severe, self-control can seldom be mustered even by persons of unusually strong will power. These unhappy efforts of the sufferer to relieve himself result in the formation of bumps and infection as a result of the entrance of bacteria through self-inflicted wounds. Often the irritation is far more acute at night than during the day, and sleep becomes a thing of the past.

The causes of itching are many. In some instances it may be as simple as contact with a new soap, shaving lotion, hair tonic, or the like. In other instances it may be due to infection with some germ or parasite. Occasionally it may be a symptom of a severe underlying disease such as diabetes. Obviously, then, the only intelligent approach to the treatment of itching is to find out what has caused the symptom. To a trained observer, this may prove to be a simple problem, although, on the other hand, it may require an extremely careful medical and laboratory investigation.

The occurrence of itching is divided about equally among men and women, and, while no age level is exempt, there is a tendency for it to be more frequent after forty. Adults with dry skins often develop itching during the winter, especially if they bathe frequently and use more than their share of soap. It may also make its appearance during the menopause and result in itching of either one portion of the body or the entire body surface.

If the itching is due to a specific cause, removal of the offending substance will result in prompt and speedy relief. This relief will be increased by the use of cold wet dressings and soothing lotions. Within recent years new antihistaminic drugs have been found extremely effective in controlling sensations of itching, whatever their cause. Of course, these drugs should be taken only under the supervision of a physician. Unfortunately, the tendency at present is to employ them as a cure-all for all itchy skin diseases, but, as might be expected, they will not perform miracles.

Itching of the skin may also be due to an associated nervous disorder, and the treatment of a difficult emotional situation may sometimes result in relief from that extremely uncomfortable and maddening itch. Where an itching condition has persisted for any period of time, do not attempt to treat the condition yourself but consult your physician.

INFECTIONS OF THE SKIN

BACTERIAL INFECTIONS

Impetigo is the commonest of all skin infections and one of the easiest to cure. It is most frequently seen in children and is caused by pus germs, the streptococcus and staphylococcus. In the newborn baby, it can be serious because the baby has no immunity to the infection and it is fatal in approximately 25 per cent of all cases. For this reason children are not permitted to visit the maternity floor of the hospital. The disease is highly communicable and spreads rapidly from child to child. It can usually be recognized by the appearance of honey-colored crusts which look as though they were stuck on the skin. Impetigo prefers to attack children, and the face is the favorite site. The scalp is not uncommonly involved, especially in children with head lice.

The treatment of impetigo is based primarily on the use of antiseptics and general cleansing with soap and water. If the crusts do not come off easily, the application of a wet dressing or a soap poultice will serve to take them off in short order. Following removal of the crusts, the application of any one of several antiseptic ointments, such as those containing ammoniated mercury, or some of the newer antibiotic agents is extremely effective. Where the condition is widespread and serious, it may be necessary to employ one or several antibiotics, such as penicillin or tetracycline, by mouth or by injection.

Folliculitis is similar in nature to impetigo, but the infection is in the hair follicle rather than on the surface of the skin. In other words, the infecting germs, either the staphylococcus or streptococcus, penetrate the deeper parts of the skin, usually through the mouth of the hair follicle or pore opening. Within a short time the skin surrounding the hair follicle becomes inflamed, sensitive, and tender and discharges pus. As with impetigo, the infection spreads rapidly from one hair follicle to another, most commonly on the beard or in the scalp. The infection sometimes is transmitted from unclean instruments or unsanitary procedures in the barber shop, and is more common in people with diseases such as diabetes. Even if true diabetes is not present, persons whose blood sugar or skin sugar content is high show a particular tendency toward the development of pus infections of the skin such as folliculitis, boils, and carbuncles. Recurrent attacks of these conditions are often successfully treated by a low sugar and starch diet in combination with proper hygiene, antiseptic agents, and both local and internal antibiotic therapy.

Boils. When the same pus-forming bacteria that produce impetigo and folliculitis dig farther in and attack the deeper parts of the follicles and the oil glands, a deep, round, inflamed mass develops. The result is a boil.

Boils are common enough to be considered slightly amusing by everyone except their victims. They are painful, hard, red lumps like marbles surrounding each hair follicle. Some tend to soften and form a soft, pus-discharging core. That is, the center around the follicle discharges the pus and the rim remains hard and bright red. When the center has softened sufficiently, it may be removed. A pus-discharging ulcer is then left, which empties itself and heals, often leaving a scar.

Boils are quite frequently the accompaniment of constitutional disorders. Almost invariably they indicate a run-down condition, if not a serious disease. Diabetes is often accompanied by boils. Frequent boils should send the patient to a physician for a general examination and treatment.

When the rim or wall of a boil is soft—because of a poor general resistance—the infection is not well confined and tends to spread and invade the blood. Abscesses may develop in other parts of the body, such as around the kidneys, and general blood infections may result. Sometimes these infections are fatal.

In certain occupations in which the skin is likely to be injured or exposed to dirt, tar, petroleum, or other chemicals, there is a constant danger of contracting boils. Bromides and iodides taken internally may produce boils and folliculitis. Both boils and folliculitis may affect any part of the face and neck. Folliculitis, of course, is more likely to occur on the bearded parts of the face. It is more chronic and obstinate, but boils are more painful.

A boil on the upper lip or in the nose is especially to be watched. It is extremely dangerous and may cause death. This is because the blood circulation of the upper lip is extensive, and also is upward to the brain. Poisons draining from the lip, therefore, may cause meningitis and abscesses of the brain.

Carbuncles. There is a widespread confusion of ideas about boils and carbuncles. A great many people rather naturally think they are the same thing. They are distinctly different, but the difference is more in degree than in kind.

A carbuncle is larger, deeper, more destructive, and vastly more serious than a boil. It is an infection by a pus-forming germ, like the boil; but it is always accompanied by the symptoms of a severe and acute illness.

A carbuncle is a hard, rounded, inflammatory mass, extending down through the corium into the subcutaneous tissues. It goes deeper than the boil, which seldom extends below the upper part of the corium. A boil affects only one hair follicle. A carbuncle affects several, through which pus is discharged from the inflamed center.

With carbuncles may be fever, chills, loss of weight, and general discomfort. In addition, there may be symptoms of a metabolic disease, such as diabetes. Because of this, a main feature of the treatment of carbuncles is the employment of every measure that will build up the body and help it to fight the disease.

THE TREATMENT OF PUS-PRODUCING INFECTIONS (FOLLICULITIS, BOILS, CARBUNCLES)

In the treatment of folliculitis, boils, and carbuncles, the doctor finds out if any constitutional disease is present and corrects it. Even if no such disease is discovered, it is advisable to clean out the bowels, remove sweets and chocolate from the diet, and take any measures necessary to bring the system's powers of resistance up to par. Plenty of fresh air and sunlight and a great deal of water, outside and inside, are highly desirable. Irritation, dirt, and harmful chemicals should be avoided, of course.

In recent years the sulfa drugs, penicillin, tetracycline, and other potent remedies of modern science have been remarkably effective in curing episodes of these diseases. They are usually not effective in the chronic and recurrent types, although small doses carefully supervised over a period of time may prove effective. There has been a gradual increase in the number of infections (especially members of the staphylococcus family of germs) which have developed a resistance to penicillin and other antibiotics and the treatment of these infections requires very skillful medical supervision and laboratory investigation.

There are two main fallacies about the treatment of folliculitis and boils. One is that the face must not be shaved, and the other is that boils must always be cut. Actually, the face should be shaved daily. The reason for keeping hair off the face is that infection is minimized and the local applications can penetrate more readily. Boils usually need not be cut. Cutting breaks down the rim, or defensive wall that the body builds around the infection, and this opens up the blood and lymph vessels and so permits the spread of the infection. It is rarely necessary to cut boils, as a matter of fact; but when it is done, the most thorough asepsis and antisepsis must be enforced.

The main aim of treatment, indeed, should be the enforcement of cleanliness and personal hygiene and the administration of measures that will reduce and remove the infection. The boils and the skin around them should be washed several times a day with soap and water. Following the washings, alcohol and water or antiseptic solutions should be lightly dabbed on and then antiseptic dressings applied. Avoid irritating and infecting the skin around the boils.

When the boils are tense and tender, a wet dressing of a 5 per cent

Burow's solution or a 5 per cent sodium propionate solution—not a compress—relieves the pain and encourages the softening and evacuation of pus. It is a mistake to put heavy bandages, oilskin, or gutta-percha over the gauze to form a compress. The dense texture of these materials causes a retention of the heat and the pus discharge, and nurtures the growth of the germs.

Ultraviolet rays also are useful in improving some local infections. Of even greater value are a whole score of new drugs, including the sulfa drugs, penicillin, bacitracin, neomycin, and the tetracyclines and other antibiotics. These drugs may be used either locally or internally, depending on the severity of the infection.

The same sort of treatment is employed for carbuncles, but here surgery may be necessary if wet dressings and the antibiotics are not effective.

As may readily be imagined, these pus infections are not trivial. The best way to treat them is not to have them. And the best way to achieve that happy state is to keep the general constitution up to its highest tone, and to make a habit of strict cleanliness and an intelligent, balanced diet.

SPIROCHETES—SYPHILIS

Syphilis is no longer considered as a disease to be discussed in whispers by both younger and older generations. This is an era in which prudery has little, if any, place. We are more concerned in measures and effects that will improve the public health and which must be known by those who wish to protect themselves. We must understand the early and beginning symptoms of a disease such as syphilis, so that any suspicious symptom may be promptly investigated. At present the ease and speed of eradication of the disease depend chiefly on the early diagnosis of the condition. A disease such as syphilis does not merely affect one part of the body, but can spread to affect almost any organ or tissue in the system. Furthermore, if the initial symptoms are disregarded, the germs which cause the disease quietly dig into the internal organs and produce serious damage which cannot be remedied if it has been persistent for many years. In this chapter the purpose for describing and discussing this disease is not so that it can be treated at home. The average person is no better equipped to take care of syphilis than is the quack who preys on frightened and uninformed youngsters without a real knowledge of the proper treatment and fundamentals of medical care. If you develop any symptoms such as those mentioned under this disease, discuss them with your family physician and not with your friends or a so-called sex disease expert who may not even be a qualified physician.

The cause of syphilis is a tiny corkscrew-like germ which swims around in the fluid discharging from a syphilitic sore. It is an organism called a spirochete, and in fresh syphilitic sores the fluid literally swarms with these corkscrew-shaped organisms. This germ is rather delicate and is usually promptly destroyed outside of the body. For this reason, syphilis is usually transmitted only by direct contact with a person who is infected with the disease. Although syphilis may also be acquired and transmitted in other ways, these transmissions are quite uncommon and the disease is truthfully called a venereal disease. The germ usually requires the presence of an open wound or slightly irritated mucous membrane such as the mouth, rectum, or outer male and female genital organs, to enter the body. Although syphilis may be transmitted through the sputum, after kissing, this method of transmission is slight in comparison to sexual intercourse as the primary means of infecting another person with syphilis.

Syphilis is usually divided by the physician into three stages. During the first stage the infection usually appears as a small sore on the genital organs. This sore usually appears within two weeks following sexual intercourse. Any sore which develops on the genital region at this period of time should be examined by your physician. He can usually perform a test known as a dark field examination, which will promptly disclose the presence of spirochetes if the sore is due to syphilis. If it is not, you are better off being told that such is the case, rather than waiting to see what happens. At this stage the germ has only started to get into the blood stream and so the Wassermann test does not become positive until a later date. If this primary stage is disregarded, the sore usually heals in a few weeks and the glands in the groin, which are swollen at the time of this primary sore or chancre, usually go down. The germ is now being transported around the body, and the unfortunate victim is passing into the second stage. If the second stage is mild, the infected person may not know that he has syphilis for many years, when it will either be disclosed by the performance of a routine blood test, or by symptoms of a serious nature.

In the secondary stage of syphilis, which appears within six weeks or so, the chief symptoms are an extensive rash, a peculiar loss of hair, and often what seems to be an ordinary cold or sore throat accompanied by slight fever and achy or "grippy" symptoms. One of the unfortunate features of the disease is that the secondary stage may be mild, and the patient may feel that he merely has a slight cold. The rash may be mild enough to be overlooked, and he may be completely unaware of the fact that his entire system is going through a mighty battle in order to build up resistance against the germs which have spread to every part of the body by way of the blood stream. Another unfortunate feature of the disease is that lack of awareness of this stage means that the victim can easily transmit it. During this secondary period the saliva and all other body secretions are loaded with the organisms, and it is very easily transmitted. To get back to the rash, it may be stated that it looks like measles and is usually present on the body rather than on the face. The hair fall is of a peculiar type in that it usually consists of either a diffuse thinning of the entire scalp, or of the appearance of small bald patches. These bald patches are so characteristic, in that they look mangy or moth-eaten, that it is described in medical textbooks as the typical moth-eaten appearance of the scalp in secondary syphilis. During this stage the blood shows a strongly positive Wassermann (or other serologic) test and the diagnosis can readily be established.

After several weeks or months the secondary stage passes, and the symptoms gradually disappear. If laboratory tests have not been performed on the blood and spinal fluid, the disease may pass unnoticed until the person passes into the final or tertiary stage of syphilis. This stage may not appear for many years and it is due to the destruction of various internal tissues and organs by the spirochete which eats away insidiously at these tissues over the years. This stage persists until the end of the patient's life and may even remain undiscovered if the symptoms are not sufficiently pronounced to bring the patient to the doctor. In the ignorant and uninformed this occasionally is the case. The average person with the tertiary stage of syphilis has usually had such mild primary and secondary stages that he was never aware of the presence of the disease. At some stage in his life either a routine blood test or a general examination brings to light the presence of the disease. The symptoms of the tertiary stage may consist of extensive sores on the skin, or changes involving any portion of the body, including the eyes, ears, nerves, blood vessels and heart, the liver, and the brain. These changes are usually so extensive and severe as to shorten the life span.

The symptoms described present the picture of a serious and unpleasant disease. The disease will only be eradicated in time by early diagnosis and prompt examination following any suspicious exposure. Don't let fear keep you away from the physician! He is sworn to secrecy and will protect your privacy as well as your health. Fortunately, public health authorities have made tremendous strides in wiping out the sources of infection among prostitutes and other groups which are responsible for the constant transmission of the disease. Only with lessened secrecy and more intelligent knowledge and information concerning the disease, will it eventually disappear. Modern treatment methods are such that the disease can be completely cured and its transmission prevented if an early diagnosis is made. Even the late and severe stages of the disease can be dramatically helped by prompt and adequate therapeutic measures. The old methods of treatment with arsenic, bismuth, and other heavy metals have to a great measure been displaced by the newer drugs, especially penicillin. Whereas formerly it was necessary to treat patients over a period of years, the disease is now practically completely eradicated in weeks with massive doses of penicillin, as well as some of the other drugs. The advances of science will eventually force the disappearance of this dread disease, but this will only come about with intelligent understanding and co-operation on the part of the general public.

VIRUS INFECTIONS

FEVER BLISTERS (HERPES SIMPLEX)

Small groups of blisters break out on the face when we catch cold or get too much sun. They usually appear around the mouth or nose as tender and tense small blisters which rapidly become crusted and sore. Herpes are due to a virus and are actually an infection, difficult to transmit. Some people seem to be peculiarly susceptible to them and get herpes regularly whenever they get a cold or sore throat. Others get herpes whenever they are exposed to too much sun or wind. The blisters seem to have a favorite site for recurrence so that some people always develop them around the mouth, yet others only get them around the nose or elsewhere on the body. They also occur in association with certain severe infections or high fevers, for example, pneumonia. They also occur at the time of menstruation, but this may often be due to some drug taken for the relief of menstrual cramps.

Herpes usually dry up and disappear within one week to ten days. The healing process may be accelerated by the use of drying lotions and powders. In the initial stage spirits of camphor or tincture of benzoin may make the tender area less sensitive and hasten the drying of the blisters. Of value also is plain zinc oxide ointment containing a fraction of a per cent of menthol. When herpes simplex recur constantly in the same spot, this may be prevented by a few X-ray treatments to the affected area. Other people who develop recurrent fever blisters may be immunized against them more or less permanently by four to eight smallpox vaccinations at intervals of two weeks. It seems as though the smallpox vaccination produces some type of nonspecific immunity against the herpes virus although controlled studies do not support this observation. Virologists hope to eventually produce a really specific anti-herpes serum. Interestingly enough, herpes simplex of the eyes can be controlled by a chemical agent (IDU).

SHINGLES (HERPES ZOSTER)

Shingles is also a virus infection like herpes simplex, but is more severe in its effects. The name *zoster* is derived from the Greek and means girdle. It got that name because the virus infects part of a nerve and the eruption appears all along the course of the nerve, thereby girdling or encircling the body. Only one side of the body is involved, and so the rash appears as a group of blisters traveling from back to front along one side of the body. Because the nerve is infected, this eruption causes severe neuralgia and the pain may be very distressing. In fact, the pain often lasts long after the rash is gone, and the poor sufferer complains far more because of the neuralgia than because of the rash.

The treatment of shingles is by no means specific and not always of much benefit. In some instances, the early use of cortisone and its derivatives (by mouth) is very effective. If the herpes blisters are infected, antibiotics may also be required. In other instances, if the pain is not great, the whole process may be treated satisfactorily with drying powders, lotions, and salves. The neuralgia may be so severe that drugs like codeine and others may be necessary. The occasional severe attack may even require blocking or destruction of the sensitive and irritated nerve. Fortunately, dangerous complications of shingles are rare, and the disease hardly ever recurs.

PARASITES

VEGETABLE PARASITES (RINGWORM)

This old name of ringworm was given to the disease because of a misconception of the cause of the ring shape of the patches on the skin. It is a complete misnomer, because the disease, in most of its manifestations, is not in the shape of rings. Of course, worms have no part in producing the disease. It is due to many different cousins of the common molds which attack bread left in an open moist place. This has been known for many years by the medical profession. Only lately have the doctors realized how important and widespread these infections are.

On the feet this disease is carried between the toes of a large percentage of those who consider themselves perfectly healthy. The wonder is not that it breaks out in other parts now and then; but that this happens so seldom. So far as is now known, it is spread chiefly by walking on moist, infected floors of bathrooms, gymnasiums, and golf clubs, and in evidence of this fact is the more modern name "athlete's foot."

The treatment of these infections is often difficult and taxes the ingenuity of the physician. The hair and nail infections are most difficult of all forms to treat, and the latter is one of the important sources for the spread of the infection. Fortunately, many new remedies are now available both for control and treatment of the ringworm. The majority of these effective agents are antifungal antibiotics known as griseofulvin or derivative compounds. These drugs are especially valuable in the treatment of ringworm of the scalp and certain chronic fungus infections of the skin. They are taken by mouth and should only be administered under careful medical supervision.

Some new local agents have also been found of value in the control and treatment of fungus diseases (tolnaftate).

Treatment of most cases of ringworm should be kept up for a long time after cure has apparently been obtained. The organisms lurk among the skin cells and await an opportunity, perhaps in the form of simple moisture, to multiply rapidly and cause another outbreak.

Everyone has a pet remedy for his own case of ringworm, but the same remedy may wreak havoc on someone else's skin. If your athlete's foot or jockey itch does not get better from simple hygienic measures, don't use your friend's remedy but seek professional advice. Some of the newer drugs may actually cure that "old faithful" ringworm of yours, so don't give up hope!

ANIMAL PARASITES

1. *Lice*—The three forms of lice which feed on man obtain their nourishment from blood sucked from the hair follicles. In procuring this food they inject a poison into the skin, which causes intense itching. Among ordinary folks the best known of this disgusting family of parasites is the head louse, pediculus capitis. The children of the family too frequently bring home samples of the parasite in the hair. Its eggs, called nits, are tiny white pear-shaped bodies glued to the hair. The parent louse has a semi-translucent gray body and is not easily distinguished through the hair. Scratch marks and bloody crusts, sometimes pustules and matting of the hair are seen.

Thorough soaking of the hair and scalp with a mixture of equal parts of kerosene and sweet oil is an old method of eradicating the lice. A cap is formed of cloths soaked in the mixture and left upon the head overnight. The next morning a thorough shampoo is given, and after this hot vinegar applied to loosen the nits, which then are removed with a fine comb. Modern methods of cure are much more effective. They include the use of DDT, HCH, and similar chemicals in the form of ointments or lotions applied for comparatively short periods of time. When large groups of children are infected, powder sprays of DDT have been very effective. They kill the parasites with speed and efficiency.

The body louse lives in the clothing and only moves to the skin at mealtime. It attaches its eggs to the fibers of the underwear. To obtain blood it marches over to the skin. This explains why the bloody crusts and itchy pimples which are typical signs of this disease are found most plentiful on parts like the waist and shoulders, where the clothing rests closely upon the skin. The derelict and the hobo, as well as those who neglect cleanliness of body and clothing, harbor body lice though it must be recognized that some people are much more attractive to the louse than are others. Body lice carry typhus, a dangerous disease fortunately rare in the United States, but a great problem when our troops entered Italy during the last war. A mild form of typhus is associated with rats, possibly carried by their fleas.

"Crabs" are caused by the pubic or "crab" louse, and this nasty parasite is found clinging to the pubic hairs with its head down close to the skin. At times the parasite travels to the armpits, the chests of hairy men, or even to the eyebrows and eyelashes. Although formerly a great nuisance and difficult to eradicate, the parasites are now destroyed with ease due to the use of DDT and similar chemicals in a form suitable for application to the pubic region. What a transition from the weeks of constant observation and the shamefaced isolation endured by the victims of "crabs" in former years!

2. *The Itch* (*Scabies*)—The itch mite, a member of the spider family, is small. The male mite is smaller than the female. Living on the surface of the skin, his only purpose in life seems to be the propagation of his kind because the female often destroys him after impregnation. She then burrows into and along the upper part of the skin, depositing her eggs as she goes, producing a small canal about one fourth of an inch long. As the eggs hatch the canal loses its roof and appears as a dark, wavy silk thread, seen most easily between the fingers. Itching is more severe at night, because the female itch mite is a night worker.

The diagnosis of scabies is often difficult. A doctor should always be consulted. Much damage can be done by unsupervised home treatment of this disease and the other conditions frequently confused with it, whereas proper medical treatment employing benzyl benzoate, DDT, and sulfur may promptly eradicate the mites.

3. *Insect Bites*—Many insects use man as their source of food supply. Mosquitoes, flies, bedbugs, and fleas are some of the many insects which disturb our travels and trips to the country. They all produce somewhat similar reactions in the skin, depending upon the individual. Some people are completely immune to their bites, but the usual reaction consists of a tiny red spot at the site of the bite, followed by itching and a small, whitish swelling or bump. There are even reports of people so sensitive to these bites that fever, chills, and severe constitutional reactions may result from them.

The first problem is one of prevention and this may be accomplished by extermination of the particular pest. DDT sprays and various new insect repellents are effective with precautions taken to avoid overexposure to these chemicals by the humans rather than the insects. Thorough housecleaning and removal of dust and rubbish may also be necessary.

Treatment consists merely of soothing lotions and tinctures. Calamine lotion with 1 per cent phenol is still a useful remedy. The more severe reactions respond well to the antihistaminic drugs.

SKIN GROWTHS

CORNS

Corns are caused by pressure, as everyone knows, usually that of improperly shaped shoes. The world is slowly becoming more sensible in its dress, but tight-fitting shoes are still much in favor, and corns still flourish. The only effective treatment is protection from pressure. Removing the central horny plug with a knife, or softening with a salicylic acid preparation, followed by soaking in hot water and scraping out the plug is good treatment, but is of no lasting benefit unless the pressure is removed. Sometimes a soft felt pad may take the pressure off the callus or corn and cause it to disappear. Anything that does not yield to such treatment over a period of a few weeks is probably a wart and requires treatment for that condition.

WARTS

Because they are at first tiny, flat, skin-colored elevations that are inconspicuous, warts are often neglected until they have had an opportunity to show their ability to grow and spread. The original wart may remain single and stationary for a time, but a month or so later a new wart may appear near this spot. This property is called autoinoculability; that is, we can infect ourselves again and again. In this way whole crops of warts are raised, like dandelions, where they are least desired. It is plain, therefore, that warts should not be picked with the teeth or fingernails or pared with the pocketknife. The virus that causes warts belongs to the interesting group of "filtrable viruses," whose ability to pass through the finest porcelain filter has given them the name.

Ordinarily warts are painless; but sometimes on the fingers, and commonly on the soles of the feet, they are tender, causing exquisite pain during walking, dancing, or as a support for someone else's feet.

Ever since prehistoric time warts have been treated successfully by suggestion. Tom Sawyer's method and many others like it which are still used by boys all over the world are survivors of the ancient practice of the witch or voodoo doctor. The modern child is often too sophisticated, even at an early age, to have any faith in such practices, and other methods must be used. The only objection to the faith cures is their encouragement of false beliefs and gullibility, which is even worse than warts. Warts respond to treatment with various chemicals, and the "electric needle." Some of the newer "wart" remedies include extremely potent chemicals such as trichloracetic acid and mixtures of podophyllin. Because warts are sometimes difficult to cure even with the most modern methods, the treatment is best left to the physician. A popular home treatment is the use of nitric acid. This is mentioned only to be condemned, for it often results in unsightly scars or even keloids.

Seborrheic warts are the brown to black-topped elevations that occur on the trunk, less often on the face or scalp, of people in middle life or later. They are of no consequence except for the fact that they are sometimes hard to distinguish from senile keratoses, which are important lesions in that they may be the forerunners of skin cancer.

SEBACEOUS CYSTS (WENS)

Sebaceous cysts or "wens" usually occur on the face, back, or scalp. However, they may appear on any part of the body surface in which there are oil glands. They are a result of a blocking of the mouth of the oil gland or hair follicle with an accumulation of oily or cheesy material under the skin. The skin around this cheesy secretion develops an actual cheese bag or pocket in order to contain this material. This bag or cyst continues to grow larger until it is a large lump in the surface of the skin. Sometimes a small black pore communicates with the interior of the cyst, and some of its cheesy contents can be squeezed out through this opening. Often several cysts of different sizes are scattered about this surface of the body. They should be removed because of the possibility of infection, and in a small percentage of cases of cancer.

These cysts may be cut out surgically, but they should not be opened unless a complete removal is planned. However, the resulting scar may be small if one of the newer techniques for removal is employed. By one of these methods, an electric needle is inserted into the cyst and its contents are actually "cooked." Subsequently the cooked cheesy material expels itself with the wall of the sac. Other methods include central incision of the cyst followed by a gradual expression of its contents together with the sac wall. When performed with painstaking care, this method may result in removal of the cyst with practically no scar formation.

MOLES

Moles are birthmarks, even though, as often happens, they do not appear until adult life. The ordinary skin-colored or brown mole, whether covered with hair or not, seldom becomes dangerous except when exposed to chronic irritation. When located so that the clothing rubs upon them, or so that they are frequently cut in shaving or possibly irritated in some other way, they should be removed thoroughly by the physician. Any mole that starts to grow rapidly, bleed easily, or show any type of unusual change, should be examined promptly by a physician and as promptly removed if the doctor considers it necessary.

Blue moles, much less common than the brown kind, but not rare, are in a class by themselves. They may last throughout life without change. Consult your physician about them if there is any question as to change in the mole.

KELOIDS (OVERGROWN SCARS)

Keloids are benign tumors (tumors that practically never become malignant) which grow in scars. At times there is no history of a preceding scar; but it may have been so slight that it was not noticed. Some people have the peculiar tendency to form keloids in their scars, or these tumors may occur in some of their scars and not in others. It is possible to remove a keloid surgically but recurrence may follow even though the operation is very skillfully performed. A post-operative course of X-ray treatments may be advisable. The careful application of solid carbon dioxide ("dry ice") by the physician has also been found of value in the treatment of keloids. The local injection of insoluble forms of cortisone directly into the keloid is beneficial especially if performed shortly after the appearance of this elevated scar.

XANTHOMA (YELLOW SPOTS)

Xanthoma is the name given to the yellow tumors caused by the deposits of fat in the skin. Some of us seem to have an inability to dispose of fats in the normal way, and the skin serves as an exit station. The only form of this disease seen frequently involves the skin around the eyelids, most often the inner part of the lower lid, in the form of small yellowish elevations. They can be removed by the physician with the production of very slight scarring. They may return if the internal condition that causes them is still operative. All patients with xanthomas should undergo a general examination by their physician with special reference to blood cholesterol and their cardiac status.

VASCULAR BIRTHMARKS

Vascular birthmarks may be flat "port-wine marks," slightly elevated, flat-topped "strawberry marks," or egglike swellings composed of groups of veins in a grapelike mass. The large swellings are easily compressed, but return immediately to their original shape, and tend to become bluish and still larger when the baby cries. Often the skin over such a mark is the site of one of the flat kinds already mentioned. Some of these growths should be treated during infancy, when the skin is able to renew itself most readily and the resulting scars are smaller. Furthermore, although some of these bloody tumors may disappear, many of them grow larger rather than smaller.

The treatment of "port-wine stains" is unsatisfactory and these disfiguring marks are best left alone. However, the patient can learn to camouflage these areas with the skillful use of make-up (special heavy base). The "strawberry mark" usually disappears in time if left alone, although the occasional one requires some form of local therapy, carefully administered. The deep or cavernous type of bloody tumor is difficult to treat. Some of the methods employed include surgical removal and X-ray or radium therapy. Consult a specialist in the field before undertaking any form of treatment!

KERATOSES

Keratoses are of two kinds. The soft or seborrheic variety are brownish, velvety plaques which appear during middle age. They are of no significance and can easily be removed from the skin. They are commonly seen on the face and back.

The hard or senile keratosis is more serious in nature. It is a rough, scaly spot often found on the face and backs of the hands. People who are exposed to a great deal of sun and wind over a period of years often develop these spots. Farmers and sailors are particularly apt to develop these spots because of their constant exposure to the elements. These small scaly or warty growths must be removed because they may turn into cancers of the skin. Removal may be accomplished by cutting or burning them off. The only important fact is to make certain the removal is a complete one. People who develop senile keratoses should protect themselves from the sun and wind, following the removal of these growths.

CANCER OF THE SKIN

Cancer of the skin offers the doctor one peculiar advantage over cancer in other parts of the body in that it can be seen at its beginning and treated early. Inability to do this is the chief reason why cancer elsewhere cannot be cured as readily. Any unusual growth on or in the skin should be shown to the physician at once, without taking the great risk of home treatment or delaying treatment until ulceration occurs. The idea that cancer always causes pain is another very harmful one, for skin cancer seldom causes pain until it is in the last stage, when it is too late to save the patient's life. Home treatment is worse than simple delay, for it is like trying to put out a fire by pouring on gasoline. If anything will insure the change from a harmless to a malignant growth, or encourage one that is already malignant, the usually irritating home treatment will do so.

Scaly spots, warts, or growths on the lips and the hands should have attention early, for cancer occurring on these parts is apt to be more malignant than upon the face. The great strides made in the treatment of malignancy are due to the early recognition and removal of suspicious growths. Any "mole," "wart," or similar spot on the skin should be examined by your doctor promptly if it becomes sensitive, enlarges in size, bleeds readily, forms a crust, or ulcerates. Make certain that the wart or lump on your skin is harmless by having it examined rather than by waiting for trouble!

MISCELLANEOUS SKIN CONDITIONS

ACNE VULGARIS

Acne vulgaris is a disease of the oil glands of the skin. At puberty, along with other changes in the body, these glands develop and frequently take on excessive activity, causing the skin to become greasy and plugs to form in the pores. These plugs of grease undergo a chemical change and show as black points on the skin, commonly called blackheads, and by the doctors, comedones. These plugs cause some irritation, as do all foreign bodies in the skin (wood, glass), and nature tries to eliminate them by the formation of pus. When the pustule breaks, the comedo is forced out with the pus. Unfortunately, if the pus remains too long in the deeper lesions before being freed, the pressure and dissolving action of the pus destroys the tissue about it. This loss must be replaced by scar tissue, leaving a permanent disfigurement. If scarring does not follow the pustule, the process may be repeated many times in the same follicle. Acne tends to clear up as the patient grows older, but the risk of scarring is too great and the distress of the young person at the disfigurement too acute to justify neglect of treatment. Don't neglect the early treatment of acne if you wish to have your child develop as few holes or pits in the skin as possible. And remember, at this impressionable age the seeds of an inferiority complex are easily sown. The physician, opening the pustules with a tiny knife, is not causing scars, as many think. He is preventing them by releasing the pus before it has time to destroy tissue.

Since acne occurs usually in greasy skins, acne is benefited by the free use of hot water and soap. Children affected with the disease should not be accused of causing it by reluctance to use these measures. No amount of scrubbing can cure a real case of acne. Neither is acne a sign of sexual irregularity, as some ignorant persons insinuate. The unfortunates afflicted with the disease are embarrassed enough because of their facial blemishes without the added cruelty of such insinuations.

In mild cases pustules may be few and comedones many, forming small yellowish elevations with a yellow, brown, or black point in the center. When the horny layer of the skin forms completely over the surface, the end of the fatty plug cannot become dirty but remains as a white pearl-like body called milium, or whitehead. These remain without much increase in size until removed and do not recur as promptly as the blackheads.

Acne is not always confined to the face, but also involves the chest, upper back, and outer sides of the arms. In persons of low resistance it becomes a disfiguring, distressing, and indeed serious disease. Cold cream or other greasy applications should not be used, for the skin already has too much fat. Massage is apt to do harm because of the cream employed. Patent medicines called "blood purifiers" are apt to make acne worse, because many of them contain iodides. The acne patient does not need this type of "blood purifier."

Removal of blackheads is beneficial, as can easily be understood when the method of formation of pus pimples is considered. It should be done with care, however, not to injure the skin by too much force. Many nervous patients increase their disfigurement by too enthusiastic attempts to remove blackheads by squeezing without preliminary loosening. The face should first be washed thoroughly with hot water and soap, hot towels applied for about ten minutes and then the skin sponged with alcohol. If necessary a needle, sterilized by flaming, or a blackhead remover, a small instrument with a hole about 1/16 of an inch in diameter in one end, may be used to help remove the blackheads. After the blackheads have thus been removed, the application of hot towels should be repeated, followed by a short application of cold water and drying with a towel. This second application of heat lessens the inflammatory reaction to the pressure. Deep pustules, the kind that are most apt to cause scars, should be opened by the physician.

Care of the health is important in all children, but particularly in those who have acne. Fresh air, good food, proper exercise, and plenty of sleep are essential to good health. Strict dieting seldom cures acne and may do harm if not properly supervised. Many youngsters with this disease need restraint, however, in the matter of eating and drinking, and should be particularly warned against the bad effect of sweet carbonated drinks, nuts, greasy foods, excessive condiments, chocolate candy and ice cream. Irregularity in the eating and sleeping schedule is also harmful. Constipation should be avoided by the generous use of vegetables and fruits and by the formation of regular habits of bowel evacuation.

This somewhat lengthy discourse on acne is not intended to convey the idea that acne can be cured by home treatment. Only the mildest cases can be handled without the help of the physician. Under medical supervision, the proper use of some of the newer drugs (both internally and externally) may result in rapid improvement of the condition.

Cleanliness is essential. Soap and water are fundamental, and the face should be vigorously washed several times daily. A good astringent should be rubbed into the skin after each washing. At night salves containing chemicals such as sulfur and resorcin are left on overnight to soften the blackheads and peel off the top layer of affected skin. In addition, your doctor applies various chemicals such as a carbon-dioxide slush and various peeling pastes to accelerate the cure. Ultraviolet light performs a similar aid in treatment. Although X ray was formerly used in the treatment of many cases of acne, it is seldom used now except in the resistant and stubborn cases of acne. However, modern science has found out that certain hormones and chemicals such as the antibotics may be helpful in the treatment of acne. Even the pits and scars produced by the disease can be removed by the newer techniques of facial planing and drilling. Don't neglect your child's skin, because acne is a disease that can and should be controlled from its onset.

ROSACEA

Rosacea, or acne rosacea, is the disease that reddens the nose and cheeks, and in extreme cases causes enlargement of the end of the nose, popularly called "whiskey nose" or "grog blossom." This title is not justified, for many sufferers from this disease are strict abstainers from alcoholic drinks. The trouble is caused by a nervous reflex flushing of the sensitive blood vessels of these areas on the face as a response to internal changes or abnormal local conditions in the mouth or nose. Anything which tends to cause flushing or heating of the face should be avoided. The patient can do much to restrain its development by the avoidance of hot foods or drinks, spicy or peppery foods, and particularly alcoholic beverages. Alcohol irritates the stomach and sets up the reflex already mentioned, at the same time that it acts directly to dilate the peripheral blood vessels. After frequent dilatations, the vessels become paralyzed and remain as disfiguring red or bluish lines. The consequent slowing of the circulation is probably the chief reason for the enlargement of the end of the nose. This can be improved by treatment with proper diet and astringent, local measures including powdered carbon-dioxide "slush."

For direct treatment of the skin, a helpful measure is merely washing the face frequently. But it should be washed with soap and cold water, or rubbed with ice. This is a marvelous tonic; it peps up the muscles and blood vessels and keeps them small and contracted. It is difficult to resist the temptation to break into eulogy of water. No cosmetic ever devised can compare with plain cold water as a tonic, cleanser, and beautifier combined. The only drawback to water is its cheapness. If it could be obtained only in tiny, ornate flasks at ten dollars an ounce, it would sweep a vast amount of perfumed trash off the toilet table!

There are, however, certain preparations which help cold water in fighting rosacea. They are all astringent in nature. Rose water and boric acid solutions and emulsions containing sulphur are especially valuable. The best sulphur lotions, such as lotio alba, tend to prevent grease formation, and as they evaporate, they cool the skin, contract the blood vessels, and leave the sulphur powder on the skin.

Where there is irritation in addition to the redness, the skin should be soothed with wet dressings of boric acid (2 per cent), or zinc oxide lotions, such as calamine lotion, before the sulphur is employed. In using these preparations, some of the mixture should be poured into a saucer and applied with a piece of clean flannel cloth. The best time to apply any such preparation is at night, so that it can remain on the face until morning, when it should be washed off with cold water and soap. After this, a fine powder or a thin, invisible or flesh-colored, sulphur-resorcin type of lotion may be dabbed on.

Vinegar, witch hazel, and weak alum in solutions of less than 5 per cent are good, mild astringents. Too strong a reaction of the skin is harmful; but drugs such as resorcin, ichthyol, and camphor are sometimes used successfully.

There is a general delusion that massage of the face is necessary in treating rosacea. Barbers are apt to prescribe it, as well as operators in beauty parlors. The fact is that massage of a diseased face is injurious. It irritates an inflamed skin and spreads infection. When the skin is unhealthy, it is very easy for it to contract infection from the masseur's fingers.

Electrolysis can do much to reduce telangiectasias—the enlarged blood vessels which show as purplish streaks. The operation is the same as that for the destruction of the follicles in hypertrichosis, or superfluous hair. The electric needle is inserted along the course of the vessel and the current allowed to flow until the vessel is destroyed. The application of the electric cautery will also destroy the unsightly vessels, if done skillfully. After such treatment, cold applications and astringents are applied.

These same methods of treatment are employed for cases where the nose is tremendously enlarged or has a hanging growth; but the quickest and best method is removal of this growth by surgical operation. The growth is cut away surgically; if the bleeding is profuse, it is easily stopped by pressure and ice. Operations by this technique usually produce excellent results. Various caustics prevent the regrowth of tissue after the operation, and caustics are used to destroy the follicles which have produced the excess growth.

Rosacea is no longer a difficult problem. With proper diet and internal measures, plus effective external applications, the victim may again regain a normal complexion. It requires self-control and patience on his part, and both proper diagnosis and therapy on the part of his physician.

HIVES

Hives or urticaria affect many people. You may get it the first time you eat strawberries or peaches. Or you may spend an uncomfortable night after that delicious lobster. Or that last injection of penicillin which cured your boil shows up again one week later in the form of little swellings or wheals all over your body. The hive itself is a small whitish or pinkish bump which can appear anywhere on the body. It means that you are allergic to something or other, and if you are lucky you can quickly blame the strawberries, the lobster, or the penicillin. Alas, not all hive sufferers can find the cause of their symptoms so quickly, and a long, tedious search may be necessary if the hives keep on appearing over a prolonged period of time.

Usually the wheal is what is called evanescent. It comes and goes. It may last only for a second, or it may remain twenty-four hours. It sometimes appears so suddenly that it can actually be seen swelling. The wheals vary in size from that of a pea to a patch big enough to cover the whole face. Usually round or oval, they are sometimes irregular or ring-shaped, or they may develop like a map or become scalloped in shape.

There is usually itching, and sometimes burning or tingling or creeping sensations in the skin. Frequently the itching is intense. Another condition occurring with the hives is dermographism. This phenomenon consists in the appearance upon irritation of elevated white spots bounded by pink borders, which take the outline of the irritation that causes them. The irritation may be only slight pressure, or it may be pinching or scratching. In medical schools it is demonstrated to the students by stroking the patient's skin, or writing on it with a finger. The elevations appear wherever the finger touches the skin.

The wheal is produced by practically anything which affects the blood vessels of the skin. It is supposed to be due to a combined action of the nervous system acting on the blood vessels. The blood vessels are first closed in the central zone which results in the white area of the wheal. Those on the border are open to make the pink area.

Although hives may be produced by almost any kind of external or internal irritation, the more serious types are associated with constitutional and emotional disorders. Even when external causes are apparently the only ones, there is almost surely some disturbance or defect in the vasomotor system—the mechanism which controls the blood vessels and their nerves.

The internal disorders which produce hives fall into special groups. There are those due to allergy or to a sensitivity to proteins; those due to the taking of such drugs as quinine, aspirin, cathartics, or any other drug for which the individual has an idiosyncrasy; disturbances of the metabolism; disturbances of the blood; and nervous disorders. Still another group is due to intestinal disorders. Another group is due to the reaction from eating certain foods. Children especially suffer from this type of hives.

An attack of hives is usually of short duration. Twenty-four hours at most should cover the appearance and disappearance of the wheal. There are, however, short attacks which recur for several weeks. Other cases last for a long time. The itching is intense in the prolonged cases.

The great point is to discover the cause. In acute cases a simple diet is usually ordered and a thorough cleansing of the bowels. Large amounts of water should be imbibed–alkaline water is especially good–and a brief diet consisting mainly of tea, wheat-free cereal, lamb, and toast is advisable.

Chronic cases require a general examination and the care of a physician. Tests should be performed to determine sensitivity to various foods, pollens, and other possible causes of allergic reactions. Laboratory tests may be necessary, before the constitutional cause can be determined.

Certain drugs are of benefit in treating the hives. These include newer and potent antihistamine drugs, which work wonders in recent and acute attacks of hives. These so-called anti-allergic drugs are less effective in the chronic types which may be resistant to all measures including cortisone and its derivatives.

Adrenalin, one of the most powerful of all drugs, is also valuable in acute cases. It has the special effect of causing the blood vessels to contract, thus diminishing the formation of the wheal. Frequently adrenalin causes the immediate disappearance of the wheals and itching. Ephedrine is also given. But all these drugs are to be taken only on a physician's orders. They may have deleterious side effects and must be carefully supervised.

PSORIASIS

Psoriasis is a strange and capricious skin condition, characterized by the appearance of bright red, coin-shaped patches on the skin, especially on the knees and elbows. These bright red patches are often covered with delicate silvery-white scales. When these scales are scraped off the skin, a bright red surface with tiny bleeding spots is characteristic of the disease. Although this disease is not serious in that it does not affect the general health, it can be very annoying in that its constant appearance and reappearance, with spread to involve many different parts of the body, can be a source of great unhappiness. No one knows why this disease occurs. Strangely enough, the condition doesn't seem to bear any relationship whatsoever to various forms of internal or external illness and often affects people who are otherwise in the best of health. It is not infectious or communicable. In a small number of cases the condition may be associated with some form of arthritis.

One of the features of psoriasis has been that patients with the condition usually improve following exposure to sunshine. An old adage used to be that psoriasis does well with grease and water, soap and sunshine. This would mean, of course, the use of some drug in an ointment, following removal of the crusts by soap and water. The average patient with the condition requires a little more than the preceding if he really wants to know how to take care of the condition. Unfortunately, the permanent relief of a severe case of psoriasis cannot be promised as there is no remedy which will produce a permanent cure of the disease. However, the sufferers from this disease often find that common sense and the help of a physician who has had special experience in the treatment of this condition can get him through the severe episodes more rapidly and will often lessen the violence of a flare-up in the condition. The local measures which have been found to be of the greatest value include preparations containing cortisone and its derivatives, and to a lesser degree tar, ammoniated mercury, salicylic acid, and chrysarobin. These are strong drugs and capable of doing a considerable amount of damage unless closely supervised by the physician. This is particularly so because the concentrations of the drugs to be employed are usually high if they are to be effective. Some of these chemicals are more effective when the treated site is covered with an impervious plastic film. Continued diligent treatment will often bring about the disappearance of large patches of the disease. Specialists in diseases of the skin have also found that, in certain instances, the use of various drugs taken by mouth will be helpful in improving or controlling the condition. Again, intelligent co-operation between the patient and his doctor is of great value. At the present stage of our medical knowledge, the patient with psoriasis must learn how to live with the disease rather than to fight it constantly. This knowledge can be gained from a combination of expert medical therapy and guidance, plus an intelligent approach to the problem.

In recent years, it was discovered that certain drugs known as folic acid antagonists were helpful in the treatment of leukemia. At the same time it was noted that patients with leukemia who also had psoriasis observed that their skin disease improved greatly while on these drugs. Accordingly, these drugs have found a place in the treatment of severe, resistant psoriasis but only under the closest medical supervision as they are extremely potent and toxic.

LUPUS ERYTHEMATOSUS

This condition is an example of one of the skin diseases which can affect both the skin and the internal organs. The internal form is far more serious and may even occur in the absence of a rash on the skin. However, in the usual case it is associated with a reddish eruption involving the nose and the cheeks in what has been described as a "butterfly pattern." This form occurs most frequently in younger women and is related to overexposure to sunshine. In other words, there is a probability that a strong sunburn in a person who has had a preceding infection, or is predisposed to this disease, may be the aggravating or precipitating factor which touches off the whole process. The subsequent occurrence of changes in the heart, kidneys, and other internal organs would indicate the serious and often fatal nature of the condition. Although the disease has been treated with some success with cortisone and ACTH, these drugs usually serve merely to arrest or lessen the condition rather than result in a complete cure.

The external form is of a somewhat different type in that the victims are not necessarily sick. It also bears some relationship to preceding excessive exposure to sunshine, and is most often present on the nose and cheeks as a red butterfly-type of rash. In addition to the red rash on the face, the scalp is often involved and the skin may show patches of crusts, scars, and bald areas in the scalp. This disease is a serious one, and no attempt should be made to treat it at home. Injection of insoluble cortisone salts directly into the diseased areas may be helpful. It requires the services of a skilled physician. The use of various internally acting drugs, such as the antimalarial agents and others which may be potentially dangerous, should only be taken under constant supervision.

PEMPHIGUS

This is an extremely serious disease involving the skin. Its cause is unknown, although recent research would seem to indicate that it may be in part an infection and in part some disturbance in the general metabolism. It usually begins around the nose or mouth as a series of blisters or crusts, which get better or worse and never seem to heal completely. In time practically the entire body becomes covered with small and large blisters. These blisters may join together to form large areas of raw, weeping skin. The unfortunate victim literally leaks his life fluid through these open surfaces of the skin. In the majority of instances the disease was formerly fatal within a period of six months to several years. Within the past few years many patients have been helped and even cured by cortisone and ACTH administered in heroic doses.

SCLERODERMA

This disease is also a serious skin problem. The sufferer develops the condition gradually after having complained of previous circulatory changes in the skin. The hands and feet are cold and bluish in the beginning and eventually become hard, tight, and ulcerate easily. In time both arms and legs may become stony hard and firm to the touch, and the process may even involve the entire body. Not much is known about its cause except that the fibrous tissue and small blood vessels in the true skin have been severely damaged by an unknown toxin. Treatment is not too satisfactory, although some patients have been helped by warm climates, measures designed to improve the circulation of the skin surface, physical therapy, and some of the newer drugs such as cortisone, and ACTH. None of these measures have proved constantly satisfactory or curative.

DISORDERS OF PIGMENTATION

FRECKLES AND TANNING

These changes in the skin are brought about by exposure to sunlight. The natural reaction of the skin to light and some other forms of irritation is the formation of pigment, tanning. Some skins, notably those lacking in pigment, are not able to produce pigment as readily as the darker ones and often produce it only in spots. Freckles, therefore, are the indication of a weakness of the skin in this important function. Such skins should not be needlessly exposed to light, for they cannot protect themselves or the owner from its sometimes harmful effects, which do not appear at once, but may come to notice much later as senile freckles, liable to change to rough, scaly spots and end in cancer of the skin. These are larger and fewer than the ordinary freckles of youth and are more persistent. Such a skin should be protected as much as is possible from direct sunlight; though, of course, this is locking the barn long after the horse has been stolen, for such a skin should have been protected since early childhood. After the damage has occurred, its progress may be delayed somewhat by the daily application of a good cold cream. Treatment of senile freckles is usually not necessary unless they are disfiguring or show some tendency to become rough and horny. They should then be eradicated. The freckles of youth are best treated by preventive measures, as already stated. The mild applications suggested for chloasma may be tried if the freckles are disfiguring; but time and protection from light are the most successful measures.

CHLOASMA

Chloasma is the unequal browning of the skin of the face that occurs in women more often than in men and, like all increases of pigment, in dark-complexioned persons oftener than in blondes. Its popular name is "liver spots"; but the liver cannot be held responsible. (Apparently a hormone from the pituitary called the MSH or melanocyte stimulating hormone is responsible.—Ed.) The treatment often unsatisfactory, consists in trying to remove the surface layers of the skin by means of an inflammatory reaction produced by caustics. These, when strong enough to be effective, are hard to control and often cause too great an inflammation with most unpleasant consequences to the patient. Certain chemicals, all derived from a parent substance known as hydroquinone, are sometimes effective in lightening these patches. They must be used with caution because of their tendency to cause irritation of the skin. Another unfortunate side effect of these chemicals is their ability to lighten the normal skin immediately surrounding the brown patch with a resultant cosmetic effect that may be worse than the original condition.

VITILIGO

This disease is almost the opposite of freckling. White spots suddenly appear on the skin, usually around the face or on the backs of the hands. In time they get larger in size, and new white areas appear elsewhere on the body surface. These white spots are due to a loss of the pigment cells in the affected areas, but no one knows why they occur. They may be due to deficiencies in the glands of internal secretion, metabolic alterations, or various unknown factors. They sometimes appear at the same time as alopecia areata (see p. 782), and may be due to similar emotional problems.

The spots become more conspicuous if the surrounding skin gets sunburned—so stay out of the sun. The whitish areas may be effectively concealed by various cosmetic products. An Egyptian chemical, derived from an herb, has been reputed of value in some instances. This substance, chemically a member of the psoralen family, is of limited benefit and is not without toxic side effects.

BERLOCK DERMATITIS

This relatively common disorder appears as flat, dark brown spots, usually in a necklace or droplike appearance. It is more common in women and is due to the action of sunlight on skin previously covered with a sun oil, lotion, or perfume containing an essential perfume oil (bergamot). The usual sites are the sides of the neck, face, arms, and armpits, but any part of the body may be involved. The eruption is often produced by dripping or running down of the fluid on the skin, and this gives it the droplike appearance. It is due to light sensitivity, and the brown spots can appear with redness, inflammation, and even blistering. Treatment should consist at first of soothing creams and later of bleaching lotions. Cosmetics or other substances containing the essential causative oils must be avoided if recurrences are to be prevented.

THE HAIR

ORIGIN AND STRUCTURE

The hair is formed by a dipping down of part of the epidermis, which forms a pouch, at the bottom of which is a papilla, like that of the epidermis; but this one is a specialist among papillae in that it is able to build hair. From this a cylindrical body of skin cells forces its way up through the pouch, called the follicle, which is now long and narrow. Soon after they leave the parent papilla the cells of this cylindrical body become horny like those of the surface of the skin, and form a spine that extends beyond the surface for a distance. After the cells turn to horn they are no longer alive but form only a mechanical projection. As the hair grows by the formation of new cells in the papilla, the part above pushes out until it has attained its destined length. It then ceases to grow, unless cut off, and after a period of rest falls out, leaving the papilla in the skin to form a new hair. As already mentioned, the sebaceous duct joins the hair follicle near its upper end, filling the follicle with oil which is forced into the body of the hair. Below the gland the erector muscle of the hair joins the outer part of the follicle. During periods of excitement this muscle raises the hair from its normal slanting position to an erect one. Contraction of this muscle also helps to force out the contents of the sebaceous gland, and, during excitement or when the body is chilled, puckers the skin into the condition we call "goose flesh."

Most of the hair on our bodies is only a remnant of the hairy covering of our ancient ancestors. It is fine and consists of two layers, the cuticle, a layer of tiny flat scales surrounding the hair, overlapping one another like shingles on a roof, and the cortex which consists of long strands of spindle-shaped horn cells with tiny spaces between them, presumably for oil. These fine hairs are called lanugo hairs, from the word for wool. Coarser hairs, like those of the scalp, contain in addition to the two layers mentioned a third, a fine pithlike center filled with a few larger cells. The cortex contains the pigment of the hair in the form of granules and also as a fluid within the cells.

The average area of the adult scalp approximates 120 square inches. It is the site of a profuse growth of hairs varying in thickness, length, straightness, and color, depending upon the individual's racial characteristics and sex. As in the skin, the oil or sebaceous glands are located along the hair shaft and secrete an oily fluid which appears to supply a protective oily coating to the scalp and gives it a gloss. As has been stated previously, the secretion of the sebaceous material is stimulated especially by the male sex hormones and is most marked at the time of puberty. As the person grows older, there is less and less secretion, until in old age both the skin and the scalp are dry. One of the constituents of the sebum, or the oil secretion of the sebaceous glands, is a chemical known as squalene. Scientific study has shown that this chemical in adequate concentration acts as a depilatory on animal skin. This has led to the interesting theory that as male sex hormones are essential for the development of ordinary baldness, and the male hormones are the most powerful known stimulants of the secretion of oil, this sebaceous material may be related to baldness. However, this is only one of many theories relating to causative mechanism in ordinary baldness.

The entire body, with the exception of the palms and soles and a few small areas, is entirely covered with hair. The greatest percentage of this hair is a soft, delicate type of hair which is referred to as lanugo or fuzz and easily escapes notice by the naked eye. It has been estimated by a painstaking count that there are approximately 1000 hairs of all types per square inch of scalp. Since the average surface area of the scalp encompasses approximately 120 square inches, it requires 120,000 hairs to cover it. The finer the hair, the more numerous are the shafts present in a given area; blond hairs are usually finest, and average 140,000, and black hairs average 110,000 per scalp. It is possibly distressing to the average redhead to learn that she has the fewest hairs on her scalp, namely, approximately 90,000. When hair is allowed to grow its full length, it will measure between 22 and 27 inches and sometimes grow as long as 36 inches, but this is indeed rare. As is well known, the hair does not live forever but is shed and regrown constantly. The life span of a single hair averages from 6 months to several years, and in the instance of extremely long hair the age can be figured from the length of the hair. The rate of hair growth approximates between ¾ and 1 inch per month, so that a hair 24 inches in length may be considered to be about 2 years in age.

Another feature of the hair that is not generally recognized is the fact that hair varies in form from a straight hair to variations of curves, with the resultant kinky hair in the Negro, as contrasted with the straight or wavy hair of the white race. Hair is extremely elastic and can be stretched very considerably. If it were not for this fact, it would be impossible to wave the hair, and this is the basis of most of the so-called "permanent" waves.

EXCESSIVE SWEATING

Excessive sweating of the scalp is not uncommon and often gives rise to unpleasant odors which are increased by infrequent washing and the use of various perfumed types of hair tonic. The condition is easily remedied by proper local hygiene and frequent washing of the scalp.

GRAYING

The color of the hair is due in part to hereditary and racial factors. Its appearance to the observer is actually due to the presence of tiny pigment granules scattered throughout the shaft of the hair. These granules make their appearance at the base of the hair under the scalp and do not change once they are scattered through the hair shaft itself. In other words, once the pigmentation has formed, it cannot be changed because of internal reasons, but only through external applications such as dyes. In other words, hair does not turn white overnight, but the pigmented hair shafts are shed and are replaced in time by new hairs which do not have these tiny pigmentation specks. Few persons have hairs of an identical color over their entire scalp, and detailed examination under various lights shows that many shades of hair occur on one head. Blondes, in particular, sometimes reveal hundreds of varying shades on a single normal scalp. Graying of the hair is still somewhat of a mystery, and the exact chemical mechanism which takes place in the hair bulb just before the hair loses its pigment and becomes white is unknown. Premature graying may begin in childhood, and by the age of twenty-five or thirty the scalp has a sort of salt-and-pepper look, and by forty or forty-five the patient is completely gray. Contrasted with this comparatively rapid type of graying, normal grayness begins at thirty-five or thereabouts, with a few non-pigmented hairs around the temples and a gradual slow whitening over a period of many years. There was a great deal of publicity given to a report that gray hair might be prevented by certain substances in the vitamin field. These substances were members of the vitamin B complex family, and are known as para-aminobenzoic acid and pantothenic acid. Unfortunately, subsequent studies have not confirmed this report, and sufferers from grayness cannot expect to be cured with vitamins. At the present time the only method of changing hair color is to resort to a dye. Although comparatively harmless dyes are available, they do not impart a satisfactory color to the hair. The stronger dyes are not entirely harmless, but the process of hair dyeing has been considerably improved and is now considered a relatively safe procedure.

ENDOCRINES AND HAIR GROWTH

The glands of internal secretion, which play such an important role in the physical and emotional well-being of the human race, also influence the scalp and the hair. The problem of relationship of hair growth to endocrine secretion is a very involved one, and the problem is often to recognize which gland is the primary factor and which the secondary, as far as the hair and its growth are concerned.

The sex glands are of the greatest importance with reference to the growth of hair. The female hormones have a very specific effect on oil secretion and on the growth of hair. An excess of female hormones, either of natural origin or due to some form of administration, results in a decreased activity of the oil glands, a shrinking of the hair follicles, and a lessened formation of skin cells. Accordingly, the administration of female sex hormones is often followed by the appearance of smooth, delicate skin, dryer and fluffier hair, the lessening of dandruff, and the softening of the beard. If the woman taking female hormones is afflicted with acne, there is usually a decreased amount of blackhead formation and even the disappearance of acne pimples. Although the statement is often encountered in the medical literature that the female hormones increase or stimulate the growth of scalp hair, this cannot be stated with absolute certainty, although the weight of evidence is in its favor. On the other hand, the male sex hormones, which are primarily responsible for the growth and development of the male organs, also have a specific effect on the hair follicle and the skin surface. They are probably the greatest single factor responsible for the production of the oil secretion, and they are also responsible for excessive growth of the skin around the hair follicles, and finally, they are of primary importance in the production of ordinary male baldness. The most interesting feature of these sex gland secretions is that while the male hormones encourage the growth of body hair, they discourage the growth of scalp hair. On the other hand, female hormones encourage the growth of scalp hair and discourage the growth of body hair. Men who have been castrated before puberty, and whose sex glands have remained infantile accordingly, have scanty body hair, of a female type, and very sparse beards but thick luxuriant hair on their scalps. Such persons do not become bald. However, if these eunuchs are treated with large doses of male sex hormones, they will become bald if their family or racial background is one of ordinary baldness. Although these scientific facts are well known, these secretions cannot be used in the treatment of ordinary baldness because they have other effects which might be of a serious nature for the person concerned. However, when hair is lost following pregnancy or during the period of menopause, this loss of hair can be checked and frequently regrown by the appropriate use of the female sex hormones.

The adrenal gland also produces hormones which affect hair growth. For example, the wonder drugs cortisone and ACTH often increase facial hair while they are being given for the treatment of some other condition. In some instances, they even produce a mild degree of acne. These unfortunate side effects are usually temporary in nature and should be disregarded where the use of these drugs is necessary for the treatment of a serious disease. When the outer layer of the adrenal gland is overly active early in life, the person is frequently affected so that he appears far more advanced and older than his actual age. These "Young Hercules" often have an early growth of hair on their face and body, long before the time of puberty. When this gland becomes overactive in woman, the person begins to take on masculine features and there is often a considerable increase in body and facial hair.

The pituitary gland, especially one of its parts, also secretes hormones which affect the growth and development of hair. There is a disease which is due to a tumor of this gland and was first described by the famous brain surgeon, Harvey Cushing. It is known as Cushing's Syndrome and it affects women primarily. The women suffering from this tumor show certain color changes in the skin which look as though the skin has been bruised and stretched. In addition, these women develop a heavy beard. In other instances of disturbances of the pituitary gland there is an undersecretion of the pituitary hormones, and the individuals are known as Fröhlich types. These youngsters often have soft white skin and fat hips. They become so feminized as to even develop breasts. The face often remains free of hair, although the scalp growth is usually a good one.

As we have already learned, in connection with the skin, the thyroid gland regulates the metabolism and affects body growth. Where the thyroid gland is overactive, scalp hair is usually abundant but fine in quality and given to early grayness. In those instances where the thyroid gland does not supply an adequate amount of hormones, the skin is usually dry and puffy, and hair growth is scanty.

From the preceding brief description, it is evident that hair growth and glandular function are very closely related. At the present stage of our knowledge, no one glandular secretion can be said to be directly responsible for the growth or absence of hair. Each secretion is dependent in part on a secretion present in another gland which may either accelerate it or neutralize it, and that is why no specific gland can be definitely stated to be responsible for the sole production of hair.

NUTRITION

The relationship of diet to hair growth is of great importance, but is still a matter for speculation and future research. A few facts are available to us. The secretion of the sebaceous glands may be changed by either an excessive intake of fat or by an intake of special kinds of fat. For example, we know that certain types of fats are necessary for proper nutrition in rats, because a diet extremely low in this type of fat results in severe dandruff, scaliness, and baldness of the rats. If they are continued on this diet long enough, they will die at an early age. We also know that certain proteins are necessary for skin and hair growth. The reason for this is that these proteins contain a substance known as cystine which is found in far greater quantities in the skin and hair than in any other organ in the body. We know, too, that vitamin deficiency may affect the scalp. If the system is deficient in vitamin A, the hair loses its sheen and luster and then becomes dry and eventually falls out. Surprisingly enough, almost similar features will occur in rare instances where too much vitamin A has been supplied to the body. In other words, don't take too much or too little of any of these substances without your doctor's approval. Other vitamins have some effect on the secretion of the oil glands as well as hair growth, and these have been mentioned elsewhere.

CARE OF THE NORMAL SCALP

The care of the normal scalp and its hair is the day-to-day attention which we give our scalp and hair to maintain its health and to increase its beauty. This definition would therefore not only include the usual brushing, combing, and cleaning, but also the cutting and waving, and the application of lotions and similar preparations which have been developed to satisfy the hair fashions of the day. There are so many nonsensical theories and superstitions which have been raised about the values of the many things done to the scalp and hair that the truth and validity for their application will be briefly presented.

BRUSHING

The implement chosen to brush the hair is just as important as the manner in which the brushing is to be performed. The one characteristic which these brushes should have without fail is the ability to undergo frequent cleaning without injury. The bristles should be well spaced to allow washing to free accumulations of dirt at their base, and should be set in frames able to withstand soap and water. Lacquered or polished wood is not satisfactory because repeated immersion causes the varnish to disappear, leaving the porous grain to absorb foreign matter. Metal frames are preferable though unattractive, but best of all are the ones more recently manufactured of pastel-colored plastics which seem capable of taking all kinds of physical punishment. Brushes should be washed in soapsuds and water regularly, whether they show signs of dirt or not. Natural bristles, when immersed too frequently, may become soft and too yielding to have any value as a medium for brushing the hair. Nylon bristles are more resistant. They may be wiped dry immediately after washing, while natural bristles must be allowed to dry in the sun or near, but not too near, artificial heat. It is unnecessary to use boiling water for antisepsis of one's own brush when the scalp is a normal, healthy one and the brush has been used by one person only. When frequenting a beauty shop, however, one should insist upon the use of a sterilized brush which is brought into the booth wrapped in a sterile container. Insistence upon sterile implements is merely a normal precaution, and reputable shops have long made this a practice.

Brushing should be performed regularly night and morning, not because a hundred brush strokes each time were thought by our grandmothers to evoke luxuriant heads of hair, but because it aids combing by unknotting tousled hair in a gentler fashion than the comb, and because it temporarily affects the circulation of the scalp.

The hair should be divided into strands and brushing should begin near the bottom of each strand, which is held firmly between the thumb and forefinger. When a two- or three-inch sector at the end of the strand seems to have been freed from all snarls, the hair should be grasped several inches higher and brushed down as before. This process should continue until finally the brush is allowed to begin at the scalp and sweep down the entire strand of hair to its end without encountering any tangles. Careful treatment of this nature excludes the breaking and tearing out of individual hairs by too hasty and too violent tugging. Such procedures are, of course, for long hair. Short hair may be brushed directly from the scalp. The value of brushing is the exercise which it gives the scalp by pulling at it, no matter how gently. Recent observations claim to show that exercise which involves bending or keeping the head in a position lower than that of the rest of the body is just as effective in producing a temporary improvement in scalp circulation as brushing was thought to be. In all probability, neither procedure has any significant effect on either hair growth or the blood flow through the scalp.

Although brushing of the normal scalp is of some value, it must be modified in diseased states involving the hair. Where the hair is weakened and its attachment is less than normal, frequent and vigorous brushing may increase hair fall and result in further damage to the sick hair. Under such conditions gentle massage of the scalp and the immediate discontinuance of daily, vigorous brushing, tight rollers or curlers, and "teasing" of the hair is advised.

COMBING

Combs are employed not only for unsnarling tangled hair but also for the parting of the hair and its arrangement. No matter of what material the comb is made—whether ivory, shell, metal, or plastic—the teeth should be evenly spaced and separated sufficiently to make thorough cleaning between the teeth not too arduous a task. It is important to see that the teeth have rounded, blunt ends to avoid accidental scratching of the scalp, since we now know that many diseases of the scalp would not have been transmitted without an initial scratch or irritation which simplified the development of inflammation and infection.

Since combs are used even more frequently than brushes, both men and women carrying them about in pockets and pocketbooks, it is most important that their cleanliness be maintained and that no borrowing whatsoever be tolerated. As with brushes, soap and water are adequate cleaners. A small nailbrush may be used to clean between the teeth to be certain that all grease, dandruff scales, and city dust and grime have been removed. Sterilization may be assured by using weak solutions of alcohol or ammonia.

CUTTING

The only reason for cutting the hair is to add to one's comfort and to keep up one's appearance. The old-fashioned notion that frequent cutting of the hair and even shaving the scalp would augment its thickness has long since been completely discarded. The source of this fallacy must have been the gardener's successes at "cutting back" rosebushes and other shrubs to make them grow more successfully. The hair of the head which the naked eye discerns is fully developed, so no shaving or cutting can possibly affect the rate of its growth or influence its thickness. Painstaking research has proved that no part of the hair shaft above the surface of the scalp is capable of independent growth. All growth develops within the hair sheath.

SINGEING

When the ends of otherwise healthy hairs split, there is no cause for concern. If this is objectionable, it is only necessary to cut the hair shaft above the section which has already shown signs of separating. There is no scientific value whatsoever in singeing the hair. It is true that the flame eliminates the split end, but it also chars the hair shaft and tends to dry it higher up. Microscopic examination reveals the charring of the inner layers of the hair far above the point where the cuticle has been singed.

The unscientific notion that singeing is preferable to cutting was originally based on the erroneous belief that the entire hair is constantly nourished by a life-giving fluid which flows through a hollow canal in the hair shaft. These pseudoscientists thought that cutting would open an end of the canal and through this orifice the nourishing fluid would be lost, with resultant death of hair. Singeing, they believed, would weld the end into a closed point which would act as a stopper to the vial of nutritive elixir. Since, as stated above, the hair shaft with which we are dealing is to all intents and purposes a matured appendage beyond the scalp surface and not an animated one, this whole theory is nothing but primitive folklore.

SHAMPOOING

Shampooing was originally intended for the purpose of cleansing the hair and scalp, and this should still be its primary objective. However, when one reads the advertisements for a constantly growing list of new shampoos, and those "brought up to date," one reads not of their detergent and grease-dissolving value, but of their ability to leave the hair with a lustrous sheen. In other words, instead of just cleansing the hair shaft of all foreign matter, the advertisements brag that the shampoo adds to the glory of milady's tresses. Actually, the new synthetic detergents now being used in shampoos are such efficient cleansing agents that they actually remove the natural oils in the hair too completely. The proper treatment is to cleanse the hair and scalp first, and then, after the shampoo is completed, to add to the hair an appropriate oil to put the hair back into condition with regard to manageability and luster.

The question always arises as to how often the hair should be washed, particularly hair which is characterized as "dry." As a general rule, once every five days is ample when the hair is not excessively oily, although the more often it is washed, the better it is for the hair and the scalp. If dried properly, and subsequently treated according to the type of scalp, it is believed that the hair may be washed with impunity as many times as one has the energy to do so. Proper drying does not mean rubbing the wet hair briskly with a towel. Experimentation has shown that the tensile strength of hair when wet is considerably lessened, so, rather than risk breaking the hair, it should be exposed to heat, preferably that of the sun, although a warm current of air propelled by the fan of a hand dryer is also adequate. The inquisitional dryers which completely cover the head must be carefully regulated, since overheating will injure the hair by excessive drying, rendering it brittle, with the danger of damage when exposed to brush and comb.

The ideal shampoo should cleanse the scalp without either irritating the skin or causing excessive reduction of its natural oil. A shampoo with too alkaline a reaction or one with too great a detergency will dry the hair and make it brittle, instead of leaving it soft and lustrous. Since shampoos are designed specifically to remove all foreign matter, they should not themselves produce, either alone or in combination with water, any scum or gritty material remaining on the hair shaft. And lastly, for purely psychologic reasons, when combined with water they should evoke an instantaneous creamy lather.

All shampoos except those characterized as "dry" depend upon the addition of water. Hard water should be avoided for shampoos, or, if no soft water is available, it should be treated until it becomes soft. So-called "hard water" is water with a sufficiently high mineral salt content to interfere seriously with the lathering of soap. Usually hard water can be softened by simply boiling the water; but if chlorides and sulfates of magnesium and calcium are components, boiling is no help and the water will remain "permanently hard." When this type of water is used during a shampoo, the soap leaves a deposit on the hair shaft, thereby dulling the hair, and the scalp becomes irritated by the action of the harsh residue.

When soft water is totally unavailable, the permanent type of hard water may be softened at home by distillation. A Permutit system for home use has also been made available, but the simplest expedient is to add a 1 per cent solution of Calgon, a sodium hexametaphosphate. To test whether the water supply is soft or hard, one needs only to shake up the same amount of soap solution in two test tubes, one filled with the questionable water and the other with distilled, and compare the subsequent lathering. For the water to be sufficiently soft to use in shampooing, the lather should persist for a minimum of two minutes after agitation.

The best sources of soft water are rain, which is usually pure but may become contaminated passing through smog or being collected in unclean receptacles, and distilled water, which is the condensation of steam arising from boiling water. Water from subsurface springs becomes purified as it wells through the soil, which acts as a filter, and water from artesian wells may have varying degrees of hardness, and, whereas it is pure, treatment may be required to soften it.

The perfect shampoo should clean the scalp without producing irritation or causing excessive reduction of its natural oil. There are three types of shampoos in most popular use, and these are the soap shampoos, the dry shampoos, and the soapless shampoos. The most popular types are the soap shampoos in liquid form, and these are composed primarily of oils such as coconut oil, which have been made into a soap and then diluted in water or in a mixture of water and alcohol. The "dry" shampoos are so-called not because they are not liquid, but because they do not contain water. They are actually dry cleaners for the hair and should only be used for special reasons and indications. The soapless shampoos are a type of detergent and are very efficient cleaners. In fact, the main disadvantage of shampoos made of such substances is that they are so efficient that they actually clean the hair too well, and remove from it the last trace of oil. To get around this difficulty, it is often necessary to add substances such as egg yolk or various other oils in order to decrease this cleansing action. In some instances these soapless shampoos can be used on an irritated scalp where an ordinary shampoo might prove to be very irritating.

HAIR LOTIONS

So many nonsensical and fantastic claims have been made by manufacturers of hair lotions that there is a tendency among intelligent persons to deride their use altogether. Actually, a good antiseptic conditioning and stimulating lotion is useful in the scalp. The use of such a lotion, together with ordinary scalp hygiene, may help to keep the hair and scalp as bacteria-free as possible, as well as improve the appearance of the hair. None of the advertised lotions is capable of growing hair, for the simple reason that there is as yet no known preparation which will effect such a miracle. When applied with enthusiastic friction, they help to free the hair mechanically from dandruff, and to make the scalp less liable to bacterial infection. Persons with oily scalps may use a lotion frequently, but those with dry scalps should be careful not to increase the dryness of their scalps.

WAVING LOTIONS

For the past few years we have heard more and more about permanent waving of the hair. Unfortunately, there is no such thing as a truly permanent wave, inasmuch as only the hair which projects from the surface of the scalp can be waved. As soon as this hair grows out, the new hair will be of the same uncurled state as it was previously, according to the shape of the hair follicle under the surface of the scalp. Artificial waving has been practiced on the scalp since the earliest recorded times. There have been many methods of waving hair, varying from the simple metal and leather curlers up to the present vogue for the cold wave lotion. Although some of these lotions were considered unsafe unless used by extremely skilled operators, the passage of time has showed that intelligent application according to the directions listed in the merchandised product render the applications a safe and effective way of waving the hair.

The reverse of the permanent waving process is called the hair straightening process. Actually, it is the same procedure done in reverse, and it is very popular not only among the colored race, whose characteristic hair kinkiness is well known, but among all persons with extremely curly hair. Inasmuch as these chemical solutions are all comparatively strong, it is recommended that proper attention be paid to directions and that their use be limited to the periods of time recommended by the manufacturer.

HAIR DYES

There are four main types of hair dyes. In the first group, the dye is a vegetable color such as henna, and is of a comparatively safe type. Unfortunately, the process is painstaking, the color is not very attractive, and the results comparatively unsatisfactory. A rinse is also a hair dye, but the word is apparently more acceptable to the public than the word "dye." Nevertheless, any substances which change the color of the hair are hair dyes and not rinses. Blond hair is usually kept in its state of natural beauty by removing the dark pigment from the hair rather than by the use of a hair dye. The bleaching agent usually employed is a peroxide and ammonia mixture, although too large an amount of ammonia will impart an undesirable reddish shade to the hair. So-called platinum blond hair results from excessive bleaching and will occur if the peroxide and ammonia solution is kept in longer contact with the hair than usual. Although the average bleaching preparation is relatively safe to use, continued bleaching will result in dryness and brittleness of the hair, with resistance to permanent waving, and a generally unattractive and unflattering appearance.

Another form of dye is the metallic group, containing silver, copper, or lead. These dyes are only successful when frequent applications are made, and the desired color emerges after a series of treatments which progressively darken the hair. They are not too desirable from a standpoint of attractiveness and nuisance of application.

Far and away the most popular hair dyes are the synthetic types, containing a substance known as paraphenylenediamine, and its derivatives. The para dyes are effective in that they produce a desirable shade of hair color. Unfortunately, they have to be applied at frequent intervals and are comparatively expensive. In addition, a certain number of people become sensitive or allergic to these hair dyes, and may develop uncomfortable and annoying skin reactions. There has been a recent trend toward the use of home hair-dyeing preparations, and several manufacturers have comparatively safe and cosmetically satisfactory products on the market. Continued usage of these products may result in some degree of skin sensitivity and the user should follow the manufacturer's directions with reference to constant testing of the product before application. In the event of an allergic reaction to these dyes, consult your physician.

IRRITATION OF THE SCALP

The term "contact dermatitis" is used to describe an acute inflammation of the scalp due to the application of some chemical or other agent. Just as we have seen with the skin itself, the scalp may be considerably irritated following contact with chemicals such as shampoos, hair lotions, and hair dyes. The subsequent inflammation results in redness and itching of the scalp. In severe cases there is often an appearance of blisters and crusts throughout the scalp. Usually the entire cycle of the dermatitis is completed within a few days to a few weeks, but if the offending substance has not been discovered, a chronic eruption may result. The dermatitis of the scalp is dependent primarily on the strength of the offending agent, the condition of the scalp, and the presence of an allergic state due to a preceding contact with the same substance. If the person has already become allergic to the chemical as a result of a previous exposure, the reaction occurs quickly. The fine balance between the scalp's capacity to withstand exposure to a new substance may be upset by a variety of factors. Scalp resistance may be lowered by frequent washings with strong soaps, by excessive secretion of the oil and sweat glands, and by over-exposure to sunlight. The presence of an associated local disease such as dandruff, or extreme dryness of the scalp, may also play a role.

The diagnosis of the scalp condition is sometimes made easy by a history of an itching and burning sensation following the application of some new preparation to the hair. An acute eruption spreading down the neck and about the ears should often make the doctor suspicious of hair dyes or some recent chemical agent applied to the scalp. The tendency is for most people to deny that they use hair dyes, and some of them honestly believe that they never have because of clever advertising and promotion which allow the dye to masquerade under the name of "hair rinse" or "color restorer." However, dyes are not the only offenders. There are many other substances which will not only cause a reaction when brought in contact with the scalp, but may produce a dermatitis after a week or so. According to the Food and Drug Administration, the government agency which controls and supervises all types of cosmetic applications, the para dyes sooner or later produce skin eruptions in four out of every hundred people if they continue to come in contact with them.

Other substances which have been known to produce acute or chronic irritation of the scalp include perfumes, hair lotions, hair lacquers, hair straighteners, waving lotions, and even the ordinary skin enemies such as poison ivy and other plants. Dermatitis of the scalp and near-by skin has also resulted following contact with hat bands, rubber caps, and hat dyes.

The treatment of dermatitis of the scalp is similar in nature to the treatment of skin disorders of this type in general. The first step consists in the detection and elimination of the suspicious chemical. Sometimes it may be a simple matter to discover the cause, and then again it may be extremely difficult and even impossible. After the suspicious agent has been detected, it may merely be necessary to stop using the preparation. Where the exposure has been going on for a long time, it is also important to shampoo the suspected preparation out of the scalp or, in extreme cases, even shaving the head. The local inflammation should then be treated with mild wet dressings, such as weak boric acid or salt solution, as well as with bland and soothing ointments and lotions. Ointments containing weak dilutions of Burow's solution and mild vegetable oils are inexpensive and effective. Creams and lotions containing the various forms of cortisone may also be effective. If the scalp is extremely irritated, some of the newer drugs which have been found of value in the treatment of itching may be necessary. This, of course, is a matter for the physician to decide, although in general it may be stated that the anti-histaminic drugs are often of value, and in the extreme case both cortisone and ACTH have been found very useful drugs for the acutely uncomfortable stage of the eruption.

ORDINARY BALDNESS

The common or so-called garden variety of baldness is referred to medically as male pattern alopecia. Alopecia means baldness, and male pattern means of the typical form common to men. It is responsible for more than 95 per cent of all the cases of baldness. The loss of hair occurs with far greater frequency in men than in women, although women occasionally become bald also. In the usual case the loss of hair first manifests itself by a thinning of hair along the side margins between the scalp and forehead, and a slight moving back of the hairline over the temples. In time the hairline gradually moves itself back, and a small bald patch makes its appearance in the middle of the back of the scalp. With advancing age, the bald patches in these two areas gradually enlarge, and in extreme cases of baldness eventually meet, so that no hair is left except for a little fringe around the scalp. At this stage the victim's friends state that he has a "nice head of skin." The rate of hair loss is more or less an individual matter. In the early stages of beginning baldness hundreds of hairs may be shed in one day. After a period of time, these decrease to approximately fifty to a hundred. Because of these slowed-up periods of hair fall, advanced baldness is seldom noticed in a man before he is thirty years old. During these periods exempt from profuse hair fall there is the usual slight growth of new hair, but these are never of sufficient nature to compensate for the preceding loss. Furthermore, these newer hairs are usually of a fine and delicate type, being produced by a half-dead papilla. Their appearance is often glibly prophesied by the quack hair grower, and their actual appearance is attended by great fanfare and mutual congratulatory exchanges. Unfortunately, they rarely turn into a normal healthy type of hair. Beware of the quack who promises to grow a new head of hair for you!

Numerous theories have been advanced in an attempt to explain ordinary male baldness. According to studies performed by competent scientists, especially Dr. James Hamilton, the essential reason for the development of common baldness is an inherited racial tendency. We know that members of certain races inherit tendencies either to retain hair or to show certain definite types of baldness. Just think of different racial groups that you are familiar with, and you will realize that each group has a somewhat similar pattern of hair growth and hair loss. Another factor of importance in the production of ordinary baldness is the hormone secretions, particularly that provided by the secretions of the male and female sex glands. We know that baldness does not appear in men who for any one of several reasons did not mature sexually. Baldness can be produced in these men if they are later treated with male sex hormones, but only if their pedigrees show their families to be susceptible to baldness. And don't let the bald men use this fact as proof of their virility because it just is not so. The third reason for ordinary baldness is the simple process of getting older. Advancing age is always accompanied by an increase in the number of bald people and the extent of the usual typical baldness. These three factors—namely, an inherited racial tendency, the male sex hormones, and the aging factors—act singly and in unison to increase the tendency toward baldness. Although typical male baldness is limited to men, women may also lose their hair in similar fashion although this occurs far less frequently and is never as extensive as the advanced cases observed among older men. Other causes which have been blamed for baldness may play a small role, and some of these include tightness of the scalp, and the presence or absence of dandruff and seborrhea. In all probability, the association of dandruff, excessive oily secretions, and other local diseases are not of importance in the loss of hair, but they may be aggravating factors and may increase the extent and rapidity of hair fall. Inasmuch as baldness develops far more rapidly in the presence of circulating male sex hormones, and inasmuch as male sex hormones are the most powerful known stimulants of oil secretion, there is probably a relationship between the two which accounts in certain measure for the occurrence of baldness with greater frequency in the male sex.

At the present stage of our knowledge, there is no effective remedy for ordinary baldness, either from the standpoint of prevention or cure. Nevertheless, general massage of the scalp rarely does any harm. The local application of remedies of value in the treatment of dandruff and similar states have but little effect on the degree and extent of the baldness. It can be stated with almost complete certainty that the many so-called "scalp institutes" and "hair growers," whose advertisements fill the daily newspapers, have never been able to prevent or treat ordinary baldness with success. If you are losing your hair and you are worried about it, consult your family physician or a skin specialist if you wish to know what, if anything, can be done for the condition. Some of the newer "remedies" include hair transplants and the process called "hair-weaving."

OTHER TYPES OF BALDNESS

Although ordinary male baldness accounts for by far the greatest number of hairless scalps, the remaining examples of baldness may occur for any one of many reasons. First of all, a certain amount of baldness may occur in association with various types of scalp or skin disease, varying from the loss of hair in small patches to complete baldness involving all the hairy areas of the body. A diffuse shedding of the scalp hair often occurs following the ordinary childhood diseases if they have been associated with high fever for any period of time. This type of hair fall may occur after scarlet fever or measles and is usually temporary in nature, as the hair starts to grow in within a few weeks to a few months following the shedding. In addition to the childhood diseases, various toxic conditions, especially if associated with a high fever, may also produce a temporary or permanent loss of hair, and this has been noticed in diseases such as typhoid fever and influenza. The loss of hair is quite general over the scalp but seldom complete, that is, only a thinning of the hair occurs rather than complete baldness. These scalp changes may also occur in chronically ill people who are suffering from tuberculosis and other wasting diseases. Infections such as syphilis often produce loss of hair during certain stages of the disease. In syphilis the hair loss is fairly typical in that the hair falls out in small bald patches, giving the scalp a somewhat typical mangy or moth-eaten look. In most instances, with proper treatment, these types of baldness are followed by complete restoration of the hair.

THE SEBORRHEIC DISORDERS AND DANDRUFF

The most common malady to involve the scalp is dandruff. In this condition the scalp often becomes covered with loose dry scales or with fine branny flakes which result in a process of constant peeling of the scalp due to a flaking off of the outer layers of the skin. The scales are gray or white and fall off the scalp when they are disturbed by combing, brushing, or scratching. Much to the annoyance of the individual, they then appear in large quantities along their hairs and as "snow" on their shoulders. The scalp often feels itchy and even slightly irritated. Inasmuch as the oil secretions cannot flow freely in this condition, the hairs become dull and unruly. In the average person dandruff appears in early childhood and may persist as such for many years. However, in the majority of people the scales in time become greasier, yellowish, and more numerous. At this stage, the underlying scalp is apt to be more irritated and there are occasional crusted areas in the scalp which may even extend down the forehead. In other cases the scalp becomes excessively oily, and the face, especially around the sides of the nose, may show a similar extremely excessive oily condition. This profuse secretion of oil bathes the hair and the scalp and contributes to the glossy, greasy appearance of the latter. At times the secretion is so pronounced that drops of oil form and have to be wiped off. This is usually referred to as "oily seborrhea." These conditions are related in part to certain germs, to changes in glandular secretion, and to various general factors such as poor nutrition, chronic intestinal disturbances, and various unknown mechanisms.

The treatment should be managed by the physician, but the patient must expect to co-operate fully if he wishes to achieve a result. The main features of the treatment consist in the frequent shampooing of the scalp, and the constant use of ointments and lotions applied with massage, without neglecting the massage of daily brushing. There are various other methods which should be suggested by the physician, but the chief points in treatment are the patience and persistence of the individual with the scalp condition. The state of the general health has much to do with the recurrence of the different types of seborrheic conditions. Over-fatigue, worry, emotional disturbances, and loss of sleep are some of the causes of lowered resistance which may play a role in the continuance of these disturbances. It should also be mentioned that there are several preparations which have been found effective in the external treatment of these conditions. Some of these include selenium sulfide in a shampoo suspension, various new drying agents incorporated in defatting preparations, and some of the newer and more drying and degreasing types of shampoo.

The very oily forms of seborrhea require even more skillful treatment. If local measures are going to be effective, the scalp must first be freed of its fatty covering by bathing it in softening solutions such as olive and almond oil, with a small amount of glycerin. Even when the oily secretions are unusually large and crusted, soap and water will free the scales and cleanse the oily surface of the scalp. After this cleansing operation has been completed, alkaline rinses may be used to lessen the oiliness, and this would include mixtures of borax and ammonia carefully diluted to proportions harmless to the scalp itself. It is important to use an oily application immediately after such a mixture in order to prevent possible irritation of the scalp, and vegetable or mineral oil are usually effective for this purpose. Here again, measures which will improve the general health are very important. In many instances it has been found that people working indoors are most apt to suffer from these oily forms of seborrhea and they are often helped by fresh air and exercise in addition to the local measures.

SEBORRHEIC DERMATITIS

This disease usually follows the preceding local scalp disturbances such as dandruff and the oily forms of seborrhea. It is a more severe form, and usually shows, in addition to the features of the conditions mentioned, a considerable degree of greasy scaling, crusting, and redness involving both small and large areas throughout the scalp. In some instances the condition becomes so extensive and severe that it may spread to involve the face, ears, and many other parts of the body. In such instances it becomes a serious and difficult skin disease to treat and requires the services of a skilled dermatologist.

The ordinary forms of seborrheic dermatitis are considered due to the same causative mechanism that produces dandruff and the oily forms of seborrhea. The excessive flow of oil on the surface of the scalp depends in turn upon the production of excessive amounts of male hormones by the gland of internal secretion. The question as to whether or not the process is also related to secondary infection is still undecided. There has also been considerable research to show that poor nutrition plays a role, as do certain hereditary factors, chronic intestinal conditions, inadequate personal hygiene, and various emotional disturbances.

The treatment of the chronic type of seborrheic eczema or dermatitis is difficult. It may be helped by proper diet and the administration of vitamin B complex, combined with crude liver extract. No matter what therapeutic measures are advised, it is necessary for all the victims of this condition to follow an intelligent daily routine with regular periods for rest and sleep, frequent bathing, the use of soap substitutes if soap proves to be an irritant, a diet high in protein and low in fats and carbohydrates, and the elimination of alcohol. In the acute stages of the condition it is often necessary to resort to wet dressings in order to lessen the inflammation. After the condition improves, a soothing ointment or lotion is of value. In the scalp the most useful preparations contain chemicals such as sulphur, salicylic acid, and resorcin. If infection is present, it is often necessary to add an antibiotic such as neomycin. This, of course, is only done under the supervision of a physician, as it is recognized that any of these preparations is capable of acting as an irritant to the skin and scalp and that they must be watched with great care. The very acute and severe forms of seborrheic dermatitis may even require hospitalization and intensive treatment with the steroid hormones. I routinely advise a low fat and low carbohydrate, high protein type of diet, with the elimination of alcohol and excessively hot foods and drinks. In the heavy and red-faced individual, it is often necessary to make sure that the mundane pleasures of steam cabinets, Turkish baths, and daily massage are not indulged in. These simple measures are important only in combination with more specific medical treatment.

INFECTIONS OF THE SCALP

The same bacterial infections that involve the skin may also appear on the scalp. Impetigo, boils, and carbuncles occasionally occur in the scalp and are similar in appearance to the condition when it involves the skin. In impetigo the scalp shows typical honey-colored crusts scattered throughout the hair, often in children having head lice. Boils start as an infection in the hair follicle, with swelling and discharge of pus. In neglected cases they may spread throughout the entire scalp. This is especially true when the boil starts in the back of the neck, and rubbing and friction from the collar cause it to spread. These conditions all respond promptly to both local and internal measures including wet dressings, antiseptics, and antibiotics such as neomycin (externally) and penicillin and the tetracyclines (internally).

It is of the utmost importance to exercise proper local hygiene if a recurrence is to be prevented. Such measures include frequent washing and shampooing of the scalp and adjoining skin, the wearing of clean, soft collars, and a proper diet, including the avoidance of excessive sweets, starches, fatty and greasy foods.

Ringworm of the scalp is a far more serious condition and is due to the attack of the hair and scalp by a fungus. This organism primarily occurs in children before the age of puberty. It is characterized by the appearance of scaly, bald patches, sometimes covered with brittle and broken hair stubs, and in certain cases with small pustules. Any bald patch in a child's scalp should be considered as a possible ringworm infection until the doctor rubs it out. The disease is highly communicable and may be spread from animals to humans, or, depending upon the type of ringworm, from children to other children. In the epidemic that occurred during the last war it was found that the backs of theater seats and barber shops were often a source of contagion. Insist that your barber clean his instruments before cutting your child's hair, and you may save yourself a serious problem. Also, if your youngster loves to go to the movies and rest his head on the back of the seat, tell him to put his handkerchief on the seat or bring along a little paper towel that he can put on the seat before sitting back and relaxing.

The most common type of ringworm of the scalp is a so-called "gray patch" or human type. In this variety the diseased area is usually round and bald except for a few hairs which have been broken off above the surface of the scalp. It may be impossible to see any bald areas in the scalp, the only sign of infection being the presence of a few scaly or crusted scabs in the scalp. In these instances a doctor should be consulted so that the child can be examined under a special light known as a Wood's filter. Under this very helpful light, the infected areas show up as bright green fluorescent hairs which are immediately both typical and diagnostic. This little gadget has been of great help in screening the scalps of hundreds of school children and in preventing the spread of epidemics of the disease. It is also of value in diagnosing other forms of ringworm, although certain unusual types of the disease do not cause the hair to fluoresce under the light.

The second type of ringworm most commonly encountered is that which is transmitted not only from child to child, but by domestic animals such as dogs or cats. It differs from the simple gray patch type of ringworm because there is a certain amount of inflammation and pus formation present. These are the two most common types of ringworm, although there are many other less common forms observed in different parts of the world. The doctor has a rule that any child showing scaly or bald patches on the scalp must be considered as having a ringworm infection until the Wood's filter and the examination of the hair shows it to be otherwise. In addition to the Wood's light as a means of diagnosis, it is also of importance to the doctor to examine the hairs directly under the miscroscope and, in suspicious cases, to attempt to grow the organism from the hair by planting the hair in some type of culture medium.

The treatment of ringworm of the scalp depends upon the type of fungus producing the disease. When the organism is of the so-called animal type, which results in infection of the scalp, the use of local remedies such as sulphur, ammoniated mercury, and some of the newer chemicals, combined with frequent shampooing, is usually effective. The reason for this is that the infection around the hair loosens the hair and causes it to be shed from the surface of the scalp. Unfortunately, in the other types of ringworm, where no infection is present, the infected hair is held tightly in the scalp and any attempts to pull it out only result in breaking the hair and the continuance of the infection in the hair under the surface of the scalp. Fortunately, the treatment of all types of ringworm of the scalp has been greatly simplified by the development of an antifungal antibiotic known as griseofulvin. This drug is administered by mouth over a period of four weeks or longer and invariably results in a cure of this disease. In former years, many youngsters required an X-ray treatment to the scalp in order to cause a falling out of the hair and this was a very exact and tricky form of treatment. Fortunately, griseofulvin has all but eliminated the need for this form of therapy.

HEAD LICE

The head is frequently infected in young children by the head louse referred to medically as pediculosis capitis. The head louse is a small animal approximately 2 mm. long, of a gray color and with black spots around the margins of its body. It inhabits the scalp, especially in children of both sexes and of questionable cleanliness. These lice set up severe itching of the scalp, due to the fact that they feed on and bite the scalp surface. As a result of itching, the child scratches the scalp and often produces a secondary infection. This infection may be so severe that the occasional child develops large glands of the neck due to drainage from the infected areas. Where the social environment is one of absolute neglect, an occasional child may be found to have the head covered with a hairy mess teeming with lice and covered with hundreds of eggs (nits). This combination, plus secondary infection and crusts, leads to a nauseating odor and the accumulation of pus and infected debris on the scalp. Fortunately, these conditions are rare at the present time, although an occasional refugee or neglected child may be seen with such an extreme degree of lousiness. The eggs look like tiny white or grayish grains stuck to the hairs, near the surface of the scalp. In many instances the duration of the infection can be determined by the distance from the egg to the hair shaft, inasmuch as the egg is deposited at the scalp margin and grows out with the hair shaft. In other words, if the egg is approximately one inch from the scalp, the infection would be approximately one month old, inasmuch as hair grows at the rate of approximately one-half inch every two weeks.

There are many local remedies which bring about a speedy and rapid cure of pediculosis capitis. First, it is necessary to remove all sources of the infection and to observe the normal rules of cleanliness if a recurrence is to be prevented. This means that hats, combs, and brushes which have been recently in contact with the scalp should be cleaned very thoroughly or thrown out. The present methods of treatment include the use of DDT in various powders or ointment forms, as well as killers of animal parasites, including benzyl benzoate and benzene hexachloride.

The eggs can be removed from the hair shaft with scalp rinses of vinegar or similar substances, and then simply eased off the hair shaft with tweezers.

ALOPECIA AREATA

Alopecia areata is a fairly common disease of the hair, occurring more often in children than in adults but not uncommonly in the latter. Often without warning, a bunch of hair may be found upon the pillow in the morning, or a small completely bald patch suddenly noticed in the scalp. There may be only one small spot, but frequently others appear and join to form large, queerly shaped areas. In rare cases this hair loss progresses until all the hair upon the body has disappeared. Such cases are difficult to cure, but to the ordinary case with a limited amount of baldness of the scalp a much more cheerful outlook can be given, for they usually clear up after some months of treatment. In the bald patches the hair may grow in blond at first, even in dark-haired persons; but this usually changes to the normal color later. In those of middle age the hair may come in white and remain so. The afflicted one need not be frightened if the first growth of hair falls out, for continuation of treatment is usually successful in causing a permanent growth. The cause of the disease is not known, but bears a definite relationship to various psychosomatic factors. Resistant cases of this disease have been successfully treated with injections of insoluble forms of cortisone directly into the bald patch. This treatment must be carefully supervised. It is most effective in recent rather than in old cases of alopecia areata. A more permanent cure may depend upon a thorough understanding of the physical and mental causes of the disease.

SUPERFLUOUS HAIR

Undesired hair on a lady's face is a greater trial even than the lack of it upon the head of her husband. This common form of irregular hair distribution often begins in early adult life and causes great mental distress. The mild form appears as lengthening and darkening of the ends of the mustache or groups of long hairs on the sides of the chin; but in severe cases the beard is complete and fairly thick. Efforts to relieve this condition have been made since time immemorial, and the old methods are still in use: the razor, the depilatory, and the resin-wax method. Shaving and the use of depilatory creams and lotions are alike in removing only that portion of the hair which projects from the follicle. After their use the hair grows out stiff. The resin-wax method pulls out the whole hair, and it grows again only after a considerable time and then as a young hair, pointed at the end.

When X rays were first studied, it was thought that they might be the long-desired means of wholesale removal of hair; but it was soon found that it could not be done by this method without great danger of injury to the skin. That such injury might not make itself known for months or years after the treatment did not make it any less serious. All reputable dermatologists have agreed that this method is unsafe. The only permanent and safe method of hair removal is electrolysis. It is slow and tedious; but safe, certain, and not very painful.

If fine hairs become dark-colored, they can be made less conspicuous by bleaching with peroxide solution, to four parts of which one part of ammonia water is added just before applying it on a cotton pledget. This should not be used often enough to irritate the skin.

THE NAILS

The nails are horny plates designed for protection of the ends of the fingers and toes and also for weapons of defense and offense. These latter uses have to some extent gone out of style, although some women are unaware of that fact. These plates are produced by the epidermal cells much as are the hairs. Normally they are smooth, curved from side to side, and very slightly curved in the long axis. At the base is a light-colored oval area where the active growth of the nail is going on, and over it, next the fold of skin under which the nail grows, is a special membrane, popularly referred to as the "cuticle." As the nail grows, the free end wears off in those doing rough work, or in those who have itching skin disease and keep their nails worn short and highly polished from constant scratching. Nervous individuals often keep their nails short by biting. When protected from friction and injury, the nail may grow several inches long, a good sign of inactivity and the so-called "leisure class."

HYGIENE OF THE NAILS

They should be kept cut fairly short. Fashion decrees at times that they should be trimmed so that they are pointed. This does them no harm. Neither does the polishing, if it is done in a way to avoid infection, nor the various colored nail polishes in popular vogue. Careful pushing back of the cuticle is also harmless if gently done with a smooth, clean instrument, preferably of wood. The manicurist should have some knowledge of cleanliness and should sterilize her instruments by boiling after each use. The polishing pad has gone out of style, and the present-day use of a liquid polish is much more sanitary. After trimming off hangnails, the little tags of skin that become loosened along the sides of the nails, the spot should be touched with an antiseptic. Do not bite or pick hangnails, for these methods favor infection, especially an infected swelling called paronychia or "run-around." Cleansing of the nails should be done after thorough washing, that the dirt under the free edge may be well loosened. A sharp instrument should not be used for this, because it will roughen the inner side of the free portion, dirt will adhere more tightly, and more scraping will be necessary to dislodge it. If the skin of the hands is dry, the nail folds should receive special attention in applying cold cream, for deformities of the nail may result from lack of oil. Dry and brittle nails are common complaints. The causes of nails of this type are not completely known, although in specific instances the reasons are definite. For example, a certain type of nail polish was only applied to the nails after a so-called "base-coat" had been applied first. Many women were allergic to this particular base-coat and their nails became dry, brittle, and deformed. In some cases the reaction was so severe that they lost their nails. Fortunately, the cause was detected and the base-coat taken off the market. In other instances dry and brittle nails may be due to a vitamin deficiency (especially vitamin A), a mineral deficiency (especially calcium), a protein deficiency (especially cystine), or a glandular deficiency (especially thyroid). Don't attempt to be your own doctor, but get professional advice if you are worried about your nail condition. It may be as simple as stopping your nail polish or avoiding soap and water to the best of your ability!

Transverse grooves appear in the nails commonly after illness, sometimes after so trivial a disorder as seasickness, and gradually disappear by growing out to the free end. Any disturbance to the nutrition of the nail may cause this deformity. Even overenthusiastic care of the nails—such as pushing down the cuticle too roughly, cutting it, or injuries received in other ways—may lead to nail deformities. The same is true of other deformities of the nails—longitudinal ridges, pitting, splitting—and often it is impossible to find the cause of these irregularities of growth because they are so slight that the nail changes are the only evidence. Loosening of the nails at the sides may occur in the absence of any other sign of disease; but is usually only temporary. Spoon-shaped nails and other abnormal changes may be hereditary, with accompanying hair and tooth deficiencies, or may result from malnutrition or anemia.

White spots on the nails, "gift spots," may be caused by general disease or local injury. They are the result of imperfect formation of the horny plate as the nail grows and usually disappear in time.

Thickening of the nails may be caused by nutritional disorder, skin disease, or more frequently by ringworm infection of the nail. It occurs most often on the nail of the big toe, and if not due to infection may be kept in check by paring and scraping. Ringworm of the nails is important because, owing to the fact that it is unobtrusive in its manifestations, it is often not noticed, and if treated is very difficult to cure. Therefore, it is likely to remain as a focus of the disease from which infection is spread to other parts. The most successful treatment entails oral administration of the antifungal antibiotic, griseofulvin, over long periods of time plus scrupulous removal of diseased nail tissue. These severe nail changes are not hopeless, but take time and skill if a cure is to be obtained.

Ingrowing toenails are caused by improper nail cutting, tight shoes, or local injury. They can be cured, before they become severely inflamed, by carefully cutting out the ingrowing part at the sides of the free border of the nail and preventing regrowth in this direction by padding with wool. This procedure should be performed with the utmost attention to cleanliness in order to minimize infection. Once infection has occurred, wet dressings and some of the newer antiseptics result in rapid cure under medical supervision.

ACKNOWLEDGMENTS

Acknowledgment is hereby given to the following articles and books which were used as a source of material and actual text matter in the preceding chapter.

1. *The Modern Home Medical Adviser* edited by Dr. Morris Fishbein. Chapter 25—The Skin—by Dr. Arthur W. Stillians, 1937.

2. *Your Skin and Its Care* by Dr. Howard T. Behrman and Dr. Oscar L. Levin. Emerson Books, Inc., New York, 1951.

3. *Your Hair and Its Care* by Dr. Oscar L. Levin and Dr. Howard T. Behrman. Emerson Books, Inc., New York, 1947.

4. *The Scalp in Health and Disease* by Dr. Howard T. Behrman. C. V. Mosby Co., St. Louis, 1952.

5. "Eczema" by Dr. Howard T. Behrman was reprinted in part from *Hygeia Magazine* (Today's Health), American Medical Association.

CHAPTER 28

The Eye

MANUEL L. STILLERMAN, M.D.
VICTOR ABRAMSON, M.D.

The eyes are man's window to the world. The newborn baby begins to recognize his family and toys, and as he grows older, he uses his eyes constantly to protect himself and to acquire more complicated physical and mental skills. Failure to develop useful vision, or early blindness, may result in inadequate emotional, intellectual, and even bodily development in the growing child. Blindness later in life may force a drastic change in the person's pattern of existence, and often deprives him of the means of earning a livelihood. An understanding of the structure and function of the eye is important, as is the realization that the eyes may be involved in diseases that affect other parts of the body.

HOW WE SEE

The human eye is roughly globe-shaped and about one inch long. It is an exquisitely sensitive instrument that has been compared with a camera. The healthy eye has a clear front window (the cornea) which fits over the colored part of the eye (the iris) and the pupil, as a crystal covers the face of a watch. Back of the pupil, which is really an opening in the iris, is a second clear window (the lens). In a perfectly constructed eye, light enters through the cornea, pupil, and lens and is focussed on the retina to form a clear image of an observed object. The light striking the healthy retina sets off a chemical and electrical reaction which is transmitted through the optic nerve and pathways to the visual center at the back of the brain. Most of us are blessed with two eyes which send slightly different pictures to the brain center. The ideal situation is for the brain to put these two pictures together (fusion) to form a single three-dimensional image. The teamwork necessary to bring this about depends on good vision in each eye, normal muscles to move the eyes together, and a healthy nervous system to receive the signals.

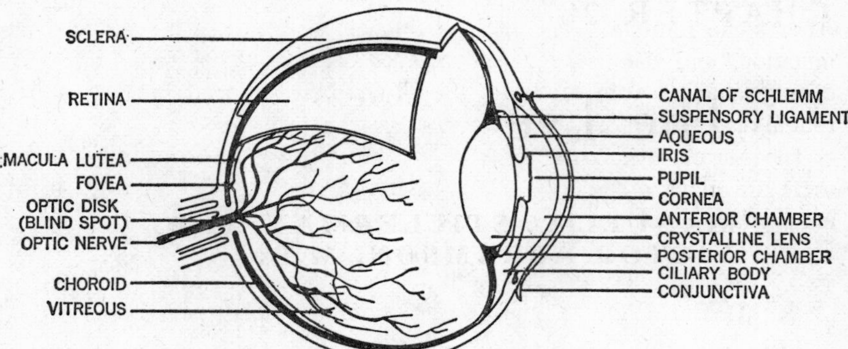

Fig. 71. If a person's eyeball is too long and the image in focus falls in front of the retina, he will be nearsighted. If the eyeball is too short and the image falls behind it, he will be farsighted. If the cornea has an imperfect curvature, he will have astigmatism. Heavily prescribed eyeglasses or contact lenses are the only means of correcting these visual faults. By courtesy of the National Society for the Prevention of Blindness, Inc.

Not all normal eyes see clearly, because few human eyes have the exact dimensions to simulate a sharply focussed camera. These differences in size and shape make certain eyes nearsighted, others farsighted, and still others astigmatic. This requires the wearing of glasses or contact lenses to obtain clear vision. The eye specialist measures the vision with charts, and determines with other tests whether corrective lenses are necessary to provide clear and comfortable vision.

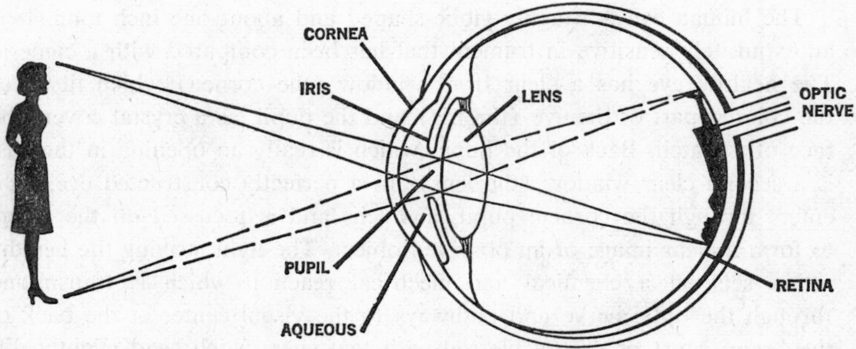

Fig. 72. Vision is a function that requires more than the eye alone. In order for the eye to do the job completely, there must also be light to see by and the brain to define what is seen. As light strikes an object in a person's field of vision—a girl, for example—the light rays are reflected from the girl to his eyes.

The eye has great adaptability with regard to seeing objects which are greatly different in their brightness. A person may see objects well in bright daylight, but if he enters a darkened room, the vision is, at first, poor. After some minutes, the healthy retina adapts itself to the reduced illumination, and the person begins to see objects which were initially indistinguishable. This adaptability is frequently reduced or lost in such retinal disorders as retinitis pigmentosa.

The normal eye not only distinguishes form, but also color. Although there are many areas of dispute with regard to color vision, some people are partially or wholly color blind.

THE IMPORTANCE OF PRESERVING OUR SIGHT

This country has 385,000 legally blind persons, and many more with such poor vision that they are unable to hold regular jobs or lead independent lives. Perhaps half of the new cases of blindness in the United States could be prevented by the combined efforts of patients and physicians to prevent accidents, achieve early diagnosis and institute prompt treatment. Over two-thirds of the known blind in the world might still have useful vision today had they benefited from modern preventive medicine and surgery. The hope for reducing needless blindness in the future lies in continuous education of the public plus the teamwork of local governments, sight-saving agencies, and the World Health Organization. Even so, many people would lose their sight because science has not solved all the problems of aging and such systemic disorders as diabetes, hardening of the arteries, high blood pressure, and nephritis. The need for continued research in these areas is evident.

HOW WE RECOGNIZE THAT AN EYE PROBLEM EXISTS

About seven million children in the United States receive improper eye care because their parents and teachers do not realize that there is a problem. Certain clues point to a possible visual or ocular defect that requires

---

The rays pass through the *cornea* or clear front window, the *aqueous,* or watery liquid behind the cornea, the *pupil,* or opening in the colored *iris,* and the *lens.* The lens of the eye bends the light rays as they pass through it, and focuses them on the retina, or rear inner lining of the eye which contains optic nerve cells. The lens operates much as a camera lens focuses light rays on film. The retina then relays the light ray image through the *optic nerve* to the brain. Though the image is received upside down because the lens has inverted it, the brain interprets it correctly and the viewer sees the girl right side up. By courtesy of The National Society for the Prevention of Blindness, Inc.

evaluation by an eye physician. Unusual events during the pregnancy or delivery of the baby, strange behavior of the infant, or abnormalities noted by the parents may suggest the need for eye examination.

For example, every mother who has had German measles or any other virus infection during the first three months of her pregnancy should have her baby's eyes studied after birth by a medical eye specialist (ophthalmologist or oculist). These infants are frequently born with cloudy lenses, and are said to have congenital cataracts which prevent development of good vision.

Babies born prematurely, especially if they weigh three pounds or less, should be observed closely during the early days and months of life by both the pediatrician and the oculist. These children are prone to develop a sight-destroying disease called Retrolental Fibroplasia (R.L.F.) if they are given uncontrolled amounts of oxygen in the immediate period after birth.

Other signs of trouble may be noted. The child who digs his fists into his eyes as if in pain, or whose eyes are sensitive to light and water profusely, should be suspected of having increased pressure in the eyes (congenital glaucoma). Tearing might also mean that the tear passages are obstructed, but if accompanied by reddened eyes or secretion, should suggest an infection.

Any baby older than six weeks of age that doesn't show signs of recognizing objects in his environment should be suspected of having some ocular problem. Any child who squints, closes one eye, or tilts and turns his head, trying to see better, should have professional evaluation. A child with eyes that cross, turn out, or deviate from the "straight" position, will seldom if ever outgrow the condition. Any child over six months of age with eyes that do not "track" together should be seen by the oculist.

Any evidence of poor vision at any age should be investigated. Sitting too close to the television set, or holding pictures or print close to the face, may not mean that the vision is poor. Many boys and girls do this, because of poor reading habits, but it could be a warning sign. The school child that has difficulty reading should have a sight test. Most of the reading difficulties, however, are not due to poor vision, but to deficiencies higher up in the nervous system which require remedial reading training.

When should you have your child's eyes examined for the first time? Certainly, before the youngster enters the first grade. Many authorities think that the first eye test should be done by three and one-half to four years of age. The reason is that two to three per cent of children without signs of visual defect may be doing all their seeing with one eye, while the other eye sees poorly. Early detection may allow the eye doctor to patch the good eye and force the poor eye to develop useful vision. If this situation is discovered at six years of age, it is virtually impossible to make the child wear the cover over the good eye because of social or emotional reasons. As a result, such a child may grow to adulthood with poor vision in one eye. This could be a handicap if the good eye were to be injured in the future.

WHAT TO DO FOR CERTAIN COMMON EYE EMERGENCIES

FOREIGN BODIES IN THE EYE

Most of these are lodged on the under surface of the lids or somewhere on the surface of the eye. Dr. Morris Fishbein has pointed out that there are hundreds of superstitions as to how these particles should be removed. It was an old custom in Russia to remove them with the tip of the tongue (the doctor's, not the patient's). Other techniques involve making the patient sneeze, rub his other eye, pulling on the upper lid and spitting three times. None of these is recommended, and certainly the eye with the foreign particle should not be rubbed lest the material be embedded deeper in the tissues. We are constantly amazed by patients who allow pharmacists, grocery clerks, shoe salesmen, and mere passers-by to attempt to remove cinders from the eye. People who understand how to remove foreign bodies are exceedingly careful to make certain that their own hands are clean, and that every instrument, solution, or other material introduced into the eye is clean or sterilized. Gentleness in handling the lids is imperative. The patient is requested to look up, and the lower lid and surface of the eyeball are inspected with a bright light.

The patient next looks downward, and the upper lid is turned over gently and inspected. If the offending particle is not discovered, the surface of the globe is explored with the light. If the foreign body lies on the surface of the cornea (the clear window over the colored part of the eye), one might try to wash it out using an eye cup and some sterile boric acid or normal saline solution. If it does not wash out, cover the eye with a clean handkerchief or a sterile pad. Do not allow anyone but a qualified eye physician to remove the particle. In industry it should be a rule that under no circumstances should an untrained or inexperienced employee attempt to remove any foreign body from the eye.

The oculist will introduce a local anesthetic solution into the eye and painlessly remove the foreign body. He is careful not to introduce infection, and will usually request a follow-up examination to be certain that there are no secondary infections, ulcerations, or other sight threatening complications. The doctor will often patch the eye and introduce antibiotic eye drops periodically until the area is healed.

Certain accidents occur in and around the household. A person lighting a cigarette may strike a match and part of the flaming head may fly into the eye. This may not only burn the eye or lids, but may also cause foreign material to lodge in the eye. The eye may be inspected as described, but it is wise not to instill any drops, ointments, or other material in the eye without consulting the eye physician as soon as possible.

Other injuries which require the same type of care are the eyes poked by a child's finger, a branch of a tree, or other foreign object.

CHEMICAL BURNS

These injuries may be devastating to the eye and may result in blindness. Although the chemicals and circumstances of injury may differ, the first-aid treatment is the same. Flush the chemical out of the eye and off the lids with copious amounts of tap water. If necessary, have someone hold the lids apart and put the patient's head and eye under the faucet. Do not take the time to find out if the chemical is an alkali, acid, or detergent, and do not worry about finding a specific antidote to neutralize the chemical in the eye.

In the industrial situation, the emergency flushing out of the eye is the same as already described. If a sterile boric acid or normal salt solution is at hand, it should be used, but time is important. Use tap water rather than go to another room to look for the sterile solutions. The person whose eye is involved should be sent immediately to the physician who is in charge of such cases. If the factory or workshop does not have a first-aid department, arrangements should be made with some nearby hospital or clinic to give prompt attention to such cases. This will avoid unnecessary blindness and will make the period of disability shorter than is otherwise the case.

MISCELLANEOUS INJURIES

Hair spray, eye-liner cosmetic pencils, false eyelashes, and other beauty aids may cause ocular injury. They should be kept out of the eyes, of course, but if they do get in, they should be dealt with in the same fashion as any other foreign body.

BLUNT INJURIES: THE "BLACK EYE"

Any blunt injury, whether delivered to the eye and its surrounding structures by a fist, baseball, squash racket, door, etc., results in the familiar "shiner." If the injury merely causes bleeding from small, superficial vessels in the "white of the eye" or in the soft tissues of the lid, there is more embarrassment than danger. Many times, however, there may be associated fractures of the bones around the eye. Such "blow-out" fractures of the orbital floor may allow the eye to drop down lower than its fellow eye and produce double vision. Early surgery is indicated to elevate the depressed bone to prevent permanent double vision. The eye itself should be examined carefully to make certain that internal injury has not resulted from the blow.

PENETRATING INJURY

Even more dangerous to the eye itself than a blunt injury is the type in which the eye is penetrated by a sharp wire, flying particles of glass, steel, or other foreign materials. Not only may the eye be damaged by the force of the entering object, but the eye can possibly be lost from infection. Even if infection can be prevented by the use of antibiotics, certain substances, such as iron, zinc, and copper, if retained in the eye, will slowly release chemicals into the eye that can destroy it. Inert substances like glass may remain inside the eye for years and not cause trouble. However, all foreign material should be removed if it can be done without destroying the eye in the process.

The removal of foreign substances is difficult, and only a skilled eye surgeon should attempt it. The X ray is of great aid in detecting and localizing opaque foreign bodies, but it is worthless for finding such particles as wood, certain forms of glass, dirt, and vegetable matter. If the foreign substance is magnetic, the surgeon may use a powerful magnet to remove it after the X rays and a localizer (similar to the mine detectors used in war) have found the exact position of the particle.

In the event that you suffer such an injury, get to an eye specialist as fast as possible. Minutes and hours are important. Early treatment may mean the difference between saving and losing an eye.

SYMPATHETIC OPHTHALMIA

Most serious in connection with any penetrating injury of the eye is the inflammation that may occur in the other eye. This is known as sympathetic ophthalmia. It may occur as early as nine days after the injury to the first eye. Most frequently the second eye becomes involved four to six weeks after the injury, but sometimes it may occur many months or years later. If the first eye is hopelessly destroyed and sightless, it is best that it be removed immediately. If sight remains in the injured eye, but it remains soft, irritable, red, and inflamed despite the use of systemic antibiotic and steroid (Cortisone-like) drugs and local medication, it is good judgment to remove the first eye before the second becomes affected. *Once the second eye develops sympathetic inflammation, removal of the injured eye will not help, and the patient may lose both eyes.* The eye surgeon has the responsibility of deciding whether it is safe for the patient to retain the injured globe, or whether it is best to remove it.

COMMON EYE DISORDERS

GLAUCOMA

One of the leading causes of blindness in the United States is glaucoma. It is responsible for 30,000 completely blind people in this country, and for another 130,000 that are blind in one eye. Glaucoma is actually not a single disease, but the term describes any eye condition in which the pressure within the eye is higher than normal. The most common type of glaucoma (chronic simple) causes a gradual, painless loss of the side vision in its early stages. It produces damage to the delicate visual nerves so gradually that the patient is unaware of the danger to his sight. This explains why it is important for every adult over thirty-five to have an eye examination by a medical eye specialist at least every two years. The measurement of the pressure within the eye is painless, and may detect glaucoma early enough to preserve the patient's vision.

A less frequently observed form of glaucoma (acute narrow angle type) gives the patient warning that something is amiss because it often causes severe pain in the eye and forehead, blurring of vision, watering of the eye, and occasionally nausea and vomiting. The sudden rise in pressure within the eye is due to a closing off of the drainage passages so that the fluid within the eye cannot escape. Fluid accumulates in the cornea and may result in the patient's seeing colored halos or rainbows. Persistent symptoms of this type should never be neglected. Vision may be lost in a matter of hours unless emergency treatment is instituted.

Of the two types of so-called primary glaucoma described, the latter (acute) requires earlier and more vigorous treatment if sight is to be preserved. Even if the patient's pressure can be lowered to normal ranges after a sudden attack by use of various eye drops and systemic drugs, most eye surgeons recommend a corrective operation. The surgery for the acute type of glaucoma, if performed early enough, may actually cure the condition. This is not true of chronic glaucoma in which surgery is seldom an emergency, but is usually only a controlling measure.

A third type occurs in infancy and childhood (congenital glaucoma). Persistent irritation of the eyes, tearing, redness, or signs that the child is in pain should send the patient to the oculist as soon as possible. Failure to seek early help will result in a blind, disfigured, and painful eye. These children *always* require surgical correction to salvage vision.

Glaucoma may also occur secondary to a blunt injury or deep inflammation in the eye. These forms may cause pain and changes in vision if uncontrolled pressure exists over long periods of time. The treatment of these cases differs from the primary types noted. Only the ophthalmologist can differentiate the various types of glaucoma and specify the proper treatment. Most prefer to treat the more common chronic type of glaucoma conservatively as long as the patient can be controlled in this manner. If signs indicate that the pressure is not in a safe range with this management, surgery is performed to create new drainage channels to lower the tension.

Once and for all, let us put to rest some of the false ideas about glaucoma that circulate around the canasta, bridge, and sewing circles.

First: GLAUCOMA IS NOT *CANCER,* or any other kind of malignancy.

Second: HAVING GLAUCOMA DOES NOT MEAN INEVITABLE BLINDNESS. People go blind only if the condition is not detected, or having been detected, is neglected.

Third: THE GLAUCOMA PATIENT WHO USES EYE DROPS IS NOT NECESSARILY "SAFE." The drops may be inadequate to control the disease. It is necessary to have the vision, ocular pressure, and visual fields checked at regular intervals by the eye specialist for the rest of the patient's life.

STRABISMUS (CROSSED EYES, WALL EYES, OR SQUINT)

At birth the eyes may not be perfectly coordinated, but within 8 to 20 weeks they work together as a team with both eyes focusing simultaneously on an object. If for any reason the eyes do not work together, strabismus is said to be present. There are various kinds of strabismus. Eyes that turn inward are called "crossed eyes." Eyes that turn outward are called "wall eyes." If one eye is higher than the other, a vertical deviation is said to exist.

There are many underlying causes for crossing of the eyes. Each case must be assessed as early as possible by an eye specialist in order to start proper therapy. Heredity, farsightedness, nearsightedness, prematurity, and disturbances of the nervous system, as well as other factors, may be causes for failure of the eyes to work together. Only careful evaluation and attack on all possible factors can lead to successful treatment.

When the eyes of an adult are suddenly crossed, double vision is produced. This is disturbing. In a young cross-eyed child, who is unable to explain this to his parents, the brain automatically overcomes the disturbing double vision by shutting off the visual message from the crossed eye. If the visual messages are shut off for too long a period, the eye may never develop normal vision. Even if the eyes are ultimately straightened by surgery, the crossed eye may suffer from permanent poor vision ("lazy eye"). To prevent this, the good eye is covered in order to force the use of the crossed eye in an effort to develop a useful level of vision.

The treatment for crossed eyes is influenced largely by the cause. Glasses, eye exercises, various eye drops, patching of the better eye, and surgery may be necessary. Competent medical eye specialists are convinced that children with eyes that do not track together should receive treatment as early as possible. This tends to avoid visual loss and to correct the cosmetic defect before the child becomes self-conscious about his appearance. Disregard the fable that your child will outgrow his crossed eyes. It almost never happens and to neglect the condition is to do great disservice to your offspring.

CATARACTS

In order to see normally one must have "clear windows" through which light may enter the eye. The second window, the lens, must be crystal clear in order for light rays to focus on the retina. If the lens becomes clouded, the condition is called a cataract. Looking at an object through a cataract may be compared to looking through a frosted glass. Objects appear fuzzy and distorted. If the cataract is dense enough, vision may be so poor that the subject may be capable only of seeing light.

The most common cause of cataract formation is a chemical change associated with the aging process. This is why cataracts are usually seen in people past middle age. At times cataracts are seen in babies as a result of hereditary factors or such conditions in the mother as German measles. Inflammations, specific diseases, certain forms of radiation, and injuries may also produce a cataract. Long-term or large-dose therapy with Cortisone has been shown to cause cataracts. Triparanol, a cholesterol mobilizing drug, has also caused clouding of the lens.

The only meaningful treatment is surgical removal of the cloudy lens. In recent years many advances have been made in cataract surgery so that now 95 per cent of these operations are successful.

Formerly the surgeon insisted that the patient wait until the lens become completely clouded before undertaking surgery. With the use of an enzyme to dissolve the fibers that hold the lens in place, a technique first discovered in the 1950s and with better surgical materials available, the eye surgeon will remove an immature cataract as soon as the vision is reduced to the point where the patient is unable to carry on his daily chores. Only the eye physician can decide the proper time for surgery.

Removing the cataract does not restore the vision to useful levels unless corrective lenses are fitted after surgery. These may be either spectacle or contact lenses. The surgery for children's cataracts is different from that of the adult because the "guy-wires" that hold the lens are much tougher in the child. This necessitates a different approach to removing a cataract in children. The commonly held idea that the cataract is on the surface of the eye and may be "peeled off," is incorrect. The cataract is inside the eye and requires a sizable incision around the cornea for successful extraction. The public should also know that special diets, drops, and injections of various substances cannot dissolve cataracts. Many people, seeking a non-surgical cure for cataracts have been bilked out of thousands of dollars by quacks promising miracle cures. If you are experiencing a gradual loss of vision without pain, see a medical eye specialist at once.

INFECTIONS OF THE EYE AND LIDS

The lids and the external covering layers of the eye may be attacked by many of the germs that affect other parts of the body. Great progress has been made in the prevention and treatment of bacterial eye infections by the use of antibiotics in the form of locally applied drops or ointments. Viral inflammations are more difficult to control, but even here, progress has been made. The new antiviral drug, IDU, has been effective against some cases of corneal infection by the "cold-sore" virus, herpes simplex.

In severe inflammations of the surfaces of the lids and eyes, as well as in intraocular infection after surgery or penetrating injuries, oral or intravenous antibiotics or chemotherapeutic agents like the sulfa drugs have been helpful. Some eye doctors inject these drugs under the covering layers of the eye, or directly into the eye as sight-saving measures.

Cortisone and some of its derivatives, originally developed to treat arthritis, has been effective in minimizing certain inflammations in the cornea, iris, choroid, and retina. These are potent drugs with many side effects throughout the body, and are specifically contraindicated in certain bacterial and viral infections of the eye. The drugs should be used in the eye or systemically only on the advice of the physician. They are particularly dangerous if the patient has a history of diabetes, high blood pressure, peptic ulcer, or tuberculosis.

Lid Infections: Stys and Chalazion

Numerous small glands in the skin and deeper tissues of the lid may become infected. The most common is the sty, which is a red, painful, and tender swelling near the lash border. It is usually filled with pus, comes to a head in a few days, and may open and drain. It may result in a thickened, inflamed lid for a long time. Once the infection starts, apply warm, moist dressings to the area three or four times a day, and antibiotics may be necessary. If stys are not treated vigorously, the pus may spread the infection to other parts of the lid and crops of stys may result. Patients who have frequent infections should be examined to be sure they do not have diabetes. Cleanliness is a "must," and children should be instructed not to finger or rub their lids for fear of starting or spreading these infections.

If some of the deeper lid glands are involved, a lump may appear under the skin or on the inner surface of the lid. This cystlike mass is called a chalazion. Although some of these gradually disappear, they frequently have to be opened and emptied by the eye surgeon. The most common cause of the lid infections is the germ staphylococcus, the organism responsible for pimples and boils.

Conjunctivitis

Any inflammation of the tissue that covers the inner surface of the lids and the surface of the eyeball is called conjunctivitis, or pink eye. The eyes may feel sandy. They may smart or burn. They become bloodshot, and varying amounts of mucus and pus may accumulate in the corners of the eyes and on the lids. The person may find the lids stuck together in the morning on arising. Tearing of the eyes and sensitivity to light are noted during the day. These conditions can be transmitted from one eye to the other, or may be transferred to other people if common towels or tissues are used. Antibiotic eye drops or ointments plus scrupulous hygiene control most of these infections in a few days. The virus conjunctival infections are less successfully treated by these drugs.

The most severe infections are caused by the gonococcus and meningococcus germs. The latter also causes meningitis, and often the eye infection may be associated with meningitis. These cases, of course, require hospitalization for systemic as well as ocular treatment.

Trachoma is a specific virus infection of the conjunctive and cornea. It is not a serious problem in the United States, but it is the number one cause of serious and progressive loss of sight, leading to blindness, in all the world. The World Health Organization has calculated that five hundred million people, one-sixth of the world's population, are affected by trachoma. Sulfa drugs and antibiotics given orally have reduced the threat of this disease, and certain vaccines have been developed for use for some strains of trachoma. Some of these vaccines have been administered to children in Formosa and to a group of American Indian children. Although the results appear promising, according to the U. S. Department of Health, Education, and Welfare Public Health Service, several years may be needed to determine how effective the vaccine has been.

Infections of the Tear Passages

Tears keep the surface of the eye moist and the surface of the cornea lustrous. If too little tears are formed by the tear gland in the outer corner of the upper lid, the delicate eye tissues dry and become more susceptible to infection. The tears drain out of the eye through a little hole in the inner edge of the lower lid. They pass through a fine duct into the nose. Hence, whenever the person cries or his eyes water, his nose runs simultaneously. If for any reason this drainage passage is narrowed or obstructed, the patient's tears run down his cheek. If the obstruction is not relieved, the tear sac may become infected, swollen, filled with pus, and be painful. This reaction is often so intense that an abscess forms that either opens and drains itself or must be incised by the surgeon. The two most common situations in which this happens is in infancy (due to failure of a thin tissue between the nasal duct and the nose to open as it usually does at birth), and in adults, if the passage is plugged by foreign bodies, lashes, infected material, or due to the changes associated with aging. Gentle dilation of the tear openings, irrigation of the passages with sterile salt solution, or probing with special silver instruments may relieve the block. This must be done by the eye physician with gentleness and respect for the involved tissues.

Infants should be treated with antibiotic eye drops and a technique of massage during the first six months of life when possible. If the obstruction is not relieved by this time, probing of the duct should be performed, preferably under general anesthesia. This usually cures the condition. In adults with repeated infection that cannot be controlled by conservative means, an operation is necessary to create a new opening between the tear sac and the nose. Relieving the obstructed tear passage may stop annoying tearing but the most important reason for opening up the tear passages is to prevent infected material from contaminating the eye. If the eye is scratched in the presence of pus from the sac, a deep infection may result and the eye may be lost.

Infections of the Cornea

Inflammation of the cornea produces a condition called keratitis. Some of the causes are similar to those external factors which cause conjunctivitis, but systemic infections such as syphilis or tuberculosis may also cause keratitis from within the eye. Keratitis is more serious than conjunctivitis because scarring of the cornea can cause serious loss of vision.

Several forms of corneal inflammation may form an ulcer. These may be due to various bacteria, but may be caused by the cold-sore virus. Any erosion of the corneal surface may result in an ulcer which may become secondarily infected. A scratch, a foreign body, or a contact lens may all cause such a sequence of events.

Intensive antibiotic treatment is necessary to minimize the scarring of the cornea when it heals. Cortisone-like preparations should not be used in any ulcer of the cornea if the cold-sore virus is suspected to be the cause.

It can lead to a fungus complication or a worsening of the virus disease, both of which can be visually destructive.

Inflammation of the Blood Vessel Containing Layers of the Eye (Uveitis)

The colored part of the eye that surrounds the pupil, the ciliary body, and the choroid may be involved by inflammations due to invasion by bacteria, protozoa, and viruses. These tissues may also become inflamed from infection in such distant areas of the body as the teeth, sinuses, prostate, gastrointestinal tract, or lungs. Various inflammations of the connective tissues such as arthritis and certain allergic states may affect this part of the eye. Pain, blurring of vision, light sensitivity, and redness are signs and symptoms of involvement of the iris and ciliary body. If the choroid is involved, the eye may be pale and free from pain, but the vision may be hazy.

Treatment depends on the underlying cause. Local and systemic steroids, atropine drops to dilate the pupil, and antibiotics are often used with success.

DISEASES OF THE RETINA

The cavity in the back two-thirds of the eye is filled with a clear, gelatinous material called the vitreous. This substance normally allows the light to pass through unimpeded to strike the sensitive cells in the retina which initiate the sensation of vision. If the vitreous undergoes any degenerative change, particles may settle out in the liquefied portion and cast their shadow on the retina. The patient may see these as floating specks. "Floaters" due to this process are usually harmless, but annoying. Certain "floaters" are more serious when they are due to retinal disorders.

When the latter occurs, the patient will complain that he sees flashes of light, floating particles, and finally a curtainlike shadow that falls over part of his field of vision. The surgeon may look into the eye and see a tear or hole in the retina with the retina pulled away from the back of the eye. When fluid enters the holes and strips the retina away, a retinal detachment is said to exist. The retina must be repaired by operation at the earliest possible time, and even so, the retina may not regain its full visual potential. If the retina cannot be repositioned, the eye undergoes a series of deteriorating changes which lead to blindness.

Advances in retinal surgery using various plastic materials to shorten the eye and pull the outer walls of the eyeball closer to the detached retina have resulted in a higher number of surgical successes than was possible with the older methods of treatment. The surgeon not only attempts to shorten the eye, but tries to seal off all the retinal holes. New instruments to close certain types of retinal holes without surgery are the photocoagulator and the Laser apparatus. These devices will not replace surgical correction, but may be important aids in the future.

Certain drugs have been found to produce severe degeneration of the retina. Chloroquine is a drug used to treat certain connective tissue disorders that may cause permanent severe impairment of sight. Other ocular effects of the drug may reverse themselves when the drug is discontinued, but the retinal changes have been permanent. All patients receiving this drug should be examined regularly by the oculist.

EYE EXERCISES

Various attempts have been made to get people to improve the strength of their eyes with so-called visual training or eye exercises. The original slogan was: "Throw away your glasses and have perfect sight."

Most competent professionals in the field of eye care believe that it is not possible to obtain meaningful or lasting improvement in vision with any of these exercise routines.

The nearsighted person can be taught to interpret his blurred images more effectively, and color-blind patients may be helped to discriminate between colors more effectively by psychological educational processes, but neither condition can be cured by these techniques. In short, nearsighted, farsighted, or astigmatic people require either spectacles or contact lenses with which to see clearly. Poor vision due to scarred corneas, cataract, or diseases at the back of the eye cannot be influenced in any way by exercise.

The area where orthoptic training, as the ophthalmic physician calls it, is valuable in the management of some children with cross-eyes or walleyes. This process is not "exercise" in the sense that a weight lifter builds up his body muscles, but is really a method of stimulating some of the higher visual centers in the brain that are concerned with combining the images from the two eyes. This training does not help every child with an eye-muscle-balance problem. If the brain does not have any basic "fusional" ability, no amount of eye exercises will improve the function. The decision as to whether a child should be exposed to orthoptic exercises should be made by an ophthalmologist.

TRANSPLANTATION OF THE CORNEA

One of the most highly publicized surgical procedures has been the replacement of part of a scarred cornea by a clear graft taken from a donor eye. Not all patients with poor vision or blindness can be benefited by such corneal transplantation. The surgeon must choose the cases according to a wide variety of considerations. There are many diseases of the eye in which the scarring of the front window is simply one of many ocular disorders, and corneal grafting would not help to improve vision. Even if it is thought that the remainder of the eye is relatively healthy, grafts in certain eyes do not remain clear. Severe corneal scars with large blood vessels in them and virtually no healthy supporting tissues around the site of the proposed graft make the outlook for a successful transplantation very poor. In eyes like this, there may be some hope in the future for using artificial plastic corneal windows instead of a natural graft. At present it is considered to be in the experimental stages.

The corneas scarred by degenerative conditions, cold-sore virus infection, localized injuries, and infections of various types have the greatest chance for success. Corneas injured by refrigerant gas or lime burns have a poorer prognosis. If one graft fails, others may be attempted, occasionally with success. Transplantation is usually not attempted in eyes with glaucoma or infection. Abnormalities or infections of the eye lids may not only doom the grafted corneal button, but might cause loss of the eye from the post-operative complications.

Fresh corneas are preferred for most transplants, and are best in the first 24 to 36 hours after removal. The care and preparation of the tissue to be used for transplant is important, because secondary infection or use of damaged cornea results in certain failure.

EYE BANKS

A federation of 35 eye banks has been organized in this country to collect, preserve, and store eyes willed by generous contributors. These centers provide the surgeon with the donor material necessary for the corneal-transplant operation. Donations of human eyes are needed because experiments have shown that animal corneas grafted into human eyes do not remain clear. It is not enough to express the wish to donate eyes in a will, because in order for the donor eye to be useful, it must be removed within six hours after death. Wills are not usually read early enough to make the patient's wishes known. A recent Public Health Service publication points out that next of kin should be informed of the dying person's wishes so that proper arrangements can be made in time to save the valuable tissue to give a blind person the chance to see again.

CHAPTER 29

The Ear, Tongue, Nose, and Throat

MORRIS FISHBEIN, M.D.

DISORDERS OF THE EAR

The outer ear differs but little from other external portions of the body in the disturbances which may affect it. Small tumors must be removed if they show the slightest tendency to growth or irritation. Sometimes cysts form that are nonmalignant tumors but that continue to swell and grow as long as the opening is blocked. These should be opened and the wall of the cyst removed, if there is not to be a recurrence.

ERYSIPELAS OF EAR

Erysipelas of the ear which was not uncommon in the past is now rare. The ear would swell to tremendous size. Sulfonamides and antibiotics now control such infections. In frostbite of the ear, it should be gradually warmed until the circulation returns. Then the skin must be protected to prevent infections.

TIN EAR

One of the most common forms of injury to the ear is what is commonly called "cauliflower" or "tin ear" of the pugilist. Repeated blows on the ear result in the pouring out of blood between the cartilage of the tissue and its surrounding membranes. At first such swellings are bluish-red; they feel like dough, and they are opaque, so that light will not pass through. In some instances, it may be advisable for the surgeon to open the tissue and to remove the clot of blood, and, in that way, to prevent permanent thickening and swelling. It is sometimes necessary to plan the use of bandages which mold the ear and hold its shape while such surgical treatment is being undertaken. Enzymes may be used to hasten breaking up of blood clots.

Modern ideas of beauty demand that the ear lie fairly close to the head and that it be relatively small. Hence the plastic surgeons try operations to hold the ears back or to lessen their size. Such operations are of established value in competent hands. They should never be undertaken unless the person's occupation is such as to make slightly protruding or large ears a menace to earning a livelihood or may damage the personality.

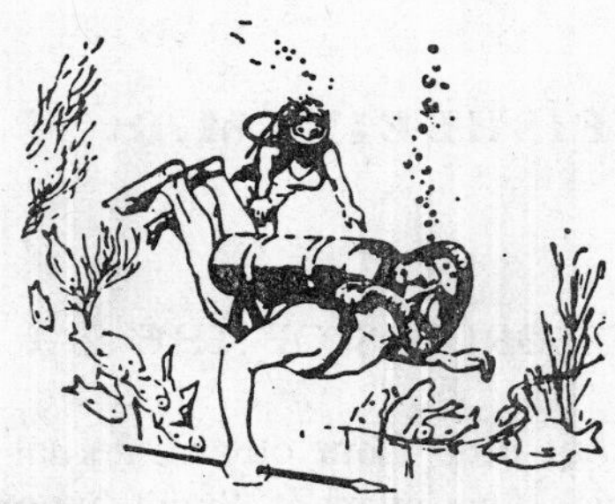

Fig. 73. Skin diving—an unusual stress cause. Navigating under water is heavy exertion and those with respiratory problems or heart and blood vessel disease should not attempt it, says *Today's Health,* the magazine of the American Medical Association. Skin diving is ruled out for those with perforated eardrums. Ear plugs are for surface swimming only and should not be used for diving because of water pressure. The depth changes also require that sinuses and ears be in good shape to equalize the pressure. Asking your doctor to evaluate your fitness for diving is a precaution that will pay dividends. *Health and Safety Tips,* American Medical Association.

INFECTION OF EAR CANAL

In addition to the diseases that may disturb the outer ear, some disturbances affect the canal up to the eardrum. Almost any infection may involve the outer canal of the ear. Under such circumstances it is necessary to remove the infection and to prevent its recurrence by the use of proper antiseptics which a physician can supply and which should be used only after he has given proper instructions. Here also antibiotic drugs are successful.

There is a good rule in medicine: namely, never put anything in the external ear any smaller than the elbow. The tissues are most delicate and may be seriously harmed by the use of wires, toothpicks, earspoons, or similar irregular or unsterilized devices. A scratch of the lining of the canal may result in the formation of a boil, which is exceedingly painful and which is difficult to handle in such an inaccessible part of the body.

HARD WAX

The cerumen or wax of the ear is easiest removed, when it becomes hardened, by the use of a syringe with slightly warm water. This need not be done often, and harm can be done by needless or too frequent syringing. The syringe should always be sterilized by boiling before using, and the water should be previously boiled and then used warm. Before a person attempts to syringe an ear for himself or for a child, he should learn the technique.

The person whose ear is to be syringed usually sits in good light. It is customary to put a towel or cape around the neck and tuck it in over the collar to prevent soiling of the clothing. A kidney-shaped pan is held at the edge of the ear so that the fluid returning will run in the basin and not down the neck. In an adult the ear is pulled up and backward in order to straighten out the passage. Then the nozzle of the syringe, which has been filled and had all the air expelled, is placed just inside the outer opening. The water is then projected along the back wall slowly and without too great pressure, so as to permit return of the flow as the water goes in.

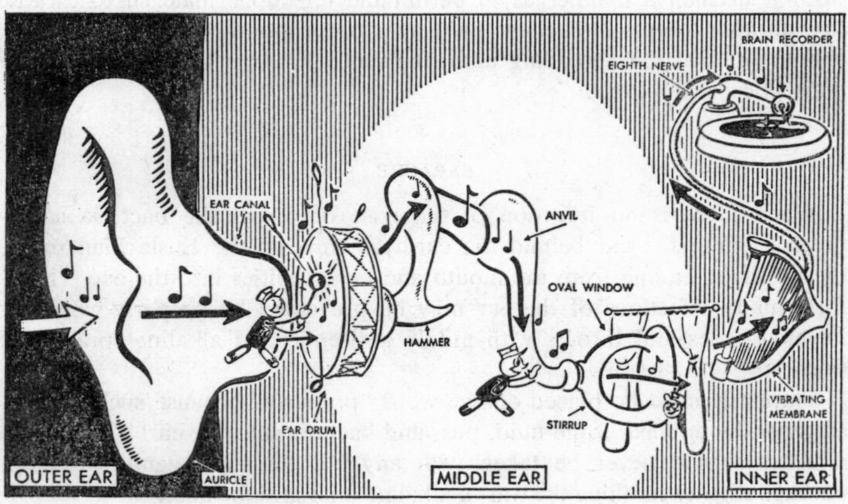

Fig. 74. How We Hear. Courtesy Sonotone Corporation.

After the ear has been washed, the head may be turned on one side and the extra fluid allowed to run out. A person who understands the technique may then wipe out the canal with a small wisp of cotton. If a permanent antiseptic, softening material, or lotion is to be used, the physician can prescribe the proper one, and this is held in place with a little wisp of cotton, never inserted under pressure.

A foreign body in the external ear will seldom cause much discomfort unless it is a living insect. Cases are on record in which living insects have entered the ear and remained for many years, gradually being surrounded by hardened wax or cerumen, to the point at which a person lost his hearing entirely. The damage from foreign bodies in the external ear lies in rough attempts to remove them. If a living insect gets into the outer ear, a physician can destroy it by the use of a suitable vapor or solution, under which circumstance the insect will either come out of its own accord or be killed and removed by a syringe.

It is not well for anyone to attempt to remove a foreign body from the outer ear if it cannot be syringed out, unless he has had special training in this type of work. Several interesting techniques have been developed for removing foreign objects, one being the use of a device with an adhesive material at the end which sticks to the body that is to be removed. It is then gradually withdrawn.

A foreign body that is infected may produce irritation and serious infection with the formation of boils or abscesses which, in the external ear, are a menace frequently to life itself. A boil in the external ear demands the immediate and competent attention of an expert, who can arrange to open it in such a manner as to permit the infectious material to escape, to withdraw the pus, to relieve pain by a prescription of proper remedies, and to prevent the spreading and recurrence through the use of suitable antiseptic preparations.

EARACHE

When there is an infection of the nose or throat the bacteria sometimes get into the ear behind the eardrum through the Eustachian tubes, the passages leading from the mouth and nose cavities into the ear. Therefore, many infections of the ear may be prevented by properly cleansing infected noses and throats with mildly antiseptic and alkaline sprays and washes.

Emphasis must be placed on the word "properly" because such washes, as generally applied, force fluid, pus, and bacteria into the ear. These nasal douches should never be taken with any but the most gentle pressure, perhaps slightly snuffling the warm, alkaline fluid into the nose.

The early diagnosis of infection of the ear is important, if inflammation of the mastoid bone, behind the ear and contiguous to the brain, is to be prevented. The ears should always be examined if a child is ill and has fever. The presence of fever, bulging drum, and the symptoms mentioned are sufficient reasons for the physician to incise the eardrum to save the hearing of the child and to prevent burrowing of the infected pus into the mastoid region. When the diagnosis and the proper treatment of an infected ear are delayed, the results are likely to be extremely serious.

The first symptom of an infection in the ear is usually pain in the ear, and in some cases this is the only symptom. It must be remembered, however, that pains in the ear also are found in connection with presence of boils in the ear canal. Sometimes a pain in the ear may be associated with an unerupted wisdom tooth and inflammation of the joints of the jaw and severe tonsillitis or an infection of the sinuses around the nose.

OTITIS MEDIA

The doctor makes up his mind as to the presence of an acute infection of the ear by taking the temperature, which in these cases usually is high. However, special examinations in such cases of acute infections of the ear are made by direct inspection of the eardrum, using a magnifying device and a light. This device is called an otoscope, meaning a device for seeing the ear.

In most instances, a physician called to such a case and making a diagnosis of severe infection within the ear will arrange to open the eardrum promptly. This not only relieves the pain, but also makes it less likely that the infection will spread to the mastoid.

Application of heat often brings relief. For persistent infections the antibiotics in powder form have been helpful. Infections of the middle ear are being tremendously reduced by treatment of infectious diseases with antibiotic drugs. Moreover, early detection permits immediate injection of such drugs and prevention of ear infections sufficient to require opening of the eardrum.

MASTOIDS

If the condition spreads into the mastoid, mastoiditis develops and constitutes a much more serious condition than infection of the internal ear alone. When the infection spreads to the mastoid, great tenderness will be found in that region, and also pain on pressure. The physician watches carefully this development. From the very first, the mastoid bone may be tender on pressure because of the swelling on the inside. Whenever pain is severe and there is fever, the physician knows that the infection is serious, and he is likely to recommend immediate incision of the eardrum. The operation is not difficult and, if performed soon enough, is likely to prevent more serious complications.

People have strange notions about perforation of the eardrum, believing that this will interfere with hearing and cause other damage, whereas actually the eardrum heals promptly after the infection disappears, and hearing is likely to be just as good as it was previously. It is far less dangerous to hearing to incise the eardrum than to postpone the incision too long.

Mastoid infections were frequent until discovery of the antibiotic drugs which control infections of the nose and throat before infection can reach the internal ear and the mastoid.

THE TONGUE AND ITS DISORDERS

The tongue is an organ which has always aroused the interest of the medical profession. Doctors of an earlier day used to pay a great deal of attention to the appearance of the tongue because of the relationship of such appearances to disturbances of the rest of the digestive tract.

Occasionally the tongue is abnormal in its construction at birth so that the condition of tongue-tie is produced, and there are other cases in which that portion of the tissue holding the tongue is abnormally long, permitting actual swallowing of the tongue with occasional asphyxiation. In some conditions the tongue becomes too large for the mouth and protrudes beyond the lips. This is particularly the case in the large tongue of the child that has deficient thyroid secretion with the development of cretinism.

GEOGRAPHIC TONGUE

Sometimes the surface of the tongue is marked by long, deep furrows instead of being smooth. There is a common condition called "geographic tongue" because the surface of the tongue looks like a relief map. In this condition there are grayish thickened patches on the surface. Apparently it is a mild inflammatory disorder which tends gradually to improve, the treatment usually including merely the washing of the mouth at fairly frequent intervals with mild antiseptic and alkaline mouth washes.

INFLAMMATION OF TONGUE

The tongue may be suddenly inflamed from a number of different causes, such as injuries, burns, insect bites, and occasionally association with such serious infectious diseases as scarlet fever, typhoid fever, or smallpox. Whenever the tongue is infected, the lymph glands in the region also become infected and swollen. In very serious cases death may result from such inflammation of the tongue, but in the vast majority of cases mild treatment tends to lead to recovery.

There are many nervous disorders or conditions affecting the nervous system in which there is pain in the tongue or burning of the tongue without any visible evidence in the neighborhood of the tongue itelf. This condition sometimes occurs in locomotor ataxia, in hysteria, and in all sorts of nervous upsets of one type or another. Under such circumstances a physician may make sure that the condition is functional and not due to any destruction or inflammation of the tissues concerned. If he discovers actual disease of the nervous system, the case is treated by the well-established methods. If such disease is not discovered it may be necessary to use psychologic methods in controlling the symptoms, not only as they affect the tongue, but probably as they affect other parts of the body as well.

The tongue is primarily responsible for the sense of taste which is, at the same time, a composite of the sense of smell and the feel of food on the tongue. Loss of the sense of taste may result from inflammation or swelling of the tongue; it may be associated with hysteria. In the same way there may be exceeding sensitivity to tastes so that a person is constantly tasting sweet, sour, salt or bitter; and in other instances foods taste different from what they should.

In every such case it is necessary to make a most careful study of the entire patient, his surroundings and environment, and particularly his emotional condition.

THE NOSE

The nose is, in general, the least ornamental of the features of man. It is the mark for more insults and injuries than any other adornment of the human countenance. It is unnecessary to locate it geographically, since it presents itself. Remarkably, however, modern living conditions have made the nose, in more ways than one, a center of interest.

Actually, there is not much to the organ itself. It is composed of some small bones and cartilages and certain soft tissues which go to surround the two cavities. Of equal importance with the nose and inevitably to be considered with it are the nasal sinuses. These sinuses are cavities in the bones in the head which connect with the inside of the nose by means of small openings. Nerves take care of the motor and sensory functions of the tissues and may be involved in any condition affecting the nose.

The most important of the structures in the nose from the point of view of disease is the mucous membrane or tissue which lines the cavities. It is one of the most sensitive tissues in the body, and when bruised or hurt in any way may respond with considerable trouble for the possessor. Not infrequently, minor infections occur, particularly in the hair follicles or in the roots of the hairs which are in the nose. These hairs have the purpose of filtering out dust or infectious material which comes into the nose with the air.

Common pus-forming germs, such as staphylococcus and streptococcus, are widespread and easily get into the human body whenever they come in contact with a tissue that has been damaged in any manner. They may set up an infection which eventually may spread throughout the body. The pernicious habit of picking the nose, pulling out the hairs, or trying to squeeze out pimples or other infections may result in most serious inflammations or other disorders.

HYGIENE OF NOSE

The right way to take care of the nose is to remove carefully, by proper use of a handkerchief, such materials as can be reached easily. Those which cannot be reached may be washed out by the use of a mild spray, without pressure. There are now generally available all sorts of mild sprays of inert oils and small amounts of camphor, eucalyptus, or menthol, which serve this purpose conveniently. Under no circumstances should such materials be put in the nose under high pressure. If a spray is not convenient, the simplest method is to drop one or two drops into the nose.

An infection in the lining of the nose manifests itself by redness, swelling, discomfort, and pain, which increase steadily. The tip of the nose becomes swollen, and sometimes the swelling may even extend up to the eyelids. In the presence of any serious swelling involving the nose, it is well to have an inspection by a physician, who will determine the presence or absence of a localized spot of infection such as a boil or pimple, who can arrange to cause the infectious material to be released, and who will provide suitable dressings of warm antiseptic or saline solutions tending toward recovery.

When for any reason the nose is lost entirely, the facial expression naturally suffers. When the bridge of the nose disappears, as sometimes occurs in certain forms of disease, a saddle nose is caused which is anything but beautiful. The frequency of automobile accidents has resulted in damage to many a proboscis. Falls, industrial accidents, railroad wrecks, and gunshot wounds also produce damages that require medical attention, and the results of pugilism are a constant source of income to specialists in nasal reconstruction.

Mother Nature brings many a break into prominence by bestowing upon it a hump, a knob at the tip, or a deviation to one side or the other. In street fights anything can happen to a wayfaring nose, and medical literature records several instances in which the tip of one has been bitten off by an agitated opponent—male or female.

Forms of the nose have been described as long and short, upturned and downturned, humped and flat, wide and narrow, pointed and saddle-shaped. It is just as well that people do not worry too much about their particular type of nasal appearance. As soon as they get their minds fixed on this, they look into the looking glass until it gets tired of reflecting their appearance. The experts find that almost any amount of repairs and reconstruction is never satisfactory to the person who once embarks on the paths of nasal improvement.

PLASTIC SURGERY OF NOSE

If the loss of tissue or destruction of tissue causes damage to the health of the person concerned, the case certainly demands surgical attention. There are many ways of building up a broken-down or absent bridge. Some surgeons transplant bone and cartilage, some use celluloid, and others use ivory. Humps are removed by dissection and scraping or cutting. The best way to take care of a deformity from an accident, however, is to give it the best possible attention immediately after the accident. It is much easier to secure a good result if such care is given at that time than to attempt a complete rebuilding operation when tissues have healed in the wrong manner.

FOREIGN BODIES IN NOSE

Children not infrequently push all sorts of things into the nasal cavity. The character of things pushed into the nose is limited only by the size and the possibilities. Insane people also occasionally indulge in a similar performance. Among some of the common substances that have been found by physicians are chalk, buttons, seeds, and pieces of wood.

Occasionally the nasal cavity becomes infected with worms. Among others are maggots and screw worms, and indeed almost any of the worms which can live in the human body. Worms are seldom found in a normal nose. However, in the presence of any disease with an associated odor, flies are attracted which may lay eggs or in other ways convey the larvæ of the worms to the nasal cavity. Among the first signs of infestation of the nose by worms are irritation, sneezing, and an increased amount of discharge usually streaked with blood. The removal of worms from the nose is not a serious matter. The nose may be washed repeatedly with solutions containing proper antiseptic substances.

The removal of inanimate foreign bodies not infrequently requires the greatest skill of a competent specialist. It may be necessary to use an anesthetic, to apply various solutions which will constrict the tissue of the nose, to employ the X ray to localize the foreign body exactly. Once this is done, the doctor merely grasps the foreign body with a forceps and withdraws it, endeavoring to cause as little damage to the soft tissue as possible.

POLYPS IN NOSE

Sometimes growths in the nose, like polyps, are difficult to distinguish from foreign bodies. Usually the discharge coming from the nose as a result of the presence of a foreign body comes only from one side. Sometimes the removal of polyps or similar tumors is followed by the disappearance of chronic infection in the nose and sometimes also by the removal of asthmatic symptoms. It is not possible for the average person to diagnose the presence of nasal polyps for himself. The condition can, however, be diagnosed by a physician following an examination of the nose, in which he looks directly into the nasal cavity.

NOSEBLEED

There are many causes of bleeding from the nose, because the blood supply to the tissues is generally rich and the tissues themselves quite delicate. In many diseases in which the tendency to bleed is great, such as hemophilia and purpura, two conditions in which the elements of the blood are so altered that bleeding occurs frequently and coagulation of the blood takes place with difficulty, bleeding from the nose is a common symptom.

In the presence of severe infection and in the condition called scurvy, which is due to a deficiency of vitamin C, bleeding of the nose also occurs frequently. In practically all of the conditions which produce severe anemia, nosebleed is not unusual. In cases of hardening of the arteries with exceedingly high blood pressure there may be rupture of a small blood vessel in the nose with severe nosebleed for some time. The bleeding from the nose and the loss of blood serve to lower the blood pressure.

Any blow on the nose or any bruise which breaks a blood vessel will result in bleeding. There are also cases in which tumors within the blood vessels cause hemorrhage. In ordinary cases of nosebleed, if the person is at once placed in a horizontal position so that the blood pressure is lowered, and if he is kept cool, he tends to recover, since in most instances the bleeding will stop promptly.

There are many superstitions about stopping nosebleed, such as dropping a key down the back, pressing on the hard palate, and similar performances. However, there is no efficacy in such measures, except that they serve to distract the attention of the person whose nose is bleeding and keep him from being too much frightened during the short interval that usually elapses before the bleeding stops.

In more serious cases, however, physicians use measures which have a greater degree of certainty, such measures including the packing of the nose with sterilized gauze, direct inspection with pinching of the bleeding vessel, cauterization with some substance like silver nitrate or chromic acid, and the use of various solutions which temporarily constrict the blood vessels, giving the blood opportunity to clot. In general, physicians avoid leaving packing in the nose for long periods of time because of possible dangers to the ears through blocking of the tubes that pass from the nasal cavity to the ears, and because of possible effects from blocking the nasal sinuses.

Bleeding from the nose is not in itself a disease, but rather a symptom of disease; it may be the warning sign for the onset of a serious disorder, such as a change in the blood, or even a tumor of the adrenal glands. On the other hand, it may merely be due to increased mental or physical excitement or any other condition that suddenly raises the blood pressure. In most cases the amount of blood lost is small, but if the person has repeated hemorrhages the amount lost may be sufficient to cause anemia and to demand special treatment for restoring the blood.

Sometimes hemorrhage from the nose in children is overlooked, because the blood goes back in the throat and is swallowed. In most cases of bleeding from the nose, even severe cases, the hemorrhage stops of itself in approximately ten minutes. If the hemorrhage continues longer, or if it is repeated, the condition is most serious and demands efficient attention. Especially important: do not blow the nose after the bleeding has stopped, because that will dislodge clots and start the bleeding over again.

New blood coagulating remedies have been discovered which the doctor can apply in plenty of time to prevent loss of serious quantities of blood.

SINUS DISEASE

The sinuses are air spaces surrounding the nose. Because of their direct contact with the exterior, they frequently become infected with the common pus-forming germs. Because they do not drain easily, the infections tend to become chronic. Associated with such infections are feelings of tiredness, loss of appetite, pains in the joints and limbs.

The mucous membrane of the nose becomes deranged from a variety of causes, either by a bad diet which is deficient in vitamins, by sensitivity to various protein substances, or by some disorders of the glands of internal secretion.

The changes that take place in the mucous membranes make it possible for germs to invade them easily, and then infection begins. In cases when there is sensitivity to various food substances, the mucous membranes swell and are much more likely to be invaded by germs. In the same way, disorders of the glands of internal secretion are reflected by changes in the mucous membranes.

If the underlying cause is removed, the infection may be brought under control, but in the vast majority of cases correct treatment involves not only control of the underlying cause but also treatment of the infection. If the vitamins are insufficient, they may be supplied through giving a well-balanced diet. For the sensitivity, it is necessary to make diagnostic tests, which will indicate the special substance to which the person may be sensitive.

Disorders of the glands of internal secretion must be carefully investigated. There are some cases, for instance those in which the thyroid is deficient, in which it is possible to supply the deficiency through proper preparations.

Persons who work indoors in crowded rooms where the air is bad and the temperature too low or too high are more likely to develop infection of the sinuses than those who spend a good deal of time outdoors.

A constant discharge from the nose, particularly a discharge of pus, is one of the most certain indications of infection in the sinuses. Sometimes when discharge from the sinus becomes blocked there is swelling of the forehead, dizziness, and even ringing in the ears. There are several sinuses, each of which must be studied individually by the physician in order to determine the extent and nature of the infection. Such a study involves a thorough examination through the nose of the openings of the sinuses into the nose, washing of the sinuses to obtain the discharge, transillumination in a dark room which indicates whether or not the sinuses are clear, and the use of the X ray, which indicates whether or not there is thickening of the walls of the sinuses or any amount of material present in the cavity.

People with chronic sinusitis never recover without treatment. Many of them have low-grade infections in which surgical treatment is not advisable, and these patients can be helped by drainage, frequent washing, and the application of various antiseptic substances.

Infected sinuses may be treated with forced inhalations of mists of penicillin and streptomycin and forced evacuation of the sinuses simultaneously by a negative pressure device. This method of treatment, developed by Alvin Barach, is perhaps the most promising of any yet discovered. Many patients with sinus disease improve by changing from moist, cold climates to warm, dry climates. Use of aerosols of antibiotics has increased rapidly but all these methods must be prescribed or administered for the individual by the doctor.

In other cases, however, the infection of the sinus persists to such an extent that it involves danger to surrounding tissues. Cases are known in which the sight of an eye has been lost because of infection in a neighboring sinus. There are other instances in which the infection extends from the Eustachian tubes to the ear and thus involves the mastoid process. The constant inhalation of pus may set up bronchitis or pneumonia. The continuous slight fever results in a loss of vigor and in disturbances of digestion.

There are even cases in which loss of memory or neurosis has occurred because of the constant infection and irritation. An infection in the nose may be carried by the blood to other parts of the body, resulting in serious inflammations of joints, infection of the heart and the kidneys, and even meningitis.

In children, chronic infection of the sinuses may be associated with enlarged adenoids and tonsils. The removal of the adenoids and tonsils may eliminate the source of the infection and end the trouble. At the same time, it should be emphasized again that correction of the diet to include a proper amount of vitamins A, B, C, and D is of importance.

A child may have an enlargement of the tonsils and adenoids, and associated with this a sensitivity to various protein substances. Obviously attention to both conditions is necessary if complete recovery is to be secured.

In older people, when the antrum is involved, the large sinus on each side of the nose, it may be necessary to remove all infected teeth in relation to the antrum and to clean out the infected bone at the roots of the teeth. An opening into the antrum from the mouth permits drainage and the healing of the diseased membrane. If such measures fail, it is possible to employ a surgical procedure, which involves a wide opening of the sinuses or even complete obliteration; such methods are, however, so delicate that they should be undertaken only by those especially competent, and then after the most careful consideration.

THE SENSE OF SMELL

Some odors are pleasant and others disagreeable. In many instances the sense of pleasure or of discomfort is associated with some previous experience of the person concerned. For instance, the perfume called attar of roses is generally much more pleasant than that of asafetida. There are persons, however, to whom the smell is not altogether pleasant. Some odors seem exceedingly pleasant at the first whiff and then tend to become more unpleasant the longer they are present.

In the University of Edinburgh, Dr. J. H. Kenneth examined twenty-nine men and thirty-four women as to their response to odors of many different substances and combinations of substances. The state of health of the person concerned seems to have something to do with the enjoyment of odors or with disagreement.

Psychological study was also made of associations with various smells. One man who was given camphor to smell immediately felt distressed and visualized the odor of a wardrobe and then had a feeling of suffocation or being in the dark. The odor reminded him of an incident in 1892 when he was placed in a closet because of some youthful misdemeanor. In the closet were clothes which had been supplied with camphor as a moth preventive.

A girl who smelled xylol visualized herself on board a vessel in a harbor in Ceylon. The odor of xylol resembles that of benzol which comes from harbor launches. The odor of cedar-wood oil was associated with a summer evening on the Norwegian coast, with a cigar box in which money had been placed, with a road in the country. Later investigation indicated that the person had been in the habit as a child of walking along this road chewing the end of a cedar-wood pencil.

To one woman the odor of cedar-wood oil brought up the idea of spring cleaning and the cleaning of floors with a cedar-wood mop. Another girl told of the playing of the music of Chopin when she smelled vanilla; another thought of Ireland's song, "Sea Fever," when smelling pine oil.

The usual thought associated with asafetida was garlic or onions. One person thought of a street car in Edinburgh, and it was discovered that these cars were formerly lighted by acetylene gas which gives off a similar odor. The odor of orris root brought to one girl the idea of smelling an elephant at a distance. These investigations are of the greatest importance as an aid in the psychologic studies of the human reaction. They seem to offer further opportunity for more of the interesting home psychological games in which so many people now indulge.

The nose, like many other organs of the body, is lined with tissue called mucous membrane that secretes mucus. Sometimes these cells over-grow, and when they do, little tumors are formed which hang down into the nose and interfere with breathing; also by the obstruction they cause they may aid in setting up infection. Hence, it is desirable that they be removed. Sometimes even after they are removed they return, and since the exact cause of such tumors is not known, there is nothing to do but keep on removing them.

In general, the causes of tumors are not definitely known, although certain contributory factors are recognized. Several observers believe that polyps never occur except in the presence of infection, although others are convinced that the infection follows the polyps.

The use of radium following the removal of tumor cells may prevent the formation of additional tumors. Hence, it has been suggested that the removal of nasal polyps be followed by mild treatment with radium element in order to prevent their return. The radium is usually applied in the form of a screen container several days after the polyps have been removed, when the inflammation due to the surgical procedure has subsided. Sometimes the polyps form in the sinuses rather than in the nasal cavity itself. Under such circumstances, a physician can detect their presence by injecting into the sinus a substance which is opaque to the X ray, such as lipoidal. Then an X-ray picture is taken, and this reveals the presence of the tumor or growth inside the sinuses, preventing their filling completely.

THE THROAT

General inflammations of the throat are associated with redness, swelling, and excessive discharge of mucus. Most common is exposure to cold, an extension of inflammation from the tonsils, the adenoids, or the nose. Excessive use of tobacco; excessive exposure to dust, smoke, irritating fumes, and sudden changes in temperature; excessive dryness, and similar atmospheric conditions may cause irritation of the throat. People who are sensitive to certain food substances sometimes react with blisters on the tissues of the throat, which become secondarily infected and produce irritations and inflammation.

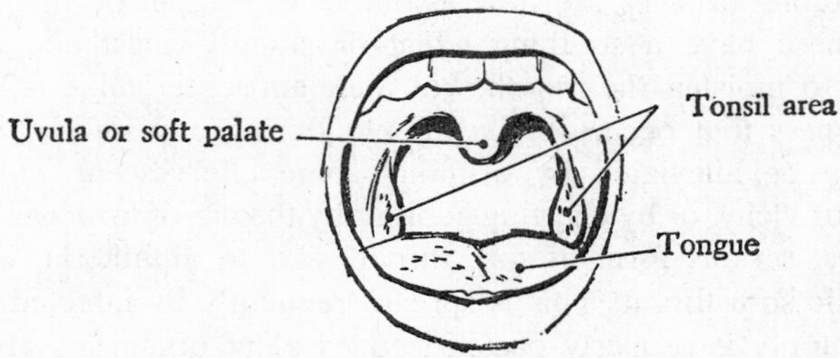

Fig. 75. Throat opening. American National Red Cross illustration from *First Aid Textbook.*

There may be severe pain associated with swelling and inflammation of the throat, including pain in the ears because of blocking of the tubes which lead from the nose to the ears; there may also be a sense of fullness or obstruction, with much hawking and spitting.

If the condition happens to be due to diphtheria, prompt action is necessary, including the giving of diphtheria antitoxin. If, however, it is due to some other type of germ, other methods of treatment are employed.

SORE THROAT

The pain of an inflamed throat is best relieved by use of an ice bag filled with cracked ice. Most doctors are now convinced that gargles seldom go deep enough in the throat in sufficient quantity or strength to permit them to have much effect in killing germs. They have the value of washing out everything they reach. They serve to relieve some of the dryness of the mouth and throat that is usually present with inflammation. They sometimes substitute a good taste in the mouth for a bad one, although some of the gargles themselves taste so bad that they make a bad taste worse. To have a definite effect from any antiseptic in the throat, it must be applied directly to the infected or inflamed part. This is best done by spreading material with a cotton swab or by using an atomizer properly. In order to get the antiseptic into the back of the throat, it may be necessary to hold the tongue or to use a tongue depressor.

MOUTH WASHES AND GARGLES

The primary purpose of a mouth wash or throat wash is to clean and soothe. Most mouth washes and gargles sold in drug stores contain water, salt, baking soda or boric acid, with flavoring material and dye substances of various kinds. Many of them contain alcohol. Alcohol is astringent, cleansing, and somewhat antiseptic. Ordinarily, mouth washes may contain one part of alcohol to four or five parts of water.

Innumerable lozenges are now available which can be dissolved on the tongue. These have a soothing effect or slightly anesthetic effect. They also serve to moisten the mouth, but their antiseptic value is little, if any.

The dryness that occurs in the mouth during any inflammation of the throat may be alleviated by drinking some effervescent water, such as ginger ale or vichy, or by chewing gum, or by the use of lozenges.

The most serious form of sore throat, next to diphtheria, is called epidemic septic sore throat. This is spread frequently by infected milk. When the milk supply is properly pasteurized, virulent organisms are destroyed. If, however, there is any carelessness whatever in the process of pasteurization, the germs causing septic sore throat may get by and infect considerable numbers of people.

This germ is a streptococcus. It is found on the udders of the infected cows and infects all the milk that comes from the infected cow. Sometimes the udder of the cow may not be infected, but the milker may have a sore throat. The milk that has become infected is then mixed with the general milk supply, and anyone taking part in the consumption of the infected milk supply is likely to develop septic sore throat.

Milkers should invariably wash their hands thoroughly before milking cows, and it will do neither the milk nor the milker any harm if the hands of the milker are washed frequently during the whole milking process. This will protect not only the milk and the consumer, but also the cow.

Infections of this type in the throat may spread gradually through the throat, involving the rest of the body. Septic sore throat usually begins with fever, chills, and a rapid pulse. These, however, are equally the symptoms of numerous other disorders of an infectious character. The fact that there are numerous other cases in the community at the same time helps to indicate the epidemic character of the disease. In most instances, investigation by the health department will serve to indicate that practically all the cases occur on the route of one distributor of milk. The study is then made to find which of the employees concerned is himself infected. An examination is also made of the herds of cows to determine whether or not any of the animals have infected udders. Not infrequently epidemic sore throat is mistaken for influenza. One epidemic has been described in which the condition was traced to infected ice cream rather than infected milk. Such epidemics are becoming infrequent. The antibiotics quickly control the streptococcus of epidemic sore throat.

TONSILLITIS

No one has ever determined certainly exactly why we have tonsils. Apparently they serve some purpose in taking care of the infectious organisms that come into the throat. However, their response to infection is prompt swelling and inflammation with pain, soreness, difficulty in swallowing, swelling of the glands in the throat, high fever, a rapid pulse, a general weakness, and serious illness generally. Not infrequently the germs which develop in the tonsils are carried by the blood to other parts of the body and there set up inflammations, the regions particularly affected being the joints, the heart, and the kidneys.

The germ that is most frequently responsible for tonsillitis is the streptococcus, which is also responsible for various forms of heart disease, for erysipelas, and for similar conditions. When the tonsils have once been seriously affected, they apparently are likely to become infected again and again.

In children particularly make sure that the condition is tonsillitis and not diphtheria. Tonsillitis produces a throat that is purplish-red and swollen, whereas diphtheria produces a grayish-white membrane. The control in diphtheria depends on early diagnosis and the proper administration of a sufficient amount of suitable antitoxin.

The patient with tonsillitis should go to bed promptly. A physician will usually apply directly to the place of infection suitable antiseptics to destroy the germs that are on the surface. He will also control the fever and provide medication which may be helpful. The application of an ice bag or hot packs will give relief from the pain and soreness. A gargle with a small amount of baking soda helps to clear out the adherent mucus.

Chronic tonsillitis is especially dangerous because of the secondary effects. For this reason, physicians advise surgical removal of the tonsils when frequent infections occur. Tonsillitis itself is seldom fatal, but the possibility afterward of an infected ear, or infected joints, or heart disease is so serious that a sore throat should never be neglected. Many years have passed since the medical profession first recognized the importance of removal of infected tonsils because of their relationship to disease. Tonsils are sometimes removed simply because they are so greatly enlarged as to interfere with swallowing and breathing. Between this simple enlargement and the severe states of infection in which the tonsils are filled with pus a wide variety of possibilities may develop.

Much investigation has been done to prove that the infection in the tonsils may be carried by the blood to other parts of the body and there set up secondary infections which threaten life. Well-established cases have been reported in which infection of the tonsils was followed by infection of the heart, of the kidneys, and even of the peritoneum, resulting finally in fatal peritonitis. There is also considerable evidence to indicate the relationship of infected tonsils to colds, infected ears, fatigue, nervousness, and rheumatic symptoms.

If it could be definitely proved that removal of the tonsils early in life would entirely prevent or greatly diminish these diseases, routine removal of the tonsils would be advised by all physicians. Unfortunately absolute proof of this fact cannot be provided.

There are many other possibilities for the production of colds, of nervousness, and of fatigue besides infection in the tonsils. Furthermore, the tonsils are not the only glandular structures involved in the upper respiratory tract. The adenoids, which lie in the postnasal cavity, may also be seriously infected and transmit infection to other parts of the body. Hence the combination "tonsils and adenoids" is just as well known as are the combinations of ham and eggs and Amos 'n' Andy.

The wholesale removal of tonsils, whether diseased or related to disease, is not warranted. In certain conditions they may be removed for definite effects, which experience has shown may certainly be secured. At present, the vast majority of physicians are convinced that the correct method for removal of the tonsils is complete surgical removal rather than the use of slow destruction by electricity or any other recently introduced method.

CHAPTER 30

The Venereal Diseases

MORRIS FISHBEIN, M.D.

The venereal diseases have been among the most common that afflict mankind. They spread from person to person in response to satisfaction of the biologic demand of the glands of man, but also occasionally through perfectly innocent sources, such as contaminated utensils, towels, and other appurtenances intimately used by people.

Both major venereal diseases, syphilis and gonorrhea, are caused by infectious organisms. The germs must be transmitted in order to transmit the disease. Every case of either one of these diseases comes from another case. Until a patient with one of these diseases is satisfactorily treated and his infection brought under control, he is a menace to everyone around him, including his wife–if he is married–his children, his friends, or associates. In a case reported in 1965, an infection with syphilis was traced from person to person. Ultimately more than a hundred were involved, one third of them teenagers.

The diseases are not new with man. They have probably existed since the earliest times, certainly since the Middle Ages. Everyone should have knowledge of the nature of these diseases and means of transmission, means of prevention, and correct method of treatment. Proper dissemination of such knowledge seems to be the only hope for their ultimate control.

SYPHILIS

Whether or not syphilis existed previous to 1493 is not established with certainty. About that time it appeared in Barcelona among Spanish sailors who had returned from Haiti. It reached Italy with the army of Charles VIII, and from Italy spread throughout Europe. At first it was called "Neapolitan disease" or the "French pox." The name syphilis was given to it in 1530 by a writer named Fracastorius. Since that time, physicians have studied the disease constantly. Even before the modern era,

TABLE 1
REPORTED VENEREAL DISEASE CASES AND CASE RATES PER 100,000 POPULATION* UNITED STATES
(Known Military Cases Excluded)
Fiscal Year 1966

State	Syphilis				Gonorrhea		Other Venereal Diseases	
	All Stages		Primary and Secondary					
	Cases	Rates	Cases	Rates	Cases	Rates	Cases	Rates
Alabama	1,928	56.1	1,252	36.4	4,056	118.0	45	1.3
Alaska	32	14.6	7	3.2	1,040	470.6	0	-
Arizona	561	35.4	201	12.7	3,158	199.1	10	.6
Arkansas	1,257	64.5	152	7.8	6,064	311.0	11	.7
California	11,726	64.1	1,768	9.7	40,243	220.0	77	.4
Colorado	509	26.4	59	3.1	2,195	113.6	5	.3
Connecticut	644	22.8	103	3.7	2,762	97.9	3	.1
Delaware	517	104.0	46	9.3	1,100	221.3	3	.6
Dist. of Columbia	1,473	186.7	468	59.3	9,941	1259.9	381	48.3
Florida	6,320	110.6	2,103	36.8	10,619	185.9	265	4.6
Georgia	2,526	59.2	1,014	23.8	12,149	285.0	117	2.7
Hawaii	130	20.1	35	5.4	402	62.0	5	.8
Idaho	17	2.4	9	1.3	1,049	152.9	2	.3
Illinois	7,188	67.8	1,260	11.9	31,153	294.0	12	.1
Indiana	1,075	22.0	76	1.6	4,540	93.1	4	.1
Iowa	851	30.9	72	2.6	2,873	104.2	5	.1
Kansas	977	44.5	62	2.8	2,798	127.5	2	.1
Kentucky	1,723	54.8	125	4.0	3,455	110.0	16	.5
Louisiana	2,869	81.8	649	18.5	5,509	157.4	63	1.8
Maine	279	28.6	4	.4	402	41.2	0	-
Maryland	3,243	93.7	555	16.0	6,741	194.7	13	.4
Massachusetts	1,787	33.6	331	6.2	4,401	82.9	5	.1
Michigan	5,784	70.7	1,057	12.9	14,765	180.1	130	1.5
Minnesota	204	5.8	56	1.6	2,187	61.6	2	.1
Mississippi	951	41.3	647	28.1	4,401	191.3	35	1.5
Missouri	3,503	78.4	214	4.8	8,622	192.9	54	1.2
Montana	145	20.8	35	5.0	473	68.0	2	.2
Nebraska	373	25.6	78	5.3	1,080	74.0	1	.1
Nevada	231	53.5	32	7.4	687	159.0	1	.2
New Hampshire	79	11.9	14	2.1	296	44.7	5	.8
New Jersey	3,943	58.5	828	12.3	4,016	59.6	13	.1
New Mexico	942	93.5	101	10.0	1,567	155.6	2	.2
New York	18,866	104.7	3,329	18.5	37,889	210.2	98	.5
North Carolina	2,242	46.5	976	20.2	10,318	214.0	87	1.8
North Dakota	19	3.1	5	.8	422	69.1	0	-
Ohio	4,277	41.9	623	6.1	14,527	142.1	26	.3
Oklahoma	1,204	49.3	110	4.5	3,446	140.8	8	.3
Oregon	362	19.2	55	2.9	2,532	133.7	3	.2
Pennsylvania	4,961	43.1	567	4.9	8,790	76.4	23	.2
Rhode Island	348	38.9	31	3.5	359	40.1	0	-
South Carolina	1,742	70.0	882	35.5	7,121	286.2	22	.8
South Dakota	115	16.5	36	5.2	659	94.7	1	.1
Tennessee	1,389	36.4	342	9.0	9,962	261.1	36	1.0
Texas	5,528	53.2	1,544	14.9	28,560	275.0	105	1.0
Utah	139	14.1	18	1.8	427	43.4	0	-
Vermont	21	5.3	2	.5	208	52.4	2	.5
Virginia	1,972	45.9	296	6.9	8,060	187.7	28	.7
Washington	251	8.6	48	1.6	3,449	117.8	5	.2
West Virginia	1,436	79.2	100	5.5	934	51.6	3	.2
Wisconsin	1,368	33.1	89	2.1	2,362	57.1	3	.1
Wyoming	101	30.2	7	2.1	160	47.8	0	-
United States Total	110,128	57.1	22,473	11.6	334,949	173.6	1,739	.9

* Rates less than .05 not shown.

Reported Venereal Disease Cases and Case Rates per 100,000 Population, United States. *VD Fact Sheet 1966,* National Communicable Disease Center, Bureau of Disease Prevention and Environmental Control.

doctors had learned to treat syphilis with a fair degree of success with mercury. However, it was the discovery of the organism of the disease, and later the discovery of specific methods of treatment, that offered the first promise of complete control. The organism of syphilis, known as "spirochaeta" or "treponema," was definitely established as the cause of the disease by the investigator Schaudinn in 1905. The organism is seen only with the microscope, and is found in the sore which is typically the first sign of infection with this disease.

TRANSMISSION OF SYPHILIS

In the vast majority of cases syphilis is transmitted from one human being to another during sexual relations. There are, however, records of accidental infection, such as those which occur on the hands of surgeons and midwives who have not properly protected their hands during their work; such as occur on the lips from infection through kissing, and such as occur occasionally on the breasts of wet nurses. Occasionally also the child may be infected before birth from its mother, in instances even when the mother herself is not actively diseased.

These facts should not frighten anyone into a phobia or constant fear of syphilis, since the disease is not transmitted as easily as the description may seem to suggest. Hotel beds, public lavatories, bathtubs, door knobs, books, utensils used in public eating places are not easily infected. Moreover, the germs do not live easily in the presence of dryness. Finally, it is necessary for the organism to get into a sore or an easily infected spot in order to invade the body. In most instances, thorough washing with soap and water does much to remove danger of infection. When it seems likely that one has been directly exposed to the development of the infection with syphilis, the rubbing of mercury ointment into the exposed area has been proved to be a protective measure of great value. It is well, however, to emphasize again that syphilis is rarely acquired by those who observe the elementary laws of personal hygiene and who have sexual relations only with those who are free from the disease.

FIRST SIGNS OF SYPHILIS

The first sign of syphilis is usually the appearance of a sore on the genital area or on the finger or wherever the germs gain entrance into the tissues. These sores develop slowly. At the same time the lymph glands in the region near by become swollen. A physician who sees such a sore makes his diagnosis certain by taking some of the fluid from the sore and studying it under what is called the dark field microscope. By reflected light he is thus able to see the spirochetes wriggling in the fluid. He may also spread some of the secretion on a glass slide and stain it with suitable stains which make the organisms visible with the ordinary microscope.

TEENAGE DOUBLE TROUBLE

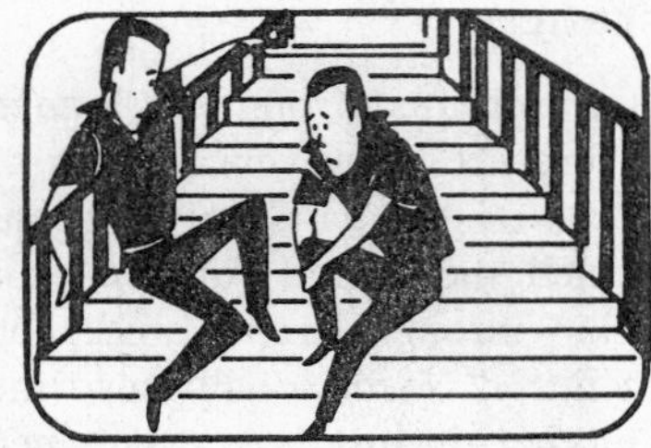

ED: What's bugging you, Joe?

JOE: I'm OK. I'm OK if it don't get worse.

ED: Ask the man at the drugstore. Maybe he's got something for it, cheap.

JOE: Yeah—let's go.

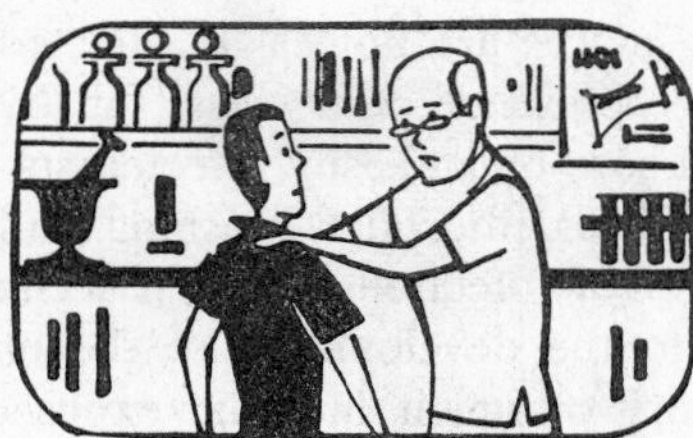

DRUGGIST: Look, Joe, if you have syphilis or if you have clap, don't take chances. See a doctor. Syphilis is big trouble, Joe. If you don't get it out of your blood, it can ruin your health.

JOE: What'll it cost, I haven't got a job. I'd sure hate to ask my pop for money for something like this.

DRUGGIST: There are treatment centers where you can go for free. The City runs them. They want you to get help before you give the same thing to somebody else.

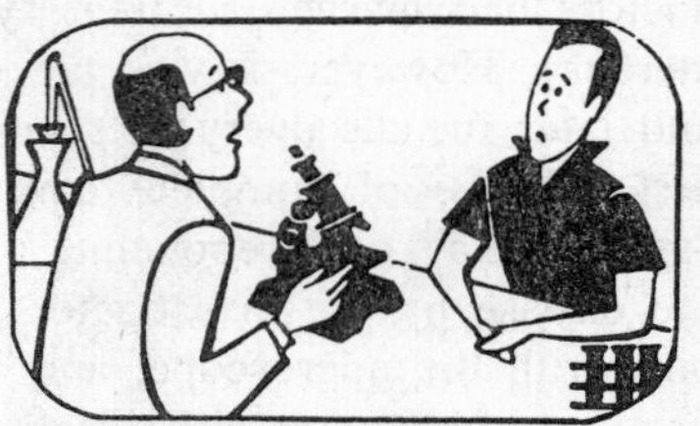

DOCTOR: Joe, you've got syphilis, all right. You know the little drop I took from the sore? It shows you have syphilis. You can see for yourself. Here, take a look.

JOE: OK, Doc. I get the idea. Can you do something to keep that from happening to me?

DOCTOR: Yes, Joe. We've got powerful drugs that will soon stop the germs from growing inside your body. Now, I'll give you a shot of penicillin. And I expect you to come back for a check-up.

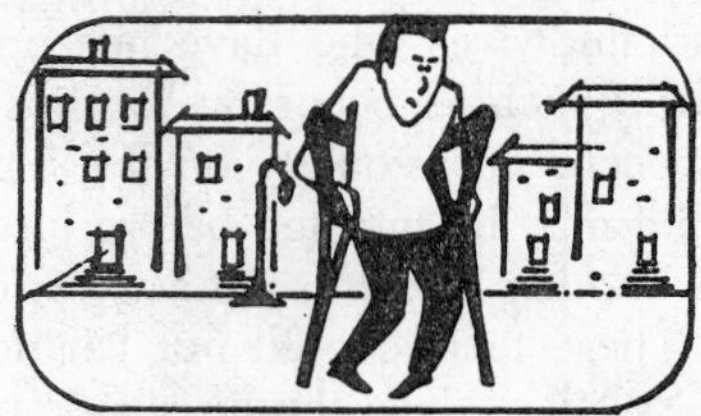

DOCTOR: Here's what syphilis did to a man who didn't get medical help soon enough.

DOCTOR: You were lucky, Joe. You came in to get help. The guy who tries to cure himself is just a square. He's headed for double trouble. Like a man playing against loaded dice. He's the one you're likely to see standing on the street corner some day—with a cup and a cane.

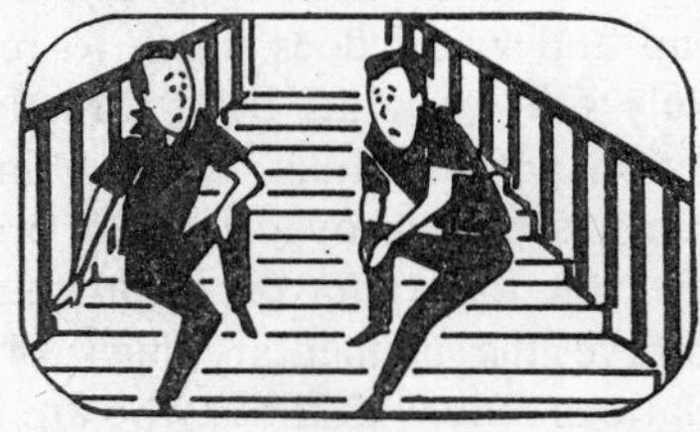

ED: Hey, Joe. How'd you make out with the doctor?

JOE: Okay, Ed. The doctor said I'm going to be all right. That doc is okay. He says anybody who fools around with VD is real square. And, he's right. All you have to do to get help for VD is see a doctor or call the nearest Health Department VD clinic.

Fig. 76. Strictly for teen-agers. Young persons under twenty years of age are responsible for one out of four reported cases of venereal disease—syphilis and gonorrhea. Venereal disease attacks one teen-ager every nine minutes, and accounts for nearly half of all the reportable communicable diseases in adults. The only way to conquer VD is through frank public discussion and education. Since attitudes and standards toward sex and sex conduct are developed as teen-agers, developing proper attitudes is the most important contribution to the prevention of VD. Venereal diseases are transmitted only through sexual intercourse. They can only be detected through medical examinations and laboratory

The healing of the primary sore or its removal will not, however, prevent syphilis from invading the body. Usually, by the time the organisms are found freely in the sore, the body has already been quite fully invaded and it is necessary to give general treatment to control the condition. If immediate treatment is given before the appearance of the secondary symptoms, these are not likely to appear. Hence, the physician urges emphatically that every case of syphilis be treated at the earliest possible moment; in fact, that every case diagnosed from the symptoms be treated even before getting the results of the Wassermann test, so as to be certain that the control will be brought about at the earliest possible moment.

The test known as the Wassermann test, and a similar test, known as the Kahn test, are means of examining the blood so as to determine whether or not it contains a substance opposing syphilis, which is present only if syphilis has invaded the body. These tests are positive in more than 95 per cent of cases in an early stage. By their nature they enable the physician to determine whether or not improvement is taking place, and later whether or not the patient has been cured.

Venereal diseases can be cured, provided treatment is given sufficiently early and with sufficient intensity and for a long enough period of time. Modern treatment is based on use of adequate amounts of penicillin or other antibiotic drugs.

The secondary symptoms of syphilis appear about the time when the first sore is disappearing. These symptoms represent invasion of the body as a whole. Now the person is usually sick, he may be jaundiced, and eruptions may appear about the body. Frequently the hair falls out in spots, and occasionally serious sores develop on the skin. There may even be inflammation of the eyes, of the mouth, of the joints, or of the nervous system in this stage of syphilis. Because these symptoms may come and go, some patients are inclined to neglect treatment in the second stage of syphilis. This, however, should never be done. It is easier to treat the condition in this stage than in the third stage, in which the brain and nervous system become involved.

In the secondary stage there has seldom been destruction of the tissues of the body, so that treatment in this stage is more likely to be effective. Under no circumstances should the patient believe that the gradual disappearance of the symptoms represents cure of the disease. He should have a definite statement by a competent physician after that physician

---

tests and cured by a licensed physician, qualified to treat them. Unfortunately, there is no immunity to VD—you can have a venereal disease any number of times. Anyone who suspects he has a VD should visit a physician or the Health Department Venereal Disease Clinic—at once. Department of Health, The City of New York. Adapted from *Teen-Age Double Trouble,* Department of Health Treatment Center for Venereal Disease, The City of New York.

has made sufficient laboratory tests to venture an opinion with reasonable certainty.

In the third stage of syphilis, there occur not only destruction of tissues, but growths within various organs of the body, inflammations of the blood vessels, hardening of some of the organs, and other serious changes. In fact, the lesions of this disease are so varied that Sir William Osler once said that one who knew all of syphilis really knew all of medicine. The third stage grows constantly worse unless sufficiently treated. Fortunately, the third stage of syphilis is not likely to be as dangerous to other people as are the first and second, because in this stage the lesions are buried deeper within the body, so that the organisms are not so easily transmitted outside the body.

In the later stage of syphilis, it affects the nervous system. As a result come those two exceedingly serious diseases which are responsible for much disability and death: locomotor ataxia or tabes dorsalis, and paresis, also called general paralysis of the insane and dementia paralytica. In these conditions, other methods of treatment are required besides those commonly used for syphilis in the early stages. It may be necessary to apply treatment directly to the spine or to the brain. It may be necessary to infect the patient with malaria, which has been found to have special virtue in the attack on general paralysis, or to use the heat treatment, which has come to be well established as a useful method.

FACTS ABOUT SYPHILIS

Among certain facts which should be known to everyone relative to syphilis are the following:

This disease does not cause pimples.

It does not cause itching conditions of the skin.

It may cause ulcers of the legs, but more frequently these are due to varicose veins.

It may be responsible for failure to produce children, but there are also other conditions which may produce such failures.

It is not a form of blood poisoning, but testing of the blood will show whether or not the patient has syphilis.

It is not responsible for the vast majority of cases of baldness, but some cases of loss of hair not only of the head but of the entire body may be due to syphilis.

It has not been established in any way that syphilis is the cause of cancer or that these two conditions are in any way related.

INSTRUCTIONS FOR THOSE WITH SYPHILIS

If you have any sore on your genitals, no matter how small, or if you think you have syphilis, consult your physician. Do not under any conditions rely on the "blood medicines" that promise to eradicate syphilis, and do not be caught by advertising doctors—quacks—who try to get your money by promising to cure you quickly. Do not let druggists prescribe for you; they are not qualified to treat syphilis.

Do not hesitate to tell your doctor or dentist of your disease. Later in life if you get sick at any time, you should tell your doctor that you have had syphilis, since this fact may furnish a clue to treatment on which your cure depends.

Live temperately and sensibly. Do not go to extreme in any direction in your habits of life.

Try to get a reasonable amount of sleep—eight hours is the amount needed by the average person. And as a safeguard to others, sleep alone. Avoid possible contamination of others by contact with your secretions or excretions.

Absolutely do not use alcoholic liquors. All experience shows that drinking—even moderate drinking—is bad for syphilis.

Take good care of your teeth. Brush them two or three times a day. If they are not in good condition, have them attended to by a dentist. But when you go to him, tell him that you have syphilis.

Do not have sexual intercourse until you are told by your physician that you are no longer contagious. It will interfere with the cure of the disease, and it is criminal, for it is likely to give the disease to your wife.

You must not marry until you have the doctor's consent, which cannot be properly given until at least two years have passed after cure seems complete. If you do, you run the risk of infecting your wife and your children with syphilis.

Early in the course of syphilis, while it is contagious, the greatest danger of infecting other people is by the mouth. Because of this danger, do not kiss anybody. Particularly, do not endanger children by kissing them.

Do not allow anything that has come in contact with your lips or that has been in your mouth to be left around so that anybody can use it before it has been cleaned. This applies to cups, glasses, knives, forks, spoons, pipes, cigars, toothpicks, and all such things. It is better to use your own towels, brushes, comb, razor, soap, etc., though these are much less likely to be contaminated than objects that go in your mouth.

If you have any open sores—you will not have any after the first week or two, if you are treated—everything that comes in contact with them should be destroyed or disinfected.

To live up to these instructions will only require a little care until you get used to them; after that, it will be easy. If you do live up to them, there is a good prospect that syphilis will not do your health permanent harm or cause injury to others; and you will have the satisfaction of knowing that, after your misfortune, you have acted the part of an honest man in your efforts to overcome it.

Remember, the antibiotic drugs, particularly penicillin, are now known to be efficient in controlling syphilis. Often the condition is fully controlled in a few weeks. The number of cases has dropped to one-tenth what it used to be. To insure future safety, treatment must be continued until every evidence of the disease has disappeared. For your own good, you must see to it that you do not neglect your treatment after the first few months.

Penicillin, terramycin, and aureomycin are most important in the treatment of syphilis. By intensive treatment, patients may be free from the danger of infecting others in a few days. In early cases, the disease is apparently brought under full control within a week or ten days. Treatment demands, however, complete control by the physician during the period of treatment. Penicillin taken by mouth or in other ways is not safe or efficient. Patients must return frequently for repeated examinations and tests to be sure the condition is completely controlled.

WHEN PEOPLE WITH SYPHILIS MAY MARRY

One of the questions most frequently asked by a patient with syphilis is whether or not he may marry. Most physicians are convinced that a patient should be free from all syphilitic symptoms for at least two years before marriage should be contemplated. In most American states the bridegroom is compelled to furnish a medical certificate to show that he has been examined and found free from venereal disease. However, fewer states require a certificate from the prospective bride. The marriage of a person who has a contagious venereal disease has been forbidden in Delaware, Indiana, Maine, Michigan, Nebraska, New Jersey, Oklahoma, Pennsylvania, Utah, Vermont, Virginia, and Washington.

The treatment of this condition is one of the most intricate problems that can confront a physician. He must use his remedies in relationship to the reaction of the patient and the response of the patient to them. No one with the disease should ever discontinue treatment until he is pronounced by a competent physician free from danger of transmitting the disease and cured to the extent that the condition is brought absolutely to a halt in his body. Persistence in the use of the new remedies that are available under proper control will yield a successful result in the vast majority of cases.

GONORRHEA

Gonorrhea has existed certainly since Biblical times. Although it is a widespread and serious disease, it is not a killing disease. As a cause of ill health, it ranks among the leaders, but as a cause of death it is not especially prominent. Many people believe that gonorrhea concerns only the sex organs, whereas the germ which causes it, described by the investigator Neisser in 1879, may invade any part of the human body. Like syphilis, it is spread mostly by sexual contacts. However, there are infections of the eyes sustained during childbirth or in other ways which attack mostly infants at birth. There are infections of the tissues in women associated with the use of bathtubs and toilet devices not properly cleansed, which are accidental infections with this disease. Little girls are occasionally infected by soiled hands of mothers or nurses.

Gonorrhea is responsible for a considerable percentage of all cases of blindness. It is one of the common causes of infection in the female abdomen, resulting in necessary surgical operations and occasionally removal of the female organs. It is responsible for a considerable amount of sterility in men due to infections of the various parts of the sex tracts. It is found not only among the poor but in all classes of society.

FIRST SIGNS OF GONORRHEA

From three to five days after a sex contact with a person who is infected the first signs of the disease may appear. These usually are a feeling of burning or stinging at the time of urination, associated with redness and soreness, and associated also with the formation of pus or matter which drips from the sex organ. This material is highly infectious and should not be allowed to come in contact with the eyes or sex organs of any other person.

If a physician is consulted immediately, he may be able to stop the disease in these early stages, when it is confined to the lower portion of the sex organs. If, however, it is not stopped at this time, the germs get farther back into the glands of the male and into the organs and tissues of the female. To the extent to which these organs and tissues are involved, gonorrhea is a serious disorder. The physician may make his diagnosis by an examination of the matter under the microscope, in which case he can actually find the germs, and also by tests of the blood. Occasionally the condition affects the joints, and it is also largely responsible for painful heels, causing outgrowths on the large bone of the heel.

TREATMENT OF GONORRHEA

In treatment, the physician uses many types of remedies, including antibiotics such as penicillin and terramycin given by injection into the muscles or blood stream. Gonorrhea is now controlled in 48 hours. Military authorities prevent gonorrhea by giving penicillin to men going on leave.

ADVICE TO THOSE WITH GONORRHEA

Persist in treatment until your doctor tells you you are cured.

Do not try to treat yourself.

Do not use a patent medicine or some "sure shot" that may stop the discharges but will not cure you.

Do not let an advertising doctor—a quack—get your money, and do not let a drug clerk treat you.

If you have had gonorrhea and you suspect that it is not cured, report to your medical officer.

During the acute stages keep quiet and take little exercise. As long as you have any discharge avoid violent exercise, especially dancing.

In order to avoid chordee, while the disease is acute, sleep on your side, urinate just before going to bed, and drink no water after supper.

Never "break" a chordee. To get rid of it wrap the penis in cold wet cloths or pour cold water on it.

Except at night, drink plenty of water—eight or ten glasses a day.

Do not drink any alcoholic liquors; they always make the disease worse and delay its cure. Also avoid spicy drinks such as ginger ale.

Do not eat irritating, highly seasoned, spicy foods, such as pepper, horseradish, mustard, pickles, salt and smoked meats, or fish.

Always wash your hands after handling the penis, particularly in order to protect your eyes. Gonorrhea of the eyes is very dangerous; it will produce blindness if not at once treated, and the infection is easily carried to the eyes on the fingers.

Keep your penis clean. Do not plug up the opening with cotton or wear a dressing that prevents the escape of the pus from it. Wash the penis several times daily.

Burn old dressings, or drop them into a disinfecting solution.

Never use anybody else's syringe or let others use yours. While you are using a syringe keep it clean by washing it in very hot water, and, when you have finished with its use, destroy it.

Avoid sexual excitement. Stay away from women. Do not have intercourse. It will bring your disease back to its acute stage, and it is almost sure to infect a woman. Sexual intercourse while you have gonorrhea is a criminal act.

You are likely to obey instructions while your gonorrhea is acute, because it causes so much pain. Persist in them after pain is gone; by so doing you will prevent relapses, make your cure much easier and more certain, and expose no one else to the disease.

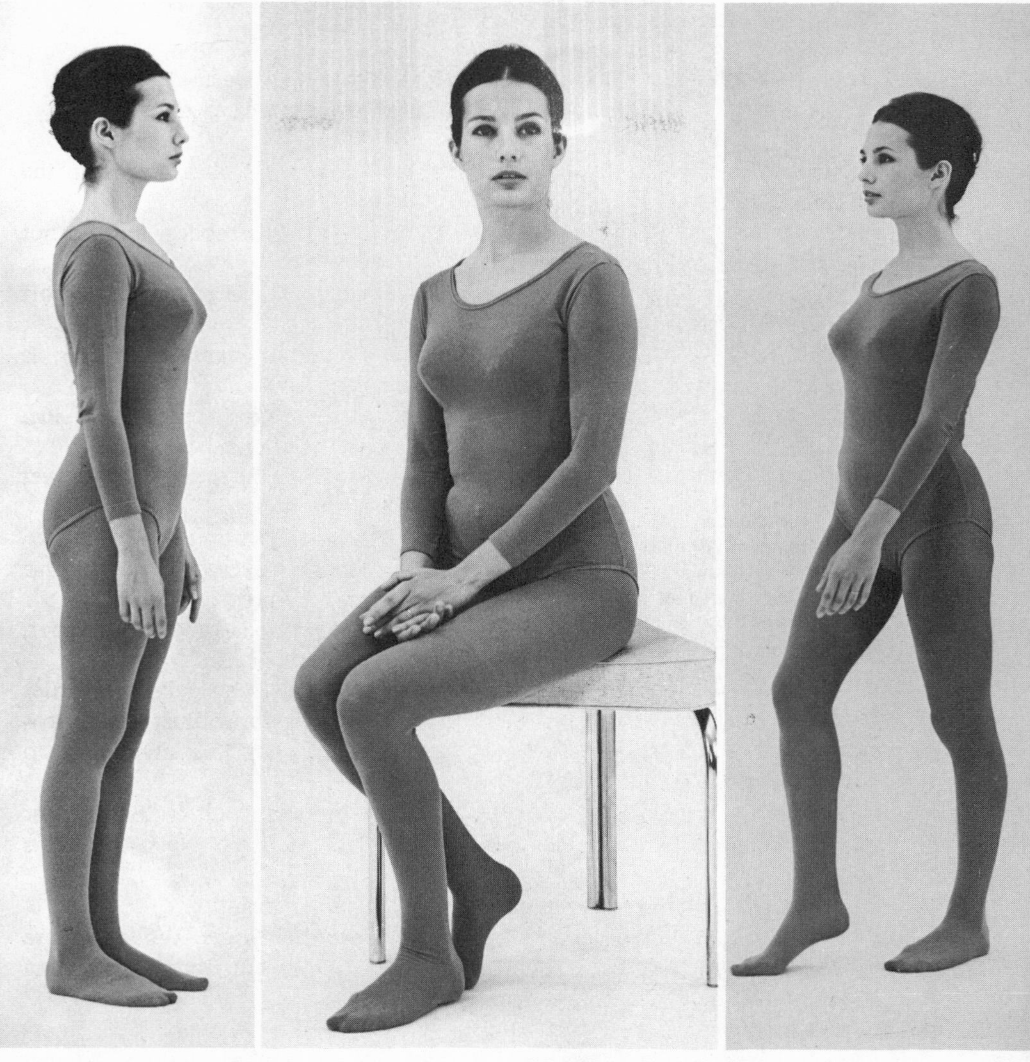

Proper posture positions. PLATE **83.** Standing. (1.) Feet parallel, about six inches apart. (2.) Head high, as if balancing a book. (3.) Chest out. (4.) Stomach and hips firm. (5.) Abdomen and back as flat as possible. (6.) Knees very lightly flexed—not stiffly locked. (7.) Weight evenly distributed on both feet—most of it on the balls of the feet. PLATE **84.** Sitting. (1.) Sit tall and back, with hips touching the back of the chair, feet flat on the floor. (2.) Chest out, back of neck nearly in line with upper back. (3.) Lean forward from the hips so you keep head and shoulders in line.

PLATE **85.** Walking. (1.) Knees and ankles limber, toes pointed straight ahead. (2.) Head and chest high. (3.) When walking, lean forward from the hips so you keep head and shoulders in a line. (4.) Swing legs directly forward from the hip joint. (5.) Push feet off the ground—don't shuffle. (6.) Swing shoulders and arms freely and easily. *(From "About Physical Fitness," a program for men and women, prepared by the President's Council on Physical Fitness. Photos by Dunlap Photo Service.)*

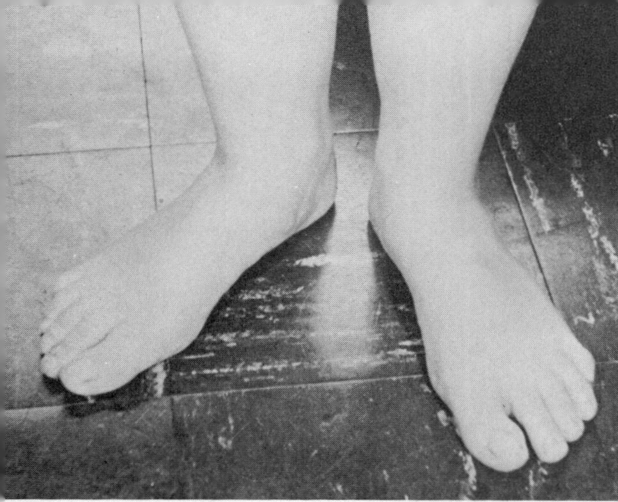

PLATE **86.** Wrong standing position. The foot consists of twenty-six bones bound together by ligaments, propelled by muscles, and supplied with blood vessels and nerves. It is subject to much strain and injury. *(Photograph courtesy of the American Podiatry Association.)*

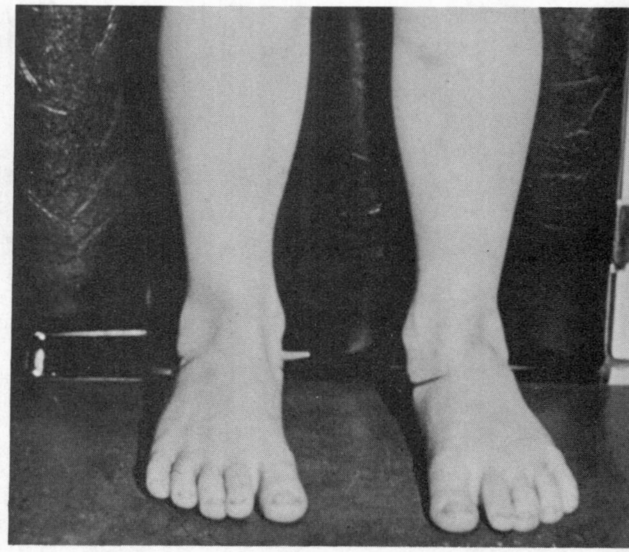

PLATE **87.** Correct standing position —feet parallel. Teach children to toe straight ahead when walking. Toeing in or out weakens the feet and throws the entire body out of alignment. *(Photograph courtesy of the American Podiatry Association.)*

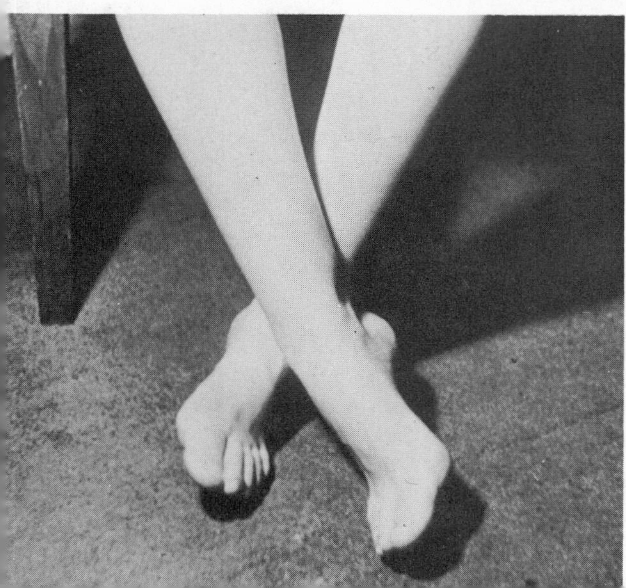

PLATE **88.** Correct position of the feet when seated. *(Photograph courtesy of the American Podiatry Association.)*

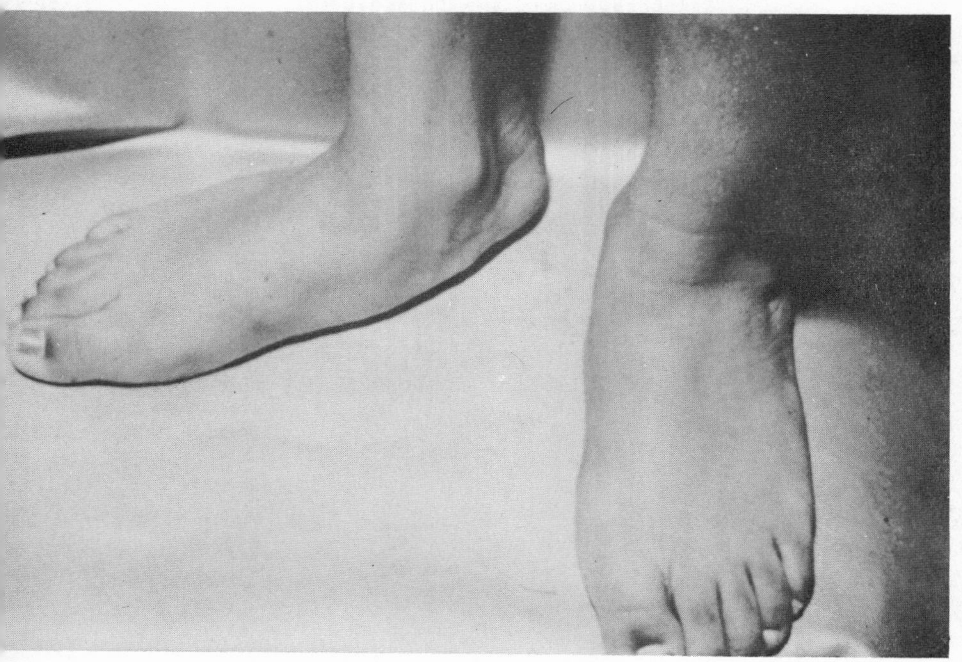

PLATE **89.** Classic flat foot. PLATE **90.** *(below)* A typical case of pronation–rear view. *(Photograph courtesy of the American Podiatry Association.)*

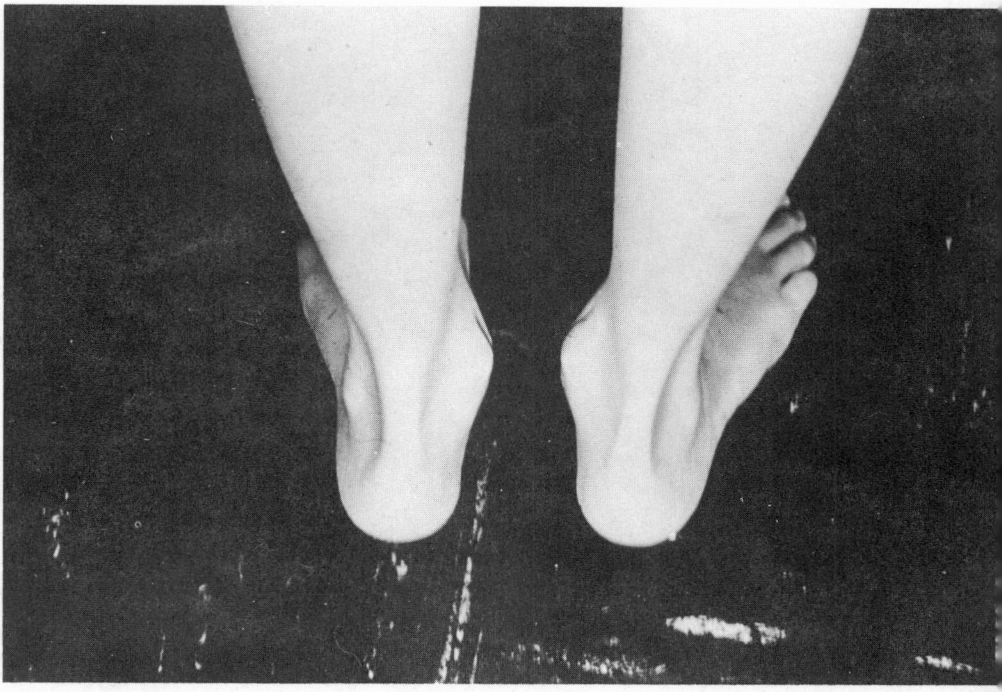

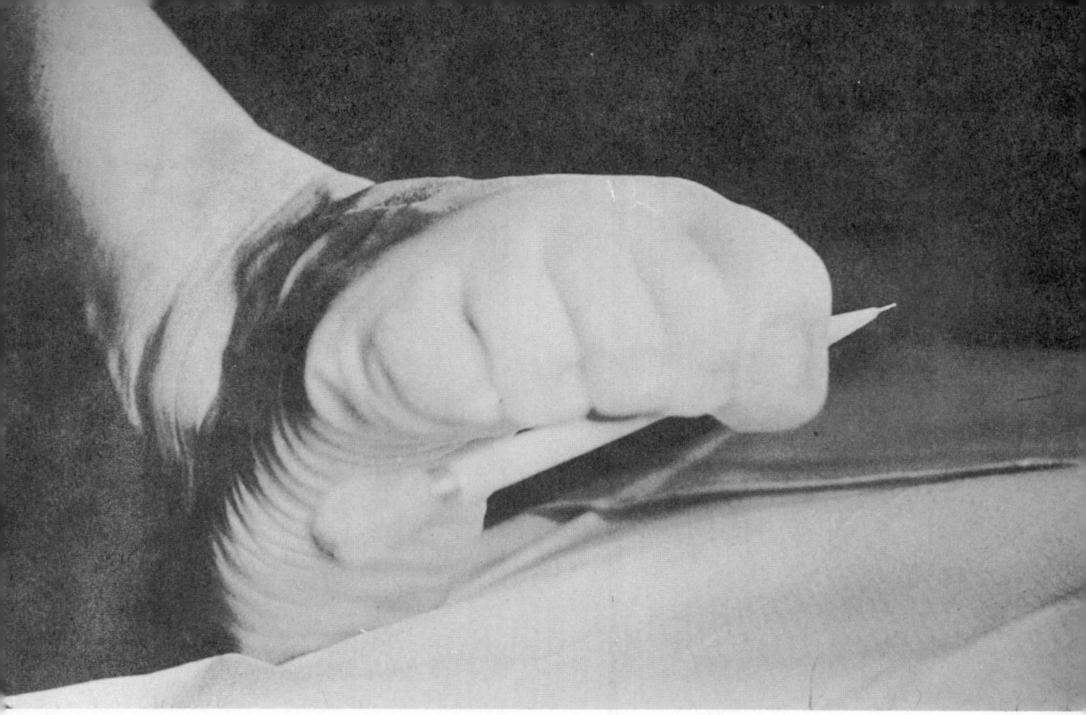

PLATE **91.** Exercises can be very helpful in keeping your feet healthy. Exercising with pencil strengthens arch and muscles. *(Photograph courtesy of the American Podiatry Association.)*

PLATE **92.** Correct trimming of toenails. Nails should be trimmed straight across without rounding of the corners. *(Courtesy of the American Podiatry Association.)*

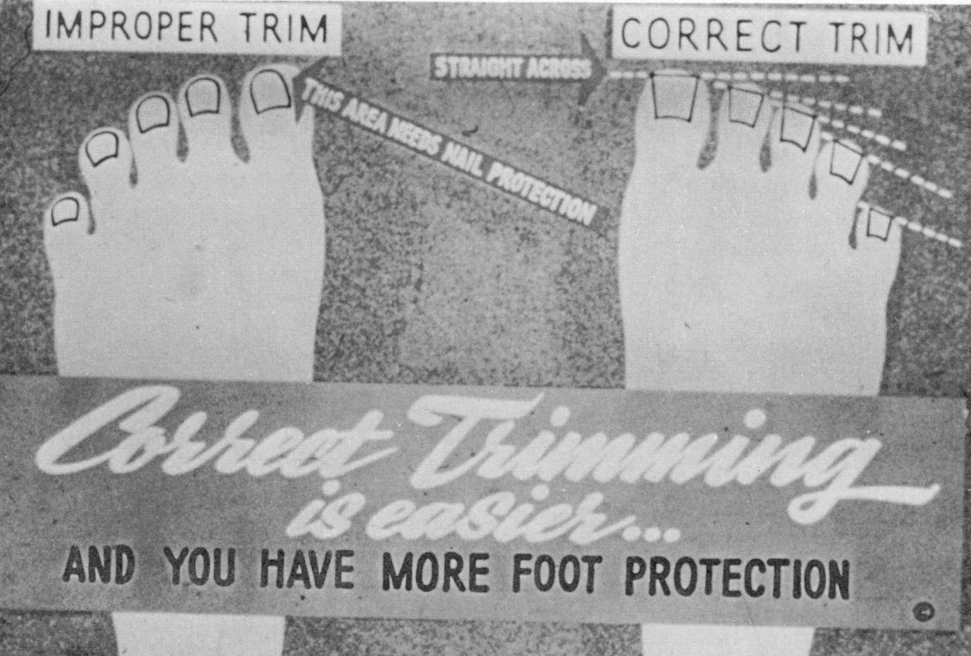

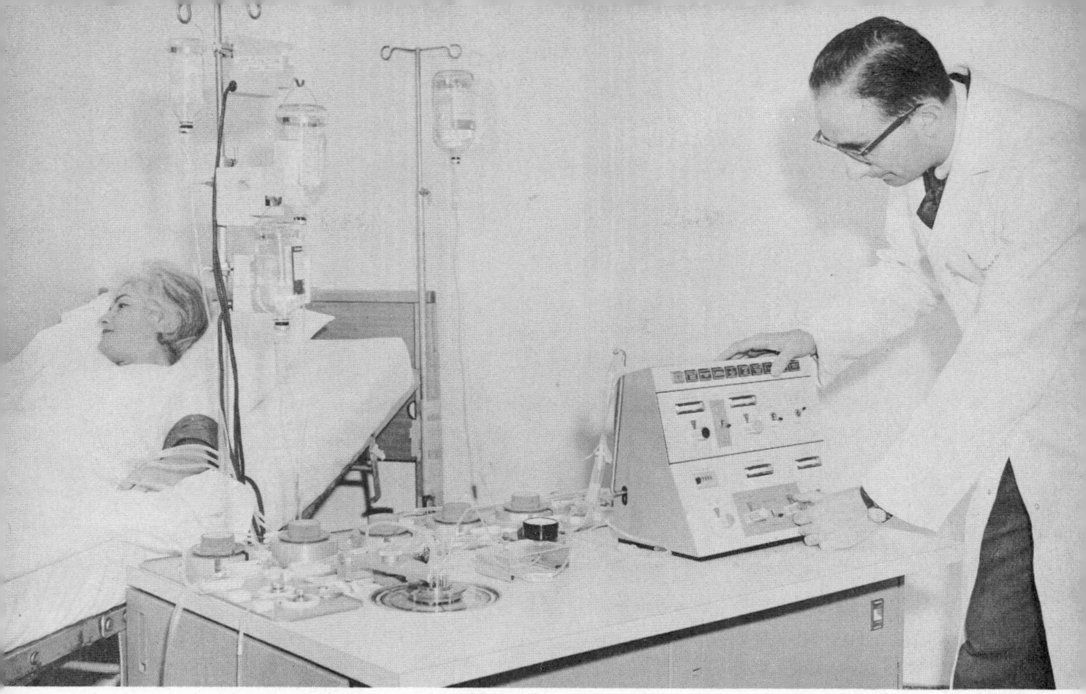

PLATE **93.** Dr. Robert K. Ausman, Chief of the blood-cell separator programs at Roswell Park Memorial Institute in Buffalo, demonstrates a new medical instrument which automatically separates whole blood into its major fractions. Developed jointly by the National Cancer Institute and International Business Machines Corporation, the blood-cell separator is being used at Roswell Park to collect white blood cells for cancer research. *(International Businesss Machines Corporation.)*

PLATE **94.** After plasma is expressed, packed red cells remain in bag 1; platelet-rich plasma is now in bag 2, which is then processed by centrifuging, separating, freezing and thawing and can be further fractioned in the production of plasma proteins. *(Courtesy of the New York Blood Center.)*

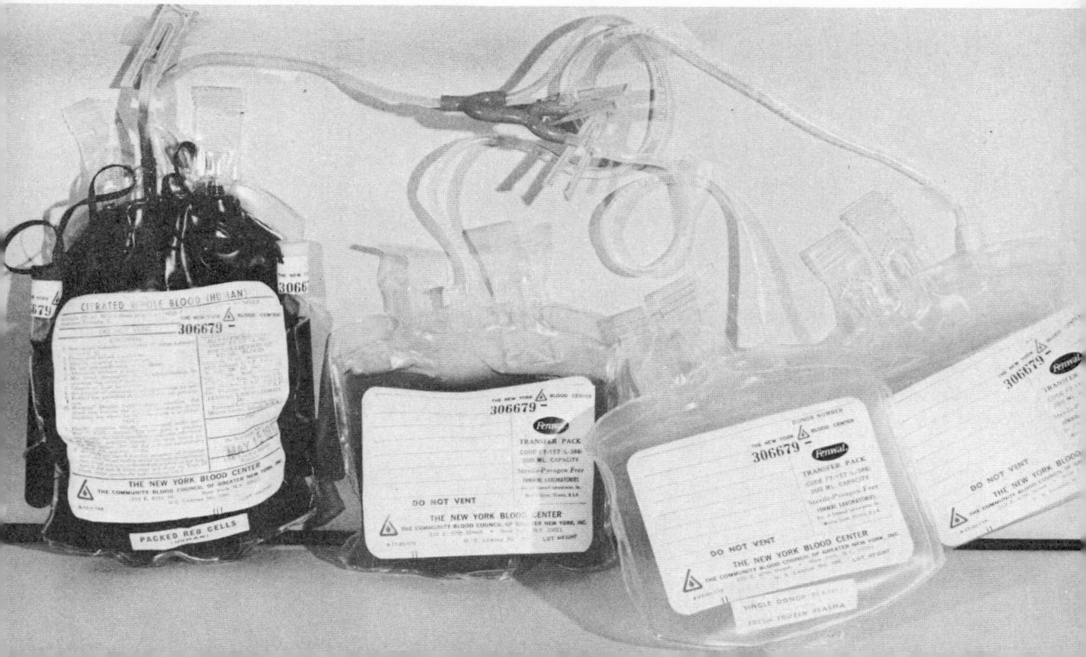

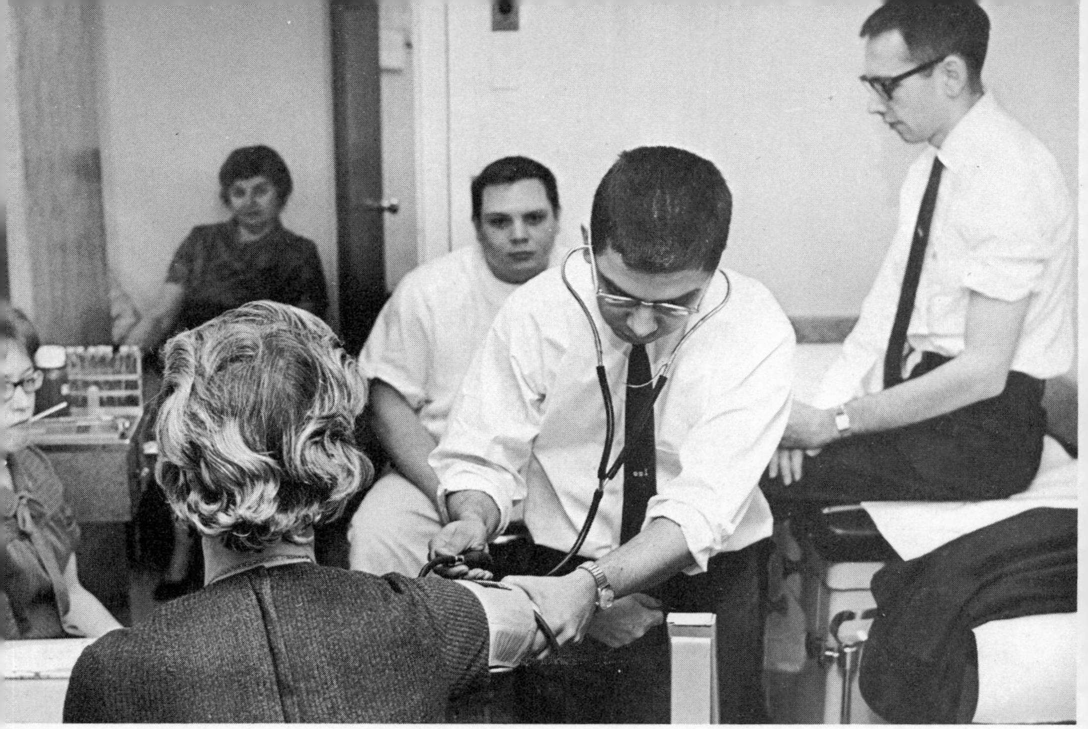

PLATE **95.** Montefiore employees who have volunteered to supply fresh blood (no more than six hours old) for a child about to undergo open-heart surgery report to the hospital's blood bank where they are given a final check-up before blood is drawn. *(Courtesy of Montefiore Hospital and Medical Center, New York, and Wagner International Photos.)*

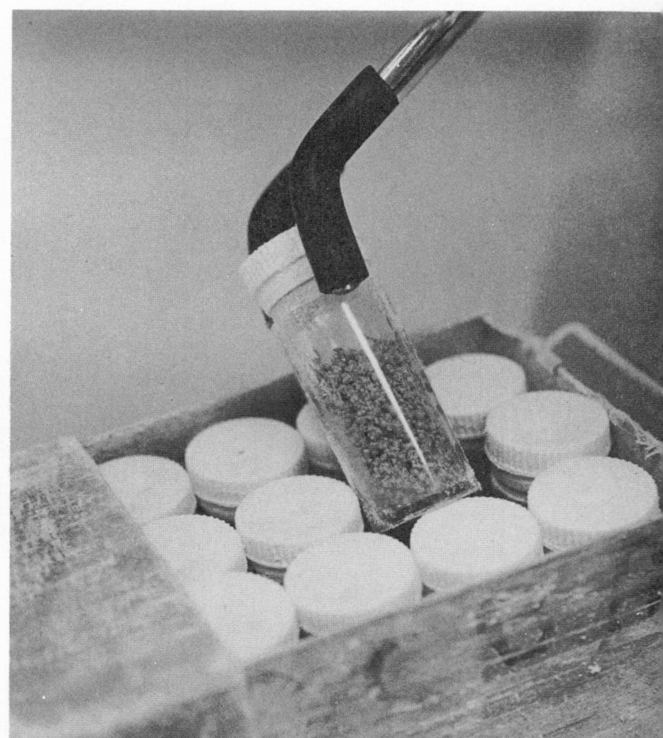

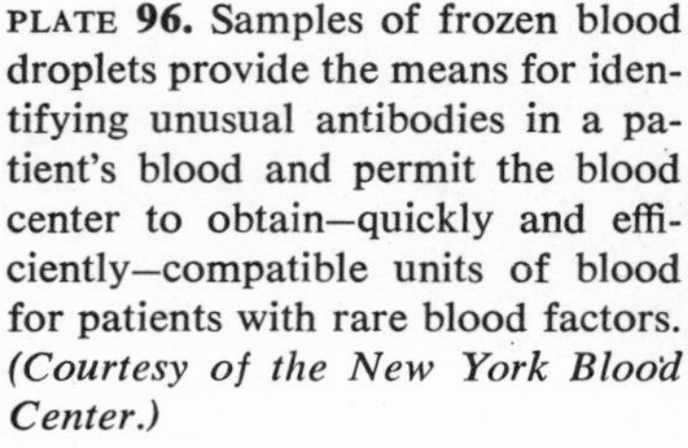

PLATE **96.** Samples of frozen blood droplets provide the means for identifying unusual antibodies in a patient's blood and permit the blood center to obtain—quickly and efficiently—compatible units of blood for patients with rare blood factors. *(Courtesy of the New York Blood Center.)*

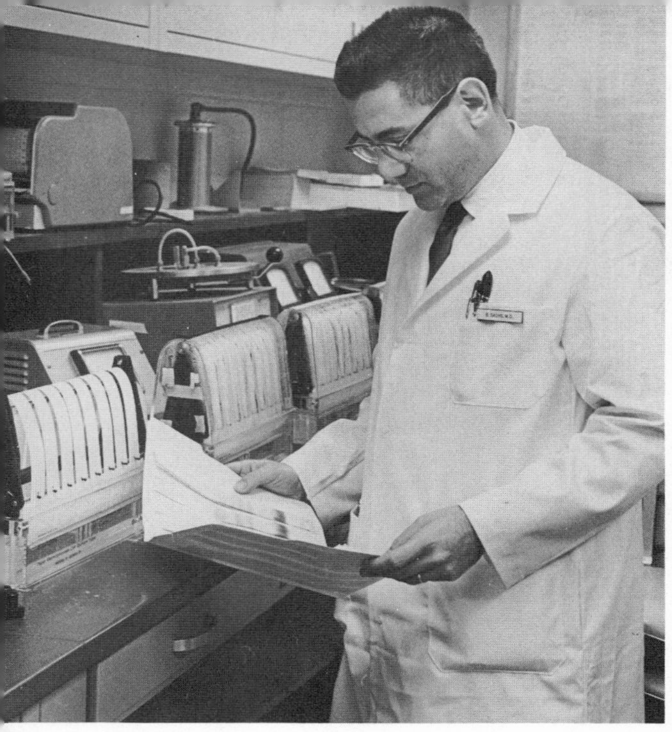

PLATE **97.** Dr. Bernard A. Sachs, head of Montefiore's Endocrine Service, at work in the laboratory where he is currently engaged in research on the effects of cholesterol-reducing drugs in helping to protect coronary patients against recurrent attacks. *(Courtesy of Montefiore Hospital and Medical Center, New York, and Ed Bagwell.)*

PLATE **98.** A registered nurse takes a prospective blood donor's blood pressure as part of the medical checkup he is given before being allowed to give blood. *(American National Red Cross.)*

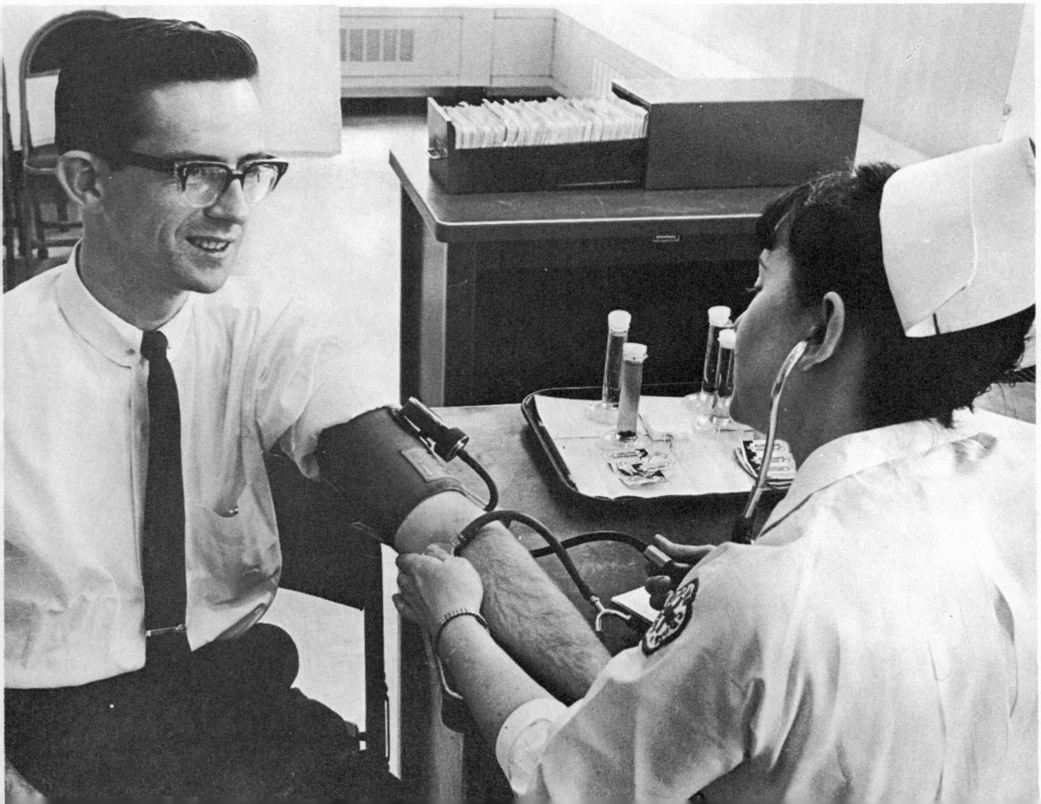

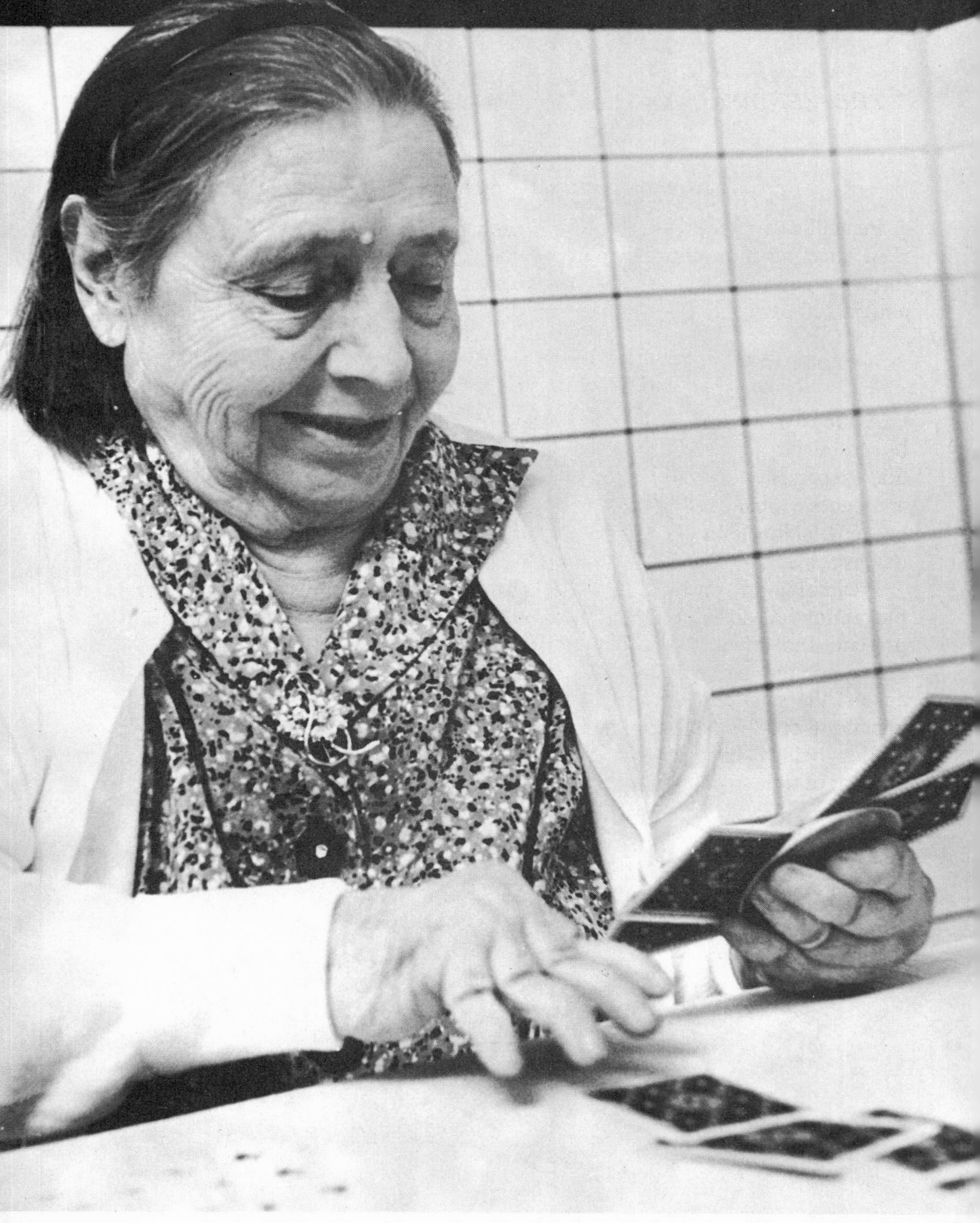

PLATE **99.** The arthritic or rheumatic person who, with the help of his physician, utilizes to the fullest every advantage indicated to improve his condition can be well repaid for his efforts by a happy and relatively active life. *(New York Chapter, the Arthritis Foundation, Inc.)*

MODERN TREATMENT OF GONORRHEA

Penicillin is effective not only in venereal gonorrhea but also in gonorrhea affecting the eyes, the joints or the heart. Whereas this disease was formerly considered well nigh incurable, with penicillin cures seem to be almost 100 per cent.

MARRIAGE AFTER GONORRHEA

As regards marriage after an attack of gonorrhea, the patient should be examined at weekly intervals to determine whether or not any infection is present following treatment. The results should be negative three consecutive times before he can be considered definitely cured. It should be remembered that self-treatment with drug-store remedies is just as dangerous as complete neglect of treatment.

Prevention in gonorrhea is far better than cure. The chief factor in prevention consists in the avoidance of sex contacts when infection is present, and infection is likely to be present in any promiscuous woman, either commercial or private. There are various methods of protection against the possibility of infection, such as the use of rubber devices and injections of various antiseptics immediately after sex contact, these antiseptics being held in the organs until the antiseptics have sufficient amount of time to act.

CHAPTER 31

The Care of the Teeth

MORRIS FISHBEIN, M.D.

THE CARE OF BABY'S TEETH

The first attention to the teeth of the child must begin before it is born. The mother should visit the dentist early, keep her teeth clean and well cared for, and eat the proper food so that the child's teeth will have materials necessary for growth. The proper foods include plenty of milk, fresh vegetables, eggs, fresh and cooked fruits, the coarser cereals, and a sufficient amount of calories to provide energy. Foods to be avoided are the sweets in excess, meat in excess, pastries, and highly seasoned foods.

During the early months the expectant mother need not eat more than her usual amount of food, but during the last four months the amount of food must be increased slightly in order to provide a sufficient amount of material for building the tissues of the child.

A notion used to prevail that it was not safe for a prospective mother to visit her dentist, but it is now realized that the dentist can do the necessary dental work without serious harm or shock, and that it is better to take care of the teeth immediately than to permit bad conditions to go on for months.

Of special importance for building sound teeth are vitamins C, D, and A. Vitamin C is found plentifully in orange and tomato juice and in the fresh vegetables; vitamins A and D particularly in cod-liver oil and egg yolks. The physician should see the prospective mother just as soon as she knows that she is going to have a child and advise her regarding the taking of dietary supplements.

The baby that is nursed by its mother gets the best food a baby can get. If it is not nursed by the mother, it will have to have a diet arranged so as to include the necessary substances. The basis of all baby diets is milk, but milk is deficient in certain necessary substances, and these the doctor can provide through modifications of the diet. He will tell the mother when the baby is to have orange and tomato juice and cod-liver oil and the amount of each it should have. The vegetables are the first foods to be added to the baby's diet, and they should be started slowly in very small quantities. By the time the child is one year of age it can eat most vegetables; it can also be having fresh milk, fruit, and Zwieback or toast.

Many physicians and dentists believe that coarse foods strengthen the jaws and help in hardening the gums. When a new tooth is about to come in, the coarse foods serve as a resistance against which the gums may work in order to permit the tooth to cut its way through. If the child is excessively irritable when the teeth are coming in, it is wise to have the advice of the dentist or family physician.

The first teeth come in at the front of the mouth between the fifth and eighth months, as a rule. If they happen to be a little early or late, there is no cause for worry. The next teeth come in between the eighth and tenth months, and the others about the time of the first birthday. Until the first teeth appear, the mouth of the child does well if let alone. After the first teeth appear, the gums and teeth may be wiped daily with a soft clean cloth dipped in water to which a little salt has been added. It is well to be exceedingly gentle.

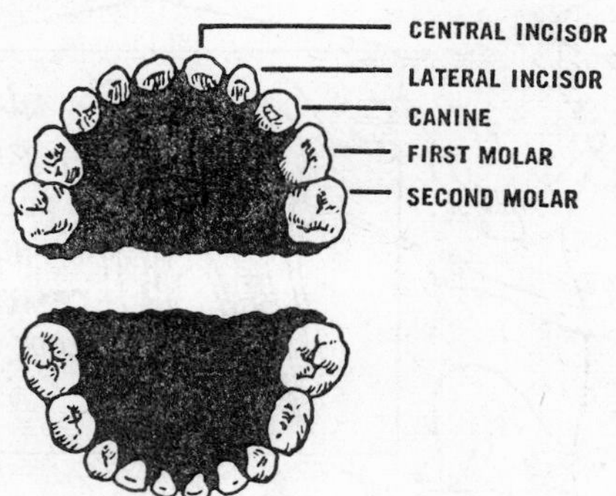

Fig. 77. Eruption of primary teeth. The first teeth are called primary, baby, or milk teeth. There are 20 of them and their presence in the mouth is essential until the permanent teeth are ready to take their place. At about 6 months of age, the first baby teeth will appear. These will be followed at more or less regular intervals by the upper front teeth, the back teeth, and the cuspids. With the cutting of the 2-year molars or back teeth, usually by the age of 30 months, a child has all 20 of his primary teeth. *Healthy Teeth,* Division of Dental Health, U. S. Public Health Service.

About the eighteenth month a soft toothbrush may be substituted for the soft cloth, and as soon as the child is old enough it should learn to brush its teeth for itself. If the child likes the taste of toothpaste, it may have toothpaste. Most physicians and dentists are convinced that a toothpaste is of service and the recommendation of fluoride in drinking water and in toothpaste for preventing dental caries is almost unanimous.

The chief reason for preserving the baby teeth is to keep the mouth in the right shape for the second teeth. All of the twenty teeth that are called primary teeth are usually in the mouth by the time the child is three. Behind the first set is the second set. In order to have the second set properly developed, the food must be right and the mouth free from infection. The only established way to control infection is to have dental attention.

The most important permanent tooth comes in between the fifth and sixth year of life and is known as the six-year molar. It comes in six teeth back from the one in the front of the mouth in center.

There are four six-year molars, one on each side of the upper and lower jaws. They should have the most careful attention. Once gone, they are not replaced except with artificial teeth. If they decay and are removed without proper dental attention, the entire expression of the face and of the mouth may change. In the absence of the proper molars, food is not sufficiently ground before entering the stomach.

Every child should see a dentist following the appearance of the six-year molars. The child should see the dentist at age 2½ to 3 and regularly

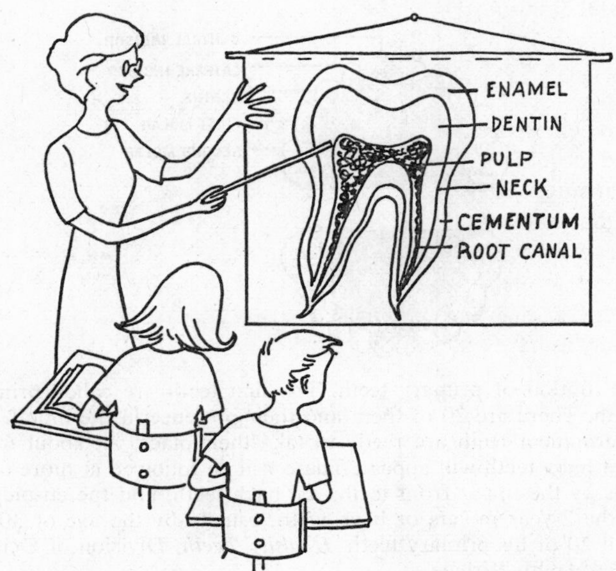

Fig. 78. Tooth structure. Only about a third of the tooth—the crown—projects beyond the gums. The crown is covered with a layer of enamel, the hardest of all body tissues. Underneath this are layers of a softer substance called dentin. The roots, which extend into jawbone, are covered with cementum, a material harder than dentin but softer than enamel. Inside the dentin is the pulp chamber, which contains tiny blood vessels and nerves that extend through a canal to the end of each root, where they join larger blood vessels and nerves. *Healthy Teeth,* Division of Dental Health, U. S. Public Health Service.

—as often as the dentist suggests—from that time. Only a generation has passed since dentists first began to give special attention to the teeth of the child. Many dentists specialize exclusively in children's teeth. They are concerned with seeing that all of the teeth are straight, that they fit properly against the opposites in the other jaw, that they do not grind off surfaces that are meant to stand, and that they remain firmly and are not pushed into the wrong positions.

With the help of the X ray, the dentist is able to see that the teeth are sound at their roots. By personal inspection he finds tiny spots which indicate the beginning of decay. These can be filled and polished and their decay stopped. The additional cost of the X-ray pictures means future saving. Preventive dentistry done early is rewarding. Curative dentistry, done after decay has proceeded far, after the teeth have gotten into wrong positions, after some teeth have been lost, may be expensive and can be prevented.

Many communities are now adding fluorides to the community water supply as a means of preventing dental caries. There seems to be no doubt that this helps prevention though other causes persist and cases appear even when all children get fluorides.

ORTHODONTIA

Within recent years a new specialty has arisen in dentistry and in medicine called orthodontics. The word means "straight teeth." It means literally to arrange crooked teeth in a more harmonious and symmetrical curve so that they will function better and improve the facial appearance. It is, of course, necessary to realize that back of all health are proper nutrition and growth. Unless the child has a diet which contains a sufficient amount of calcium, phosphorus, vitamins A, C, and D particularly, it is not likely to have good teeth.

Unless the baby teeth have been suitably controlled and well taken care of, the teeth that come in thereafter are less likely to be properly developed and distributed. Dentists are convinced that there are a considerable number of bad habits that are associated with development of malocclusion, which means improper closing of the teeth and jaws. Breathing through the mouth, sucking the thumb, and similar bad habits may be associated with bad formation of the teeth, the bones of the jaw and the muscles which control them.

The twenty baby teeth of infancy begin to disappear around the age of six, at which time also the four big six-year molars appear. Unless there is a full number of healthy teeth in the mouth at each age, they may not be properly arranged nor will they close properly. Each tooth depends on the one next to it for support. If any groups of teeth are pushed out of position, the whole set becomes irregular.

The orthodontist is a specialist in producing regularity of the teeth. Through gradual changes exercised at certain points the teeth are brought into proper position. This is done by the use of wire and other appliances, and must be done slowly and carefully so as not to destroy the teeth in the process. It is a specialty within dentistry. It is no longer necessary for any girl to appear in public after she has grown to mature age with teeth crossing over one another or with the protruding snaggle teeth that gave so many women a comical appearance in the past. Science in this way does much for human happiness.

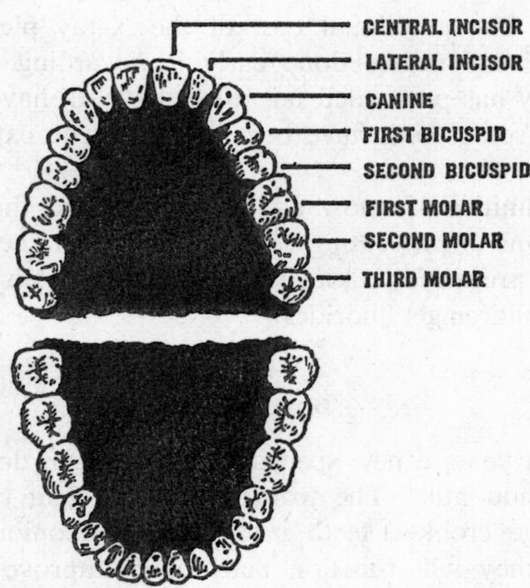

Fig. 79. Eruption of permanent teeth. The first permanent teeth to appear are the four 6-year molars, one on each side of the upper and lower jaws. The permanent teeth erupt into the mouth in approximately this order: the first molars (at the age of 6 or 7); the central incisors (7–8); the lateral incisors (8–9); the bicuspids (10–12); the canines (11–12); the second molars (12–13); the third molars ("wisdom teeth," 17–21). *Healthy Teeth,* Division of Dental Health, U. S. Public Health Service.

THE CARE OF ADULTS' TEETH

The care of the teeth in the adult involves not only a suitable diet, but also a certain amount of simple dental hygiene. The popular slogan that a clean tooth never decays is probably correct if associated with the right definition of a "clean tooth." Actually millions of unclean teeth never decay. Unclean teeth are not desirable, because they permit the growth of bacteria that are usually associated with foul breath, they are unesthetic in appearance, and they are associated with irritations of the gums, cheeks, and tongue that may be serious.

About 1890 it was shown that certain acids formed by the action of mouth bacteria on a substance containing sugar when held in contact with enamel of the teeth would cause the enamel to break and open the way to destruction of the softer dentin substance beneath. Since the acid must exist in concentrated form in order to do such work, the process usually goes on only in the tiny pits, fissures, or other defects in the enamel, or in the spaces between the teeth. The exposed surfaces of the teeth seldom decay because the natural movements of the lips, cheeks and tongue help to keep them clean.

Associated with the cause of tooth decay are errors in the diet. Once decay begins, once the enamel of the tooth is broken down, bacteria, constantly present in the mouth, aid the destruction. Chemical changes occur that are disastrous. The most that anyone can do is to keep teeth clean by the best methods possible, and to see that the diet is of the proper nature to keep the teeth in a state of satisfactory nutrition.

TOOTH DECAY

The University of Chicago summoned four experts who have been devoting themselves to research on teeth to discuss the problem of constant decay of the teeth which is a disease of our modern civilization. Apparently people who live in remote areas of the globe under native or natural conditions are more free from tooth decay and have fewer cavities than do civilized men. When these people come into contact with the civilization of the white man and adopt his manner of living and his diets, their teeth begin to decay immediately and apparently tooth decay progresses rapidly.

The United States now has a national institute of dental research which is under the direction of the United States Public Health Service. The director of this institute of dental research says that the acids of the mouth have a great deal to do with the amount of decay. However, modern medicine and dentistry have apparently failed to find any specific method of changing the reaction of the material around the surfaces of the teeth or of making the surfaces of the teeth more resistant to the actions of the acids. Several methods have been suggested, including various techniques for getting rid of the bacteria in the mouth, but apparently none of these is yet well established.

TOOTHBRUSH

In cleansing the mouth a good toothbrush is necessary. Many of the toothbrushes sold are too large for efficient brushing. All sorts of shapes are available with many strange distributions of bristles, but so far as is known it is impossible to make a toothbrush that will conform exactly to the shape of the dental arch inside and outside. Some toothbrushes are made with bristles higher in the center and low at the ends, some with the bristles high at one end and low at the other end, some with bristles lower in the middle and high at both ends.

This seems to make little difference, the only necessity being that the brush be small and that the handle be such that it can be manipulated so that the bristles will reach the front, back, and sides of every tooth. The toothbrush demands proper care to give it long life and to prevent its acting as a carrier of infections rather than as a preventive.

When a toothbrush is split, when bristles begin to break off and come out, the toothbrush should be thrown away. Cold water should be used to moisten the brush before using and to rinse it thoroughly after the teeth are brushed. The brush should then be hung in the open air in such position that the bristles will not come in contact with anything else for twenty-four hours before the brush is used again.

Obviously, therefore, persons should have two brushes, one for morning and one for evening use. If a toothbrush is kept moist for too long a period of time or kept in an airtight container, the bristles are quickly destroyed. Most important, however, is the fact that bacteria grow on warm, moist toothbrushes, and that the use of the brush before it has dried thoroughly will merely add new bacteria to those taken from the mouth in the previous washing.

TOOTHPASTES, MOUTH WASHES, AND TOOTH POWDERS

One of the most debatable questions in medicine and dentistry concerns the exact value of toothpastes, mouth washes, tooth powders, and similar mixtures for the health of the mouth and the teeth. Many physicians and dentists are convinced that the most any toothpaste can do is to help keep the teeth clean and polished, and that therefore any good soapy preparation that tastes good serves the purpose. However, the preparations that are available are complex in their formulas and extraordinary in their claims.

Often a preparation is sold with the argument that it duplicates normal saliva and that the presence of normal saliva prevents tooth decay. It has been shown that sugar helps to cause decay of the teeth and that food particles between the teeth increase dental caries. The disadvantage associated with food particles and sugar is that these provide mediums on which bacteria grow and that bacterial products are injurious to the teeth.

Some toothpastes are sold with the special claim that they kill the germs in the mouth on contact, but most physicians realize that the first mouthful of food or the first breath of air will bring new germs into the mouth. Some toothpastes have contained abrasive substances which scratch the enamel, and this is bad, since anything that makes a scratch or an abrasion may produce a spot in which germs may enter more easily.

Another toothpaste was sold with the claim that it contained a substance which digests away food particles and mucus, and another was sold with the claim that it contained enough of certain antiseptic to sterilize the gums and keep them sterile. The important thing for the average person to remember is the fact that most of these preparations are kept in the mouth not longer than a few seconds and that any effects which they may accomplish are quite temporary.

Some additions to toothpastes are ammonia preparations for preventing decay and chlorophyll for preventing odors. The evidence in support of these additions is not generally convincing to most scientists.

PYORRHEA

Pyorrhea means a flow of matter. However, the flow of matter or, to speak of it scientifically—pus—is not the most significant thing about this disturbance of the mouth and teeth. The important fact is that the condition becomes chronic and that as a result of this the tissue of the gums separates from the roots of the teeth. When they have once separated they are not likely to become attached again without proper treatment. Moreover, a constant presence of infectious matter leads to secondary disturbances in the body which may be exceedingly serious.

The blood picks up the germs from the pus pockets around the teeth and carries them to other parts of the body, where they may set up new infections. Because the teeth are loose and the mouth is foul, the person with pyorrhea is likely to lose his appetite. He is unable to chew food satisfactorily, his digestion is interfered with, and he becomes in general much sicker than he would be with a clean mouth cavity.

Because the mouth is easy to get at, because the gums are tough, and because the saliva keeps the mouth constantly lubricated, the tissues stand a great deal of punishment before the condition becomes so severe that it is impossible to delay attention. For this reason, pyorrhea is usually a chronic rather than an acute disease.

For this reason also it is necessary to remind people again and again that the mouth should be looked at by a competent dentist at least once in every six months in order that such conditions may be detected early and given adequate care before they become so serious that the only hope lies in removal of all of the teeth, surgical attention to the gums, and the provision of artificial dentures or plates.

Among the causes of infections of the gums are continuous irritation from the edge of rough crowns or of fillings. A good dentist will see to it that a crown or a filling is absolutely smooth and continuous with the surface of the tooth to which it is applied.

Food particles may accumulate between the teeth and set up spots of local irritation and decay. The regular use of the toothbrush and of dental floss is necessary to prevent such an occurrence. Toothpicks, and especially pins, knives, forks, or other objects used in lieu of toothpicks, do severe damage to the delicate tissues when manipulated by a careless hand.

Tartar deposits are just as irritant as rough fillings. Moreover, they are easily susceptible to the accumulation of bacteria. Pyorrhea is one of the most menacing diseases known to man, and its prevention depends on constant vigilance.

Antibiotic drugs, applied locally to infected mouths and also taken internally, may help to eliminate pyorrhea.

HALITOSIS OR BAD BREATH

Bad breath, now politely referred to as halitosis, is offensive. There is little excuse for anyone to permit himself to become obnoxious for this reason to everyone around him, since it is possible to prevent the presence of such odors. The most frequent cause is related to the teeth, which may be subject to cavities or which may simply be surrounded with accumulations of decaying food products. Cavities should be filled and tartar deposits should be removed at least once every six months. The teeth may be kept clean by the use of dental floss and by the regular use morning and evening of a toothbrush with proper powder or paste.

There are innumerable mouth washes containing antiseptics, alkalis, or acids, that may be used after the teeth have been brushed. Weak hydrogen peroxide solutions are sometimes of value. It is best to use strong solutions only on the advice of a competent physician or dentist.

After the teeth as the cause of bad breath have been eliminated, the tonsils must be examined as to the presence of infection. Another frequent cause of bad breath is infection in the nose or in the space behind the nose. The formation of crusts and of accumulations of infected material is bound to produce foul odor of the breath. Halitosis may also result from chronic disturbances of the stomach and of the intestines. If the tongue is constantly coated, if there is eructation of sour material from the stomach, the person concerned should consult a physician. Claims are now made that chlorophyll preparations control all sorts of body odors. Most recent evidence fails to support the claims for chlorophyll.

FALSE TEETH

The person who is compelled to wear any form of removable appliance in the mouth to replace natural teeth has special problems to which dentists have been giving concern. False teeth, artificial teeth, removable bridges, and plates are included in this category.

The person who is going to lose his natural teeth by extraction because of infections or due to any other cause should have a thorough study by a dentist who will probably employ X-ray pictures before any natural teeth are removed. The dentist who is going to make the artificial denture can then advise intelligently which teeth may be saved and which should be extracted. This is particularly important because he wants to restore the patient's natural appearance, and he wants to retain everything possible to permit the making of the most suitable denture.

To do this, he takes impressions of the mouth, makes a record of the patient's profile and facial contour, studies the natural color of the teeth and similar factors. It is sometimes possible in making an artificial denture to correct deformities or abnormalities of the lower portion of the face. When a person is fitted with an artificial denture his experience is similar to being fitted with a suit or a dress. It may not be exactly right the first time, and some adjustments may be necessary.

When the work is completed the patient should not assume that it is permanent. The human body is a growing and changing organism which differs from year to year. This means that dentures should be studied from time to time if they become uncomfortable so that old ones may be refitted or new ones substituted. If this is not done there actually may be changes in the appearance of the face, deep lines and wrinkles being associated in some instances with the constant wearing of unsuitable dentures.

Artificial dentures must be given cleansing care as with natural teeth. They should be brushed carefully and thoroughly after each meal and on going to bed at night. In this cleaning, cold or lukewarm water should be used—never hot water. It is just as important to be careful about handling dentures as handling expensive eyeglasses. The dentists suggest that when removing the dentures from the mouth the wearer should lean over a washbowl filled two-thirds full of water and hold the plates close to the water when brushing them. Then the water will break the fall if he happens to drop the artificial plate.

It is not advisable to try to crack nuts with artificial teeth. Biting threads, eating hard candy, and chewing on bones are sometimes responsible for ruining expensive dentures.

Just as soon as the teeth are secured, the person will do well to go into a private place and practice reading aloud in order to get used to the feel of the teeth and to their weaknesses. When the false teeth are first inserted, the facial expression may seem to be changed, but this is due to the effort of the muscles to take care of the plates. Just as soon as the false teeth become properly adjusted, the effort will disappear, and the expression will become natural again.

Naturally, the hardest thing to do with the false teeth is to eat. The person who has the teeth thinks that he has to manipulate both the teeth and the food. He will, therefore, do well to begin with food that requires little chewing and to avoid steaks and chops for the first few days. Small bits of food chewed slowly will easily be taken care of. Big masses of food may cause trouble. Until one learns to manipulate the teeth, and until the gums and the ridges have become hardened, one need not expect to eat everything and anything that is offered. If there are spots in the gums and the ridges have become excessively sore, the dentist should be consulted immediately to make the necessary changes and to prescribe the necessary treatment.

Artificial teeth, when out of the mouth, should be kept moist. The best arrangement is to put them in a salt-water solution, boric acid, or some favorite mouth wash.

CHAPTER 32

Advice on the Diet

JOEL F. PANISH, M.D.

INTRODUCTION

The phenomenal increase in American living standards over the past twenty-five years has led to changes in our dietary habits. Nutritional standards have been altered because of the decrease in physical activity which has accompanied increasing automation in industry. This chapter will attempt to set forth basic principles whereby normal nutrition (e.g., optimum intake of calories, protein, fat, carbohydrates, vitamins, minerals, fluids, acids and bases, and bulk) may be achieved.

To understand the problems of modern "normal" nutrition some of the factors responsible for our changing dietary habits must be understood. The increased availability and consumption of meat and dairy products has resulted in fat providing about 45 per cent of our caloric requirements as opposed to 25 per cent twenty years ago. Foods once considered regional or seasonal, or even national, are now available any place, anytime, through improved freezing techniques. Staples, such as bread and milk, are routinely fortified with vitamins so that vitamin deficiency diseases such as pellagra and beriberi are uncommon, and scurvy and rickets present only minor problems. The ready availability of commercial vitamin preparations and the popularity of various fad diets has led to new diseases secondary to overindulgence in vitamins.

The major dietary problem at present is not undernutrition (not enough food), or malnutrition (not enough of the right kind of food), but overnutrition (too many calories). New standards of height and weight have been established (*See* Table 1), and due to our decreased physical activity there has been a decrease in our estimated minimum daily caloric needs (*See* Table 2).

DIETETICS AND DISEASE

Many changes have developed in our concepts concerning dietary treatment in some specific diseases. Deletion of gluten (a protein found mainly in grains) from the diet results in control of nontropical sprue. The rigid milk and cream diet for the patient with peptic ulcer is losing favor to the idea that frequent feedings of any nutritious food together with vigorous antacid treatment is more physiologic. Whereas people with liver disease used to be put on low-fat, high-protein diets, it is now recognized that fat is not harmful and that protein may be injurious to patients with severe liver damage. A low-salt diet was formerly a mainstay in the treatment of high blood pressure; because of improved drugs, this is no longer a major factor in treatment. These are only a few examples to illustrate the rapid changes which are constantly taking place.

NECESSITY FOR FOOD

Food provides fuel for energy and raw material for rebuilding tissues that break down during daily activities. Just as an automobile requires gasoline to operate, we require fuel to provide energy for activity. Even when we sleep, our body expends energy to keep bodily processes functioning. This energy is supplied by food and the "energy value" of food can be equated to the number of calories it supplies. Calories represent the fuel value of anything that is burned up, be it gas, oil, coal, or food. Every food has a caloric value (some may be zero) and this has been tabulated (*See* Tables 3 and 4). Calorie needs vary with age, activity and each person's metabolism. However, minimum caloric intake standards have been established according to height, weight, age and activity (*See* Table 2).

If caloric intake equals energy expenditure, body weight remains constant. As physical activity increases, the caloric need rises proportionately. These established concepts are still probably true, but may be modified by experimental work currently in progress. Recent investigations are questioning whether or not people utilize calories in the same manner and at the same rate. Perhaps our methods of measuring metabolic processes are too crude to differentiate certain important alterations.

Protein and carbohydrates provide 4 calories per gram, while fat provides 9 calories per gram (*See* Table 5 for weights and measures). Thus, fat provides more energy source per weight than the other two main dietary constituents; however, the calories from carbohydrates are more readily available. Protein, although partly utilized as an energy source, is most important in providing the basic units necessary for repair of body tissues.

PROTEINS

Proteins are made of smaller constituents called amino acids. The nature of a specific protein depends on the kinds and amounts of amino acids and the manner in which they are combined. Certain amino acids are important to good health and must be included in the diet; these are called essential amino acids. Animal matter (meat, fowl, fish) contains a greater amount of the essential amino acids. In addition to meat, eggs, dairy products, grains, and vegetables also contain some protein. Table 6 shows the protein values of some commonly used foods. There is fundamentally no difference in the amount and type of protein derived from meat, fowl, fish, or eggs. In other words, it does not matter which of these serve as the main source of protein; they are all interchangeable. This is how we can achieve such variety in our diet and still maintain good nutrition. Cereals contain 7 to 15 per cent protein and are a good secondary source. By proper selection, a completely vegetarian diet, if supplemented by the proper synthetic proteins, may provide all the essential amino acids. However, one should not adhere to a strictly vegetarian diet without competent advice. Recommended daily allowances for protein are: 1 gm/kg for adults; 3.5 gm/kg for infants; 1.6 to 3.3 gm/kg for children, decreasing with age; 80 gm/day during the last trimester of pregnancy, and 100 gm/day during lactation.

CARBOHYDRATES

Carbohydrates are the starch or sugar parts of food. Cereals, milk, fruits and vegetables are the main sources (*See* Table 7). Table sugar is the most concentrated form of carbohydrate commonly used. Starches are sugars in various combinations and are the major ingredients of cereals. Most grains contain approximately the same amount of carbohydrate. There is no minimum daily allowance of carbohydrate. Since its main function is to supply energy, the daily requirement depends on the person's caloric requirement and is calculated after protein and fat rations are decided upon.

FATS

The common sources of fats are meat, oils, dairy products, and eggs (*See* Table 8). The great nutritional controversy of today centers upon fats. A number of people believe that the American diet of today, which obtains 40 to 45 per cent of its caloric value from fats, is too high in its fat content and should be reduced to about 33 per cent. They also believe that too much of the fat is of the saturated variety. Roughly, saturated fats are found in meat and dairy products, whereas unsaturated fats are mainly vegetable fats. The reason for this concern is that some research workers believe that this high intake of saturated fat is related to the development of heart disease, strokes, and blood clots. Although a final decision has not been reached, the AMA Council on Nutrition has recommended that people suffering from arterial disease or obesity, or who have a family history of arterial disease, high blood pressure, or diabetes, should decrease their intake of saturated fat and increase the percentage of unsaturated fat in the diet. Many years may pass before a final answer is reached. Although 80–120 gm fat/day is the recommended intake, diets containing as little as 40 gm/day appear to maintain normal health.

FLUIDS, ELECTROLYTES AND BASES

Electrolytes denote a group of inorganic chemical substances which maintain the acid-base balance of the body. Salt is the commonest example. The daily requirement for fluids and electrolytes is that amount which replaces daily losses. This does not present a problem in normal people and is automatically regulated by the normal physiologic functions of the kidneys, lungs and sweat glands. Imbalance can result from abnormal losses or retention, defective absorption, and abnormal distribution. These conditions result from certain disease states and are dealt with in other chapters in this book. Remember that water comprises 70 per cent of our lean body mass. The average daily loss of fluid amounts to 2000 to 2500 cc. daily; this equals 4.2 to 5.2 pints.

VITAMINS

These are complex organic substances that are necessary for vital bodily functions, deficiencies of which result in specific diseases. The essential vitamins and their minimum daily requirements are listed on page 850. There are other vitamins, but their actual requirements are unknown. The daily requirements necessary for good health are small and will be met by any diet with an adequate content of meat, cereals, fresh fruit and vegetables. Vitamin preparations do not offer advantage over those obtained naturally in the diet and vitamin supplementation is not needed except in specific vitamin-deficiency diseases. However, supplementary vitamins may be used during childhood, pregnancy, following debilitating illnesses, and during severe dietary restrictions. Diseases can also occur as a result of excess vitamin intake.

MINERALS

Minerals are simple inorganic chemicals necessary for certain bodily functions. Most important are calcium, phosphorus, iron, copper and iodine. Others, called trace elements, such as zinc, cobalt, magnesium, manganese and selenium are thought to be important, but actual requirements have not been delineated. A normal diet includes more than enough of all these elements.

BULK

Fruits, vegetables and cereals such as bran, in addition to being good sources of carbohydrate and minor sources of protein also provide bulk. Fruits and vegetables contain fiber which is undigestible and nonabsorbable. As it travels through the intestines, it stimulates intestinal activity which is helpful in formation and maintenance of normal bowel habits. It is not a dietary requirement in the sense of a nutrient, and in fact, is contraindicated in certain diseases. However, at least one daily serving of a bulk-containing food should be included in the diet of a normal person.

THE NORMAL DIET

A single normal diet cannot be constructed for everyone. People's dietary habits differ because of national origin, geographical location, religious beliefs, economic level, availability of foodstuffs, and family influences. The basic dietary needs of any person may be outlined and then selection made from among the edibles that he fancies an adequate diet. The most carefully prescribed diet will not be followed if the food is not carefully and tastefully prepared.

The prime requisite is energy supply. Referring to Table 2, the basic caloric need for a person according to height, weight, age, and physical activity may be ascertained. The next requirement is for adequate protein. Since the adult requirement is 1 gm/kg, 70 gm protein per day is the average requirement. Seventy gm protein supplies 280 calories, so the remainder must be supplied by carbohydrate and fat. An average normal diet should include 100 gm fat, which results in a most palatable diet and supplies 900 calories. The remainder of the caloric need can be met by carbohydrates.

A FOOD PLAN FOR GOOD NUTRITION

Quantities for one week

Kinds of food	For children 1 to 6 years	For children 7 to 12 years	For girls 13 to 19 years	For boys 13 to 19 years	For women		For men, all ages	Total suggested for your family
					All ages	Pregnant and nursing		
Milk, cheese, ice cream (milk equivalent)[2]	6 quarts	6–6½ quarts	7 quarts	7 quarts	3½ quarts	7–10 quarts	3½ quarts	
Meat, poultry, fish[3]	1½–2 pounds	3–4 pounds	4½ pounds	5–5½ pounds	4–4½ pounds	4–5 pounds	5–5½ pounds	
Eggs	6 eggs	7 eggs	7 eggs	7 eggs	6 eggs	7 eggs	7 eggs	
Dry beans and peas, nuts	1 ounce	2–4 ounces	2 ounces	4–6 ounces	2 ounces	2 ounces	2–4 ounces	
Grain products (flour equivalent)[2] Whole-grain, enriched, or restored	1–1½ pounds	2–3 pounds	2½–3 pounds[4]	4–5 pounds	2–2½ pounds	2–3 pounds	3–4 pounds	
Citrus fruits, tomatoes	1½–2 pounds	2½ pounds	2½ pounds	3 pounds	2½ pounds	3½–5 pounds	2½–3 pounds	
Dark-green and deep-yellow vegetables[5]	¼ pound	½–¾ pound	¾ pound	¾ pound	¾ pound	1½ pounds	¾ pound	
Potatoes	½–1 pound	1½–2½ pounds	2 pounds	3–4 pounds	1–1½ pounds	1½–3 pounds	2–3 pounds	
Other vegetables and fruits	3½ pounds	5½ pounds	6 pounds	7 pounds	4–6 pounds	6–6½ pounds	5–7 pounds	
Fats, oils	¼–⅓ pound	½–¾ pound	¾ pound	1–1¼ pounds	½ pound	½–¾ pound	¾–1 pound	
Sugars, sweets	¼–⅔ pound	¾ pound	¾ pound	1–1¼ pounds	½–1 pound	¾ pound	1–1½ pounds	

[1] When a range is given, unless otherwise noted the smaller quantity is for younger children, for adults over 55, or for pregnant women.
[2] For explanation of milk-equivalent and flour-equivalent foods see pp. 16 and 17.
[3] To meet the iron allowance needed by children 1 to 6 years, girls 13 to 19, and pregnant and nursing women, include weekly 1 large or 2 small servings of liver or other organ meats.
[4] The larger quantity is for the younger girls.
[5] If choices within the group are such that the amounts specified are not sufficient for the number of servings suggested on p. 18, increase the amounts and use less from the "other vegetables and fruits" group.

Fig. 80. A food plan for good nutrition (quantities for one week). From *Nutrition—Up To Date, Up To You,* U. S. Department of Agriculture, Agricultural Research Service.

Example: A moderately active 25-year-old man weighing 154 lbs. should have a daily caloric intake of 2900 calories (*See* Table 2).

$$\begin{aligned} \text{Protein} \ldots\ldots\; 70\ \text{gm} \times 4 &= 280\ \text{cal.} \\ \text{Fat} \ldots\ldots\ldots\; 100\ \text{gm} \times 4 &= \underline{900\ \text{cal.}} \\ \text{Total} &= 1180\ \text{cal.} \end{aligned}$$

2900 cal. − 1180 cal. = 1720 cal., which remain to be obtained from carbohydrate. Since there are 4 cal/gm carbohydrate, $\frac{1720}{4} = 430$ gm carbohydrate that must be included to meet caloric requirements.

Now we must select the types and amounts of foods that will fulfill the above requirements.

Utilizing the various tables in this chapter, that is, by becoming familiar with the relative values for protein, carbohydrate and fat in different types of foods and knowing the amounts present in average served portions, each person's theoretical diet can be easily constructed.

However, everyone's taste in foods differs; we also tire of eating the same meals day after day. Here the concept of food exchanges is useful. This is a system whereby one food can be exchanged or substituted for another because it has the same caloric, protein, carbohydrate, and fat value per serving. Table 9 is a list of food exchanges. In other words, if one did not wish meat for dinner, 1 ounce of fish, or ¼ cup tuna, or 1 ounce cheese or ¼ cup cottage cheese could be substituted for every ounce of meat that was to have been used. Similarly, if bread was not desired, ½ cup cooked cereal or 1 white baked potato could be substituted instead of one slice of bread. In this way, nutritional values remain the same and a wide range of individual tastes can be satisfied.

If the diet is selected according to the precepts outlined, requirements for vitamins, minerals, electrolytes, and fluids will automatically be fulfilled and the person need not worry about artificial supplementation.

OTHER DIETS–FADS AND FANCIES

Reducing diets are the most common dietary problem for which people seek help today. They have been offered pills, injections, liquid diets, high-fat diets, low-fat diets, and starvation diets. One fact still remains: To achieve a normal weight, the person must reduce his caloric intake below that which is calculated to maintain his ideal weight. The rate at which he reduces will depend upon how much less than his normal requirement he ingests. As weight is lost, the rate of loss will decrease if caloric intake is maintained at a constant level. All other manipulations are secondary.

RECOMMENDED DAILY DIETARY ALLOWANCES [1] [2]

Designed for the maintenance of good nutrition of practically all healthy persons in the U.S.A.

[Allowances are intended for persons normally active in a temperate climate]

Persons	Age in years [5] From	Age in years up to	Weight in pounds	Height in inches	Food energy [3]	Protein	Calcium	Iron	Vitamin A	Thiamine	Riboflavin	Niacin equivalent [4]	Ascorbic acid	Vitamin D
					Calories	*Grams*	*Grams*	*Milligrams*	*International units*	*Milligrams*	*Milligrams*	*Milligrams*	*Milligrams*	*International units*
Men	18	35	154	69	2,900	70	0.8	10	5,000	1.2	1.7	19	70	
	35	55	154	69	2,600	70	.8	10	5,000	1.0	1.6	17	70	
	55	75	154	69	2,200	70	.8	10	5,000	.9	1.3	15	70	
Women	18	35	128	64	2,100	58	.8	15	5,000	.8	1.3	14	70	
	35	55	128	64	1,900	58	.8	15	5,000	.8	1.2	13	70	
	55	75	128	64	1,600	58	.8	10	5,000	.8	1.2	13	70	
Pregnant (second and third trimester)					+200	+20	+.5	+5	+1,000	+.2	+.3	+3	+30	400
Lactating					+1,000	+40	+.5	+5	+3,000	+.4	+.6	+7	+30	400
Infants [6]	0	1	18		lb. x 52±7	lb. x 1.1±0.2	.7	lb. x 0.45	1,500	.4	.6	6	30	400
Children	1	3	29	34	1,300	32	.8	8	2,000	.5	.8	9	40	400
	3	6	40	42	1,600	40	.8	10	2,500	.6	1.0	11	50	400
	6	9	53	49	2,100	52	.8	12	3,500	.8	1.3	14	60	400
Boys	9	12	72	55	2,400	60	1.1	15	4,500	1.0	1.4	16	70	400
	12	15	98	61	3,000	75	1.4	15	5,000	1.2	1.8	20	80	400
	15	18	134	68	3,400	85	1.4	15	5,000	1.4	2.0	22	80	400
Girls	9	12	72	55	2,200	55	1.1	15	4,500	.9	1.3	15	80	400
	12	15	103	62	2,500	62	1.3	15	5,000	1.0	1.5	17	80	400
	15	18	117	64	2,300	58	1.3	15	5,000	.9	1.3	15	70	400

[1] Source: Adapted from Recommended Dietary Allowances, Publication 1146, 59 pp., revised 1964. Published by National Academy of Sciences—National Research Council, Washington, D.C., 20418. Price $1.00. Also available in libraries.

[2] The allowance levels are intended to cover individual variations among most normal persons as they live in the United States under usual environmental stresses.

[3] Tables 1 and 2 and figures 1 and 2 in Publication 1146 (see footnote 1) show calorie adjustments for weight and age.

[4] Niacin equivalents include dietary sources of the preformed vitamin and the precursor, tryptophan. 60 milligrams tryptophan represents 1 milligram niacin.

[5] Entries on lines for age range 18 to 35 years represent the 25-year age. All other entries represent allowances for the midpoint of the specified age periods, i.e., line for children 1 to 3 is for age 2 years (24 months); 3 to 6 is for age 4½ years (54 months), etc.

[6] The calorie and protein allowances per pound for infants are considered to decrease progressively from birth. Allowances for calcium, thiamine, riboflavin, and niacin increase proportionately with calories to the maximum values shown.

NOTE.—The Recommended Daily Dietary Allowances should not be confused with Minimum Daily Requirements. The Recommended Dietary Allowances are amounts of nutrients recommended by the Food and Nutrition Board of National Research Council, and are considered adequate for maintenance of good nutrition in healthy persons in the United States. The allowances are revised from time to time in accordance with newer knowledge of nutritional needs.

The Minimum Daily Requirements are the amounts of various nutrients that have been established by the Food and Drug Administration as standards for labeling purposes of foods and pharmaceutical preparations for special dietary uses. These are the amounts regarded as necessary in the diet for the prevention of deficiency diseases and generally are less than the Recommended Dietary Allowances. The Minimum Daily Requirements are set forth in the Federal Register, vol. 6, No. 227 (Nov. 22, 1941), beginning on p. 5921, and amended as stated in the Federal Register (June 1, 1957), vol. 22, No. 106, p. 3841.

Fig. 81. Recommended daily dietary allowances designed for the maintenance of good nutrition of practically all healthy persons in the U.S.A. From *Nutrition —Up To Date, Up To You,* U. S. Department of Agriculture, Agricultural Research Service.

Certain medications can help curb appetite, but do not promote weight loss if the patient continues his usual eating habits. Various medications may help rid the body of fluid but this is actually not tissue weight loss. Humans can subsist on nothing but noncaloric liquids plus vitamins for as long as six months under hospital supervision, without any damaging side effects. These dietary programs are still experimental and used only in cases of extreme obesity. Although examples of reducing diets are listed at the conclusion of this chapter, competent medical advice should be sought by anyone desiring to reduce.

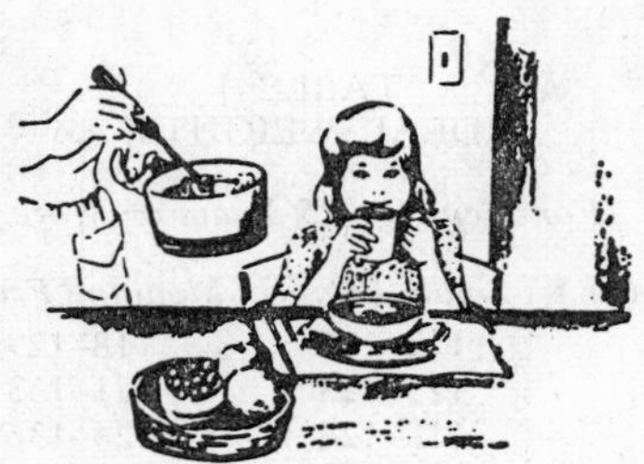

Fig. 82. In children—obesity is a health risk. Faulty eating habits started in early childhood often are the cause of overweight adults in later life, says *Today's Health,* the magazine of the American Medical Association. That plump, healthy, happy youngster may grow up to be a fat, unhappy, unhealthy, older child, and later into a fat adult who is prey to all of the physical ailments that are a part of obesity. The parent is not the one to decide whether the child should lose weight and how he should lose it. The doctor should be consulted. *Health and Safety Tips,* American Medical Association.

Low-cholesterol, low-fat, unsaturated-fat diets: This is the second major nutritional concern in America today because of its possible relationship to vascular disease. Cholesterol is only one type of fat, and because it was found to be elevated in many people with heart disease, is believed by many to be a causal factor. Many other people feel that it may just be a reflection of disordered fat metabolism just as blood sugar is a reflection of disordered carbohydrate metabolism in diabetes. A low-cholesterol diet is not the preferred diet in vascular disease. Probably more important is limiting total caloric intake, reducing the total amount of fat, and having a balanced saturated/unsaturated fat intake. Examples of a low-fat diet and sources of unsaturated fats are listed in tables at the conclusion of this chapter.

Examples of bland and soft diets are listed because they are useful during the common gastrointestinal disturbances encountered by everyone. Also listed are essentials of a normal diet and examples of reducing and high-calorie diets.

CONCLUSION

The science of nutrition is expanding and progressing as rapidly as other fields of medicine. The principles set forth in this chapter will shortly be supplanted, added to, modified, and refined, so that what is written here must not be looked upon as final and absolute. Following these simple rules should, however, enable everyone to achieve and maintain good health insofar as optimum nutrition can serve this purpose.

TABLE 1
IDEAL WEIGHTS*

For Men Age 25 Years or More

Height in Shoes (in.)	*Small Frame*	*Medium Frame*	*Large Frame*
62	112–120	118–129	126–141
63	115–123	121–133	129–144
64	118–126	124–136	132–148
65	121–129	127–139	135–152
66	124–133	130–142	138–156
67	128–137	134–147	142–161
68	132–141	138–152	147–166
69	136–145	142–156	151–170
70	140–150	146–160	155–174
71	144–154	150–165	159–179
72	148–158	154–170	164–184
73	152–162	158–175	168–189
74	156–167	162–180	173–194
75	160–171	167–185	178–199
76	164–175	172–190	182–204

For Women Age 25 Years or More

Height in Shoes (in.)	*Small Frame*	*Medium Frame*	*Large Frame*
58	92–98	96–107	104–119
59	94–101	98–110	106–122
60	96–104	101–113	109–125
61	99–107	104–116	112–128
62	102–110	107–119	115–131
63	105–113	110–122	118–134
64	108–116	113–126	121–138
65	111–119	116–130	125–142
66	114–123	120–135	129–146
67	118–127	124–139	133–150
68	122–131	128–143	137–154
69	126–135	132–147	141–158
70	130–140	136–151	145–163
71	134–144	140–155	149–168
72	138–148	144–159	153–173

* Metropolitan Life Insurance Company, Stat. Bull. 4D:1–12 (Nov.-Dec.) 1959.

TABLE 2
AVERAGE CALORIC REQUIREMENTS*

Sex	Age	Wt. (lbs.)	Ht. (in.)	CALORIES-ACTIVITY Sedentary	Moderate	Heavy
Male	25	154	69	2400	2900	3600
	45	154	69	2100	2600	3400
	65	154	69	1700	2200	2900
Female	24	128	64	1800	2100	2600
	45	128	64	1700	1900	2400
	65	123	64	1300	1600	2100

Pregnant (2nd half) + 200
Pregnant (lactating) + 1000

* Modified from Food and Nutrition Board, National Research Council, 1964.

TABLE 3
CALORIC VALUES OF FOODS

Food	Measure	Calories
Pork	4 oz.	402
Beef	4 oz.	369
Lamb	4 oz.	367
Fowl	4 oz.	269
Lean meat	4 oz.	210
Veal	4 oz.	186
Liver	4 oz.	177
Fish	4 oz.	177
Milk (whole)	8 oz.	166
Milk (skim, butter)	8 oz.	87
Lard	½ oz.	126
Butter, margarine	½ oz.	107
Beans, peas	1 oz.	103
Nuts	½ oz.	100
Vegetables (fresh)	3½ oz.	89
Cereals	¾ oz. (½ cup)	78
Bread	1 slice	76
Eggs	1	75
Sugar	1 level tsp.	16

TABLE 4
CALORIC VALUES OF "SNACKS"

Food	Measure	Calories
Beverages		
Carbonated	1 6 oz. bottle	80
Chocolate malt	1 avg.	500
Chocolate milk	1 cup	240
Cocoa	1 cup	190
Beer	1 12 oz. bottle	170
Martini	1 avg.	145
Whisky	1 jigger	105
Wine	1 wine glass	85–160
Desserts		
Cake	1 avg. slice	150–300

TABLE 4
CALORIC VALUES OF "SNACKS" (*cont'd*)

Food	*Measure*	*Calories*
Deserts (cont'd)		
Candy	1 avg. bar	270
Cookies	1 piece	100–150
Crackers	1	15–25
Doughnut	1	120–250
Pie	1 avg. slice	250–350
Ice cream	⅓ cup vanilla	145
Fruits		
Apple	1 avg.	75
Banana	1 avg.	90
Grapes	40	105
Orange	1 avg.	70
Sandwiches		
Hamburger	1 avg.	330
Egg salad	1 avg.	280
Ham	1 avg.	280
Peanut butter	1 avg.	330
Soups		
Beef	1 cup	100
Chicken	1 cup	75
Tomato	1 cup	90
Vegetable	1 cup	80
Miscellaneous		
Cheese	1 oz.	75–150
Potato chips	10 avg.	110
Popcorn, unbuttered	1 cup	55
Waffles	1 avg.	215

TABLE 5
WEIGHTS, MEASURES, EQUIVALENTS

Measure	*Equivalents*
4 oz.	¼ lb.
16 oz.	1 lb.
2 cups	1 pint (16 oz.)
4 cups	1 quart
28.35 gm	1 oz.
1 kilogram (1000 gm)	2.2 lbs.
454 gm	1 lb.
1 liter	33.8 oz. (2.1 pts.)

TABLE 6
PROTEIN CONTENT OF FOODS

Food	*Protein per 100 gm (3½ oz.)*
Pork	14.9
Beef	17.5
Chicken	18.0
Fish	18.8
Eggs	11
Milk	3.5
Cheese	34
Wheat	11.7
Potatoes	1.7
Fruits	0.5
Peas, beans (dry)	22.2

TABLE 7
CARBOHYDRATE VALUES OF FOODS*

VEGETABLES

3 Per Cent	*6 Per Cent*	*15 Per Cent*	*20 Per Cent*	*25 Per Cent*
Asparagus	Beans, string	Artichokes	Beans, lima	Rice
Bean sprouts	Beets	Beans, kidney	Corn	Yams
Broccoli	Brussels sprouts	Hominy	Potato, white	
Cabbage	Carrots	Parsnips		
Cauliflower	Eggplant	Peas		
Celery	Onions			
Cucumber	Peppers, red			
Pickle	Pumpkin			
Lettuce	Turnips			
Mushroom				
Peppers, green				
Radishes				
Spinach				
Squash				
Tomatoes				

FRESH OR FROZEN FRUIT

5 Per Cent	*10 Per Cent*	*15 Per Cent*	*20 Per Cent*
Cantaloupe	Apricots	Apples	Bananas
Rhubarb	Blackberries	Blueberries	Figs
Strawberries	Cranberries	Cherries	
Watermelon	Grapefruit	Grapes	
	Honeydew melon	Pears	
	Lemons	Pineapple	
	Limes		
	Oranges		
	Peaches		
	Plums		
	Raspberries		
	Tangerines		

* Per Cent refers to per cent by weight; e.g., if an apple weighs 100 gm, it contains 15 per cent or 15 gm carbohydrate $\times$ 4 = 60 calories.

TABLE 8
FAT CONTENT OF FOODS

Food	*Measure*	*Fat (Gm)*
Milk, whole	8 oz.	9.5
Milk, skim, butter	8 oz.	0.2
Eggs	1 boiled	5.5
Bread	1 slice	Under 1
Cereal	1 cup	Under 1
Butter	1 pat	5.7
Cheese	1 oz.	About 10
Cheese, cottage	1 cup	1.1
Lard, oil, margarine	1 tbsp.	10–15
Fish, broiled	1 avg. serving	5–20
Fruits	1 avg. serving	Under 1

TABLE 8
FAT CONTENT OF FOODS (*cont'd*)

Food	*Measure*	*Fat* (Gm)
Meats		
Hamburger	1 med. patty	20.4
Steak	1 large	32.4
Hot dog	1	10
Ham	1 slice	10
Lamb Chop	1 med.	15
Liver	1 slice	3.6
Pork Chop	1 med.	18.2
Veal Chop	1 med.	9.4
Chicken, roasted, broiled	1 avg. serving	10–20
Vegetables	1 avg. serving	Under 1

ESSENTIALS OF A NORMAL DIET

1. MILK GROUP:

Children	3–4 cups
Teen-agers	4 + cups
Adults	2 + cups
Pregnant Women	4 + cups
Nursing Mothers	6 + cups

Cheese and ice cream can replace part of the milk.

2. MEAT GROUP: 2 or more servings
   Beef, veal, pork, lamb, poultry, fish, eggs; dry beans, peas and nuts as alternates.

3. VEGETABLE-FRUIT GROUP: 4 or more servings
   Including a dark green or deep yellow vegetable for Vitamin A, at least every other day. Citrus fruit daily for Vitamin C.

4. BREAD-CEREALS GROUP: 4 or more servings
   Whole grain, enriched, restored.

The above represent essential minimums; to achieve an optimum, greater amounts have to be used plus the use of butter, margarine, other fats, oils, sugars and unenriched, refined grain products.

TABLE 9
DIETARY EXCHANGES

List 1: Milk Exchanges

Carb. – 12 gm, prot. – 8 gm,
Fat – 10 gm, calories – 170

*Milk, whole	1 cup
Milk, evap.	½ cup
*Milk, powd.	¼ cup
*Buttermilk	1 cup

*Add 2 fat exchanges if fat-free.

List 2: Vegetable Exchanges

A. May be used as desired in ordinary amounts. Carbohydrates and calories negligible.

Asparagus	Cabbage
Broccoli	Cauliflower
Brussels sprouts	Celery

TABLE 9
DIETARY EXCHANGES (*cont'd*)

List 2: Vegetable Exchanges (cont'd)

Chard	Mustard
Chicory	Okra
Collard	Pepper
Cucumbers	Radishes
Dandelion	Rhubarb
Escarole	Sauerkraut
Eggplant	Spinach
Kale	String beans
Lettuce	Summer squash
Mushrooms	Tomatoes

B. 1 serving = ½ cup = 100 gm
carb. – 7 gm, prot. – 2 gm,
calories – 36

Beets	Pumpkin
Carrots	Rutabaga
Onions	Squash, winter
Peas, green	Turnips

List 3: Fruit Exchanges

Carb. – 10 gm, calories – 40

Apple	1 sm. (2″ diam.)
Applesauce	½ cup
Apricots, fresh	2 med.
Apricots, dried	4 halves
Bananas	½ small
Blackberries	1 cup
Blueberries	⅔ cup
Cantaloupe	¼ (6″ diam.)
Cherries	10 large
Dates	2
Figs, fresh	2 large
Figs, dried	1 small
Grapefruit	½ small
Grapefruit juice	½ cup
Grapes	12
Grape juice	¼ cup
Honeydew melon	⅛ (7″ diam.)
Mango	½ small
Orange	1 small
Orange juice	½ cup
Papaya	⅓ cup
Peach	1 med.
Pear	1 small
Pineapple	½ cup
Pineapple juice	⅓ cup
Plums	2 med.
Prunes, dried	2 tbsp.
Raisins	1 cup
Raspberries	1 cup
Strawberries	1 cup
Tangerine	1 large
Watermelon	1 cup

List 4: Bread Exchanges

Carb. – 15 gm, prot. – 2 gm,
Calories – 68

Bread	1 slice
Biscuit, roll	1 (2″ diam.)
Muffin	1 (2″ diam.)
Cornbread	1 (1½″ cube)
Flour	2½ tbsp.
Cereal, cooked	½ cup
Cereal, dry	¾ cup
Rice, grits (cooked)	¾ cup
Spaghetti, noodles (cooked)	½ cup
Crackers, graham	2
oyster	20
saltine	5
soda	3
Vegetables:	
Beans, Peas (dried, cooked)	½ cup
Baked Beans	¼ cup
Corn	⅓ cup
Parsnips	⅔ cup
Potatoes, white (baked, boiled)	1 (2″ diam.)
(mashed)	¼ cup
Potatoes, sweet	¼ cup
Sponge cake	1 (1½″ cube)
Ice cream (omit 2 fat exchanges)	½ cup

List 5: Meat Exchanges

Prot. – 7 gm, fat – 5 gm,
Calories – 73

Meat, Poultry (med. fat)	1 oz.
Cold Cuts (4½″ sq., ⅛″ thick)	1 slice
Frankfurter	1
Fish	1 oz.
Salmon, tuna, crab,	¼ cup
oysters, shrimp, clams,	5 small
sardines	3 med.
Cheese	1 oz.
Cottage cheese	¼ cup
Peanut butter (Limit use or adjust carb.)	2 tbsp.

TABLE 9
DIETARY EXCHANGES (*cont'd*)

List 6: Fat Exchanges

Fat – 5 gm, calories – 45

Butter or margarine	1 tsp.
Bacon, crisp	1 slice
Cream, light, 20%	2 tbsp.
Cream, heavy, 40%	1 tbsp.
Cream cheese	1 tbsp.
French dressing	1 tbsp.
Mayonnaise	1 tsp.
Oil or cooking fat	1 tsp.
Nuts	6 small
Olives	5 small
Avocados	1/8 (4" diam.)

Foods to be Used as Desired

Coffee
Tea
Clear broth
Bouillon (without fat)
Gelatin, unsweetened
Pickles, sour
Pickles, dill
Cranberries

Condiments to be Used as Desired

Parsley
Garlic
Celery
Mustard
Pepper
Lemon
Mint
Onion
Nutmeg
Cinnamon
Saccharin
Vinegar

SOFT DIET

Breakfast

Strained orange juice	½ cup
Farina	½ cup
Soft-cooked egg	1
White Toast	1 slice
Butter	1 tsp.
Coffee	1 cup
Half and half	⅓ cup
Sugar	½ tbsp.

Lunch

Ground beef patty	2 oz.
Mashed potato	½ cup
Vanilla ice cream	⅓ cup
Milk	½ pt.
White bread	1 slice
Butter	1 tsp.

Dinner

Cream soup	½ cup
Meat, ground	4 oz.
Potato, boiled	1 med.
Banana	1 med.
Half and half	3 tbsp.
Milk	½ pt.
White bread	1 slice
Butter	1 tsp.
Sugar	1 tbsp.

BLAND DIET

Breakfast

Grapefruit	½ med.
Whole-grain cereal, cooked	½ cup
Boiled egg	1
White toast	1 slice
Butter	1 tsp.
Coffee	1 cup
Half and half	⅓ cup
Sugar	1 tbsp.

Lunch

Roast beef	2 oz.
Gravy	¼ cup
Mashed potato	½ cup
Buttered beets	½ cup
Tomato	½ med.
Vanilla ice cream	⅓ cup
Milk	½ pt.
White bread	1 slice
Butter	1 tsp.

Dinner

Cold sliced ham	2 oz.
Baked potato with butter	1 med.
Buttered green string beans	½ cup
Banana	1 med.
Half and half	3 tbsp.
Sugar	½ tbsp.
Milk	½ pt.
White bread	1 slice
Butter	1 tsp.

LOW FAT DIET
(40 Gm)

Breakfast

Grapefruit	½ med.
Whole grain cereal	½ cup
Soft-cooked egg	1
Whole wheat toast	2 slices
Butter	2 tsp.
Coffee	1 cup
Skim milk	½ cup

LOW FAT DIET (*cont'd*)

Breakfast (cont'd)

Sugar	1 tbsp.
Jelly	1 tsp.

Lunch

Lean roast beef	3 oz.
Boiled potato	1 lge.
Cabbage	½ cup
Tomato	½ med.
Sherbet	⅓ cup
Skim milk	½ pt.
Whole wheat bread	2 slices
Butter	2 tsp.
Jelly	1 tsp.
Pineapple juice	1 cup
Sugar	1 tbsp.

Dinner

Lean chicken	2 oz.
Baked potato	1 lge.
Green string beans	½ cup
Celery, carrot sticks	3–4 each
Sliced banana	1 med.
Skim milk	½ pt.
Whole wheat bread	1 slice
Butter	1 tsp.
Jelly	1 tsp.

DIET HIGH IN POLYUNSATURATED FATTY ACIDS

Dietary Pattern	*Sample Menu*	*Measure*
BREAKFAST		
Fruit	Grapefruit	½ med.
Cereal	Whole grain cereal	½ cup
Bread	Whole wheat toast	1 slice
Unsaturated fat	Corn oil	2 tbsp.
Beverage	Coffee	1 cup
Skim milk	Skim milk	½ cup
Sugar	Sugar	1 tbsp.
Jelly	Jelly	1 tsp.
LUNCH		
Lean meat	Lean roast beef	3 oz.
Vegetable	Cabbage	½ cup
Salad	Tomato	½ med.

DIET HIGH IN POLYUNSATURATED FATTY ACIDS (*cont'd*)

Dietary Pattern	*Sample Menu*	*Measure*
LUNCH (*cont'd*)		
Dessert	Sherbet	⅓ cup
Skim milk	Skim milk	½ pt.
Bread	Whole wheat bread	1 slice
Unsaturated fat	Corn oil	2 tbsp.
Jelly	Jelly	1 tsp.
DINNER		
Lean meat	Lean roast chicken	2 oz.
Vegetable	Green string beans	½ cup
Salad	Celery, carrot sticks	3–4 each
Dessert	Banana	1 med.
Skim milk	Skim milk	½ pt.
Bread	Whole wheat bread	1 slice
Unsaturated fat	Corn oil	2 tbsp.
Jelly	Jelly	1 tsp.

HIGH (3500) CALORIE DIET

Breakfast

Grapefruit	½ med.
Whole grain cereal	½ cup
Boiled egg	1
Bacon	2–3 slices
Whole wheat toast	2 slices
Butter	3 tsp.
Coffee	1 cup
Half and half	⅓ cup
Sugar	1 tbsp.
Jelly	1 tsp.

Lunch

Cream soup	½ cup
Cold ham	3 oz.
Mashed potato	½ cup
Buttered cabbage	½ cup
Tomato	½ med.
Mayonnaise	1 tbsp.
Ice cream	⅓ cup
Half and half	½ pt.
Whole wheat bread	2 slices
Butter	2 tsp.
Jelly	1 tsp.

HIGH (3500) CALORIE DIET (*cont'd*)

Dinner

Cream soup	½ cup
Roast beef	3 oz.
Gravy	¼ cup
Baked potato with butter	1 med.
Buttered green string beans	½ cup
Celery, carrot sticks	3–4 each
Chocolate pudding	½ cup
Half and half	½ pt.
Whole wheat bread	2 slices
Butter	2 tsp.
Jelly	1 tsp.
Between meals—chocolate malted milk	1 cup

LOW CALORIE DIET

FOOD	MEASURE 800 Calories	MEASURE 1000 Calories
Breakfast		
Grapefruit	½ med.	½ med.
Boiled egg	1	1
Whole wheat toast	½ slice	1 slice
Butter	0	1 tsp.
Coffee	1 cup	1 cup
Lunch		
Cold ham	1½ oz.	2½ oz.
Cabbage	⅔ cup	⅔ cup
Tomato	⅔ med.	⅔ med.
Orange	1 med.	1 med.
Skim milk	½ pt.	½ pt.
Whole wheat bread	0	1 slice
Butter	0	1 tsp.
Dinner		
Roast beef	2½ oz.	2½ oz.
Green string beans	⅓ cup	⅓ cup
Celery, carrot sticks	5–6 each	5–6 each
Banana	½ med.	½ med.
Skim milk	½ pt.	½ pt.

LOW CALORIE DIET

FOOD	MEASURE 1200 Calories	MEASURE 1500 Calories
Breakfast		
Grapefruit	½ med.	½ med.
Boiled egg	1	1
Whole wheat toast	1 slice	2 slices
Butter	2 tsp.	2 tsp.
Coffee	1 cup	1 cup
Lunch		
Cold ham	2½ oz.	2½ oz.
Green string beans	⅓ cup	⅓ cup
Cabbage	⅔ cup	⅔ cup
Tomato	⅔ med.	⅔ med.
Orange	1 med.	1 med.
Skim milk	½ pt.	0
Whole milk	0	½ pt.
Whole wheat bread	1 slice	1 slice
Butter	1 tsp.	1 tsp.
Dinner		
Roast beef	2½ oz.	2½ oz.
Mashed potato	0	½ cup
Celery, carrot sticks	5–6 each	5–6 each
Banana	½ med.	½ med.
Skim milk	½ pt.	0
Whole wheat bread	1 slice	1 slice
Butter	1 tsp.	1 tsp.
Whole milk	0	½ pt.

CHAPTER 33

Posture

MORRIS FISHBEIN, M.D.

Good posture will cure some conditions and certainly prevent many others. In infancy its preventive value has the greatest influence on the ensuing life of the baby, though much can be done, by means of persistent exercise, to overcome faults of posture in later life.

The home and school can cooperate effectively in training children to observe the rules of correct posture. In the school, however, most can be done in providing desks and seats of correct height and size, as well as the instruments for gymnastic exercises.

The need for proper seating cannot be too greatly emphasized, because of its direct effect on the spine. Desks should be designed to fit the abnormally large or small, as well as the normal-sized child. The seated pupil should not use a seat so low that his shoulders perforce become rounded, his head droops, and his chest is flattened. The elbows should be able to rest on the desk without stooping or unduly elevating the shoulders, and the edge of the desk should overlap the edge of the seat. Many schools have a certain number of specially adjustable desks and seats for the express use of children who are above or below the average size.

Perfectly fitting seats are not everything. A child cannot sit still long. It is not in his nature to do so. He will become weary unless sufficient opportunity is allowed for exercising and changing the posture during school hours. If he sits too long, the upper part of the body leans forward on or against the desk, constricting the chest, crowding the abdominal organs, and impeding the circulation in the veins. The weight is supported by the arms, and the head, neck, and spine hang by the muscles of the shoulder blades in abnormal curves. To relieve this overstrain of the back and shoulder muscles the pupil slumps back until his weight rests on the shoulder blades and lower end of the spine, leaving the center of the back unsupported. The back sags down in a single long curve, the chest contracts, the breathing is made shallow, and the circulation slows up. This position stretches the muscles and ligaments of the spine, rounds the back and shoulders, and shoves forward the chin.

CORRECT SITTING POSTURE

The correct sitting posture is one in which the pupil sits erect, the pelvis resting equally on the seat, with the arms beside the hips and the head poised so as to bring the center of gravity within a line joining the seat bones. This posture makes a minimum demand on muscular energy, and is most conducive to correct carriage. But the demands of school life do not permit the pupil to keep it long. Reading, writing, and drawing are exercises that require deviations from the ideal. If we add to these requirements ill-fitting desks and long periods of sitting, in which bad posture becomes habitual, the mischievous result cannot long be in doubt. The work of the school day should be arranged with these things in mind. The first year of the child's school life should not have more than one third of the time in confinement at the desk.

KINDERGARTEN TRAINING

Short periods of sitting, followed by double that time spent in muscular activity out of the seat, should be the rule. This activity may in most cases consist of movements correlated with intellectual exercise. In the kindergarten exercise is admirably combined with mental culture by the teaching of imitative games in which the large muscle groups are exercised in hopping, jumping, and running, and in imitating with the arms the flight of birds and insects. The circulation is stimulated and postural faults are prevented, while at the same time the child is taught valuable lessons in natural history in which his interest never flags.

TRAINING IN HIGHER GRADES

The school day of children in the higher grades should have two five-minute periods of corrective exercise at least, in addition to the games of the recess, previously described. These exercises should be designed to promote quick, strong, muscular control; to expand and enlarge the chest by deep breathing; to bring the blood from the abdomen out into the extremities; to correct spinal fatigue, and to teach the proper carriage of the body.

It is not possible for a child to remain long at rest with the weight equally on both feet, because the tension on both legs being the same, the muscles rapidly tire. The pupil instinctively rests his weight on the right, placing his left leg with bent knee out to the side as a prop. This resting position lowers the right shoulder, curves the spine, and may start the first stage of a permanent scoliosis. The best resting pose to teach is that recommended by Dr. Eliza Mosher, in which the inactive foot is placed in front instead of at the side. In this the feet can be changed as the weight-bearing leg tires.

BAD POSTURE

What are the best rules and exercises for correct posture?

There is a test now widely used by which even the untrained teacher may form an accurate estimate of a child's posture. The first part of the test is designed to find the pupil's ability to take the erect attitude. The long axis of the trunk should continue the long axis of the head and neck. To assist the eye of the observer, a vertical line may be dropped from the front of the ear to the forward part of the foot. In poor posture the axes of the head, neck, and trunk will form a zigzag instead of a straight line.

Another simple way to estimate the extent of the deformity is to stand the child beside an upright pole or rod. The variations from correct posture are three: the so-called fatigue, or gorilla type, in which the head is thrust forward, the chest sunken, and the abdomen protruded; the round-back posture, in which the hollow at the small of the back is obliterated, a posture cultivated by faults of seating already described; and the bantam, or pouter-pigeon type, in which the chest is pushed forward and upward, and the lower spine over-extended, forming a marked exaggeration of the natural lumbar curve. This posture is always the result of faulty teaching and is an exaggeration of the correct standing posture caused by the mistaken efforts on the part of the teacher to overcorrect the first two faults.

ENDURANCE TEST

A child who can assume a good posture may not be able to sustain it. Some kind of endurance test is therefore an aid whereby faults of posture may be discovered and eliminated by having the children march. As the march proceeds, old muscle habits reassert themselves, and many pupils who could hold the correct posture for a few minutes fall back into habitual faults. Heads will drop forward, shoulders droop, and chests sink, as they march. As these faults appear, the child is taken out of the marching line. Those who pass the standing and marching tests are then put through the third test, designed to show the action and endurance of the muscles of the spine and shoulders that are usually the first to yield to fatigue. When the arms are raised upward these postural muscles, if weak, allow the chin to come forward and the chest to sink backward, so that a few minutes spent in raising the arms forward and upward fully extended, lowering them sidewise and downward to the position at the start, will bring this weakness to the surface.

PHYSICAL TRAINING

Physical training is not only a matter of health. It is necessary for the education of the fundamental nerve centers of the body and the building of character. During the whole of childhood these centers are developing, and their growth is not completed until adult life. For this reason not less than one hour in five should be devoted to training the motor area of the brain, in addition to the time allowed for free play. This should take the form of both gymnastics and athletics. Gymnastics, in addition to their corrective or medical character, have a value in discipline and also in the accurate application of exercise for a given purpose; they are less diffuse than athletics, more concentrated, and for this reason they cannot be applied closely or for long to the very young, except in the guise of play. For girls, the exercises most popular are the peasant dances of Ireland, Scotland, Spain, and Sweden, in which good posture is an integral part of the dance, and agility and grace are developed.

POSTURE OF STUDENTS OF COLLEGE AGE

The necessity for good posture at college age is a logical sequence to the valuable habits learned in childhood. The college student's remediable defects must be corrected, and his physical powers trained to the highest point of efficiency. He must be taught that graceful carriage characteristic of the well-bred man. His powers of self-preservation and efficiency must be increased. If he has not learned it already, he must be given the opportunity for physical recreation through a knowledge of sports and games, for athletic activity should be the safety valve of a sedentary life, and should also teach, in addition to those social and moral qualities which can be cultivated so well in no other way, the lesson of gracefully carrying the body. That is why a university course in physical education should begin with a careful examination to find the exact bodily condition of the student and so to give an intelligent foundation on which to base advice and instruction. Nor is the examination of the student complete without a test of his ability to accomplish certain muscular feats that cover the main activities of the body, in exercises of maximum effort and of endurance.

PHYSICAL EDUCATION FOR WOMEN

Physical education for women too often follows slavishly the scheme planned for men, not because it is best for women, but because it is the same. This is a deplorable mistake, because bodily training of the two sexes must differ radically in order to fit each for its own future life and environment. It cannot, with impunity, ignore the psychologic and physiologic differences between the boy and the girl and between man and woman.

In these days of professional freedom for women, with its consequent demand on their efficiency and endurance, there is much reason for women to practice good posture. Many women suffer from the effect of faulty attitude with its direct relation to pain, like backache and headache.

The first twelve years of a girl's life need differ little from that of a boy's in physical activity. She may lead the same outdoor life, climbing, swimming, running, playing ball, and nothing will prepare her so well for the great physical and mental change which takes place with the attainment of puberty. Outdoor games and exercises establish nervous stability and poise and give the best possible foundation on which to build her future womanhood.

GAMES FOR WOMEN

Women cannot stand prolonged physical or mental strain as well as men, but with frequent rests they can in the end accomplish almost as much. Certain games, such as football, boxing, pole vaulting, and heavy gymnastics, are obviously unsuited to them; but in dancing, swimming, calisthenics, archery, skating, and fencing they come much nearer to competing with men on equal terms. While they are less adapted to arduous muscular work, their vital endurance is better; so that the disadvantage they have in other activities is made up for by this greater tenacity to life. With a few exceptions, girls accustomed to athletics and gymnastics can continue exercise without detriment during menstruation, though they should refrain at that time from too exhausting contests or competitions.

Swimming is one of the best exercises for women, calling into action most of the muscles of the body, but sparing those of the back so generally overworked in standing and sitting postures.

Finally, it is quite as important to take occasional hours of absolute rest, in the recumbent position, as it is to exercise, especially when the nervous and muscular system is overwrought.

POSTURAL EFFECT OF CLOTHING

The importance of proper clothing for men, women, and children has a high place in the promotion of good posture that cannot be overemphasized, although in these days of greater freedom and simplicity in dress there is not so much need to belabor the point as there was a few generations ago. Any tendency to return to the constricting, overweighted, and too numerous garments of a few decades past should be greatly deplored.

Proper shoes have a definite effect on posture, in both children and adults. It has been found that the ground plan of the human foot varies so that it may be straight, inflared, or outflared; therefore, no one type of shoe will be suited to all types of feet. Deformities of the feet, either from the construction of the footwear or from the breaking down of the longitudinal and lateral arches of the feet, have a vital influence on posture. The balance of the foot, either flat or on a high heel, also affects the posture, although this is not so serious as was formerly supposed, if the shoe is so made that the weight rests on the heel instead of slipping forward and crowding the toes into the forward part of the shoe.

The advantage of the upright position is somewhat offset by the frequency of deformities due to a yielding of the structures concerned with support. The body may yield at the spine, at the knee joints, or at the arch of the foot, which becomes broken down and flattened, causing the deformity known as flat-foot. A typical case of flat-foot shows a turning out of the line of the heel, a convexity of the inner contour of the foot, and a concavity of its outer margin. A tracing of the foot would show no instep. The great majority of such cases are what might be termed static and are found in nurses, clerks, waiters, barbers, motormen, and all others whose long hours of continued standing keep the muscles and ligaments of the foot constantly on the strain. The pernicious habit of standing with the toes turned out always makes it worse. Flat-foot is also found in the very fat, whose weight is too much for their ligaments. Bernard Roth, in his series of 1,000 cases of twisted spine, found flat-foot in 76 per cent of them. In an examination of 1,000 supposedly normal students I have found it in 217 cases. Lovett has found many cases among hospital nurses, who are peculiarly susceptible to it. The symptoms are varied. A considerable degree of flat-foot may be present without causing much irritation, and again great pain may be caused by a comparatively slight degree of this deformity. In any case, the close association between footwear and posture must always be kept in mind. The Posture League has designed shoes of the straight, inflared, and outflared types, providing for this natural variation in the normal foot, and at the same time correcting or preventing a position which would tend to drop the arches and produce pain or deformity.

CLOTHING AND ROUND SHOULDERS

Another frequent postural deformity caused or aggravated by improper clothing is round or uneven shoulders. Clothing which is supported by suspenders bearing on the points of the shoulders tends to pull them downward and forward. It is a common deformity among school children, and occurs in almost 20 per cent of university students uncomplicated with other postural defects. It is frequently discovered in girls about the age of puberty, when especial attention is apt to be paid to their figure and carriage. Round shoulders are not likely to be outgrown, and patients usually become permanently and structurally set in the faulty posture, with flattened chest walls and distorted figure.

The clothing should be examined, and when found to be supported from the tip of the shoulders the garments should be altered to bring the pressure in toward the root of the neck, instead of out on the shoulders. It has been pointed out that the cut of most ready-made clothing causes pressure on the back of the neck and tip of the shoulders, constantly tending to produce this deformity. Such clothing, especially men's and boys' suit coats, and men's, women's, and children's top coats, should be bought with particular care that the fitting of the shoulders and backs of these garments does not have a tendency to encourage poor posture.

EXERCISES FOR FAULTY POSTURE

The following six exercises are recommended for the correction of the ordinary case of faulty posture:

1. With the patient standing in his habitual faulty position, place the hand about one inch in front of the sternum and tell him to raise the chest and shove it forward to touch the hand without swaying the body. He will at first try to draw the shoulders back, but this fault must be overcome at the very beginning, and the shoulder muscles must be kept relaxed. Gradually increase the distance to which he can bring the chest forward, repeating it again and again until he can take the position without difficulty and without contracting the muscles of the back. While in this position make him breathe deeply five times and then relax. This should be done before a mirror, so that he will recognize the feeling of the correct posture and associate it with the proper attitude as seen in the glass. He should then try to take it without looking at the mirror. This posture should be drilled into him until it becomes habitual and until he can maintain it without discomfort. R. J. Roberts, of Boston, used to tell his young men to press the backs of their necks against

the collar button, considering this as the keynote of the position. In whatever way it is accomplished, the object is to get the proper relation between the thorax and the pelvis.

After repeating Exercise 1 twenty times, take:

2. Arms forward raise, upward stretch, rise on tiptoes, inhale. Sideward lower, slowly press the arms back, and exhale. This exercise, when done correctly, expands the chest, bringing in all the extensors of the back and levators of the shoulders.

3. The patient stands, arms downward and backward, fingers interlocked and palms outward. Extend the neck, roll the shoulders backward and forearms into supination, the palms being first in, then down, and then out. Reverse to starting position and relax. This exercise is valuable for projecting the chest forward, stretching the shortened ligaments, and drawing in the abdomen. Care should be taken to have the chin pressed backward when the arms are brought downward and turned outward. In resistant cases, where this exercise cannot be done with the fingers interlocked, a handkerchief tied in a loop may be substituted and held in the fingers.

4. Patient stands with the arms at the sides. Arms sideward raise, upward stretch, inhale, forward bend, and rise. Arms sideward, lower, exhale. In this exercise the lungs are filled when the chest is in the most favorable position for expansion. The breath is retained when the trunk is flexed, forcing the air into the cells of the lungs under pressure. The bending and rising bring into powerful action the extensors of the back and neck and the retractors of the shoulders.

5. Patient lies prone on a couch with the feet strapped, or upon the floor with the feet caught on the edge of a bureau or other article of furniture. Hands clasped behind the head. Raise the head and extend the spine, pressing the elbows backward. This exercise is a severe one on the back and shoulders. Follow with a deep breathing exercise.

6. Patient lies in similar position as in Exercise 5, arms at the sides. Raise head, bring arms forward and imitate the breast stroke.

In this exercise the spine is kept in static contraction, while the retractors of the shoulders are alternately contracted and relaxed.

ADDITIONAL EXERCISES

Here are some simple exercises which help to strengthen the muscles of the back and abdomen and thus improve posture:

1. Lie on the back, hands back of the neck. Take a deep breath and raise chest high; keep chest up and exhale by pulling abdomen in. *2.* Same position; knees bent, feet pulled up. Pull abdomen in hard and then relax part way. *3.* Sit in a chair, trunk bending forward. Incline trunk forward from the hips, keeping spine straight. This exercise may be done standing. *4.* Standing; abdominal retraction. Stand with the heels four inches away from the wall but with the hips, shoulders, and head touching the wall; flatten the lower part of the back against the wall by pulling in the abdominal muscles. Holding this position, come away from the wall with the weight well forward on the balls of the feet. *5*. Standing; leg raising. Stand with hands on hips, back flat, and chin in; raise leg forward without bending the knee; lower it; repeat with other leg. This exercise teaches how to hold the back flat. *6*. Carrying the head forward; clasp hands behind the head. Force the head back against their pressure, keeping chin in. This strengthens the muscles of the back of the neck. *7*. Spinal curvatures. "Stand tall," holding the back straight. Rise on the toes with the arms extended forward and up, stretching the arms and the body. *8*. Distended abdomen. This condition may be prevented and largely overcome by doing exercises 2 and 4.

CHAPTER 34

The Foot

ROBERT D. MOORE, M.D.

INTRODUCTION

Man, in his evolution from earlier mammalian forms of life, which first enjoyed the privilege of supporting their body and moving themselves about the earth's land surface supported by all four extremities, received a tremendous boost to his ability to adapt functionally and to control his environment with the assumption of an upright posture. The functions of body support and locomotion were delegated to only the two lower extremities. This accomplishment was further accompanied by the evolution of structural and functional capacities in the upper extremity, in particular, the hand, which modern man now takes for granted in his ability to perform fine and intricate movements. Thus he discriminates fine differences of tactile and temperature sensation so vital to his regulation of the environment in which he lives and his protection from adverse effects. By contrast, the foot, though participating beautifully in many functions and activities of the human body, has remained largely a structure providing support and the ability to move from place to place at will. This is apparent when one considers one's inability to pinch or grasp with the foot, the lack of individual coordination of movement of one's toes, and the relative shortness of the digits of the foot when compared with the hand. Nevertheless, survival of man in his environment is as dependent upon his ability to support his body weight comfortably and to move about, as it is on his ability to use his hands in a productive or creative manner.

As a consequence, however, the evolution of man from a quadrupedal or four-footed gait to a bipedal or two-footed posture has in a sense doubled the functional demand on the foot insofar as weight and locomotion are concerned. Unfortunately, the patterns of biological evolution have never been perfect. The assumption of an upright posture has not only been accompanied by static and dynamic malfunctions of the upper extremities and the spine, but of the foot as well. To this has been added the use of protective coverings of the foot which of themselves in many instances add further to the stresses and strains imposed upon the foot by our upright posture. An understanding of the nature of diseases and deformities of the foot, their prevention and proper care of the foot, is therefore essential to our comfort, our welfare, and our self-sufficiency in daily life.

BIRTH DEFECTS AND DEVELOPMENTAL DEFECTS OF INFANCY AND CHILDHOOD

DEFORMITIES INVOLVING ONLY THE FOREPART OF THE FOOT

Splayfoot, or Prominence of the First Toe. Deviation of the first toe, and in some instances the entire forepart of the foot, inward toward the midline, is perhaps the most common deformity of the forefoot seen in infancy. The mother of a first child, who has not had the opportunity to see this condition correct itself following the onset of walking and the use of shoes during the second year of life, may be concerned about this deviation. It is thought to be due to a prolonged intra-uterine position of the baby in the breech position with the feet enfolded during the later stages of intra-uterine development. The deformity may be perpetuated following birth by the child's sleeping in a position with the buttocks elevated and the lower limbs drawn up in a position of flexion with the feet folded inward. As the child learns to sleep on its back, side, or with the lower extremities extended, the deforming forces no longer exist. With ambulation and with proper footwear, the toe returns to its normal position. Should the habit of sleeping with the limbs folded beneath the baby persist for an unusually long time, it may be advisable to have the deformity corrected by the application of plaster casts over a 2 to 4 week period. This may be followed with the use of special flair-out pre-walker shoes in which the toe of the shoe is curved outward. These should be worn both during waking and sleeping hours until the child learns to walk, when normal shoes may be worn. This deformity may occasionally be confused with clubfoot, a more serious deformity involving the entire foot and calf. However, examination by a competent pediatrician or orthopedic surgeon will readily distinguish the two. Persistence of a splayfoot condition after the second year of life, should lead one to suspect that a rare, truly congenital type of a deformity exists. Corrective surgery may be necessary about the time growth is complete in adolescence.

A second common deformity of the forepart of the foot, *overlapping of the fifth toe,* frequently leads to more concern than is justified. Early concern by a mother of a child with such deformity is usually based on a desire for cosmetic perfection. The only disability that may ensue is the development of a callus or corn on the prominent fifth toe if tight-fitting footwear is worn in later life. Since this deformity is usually associated with contracture of the skin and tendons on the upper surface of the toe, as well as with a degree of fixed internal rotation of the toe, plastic surgery involving all three components is usually necessary after the child is older to obtain permanent correction.

A third but far less common forefoot deformity is *webbing of the toes.* In this condition the cleft between the toes is shorter than normal, and occasionally may not exist. This deformity may only involve the skin of the toes, or the underlying bones and joints may be involved as well. Frequently a similar condition of the fingers, where the deformity is much more disabling, may be associated. Since there is little demand upon the toes for fine individual function, as in the fingers, there is little need for correction of the webbing, and normal function of the foot may be anticipated. The webbing is usually inconspicuous and correction by plastic surgery is only justified for cosmetic reasons.

DEFORMITIES INVOLVING THE ENTIRE FOOT AND THE LOWER PART OF THE EXTREMITY

Clubfoot is a not uncommon congenital deformity involving the entire foot and frequently the bones and muscles of the leg. Its cause has been a subject of much controversy. It is thought that a recessive hereditary trait exists which appears about twice as frequently in males as females, although other factors of the intra-uterine environment undoubtedly play a role. The defect consists of marked inversion of the entire foot which is pointed downward with the heel elevated. Usually associated is shortening of the heel cord, the foot may be somewhat shorter than its partner when the deformity is one-sided, and the muscles of the calf on the affected side may be smaller than the opposite normal member. The affliction will be readily recognized by the obstetrician or pediatrician who first examines the baby and early, intensive, and persistent treatment is mandatory from the time of birth on. The deformity may be easily corrected in some cases by manipulation and the application of plaster casts, and further treatment will not be needed following the first few months of life. In these mild instances a relatively normal foot and calf may be expected, and prolonged treatment is unnecessary. However, the changes in the calf and foot may be extensive, the foot may be quite rigid, and prolonged treatment and surveillance by a competent orthopedic surgeon may be necessary during the entire growth period. Some residual difference in the size of the foot and calf when compared with the normal side must be anticipated in this severe form. Much patience and faithful adherence by the parents to recommended treatment is necessary for several years if good function and a relatively normal gait is desired.

A second though less serious deformity involving the entire foot is *reverse clubfoot* or a deformity in which the heel points downward and the forefoot and ankle may be opposed to the forepart and lateral aspect of the lower shin. This affliction, as with a deformity of the first toe (already mentioned), is again thought to be due to persistent holding of the foot in such a position for prolonged periods during intra-uterine life. As with the deformity of the first toe, reverse clubfoot is a self-correcting deformity during the first 6 to 8 weeks of life and vigorous treatment is not needed. There may be some persistent flat-footedness on the involved side for a year or two; however, this usually corrects itself with the use of proper footwear.

Among the more common deformities of the foot which lead to an abnormal gait are those due to dynamic forces affecting the growth of the bones of the leg below the knee which lead to *pigeon toes,* or *toeing in* or on the contrary, a *duck-foot* gait with the toes pointed outward. Contrary to popular belief even among some physicians, these abnormalities of gait are not due to intrinsic deformities of the foot, but are rather due to torsional twists imposed on the bones of the leg—in some instances during intra-uterine life, but frequently the result of positions the child assumes in sleep during infancy or the first year of life, with the buttocks elevated and the leg or foot internally rotated and with the feet crossed. External rotation of the limb with the feet pointed outward may be perpetuated by sleeping on the abdomen with the limbs rotated in the opposite direction. Such torsional stresses imparted on the rapidly growing long bones of the leg in the infant, who may sleep in such postures for ½ to ¾ of the time during the first year of life, lead to remodeling of the shape of the long bones in a manner similar to that seen in a growing tree where the trunk may be bent by such persistent imposed forces. Much misguided effort has been directed toward the correction of such deformities by the insertion of wedges, special heels, and pads in the shoe without avail. Again, these deformities may be associated with a degree of knock-knee or bowleggedness and be suggestive of rickets—even in the child who has had an adequate Vitamin D intake. The bowing deformities and torsional deformities of the leg for the most part correct spontaneously as the child grows and assumes more normal and changeable positions of sleep. Progress of the deformity may be halted or correction may be obtained by the application of a short metal bar to foot plates on pre-walker shoes which hold the foot in the opposite corrective position, thus preventing the assumption of positions in sleep which tend to perpetuate or increase the deformity. After the onset of walking at 10 to 14 months of age, the apparatus may be worn as a night splint if the child persists in such habits. The vast majority of such cases will undergo spontaneous correction without treatment by the age of 6 to 7 years, and the use of corrective shoes alone will not provide relief and may be detrimental.

FOOT DEFORMITIES OF CEREBRAL PALSY

The unfortunate child who is the victim of *cerebral palsy* may develop deformities of the feet incident to the imbalance of various muscle groups responsible for motions of the foot necessary for a well-balanced gait. The most prominent of these deformities is that in which the child is unable to approximate the heel to the floor surface due to a contracture of the powerful calf muscles unopposed or weakly opposed by muscles which normally lift the forepart of the foot in a normal gait. A second common deformity is a severe flat-foot deformity due to abnormal pull of the muscles affecting the outer portion of the foot with corresponding weakness of muscles supporting the inner aspect of the foot. A less common deformity is the opposite in which the muscles supporting the inner portion of the foot are in spasm while those responsible for eversion of the foot are weakened. These deformities generally become most evident at the time the parent normally anticipates the child will commence walking—usually at about the end of the first year of life. In the child with cerebral spastic palsy such motor activities will usually be delayed many months, and deformities of the foot which may lead to permanent contracture of such structures as the heel cord should be attended to early in order that gait training and the attempts of the child at ambulation are not inhibited by such fixed deformities. Since the affliction is due to damage or destruction of motor cells and tracts in the brain which are responsible for the activity of the motor units or muscles involved in walking, corrective measures directed toward the functional units in the extremity will not have any effect on the underlying damaged brain, but may aid the child in making progress within the limits of his own capabilities. The early care of such deformities therefore entails the use of proper bracing to ensure as near normal functional position of the foot as possible without encumbering the child with an excessive amount of apparatus which of itself may inhibit gait development. Such bracing may be discontinued by well-advised release of taut muscles or by stabilization of joints within the foot at an appropriate age. Deformities due to such abnormal muscle tension may recur during the growing period when surgical procedures are performed at an inappropriate time. The advice of a competent bone-and-joint surgeon should be sought in this regard.

FLAT-FOOT

Flat-footedness, or a flattening of the longitudinal arch of the foot which allows the inner border of the foot to approximate or come in contact with the floor, is a common affliction of mankind. Usually hereditary in nature, the condition usually persists from childhood into adult life in spite of all attempts at prevention or treatment.

Flat-footedness in the child. Almost all children reveal a variable degree of flat-footedness during the first 2 to 3 years of life. This may be in part more apparent than real due to an abnormal accumulation of fat in the sole of the foot beneath the long arch which disappears with development of the foot during the second or third year. In others it becomes apparent at the time of ambulation—due to incoordination of muscles arising from the bones of the leg and foot which together with the ligaments of the smaller bones of the foot, provide support, and produce the normal contour of the foot. In such cases by the end of the third year, the normal ambulatory activities of an active child lead to increasing power and balance of the musculature supporting the foot, and the deformity disappears. In other children in whom the affliction is hereditary and persists beyond the early developmental years, all the joints—including the joints of the hand, wrist, elbow, knee, and ankle—reveal an abnormal degree of mobility due to excessive laxity of supporting ligaments. Such persons are frequently known as being "double jointed." This *flexible form of flat-footedness* in childhood seldom if ever produces symptoms and does not require treatment. In fact, foot development in the young child is apt to be more normal if the child is permitted to go barefoot when indoors during the winter months, or even out of doors during the warmer weather. Motions of the foot in running and dancing are thus uninhibited by footwear, and the development of normal muscle tone and balance is encouraged. Indeed, when symptoms prevail in a child who is flat-footed, they are usually associated with previous use of arch supports, wedges, and special heels applied to footwear which disturb the balance of gait and may throw excessive strain on the muscles of the leg which support the foot. In such instances, symptoms of strain in childhood are usually relieved following the use of adequate arch-support lasts with a special heel. Additional supports inside the shoe are apt to lead to trouble.

Doctors, podiatrists, and chiropodists are frequently coerced by mothers who are overly anxious for perfection in the child to apply such corrective shoes to relieve the mother's concern. If the condition has been without symptoms before, such modifications of footwear may produce symptoms and lead to an abnormal focus of the child's attention on his feet. Likewise the child becomes instinctively aware of the mother's overconcern with a part of his body, and may then register complaints where discomfort does not exist in order to gain the mother's attention whenever the child feels it is needed. Such responses often lead to the development of bizarre behavior patterns which compound the parents' concern over the child and only perpetuate the vicious cycle.

In the older child one not infrequently encounters a *spastic* or rigid flat-foot deformity which requires conservative, or in some instances surgical, treatment. The flat-footed deformity occasionally seen in *cerebral palsy* has been mentioned in a previous section. Such a deformity usually requires bracing during the early years of life and at an appropriate period in adolescence, surgical correction and stabilization of the foot will usually permit the brace to be discarded. A not uncommon cause of spastic flat-footedness in the adolescent is obesity. Such accumulation of excess fat before full muscular development has occurred may produce considerable strain on the foot leading to pain in the calf and spasm of the muscles of the outer side of the leg and foot which contract and roll the foot inward. Such a condition requires professional help and weight reduction is mandatory. Muscle spasticity and imbalance may be resistant to conservative care and on occasions manipulation of the foot under anesthesia and immobilization in a plaster cast for a period of time becomes necessary. A Whitman metal plate supporting the arch in the corrective or normal position may be worn within the shoe for some period thereafter to prevent recurrence. A third cause of spastic flat-footedness in childhood, which may reveal itself at any period from 6 years through adolescence is a birth or developmental defect manifested by a fusion or coalition of two or more small bones of the mid-portion of the foot. Such a condition interferes with a normal range of motion of the foot and imparts exceptional stress on other joints leading to chronic strain, muscle spasm, and imbalance of the musculature supporting the foot. This condition can be detected only by adequate X-ray examination of the foot. The treatment is usually surgical.

Flat-footedness in the child who has been the victim of poliomyelitis is much less common today than in former years; it is due to weakness of the muscles supporting the innerside of the foot. This condition usually requires protection with a brace during the early period of growth, followed by surgical stabilization of the foot at 5 or 6 years of age, or later in adolescence, to do away with the need for bracing.

Flat-footedness may be associated with late adolescence or adult life. In such instances the person is usually overweight, has been wearing inadequate footwear such as "loafers" or other soft footwear, or has been employed in occupations requiring prolonged standing in one position on hard surfaces. Every attempt should be made to reduce or eliminate such underlying causal factors. If this is impossible, relief may be obtained by the use of well-constructed orthopedic shoes in which the last is usually straight and the shank of the shoe is reinforced with a special heel, referred to also in flat-footedness in the child. The special heel is known as a Thomas heel, which extends farther forward on the inner side and on the outer side of the shoe, thus providing adequate support for the inner aspect of the foot. In some resistant cases, the use of custom-built footwear made over plaster molds of the foot is a worthwhile investment.

FOOT INJURIES

The most common injury of the foot in youth or adult life is *sprained ankle*. Such an injury is invariably associated with tearing of soft parts—principally ligaments—which support the foot on the lower part of the leg. The injury should not be taken lightly if chronic disability is to be avoided, and the services of a physician should be obtained. If a physician is not immediately available, the injured member should be elevated and an ice pack applied. The use of heat in an acute injury of this type leads to an increase of extravasation of blood and blood fluids in the damaged soft tissue, causes greater swelling and pain, and should be avoided at all costs. If adequately protected, the soft parts will usually heal within a period of 2 to 3 weeks and the part will be as strong as ever. Depending upon the extent of the injury—determined by adequate inspection and examination of X-ray films to rule out the presence of associated bony injury—the limb may be protected by adequate strapping followed by partial weight bearing with crutches or a cane. In cases in which there is evidence of more extensive ligamentous damage, the application of a plaster cast boot for a period of 2 to 3 weeks will assure a stable ankle. The injection of novocaine for the relief of pain, freezing the skin with volatile solvents, or the use of digestive enzymes are illogical and should be avoided.

Fractures of the small bones of the toes are the most common injuries involving the bony components of the foot. The fifth toe is the usual victim of a collision with legs of furniture on attempting to reach the bathroom without turning on the lights during the middle of the night. Again, heat should never be applied to such an injury, and an ice pack will alleviate some of the discomfort. If the skin of the toe becomes discolored, there is usually a fracture of one of the small bones of the toe. With such fractures the physician will tape the injured member to the adjacent toe and advise that the last over the outer toes be cut out of the shoe to relieve pressure. He may likewise advise that a leather metatarsal bar be applied to the sole of the shoe to provide additional comfort in walking. Such injuries usually require 2½ to 3 weeks to heal, and do not lead to disability.

A second common fracture of the foot is that at the base of the longer bone of the fifth toe. The mechanism of this injury is similar to that experienced in a sprain of the ankle; however, the pain and swelling will be localized to the outer border of the mid-portion of the foot. A plaster boot cast applied for a period of 2 to 3 weeks to permit healing may be necessary for reasonably comfortable ambulation.

A third, but much less common fracture of the forefoot is known as a "march" or "stress" fracture usually of the long bone of the second toe. This fracture is not the result of a direct injury and the symptoms usually appear insidiously. It usually occurs in those with delicate bones who have been subject to prolonged marches with heavy packs in military service, or in women from prolonged walking or standing in high-heeled shoes. This injury again requires protection for a period of 3 to 4 weeks in a plaster boot. Injuries to the other small bones of the mid- and hind-portions of the foot are usually due to severe forces such as those occurring in a fall from a height or an automobile accident. Instances of this kind are usually complicated by the involvement of joints or associated dislocations, and require the care of a specialist if permanent disability is to be avoided.

Prolonged pressure or strain on the heel bone may lead to a condition known as *painful heel* in childhood or adult life. In the former, pain is usually localized to the hind part of the heel in the region of the attachment of the powerful heel cord. This is generally observed in boys, at the time of puberty or early adolescence, who are active in competitive sports. It is due to excessive strain on a yet unfused portion of the heel bone to which the powerful heel cord is attached, and is usually relieved by a respite from participation in sports for a period of a few weeks. A ½-inch elevation of the heel contributes to the relief of the symptoms by reducing the tension of the heel cord on the afflicted part.

In adult life, pain in this region is almost invariably due to irritation of a bursa or small sac lying between the heel cord and the heel bone which has been irritated by an ill-fitting shoe last or from some minor injury. Relief is usually obtained by injection of a cortisone preparation into the bursa which counteracts the inflammation in the lining of the sac. A similar condition is found on the bottom of the heel which has been traditionally referred to as "policeman's heel." This is a sterile inflammation of the tendinous portions of the short muscles of the foot arising from the weight-bearing portion of the heel, and is usually brought on by prolonged standing on hard surfaces. It is best relieved by local injection of a cortisone preparation by one experienced in the localization of the affliction and the structures involved.

Other afflictions of the foot occasioned by chronic irritation or repeated minor injury are those involving the tendons as they pass over or through bony grooves below the ankle. Most commonly this is noted beneath the inner prominence of the ankle joint, and is due to inflammation of the sheath of the tendon supporting the long arch of the foot as it passes through a groove in this region. On occasion, the large heel cord may be similarly inflamed and both conditions respond effectively to the local injection of an appropriate cortisone preparation.

AFFLICTIONS OF THE SKIN AND NAILS OF THE FOOT

Ringworm of the feet, or "athlete's foot," is a common disorder of the skin caused by a variety of fungi or mould-like organisms. Such fungi normally exist in a harmonious balance with other normally occurring bacteria of the skin without causing trouble unless the balanced environment is upset by a change in the surface acidity of the skin toward the alkaline side, together with a local accumulation of moisture. Excessive perspiration of the feet, uncleanliness, ill-fitting shoes, or shoes impervious to the dissemination of moisture such as tennis shoes are important factors in acquiring the disease. The condition is seen most commonly in males engaged in athletic pursuits or those employed in occupations where excessive perspiration or daily exposure of feet to damp conditions are contributing factors. For these reasons, it is also seen much more commonly during the hot summer months or in the tropics where heat and moisture co-exist throughout the year. The onset is usually characterized by the appearance of small, itching, watery blisters between the toes or along the longitudinal arch of the foot. This is followed by thickening, fissuring, and peeling off of superficial layers of the skin. If improperly treated, secondary complications such as local allergies, secondary infections, and involvements of the nails may follow. An allergy from absorption of fungi or their toxic products may manifest itself in the hands and fingers, known as an "id" eruption which may be troublesome and difficult to eradicate. The treatment, therefore, of a serious fungus infection of the feet, lies in the realm of a competent dermatologist, and indiscriminate use of ointments and proprietary medications is to be discouraged. Treatment of the mild or early form of the disease and prevention of reinfection is largely a matter of immaculate personal hygiene and foot care. The feet should be washed twice daily with soap and water followed by thorough drying, particularly between the toes. The nails should be kept clean and any scales of skin removed from the nail edges. This should be followed by the application of astringent acid powders such as boric acid, salicylic acid, or undecylenic acid found in many commercial foot-powder preparations. Cotton socks should be worn and changed daily. In women, open-toed shoes may be beneficial in maintaining dryness of the feet and shoes should never be worn on two successive days. When not worn, shoes should be kept in a well-ventilated area so that thorough drying occurs between periods of use. Scuffs or wooden clogs should be worn by persons using common shower facilities in a gymnasium or dormitory. A cure is effected when there is cessation of itching and absence of skin scaling and watery blister formation.

Hyperhydrosis is a disturbance of the skin of the feet caused by excessive perspiration which leads to the accumulation of moisture in the socks and shoe leather. Commonly this is a predisposing factor to the development of ringworm of the feet. It is a functional disturbance of that part of the nervous system responsible for the secretion of sweat glands, tone of blood vessels, and functions of the internal organs which are not under voluntary or higher brain-center control. Not uncommonly such sweating is seen in those living under chronic emotional tension or with unresolved personal conflicts. Consideration of these factors as well as a search for local causes such as poor foot hygiene, faulty footwear, or foot strain must be made if relief is to be obtained. Local care requires changing shoes and hose twice daily, and thorough drying of footwear between periods of use. Astringent solutions or powders prescribed by a dermatologist may be of assistance. The local use of X-ray therapy to suppress sweat-gland activity is not justifiable and may be dangerous in view of the damage to other elements of the skin. The use of recently introduced drugs which suppress the nerve endings of that portion of the nervous system controlling sweat production inhibits hyperhydrosis, but is usually objectionable because of associated side effects such as dryness of the mouth, visual blurring, and difficulties in urination.

Fungus infections of the nail comprise some 20 per cent of all diseases of the nails. This is characterized by a cloudy patch occurring at the edge of the nail which extends gradually toward the nail root. Usually thickening beneath the nail occurs in the involved area, and is a notoriously resistant affliction to treat because of the inaccessibility of the diseased tissues. Anti-fungal drugs which may be taken by mouth such as Fulvian® have proved effective when taken for months at a time; however, in some resistant cases, surgical removal of the nail and the use of topical medication may be necessary.

Ingrown toenail. By far the most common cause of ingrowing toenail is improper trimming of the nail of the first toe, together with the use of pointed footwear which imposes excessive stress on the top of this nail. The toenail subject to pressure from shoes should be cut straight across, leaving the edges of the nail projecting beyond the underlying soft parts. The mid-portion of the nail may be cut shorter than the outer edges which will further relieve direct pressure on the convexity of the nail. When toenails are trimmed in the fashion commonly practiced with the fingers, a sharp spike left at the edges of the nail may penetrate the flesh with growth leading to puncture of the tissues which with chronic irritation usually becomes secondarily infected. In the early form without infection, elevation of the edge of the nail with a firm cotton packing soaked in a household antiseptic—such as Mercurochrome®—elevates the edge of the nail and if maintained for a sufficient period of time permitting growth of the edge of the nail beyond the bed, will bring relief. With severe cases or those complicated by secondary infection, surgical measures may become necessary.

CALLUSES AND CORNS

Calluses are circumscribed areas of skin occurring on the heel or soles of the feet which are due to constant friction and pressure. They are unlike corns in that they do not contain a central core, but must be differentiated from warts on the weight-bearing portion of the foot. They are invariably due to poor fitting shoes or to the pressure of abnormal bony prominences such as the heel, incident to the wearing of high-heeled shoes or to deformities of the foot caused by diseases such as arthritis or neurological disturbances affecting the functions and structure of the feet.

The treatment of calluses by repeated shaving or the application of desquamating chemicals is rarely successful unless the underlying cause is removed. In some instances where faulty footwear is the cause, the use of well-fitted orthopedic shoes may alleviate pressure and friction with beneficial results over a period of time. In other instances, surgical correction of stress- and pressure-point abnormalities of the foot or the relief of bony prominences may be necessary.

Plantar warts are calluslike growths which occur singly or multiply on the sole or heel of the foot, as well as the sides of the toes. The causative agent is a virus and the lesion must be distinguished from an ordinary callus due to friction by a competent dermatologist or foot specialist if successful treatment is to be carried out. The lesion may vary from the size of a pinhead to that of a quarter, and is usually characterized by a central cluster of dark spots. These afflictions are most resistant to the local topical application of drugs or chemicals and the most successful form of treatment is that by irradiation therapy in the hands of a skilled X-ray therapist. Cure may usually be expected in from 3 to 6 weeks, and if the lesion recurs, the base may be removed by electrocautery. Surgical removal of such warts is contraindicated in view of the resultant painful scar which may ensue on a weight-bearing surface of the foot which may be tender to pressure of a shoe.

ACQUIRED DEFORMITIES AND DISEASES OF THE ADULT FOOT

The most common affliction of the forepart of the foot seen in adult life is known as *bunion*. This is a deformity characterized by lateral deviation of the first toe which may be overlapped by the second toe with a bony prominence appearing over the inner and upper point of the angulation of the toe. This bony prominence is usually overlain by bursa or protective sac and considerable callus formation of the overlying skin. This affliction is almost invariably the result of the vagaries of fashion and vanity in the high-heeled, pointed-toe design of footwear to which women are subjected. Too much cannot be said in condemnation of such footwear design, but the custom of centuries of use would indicate that the slenderized ankle and foot is here to stay. The concentration of body weight on the forepart of the foot when high-heeled shoes are worn, leads to pressure and stress on the joints at the base of the toes which is followed by muscle spasm leading to progression of the deformity of the first toe and angular deformities of the remaining toes of the foot. Localized pressure of the shoe last on such angular bony prominences is followed by the development of calluses on the weight-bearing portion of the forefoot and bunions or corn on the tops of the toes. These in turn become painful and further contribute to foot discomfort. The correction of such deformities is usually surgical, and if prolonged disability of the foot is to be prevented following surgical correction, sensible shoes must be worn. If surgical correction is contraindicated or inadvisable, some relief may be obtained by the use of custom-built shoes in which the last is made from a mold obtained from a plaster impression of the deformed foot. Such footwear is expensive, however, and is often cosmetically objectionable.

Rigid first toe is a condition in which the joint of the base of the first toe becomes stiffened due to chronic wear-and-tear changes in the joint surfaces. It is seen as frequently in men as in women, and causal factors are not always in evidence. Frequently it is accompanied by extensive callus formation on the inner aspect or weight bearing surface of the first toe. Discomfort may be conservatively relieved in some instances by the application of a leather bar on the sole of the shoe behind the affected joint. This prevents stress on the joint when walking by eliminating the break or bend in the forepart of the sole. When symptoms are severe, surgical intervention may be necessary.

Arthritis of the foot may be of the *rheumatoid* or deforming type, *degenerative* or that due to wear and tear and aging of the joint, or to *gout* which is characterized by the deposition or precipitation of crystalline metabolic end products within the bony or ligamentous supporting structures about a joint. *Rheumatoid arthritis* in general leads to deformities similar to that already noted in our discussion of deformities of the forefoot occasioned by faulty footwear in women, in other words, bunion and deformity of the toes. Such deformity, when observed in the male, is usually preceded by this disease. Considerable relief of deformity and associated pressure complications such as calluses and bunions may be obtained by properly timed, appropriate surgical procedures. The degenerative or wear-and-tear form of arthritis is that seen in rigid first toe and may likewise occur in the joints at the base of the other toes of the foot when these become prominent on the weight-bearing surface of the foot. Relief of pain from such afflictions may be dramatic following the installation of cortisone preparations within the joint and subsequent relief of pressure by adequate alterations in footwear. *Gouty arthritis* characteristically involves the first toe and is rather sudden in onset. It is characterized by redness and swelling at the base of the first toe, and extreme sensitivity such that the pressure of a sheet may considerably aggravate the local pain. Pain and swelling generally subside after a few days of appropriate rest and elevation of the foot; however, periodic relapses are to be expected unless the underlying metabolic disturbance is modified by proper diet and medication.

A not uncommon and frequently unrecognized affliction of the forefoot is known as *Morton's Toe*. This is a painful affliction, usually localized between the second and third toes, but not infrequently between the third and the fourth toes which has the lancinating character of nerve pain, usually coming on after prolonged periods of standing or walking for a given distance. The afflicted person frequently finds it necessary to stop and remove the shoe and to massage the foot to obtain relief. It is seen more commonly in women than in men, and the affliction is again thought to be related to abnormal stress imposed on the forepart of the foot by high-heeled shoes. The root of the affliction is found in a thickening of the sheath of small nerves which pass between the toes in the ball of the foot caused by chronic pressure, tension, and irritation. As the thickening of the nerve sheath increases, symptoms become more marked and sensation in the skin between the toes may be diminished. Conservative measures are usually of little avail and surgical excision of the thickened nerve and its sheath is necessary to obtain permanent relief.

CARE OF THE DIABETIC FOOT

True diabetes mellitus, fully discussed also in another chapter, is a disease of the human pancreas in which small clusters of cells responsible for the internal secretion of a hormone, *insulin,* undergo degeneration, leading to faulty utilization of fat and sugar in the body. If undetected for a long time, or if inadequately controlled by proper dieting and substitution therapy, the defective metabolism of fats leads to the premature deposition of by-products of fat metabolism in the walls of the larger arteries and small arterioles which transport nutritional materials to the tissues of the body. These blood vessels are responsible for the removal of metabolic waste products via the veins into which they empty through the minute capillaries. Such deposition of fatty materials in the wall of the arterial system lead to narrowing of the openings of such vessels and loss of elasticity of the walls, thus seriously impairing the nutrition of the tissues that they supply. All of the tissues of the extremities, such as nerves, muscles, bones, and ligaments may be thus affected leading, in the diabetic, to conditions of the foot which may involve sensation in the skin as well as protective stretch sensations in the ligaments supporting the joints in the foot. Due to the gradual obliteration of small arterioles supplying nutrition to the nerves of the extremity, such changes involving the blood vessels supplying nutrition to the skin, or underlying soft tissue and bony structures, may in the untreated case eventually lead to progressive failure of the blood vascular system to provide nutriments and to remove waste products of metabolism of such tissues. The local defense mechanisms of the tissues against invasion of bacteria from the external environment, may be seriously impaired and infection of the soft parts or joints may occur. If the changes in sensation incident to similar impaired nutrition of the nerve makes such a diabetic person more prone to superficial breaks in the continuity of the protective skin surface, the invasion of bacteria normally present on the skin surface may be hastened. The major afflictions of the foot in the untreated or inadequately treated diabetic therefore fall into four categories, namely (1) infection of the skin or soft parts, (2) trophic ulceration or pressure ulceration due to loss of sensation in the skin, (3) gangrene of the soft tissue or bony structure due to progressive and final obliteration of the blood vessels supplying such parts, and (4) gradual painless destruction of joints of the mid-portion of the foot due to loss of normal stretch sensation in the ligaments supporting the bony structures of the foot. Diabetes whether mild or severe should be brought under complete control, and thereafter be carefully maintained under control throughout the balance of the life of the diabetic person. In the advanced diabetic stage or in the long unrecognized case, meticulous care of the feet is vitally important if secondary complications due to nerve or soft tissue and joint involvement are to be avoided.

The diabetic should purchase footwear of only the best quality. Shoe lasts should be ample in size, but not poorly fitted, in order to avoid friction and localized pressure on bony prominences or toenails which might further impair nutrition and oxygen supply by pressure of the shoe itself. Toenails should be cut properly and kept short in order to avoid ingrown toenails or laceration of adjacent toes by the edges of uncut nails. One should observe care, however, to avoid cutting the nail back to the nail bed where bleeding may occur, and the skin be broken if the nail is cut too short. The edges of the nails should be kept free of desquamated surface skin and the feet should be kept meticulously clean by daily bathing. Calluses and corns should preferably not be trimmed, and are better softened by drugs prescribed by a physician. Any evidence of infection such as redness or swelling should be immediately brought to the attention of a physician and the foot should be elevated until all signs of infection have subsided. The local use of heat is to be avoided at all costs, in view of the increased metabolic needs of the tissues incident to its use. Such infections may not be painful in view of the impaired sensation of the skin associated with nerve involvement as well. Infection may seriously affect control of the diabetes and conversely, lack of control of the diabetes seriously interferes with the body's ability to control and localize infection. The treatment of such complications is therefore best performed in a hospital under close surveillance by a physician.

CHAPTER 35

Diseases of the Nervous System

MORRIS FISHBEIN, M.D.

The nervous system, which includes the brain, the spinal cord, and the nerves associated with them, which spread throughout the body, is concerned with both physical and mental disorders. For purposes of reference, the nervous system includes the brain, the special nerves of sensation such as those going to the eye and the ear, the autonomic or sympathetic nervous system, and all of the peripheral nerves which branch out through the body.

PARKINSON'S DISEASE

The condition called Parkinson's disease has been known also as shaking palsy and as paralysis agitans. Dr. James Parkinson of London described this condition first in 1817 in a classical essay which carefully listed the symptoms and the progress of the disease. Parkinson's disease affects principally older people; most cases of patients with this disease of long duration are people in their sixties and seventies. Some cases occur after inflammations of the brain called encephalitis.

Paralysis agitans ordinarily affects first a single arm or leg, then the second limb on the same side, and finally those on the other side. Often an arm first betrays symptoms by losing the typical swing that accompanies walking, and the face begins to lack its customary expressiveness and changes slowly or not at all with passing moods. Involvement of the limbs is followed by that of the trunk muscles, which gives the body a stooping posture. Steps become shorter and more rapid and develop into a combination of a shuffle and run. The rate at which the disease advances varies in different persons. Often it progresses slowly, leaving the health good in other respects. Intervals as long as a year may occur between the phases of development from one limb to another.

Changes in the brain, in other nerve tissue, and in blood vessels of the brain have been observed in association with paralysis agitans. Although exact knowledge as to its cause is not known, special or direct relationship to either brain hemorrhage or high blood pressure is doubtful.

Treatment of paralysis agitans is usually limited to relief of symptoms, to efforts to keep the patient comfortable, to maintaining his general health and thus to endeavoring to retard the progress of the disease.

Drugs of the belladonna type reduce rigidity; they may be administered in various ways to give relief. Baths and massage relieve the tensions in the muscles and are soothing to the skin.

Operative procedures have been developed which diminish the circulation of blood to the areas in the brain concerned with the tremors. Success has been reported in many cases of paralysis agitans.

Recently Dr. Irving Cooper, New York, developed a procedure for treating Parkinson's disease by eliminating surgically a section of the brain from which the impulses to the tremors arise. After the surgical method was developed, the technique proceeded to using chemicals injected into the area to produce the necessary destruction, and during the last few years a device has been developed which freezes the area—this being apparently most important of all the methods thus far discovered.

As has already been said, Parkinson's disease affects mostly older people but may occur as early as 30 years of age. Ths most common age of onset is 45 to 55. Estimates indicate that at any one time over one million people in the United States suffer from this disease. Cases are likely to increase because of the increasing number of older people with the increase in life expectancy at birth.

The exact cause of Parkinson's disease is not known but various views suggest that circulatory disturbances or abnormalities of chemical changes in the body may play a role.

When a person has Parkinson's disease, proper treatment in the early stages may prevent serious complications, retard the progress of the disease, and permit the person to continue active for years without becoming totally disabled. In such medical care, rehabilitation centers where physical therapy, psychotherapy, and occupational training are available, play a great part.

Parkinson's disease is not inherited and is not contagious. Once the condition has begun it slowly progresses. However, many patients have stationary periods of 5, 10, or more years. The minds of people with Parkinson's disease are not affected as far as intelligence is concerned. The muscles do not waste away as in some forms of infantile paralysis or meningitis. Seldom is the hearing, speech or vision disturbed in patients with Parkinson's disease.

When the patient with Parkinsonism first comes to the doctor, studies may be made using such important equipment as the electroencephalogram (EEG), the electromyelogram (EMG), and other devices and tests to determine the exact nature and extent of the disease. Such studies enable the neurologist to determine with certainty that the condition is Parkinsonism and not some of the various other conditions that may be confused with it.

Much research continues to be devoted to Parkinson's disease in many centers throughout the United States. In one study of 800 people with Parkinson's disease, 25 per cent progressed so slowly that changes were hardly noticeable after five years. Another 25 per cent developed progression only after six or more years. Two-thirds of all the patients were well able to get about and to care for themselves. Only 20 per cent were totally invalided. With modern neurosurgical methods, good results are obtained in 80 per cent of selected cases; however, only about 2 per cent of all patients with Parkinson's disease are considered suitable for this modern type of surgery. People with only one side affected are considered most suitable for the use of modern surgical methods.

The greatest hope that lies ahead for patients with Parkinson's disease is the fact that drugs are now known which are most useful in controlling the symptoms even though they do not produce cure of the disease.

MULTIPLE SCLEROSIS

Multiple sclerosis was first described scientifically in 1868. The total number of persons afflicted with this disease in the United States is not known but estimates in 1960 indicated about 500,000 people in the United States suffering from multiple sclerosis and other similar conditions in which the myelin sheaths of the nerves in the spine are destroyed.

Multiple sclerosis is a chronic disease which progresses and which strikes usually people in the 20 to 40 year age range. The condition occurs more frequently in northern than in southern latitudes. Investigators have not found any ethnic, occupational, social, or economic reasons related to the appearance of this disease. Unfortunately the condition is difficult to diagnose in its earliest stages. When the symptoms have progressed sufficiently to produce disability, the diagnosis becomes clear. Thus far a laboratory test which would diagnose the condition specifically has not been discovered.

The usual early symptoms are mild, including perhaps some numbness in an arm or a leg, a blurring of vision or double vision, and excessive fatigue. These symptoms may come and disappear, only to return again. As the disease progresses, movements may become uncoordinated, walking unstable; the legs may become spastic. Ultimately the paralysis may extend even to failure to control the excretions of the body.

Examination of the brain and the spinal cord shows that there are areas in which the myelin, which sheaths the nerve fibers and appears to act as an insulator, has begun to disappear. As a result, nerve impulses are distorted, much as destruction of insulation in a telephone cable would result in short circuits and blocking of electrical impulses. As the condition progresses, the body forms scars where the myelin has been lost. This may further disrupt the nerve impulses. A not infrequent symptom of multiple sclerosis is the slowing down of speech. The person may talk in a monotone and utter syllables with difficulty. Fortunately there are no serious mental disturbances although some people become emotionally or mentally disturbed or depressed.

The rate of development varies in all cases. However, eventually the basic functions, such as sight, hearing and digestion, are involved, and constant nursing becomes a necessity. Sometimes this point is not reached for many years.

As yet, nothing is known that will arrest or cure the disease. Nevertheless, the adequacy of the care given can make a real difference. General and medical care must be properly given in order to secure any relief. Also, the patient can be protected from those conditions which are especially threatening to his condition. Only with such meager methods can the effects of the basic disorder be held to the minimum at this time.

Recently the view has been expressed that multiple sclerosis represents a sensitization of the body to its myelin substance whereby that myelin substance is destroyed. Hence efforts have been made to arrest progress by the use of the strongest desensitizing substances known, among which are, of course, ACTH and the cortisone derivatives. Apparently an insufficient amount of the product can reach the myelin by giving the drugs either by mouth or intravenously. However, attempts have been made to treat the disease by injecting these drugs directly into the spinal fluid. Optimistic reports have appeared from some of the greater clinics as to the results of this method of treatment.

Medical researchers are still working to determine whether or not a virus infection or inflammation coming from some toxin is responsible for multiple sclerosis. No organism has yet been found to which it can be attributed. There are instances in which the disease makes its appearance after childbirth or a major operation, but apparently this is a matter of coincidence. No special hereditary factors seem to be involved. It generally appears before the age of forty.

Among the most important recent efforts has been the development of results under the auspices of the National Multiple Sclerosis Society to prove that the allergic autosensitization processes are at the basis of the disease.

MYASTHENIA GRAVIS

This chronic disease of the nervous system is actually a disturbance which primarily affects the muscles, making them weak and easily exhausted with use. The exact cause of this condition is not known although there are many theories as to its causation, some concerned primarily with glands, some with nerves, some with the metabolism of the muscles.

In myasthenia gravis the muscles of the eyes, face, neck, tongue, throat, and lips are especially involved. The muscles of the arms and legs may be affected later. Sometimes the person with myasthenia is so exhausted that he cannot hold anything in his hands, keep his eyes open, or even feed himself.

Myasthenia gravis comes on gradually but sometimes suddenly. The earliest symptoms are the symptoms of weakness. The muscles concerned are not the involuntary muscles such as those of the heart and the intestines over which there is little conscious control; they are the voluntary muscles which can be moved at the will of the person. Double vision, difficulty in swallowing, chewing and talking may ensue. The condition usually begins in adulthood but cases affecting babies have been reported. Women with myasthenia gravis usually develop the condition in the early thirties and before the age of 40. In men the condition may occur later in life.

The exact cause of this condition, as has already been mentioned, is not known. Recently people with enlarged thymus glands have been found with this disease and some investigators have associated it with overactivity of the lymphatic tissues of the body, particularly the thymus. Some physicians have, therefore, recommended either removal of the thymus gland by surgery or invalidation of the action of this gland by submitting it to X ray.

Fortunately most cases of myasthenia are helped by a drug called prostigmine or neostigmine which the physician may inject directly into the veins or prescribe to be taken by mouth. In many instances treatment designed to strengthen the muscles by activity is attempted. The physician will also prescribe other drugs depending on the symptoms.

NEURALGIA

Neuralgia means simply a pain in the nerves which, however, may not represent a disease which primarily concerns the nerve itself. The pain is felt along the nerve or in the part of the body which is supplied by that nerve. Various forms of neuralgia may develop into what is called neuritis or inflammation of the nerves.

Many different types of neuralgia are recognized, depending on the nerve involved. Nerves especially apt to become irritable and produce severe pain are the brachial nerve in the arm, the intercostal nerves running between the ribs, the nerves of the scalp, and the sciatic nerve. The fifth cranial nerve, also known as the trigeminal nerve, which supplies the forehead, face, and jaw, is most often affected with neuralgia. The nerve may be so sensitive that even a cold current blowing on the face or a light touch of a finger to the face causes stabbing pain.

In severe cases of neuralgia, or when medical treatment fails, a surgical operation which destroys the nerve roots usually gives permanent relief and involves little risk, even for elderly persons. In neuralgia affecting any nerve, the doctor first determines the nerve area involved and then takes steps to prevent the sensation of pain from traveling along that nerve. To do this, he may use sedative drugs, inject local anesthetics or alcohol, or treat the nerves with X rays. Diagnosis is more difficult in those cases in which the sensations of pain are mental rather than physical in origin.

NEURITIS

When a nerve or the sheath that surrounds it becomes inflamed, the condition is called neuritis. In neuritis, the pain and tenderness are felt definitely over the area supplied by the particular nerve that is involved. If more than one nerve is involved, the condition is called multiple neuritis or polyneuritis. Neuritis of the optic nerve which supplies the eye or of the otic nerve which supplies the ear, for instance, would cause temporary or even permanent disability of the organs concerned.

A frequent form of neuritis is sciatic neuritis which involves the sciatic nerve and its branches. This nerve, one of the largest in the body, supplies the muscles of the thigh, leg, and feet and the skin of the leg. It runs entirely down the back of the leg and thigh with many branches and subdivisions.

The word sciatica is often applied to cover a variety of ailments which do not involve the sciatic nerve. True sciatica is sciatic neuritis, and pain is felt in the thigh and other areas associated with the sciatic nerve. Sciatic pain accompanies numerous conditions, and may be due to a number of factors which adversely affect the sciatic nerve.

The part of the spinal cord where the nerve originates may be disturbed, for example, by a slipped or ruptured disc, or by an inflammation in the vertebral bones. An abnormal condition in a nearby blood vessel may cause it to press on the nerve. Acute and prolonged constipation is sometimes responsible because the accumulation in the bowel exerts pressure on the nerve or because the body absorbs unexcreted toxic substances to which the nerve reacts. External conditions or occurrences may precipitate a sciatic disturbance, such as a bad fall or severe contortion of the body, or prolonged exposure to cold and dampness.

Because of the number of possible causes and the numerous possible ramifications which sciatic neuritis may have, it is, like headache and backache, an apparently simple discomfort which masks a potentially complicated situation. Diagnosis of the specific cause of a particular case of sciatic neuritis demands the attention of a skilled physician. The pain is only a symptom and the source of it must be determined before proper treatment can begin. The physician will first ascertain whether the pain involved is due to a sciatic condition or some other cause. He will check the sacroiliac joint, the spine for curvature, the back for bones out of position, the legs for muscle spasms or disordered muscles and tissue.

Treatment may begin with simple measures to relieve the immediate discomfort: bed rest, placing the body in the position with the least possible strain on affected parts, or use of heat to reduce pain. The doctor will examine the patient's diet and his daily activities, making sure that the diet is nutritionally adequate and that the patient's job, exercise, and general environment do not aggravate his condition. He may, for example, recommend that a patient who works in a cold damp place change his job. Injection of one of a variety of medicinal substances into the sciatic nerve or the surrounding areas is sometimes advisable and may bring good but not permanent results. Other measures are available for specialized treatment.

Sometimes the condition called sciatic neuritis is actually pressure of one of the bones of the spine on the nerves which come to the sciatic. This condition is frequently called slipped disc.

EPILEPSY

Epilepsy is among the most misunderstood of all human afflictions. Known to the ancients as the falling disease, it has also been described simply as "fits." Until people understood the nature of epilepsy, victims were avoided, feared, scorned, and even burned at the stake. The ancients thought that some evil spirit had gotten into the skull. Sometimes they opened the skull by the procedure called trephining and because nothing was then known about the prevention of infections, the majority of those exposed to such operations died.

Epileptics are subject to seizures, temporary loss or alteration of consciousness, with or without convulsive movements. Five or more types of seizures are known, but only one, the *grand mal,* has the characteristics of the popular conception of a "fit" or convulsion. Even a violent *grand mal* seizure rarely lasts much longer than a minute, though it will probably seem much longer to an observer. After a seizure, the person may sleep for a few hours or resume normal activity within a few minutes.

Contrasted with the *grand mal* is the *petit mal* seizure, a momentary blackout, with or without a twitching of the eyelids or of other facial muscles. Its manifestations, however, are so slight that it may go unnoticed even in a crowd.

Little can be done while a person is having a seizure. At the beginning of an attack he may be lowered to the floor, well away from hard objects against which he might injure himself. Any tight collars or belts should be loosened, and a folded handkerchief inserted between the back teeth to prevent biting of the tongue. The patient should be turned on his side to permit saliva to flow from his mouth.

Science has made great progress in diagnosing and treating epilepsy through the use of an instrument, the electroencephalograph, which magnifies and records the electric impulses from the brain, much as an electrocardiograph checks the heart. An electroencephalogram, the written record, is unique for each person, like a fingerprint. This record is a significant clue to the type of medication most likely to be successful.

At present, approximately 0.5 per cent of the population of the United States is afflicted with epilepsy. Seizures begin prominently in early childhood and in adolescence, but many persons are subject to them after the age of twenty-one. The number of males and females who suffer from epilepsy is almost equal. The true cause of epilepsy is not as yet known. Epilepsy is known to be related to damaged brain tissue, or to a brain tumor in some cases, but it may be present when such conditions do not exist. Tension, although it does not cause seizures, may precipitate them. A well-adjusted person who is physically and mentally active will have fewer seizures.

One of the nation's leading authorities on epilepsy, Dr. William G. Lennox, in his book *Science and Seizures,* compares the electric impulses to a stream with a moderate flow, controlled by an adequate dam. In the case of a person with epilepsy, the level at times rises and spills over the dam and a seizure results. The level overflows when the predisposition to epilepsy combines with minor body or emotional disturbances which most people experience without ill effects.

The hereditary cause of epilepsy is more significant than the acquired one. Among near relatives of epileptics, the illness is about three times more frequent than among the population as a whole. Certain disorders which may bring about epilepsy are thus acquired causes. Among these are (1) congenital defects of the central nervous system—as, for example, degeneration of the nervous system, congenital mental defect, and scarring of nerve tissue; (2) changes in the development of the brain after birth—as, for example, various types of meningitis, multiple sclerosis, general paresis, tumors, hemorrhages, cerebral abscess, arteriosclerosis, and senile degeneration; (3) general diseases such as uremia, toxemia of pregnancy, fluid swelling of the brain, pernicious anemia, asphyxia, protein shock, acute fever in children, hypotension, insulin or electric shock; (4) effect of convulsant drugs—for example, camphor, caffeine, ergot, epinephrine, cocaine, magnesium sulfate, and sulfathiazole.

According to the Foundation to Combat Epilepsy, the incidence of epilepsy because of acquired causes is variable. The incidence related to convulsant drugs and brain tumor is not larger than 15 per cent, abnormalities at birth around 9 per cent, infections about 5 per cent, brain tumors about 1.5 per cent, cerebral circulatory defects about 1.2 per cent, and postnatal brain trauma about 6 per cent. In approximately 77 per cent of the patients, evidence of antecedent organic diseases of the brain does not exist.

A specific cure for epilepsy is not known, but medication can reduce the frequency of seizures or eliminate them completely in about 85 per cent of those affected. Many drugs and combinations of drugs are effective when taken under the guidance of a physician. Seizures can be completely controlled—that is, prevented from occurring—in about one-half of all persons with epilepsy. An additional 35 per cent under medication have the frequency of their seizures reduced by half or more, and the remaining 15 per cent of epileptic patients are not helped by medication.

A person with epilepsy should never try to treat himself, since the drugs and dosage needed vary from person to person and only a physician, specially trained, is competent to prescribe. Mail-order remedies should never be used. For most persons with *grand mal* or psychomotor seizures, the doctor employs, among other drugs, phenytoin sodium or Dilantin; and, if this drug is not fully effective, phenobarbital may be added. Another drug, Mesantoin, can be tolerated in larger amounts by some patients than others. These drugs can be obtained only by prescription and changes and directions in dosage must be supervised properly to be effective. For convulsions, the physician may employ first phenobarbital or Mebaral. Bromides, although now replaced by newer drugs, are still useful in some circumstances. In cases of *petit mal,* tridione, paradione, Milontin, and phenurone have been successfully used in many cases.

The person subject to epilepsy must take his medicines regularly, avoid alcohol, emotional upsets, and fatigue and live as regular a life as possible. He should not be overprotected by his family, but should be encouraged to lead a full life. Children should not be kept out of public schools and should play with their friends as usual. The epileptic must never be put into a position of feeling that he is "different."

In prevention of epilepsy as regards marriage and having children, each patient must receive individual consideration. Only the predisposition to epilepsy is inherited, not the disease itself. The chances that a child of epileptic parents will have epilepsy are about 1 in 40; and that a child will have more than one convulsion during childhood about 1 in 70. If an acquired cause is responsible for epilepsy in parents, these changes are greatly reduced.

If the number of cases of infectious diseases that involve the brain were reduced, a great step toward controlling acquired epilepsy would be made. Many of these diseases are the result of traffic accidents, occupational accidents, and war injuries. Concentrated efforts to reduce asphyxia and injuries at birth should be made.

Psychologically the illness may have a great effect. Approximately 80 per cent of all victims of epilepsy are capable of leading normal lives; those persons about them should recognize that epilepsy is not communicable and not a sign of insanity. Unfortunately, through misunderstanding of the disease, a person with epilepsy may find himself shunned by other people and discriminated against in employment. Concealment of the disease may deny many epileptics the advantages of education and marriage. Not only must the public be educated about epilepsy but the epileptic himself must learn to have self-confidence and courage.

Many people with epilepsy have achieved great heights of accomplishment—for example, Richard Wagner, Algernon Swinburne, Vincent van Gogh, and Hector Berlioz. A new organization, Epilepsy: Self-Help, sponsored and financed by the Variety Club Foundation to Combat Epilepsy, has been organized for people with epilepsy to meet for mutual association, understanding, and encouragement. The self-confidence of the epileptic can be strengthened when he has an opportunity to discuss his problems with persons who understand them. For information about epilepsy, write to the National Epilepsy League, 130 North Wells Street, Chicago, Illinois.

MUSCULAR DYSTROPHY

Many different conditions can affect the muscles of the body since they are intimately associated with the bones, the metabolism of the body, and its general structure. However, certain serious diseases of muscles have become of great concern. All of them involve muscular wasting and paralysis. Any tissue of the body that is not used tends to waste away. Therefore paralysis of the nerves supplying muscles or of the blood circulation to the muscles might result in wasting of the muscle. However, a number of conditions called muscular dystrophies are quite different both in origin and scope from ordinary instances of muscle wasting or atrophy. Physicians have classified various dystrophies in many different ways, depending on the muscles concerned and the changes that are seen when the tissues are studied under the microscope. Some classifications divide these conditions into the age epochs in which they occur. Thus there is a childhood type, a hereditary type, and others which affect mostly the muscles of the hands and the feet. In each of these conditions the person should have a most careful examination, if possible not only by the family doctor but also by doctors who specialize in orthopedic surgery and in neurology. This is emphasized because the ultimate decision as to what to do to secure the most benefit will depend on a fairly accurate determination of exactly what is wrong.

An organization called the National Foundation for Neuromuscular Diseases, Inc. (250 West 57th Street, New York, New York 10019) is concerned with all of the conditions of this type, including some related conditions. They have described so well the disorders included under these classifications that their report is presented herewith:

TAY-SACH'S DISEASE

"Affects infants before first year of age. Progressive mental deterioration and amaurosis (blindness) usually complete by second year; idiocy, usually in extreme degree. Motor paralysis and spasticity are usually manifest and, toward the end, a decerebrate rigidity may be observed. This is a progressive disease. Death occurs before the third year of life."

RHEUMATOID ARTHRITIS

"A chronic disease which may begin at any age, runs a relapsing course, and ultimately can result in severe crippling and muscular atrophy."

AMYOTONIA CONGENITA

"A disease of unknown origin characterized by flaccidity and weakness of the muscles, noted either at time of birth or during first few months of life. About one third striken die the first year. Most die within five years, usually from pneumonia. The underlying defect is thought to be absence of muscular development, due to degeneration of the anterior horn cells. Condition is often familial. No known cure."

FRIEDREICH'S ATAXIA

"A hereditary, degenerative condition which develops gradually in the first or second decade of life. Although a familial incidence is most common, dominant and recessive types of hereditary transmission have been reported, as well as sporadic cases. Attacks both spinal cord and certain parts of the brain. Affects lower limbs, the stance is unsteady, there is tremor and blurred speech. Typical case has onset between six and fourteen years of age. By second decade there is incapacity, and life expectancy rarely exceeds twenty years from date of onset. Intercurrent infection is the usual cause of death. Origin unknown. Cure unknown."

DERMATOMYOSITIS

"A disease of the connective tissues, which affects the muscles directly. An acute, subacute, or chronic disease of unknown origin characterized by a gradual onset. Premonitory symptoms are followed by edema, dermatitis, and multiple muscle inflammation. The common denominator of this syndrome is acute or subacute degeneration of the skeletal muscles.

"(a) Acute, more commonly seen in children.

"(b) Chronic polymyositis, begins in the peripheral limb muscles and is associated with dermal (skin) involvement. Chronic stage characterized by atrophy and fibrosis. Both dermal and muscular involvement. Cutaneous lesions and muscle dysfunction. Discoloration, resembling psoriasis.

"The course is progressive in about fifty per cent of the cases. Death due to cardiac failure, respiratory inefficiency or pneumonia. Some victims die in first year, but others survive with varying degrees of crippling."

WILSON'S DISEASE

"A familial, coarsely nodular cirrhosis of the liver, associated with progressive damage to the nervous system, resulting in tremor, rigidity and marked incoordination of speech, swallowing, and all movements. Onset in childhood. The disease is progressive and ultimately fatal."

AMYOTROPHIC LATERAL SCLEROSIS

"A disease of unknown origin with a rapidly progressive course; combination of anterior horn cell and pyramidal tract disease, the former involving both the spinal cord and brain stem. Drastic reduction of A.H. cells in the spinal cord; cells of medulla (brain stem) are diseased; cervical cord most affected. Onset comes with weakness of hands and arms, then bulbar symptoms, difficulty in talking and swallowing, followed by weakness and spasticity of legs, or combinations of all these symptoms. Always fatal, death usually occurs in a few years. No known treatment."

BRAIN TUMORS (CERTAIN FORMS)

"General symptoms are headache, vomiting, crossing of the eyes (diplopia), focal symptoms depend upon the location of the tumor. Four thousand deaths annually. Treatment is by surgical removal. In many cases in childhood the tumor may be completely removed."

PROGRESSIVE MUSCULAR ATROPHY

"This disease, strongly hereditary, but occurring in isolated forms at times, is characterized by progressive weakness involving the feet and legs, with eventual extension to the bones and arms, associated with muscular atrophy, reflex loss, and sensory disturbance. There is a widespread involvement, damaging muscles, peripheral nerves, anterior roots, and horn cells. The process develops early in childhood. Difficulty in walking; pains and burning or stinging sensation in the legs common and manifested early. Examination reveals atrophy of the foot muscles, development of claw foot; hand muscles become involved, causing atrophy, claw hand, and thinning of forearms. The disease runs a slow, progressive course. Treatment is symptomatic, with drugs, analgesics, therapy. No known cure."

CHAPTER 36

Mental Disorders

LOUIS D. BOSHES, M.D.

Mental illness has always occurred among people in one form or another and in varying degrees; in recent years these have become among the most important health problems. The unusual rise is probably associated with many new and vast social changes characteristic of our times. About 10 per cent of our population or about 20,000,000 people in the United States suffer from some form of mental illness or personality disturbance. Of this total, some 4,000,000 are suffering from specific mental illness, while the other 16,000,000 have various forms of personality disturbance.

Estimates indicate that 3 per cent of the people in the United States or about 6,000,000 persons are affected, some mildly, with mental retardation. About 500,000 are so retarded that they require constant care and supervision. They may be limited in their ability to take care of themselves or engage in any type of productive work or activity. The 5,500,000 others are persons of only mild or moderate disability. At the present rate of prevalence perhaps 150,000 babies born each year will be regarded as mentally retarded at some time in their lives.

About 950,000 patients are in institutions, 700,000 for mental illness and over 300,000 for mental retardation. Each year nearly 2,000,000 people receive treatment in institutions for the mentally ill and mentally retarded. Until 1955 the number of patients entering mental hospitals and the rate for 100,000 population had both risen uninterruptedly since early in the century. In recent years the trend has somewhat reversed. While admissions have continued to increase, the probability of early or eventual release has also increased, because of a new concept and philosophy of the management of mental illness. Second or readmissions have risen at a much faster rate than first admissions.

Up to 65 per cent of patients who are admitted to general hospitals and up to 70 per cent of patients who are seen on an office basis by their private physicians are afflicted with emotional illness and other personality disturbances. Mental illness and these personality disturbances are usu-

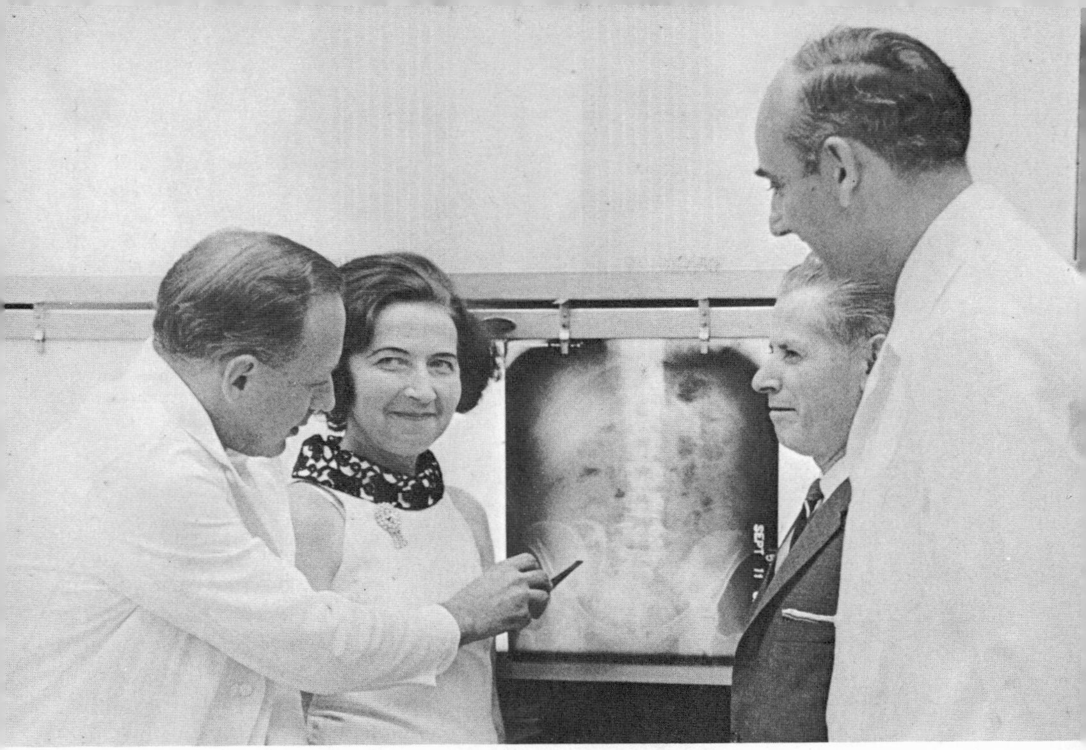

PLATE **100.** Mrs. Kaufman Russek, Montefiore's first kidney transplant patient, is shown an X-ray picture of her new kidney by Dr. Marvin Gliedman, Chief of Surgery, who performed the operation. Looking on are Mr. Russek and Dr. Robert Soberman, head of Montefiore's Renal Services. *(Courtesy of Montefiore Hospital and Medical Center, New York, and Ed Bagwell.)*

PLATE **101.** Patient suffering from chronic kidney failure undergoes treatment with artificial kidney machine under supervision of specially trained nurses, Margaret Houlihan (left) and Janet Carrelle. *(Courtesy of Montefiore Hospital and Medical Center, New York, and Ed Bagwell.)*

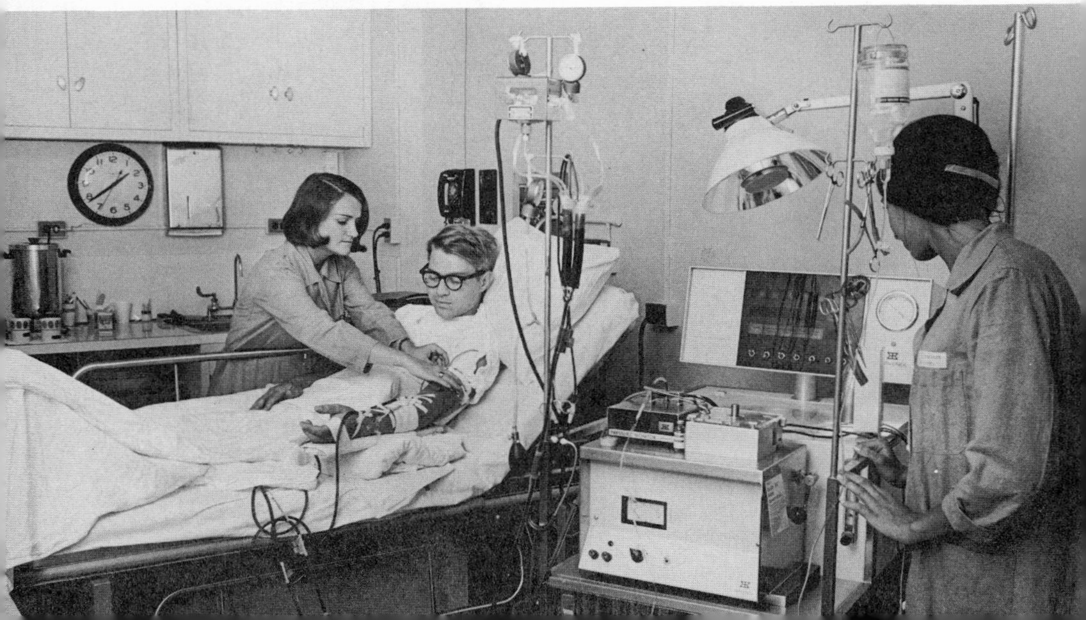

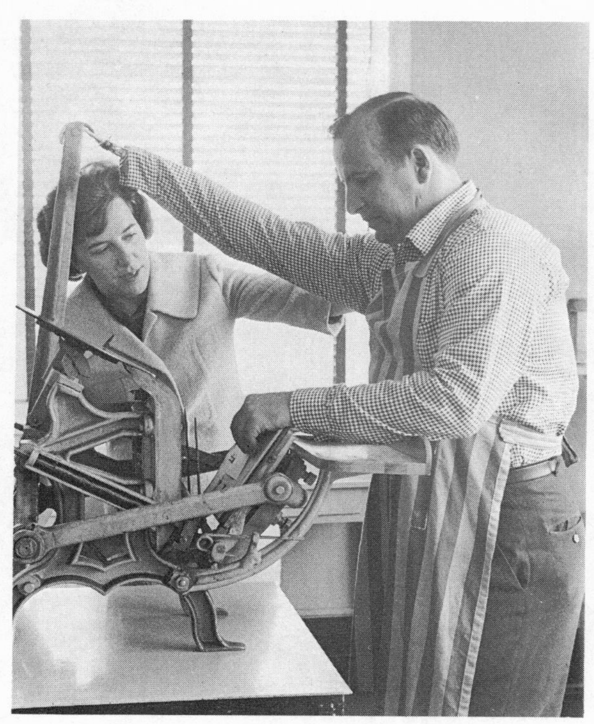

PLATE **102.** New hand, new skills. After losing his arm, he needs self-confidence and faith in his ability to do useful work. Operation of a printing press in the work-oriented occupational therapy department of the ICD gives him the strength and skills to use the arm made for him by the Institute's Prosthetic and Orthotic Laboratories. *(Institute for the Crippled and Disabled, New York City.)*

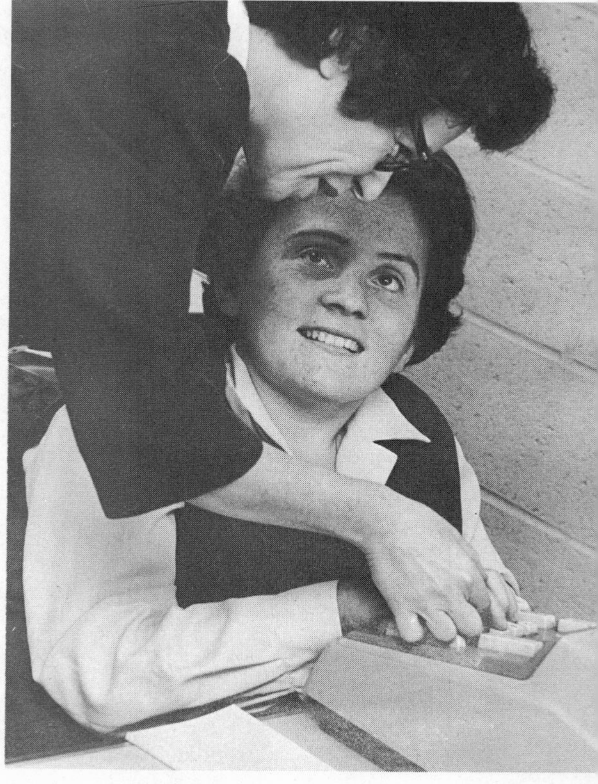

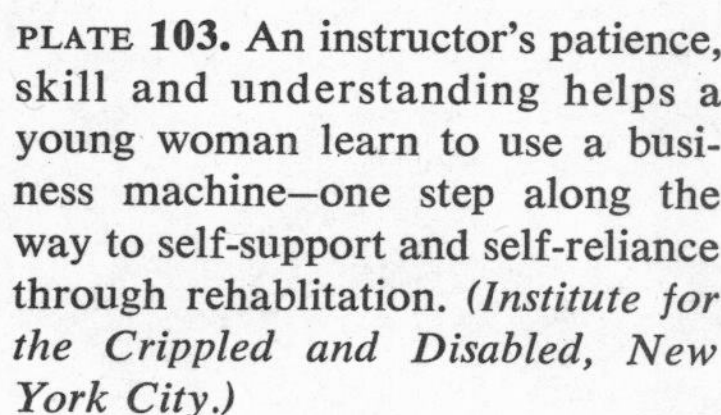

PLATE **103.** An instructor's patience, skill and understanding helps a young woman learn to use a business machine—one step along the way to self-support and self-reliance through rehablitation. *(Institute for the Crippled and Disabled, New York City.)*

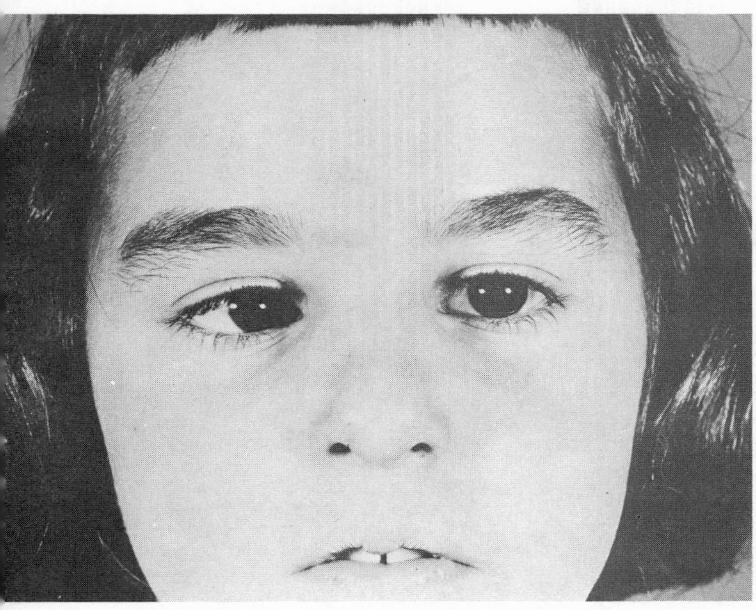

PLATE **104.** Strabismus, otherwise known as "crossed eyes."

PLATE **105.** With corrective treatment, cross-eyed children can get back normal sight. *(Courtesy of the National Society for the Prevention of Blindness, Inc.)*

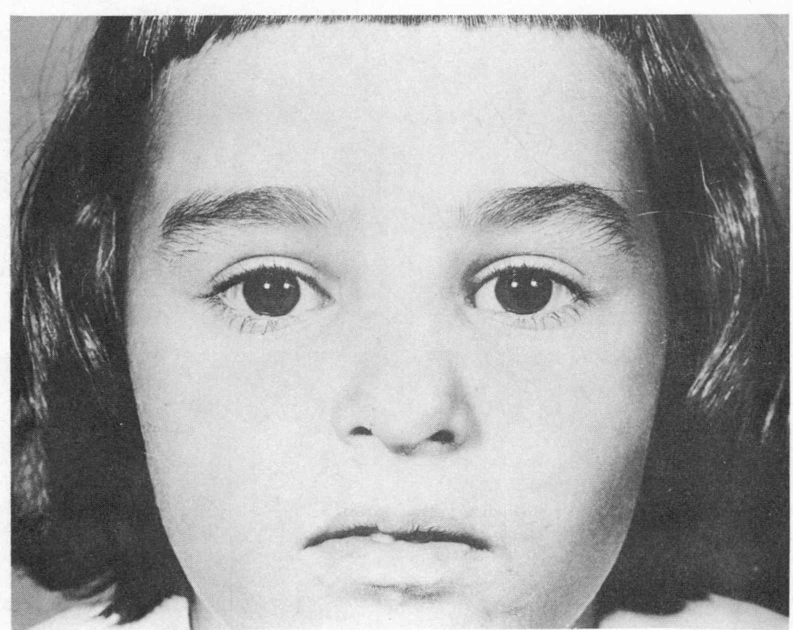

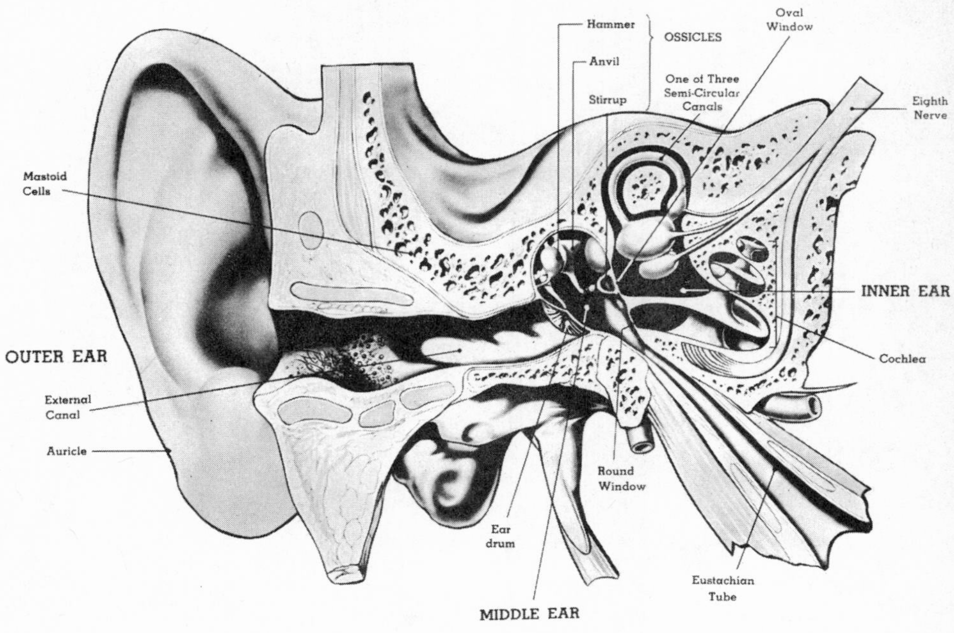

PLATE **106.** Anatomical construction of the ear. *(Courtesy Sonotone Corporation.)*

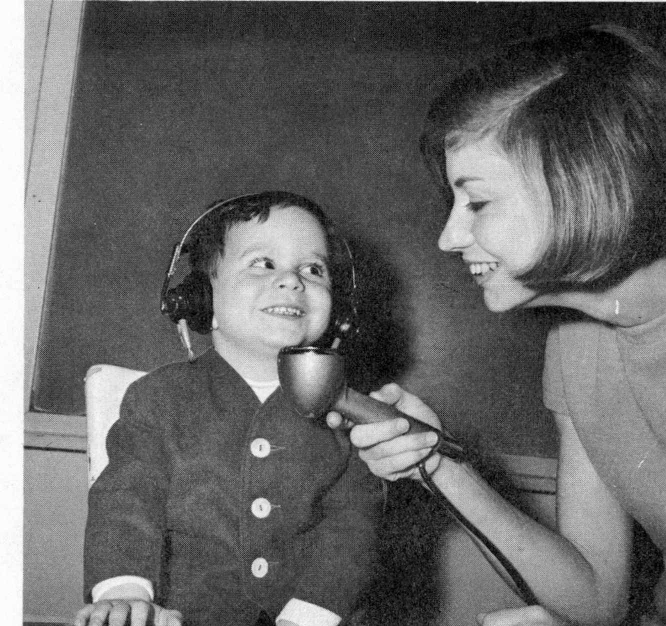

PLATE **107.** Hearing and speech therapy begun at an early age (2 to 3 years) helps the child with impaired hearing to develop his speech and language abilities so that he may be able to attend a regular school. *(New York League for the Hard of Hearing.)*

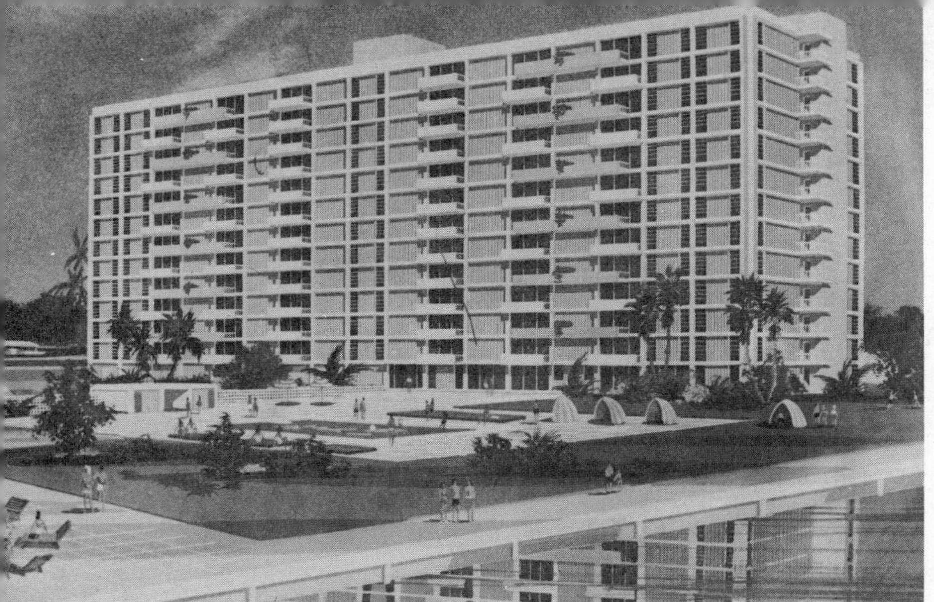

PLATE **108.** Parkinson's Disease has been one of the neglected medical problems in our country. It is only in recent years that an awareness of the tremendous number of patients involved has developed. Parkinson's disease is considered one of the major medical problems because one and a half million people are involved. The National Parkinson Foundation's M. L. Seidman Tower of Hope, located in Miami, Florida, is a fifteen-story building dedicated to research and rehabilitation—the only facility of its kind in the world. It is now possible to have patients and their families as well as staff members and visiting medical specialists under one roof. The purpose of this new facility is chiefly focused toward research and the development of new techniques in rehabilitation. *(National Parkinson Foundation, Inc.)*

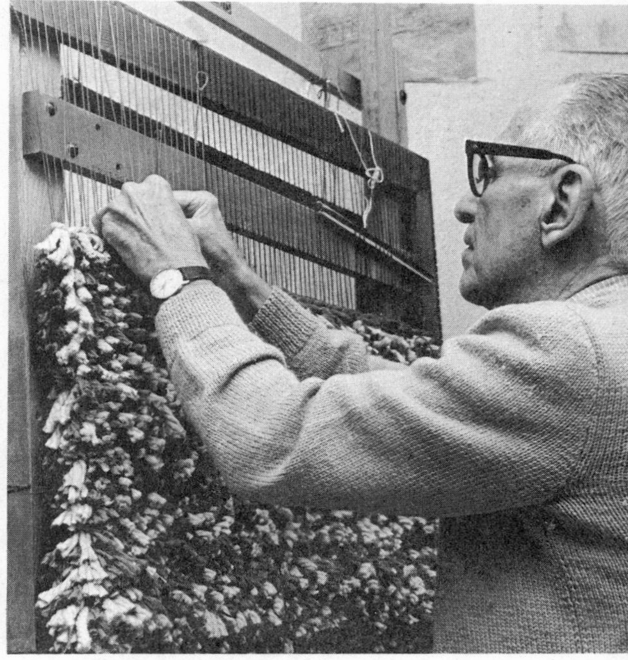

PLATE **109.** The problems most commonly incurred by the Parkinson patient are rigidity (stiffness); tremor (shaking); bowels and walking difficulty; slowness of movement; and stooped posture. To offset these disabling problems, specific treatment needs and therapeutic aims are formulated for each patient. He then participates in a program of activities designed to retrain him to the fullest extent of his capabilities. For improved coordination and dexterity of finger movements, patients learn to use the upright loom for rug making. *(National Parkinson Foundation, Inc.)*

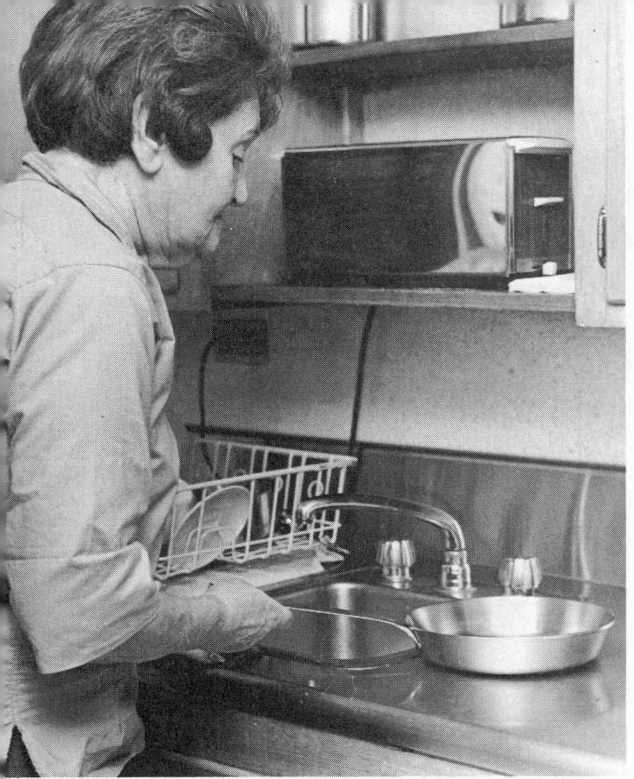

PLATE **110.** Effective therapy for these patients lies in a special framework of individual medical evaluation and prescription. Parkinson patients indulge in various purposeful activities to improve their coordination, speed, strength, and endurance. Kitchen activity stimulates independence in self and family-care ability. *(National Parkinson Foundation, Inc.)*

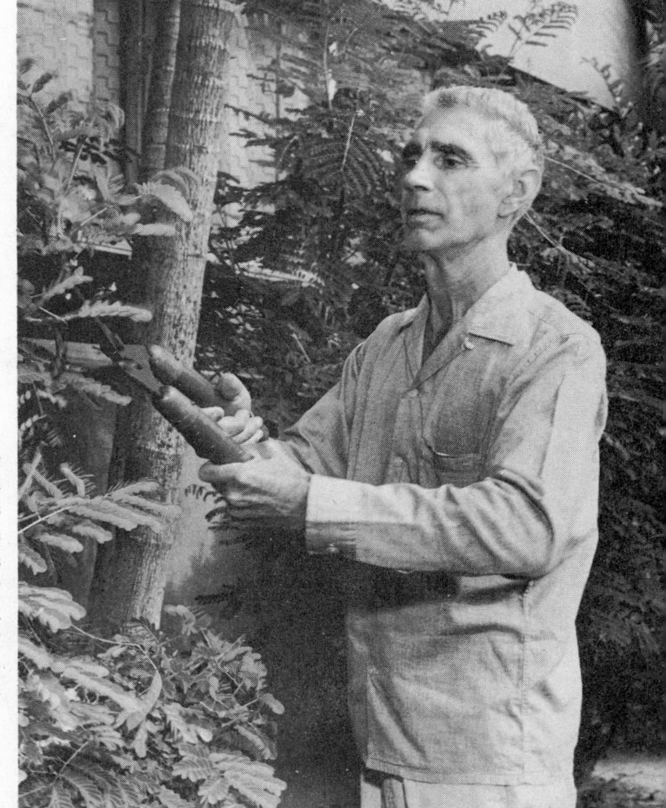

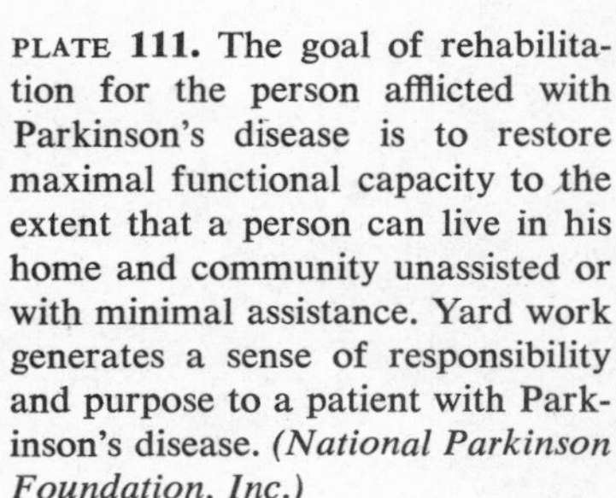

PLATE **111.** The goal of rehabilitation for the person afflicted with Parkinson's disease is to restore maximal functional capacity to the extent that a person can live in his home and community unassisted or with minimal assistance. Yard work generates a sense of responsibility and purpose to a patient with Parkinson's disease. *(National Parkinson Foundation, Inc.)*

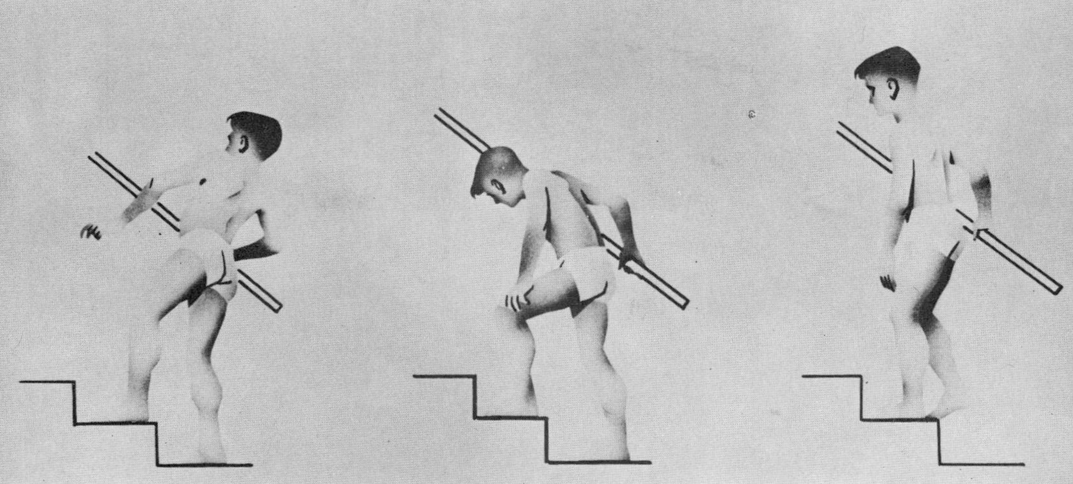

PLATE **112.** Difficulty in climbing stairs may be one of the early symptoms of muscular dystrophy. (1) The railing is grasped for support and used to pull body up. The leg is lifted by tilting the body, and using all possible muscles. (2) The leverage afforded by placing the hand on the knee assists in resting the body and dragging up the other leg. (3) The ascent is made one step at a time, one foot does not pass the other. *(Muscular Dystrophy Associations of America.)*

PLATE **113.** A probing six-year investigation by the Institute for the Crippled and Disabled, which enlisted the financial support of the United Cerebral Palsy Association of New York City, Inc. has revealed additional types of work that CP victims can do. Proof that almost half of the cerebral palsied in the program are capable of gainful employment was one of the significant results. *(Institute for the Crippled and Disabled, New York City.)*

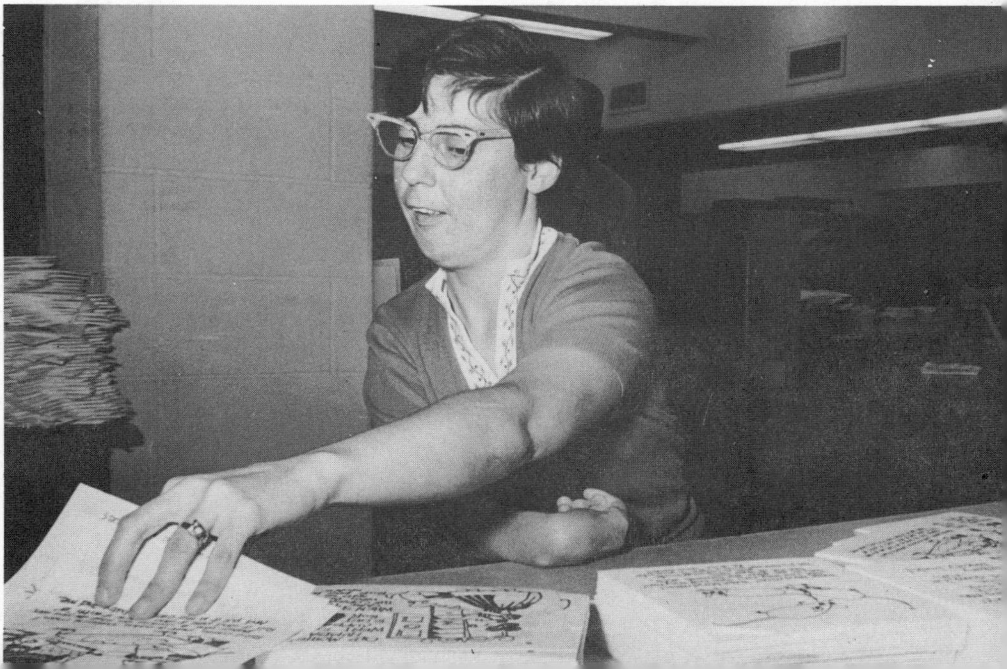

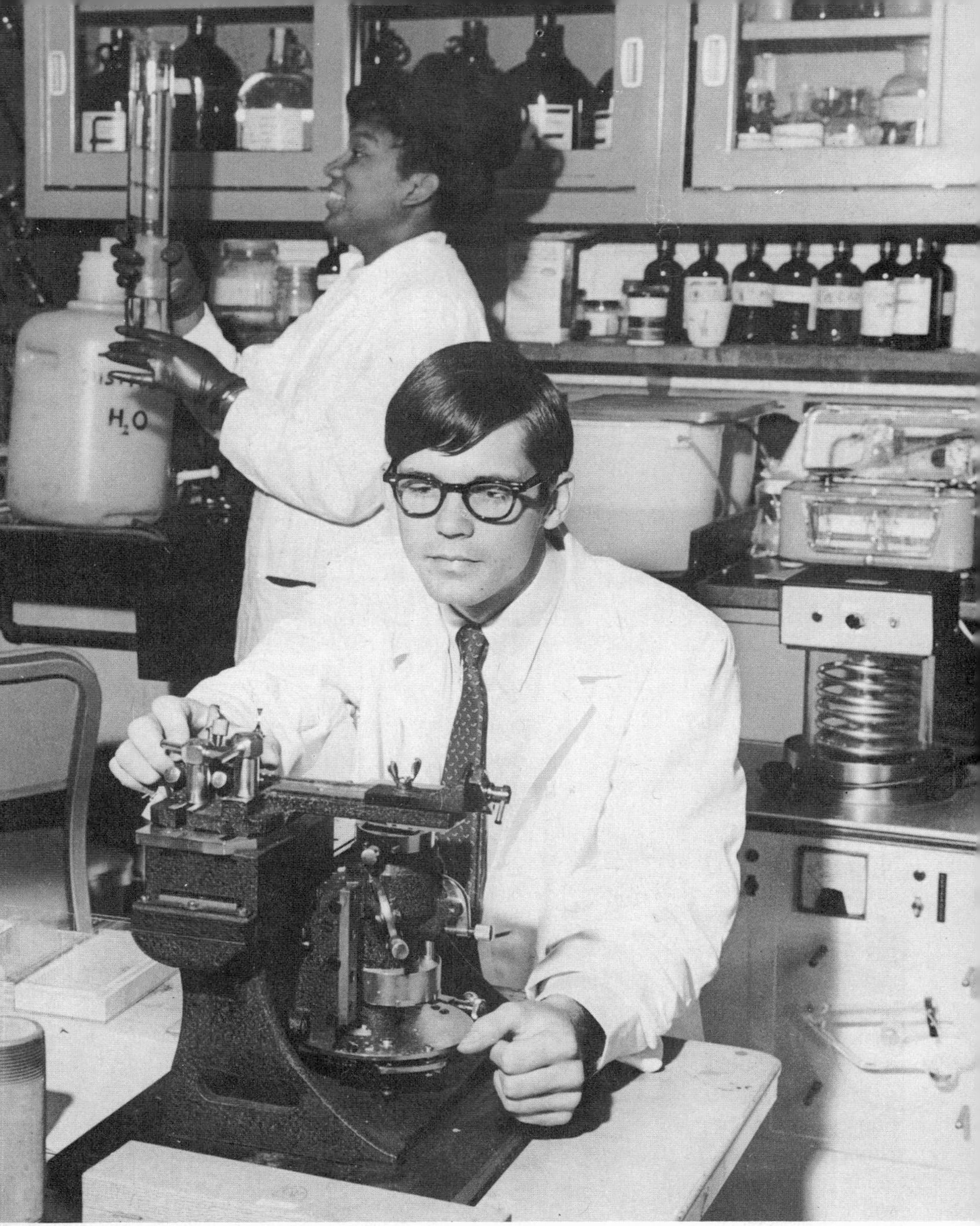

PLATE **114.** A technician processes slides of brain tissue. Research is under way in many areas relating to diseases of the central nervous system, as well as muscle disorders. *(Institute for the Crippled and Disabled, New York City.)*

ally significant in people with criminal behavior, such as suicidal tendencies, and even in persons seeking divorce.

Over 50 per cent of all beds in hospitals in the United States are occupied by mental patients. The chance for being hospitalized for mental illness is roughly 1 to 10 sometime during the lifetime. The chance of being released from a mental hospital within the first year is good, but the chance for a release subsequent to the first year seems to be decreasing rapidly. Well over 20 per cent of patients resident in our state mental hospitals system have been there 20 to 25 years or more, 40 per cent for ten years or more, and some 60 per cent of the total resident population has been hospitalized for five years or more.

The current cost of mental illness in the United States is estimated at about $2.8 billion a year. This figure includes both the direct costs in terms of patient care and the indirect cost of loss of earnings. It costs more than $1 billion a year to care for the mentally ill. The financial needs of the patient's family often place burdens on public welfare services, thus developing into great expenditures.

AGE OF ONSET OF MENTAL ILLNESS AND OTHER PERSONALITY DISTURBANCES

Every age group includes some mental illness or other personality disturbance. However, only a few and rare cases of psychosis occur before age 15. Schizophrenia, also known as Dementia Praecox, is the "psychosis of youth and early adult life," beginning usually between ages 15 and 30 years. The most common psychoses seen in the middle age group between ages 35 and 60 years are manic depressive psychosis, alcoholic psychosis, the paranoid state, general paresis, and a few others. The first three develop more frequently between ages 40 and 55; the last two are prevalent between ages 50 and 55 years. After 65, at which time many anatomic changes are expected in people, the common cerebroarteriosclerosis and senile psychoses appear.

Many people have minor emotional disturbances that are unrecognized but eventually become sufficiently obvious to affect the general health. Numerous people in public life, in industry, and in labor manage to get along in spite of difficulty of adjustments. A vast percentage of these will come to doctors as patients primarily because of emotional disorders, but yet these complaints are referred to various organs of the body. Phobias, anxieties, frustrations, disappointments, rejections, dissatisfactions, or other conditions may appear as functional symptoms to include headaches, dizziness, visual difficulty, gastrointestinal complaints, respiratory problems, or asthma. Treatment must therefore be concerned with the emotional as well as the physical spheres once the relationship has been established.

In the United States, people are living much longer than they did in 1900. As they grow older they go through emotional experiences which require psychiatric care. Certainly this group requires guidance from doctors or paramedical personnel who have become adept in the management of emotional illness.

One of every ten people will require some emotional advice or guidance during his lifetime. More than half of the veterans in Veterans Administration Hospitals at present are in the psychiatric classification. Almost 40 per cent of the men released from the Army for medical reasons were discharged with psychiatric diagnoses. Of all medical separations within the military service 51 per cent were due to personality disturbances.

Not uncommonly people become self-critical and self-condemnatory for reasons they do not recognize or understand. Social and cultural considerations which regulate human sex behavior are far more rigid than the biological considerations. These considerations define what is moral much more definitely than do biological and medical sciences.

In different parts of the United States, attitudes of the population vary as to the ordinary relationships between the sexes. In one part of the country a married man's having lunch with a married woman other than his wife is considered a violation of established conventions. In other areas of marital society, particularly in larger cities, such meetings are well within the ordinary pattern of everyday social existence.

When a young man moves from one area to another, a long time may be needed for him to find out what the restrictions on conduct are, and what is considered sensible and suitable within the new community. Until 1915, people paid little attention to inhibitions and did not worry much about such matters. Since then public education and psychological discussions have created fear among people to such a degree that they are becoming more inhibited. As a result, they are infantile in their emotional attitudes and are likely to become dependent on their parents or parent substitutes. In some cases the substitute will be an aunt or an uncle, a governess or a nurse. From these adults they will expect tolerance. Often men and women grow older retaining these infantile attitudes until a loss of a parent or some forceful separation from a parental figure causes a severe tragedy in their lives. They lose the strong influence and are insecure, ineffectual, and inadequate without this force. A child who was always known as a "teacher's pet" will grow to become the "boss's favorite" in his job.

If a child develops some sense of personal responsibility, he can always rid himself of this situation through an excuse. As children grow older, they maintain this childish attitude and find excuses for their failures and alibis for their weakness and inadequacies. They may tend to "pass the buck" whenever confronted with difficult situations. At other times, they will call it the "breaks," the "fates," "lady luck," or some similar term. A child who passes his period of puberty with a development of secondary sexual characteristics in his body really goes through two periods which can be called adolescence, including the early and the late types. In early adolescence, the child begins to have a drive for self-application and assertion, and begins to resent parental domination by small acts of rebellion. Just as a male animal will reveal his finest characteristics to attract the female, so will a boy in early adolescence show off and indulge in contests in which he can demonstrate his superiority to the girl he intends to impress or to his parents. His room will be filled with trophies won at the track, at the swimming pool, at bowling, or at golf, whereas the girl's room begins to be decorated with programs from dances, souvenirs from parties, and knickknacks accumulated on dates. The larger her bulletin board the more important she is to herself and, she hopes, to others.

As late adolescence develops, "dating" becomes the most important aspect of life. If this passes on to what the boy or girl will call "going steady," many difficult emotional situations may develop. The parents will try to get their opinions into this situation and try to dominate it because of purely emotional reactions or economic or religious reasons. As a result, these situations may lead to emotional disturbances in the young. They mark the life of the growing youth and have a deep effect upon him for many years thereafter. An adult is expected to have a balanced perspective in life and should be able to adjust to various social roles, but adults, much as children, still require love or affection, security, recognition, and appreciation and must have a well-established relationship with other people. However, if the child has failed to mature, he will depend heavily on the affection of others. If he requires definite signs of favoritism he is unlikely to be able to develop a satisfactory parent relationship and may react emotionally to the situations which he cannot solve and may depend upon the aid of others.

MENTAL HEALTH IN INDUSTRY

Suitable adjustments of workers to their surroundings are important. Many large industries have employment interviewers who have knowledge of the varied positions within the company. They are expected to select the type of person necessary for the job, one who will best fill the need under the most satisfactory of conditions. Through experience, and certainly by training, the experts recognize the prospective employee who is not fit to hold the job because of mental disturbance. What the employer wants is a worker who can respond to any particular problem or procedure in the job for which he is seeking employment. The executive rarely wants trouble with personality problems. He relegates these problems to his personnel director who normally is adequate to handle them.

MENTAL INSTITUTIONS

Departures from the average mentality in past centuries were usually considered to be religious or even legal problems. It was not until well into the seventeenth century that insanity was recognized as being a sickness. Not much was known about the symptoms except that the person was disturbed, and even violent and required institutionalization. For many years a doctor could only see that the emotionally disturbed patient was given humane care in a suitable institution. This institution therefore became known as an "asylum." Pinel, a great French psychiatrist, introduced warmth, kindness, and understanding into the management of patients in institutions. He brought a new concept into the management of the mentally disturbed. Mental illness was found to be not one sickness but many illnesses with many different symptoms. Some involvements were mild, others, severe. Classification of the various kinds of mental illnesses developed giving them recognizable descriptions and labels. Physicians devoted considerable attention to description, classification, and the diagnosis of the many divisions and subdivisions that were becoming recognizable. However none of this study did anything in getting the patient better.

Many physicians approached the problem as of physical illness. They looked within the physical make-up of the patient's body for motivation that underlay human behavior. In many mentally disturbed people they found physical illness or disorders of physical function that seemed to account for the symptoms. An example was general paresis, or syphilis of the brain. The patient's brain was invaded by a parasite called the Treponema pallidum or spirochete. In other abnormal mental conditions, even the most elaborate scientific study failed to produce an adequate specific physical cause.

Other doctors reasoned that if unusual displays of behavior did not have a physical cause, they would seek a cause in the thought processes. This was the first attempt to look at the person from a "whole" point of view.

The symptoms of people with various mental disorders have a close, if slightly disguised, resemblance to the personality and character that these people had for many years before they became mentally ill. The symptoms of mental illness, when properly studied and interpreted seem to be exaggerations of similar symptoms which they had since childhood. In many families such annoying behavior seems to be passed off and considered to be just the routine habits of a small child. There is however a close connection between adult mental disturbance and development of healthy "patterns" or "habits" of personality during the first few years of childhood. Often one may predict whether or not a child will become an adult who will go through life evenly. A child whose "patterns" of personality enable him to meet disappointments, rejections, and frustration in a healthy fashion will probably grow to be an adult free from mental disorder. Or a child may develop patterns that will not permit him to face disappointments, frustration, or rejection later. As a result, he is unable to adjust himself wholesomely as does the other child. He cannot face difficult situations. Instead of fighting he flees and then may withdraw into some form of mental illness.

CAUSE OF MENTAL ILLNESS

Why do people behave as they do? One patient may develop mental symptoms because he lost his job and his money. Another may have symptoms attributable to a loss in love. Many of these alleged causes are not the real causes but merely precipitating factors. The loss of money or rejection in love were only the last straws which broke the camel's back. The final strain on the adjustive capacity that had never been too strong initially resulted in mental disturbance. Everyone who has lost his money or been disappointed in love does not develop a mental disturbance. Many men and women who are faced with similar difficulties every day manage to adjust to them. In most functional mental disorders (those for which it is not possible to find a physical cause), the true basic cause is the failure of the patient to adjust to stresses or strains that may face him.

When a child is born into this world he brings with him a variety of psychological baggage. Part of this is his intellectual endowment. From the point of view of mental health, emotional tendencies inherited from his immediate ancestors including his parents and grandparents are important. Besides he inherits primitive, savage instincts and "drives" as his share of the heritage of all mankind. These so-called "drives" or primitive instinctive feelings include the instinct of self-preservation and race-preservation. In early days of man's development, a painful struggle for survival between man and man prevailed. People were uninhibited. A man would kill just to possess something: food, a woman, or a child. There was little to hinder people except the one restraint of superior physical strength. The tribal codes did not recognize feelings of compassion or civilized thinking.

As man became more civilized, he began to realize the first stirrings of finer needs not to be satisfied by physical forces. Some in the tribe yearned for the "good old days" when there were no restraints. Mental conflicts developed, a conflict between desire and duty, between savage whims of instinct that unfortunately were expressed in crude, direct form without pretense of disguising them and the dawning realization that the demands of individual and social progress called for the repression and the transformation of some of these primitive instincts into more socially acceptable ones.

Physicians know that the human still harbors vestigial remains or remnants of organs that do not have any function. They may have served a vitally necessary purpose in the human body millions of years ago. The human appendix is such an organ; no one knows of its function today. The psychiatrist feels that modern man carries within his subconscious certain vestigial remains of ancient instinct and impulses that once served a useful purpose.

A child is born with certain psychological traits deep in his unconscious that carry over from some of his primitive drives. The modern nursery school teacher insists that the young child is completely selfish (selfish, that is, when viewed from adult standards), and completely antisocial as well. The infant is accused of being the most selfish being in the world. A baby's cry will bring his parents and grandparents to his crib. During the first two or three years of life, the child wants to do what he wants, when he wants, and will not permit interference. The mental life at this period is much nearer to that of its primitive caveman ancestors than it is to his immediate generation, and he tries to act accordingly. He demands immediate and quick gratification of his desires. If he is hungry for attention, he demands to be cuddled immediately. If he is uncomfortable from a full bladder, he wets himself at once and, of course, receives attention. This little, self-centered person does not consider the feelings of others; his chief aim is to obtain pleasure at all times and to avoid pain.

As he grows older, his mother begins to train him in proper eating and toilet habits. She attempts to teach him to control his needs and his wants. He has to wait for a more correct and appropriate time for this expression. She also, lovingly, but firmly, gets across to him that he can't always have his way and that self-gratification is possible only through consideration of others or that it is dependent on the will of someone who is older and stronger. Gradually he is required to submit to the process known as "the civilization of instinct"; he becomes a more socialized creature.

One should not however be caught off guard and make the mistake of thinking that he has for all time lost these desires or that he has suddenly become altruistic because he gradually checks some of his primitive desires and shows a willingness to give in to others. True, he has learned to his advantage to make certain concessions to his mother who has power either to give or withhold pleasure or approve or punish him. He concludes that the gratification of his pleasure must come in a roundabout manner after first "placating" his mother who stands before him in a role of authority.

Thus, genuine unselfishness and altruism have their beginnings. This child learns that full gratification must require the cooperation of others; he becomes altruistic only as he begins to realize that it pays to be so. He must submit gracefully, it is true, to the "civilization of the instinct" only with a minimum of protest. The same instincts are always there under the surface of consciousness, and no matter how old he becomes, he is forever trying to shape his mental life in accordance with what we know the followers of the school of dynamic psychiatry call "the pleasure principle." Both seem to be pulling within the unconscious mind of a person in different directions. Swayed by the "pleasure principle," he seeks to act in such a way as to ensure immediate gratification of his primitive instincts and desires but to avoid as much unpleasantness in the process as is possible. In the opposite direction, he is confronted with the reality principle which tends to shape his mental life according to the demands of necessity as personified by the power of the parent and later by the demands, expectations, and customs of society. Dr. Abraham Meyerson, a Boston psychiatrist, said of these conflicts:

"Every human being is a pot boiling with desires, passions, lusts, wishes, purposes, ideas, and emotions, some of which he clearly recognizes and clearly admits, and some of which he does not clearly recognize and which he would deny. These desires, passions, etc., are not in harmony with one another; they are often irreconcilable, and one has to be smothered for the sake of the other. Thus, a sex feeling that is not legitimate, an illicit, forbidden love has to be conquered for the purpose of being religious or good, or the desire to be respected. So one may struggle against hatred for a person whom one should love—a husband, a wife, an invalid parent, or child whose care is a burden—and one refuses to recognize that there is such a struggle. So also one may seek to suppress jealousy, envy of the nearest and dearest: soul-stirring, forbidden passions; secret revolt against morality and law which may (and often does) rage in the most puritanical breast."

In the theory of the subconscious these undesired thoughts, feelings, passions, and wishes are suppressed and pushed into the innermost recesses of the being, out of the light of conscious personality, but nevertheless acting on that personality, distorting it, wearying it."

The real task of childhood is to bring a trial balance between primitive biological desires on the one hand, and the demands of society as symbolized by one's mother and father as authoritative figures on the other. If a child can bring about such a balance, we say he is well adjusted and has good mental health. However, if he cannot achieve such a balance, the degree of resulting maladjustment depends on the strength of the primitive impulse that grips him and on the severity of the social demands that are made upon him.

ADJUSTMENT OF BEHAVIOR

The ability to adjust oneself to experience that thwarts one's desires or primitive drives is an ability which is partially acquired during childhood. Heredity does play a part in certain mental disorders. The modern psychiatrist does not wholly disbelieve in the effect of heredity. However much research will be necessary before we can say definitely what traits man inherits and which ones he forms after birth as imitations of or reactions to similar traits displayed by his parents.

Modern opinion is tending to believe that the types of training a child receives from his parents during his early, elastic years when his personality is in the process of being shaped will determine greatly how successful he is going to be in harmonizing the conflicts that have been listed and how well he will adjust to them. For this reason, increasing attention is being paid to problems of mental hygiene and child guidance in groups of normal boys and girls. Parents, schoolteachers, athletic instructors, spiritual leaders, and others may help the child form habits or patterns of personality so firm and strong that these will aid him in meeting and adjusting to those inevitable frustrations in life that are bound to appear.

The formation of sturdy patterns of personality in these early years helps explain why one person is able to adjust in a healthy manner to a distressing experience such as the loss of a loved one, a job, or an inability to attain some cherished goal, while another, faced with a similar experience, cannot adjust to it and expresses his resulting maladjustment in symptoms in some form of mental disorder. A child of six may be taught by his parents to develop healthy patterns of making decisions and in finding security in the product of his own accomplishments rather than depending on the personal favoritism of others. This same child, when he grows older and passes into the adolescent stage still has these patterns remaining with him and is able to cope with the mixture of adolescent emotions (made up of a desire to grow up to be independent versus the wish to remain in the sheltered, protected state of childhood) with only a minimum of difficulty. This ease of adjustment will likely remain also in his adult years when he finds himself able to meet adult responsibilities, disappointments, rejections, frustrations, dissatisfactions, and rebuffs; he will not flee from these or handle them by developing neurotic or psychotic symptoms.

Another child of six may have a mother whose own emotional satisfactions in life can be gratified only through the realization that someone else needs and depends upon her. She may develop an overprotective and oversolicitous attitude toward the child which keeps him tied to her; he is unable to become normally independent. The physical and intellectual role in this child continues, but his emotional growth tends to remain static or even regress. He may reach the physical level of adolescence, even the age, but because his principal patterns of personality are still the dependent childish ones of an early age, he is unable to adjust to adolescent demands and expectations and thus produces a variety of symptoms to express this maladjustment. Such symptoms sometimes take the form of quarrelsomeness, defiance, or rebellion, or may be expressed in the quiet but ominous other forms of withdrawal into a seclusive, shut-in, and solitary existence in which he forsakes the discomfort of trying to adjust to the demands of the world's reality. He recedes to a daydream world of fancy and imagination.

MENTAL TRAINING IN CHILDHOOD

Correct instruction in mental hygiene in childhood, therefore, becomes important if good mental health is to be maintained and mental disorder avoided. Most vital is the process of aiding a child to form strong healthy patterns of personality and to assist him in creating a true sense of security for himself. This does not mean the feeling of physical or even economic security only but also emotional security. To feel emotionally secure, a person must develop at least two firm convictions: first, that he is recognized as an individual who is loved and valued by others, and second, that he really belongs to and is accepted and needed by the group of which he has become an integral part. Most important this implies acceptance and love by his family, later by his schoolmates, then by the neighborhood in which he lives, and finally by society. The second conviction is that he can be confident of success in doing at least one thing well. It matters little what this is, providing that the person is able to do it and do it alone through his own efforts and is not dependent for success on the favoritism of someone else. To be able to accomplish this means a feeling of true accomplishment and the poise and self-confidence that bespeak the presence of security.

DEGREE OF MENTAL DISORDER

On the left hand of the line shown here is a condition of normal or average mental health such as most of us enjoy. Toward the right side of the line some interesting changes begin to appear. Somewhere near the point on the line marked (1) an average mental health begins to show a clue of unsoundness. This may be nothing more unusual than temper tantrums or perhaps chronic timidity in a child causing it to withdraw into seclusion or possibly in an adult a constant or an habitual irritability, a feeling of "touchiness."

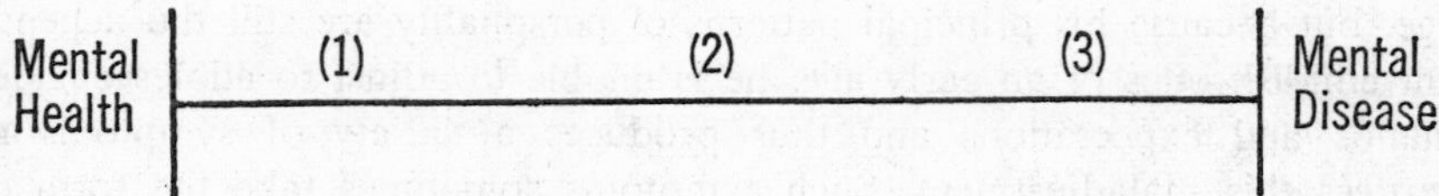

Toward the right, departures from average mental health become obvious. At (2) for instance, a person may be considered by his neighbors as "queer" in some ways. Perhaps he may become involved in religion or politics or in the healing cults. A woman, perhaps, may be considered "queer" about keeping an immaculate house; everyone in it is uncomfortable or else she may have a perpetual "chip on the shoulder" attitude, complaining that everyone is trying to get the better of her. While still retaining more or less of the good mental health with which they began, such people nevertheless show by their "queerness." They have already traveled some distance on the left to the end of the line. At the point marked (3) mental health becomes unmistakably impaired; the efficiency of the person becomes correspondently lessened and the symptoms much exaggerated. If, perhaps, these people may have complained that the world has not given them a square deal, that "lady luck frowns" on them, that they have not had the breaks, that they have been singled out always to get the short end, they have already begun to develop definite and specific ideas which become delusions of persecution. They necessarily must arm to protect themselves against their "enemies." Some curious notions have crept into this person. He becomes invalided. He cannot go outside unaccompanied or mix with crowds. He becomes agitated and disturbed when he is required to ride on a bus. He is equally uncomfortable when walking and will become severely disturbed by the idea that he is going to become dizzy, faint, or even die.

Finally, the right-hand end of the line is reached. Here mental health ends completely and mental disease takes over. Such a person is considered mentally disturbed and his pattern of adjustment has broken down entirely. Actually, a sharp or clear-cut line does not divide mental health from mental disease. The former may be considered excellent, good, fair, or poor, grading imperceptibly to the right of this line toward the point where mental disease may enter the picture. This point is extremely difficult to locate in the mind because standards differ in different groups. What may pass as merely a poor or even a fair degree of mental health among one group of persons might well be labeled a mild degree of mental disorder in another. Only when mental disease has progressed from mild to extreme are we justified in calling a person mentally ill or "insane."

INSANITY

"Insanity" is really a legal term and does not have medical standing. It means simply that a person's symptoms of mental disorder have progressed to such a degree that his sense of judgment has become so faulty that the law must step in and make it possible for others to decide for the patient what measures are necessary for his proper treatment and the safeguarding of his property. In other words, he is then considered unfit and irresponsible; also he does not know the difference between right and wrong. Many such "insane" people are in mental hospitals; no doubt thirty to forty times as many others may display some signs of maladjustment or mental disorders of a lesser type which will probably never bring them into institutionalization. While not in good health, and often considered "queer" and hard to get along with, many people are never considered by their fellow citizens, friends, or family members as being mentally ill. According to modern psychiatric conceptions of what constitutes mental disorder, the fears, worries, spells that these men and women may have actually almost approximate the signs and symptoms that patients in the psychiatric hospitals might possess.

This modern psychiatric conception of what constitutes mental disorder is explained admirably by Dr. C. Macfie Campbell onetime professor of psychiatry at the Harvard Medical School:

A disorder is a mental disorder if its roots are mental. A headache indicates a mental disorder because one is absorbing something disagreeable. A pain in the back is a mental disorder if its persistence is due to discouragement and a feeling of uncertainty and a desire to have a sick benefit instead of putting one's back onto one's work. Sleeplessness may be a mental disorder if its basis lies in personal worries and emotional tangles. In fact, many mental reactions are indications of poor mental health, although they have not usually been classed as mental disorders.

Thus, discontent with one's environment may be a mental disorder if its causes lie, not in some external situation, but in personal failure to deal adequately with one's emotional problems. Suspicion, distrust, misinterpretation, are mental disorders when they are the disguised expression of repressed longings into which the patient has no clear insight. Stealing sometimes indicates a mental disorder, the odd expression of underlying conflicts in the patient's nature. The feeling of fatigue sometimes represents, not overwork, but discouragement, inability to meet situations, lack of interest in the opportunities available. Unsociability, marital incompatibility, alcoholism, an aggressive and embittered social attitude; all these may indicate a disorder of the mental balance which may be open to modification.

How different is this conception from the older one that held that there were only two varieties of people in this world: the sane and the insane.

MENTAL DEFECT

Another kind of mental condition is not mental disease, but instead a mental defect. After talking with someone who is seriously mentally sick or "insane," many people seem astonished to find that the patient remembers many things, knows what he is talking about, and in general his intellectual faculties are not affected by his illness. This is because many types of mental sickness are disorders in a patient's feelings and emotions. His intellect remains intact. A few types of mental disease are associated with physical changes in the brain. The more advanced changes are accompanied by lessening of intelligence, but for the most part the patients ill from mental disease tend to retain much of whatever original intellectual ability they once had.

With mental defect, however, this is not entirely true. A person who is mentally defective (feeble-minded is another term meaning the same thing) is one whose intelligence has never developed adequately. Mental defect and mental disease, therefore, are quite different and should not be confused with each other.

FEEBLE-MINDEDNESS

The late Dr. Walter Fernald, one of the great pioneers in the study of mental deficiency, describes the symptoms of feeble-mindedness as follows:

> The symptoms of mental defect vary according to the degree of defect. In extreme cases the defect is observable in early infancy. The baby does not "take notice" or follow sounds or bright lights, or smile, or grasp objects with his fingers, or have vigorous muscular movements, or nurse properly, and so forth. As he grows older his teeth may not appear at the usual age, or he may learn to walk late and with an awkward, shambling gait, or he may be late in using his hands, or his untidy habits may persist for a long time. He is very apt not to talk until he is three or more years old. In general he remains a baby for a long time.
>
> In less severe cases, the above symptoms may be less marked or absent, and the defect may not be recognized until the child is found to be unable to learn in school at the usual school age, and cannot be promoted from year to year like other children.
>
> He usually shows his defect in other ways. He may not be able to get along with other children in games and sports. He is often teased and picked on by playmates of his own age, but since they do not regard him as an equal, he

usually associates with children younger than himself. He is usually easily influenced and shows poor judgment and reasoning power. In general he is not able to meet new situations.

As he grows older he is apt to be led into mischief, since he finds it hard to resist temptation. If neglected or allowed to associate with evil companions they are rather more likely than normal persons to acquire immoral or vicious habits, although this tendency has probably been overstated. Some mental defectives seem innately vicious and troublesome from early childhood, but the majority seem about as amenable to proper associations and proper bringing up as do normal children.

Whatever the cause be, inherited or acquired, medical science knows of nothing to do to repair the damage to the brain tissue that is responsible for the condition. Therefore, the patient can never be cured. In this respect, also, mental defect is not like mental disease where cure is often accomplished. However, if the condition cannot be cured, at least there is much that can be done to help the feeble-minded person to make a fair and a reasonable adjustment in life with whatever intelligence he possesses. Three degrees of feeble-mindedness are recognized: the moron, who is next to normal in intelligence, the imbecile who is lower on the scale, and lastly the idiot. In the higher grade, early recognition of this defect will assist parents and teachers to avoid making too many demands so that the child can keep up those standards set by normal children. This will help him to maintain his morale and prevent him from developing feelings of inferiority as a result of encountering nothing but failure as he goes through life. The child can be trained in good habits which will stand him in good stead when his impulsive judgment threatens to fail him. Later, training in simple trades and occupations within their capacity of accomplishment is possible for those in the moron and upper imbecile groups. Like all people with some level of mental awareness, the mental defective needs individual management. What works with one may fail with another. In each case, the child must be dealt with as a special problem requiring an individual method.

CLASSIFICATION OF MENTAL DISEASE

The following classification has been adopted by the American Psychiatric Association and involves both causes and symptoms.

Mental disorders are divided into two major groups:

(1) Those in which disturbed mental function results from or is precipitated by a primary impairment (gross or diffuse) of brain tissue;

(2) Those which result from some difficulty in adaptation by the patient.

In the first group are individuals with organic brain disorders, characterized by difficulty in judgment, intellectual functioning, memory, orientation, etc. The group is further subdivided into two other classes, "acute" and "chronic" and each has its differentiation as to symptoms, signs, course, prognosis, and treatment.

A patient may make a recovery from an acute brain syndrome such as seen in alcoholism. Either transient or permanent brain damage may result however. At the beginning the condition is usually acute, but if the symptom becomes permanent with continuing and finally persistent brain damage, the diagnosis is chronic.

Acute brain syndrome may be caused by drug poisoning or the chronic brain syndrome may be associated with chronic intoxication such as caused by alcoholism. The second group includes disorders of emotional nature without any clearly defined physical causes or structural changes within the brain. Symptoms and signs include changes in personality with disintegration, failure to judge reality, and failure to react properly to people in their work. This group is further divided into psychosis, psychophysiologic internal disorders, psychoneurosis, and personality disorders. These disorders designate a group of related psychiatric syndromes and may be labeled as "reactions."

A third category is mental deficiency which has already been described. In the American Psychiatric Association classification, mental deficiency includes cases of defective intelligence existing since birth in which an organic brain disease or prenatal cause cannot be demonstrated. The degree of intelligence defect is characterized according to the intelligence quotient (IQ) as "mild" mental deficiency where there is a score of 70 to 85 associated with vocational impairment, "moderate" mental deficiency 50 to 70 indicating functional impairment which may require special training and guidance, and "severe" below 50 which means that functional impairment in this situation will require custodial care.

I. ORGANIC BRAIN DISORDERS

In this group is impairment of brain tissue function manifested by regression, retardation, disturbances of sensorium, hallucinations, delusions, behavior difficulties, convulsive disorders which may be caused by birth injury, prenatal influences, infections, toxicity, drug or poison intoxication, cerebral arteriosclerosis, circulatory or vascular disturbances, abnormal metabolism, faulty nutrition, intracranial growths, or conditions such as multiple sclerosis and cerebral palsy.

These disorders are further classified according to the cause of brain damage.

1. Prenatal (Constitutional) Influences

The chronic brain syndrome associated with congenital abnormalities of the skull or developmental defects to include small, undeveloped brains and the results of premature closing of the skull, hydrocephalus, cerebral palsy, and mongolism.

2. Infection

Acute and chronic syndromes may be due primarily to infection inside the skull which includes meningitis, encephalitis, brain abscess, tuberculosis, syphilis, and rebella.

3. Toxins

The reversible and chronic brain syndromes which are caused by drugs such as barbiturates, bromides, or by other chemicals, including lead, mercury, arsenic, carbon monoxide, or alcohol.

Alcoholic intoxication may lead to permanent brain damage manifested in a syndrome which is characterized by disorientation, confabulation, memory defect, easy suggestibility, etc. Many chronic alcoholics will eventually show evidence of personality deterioration, inability to concentrate, defective judgment, unreliability, paranoia with a tendency to blame their own personal failure on others. Other brain injuries may be included in this group of causes.

4. Circulatory Disturbances

Circulatory disturbances include progressive mental disorders which occur in conditions of hardening of the arteries of the brain, cerebral thrombosis, cerebral hemorrhages, arterial hypertension, and other diseases originating in the blood vessels.

5. Metabolism and Nutrition

Senile and presenile brain syndromes, glandular disturbances, familial blindness, avitaminosis and its associated conditions may be associated with mental problems.

Pellagra which is now rare once accounted for at least 10 per cent of patients who were institutionalized as mental patients in the south. Another condition resembling pellagra is called kwashiorkor which is due to a loss or lack of protein in the diet.

Phenylpyruvic amentia, sometimes classified as a hereditary or familial disease, is caused by a metabolic disturbance in which severe mental deficiency is seen. This condition is easily discovered through a simple urine test which is done almost routinely in most hospitals.

II. FUNCTIONAL DISORDERS

Here is a group in whom definite physical causes cannot be found. New drug treatment has improved the possibility of these patients not only to improve but also to remain well for varying lengths of time. Several subgroups are:

1. Psychoses

These patients have disturbance of perception, regressive behavior, loss of ability to function and to relate to the realistic world. They also possess diminished or loss of control of impulses.

(a.) *Involutional psychotic reaction.* This usually occurs in the aging and degenerating period in both men and women who have not previously had psychiatric illness, and particularly not the manic-depressive state. One often finds on deeper questioning that these people have had problems previously. This condition is characterized by anxiety, tension, paranoid ideas, insomnia, agitation, and severe preoccupation with exaggerated somatic ailments.

(b.) *Affective reactions.* People with severe disorders of mood and emotion have affective reactions. Thoughts and behavior play but a secondary role. They have severe depression, severe moods change from high to low, and from low to high. They do have a tendency to become better but unfortunately this condition is known to recur. Distinct types in this group include the manic, the depressed, and the agitated-depressed state.

In the manic state, the predominating symptom is agitation, hyperirritability, elation of mood and severely increased movements. In the depressed group, the most striking symptom is lethargy and depression of mood and emotion. There is also retardation and inhibition of motions. Occasionally, these patients may have either depressed or agitated mood variations. Often these two manifestations may occur together, and occasionally they are known as the circular type when both phases alternate.

The manic-depressive psychosis represents 5 per cent or more of all admissions to psychiatric hospitals. Sometimes people in the manic state verge on the schizophrenic.

Depression may be due to various causes: psychological and physiological factors play an important role. Psychologically, underactivity of the sympathetic and the parasympathetic nervous systems may be underlying. In the retarded type of endogenous depression, the person may have a severe guilt response with feelings of inadequacy, insecurity, and ineffectuality. With loss of esteem, status, or love, he believes that he is abandoned or alone. Severe agitation, psychomotor restlessness, and expression of self-depreciation are seen in the agitated depressive state.

Physically these patients have severe fatigue, headache, fullness of the head, pressure on top of the head, tension in the back of the neck, pain or constriction of the chest, palpitation, shortness of breath, loss of weight, loss of appetite, disturbance of bowel and bladder function, decrease in sexual activity, disturbance of the menstrual cycle, muscular aches and pains, insomnia, and other symptoms.

Emotional disturbance may be seen in feelings of sadness sometimes with anxiety, obsessions, and phobias. The obsessive thoughts are likely to center around the fear of "losing my mind." As a result, the individual develops feelings that portions of his body are absent or fail to function. He will go from doctor to doctor seeking an explanation for his complaints, he usually worsens with each doctor's assurance that "there is nothing wrong with you." These patients will also have disturbed thinking including lack of concentration because they are so preoccupied with themselves. They have memory difficulties and are unable to make decisions.

Any depressed patient is a potential suicide, particularly in the early stage of his illness. There is no rule for suicide whether the patient announces he will do it or whether he does not announce it.

The reactive depression has a more favorable prognosis and is more amenable to treatment than the other types of depression. Although the onset is rather sudden, such patients have a record of emotional instability. Some triggering mechanism initiates this form of depression. These causes include loss or rejection by a loved one, financial reversal, economic difficulties, loss of employment, frustrations, disappointments, rejections, and similar disturbing incidents. Usually the depression is severe when the patient awakens and as the day progresses. The patient feels that sleep is the best treatment for him even though the pattern is disturbed.

(c.) *Schizophrenic reactions.* Schizophrenic reactions are characterized by strong tendency to withdraw from or to have an impaired sense of reality, disturbance of emotional balance, behavior and intellectual deviation, unpredictability of thought and association, regression, apathy and indifference to human relationships. Schizophrenia is one of the most common forms of mental illness; perhaps one third of the institutionalized patients in the United States are schizophrenic. The incidence has been placed as high as 8 per 1000.

Schizophrenic reactions may be divided into groups depending on the nature of their symptoms.

The characteristics of simple schizophrenia are chronic, progressive personality deterioration and loss of contact with reality, but with a lesser tendency to hallucinate and have delusions. These patients are emotionally blunted, their faces are expressionless, they may have silly or inappropriate grins, and they may be restless. Many simple schizophrenics are not in institutions because they function at a fair capacity.

Hebephrenic schizophrenics are characterized by a shallow and regressed mood and behavior. They are childish and silly; they giggle and are prone to hallucinations. Occasionally their speech becomes incoherent and unintelligible and is called "word-salad."

Catatonic schizophrenics are conspicuously immobile. They have muscular rigidity, are mute, stuporous, negativistic, and inflexible. With continuous regression, such patients become vegetablelike and are inaccessible to all ordinary means of communication. They are seen in institutions poised in one position, often unclothed, for hours and days at a time and often they require forcible feeding. This catatonic state may alternate with periods of severe agitation with wild activity, furor, destructiveness, and homicidal tendencies.

Paranoid schizophrenics have a fully systematized set of delusions often built in a logical but unrealistic form and composed chiefly of a sense of persecution, grandeur, genius, or special ability. This self-centered delusional state is expressed in the patient who may even sense himself as being God. Often included are those patients with systematized states of belief in illness and with threatening fears of attack and of dangerous "voices." They may try to shut out such imagined voices even with cotton or ear plugs. The behavior is unpredictable and often includes severe hostility and aggression.

Schizo-affectives are patients with a mixture of manic depressive reactions and schizophrenic mental content. Although they are basically schizophrenic, the predominating symptoms are disturbed emotion, sometimes elation, and more frequently depression.

Undifferentiated is a "catch-all" term for a wide variety of schizophrenic symptoms which eventually may develop into classical schizophrenia. These patients have confused thinking, emotional turmoil, are phobic, dreamy, and have dissociation of ideas with excitement or depression. In the acute state, the symptoms frequently clear within several weeks but are quite likely to recur at stated intervals.

Childhood schizophrenia is a prepubertal psychotic reaction usually autistic in behavior.

2. *Psychoneurotic Disorders*

A psychoneurosis may result from poor adaptation to "emotional conflict." Here impaired thinking and judgment occur but not as severe as in a psychosis. A minimal loss of contact with reality and less distortion of reality are characteristic. Although the personality may be disturbed, it is not disorganized. The person has been maladjusted in various degrees throughout life depending upon the special stresses and strains at different times. The chief characteristic of this condition is anxiety, which is either directly perceived as such or which is expressed through various psychological defense mechanisms. The person is uncomfortable, feels threatened, is uneasy, apprehensive, worried, either without knowing why or because of an exaggerated idea of the external cause. The means by which the neurotic patient attempts to resolve his conflict determines the type of reaction he will exhibit and is, in fact, the true basis for classification.

Acute anxiety neurosis is a form in which the patient is severely anxious and apprehensive for reasons usually unknown to him. At other times, he may project these to a specific situation. For example, he is unable to adjust to relocation of his home, or of infidelity in his wife. He is afraid of failing an examination; or he is afraid of dying. These patients have feelings of inadequacy and ineffectuality, and they worry about every little detail. They are markedly meticulous, fear to make mistakes, are indecisive and hypersensitive, and have emotional outbursts of anger. Often they have an irrational sense of impending disaster.

Physically, the people with acute anxiety neurosis have feelings of pressure in their heads, disturbed sleep, and disturbed dreams. Objectively, they have rapid pulses, elevated blood pressure, are breathless, have exaggerated deep tendon reflexes, clammy hands, and tremor of the outstretched fingers. They may have many complaints related to the heart, lungs, back, or gastrointestinal tract.

Conversion reaction is a term used to describe the patient who instead of expressing his anxiety as fears, may "convert" his painful unacceptable emotional conflict into loss of one or more functions which he normally has under good control. These may take the form of weakness of one side of the body (hemiplegia), irregular movements which include limps, tremors, or tics and there may be sensory loss to include blindness, deafness, or loss of the voice.

Dissociative reaction is a psychoneurosis characterized by depersonalization, dream states, amnesia, sleepwalking, confused states, and even stupor.

Phobic reaction is a form in which anxiety expresses itself as a persistent, overpowering, and irrational fear of an object or a situation including crossing streets, moving vehicles, high places, low places, closed places, open places, animals, infections, almost anything. There are hundreds of different phobias that such patients might have and they desperately try to control anxiety by avoiding the object or situation.

Obsessive-compulsive reaction is a form in which the anxiety is linked to a compulsion to perform specific acts in spite of the fact that the person may know that these are unreasonable. Here may be seen ritualistic patterns associated with repetitive actions to include counting slats in window blinds, taking several steps before crossing a threshold, washing the hands a certain number of times to include sevens, nines, and elevens, smelling or touching a dish before putting food on it, washing money to "remove the germs," etc. However many highly intelligent people may reveal evidence of "magical" thinking but not to the point of gross specific compulsive behavior.

Depressive reaction is a psychoneurosis in which the anxiety partially may be relieved by depression, self-condemnation, and feelings of guilt. Ordinarily, one of these reactions arises from a specific traumatic situation such as loss of a loved one, economic loss, illness, fear of loss of position. Here, suicidal possibilities are quite frequent.

3. Psychosomatic Disorders

Disturbed feelings or emotions which have been repressed and thus prevented from taking a conscious form may manifest themselves in reactions of the body. Anger or acute fear are usually accompanied by increased heart rate, elevated blood pressure, or a sensation of abnormal stomach movements. When these responses are exaggerated, they outlast the immediate emotion and therefore become chronic; thus a disease process is set in motion. Abnormal organic states which at first are considered "functional" lead to structural changes. For example, a neurosis related to the heart may result in paroxysms of rapid heart beat and elevated blood pressure. A gastric neurosis may develop into gastritis or even into the condition known as pylorospasm—a spasm of the opening at the lower end of the stomach.

Under stressful situations, the anxiety may take the form of a much greater variety of somatic complaints involving any or all organs of the body. Disturbed appetite, gastric discomfort, chest constriction, shortness of breath, palpitation, "bloated stomach," constipation, "heartburn," urinary urgency and frequency, are frequent manifestations. The dermatologist, cardiologist, gastroenterologist, neurologist, and urologist usually quickly recognize the emotional factors which are present in dermatoses, backache, myalgias, bronchial spasms, hiccups, migraines, hypertension, constipation, irritable bowel syndrome, menstrual disturbances, dysuria, polyuria, anorexia, loss of weight, general fatigue, and even convulsive disorders.

The physician, in the diagnosis of these psychosomatic disorders, first excludes any organic causes and also notes the relationship between the physical cause and the psychoneurotic conversion reaction. Ordinarily, the latter involves organs under voluntary control. The psychosomatic problem usually is involved with organs not under voluntary control.

4. Personality Disorders

Developmental defects or strange trends in the personality structure may be reflected in a classical or characteristic lifelong pattern of behavior rather than in emotional or mental symptomatology. People who are classed as inadequate personality may reveal poor adaptability, impetuous behavior, lack of physical and emotional strength, and social disharmony. The schizoid personality is withdrawn and seclusive, aloof, tearful, and avoids any situation which might become competitive. The cyclothymic personality adjusts superficially to life situations and may relate to others in a warm and friendly manner and show a ready enthusiasm for competition. However, he has alternating moods of elation, depression, euphoria, and sadness which are not warranted or related to external events.

Personality traits which may stand in the way of wholesome social functioning in reaching emotional equilibrium and stability under stress may include poorly controlled hostilities, undependable judgment, dependence, indecision, helplessness, stubbornness, and delaying tactics, but conversely also aggressive behavior and severe resentment with intense reactions to frustration. These people are overinhibited, rigid, overly conscientious, obsessive, regressed, immature, compulsive, and antisocial.

What delineates such disturbances from those of the first three groups is that they represent certain characteristics which are not readily accessible to treatments. Basic changes are rarely achieved and the development of a psychotic process under conditions of stress is an ever present danger. Just a little bit of "separation" may exist between a psychoneurotic and a psychotic state.

AIDS IN DIAGNOSIS

I follow largely from the book *Psychochemotherapy* by E. Remmen, S. Cohen, K. S. Ditman, and R. Frantz, Jr., in discussing diagnostic aids in evaluating psychiatric illness. In mental illness nothing comparable to tests such as the Kahn Test for syphilis, the basal metabolic rate, or the radioisotope studies for thyroid dysfunctions is available. As yet, there are no specific tests for schizophrenia. The psychiatrist may, however, avail himself of a number of psychological, behavioral, and psychomotor criteria to confirm his diagnosis. He may employ techniques such as the Rorschach test, utilize questionnaires, or observe vocabulary responses. Social behavior may be rated by a scale measuring such opposing traits as cooperativeness, sociability, and withdrawal. There are other comparable improved diagnostic techniques to determine the psychotic self-evaluation, time estimation, sex identification, attention span, motivation, preoccupation, ability to make decisions, perception of objects in the environment, psychomotor activity, dexterity, and reaction signs.

The willingness or the unwillingness of the patient to cooperate is an important factor. To observe the patient for significant details including his tension, anxiety, sweating, flushing, tremors, chewing of a pencil, tugging at his hair, repeating a muscle movement, the way he will stand, the way he walks or speaks, may help in his diagnosis. A patient with "free-floating" anxieties will discuss in great detail the situation or the activities which he feels are disturbing him so badly. A patient describing his depression may give many clues.

The nervous system is subject to psychosomatic malfunctioning to include weakness, fatigue, numbness, paresthesias, insomnias, faintness, ringing in the ears, hyperirritability, nervousness, cold sweats, headaches, temporary loss of sight, hearing, touch, smell, use of a limb, etc. All these are diagnostic leads.

In the physical examination, the person with acute anxiety may reveal tension, flushing, rapid pulse, high blood pressure, dilated pupils, and cold clammy hands. Laboratory tests may or may not rule out organic changes but whether the anxiety stems from situational or physiological causes, the tests are usually helpful to a diagnosis. However, one must be careful not to make too many tests because the patient may interpret them as indecision or insecurity on the part of the doctor who "is not sure of himself or of me, and must make test after test to find out what is wrong with me."

PREVENTION OF MENTAL DISORDERS

The psychiatrist is more interested in learning why the patient had to take refuge in mental disease and what his symptoms imply to him instead of merely knowing what they are.

Sigmund Freud wrote, "I should advise you to find out what is happening. When you have done that, therapy will take care of itself." With this viewpoint in mind a doctor evaluates diagnostic aspects of a situation before he begins the management.

1. Mental health and mental disease blend into one another as do colors in the rainbow and there is no sharp line of separation. This may be seen between conditions such as psychoneurosis and psychosis.

2. Since the mind affects the body, and vice versa, the patient must be studied as a whole and not just in separate parts.

3. Mental disorders rarely come on suddenly except for those caused by an acute organic deficit or illness. Most of the conditions have been

in the process of development for many years before finally appearing in a clear-cut fashion.

4. The symptoms of mental disorders usually are only the exaggerations of attitudes or traits in personality which have been present in the patient for a long time.

5. While there are many different precipitating causes for mental disorders, most of them have one basic cause in common, namely, an inability to adjust to certain inner conflicts or to the demands for conformity to the outside world.

6. The basic cause is practically always within the unconscious part of the patient's mind and he is therefore unaware of what is going on about him or what it is all about.

7. Mental defect should not be confused with mental disease. The first has to do with impairment of intelligence. The second has to do with the disturbance of emotions.

MANAGEMENT OF MENTAL DISEASE

In the management of mental disorders the treatment of children and that of adults differ. Considerable overlapping is encountered in the type of treatment selected for the type of involvement.

The parent of a child is helped to "build up a vast supply of sturdy mental health." A parent learns to recognize and actually to "nip in the bud" quickly any well-established disturbed trait or attitude which may result in some form of mental maladjustment in later years. One wishes to insure that a child will grow up with good mental health.

In the United States, mental-hygiene movements in practically every state are performing a valuable service to parents and teachers. Only recently has there been complete recognition that an attempt must be made to build strong mental health as well as to prevent mental illness. By the time a child is an adult, there is relatively little that can be done in terms of prevention of mental disorders but there is help available to keep them from growing more serious. Treatment becomes more difficult as the mental disorder becomes more deeply entrenched and involved. The observant parent or parents should recognize maladjustment of children at the start. They may be expressed in the child in many ways including temper tantrums, "fussy" food habits, shyness, withdrawal, insecurity, overconscientiousness, bed-wetting (especially in older children), sleepwalking, bullying, lying, stealing, aggressiveness, and truancy. These should be regarded as early danger signals pointing to some underlying conflict which must be sought out before anything practical can be done permanently to correct the condition. Unlike other methods of treatment in other stages or branches of medicine, the management of behavior disorders and undesirable personality defects or traits in children can seldom be successfully undertaken by directing treatment to the child alone. The combination of difficulties in child and parent must be considered at the same time. The annoying behavior of a child is a sense of maladjustment somewhere within his emotional make-up. This is usually bound in one way or another with the attitude or the emotional reaction displayed toward him by his parents. The treatment of the behavior problem will require that all parental attitudes and conditions be considered as well. Indeed, so thoroughly is this believed by mental hygienists that they have created a sixth concept to the effect that "you cannot change the child's behavior until you first change the parental attitude that causes this behavior." Treatment is primarily directed toward the parents and generally consists of endeavoring to modify, if not entirely remove or displace, the undesirable attitude that they have unwillingly adopted with even the best intentions.

The type of management directed to a mental disorder is dependent on the nature of the problem. Adult management or treatment comprises two chief varieties including the treatment of the basic personality difficulty whenever this is possible and the management of the symptoms. One should not be satisfied to restrict treatment to mental-disorder symptoms alone unless there is nothing else that can be done under the circumstances. Unhappily, in many cases of serious mental involvement or "insanity," the situation has progressed so far before there is a call for psychiatric aid that there remains but little to do except to treat the symptoms. However, with the less involved cases, for example, in the psychoneuroses with fears, anxieties, compulsions, obsessions, etc., it is possible to try to reach the root of the difficulty. In fact, these symptoms may be controlled if not "cured" by a type of management known as "psychotherapy."

PSYCHOTHERAPY

This method does not involve the use of medicine or any type of physical therapy treatment like massage, heat, or soothing baths, but relies for its effectiveness on a special emotional relationship which is established between the patient and psychiatrist. One type of psychotherapy is called "psychoanalysis." Only a comparatively few kinds of mental difficulties are suitable for psychoanalytic treatment. For special cases in the hands of a well-trained psychiatrist, psychoanalysis enables exploration into the unconscious mind of the patient. After locating his source of conflict, this is helpful in emotional re-education. As a result, the patient may be restored to an improved degree of adjustment and to practical functioning.

Other forms of psychotherapy are used for cases which do not require as deep and as prolonged an exploration into the unconscious. Thus there may be various kinds of suggestion to use, occasionally, even hypnosis. Many psychiatrists consider hypnosis at best only a temporary relief for symptoms and powerless to bring about a lasting cure. It is actually little employed by psychiatrists.

The management of more serious conditions of mental disorders such as "insanity" in whom institutional care is necessary is much more complicated. The patient in all probability has been behaving peculiarly for many months before the family or friends have become courageous enough to seek medical advice. The patient may have been depressed or even agitated. Perhaps, he has delusions of people following him, placing something in his food to poison him, voices have been speaking to him, and there are microphones everywhere in the room noting everything he has said and transmitting this to others out to "get him." As time goes on the condition worsens. Finally, a point comes where the family or friends recognize that things are not right. The family physician is consulted and he makes a careful examination both physically and neurologically to make sure there is no organic illness. Then he examines the patient mentally and either recommends that a psychiatrist be consulted by the family or that the patient should be hospitalized in either a private or public hospital where psychiatric illnesses are handled. Most of the time, he advises the family or friends to secure the services of a capable psychiatrist who will make the ultimate decision.

Assuming that the patient has been seen by a psychiatrist, few of these patients will be handled in the home. It is better for the patient and the family alike if he is removed to a hospital for this much needed attention. This is a difficult decision for relatives to make for there still exist antiquated attitudes about the management of a psychiatric patient in a mental hospital. However in many cases it is almost certain that much of the patient's underlying conflict is tangled in family relationships, and he must be removed from his well-meaning family atmosphere for a time so that opportunities for an early cure may be improved.

In many states, institutionalization merely consists of taking the patient to a private hospital and applying for his admission. If commitment is required, this is done as a legal device to safeguard the rights and interests of the patient. Application is made or the court petitioned for an order to have the patient admitted to a hospital so that he may have special treatment. In many states, commitments can be made without undue publicity and this is handled by one or two physicians who certify that "the patient is mentally unable to take care of himself and is in need of mental treatment or is in need of hospitalization."

The patient arrives at the hospital. He is first taken to a receiving ward where he remains for days or weeks for early study depending on the nature of his condition. Upon arrival at the hospital, he is given a complete physical and neurological examination and later a psychiatric interview. Also, the family or friends who are known as "informants" give a complete record to either the intern, resident, psychiatrist, or social worker. He is assigned a room and a bed and is questioned concerning his diet; if disturbed upon his admission, he may be given a sedative. This medication or even the initial interview will in many cases result in quieting the patient, but in some hospitals a sedative bath is used if he is agitated. This consists of covering the body with vaseline and then placing the patient in a sedative bath which is a large bathtub with water kept at a specific soothing temperature. A canvas sheet is placed over the tub to prevent the patient from getting out. An attendant or nurse remains at his side continuously to see that he does not do himself any harm or even attempt to slip underneath the sheet into the water.

Occasionally, the patient may require more than a sedative or a bath to soothe him. He may require drugs such as intravenous hypnotic medications or possibly even restraints. These restraints may be confined to the arms, legs, waist or the complete body; this is known as a "strait jacket." However, the use of the last measure is rare.

The patient may be seen to be depressed instead of excited: he may have complete loss of appetite and refuse to eat, or he may have delusions that he has committed a crime and that he has done many ghastly deeds for which he should be punished. He may accuse himself of having brought ruination down upon his family and himself, that he is causing all the misery in the world and that he has committed many unpardonable sins. He is severely depressed and is potentially a suicidal candidate. Several precautions are used to avoid permitting this person to make an attempt to take his own life. He must be safeguarded against self-injury. Many of these patients are clever in managing to evade nurses and aides who are constantly on the alert to prevent such attempts at self-destruction. Obviously, this is another important reason why permitting the patient to remain in the home is dangerous. Even under the most intense surveillance, a patient may elude his nurses, aides, orderlies, and others and may make attempts to cut or electrocute himself, or even swallow something which can cause severe damage.

Often the patient will refuse to eat, and other methods of furnishing him with nourishment become necessary. If his refusal of food threatens life, he may have to be fed by tube which is inserted through the nose or mouth into the stomach and into which is passed a nutritious mixture consisting of milk, eggs and other nutritional substances.

Gradually, as the patient improves, he is transferred from the receiving ward into another unit. Here he will find other patients whose behavior is like his own and who are in various stages of recovery. Seeing these patients whose conditions have improved is an incentive for any patient to continue to make progress. Presently, he is involved in occupational therapy or in activity therapy, and later he is encouraged to take walks on the grounds outside in the company of other patients or with authorized personnel. Eventually, he will make these trips on his own. He is given the opportunity to visit the activity therapy departments at frequent intervals where under skilled supervision he may re-establish habits of concentration and industry and at the same time take his mind off his troubles.

Some new and modern psychiatric hospitals have different units graded for the acceptance of mild patients, intermediate patients, or agitated patients. Some of these units have the "closed-door" policy and others have the "open-door" policy. Often these patients are evaluated carefully before being admitted into the hospital and before any unit is designated. Still other patients who have medical problems are first placed in an infirmary before being transferred to a unit which is usually the area in which they are going to remain throughout their hospitalization with little if any transfer necessary.

Eventually most patients are ready to go home. Unfortunately, this is not the usual hospital course with all patients. Some mentally sick men and women are not permitted by their relatives to enter a hospital until their illness has progressed to such an advanced stage that little active management can be given and only custodial care can be applied. Moreover, there are certain types of mental illness which are so stubborn from the beginning that a case is almost a chronic one right from the start. Nevertheless the rate of recovery is steadily increasing. About 35 per cent to 40 per cent of first admissions to mental hospitals leave completely cured, while an additional 20 per cent are able to return home and are well enough to live in the outside community even though they are not entirely recovered. About 40 per cent of patients admitted to state hospitals are discharged within a five year period. Of the patients who are discharged, about 90 per cent are regarded as improved or recovered. The most probable duration of hospitalizations for those who are mentally disturbed is six months or less. The likelihood of discharge with favorable outcome decreases sharply after two years and reaches a low by the end of five years.

In the average state hospital, about 50 per cent of all patients have been there less than a year, 25 per cent have been there between one and five years, and 60 per cent have been there from 5 to 55 years or longer.

This recovery rate depends to some extent on the kind of hospital in which the patient is treated. Most modern hospitals do not have difficulty in maintaining this rate. The less progressive ones are usually able to do little more than provide custodial care for their patients. A technical distinction is made between hospitals that treat and are known as "treatment hospitals" and the others in which only custodial care is given which are called "custodial hospitals." In the former modern forms of medical and psychiatric management are employed to help cure patients. Most of these hospitals are adequately supplied with paramedical personnel to include psychologists, sociologists, play therapists, music therapists, etc., all of whom work together to give the patient service.

PSYCHOTROPIC MEDICATION

A new era has appeared in medications which are called "psychotropic." They include central-nervous-system depressants, and central-nervous-system stimulants. A further classification divides these drugs into psychomotor stimulants, antidepressants, and energizers. Such a division has the advantage of being based on the reversal of two presenting symptom complexes, agitations and depressions.

The psychomotor stimulants or antidepressants are direct aids in the management of anxious and agitated people. They are most effective for the relief of a depressed state. Occasionally this is all that may be necessary in the management of the patient in the hospital together with his psychotherapy. However, modern psychiatry still requires other techniques listed under physical therapies to include electroshock therapy, insulin coma therapy, or other forms.

COMMUNITY HOSPITALS FOR MENTAL DISORDERS

Well-equipped and modern mental hospitals require considerable funds. The expenditure is worth while because of the high percentage of patients who are restored to health. Any community can have this high quality of service. A modern treatment hospital, whether it be private or state, is generally more effective for a mentally ill patient than a simple custodial private or state facility.

The modern state hospital deals with many thousands of patients and depends on funds furnished by the state government. Even though the salaries of its staff are usually lower than that seen in private sanitariums, the progressive scientific spirit permeates the entire atmosphere and the opportunity to utilize the most modern equipment will tend to attract better medical personnel to such an area. If costs are a serious matter for the family to consider, a state hospital will be recommended for the patient under most circumstances.

Mankind has traveled far since the days centuries ago when people with "insanity" were considered to be afflicted with evil spirits, demons, and therefore were placed into dungeons where they were chained and fettered. Pioneers such as Philippe Pinel removed these chains as they did the stigma of mental illness. The mystery of mental illness has passed.

Now it is recognized as a kind of illness amenable in great measure to skilled and intelligent psychiatric management, which may result in the cure of increasingly large numbers of people. The early recognition of presenting signs and symptoms enable prevention and will result in a better and earlier opportunity for recovery.

CHAPTER 37

Medical Care of the Aged

MORRIS FISHBEIN, M.D.

STATISTICS

The aged require hospitalization about three times as often as do people under sixty-five years of age. Estimates in 1965 indicated that there were between eighteen and nineteen million people over sixty-five years old in the United States, with an expected increase to twenty-one million by 1975.

In ancient Egypt life expectancy at birth as shown by the bodies of mummies which have been examined was about 20 years. In ancient Rome about A.D. 64 life expectancy at birth was about twenty-five years. In the United States in 1900 it was about forty-five years. In 1965 life expectancy at birth for men was seventy years and for women seventy-five. This means many more are living eighty or ninety years or even more.

An explanation is not available as to why women have a longer life expectancy than men although many theories have been suggested. Dr. Amram Scheinfeld says that the big advantages of females in longevity derive primarily from the inherited sex differences which produce in the male many more defects and make him an easy prey for most of the major diseases. These are not necessarily anatomic structural defects but may also be related to the resistance of the tissues to various environmental hazards, including infection. Men with parents who have lived long are likely to live longer than others. Among people who lived 90 years or longer, Dr. Raymond Pearl found that in seven of eight instances, two or more of the grandparents had lived long. In general, however, women take better care of themselves than do men.

Men have coronary attacks five times as often as do women. Men, naturally, do not suffer of the cancers that attack the organs of women associated with childbirth, but men have more cancers of the stomach than do women. Incidentally the cancers that affect women mostly have lower mortality rates than the cancers of the stomach and the cancers of

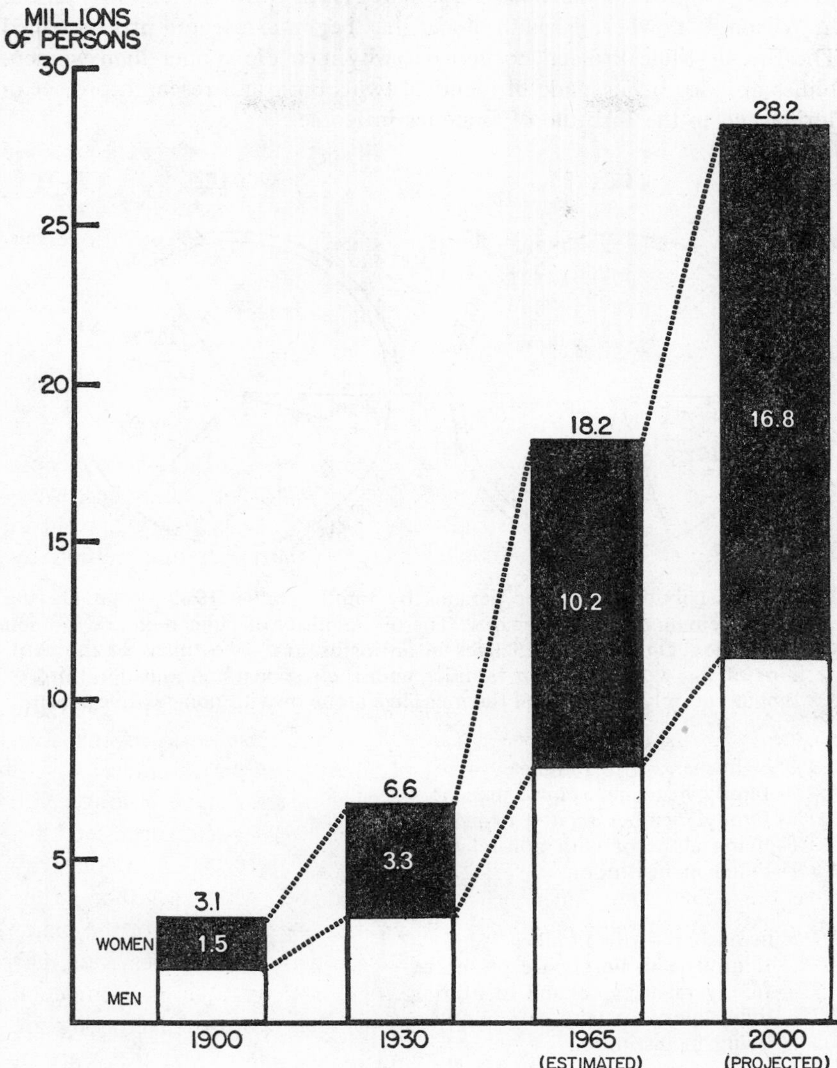

Fig. 83. Growth of U.S. population 65 and over. Bureau of the Census and U. S. Department of Health, Education & Welfare, Administration of Aging.

the lung which affect men. Cancer of the lung is about seven times as frequent in men as in women.

Women are likely to see the doctor much more often than do men. An actual record shows that women make 5.5 visits to doctors per year compared with 3.9 visits for men. After sixty-five years of age women make

7.6 visits per year to the doctor compared with 5.8 for men. In Florida, Dr. Wilson T. Sowder, a health officer, has begun a research project called "The Fragile Male Project" to find out why men die sooner than women. Studies are also being made of identical twins both in a research project in Florida and in the Institute of Genetics in Rome.

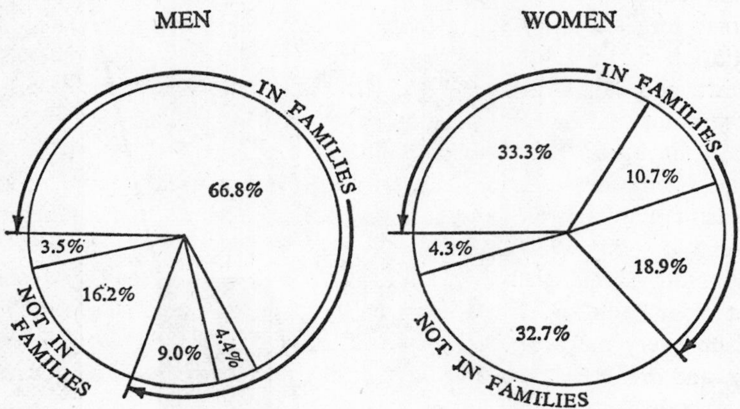

Fig. 84. Distribution of older persons by family status, 1965. What are the living arrangements of older persons? The big majority of older men and women live in families. Only one in 25 lives in an institution. Two thirds of the men, one third of the women, live in families with their spouses. About one third of the women, but only one sixth of the men, live alone or with non-relatives.

Men:
66.8% in husband-wife families.
4.4%–family head, no spouse present
9.0%–family member related to head
16.2%–living alone or with non-relatives
3.5%–living in institution

Women:
33.3% in husband-wife families
10.7%–family head, no spouse present
18.9%–family member related to head
32.7%–living alone or with non-relatives
4.3%–living in institution

FAILINGS OF THE AGED

In many surveys of the elderly that have been made, evidence indicated that ninety per cent of women and sixty-five per cent of men have trouble moving about in the dark. Because of various lessenings of special senses, the aged suffer much more than do younger people from falls and particularly from fractures of the bones of the leg and hip.

Investigations have shown that older people have difficulty in making quick decisions. This is coupled with the fact that memory for recent events is lessened—apparently a function of the temporal lobes of the brain which may be injured by changes in circulation. Older people may, for example, turn on the gas and forget to turn it off without lighting it. They may let the bathtub overflow. They may forget the roast in the oven. They may forget to relay telephone messages. They may forget a burning cigarette left on an ashtray. They may fall on stairways. They may hesitate, start, and stop in crossing streets so that many older people are injured by motor vehicles simply because of this kind of indecision.

Studies have also shown that intelligence is linked with survival. The human capacity increases from age 35 to 40; after 40 impairment begins. Impairment with age is greater in the less intelligent than in the more intelligent.

Among other frequent changes in the elderly is an increase in fatigability so that older people get tired more easily. One man of eighty-eight said, "I get up every morning feeling fine after a good night's sleep. I shave, shower, and dress. By the time I have finished breakfast, I am so exhausted I want to go back to bed."

Obviously old people as individuals differ greatly from one another. Many older people are capable of working four, five, six, or even eight hours without fatigue, but in general people over sixty-five years of age should plan to have some rest periods between periods of activity and work.

A survey made by Blue Cross insurance agencies indicated that most old people have multiple ailments. People under sixty-five years of age may, for example, receive hospital attention for such conditions as childbirth or conditions affecting the periodic functions of women, for appendicitis, tonsils and adenoids, and pneumonia. People over sixty-five may be involved in hospitalization primarily because of heart disease, heart failure, cancer, conditions affecting the blood, accidents, and in men, enlargement of the prostate gland, which includes interference with urination.

In general, elderly people suffer frequently with rheumatoid arthritis, disturbances of digestion, pruritus or itching, and various other eruptions and disturbances of the skin. One out of every two people examined was found to have some chronic disease or some disablement.

While old people constitute about nine per cent of the population, they use eighteen per cent of the general hospital beds, ninety per cent of beds in nursing homes. Two thirds of the women and fifty per cent of the men must rely on someone else other than the husband or the wife to look after them.

CHANGES IN OLD AGE

Every person over sixty must realize that his organs are functioning more slowly than in his youth and that allowances must be made for this change. The glands tend to function less in old age, so that the skin becomes dry. Even the gastric juice carries a lower percentage of hydrochloric acid, and for this reason there is difficulty with digestion. Moreover, the mucus in the intestines becomes less, so that there is a tendency to dryness of the intestinal contents and therefore to constipation.

One of the significant changes in old age is the blunting of sensibility to pain. This is important, because the breaking down of the tissues leads to sensations that are uncomfortable. For the same reason disease in old age comes insidiously.

Whereas pneumonia, heart disease, stones in the kidney or gall bladder may cause agonizing pain to a young person, they come on so insidiously in older ones they may be unrecognized until they have reached the point where help is difficult. Even cancer comes on insidiously in the aged.

The sensations of taste and smell also become weaker, so that food is not so appetizing. Everyone knows also that sight and hearing are greatly depreciated in the elderly.

One of the most interesting aspects of old age is the change in the mind and ability to sleep. Because the aged sleep less continuously, they frequently estimate the amount of sleep at much less than it really is. However, the aged are able to use much less sleep than vigorous, active people, and it is not desirable to get them into the habit of taking sedative drugs. It is likely that excessive sleep is more harmful to them than too little.

The mind becomes much more easily fatigued in old age than in middle age. Gradually the power of affection wanes in the old, perhaps because they have become habituated to the loss of relatives and friends. Possibly they are more self-centered; time passes slowly, and their minds are occupied with their own feelings.

THE BODY IN OLD AGE

In Great Britain a foundation was established to study the problem of aging and the care of old people. They point out that old age is actually a quality of mind and body and that the time of onset of old age varies from person to person. For a number of reasons old age has been taken to begin at 60 for women and 65 for men, and these figures are taken as standard in pension acts.

People in advanced years require more medical attention than do those of younger ages. Nevertheless, one-fourth of all the old people studied had gone for three years or more without seeking medical aid and in many instances had virtually never required any. More than 12 per cent of the people had gone so long since seeing a doctor that they could not remember when the last time was, and more than 7 per cent were certain that they had 20 years or more of good health.

They found relatively little undernourishment among the old people; in fact, only 3 per cent were classed as undernourished. The chief nutritional disturbance was a lack of iron, which affected about 5 per cent of the women.

It was found also that men tend to remain normal in body build as they grow old, whereas women show much growth variation in the direction of either leanness or stoutness. Twenty-five per cent of women over 85 years of age were undeniably obese.

As people grow old, they find more or less difficulty in getting around as well as they used to. Only 2½ per cent of the people over 60 years of age were confined to bed, and it was thought that the figure was low because old people who live at home have in most instances to help in looking after themselves. For that reason, if the aged find it necessary to be continuously in bed, they are transferred to institutions.

Almost one-fourth of the old people were capable of only limited getting about in their immediate districts. After 70 years of age the specific symptoms of old age are likely to become emphasized. These include weakness, dizziness, difficulty with traffic, inflammation of the back and lack of confidence.

Caring for old people at home puts a severe burden on the younger generation, many of whom carry this strain for years and years without relief.

Stairs are a particular problem when old people are concerned and when they are in poor health. At least one-third of old people have trouble getting up and down stairs or both ways. Stairs are especially a hazard when they are steep and when they lack a rail. Whenever old people are compelled to use stairs, there should be a rail to help them. Over 6 per cent of old people were unable to use stairs at all. The trouble with stairs was especially hard on old women because of their desire to participate in housework. Old people themselves recognize the special problem that is presented by stairs, and a large majority think that bungalows are the ideal type of home.

Among the medical conditions that affect old people most are rheumatism or arthritis, the effects of falls or accidents, and bronchitis.

Almost half of all old people are troubled with coughs, and men more than women. Rheumatic conditions of one kind or another affect more than half, and they vary from just twinges of pain to crippling incapacity from involvement of the joints. Women are more frequently affected than men, and this is particularly hard on them because of the nature of their work in the household.

Men have a liability to gout nearly ten times that of the women. Pain in the feet affects nearly 40 per cent of the old people and women twice as often as men. Another symptom that causes much distress is frequency and urgency of emptying the bladder. This affects one-third of all the old people. It is commoner in women than in men, and it makes shopping difficult.

Difficulties in hearing affect men more than women. Some dizziness is experienced by at least 75 per cent of the women over 85 years of age, and difficulty in getting about in the dark is a symptom for more than 90 per cent of women over 85. However, in general, old people are extremely unsteady in walking, some of it due to dizziness, some to failure to lift the feet properly.

DISEASES OF OLD AGE

Even premature senility may occur in youth. Heart disease, atrophy of the brain, and hardening of the arteries may also occur in comparatively young people. However, most of the diseases that occur in the aged are the result of gradual breaking down of the tissues. These include hardening of the arteries, heart failure, hardening of the liver, enlargement of the prostate, cancer, obesity, and indigestion. However, old age does modify any disease, so that it is different from the same condition in youth.

Measles, scarlet fever, typhoid, and diphtheria occur very rarely in old people, probably because they have been infected in youth and thereby developed immunity from these diseases. The form of sick headache called migraine usually becomes less troublesome as age advances and may disappear with increasing years. A recent conception of this disease indicates that it may be the result of sensitivity to some protein food substance, and perhaps the repeated attacks eventually bring about desensitization.

Even when an aged person is in good health, he must keep a close watch for the diseases to which his age makes him particularly susceptible. Happiness for all elderly persons is principally a matter of health, and so health must be guarded more and more closely as time goes on.

The changes that occur in the skin of the aged are due to gradual loss of activity on the part of the glands and of the tissues responsible for immunity. Because the aged are likely to be a little less scrupulous in the care of the skin, slight infections occur repeatedly. There are also bed sores. Itching is a stimulus to severe scratching and secondary infections take place in the scratches.

The blood vessels may lose their contractile power, and there are occasionally tiny hemorrhages under the skin. One of the most severe conditions that affects the aged is the reaction called herpes zoster. It is a form of shingles which develops along the course of a nerve and which in the aged may be exceedingly painful. Moreover, once the attack has passed, the pains may continue and return at intervals without the eruption. These conditions must be watched closely and treated immediately.

The aged suffer frequently with dizziness, as already mentioned, due to many possible causes. Sometimes it is due to accumulated hard wax in the ear, sometimes to changes that have taken place in the internal ear; frequently it is associated with high blood pressure, hardening of the arteries, and changes in the circulation of the blood in the brain. Sometimes the result is a difficulty of coordination between the eye, the ear, and the sense of balance, so that the aged may stagger or fall when the eyes are raised suddenly or under some similar stimulus.

One of the diseases more likely to occur in the aged than in the young is paralysis agitans, or the shaking palsy. Although this disease may occur in youth, the vast majority of cases occur in people between fifty and seventy years of age. The disease occurs twice as often in men as in women. It is marked by tremor of the hands, with a pill-rolling movement, and it tends to progress, running a complete course in from ten to fifteen years.

The aged should be especially careful to consult a good physician when any of the symptoms described in this article occur. While they may be simple results of old age, without more serious implication, they should be checked at frequent intervals by the family doctor.

Old people have particular difficulty in walking, for many reasons. First, there may be weakening in the circulation; sometimes pain in the muscles results from imperfect circulation. Often older persons walk with short steps, because in this way they are better able to control their sense of balance.

While the aged may have high blood pressure, it is not so serious as in youth.

Of course, old people suffer with disturbances of digestion because of the changes that have taken place in their secretions, and also because they have difficulty in keeping infection away from their teeth and because they do not chew the food properly. The constipation of old age is now largely controlled by the taking of mineral oil which serves the purpose of softening the intestinal mass and making elimination easy. This remedy is practically harmless and adds years of health to many older persons. Hemorrhoids are frequent in the aged and are, of course, associated with constipation.

There was a time when the teeth of the human being gradually fell out as he grew older so that he found himself, by the time he reached old age, able to take only liquid food or food that was soft. Modern dentistry has made it possible for the aged to chew steaks or vegetables of considerable fibrous content. It is for this reason that the aged must frequently resort to laxatives or to mineral oil in order to aid the weakened intestinal muscles in handling the waste material.

The aged are likely to suffer particularly with accumulations of mucous material in the lungs; with diminished power of the lungs to repair themselves, small areas of degenerated tissue break down, and the material accumulates and has to be coughed out of the lung. The continued inhalation and coughing results in disturbances such as bronchopneumonia or similar complaints.

The elderly are particularly prone to varicose veins, to inflammations of the joints, and to fixed joints which follow inflammation.

CANCER IN OLD AGE

Cancer has always been recognized by the medical profession as a disease of old age. More recently it has seemed to occur fairly frequently among younger people, and there are many explanations advanced for this fact. It is recognized that heredity plays a large part in cancer, and that inbreeding may bear some responsibility. The British statistician, Karl Pearson, found that the maximum incidence of cancer occurs at the age of forty-six in women, and of fifty-six in men. The chief cancer period is from forty-six to sixty-four years.

It is well established that cancer is associated with long continued irritation of susceptible spots in the tissue. Obviously aged people are more subject to long continued irritation than are the young. Men suffer, of course, much more frequently than do women with cancer of the lips and tongue, perhaps because of their smoking habits. Even though women have begun to smoke cigarettes regularly, it is unlikely that they will suffer as much with cancer of the lips and tongue as do men, because women are much more careful about the state of their mouths and teeth. Men suffer with cancer of the prostate; women with cancer of the organs particularly concerned with childbearing.

There have been many attempts to explain cancer in old age, but all of them are theoretical. In old age the degenerative process in the cells leads to the formation of new tissue, and the repeated demands made on the cells in this way may result in the sudden rapid growth that is called cancer. Warthin, eminent pathologist, considered cancer to be merely a sudden rapid aging of a group of cells.

Whatever the cause may be, older persons should be especially careful to treat all slight infections and to visit a physician if these irritations do not respond readily to treatment.

The chapter on cancer in this book gives the most recent and reliable information available.

THE CRITICAL AGE FOR MEN

Pediatricians say that the first year of life is the most critical. Others insist that the first 10 years are the hardest. Some call adolescence with the transition from childhood to adult life the most critical period.

The great control that is now asserted over infant mortality and the elimination of many of the diseases that used to affect youth make the majority of doctors today think that the most serious age is the period of transition from maturity to old age. Men enter the most critical period of their lives at 50. This is the time when they begin to need glasses to read the print in the telephone book. Now they begin to get tired a little earlier in the afternoon.

Occasionally, the onset of these conditions induces resentment. Many a physical culture expert or the proprietor of a health institute or a gymnasium has earned an excellent livelihood from the fact that these men take up exercise and try to prove to themselves that they are better than they really are. The wise man will realize that aging is a natural process and that the conditions that come with advancing years must be treated with respect. If the thyroid gland, the sex glands and the pituitary are less efficient, the deficiency will be reflected in the body generally. A doctor can prescribe glandular substances to overcome such deficiencies in part.

Hardening of the arteries and high blood pressure are two of the most important symptoms. Many years ago a wise physician said that a man is as old as his arteries. Incidentally, men are more frequently affected with hardening of the arteries than are women.

Arthritis is another condition that occurs many times to people after the age of 40 and which cripples and disables a good many older people.

Medicine can do a great deal for these disturbances if they are brought soon enough to medical attention. But man is not immortal and the wise man will recognize the aging process and conduct himself accordingly.

THE OLD MAN AND THE JOB

Women in the home keep on at their job of running the household and taking care of the family as long as they are able. Many of them find work ready to handle even up to seventy-five or eighty years of age. By contrast the man retired at anywhere from sixty to seventy years of age may find himself full of the desire to work and produce and to contribute to the public good and yet be shut out of his opportunity to do the work that he can do best.

The professional man who can serve as a doctor, a lawyer, a clergyman, an artist or a writer can keep on without too much difficulty. The worker in industry finds the situation much more difficult, regardless of his physical or mental age. As a man gets older he loses speed and those who operate machines find that they cannot keep up. Furthermore, the conditions of industry do not provide for continued work at a lesser wage but insist that the full wage be paid regardless of advancing years. Insufficient study has been given to the kinds of work that are especially suited to the older worker, aside from employment as a timekeeper or foreman or administrator. If the old men are kept on too long the younger men complain that there is no opportunity to rise in the establishment. Power and increased income are likely to go with promotion and few old men wish to go back to positions of less influence or income.

Many men anticipate with the greatest of pleasure the day when they are to retire from work. These are the men who dislike the job to begin with, and who have an avocation which gives pleasure and to which they can devote themselves after retirement.

Physicians are convinced that a busy rather than an aimless life is the ideal prescription for old age. Far too many instances are known of fairly young men who retired only to die within a few years from what seemed simply to be the ultimate effects of boredom and self-neglect.

A survey in Britain showed that the care of the aged for the most part rests on the family, and then the neighbors where there is real community life and spirit. In one community 57% of the burden rested on one daughter and there was little indication that multiple daughters shared the responsibility. Usually it was the youngest daughter that carried the burden, and the older ones reserved the right of criticism.

EMOTIONAL PROBLEMS OF OLDER PEOPLE

As people grow older they develop limitations on vision and hearing and a reduction of physical activity and of endurance. They also begin to have difficulties in remembering and in coordination. Fortunately the specialists in sight and hearing are now able to give great aid toward supplementing weaknesses in sight and hearing. We are also learning much about rehabilitation and measures for helping people who are failing physically.

Older people often begin to find incomes steadily reducing with expenses steadily increasing. True social security aims to help in meeting the situation but other trends incline toward putting older workers completely on the shelf.

Many older people having given up their steady occupations have failed to develop any hobbies or outside interests to which they can turn their attention. Their lives assume continuous boredom and ultimate depression.

As a husband or wife is lost the friends of the family incline to fall away from the remaining member and social contacts diminish leading to loneliness and introversion.

In ancient societies the aged were viewed with respect and came to be the Nestors, advisers and counselors. Our modern civilization drifts to an opposite extreme where all the emphasis is placed on youth.

The American Journal of Public Health says "we would do well to recognize the assets as well as the liabilities of senescence; to train ourselves in middle age for ripe and fruitful later years; to provide the medical and psychiatric and rehabilitative aids needed for healthy aging; and to regard the elderly not as outcasts but as essential and potentially valuable elements in the life of the family, the neighborhood and the nation."

CHARTER FOR THE AGED

In the early 1930s a conference called by President Herbert Hoover developed a charter for the child indicating its rights in a civilized nation. I submit the following charter as the rights of the aged in our present civilization.

1. Every older person has the right to tender loving care.
2. Every older person has the right to the most that medicine can do to provide freedom from pain and suffering.
3. Every older person has the right to ask for some interest or occupation worthy of his attention.
4. Every older person has the right to food, fuel, clothing, and shelter sufficient to his needs.
5. Every older person has the right to find happiness and contentment in his declining years.
6. Every older person has the right to the most that can be done to help him die comfortably of old age rather than uncomfortably of disease, accident, or disability.
7. Every older person is entitled to as much peace of mind and peace of soul as modern civilization can give.

Thus there are seven fundamental rights in the charter—one for each decade in the life cycle of man.

CHAPTER 38

Drugs and Their Uses

MORRIS FISHBEIN, M.D.

Modern man is protected against disease, is relieved of pain, and occasionally cured by discoveries that have been made in the professions of pharmacology, pharmaceutical manufacture, and pharmacy.

HOUSEHOLD REMEDIES

Elsewhere in this book is a discussion of the family medicine chest with a list of the household remedies that are easily available and which may be used by any person according to his own judgment. For example, the laxatives like mineral oil, phenolphthalein, cascara, and substances like agar and psyllium seed which add bulk to the excretions. Included also are such mild antiseptic substances as iodine, mercurochrome, and similar preparations. For pain relievers there are combinations of aspirin, phenacetin, and caffeine, sold under a wide variety of names, as well as simple preparations which include aspirin alone or aspirin buffered or other products related to aspirin.

Most of the potent and possibly toxic preparations prescribed by doctors are not sold over the counter without a physician's prescription. The Federal Food, Drug and Cosmetic Act regulates the labeling of drugs. It prohibits certain statements from appearing on the labels and demands warning labels for other substances which may be habit-forming or which are especially toxic. A new drug cannot be introduced into sale between the states unless an application has been made for it. This application must show by adequate scientific evidence that the drug is safe for use under ordinary conditions.

PRESCRIPTION DRUGS

The American Medical Association's Council on Drugs publishes annually a volume known as "New and Nonofficial Drugs" in which drugs are classified as to their general character. If the product is manufactured properly and the claims made for it are justified it is described in this book.

ANESTHETICS

Anesthetics are not of course easily available except by prescription and are generally used only in the hospitals and in the doctor's office. Local anesthetics are substances which may be put on the skin or injected under the skin and thus produce freedom from pain in the areas concerned. One type of anesthetic is injected into the spine to block the nerves of the spine, thus preventing pain during childbirth. When the drug is permitted to flow in gradually during the childbirth, the method is described as continuous caudal analgesia.

The general anesthetics include a wide variety of substances, such as ether, nitrous oxide, oxygen gas, ethylene, cyclopropane, and several other substances which the anesthetist gives to the patient for inhalation. Another type of anesthesia is basal anesthesia in which drugs capable of blocking sensation are injected into the veins. These are usually derivatives of barbituric acid.

ANTIHISTAMINES

During allergic reactions a substance known as histamine is released into the tissues. The antihistamines are used in such conditions as hay fever, asthma, and rhinitis because they block histamine. When these substances are used in mild hay fever, particularly in the first part of the season, they are usually effective in relieving symptoms.

The antihistamine drugs are useful also in the prevention and treatment of general reactions such as the allergic coughs, the allergic inflammation of the nose, the eruptions of hives, and the itching which accompanies other allergic diseases.

Any of the antihistaminic drugs can occasionally produce undesirable reactions in some people. The physician must be aware of this possibility. Sometimes the antihistamines produce a tendency to deep sleep. In other instances they may produce inability to concentrate, dizziness, and disturbed coordination. The worst symptoms that may result are tremors, nervousness and even convulsions. These are some of the reasons why the antihistamines in large doses should be used only when prescribed by a doctor. Several antihistamines are available in drug stores and can be purchased without a prescription. These are usually used to stop excessive secretion from the nose during the beginning of a cold and sometimes are applied in ointments for ivy poisoning or other skin reactions.

MOTION SICKNESS DRUGS

Most of the effective motion sickness drugs are now dependent on an antihistamine action. Among the most common of these are Dramamine, Bonine, Marezine, and various other preparations of antihistaminic drugs.

For years derivatives of scopolamine and hyoscine have been used effectively in preventing motion sickness.

Since all of these drugs possess the possibility of harm, they should not be taken continuously unless prescribed by the doctor. On most ships and on airplanes the attendants usually have available some of these anti-motion sickness remedies and they will give one or two doses with the understanding that the dosage is not continued and is only for immediate relief over a short period.

ANTI-INFECTIVES

Certain substances have the power to stop the action of bacteria, to impede their growth, and sometimes to destroy them. For instance certain drugs are known to be effective in controlling the germ of tuberculosis. These include streptomycin, one called PAS or para-amino-salicylic acid and also isonicotinic acid derivatives of which the one most frequently mentioned is isoniazid. There are several forms of these drugs known by various names which the physician prescribes according to his choice.

A substance known as oxyquinoline is available in various forms and is used frequently against germs or fungi.

Another drug called mandelamine has the special property of being eliminated in the urine and acting as a urinary antiseptic.

Another chemical group is known as the nitrofurans. These substances and their derivatives are effective against a variety of diarrheal disorders, infections in the urinary tract, and infections throughout the body, particularly by the pus-forming germs.

Among the earliest and most important of the anti-infective substances were the sulfonamides, discovered by Domagk, for which he received the Nobel Prize. The sulfonamides are available in a variety of forms. The ones to be used in the control of a known infection are chosen according to their established ability to stop the growth of the germs that are concerned. Among the best known sulfonamides are sulfadiazine and sulfamerazine. Another is sulfamethazine. A newer form is sulfacetamide which is available in various forms, depending on the area of the body where it is to have its effect.

The modifications of the sulfa drugs are numerous. Still another is known as Kynex or Midicel. There are varieties of gantrisin which are designed to affect specific portions of the body and to be used either in tablets, capsules, or given by injection.

ANTIBIOTICS

The antibiotics are substances derived from various living organisms which can stop the growth of germs or destroy germs. The first to receive extensive use was penicillin. Then came many others of which about twenty are in common use. Their names are streptomycin, Chloromycetin or Chloramphenicol, Bacitracin, Tyrothricin, magnamycin, Seromycin or cycloserine, Erythromycin or Ilotycin, Neomycin, Albamycin, Nystatin or Mycostatin which is used especially against monilia.

Another group includes oleandomycin which is especially active against germs like the staphylococcus, the streptococcus, and the pneumonococcus. It may also have effects in stopping the growth of the gonococcus and the meningococcus. Of this variety is Cyclamycin.

Penicillin is used in a variety of ways, either by tablets taken by mouth, or capsules, or by injections under the skin, according to what the physician thinks is best for the individual patient.

Among the variety of forms of penicillin is crysticillin (which is a combination of penicillin with a local anesthetic). Some forms of penicillin have been prepared so that they may be injected into the muscles and remain active over long periods of time.

Another new antibiotic is polymyxin, also ristocetin, and the various tetracyclines which include Aureomycin, Terramycin, Achromycin, and Panmycin. Most recent are Vancomycin and Viomycin.

Especially important is the fact that there are some two thousand possible antibiotics. One of the latest to be developed is an antibiotic which apparently can affect the growth of cancer cells. This is known as actinomycin D.

ANTIFUNGAL AGENTS

Various fungi may attack the human body, infecting the skin or the lungs or, indeed, other portions of the body. One substance which attacks them particularly is griseofulvin but there are other substances derived from chemicals such as Iso-par, Asterol, Sterisil, and Sodium Caprylate. Another is Triacetin, and one of the most frequently used is Undecylinic Acid which is commonly called Desitin.

ANTIMALARIAL AGENTS

Malaria is caused by an organism known as the plasmodium which occurs in various forms in the body. Quinine and various derivatives of quinine which have been developed act particularly against the malarial organisms. Among the important derivatives are Camoquin, Aralen, Primaquine, Daraprim, and Atabrine, which was much used during World War II. Because these drugs are so powerful they are used only when prescribed by a physician and in the manner prescribed. The drugs may be used to cure malaria or even taken to prevent malaria.

ANTIPEDICULAR AGENTS

Pediculosis is caused by three varieties of lice, which are commonly called the head louse, the body louse, and the crab louse. A number of drugs have been developed which are especially active against lice and these are called pediculocides. These drugs are applied externally and great care is taken to see that they do not get into the eyes or on the mucous membranes.

DISINFECTANTS AND ANTISEPTICS

Among the most important of all disinfectants is chlorine. An ideal disinfectant has never been discovered because such a substance would have to have the power to destroy all forms of all infectious agents and still not be injurious in any way to human tissue cells or be capable of causing sensitization in human beings. Every antiseptic must, therefore, be used in relationship to its effects not only on the organisms that are to be destroyed but also on the human body. Various antiseptics and disinfectants depend principally on chlorine, mercury, silver, peroxides, carbolic acid, soaps, and similar substances.

VERMIFUGAL AGENTS

The human being is susceptible to infestation with a great number of worms, such as the pinworm, the whipworm, the tapeworm, and hookworm, the filaria, and even such strange worms as the loa loa. Drugs have now been developed which can rid the body of these worms but as with the disinfectants and antiseptics, they must be used with great care because of the danger of toxic reactions.

ANTICANCER DRUGS

Already there are available and in use under controlled conditions in hospitals a number of drugs which can destroy the cells of cancer. These are known as cytotoxic agents. Many of them are highly poisonous and, therefore, they must be used only under completely controlled conditions. Among older drugs which have been used in this way are derivatives of arsenic and urethan, also nitrogen mustards and substances derived from folic acid which stop metabolism. X ray is used to destroy cancer cells and radioactive isotopes may be used directly in contact with cancer cells. There are also hormones like estrogens and testosterone which act against the spread of cancer cells.

AUTONOMIC DRUGS

Certain drugs act particularly against pain in the nerves, against the effects of stimuli coming along the nerves, and in the tissues of the brain. One class of these drugs is known as the autonomic drugs since they are concerned with the effects of nerve impulses coming through the autonomic nervous system. This is also known as the sympathetic nervous system.

Some drugs induce responses by the body which mimic the responses which come when stimuli pass along the nerves of the sympathetic nervous system. One of the autonomic drugs is amphetamine or benzedrine. This acts to overcome depression. Its effects are opposed to those of the sedative drugs like the barbiturates. This drug has been found useful in depressing the appetite and it alleviates sleepiness and fatigue; however, it is not desirable to eliminate fatigue by destroying the sensation. The real answer to fatigue is rest. The dangers lie in the elimination of the warning signal of fatigue in people who are overdoing. There is also the possibility of habit-formation from continued use. And finally there are possible dangerous effects on the circulation of the blood.

Other drugs of similar type are Dexedrine, Paredrine, Octin, and Isoprel. The number of possibilities is considerable and perhaps a score of drugs acting in a similar way will eventually become available.

Some drugs are used to constrict the membranes of the nose—as adrenalin and Privine. An appetite destroyer is Preludin.

ADRENERGIC BLOCKING AGENTS

Drugs have been found which can block the stimuli coming through the sympathetic nervous system. These drugs act to oppose the action of adrenalin. They lower blood pressure by causing dilation of the blood vessels and they stimulate the action of the intestines. Usually they increase the heart rate.

Among the most well known of these drugs are ergotoxine, ergotamine, piperoxan, and dipenamine.

CHOLINERGIC AGENTS

These drugs act to produce effects such as occur when the parasympathetic nerves are stimulated. They can slow the action of the heart, dilate blood vessels, and increase gastrointestinal motion and secretion. Most of these drugs are derived from a substance called choline.

DRUGS USED FOR THE HEART

Cardiovascular drugs are those whose action on the heart and other portions of the blood vessel system affect either the total output of the heart or distribution of blood to various branches of the circulation. Some of these drugs affect the rhythm and output of the heart; others dilate blood vessels, and still others may act to affect hardening of the arteries.

Most important of all drugs for the heart is digitalis and associated with it a variety of preparations and derivatives.

Many substances have been discovered which have a specific effect on high blood pressure. All of these are potentially toxic and can be used only when prescribed properly by the physician. One of the best known is hexamethonium, also Apresoline, mannitolhexanitrate, Inversine, Ansolysen, and Metamine.

CENTRAL NERVOUS SYSTEM DRUGS

Many drugs have their principal actions in depressing the central nervous system. These include anesthetic drugs, hypnotics, and sedatives. Here also come the anticonvulsants, the drugs used against cough, and the tranquilizing drugs.

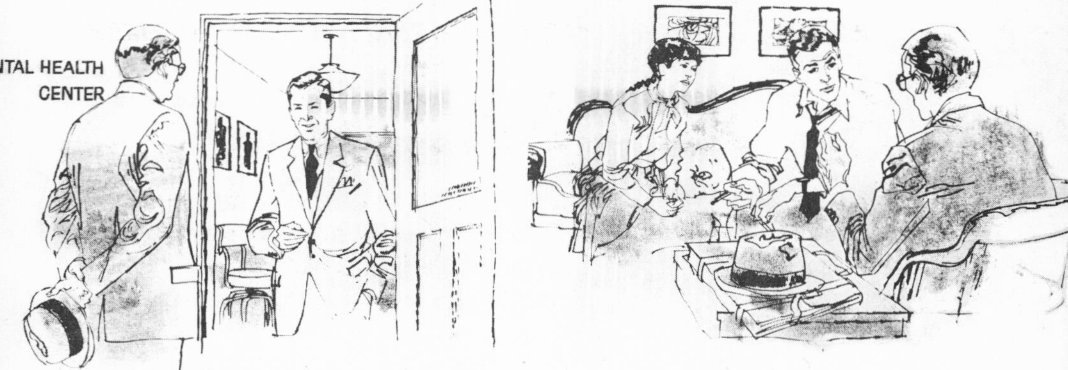

PLATES **115–116.** At least 1 person in every 10 has some form of mental or emotional illness (from mild to severe) that needs psychiatric treatment. With good care and treatment, at least 7 out of 10 patients admitted to a mental hospital leave partially or totally recovered. The family of any emotionally disturbed or mentally ill person has to understand all of the aspects of treatment and rehabilitation.

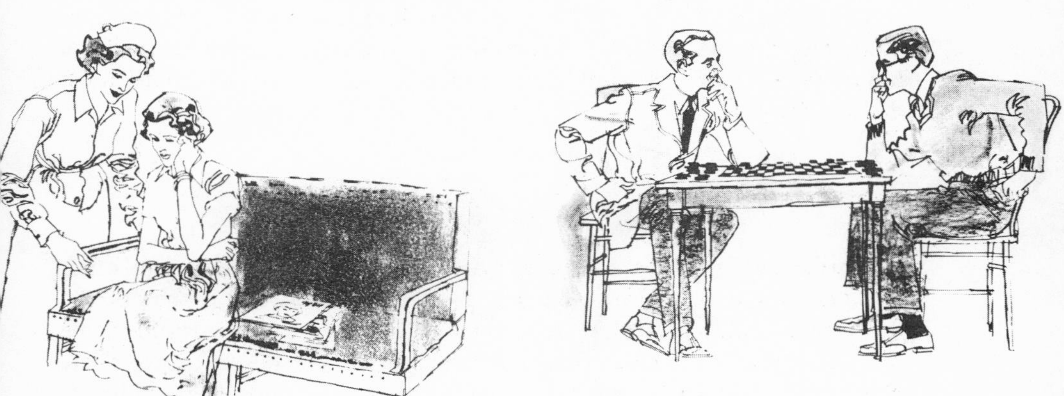

PLATES **117–118.** Mental health services should provide the patient with the best treatment possible aimed at their earliest possible return to the community.

PLATES **119–120.** Mental illness occurs at all ages, including childhood and adolescence. Half a million school-age children suffer from the most serious forms of mental illness—childhood schizophrenia and other psychoses. Only through correct diagnosis, treatment, education, and rehabilitation can they learn to lead productive lives. *(The National Association for Mental Health, Inc.)*

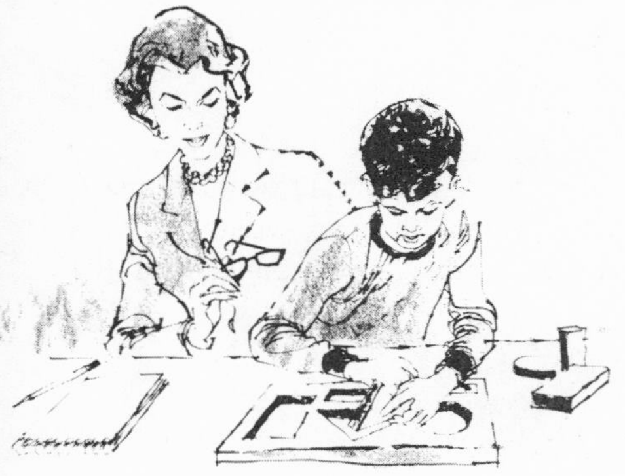

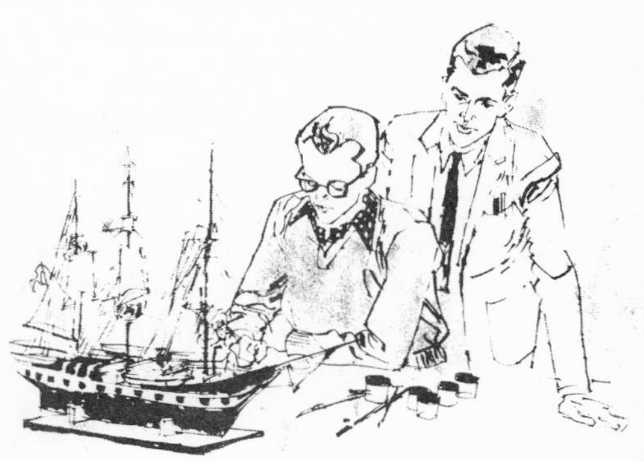

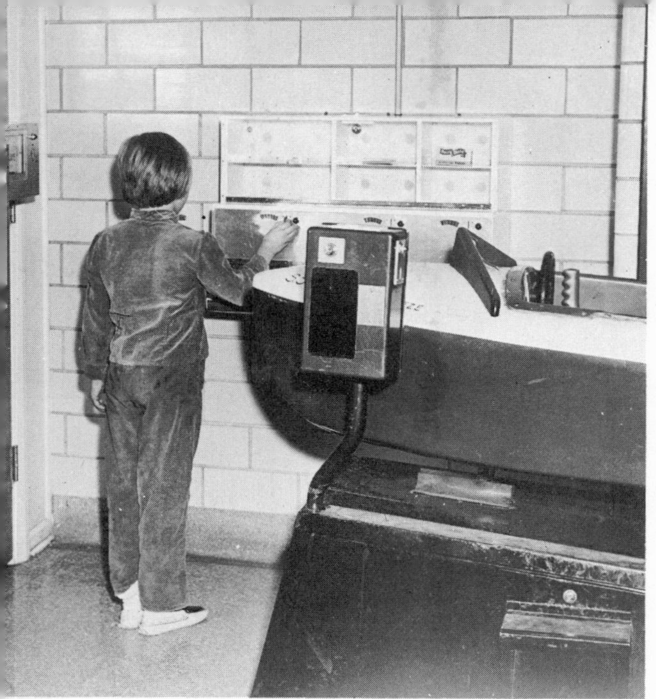

PLATE **121.** Dr. Marion DeMeyer and Dr. C. B. Ferster have studied regressed children suffering from a form of childhood schizophrenia. As a child emerges from withdrawal into fantasy and learns the small activities of daily living, he is rewarded with tokens which are used to buy trinkets or candy or a ride in a motorboat [right]. *(The National Association for Mental Health, Inc.)*

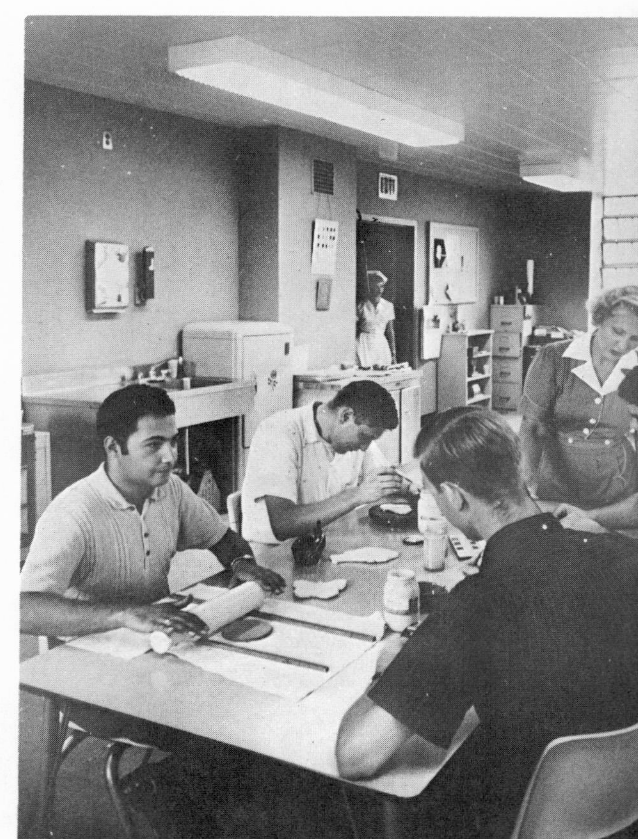

PLATE **122.** An example of the goal toward which mental-health associations have worked for years—*care* for mental patients instead of mere custody.

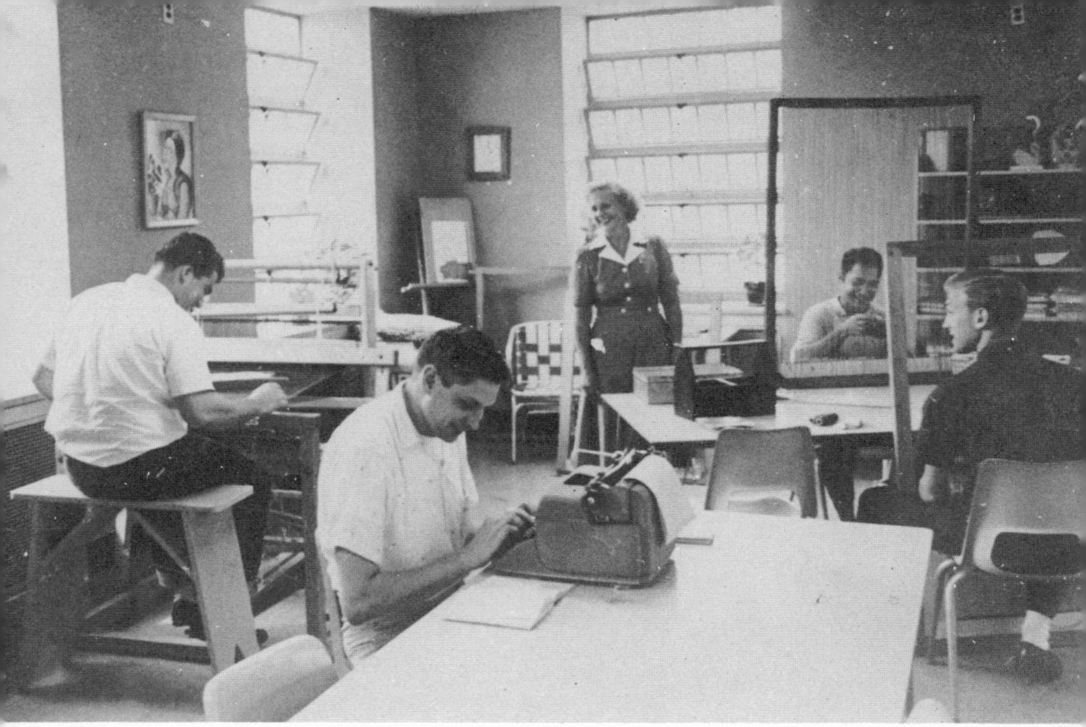

PLATE **123.** Here typing, weaving, and handicrafts are activities used in a modern mental hospital's occupational therapy program—an important supplement to medical treatment and psychotherapy. PLATE **124.** *(below)* Group therapy. *(The National Association for Mental Health, Inc.)*

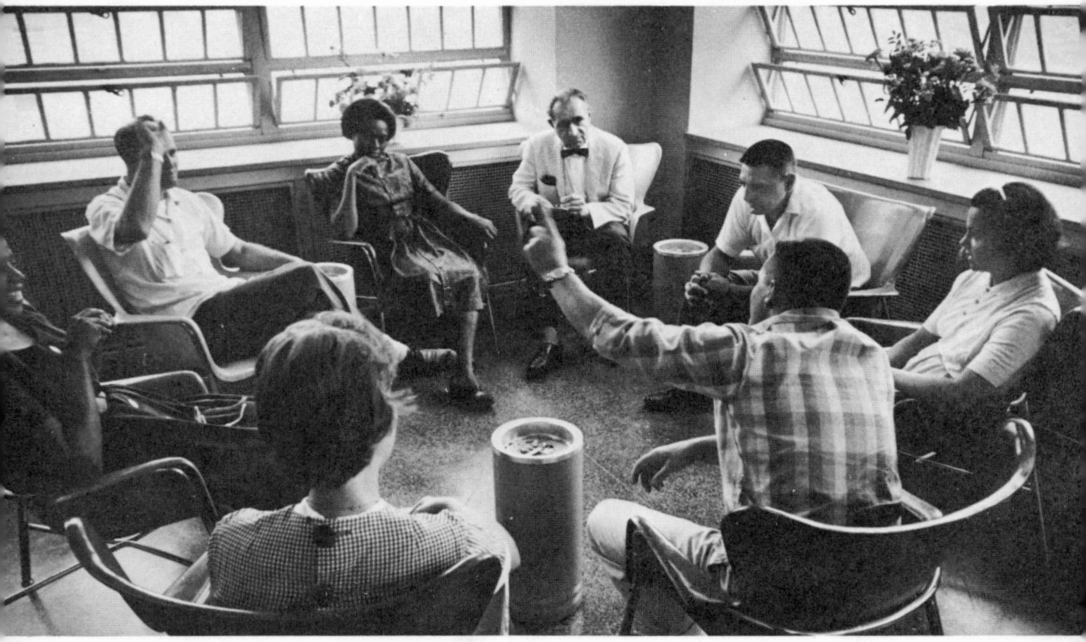

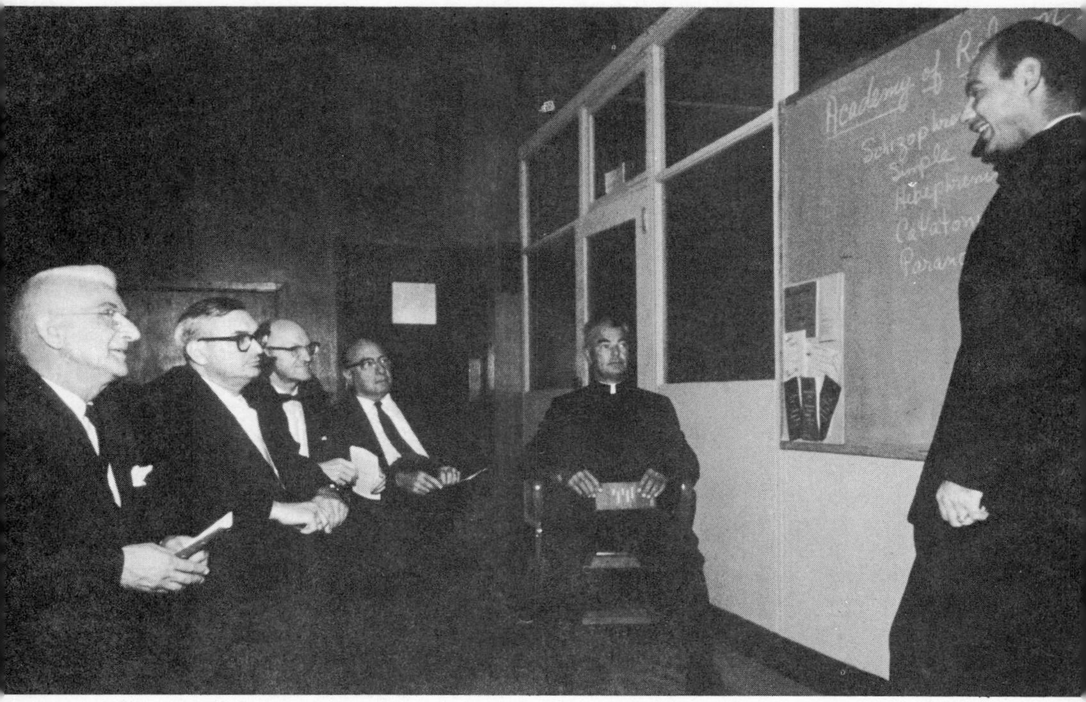

PLATE **125.** Educating the clergy about mental health. PLATE **126.** *(below)* Educating the police about mental health. *(The National Association for Mental Health, Inc.)*

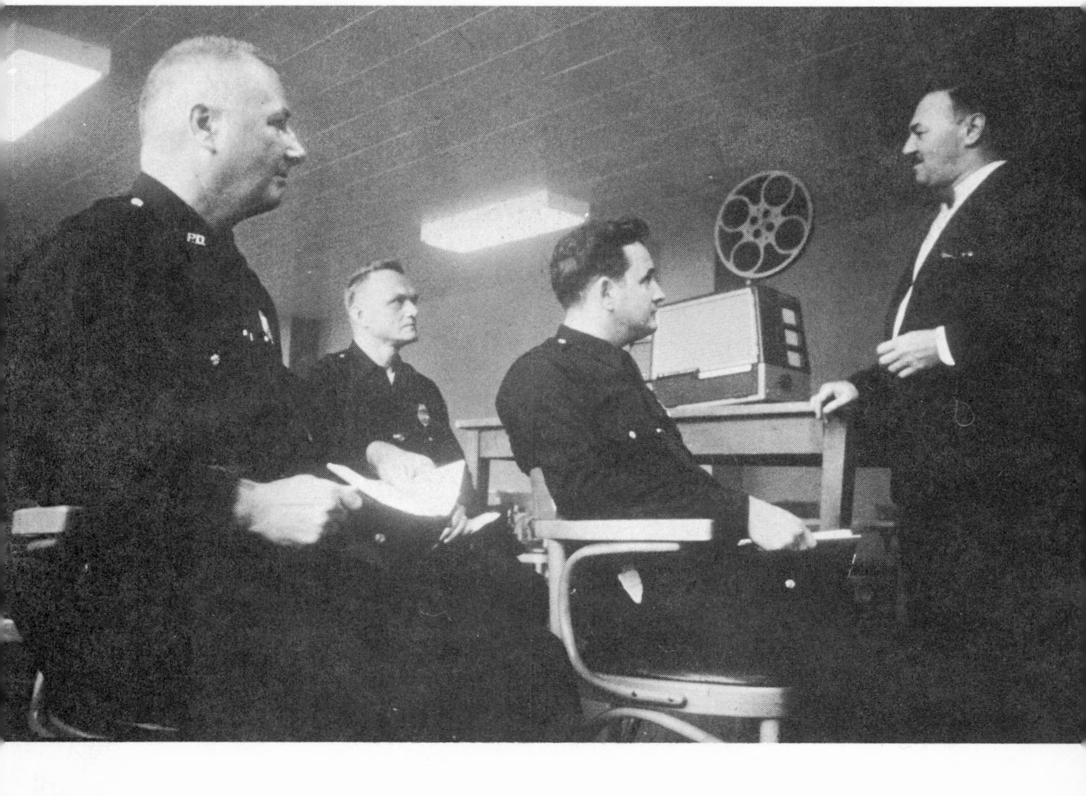

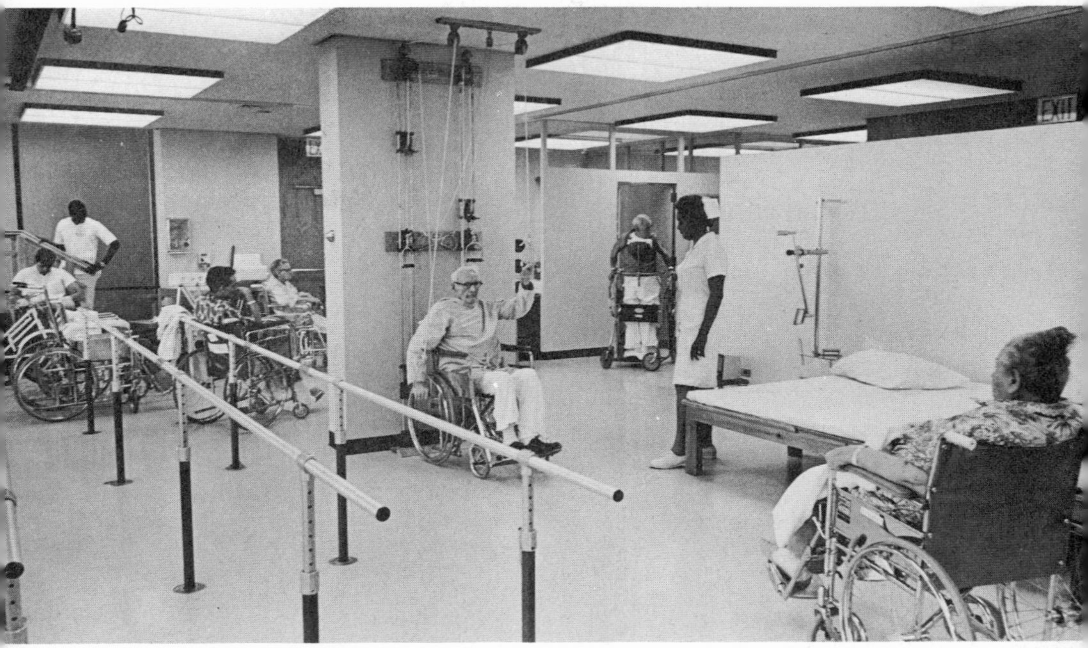

PLATE **127.** Rehabilitation medicine—physical therapy room. This is a new physical therapy room and contains the most modern facilities available. It is used by out patients as well as in patients. PLATE **128.** Dr. Ira Rubin, Montefiore cardiologist and head of the hospital's Electrocardiographic Service, visits a patient who is recovering following rare type of open-heart surgery. *(Courtesy of Montefiore Hospital and Medical Center, New York, and Ed Bagwell.)*

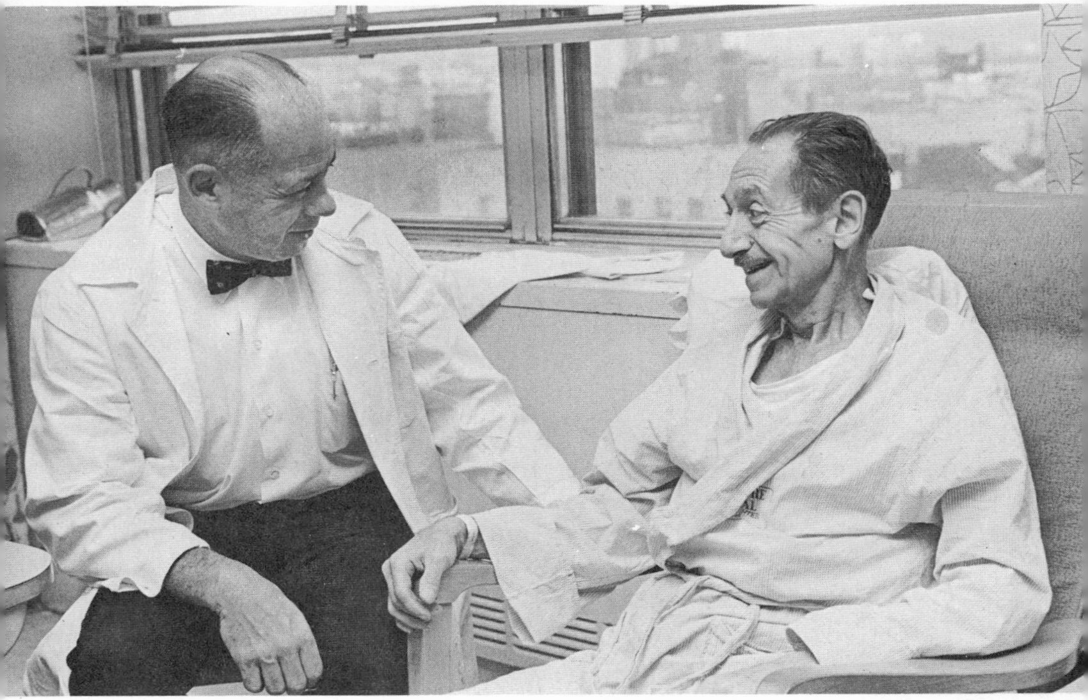

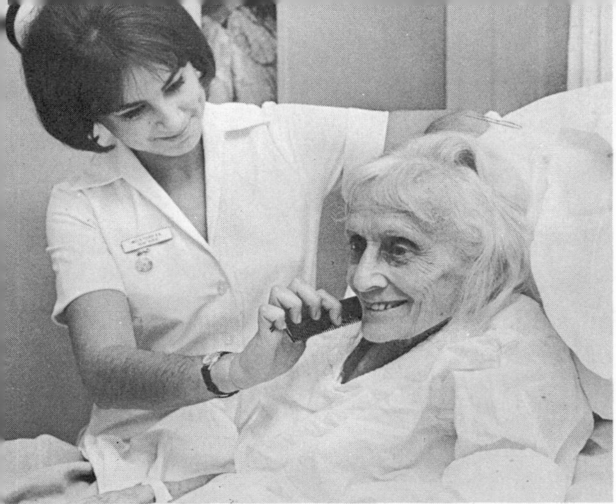

PLATE **129.** Nurse Rona Feder provides an extra measure of "tender-loving-care" for one of her patients. *(Courtesy of Montefiore Hospital and Medical Center, New York, and Ed Bagwell.)*

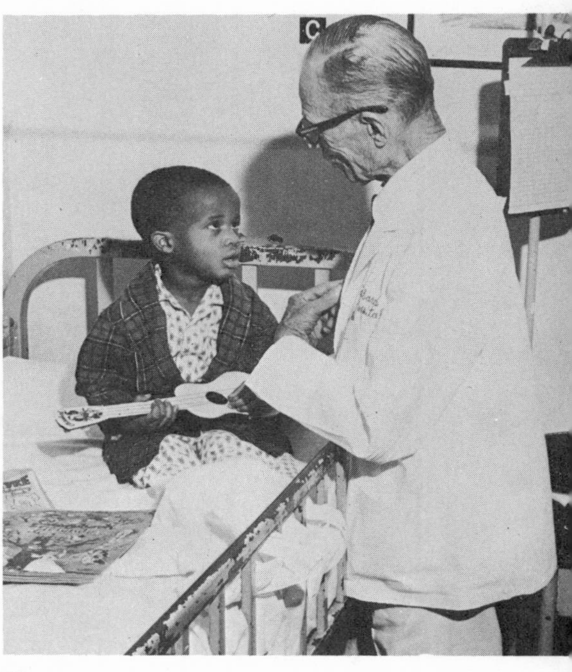

PLATE **130.** Under grants made by the Office of Economic Opportunity, foster grandparents work with mentally retarded, physically handicapped, delinquent, emotionally disturbed, or dependent and neglected children in institutions, day-care centers, and homes. These projects are supervised by the Administration on Aging under a contract with the Office of Economic Opportunity. Here, a foster grandparent talks to a foster grandson at the Hubbard Hospital in Nashville, Tennessee. The foster grandparent program recruits, trains, and employs low-income persons over 60 to serve neglected and deprived children who lack personal relationships with an adult. *(From July 1966* Aging, *U.S. Department of Health, Education, and Welfare, Administration on Aging.)*

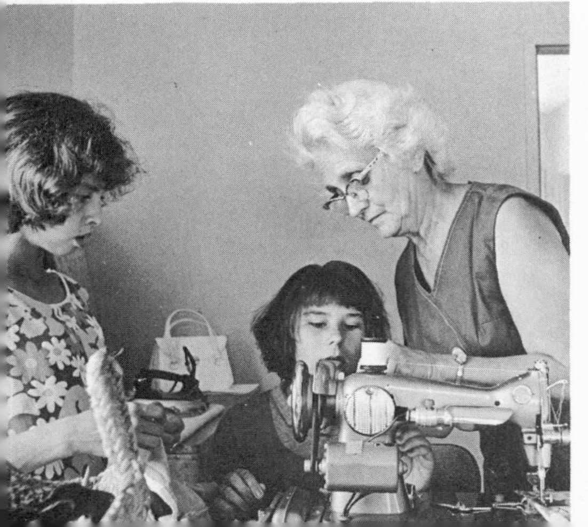

PLATE **131.** VISTA volunteer Irene Gallant, 67, conducts a sewing class for girls who often make much-needed clothes for themselves and other members of their families. Mrs. Gallant was assigned to work with the residents of a public housing project under the supervision of the Miami, Florida Housing Authority. VISTA volunteers have proved their value to their nation and its communities. VISTA was established through the passing of the Economic Opportunity Act and is governed through the Office of Economic Opportunity. *(VISTA Volunteer Magazine.)*

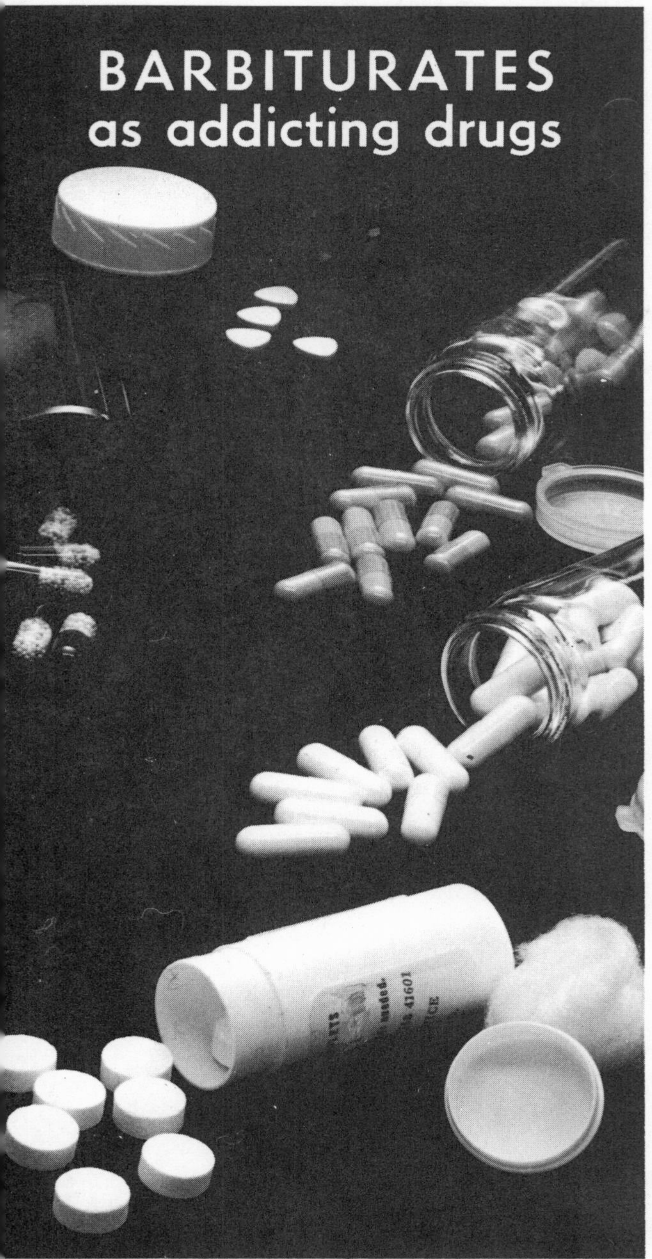

PLATE **132.** Barbiturates, commonly prescribed as sleeping pills, are useful depressants of the central nervous system, and, if taken in small amounts under the direction of a physician, cause no bad effects. Experiments have shown that when they are taken in large and uncontrolled amounts these are dangerous, intoxicating drugs—not only habit-forming but addictive. Intoxication by barbiturates produces symptoms similar to alcohol intoxication. Three of the symptoms of this addiction are: (1) A tolerance to the drugs so that the same amount produces progressively less effect; (2) Physical dependence on the drug which requires its continual use to prevent the characteristic symptoms that follow abrupt withdrawal; (3) Psychic dependence or habituation. Treatment for barbiturate addiction is complex, similar to the treatment for chronic alcoholism or morphine addiction and must always be given in a hospital. *(From "Barbiturates As Addicting Drugs," National Institute of Mental Health.)*

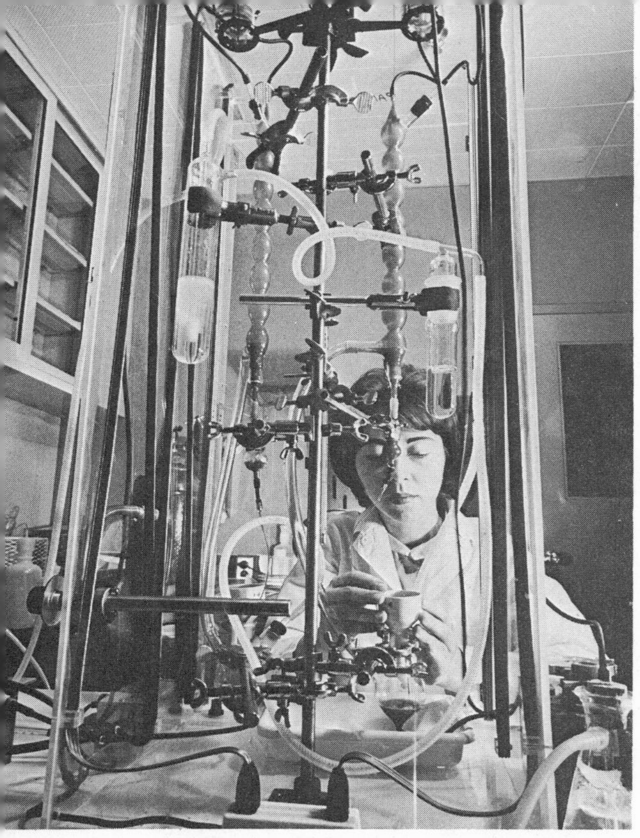

PLATE **133.** New antidiabetic drugs are studied in this test at Pfizer's Medical Research Laboratories in Groton, Connecticut. Procedure measures the effect of a new compound on glucose metabolism, giving an index of the drug's effectiveness. *(Courtesy Charles Pfizer & Company, Inc.)*

PLATE **134.** Toward the Future. In this isolation laboratory, a technician, clothed in sterile garb and face mask, examines special "test" plates which have been "seeded" with diseased germs and onto which solutions of experimental antibiotics have been planted. In this manner, the search goes on for new compounds to bring about the control of diseases not now conquered by today's medicines. *(Courtesy Charles Pfizer & Company, Inc.)*

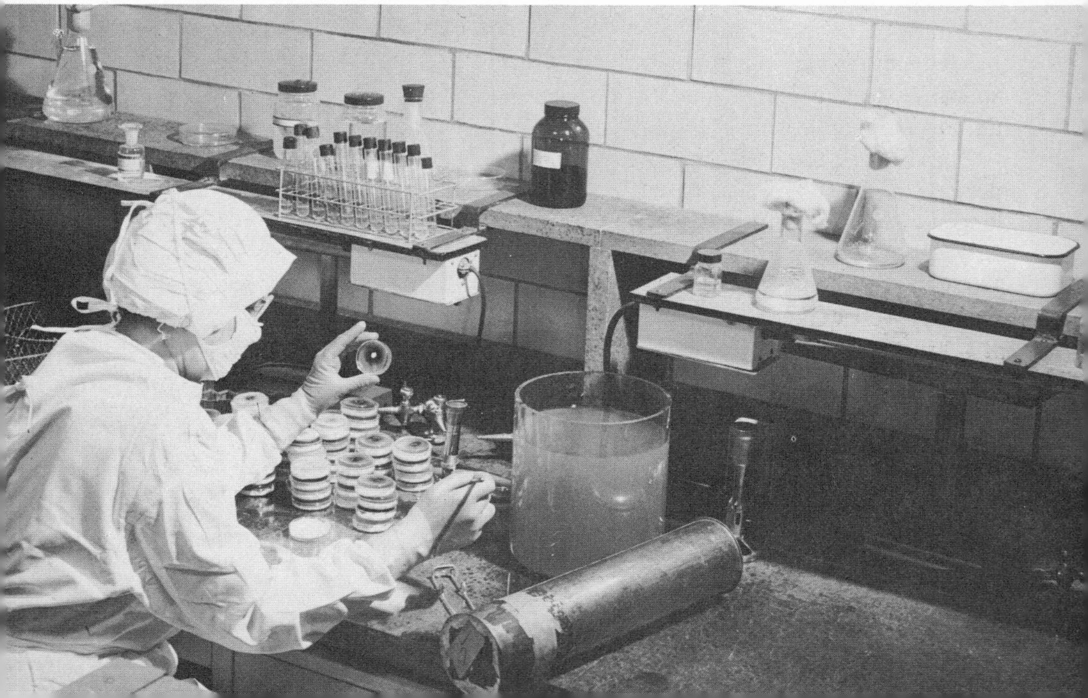

The analgesics are used to relieve pain. For this purpose morphine is best known, but similar effects are had from milder salicylates like aspirin and phenacetin. These mild analgesics do not produce addiction and are usually considered safe for sale without a prescription.

The more powerful drugs which have been developed must be sold only with a prescription.

Many modifications have been made of opium and its derivatives, including morphine. All of these substances must be prescribed only with the use of a license to prescribe under the Anti-Narcotic Act.

Many persons have become accustomed to taking sedative drugs in order to encourage sleep. There are great numbers of barbituric acid derivatives which are used for this purpose. These are effective as sedatives and are used in insomnia, hysteria, nervousness, mental disturbances, and epilepsy. They act directly on the central nervous system.

Insomnia is of several varieties: One in which falling asleep is difficult; another in which sleep comes easily but is very quickly disturbed so that the person awakes frequently during the night or exceedingly early in the morning. Drugs should never be taken routinely for this purpose. Sleep may be promoted in a variety of ways. Perhaps it is best that sleep-producing drugs be used only when prescribed and only in the manner of use prescribed by the doctor. A very small dose of a sleep-producing drug may start the sleep and thereafter the person sleeps well throughout the night.

Many sleep-producing drugs are followed by hangover which seriously interferes with the usual activities.

ANTICONVULSANTS

Many drugs have been discovered which can stop the convulsions of epilepsy or other convulsive disorders. Among the best known are Dilantin, Peganone, Phenurone, Paradione, Tridione, Mysoline, Milontin.

These drugs are of the greatest importance because today thousands of persons with convulsive disorders are enabled to go months or even longer without a convulsion through proper use. Because of their potency, only a physician who has thoroughly studied the patient and who understands the nature of the convulsive disorder should prescribe the drug of his choice according to the needs of the individual patient.

Certain other drugs which act on the nervous system may prevent cough by their local effects on the nervous system and on the tissues involved in coughing. Codeine, a derivative of morphine, is a powerful drug in preventing coughs. There are, however, other drugs not derived from morphine which prevent cough through action on the nervous system.

The tranquilizing drugs include particularly Thorazine, Pacatal, Trilafon, Compazine, Sparine, Dartal, Vesprin, and Temeril. Under this group also come the derivatives of rauwolfia which includes Serpasil, Reserpine, and similar preparations. Most widely known of the tranquilizers is meprobamate which is also known as Equanil. This, however, is a relaxant drug rather than a depressant.

NERVOUS SYSTEM STIMULANTS

There are drugs which stimulate the nervous system and which are used to overcome depressions, to energize the body, and to oppose the actions of sedatives and tranquilizers. Many of these drugs are toxic in the sense that they may raise the blood pressure, stimulate the beating of the heart, and produce great breathlessness.

For years people have known that tea and coffee, which contain caffeine or theobromine or theophylline, have the power to stimulate. Students have taken caffeine or many cups of coffee to keep awake during study. Some derivatives of choline and of xanthine have effects of stimulating the central nervous system. New psychic energizers which control endogenous depression are Nardil Catron Tofranil and many more.

CONTRACEPTIVES

Contraceptives are used to inhibit the action of the sperm cells or to prevent the passage of the sperm into the uterus. They are of many varieties and are discussed under other sections of this work.

SKIN REMEDIES

The number of chemical substances used upon the human skin runs into hundreds. These are used to protect the skin, to control blemishes, to disinfect the skin, to stop itching, to take care of scaling and oiliness, to remove the skin, and for many other purposes. In the chapter on the skin many of these remedies are thoroughly discussed.

ALCOHOL DETERRENTS

Among the new remedies recently developed are drugs like Disulfiram or Antabuse which cause the person who takes them to develop unfavorable symptoms to drinking alcohol. Such a drug obviously must be used with the greatest of care because of the possible dangers from poisoning.

ENZYMES

Within the human body there are many substances produced which act to aid the functions of the body. For instance, one enzyme called hyaluronidase can limit the spread of fluids in the body and is used to prevent scar tissue.

Another enzyme can inactivate penicillin and is used when there are toxic reactions from the use of penicillin.

Some enzymes prevent clotting of the blood and are used to dissolve clots. One such enzyme, Chymotrypsin, is injected into the eye to loosen the tissues around a cataract.

STOMACH AND INTESTINAL DRUGS

Persons who suffer from excess acid can take drugs which stop the *flow* of acid. Other drugs protect the wall of the stomach against the *effects* of acids.

BLOOD DERIVATIVES

Many substances have been derived from blood and are used in medicine. These include the whole blood itself as is used for transfusion, the serum from the blood, the liquid portion of the blood (which is called plasma), the clotting material (which is called fibrin). Other substances such as heparin, dicumarol, and Tromexan prevent the clotting of blood and are used after coronary thrombosis to prevent further clotting. Some drugs have been developed which are used to prevent bleeding. These include Thrombin, which is derived from the blood itself.

Various drugs are used to stimulate the growth of red blood cells, including particularly iron, and various forms and modifications of iron. Also there are organic substances derived from liver and from the wall of the stomach which may stimulate the growth of red blood cells.

HORMONE DERIVATIVES

The glands of internal secretion include the pituitary gland, the thyroid, the adrenal glands, and the sex glands. From all of these, substances have been derived which have powerful effects. From the adrenal glands comes cortisone and hydrocortisone, also adrenalin, and aldosterone. From the pituitary gland comes pituitrin, ACTH, and various other hormones which stimulate the action of the breasts, the sex glands, the thyroid, or the adrenals. The sex glands which include the ovaries and the testes give rise to hormones which are of great importance in the functions of the body, including the function of growth.

The pituitary is believed to contain hormones which are important in affecting the color of the body and the growth of the body.

From the pancreas comes insulin, which controls the use of sugar by the body, and trypsin which is a digestive ferment (*See* also Chapter 22, *Endocrinology*).

IMMUNOLOGIC AGENTS

By injection of various substances into the human body the blood produces substances which resist the proteins which have been injected. By such techniques we derive various serums and antitoxins. Thus there are vaccines and serums against many diseases. These vaccines are now available against influenza, whooping cough, poliomyelitis, rabies, tuberculosis, and many other disorders.

Serums may be made against almost any type of germ but they are effective only according to the response of the animal to the toxic substance.

EDEMA-REDUCING AGENTS

Among the greatest of recent discoveries are drugs which can cause elimination of fluid from the body. Among these are particularly Diamox and Diuril. These have been found to be of the greatest importance in heart failure and in various other conditions in which fluid collects in the tissues. Before these new discoveries, various mercury derivatives were used and some are still used for the same purpose. On the other hand, a drug called Benemid derived from benzoic acid serves to block the renal tubules so that a drug like penicillin is held in the body until it can have its effect.

THE VITAMINS

Many vitamin preparations are now available to provide for the effects of these important substances when they are insufficient in the diet or when the body does not use them satisfactorily. They are fully discussed in Chapter 32, *Advice on the Diet.*

CONCLUSION

Many of the drugs here discussed were first announced as miracles. Today the "miracle drugs" have become commonplace, but as a result of their use human beings have been freed from much pain and distress; lives have been saved from infections which were formerly invariably fatal.

The development of these drugs has given us a better world in which to live.

Index

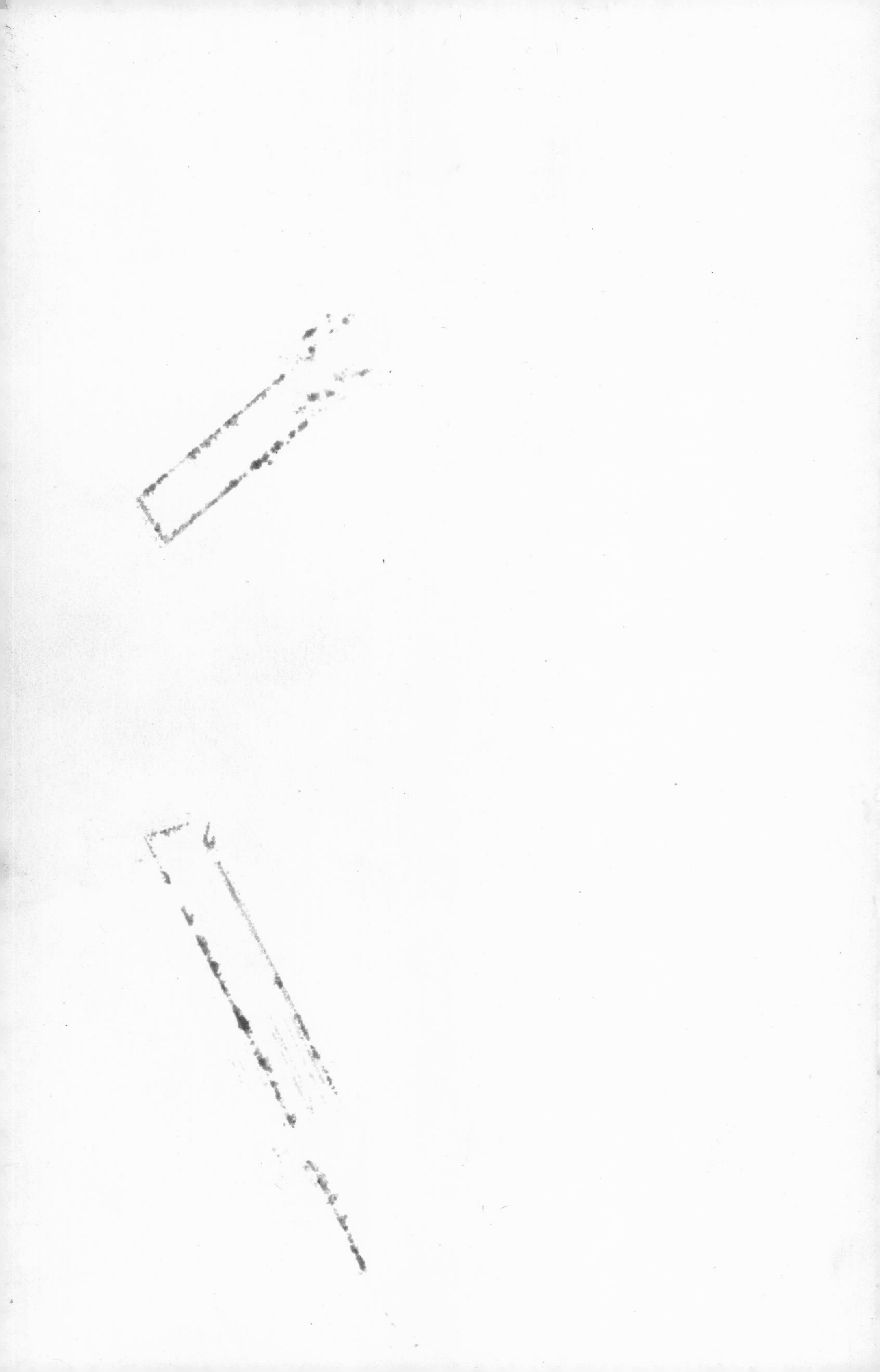